NUTRITION AND DIET THERAPY

Nutrition and diet therapy

SUE RODWELL WILLIAMS, M.P.H., M.R.Ed., Ph.D., R.D.

Chief, Nutrition Program, Kaiser-Permanente Medical Center,
Oakland, California; Instructor, Human Nutrition, Chabot College,
Hayward, California; Field Faculty, M.P.H.–Dietetic Internship
Program and Coordinated Undergraduate Program
in Dietetics, University of California,
Berkeley, California

FOURTH EDITION

with **109** illustrations

including original drawings by
George Straus

The C. V. Mosby Company

ST. LOUIS • TORONTO • LONDON   1981

MOSBY
1906 **75** 1981
YEARS

A TRADITION OF PUBLISHING EXCELLENCE

Editor: Michael R. Riley
Copy editor: Elizabeth O'Brien
Production: Gail M. Hudson
Design: Nancy Steinmeyer

FOURTH EDITION

Copyright © 1981 by The C. V. Mosby Company

Previous editions copyrighted 1969, 1973, 1977

Printed in the United States of America

The C. V. Mosby Company
11830 Westline Industrial Drive, St. Louis, Missouri 63141

Library of Congress Cataloging in Publication Data

Williams, Sue Rodwell, 1922-
    Nutrition and diet therapy.

    Includes bibliographies and index.
    1. Diet therapy. 2. Nutrition. I. Title.
[DNLM: 1. Diet therapy. 2. Nutrition. WB 400
W727n]
RM216.W684 1981   641.1   80-27219
ISBN 0-8016-5554-4

GW/VH/VH 9 8 7 6 5 4 3 2   03/B/309

To my husband

Luke

minister, helpmate, ''my other self''

and to our children

Jim, Mary, Ruth

whose constant support and encouragement

never cease to sustain me

Foreword

In this book Mrs. Williams shows her great understanding of the field of nutrition. She demonstrates strongly the concept that all of us—the nurse, the nutritionist, and the physician, that is, all who are associated with the care of our fellow human beings—work as a team. In this concept, care of the patient is the primary objective of all members of the team. Mrs. Williams stresses the role, obligations, and importance of the nutritionist and the nurse in this total picture. She emphasizes the fact that change in environment, affected by the scientific advances of our times, must be accepted and that "health is a relative concept in any culture."

Mrs. Williams has conscientiously laid out her philosophy relating to nutrition and has masterfully organized her book to focus on the needs of the patient and the health professional. It is also apparent that this book is of value to others in the health sciences and is worthy of the author's effort.

A. J. Sender, M.D.

Physician-in-Chief, Oakland Division,
Permanente Medical Group, Oakland, California

This most interestingly written book meets a very important need for an up-to-date, comprehensive, and authoritative text on nutrition as related to patient care. The reader will be quickly aware that Mrs. Williams is a highly able and dedicated person. She has a unique ability to make the subject matter actually live for the student, almost as though she were teaching the material personally to each reader.

Sufficient basic information about nutrition is provided to enable the student to become knowledgeable about the subject and to recognize and refute food faddism, which often creeps into patient care from one source or another. Students in the health professions will become very aware of the great importance of nutrition in the care of patients of all ages.

The inclusion of a nutrition course in medical and nursing education programs is extremely important. I decry the recent practice in some curricula of removing or curtailing the subject because of the pressures from other topics. A study of the contents of this book should provide proof of the primary care practitioner's need for nutrition education; this need is demonstrated by the vital interrelationships of nutrition to disease, patient care and well-being, and good health.

I highly recommend this textbook, not only for nutritionists, dietitians, and nurses but also for other professional workers interested in patient care as it relates to nutrition.

George M. Briggs, Ph.D.

Department of Nutritional Sciences,
University of California, Berkeley, California

Preface

This book is concerned with nutrition and human health. A careful reading of Chapter 1 will reveal its tone, its focus, and its form.

This book is the result of many years of teaching and clinical practice and is born of two deep feelings: my concern for students and my concern for people, or more rightly I should say persons, for we relate to individual persons, not to masses of people. Through these pages I have tried to reach not only the students' minds and intellects but also their hearts by seeking to stimulate deeper dimensions of caring for persons and their individual health needs. For this I make no apology. Learning itself involves by necessity not only the intellect but also the emotion and the will. I realize that I may have challenged some old ideas and ritualistic practices. But at the same time I hope that I may have caused some new thinking and initiated some new approaches, which are demanded of us in these rapidly changing times, to pressing human needs, to the basic role of nutrition in meeting these needs, and to the vital teaching-learning process.

In these days of burgeoning scientific knowledge and booming population growth we are beginning to hear an increased number of concerned cries for more comprehensive, less fragmented patient care, for greater awareness of individual need, of concern for the "whole person." As health professionals in the midst of this rapidly changing world we are at one and the same time charged with two responsibilities: to know our subject and to know our patient. Sound knowledge must be our tool; genuine concern for human need must be our motive. Furthermore, the realities of life must be the context of the practice of our art.

For whom, then, do I write this book? You will see that I focus primarily on nutrition in health care, seeking to provide a textbook for professional students and their teachers. Health team members, all those concerned with the integration of nutritional needs in the care of patients and families, will find here useful, practical information and direction. The book may well serve as a tool of learning for students in dietetics, nursing, and other health fields, as well as a helpful resource for busy clinicians and practitioners—physicians, nurses, nutritionists, dietitians, dentists, dental hygienists, public health workers, health educators, physical therapists, home economists, and others.

In decisions concerning organization of material, one idea has remained uppermost in my mind. I suppose the word *life* describes it best. I wanted to provide "meat" for my subject, to give it "bone and blood and sinew," to make a subject too long lifeless and colorless and irrelevant in the experience of many nurses come alive with new meaning. I wanted to help them view nutrition in terms of the very throbbing, pulsating "stuff of life" it provides and to see it applied to living persons in real life situations of daily living as well as in times of stress. To this end, two basic objectives have prevailed: clarity of content and person-centered focus. To achieve greater clarity of content, scientific and philosophic concepts are developed in more depth through discussion of key terms and relationships as well as through diagrams, illustrations, questions raised for study, outlines, boxes giving further background, and summary glossaries. To achieve a greater degree of person-centered focus, clinical application is made of all scientific principles, and increased emphasis is given to the role of nutrition in public health, in the basic health care specialties, and in clinical management of disease—all in the context of human need. The book is divided therefore into four parts: One, Foundations of Nutrition; Two, Applied Nutrition in Community Health; Three, Nutrition in the Health Care Specialty; and Four, Nutrition and Clinical Care.

In response to current trends and the growing number of health professionals practicing in specialized areas, an important new chapter has been added to the fourth edition: Chapter 31, Nutrition and Cancer—Care of the Hypermetabolic or Malnourished Patient.

Clinical case studies are now presented in selected chapters throughout the book, providing the reader with community, family, and individual patient situations that provoke and stimulate thinking about possible solutions to the problems involved. In addition, new material on dietary fiber has been included in Chapter 2, Carbohydrates, and new information on nutritional assessment is presented in Chapter 23, Principles of Nutritional Assessment and Therapy in Patient Care.

The recommended daily dietary allowances (revised 1980) of the Food and Nutrition Board, National Academy of Sciences–National Research Council are presented in Appendix M.

To facilitate the use of the book, several reference tools are used. There is considerable cross-reference throughout the text to relate similar or needed material. Appendixes provide the basic tables for simple calculations. An index provides ready access to desired material. If anything, I may have erred on the side of overindexing. Perhaps this results from my own personal irritation with a book in whose index I have to search in vain through a series of related words for reference to some needed bit of information. One thing, however, I have not included. Those looking for recipes among the references will be disappointed. I do not think that a student comes to nursing school, for example, to learn to cook.

A book of this nature emerges gradually from the work of many people. I am deeply indebted to all those persons who have helped to make this one become a reality. I owe much to Ruth Straus, scientific editor, writer, craftsman, and friend, for her constant encouragement, her sharp and discerning eye to editorial details, and her sympathetic feeling for student and patient alike. Many times her probing questions led to greater clarification of the writing. Also I am grateful to George Straus for bringing further clarification and sheer beauty to scientific concepts through his diagrammatic illustrations. In these illustrations he has contributed a freshness of view, a precision of content, and a rare artistry. The book is a better book because of the loving efforts of these dear friends.

I am also particularly indebted to my esteemed teacher and friend, George M. Briggs, chairman of the Department of Nutritional Sciences at the University of California, Berkeley, who counseled with me at the outset when the book was only the germ of an idea, who helped the idea to grow, and who gave me the courage to undertake the enormous effort to develop the material that nourished it. I am grateful for his careful reading of the manuscript's first basic science section, his discussions with me of many interesting points, and his writing of one of the book's forewords.

Many other persons made valuable contributions that shaped the course of the book. To each of the following I give my deep appreciation: the fine faculty of educators with whom

I am privileged to teach and in whom I have found the highest ideal of patient care, especially to those among them who have read various portions of the manuscript and offered helpful suggestions—Clair Lisker, Elizabeth Bridston, Betty Smith, and Marion Yeaw; my colleagues in the California Bay Area Dietetic Association, especially those close friends and fellow teachers who have encouraged my effort, reviewed material, and influenced my thinking—Claire Fry, Natalie Calhoun, Phyllis Howe, Mildred Bennett, Leona Shapiro, and Sylvia Mitchell; Pat Collins and Mary Williams of Agricultural Extension Service, University of California, for aiding in early explorations for direction and for giving many practical guides for community application; my teachers, whose examples inspired my own effort—Ruth Huenemann, Harold Harper, and Sheldon Margen; my students—past, present, and future—who always teach me much and some of whom will find familiar words on many pages; the physicians with whom I work, all of whom have contributed much to my own learning and given to me a model of professional practice, especially to Dr. A. J. Sender, our physician-in-chief who reviewed clinical sections of the manuscript and wrote a foreword; my dietetic interns, who stimulate and challenge my think-ing, and especially to Mary Blackburn and Marni Miller who helped teach me what human need means; the many authors, publishers, companies, government agencies, and world health organizations, at home and abroad, who have generously permitted me to use their materials and provided resources, illustrations, and personal encouragement; the patients and staff in our hospital and in the public health department who graciously served as models for our photographs; the typists whose unfailing assistance at various stages of the writing produced the final typescript—Aileen Simpson, Elin Carlson, Lorraine Satterthwaite, and Helen McGrath.

And finally, but certainly not least, to my family I give my love and my deepest gratitude —to my patient husband who helped to develop my insight at numerous points, to my son whose standards of scholarship and personal example of concern for human need have helped to open my own eyes of understanding, to my alert and sensitive daughters whose keen awareness and warm encouragement have lighted my way. All of these persons close to me have stimulated me enormously and have never ceased to share in this family project—''the book''!

Sue Rodwell Williams

Berkeley, California

Contents

PART THREE

NUTRITION IN THE HEALTH CARE SPECIALTY

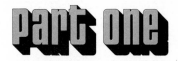

FOUNDATIONS OF NUTRITION

The study of nutrition

The thoughtful student in any one of the health professions may well ask, "What place does a knowledge of nutrition have in the practice of my profession?" This is a significant question, because ideas concerning nutrition are currently undergoing tremendous change in America as well as throughout the world. Nutrition is rapidly emerging as a vital component in health care and in our developing national health care policies to meet human needs. Indeed we are realizing increasingly that nutrition as a part of the health care professions must be viewed in the context of human need if the study of nutrition is to have relevancy and meaning. The focus of this book is just that — human need and thus patient-centered care.

NUTRITION AND HEALTH CARE

Nourishment is that which sustains life. The science and art of human nutrition both focus on nourishing human life. They do this in many ways. Human beings breathe, work, rest, play, sleep, and so on, all of which require energy. Humans must replenish that energy with food to sustain physical life. This need for food is basic to survival and is a fundamental concern of nutrition.

However, human beings are much more than mere biologic organisms, and food has many meanings for them other than simply physical sustenance. Persons in the health care professions must have a broad range of knowledge, understanding, and skills that will enable them to meet human needs. The patient needs care that helps to heal both body and spirit, and concern must encompass the patient's physical and emotional needs if valid healing care is to be provided.

Physiologic health depends on certain essential chemicals and their intricate biologic interrelationships in the body's cells and tissues. These basic chemicals are supplied by, or derived from, food. A person is literally what he or she eats.

Psychologic health depends on certain personal, social, and cultural factors that exert strong influences on each individual. Unmet needs may bring about physical illness. Medical experts generally agree that there is a psychologic component in almost all disease.

The relationship between the physical and emotional aspects of health and the pertinent functions of nutrition and health may be seen by applying the four functions of nutrition (to sustain life, to promote growth, to replace loss, and to provide energy) to the concept of health care as the nurturing and healing of patients, both physically and emotionally.

Functions of nutrition	Related emotional functions of health care
1. To sustain life	1. To sustain and support persons through times of dependence and need
2. To promote growth	2. To promote personal growth and restore health

Functions of nutrition	Related emotional functions of health care
3. To replace loss	3. To replace the loss of self-care ability and help maintain a sense of personal wholeness
4. To provide energy	4. To help provide emotional strength to cope with the total experience of illness

All these ideas are part of the evolving concepts of nutrition and human health care.

CHANGING CONCEPTS OF DISEASE AND HEALTH

Since nutrition, medicine, nursing, and other health professions are all a part of health care, the changes in the concepts of disease and health that are taking place today have profound effects on the practice of these professions.

In primitive societies disease was associated with evil spirits, mysterious supernatural powers that had to be driven out by some means. Treatment of disease therefore was in the hands of the religious leader of the group, the shaman, who acted as both priest and doctor. Gradually, as scientific knowledge increased, the biologic basis for disease became well established. Consequently, public and personal hygiene improved, treatment for specific diseases became more scientific and skilled, and many of the most lethal childhood diseases were eliminated.

Faced with the so-called gift of longer life, humankind began to view health increasingly in qualitative terms. Health concepts are moving from the wholly negative view of absence of disease (the curative approach) to a more positive view of optimal productivity (the preventive approach). This positive view was written into the preamble to the World Health Organization constitution in 1946: "Health is a state of complete physical, mental, and social well-being, and not merely the absence of disease or infirmity."

On the face of it, this is a noble goal for persons of all nations, but it is not totally realistic. Is such a complete state of health possible, and if it is possible, is it consistent with a state of social well-being? Such a goal is neither possible nor attainable, or perhaps even desirable. In reality, a human has health goals in two categories: (1) At any given time an individual may have an obvious, specific health need. (For example, the individual may need to have a broken bone set so that it will heal in good alignment, or he may need an antibiotic to help him overcome a specific disease.) (2) At the same time, whether the individual is aware of it or not, he has other needs. In some instances these other needs may even be in conflict with the need for restoration of physical health.

An example of such a conflict may be seen in the experience of two men who have each had a stroke. One is a wealthy retired financier who can readily afford to spend a year or two in a rehabilitation center and who may learn to be relatively contented when he has regained sufficient function to enable him to manage his own physical care. The other man is a 45-year-old engineer with three children in school. This man must choose between prolonged rehabilitation therapy, while earning nothing, and returning to a job offered by his employer at half his former salary—barely enough to maintain his family.

Health is a relative concept in any culture, and it must be viewed in relation to a human's total wants and needs. Health competes with other values and is relative to a culture's way of life. The kind and degree of physical health required for success as an accountant in New York differs from the kind and degree of physical health needed to succeed as a Maori hunter. This recognition of the difference in needs extends the concepts of health to include moral, religious, and philosophical dimensions.

Perhaps a more realistic goal for world health efforts would be a level of physical and mental health that would make for social well-being within the social system in which the individual must live, and that would provide opportunity for personal productivity and self-fulfillment. Health workers therefore work at three levels: (1) personal health care, (2) control of devastating epidemics, and (3) promotion and maintenance of general health levels adequate to enable individuals to achieve self-fulfillment.

A number of factors in this rapidly evolving society have contributed to changes in health values and practices.

Scientific knowledge explosion

The accelerated pace of expansion of scientific knowledge challenges the medical profession's capacity to integrate and use it. Cures for specific diseases, a wide variety of therapeutic techniques, a panoply of pharmaceutical agents, constantly increasing knowledge of the body's intricate chemistry, and use of many delicate electronic and other instruments in diagnostic and therapeutic procedures have all become a regular part of medical care. This burgeoning knowledge in each field means that few persons can gain an adequate comprehension of more than one specialty. The benefits that specialization provides are obvious. However, as anyone who has ever visited a large clinic is aware, specialization (which from the point of view of the medical worker is necessary) means to patients that services are fragmented. They feel further and further removed from their doctors and from allied workers in the health professions. They feel that no one member of the health team sees them as total persons. To the medical worker, the patient often becomes the forgotten person.

Population explosion

Already in some parts of the world the population has increased beyond the available food supply. Some years ago in their disturbing book, *Famine — 1975!,* as prophets before their time, William and Paul Paddock[1] wrote of the inevitability of famine because of the rapid increase in world population and the decrease in food production resources. They described why famine cannot be evaded in underdeveloped nations and pointed out the critical questions that the affluent nations must consider concerning the use of resources. Other scientists also involved in world hunger and food supplies reinforce this state of human need. Mayer has described the dimensions of human hunger as involving roughly an eighth of mankind,[2] a state that continues to plague many parts of the world.

Population expansion and change pose a potent social force affecting many areas of human life. Demographers and sociologists such as Davis[3] have reported that the world population of some 6 billion (an increase from approximately 3.5 billion only a decade or so ago) is multiplying so fast, especially in underdeveloped countries, that if the present rate continues, the total population will double about every 30 years. On this basis, within 200 years the world population will be approximately 230 billion or nearly 40 times the present total of some 6 to 6.5 billion people! In the past decade the population of the United States has reached about 200 to 250 million, which the last census of 1980 clarifies and describes, with estimates that our population will probably reach approximately 300 million in the next three or four decades, although the rate of growth has shown some decline in recent times.

In America this population increase has been reflected not only in total numbers but also in percentage shifts in age and location. For example, there is an increasing percentage of older people, and there is greater overall mobility. It is estimated that this increased movement of individuals and families continues to represent about 20% of the total population at present. Also, urban-suburban trends have created changes in individual psychologic patterns, in family patterns, and in community and national social patterns. All these changes affect health needs and social values.

Social revolution

Radical changes in family and community patterns have come with the development of the urban-suburban complex in a highly industrialized society. Crowded, low-income housing in the cities contrasts with sprawling, affluent suburbs that consume, at an alarming rate, open land that was once used for agriculture. While the food-eating population grows, the food-bearing potential of the land is being rapidly destroyed. Economic affluence, higher costs of living, and more emphasis on higher education (all in the face of poverty pockets in urban and some rural areas) have changed human goals, health values, and medical care programs.

Development of the social sciences

The behavioral sciences (psychology, sociology, and anthropology) are contributing insights into the concern for human behavior and response to illness, and there is a new effort within the health professions to understand and help the total patient. More time is devoted to analysis of the impact of social and cultural factors on human life. The functional illness is recognized as a very real phenomenon, and the medical profession is beginning to realize that an individual's life situation and his reaction to stress must be considered if his total health needs are to be met.

However, the recognition that the social sciences are basic to medicine and nutrition is still in the course of a slow development. It is significant, however, that an increasing number of current texts emphasize this combined approach.

EFFECT OF CHANGE AND DEVELOPMENT ON HEALTH CARE PRACTICES

Scientific and social developments, together with the changing attitudes toward health and disease, have had some profound effects on the kind of health services provided to the individual patient by physicians, dentists, nutritionists and dietitians, nurses, social workers, and other health personnel.

Four basic changes in our health care system are evolving with increasing focus and certainty:

1. Change in *focus* to include the social issues involved, without which a viable system cannot exist. This focus places value and emphasis on preventive health maintenance and promotion rather than on the exclusive traditional medical approach of curative practice.[4]
2. Changes in *systems of delivery* of health care based on two ideas:
   a. A health team for primary care — family physician, nurse-practitioner, nutritionist, and family health worker, bringing in other specialists as needed
   b. Stations for service, such as satellite clinics or health centers, surrounding a central core medical center or hospital

   The current development of Health Maintenance Organizations (HMOs) reflects these emerging patterns in the nature of health care and the changing roles of health practitioners in providing that care.[5]
3. Changes in *relations with consumers* involving them in community control, planning, and decision making. Such an active role in personal health care implies an increased need for client education.[4]
4. Changes in *payment for services* to some form of national health insurance program.

The effect of all these changes will be far reaching, and education and practice in the health professions must confront the issues involved. With the increasing complexity of our society, these issues become more difficult. For example, Mott has described such difficulties in relating health legislation, Public Law 93-641 — the Health Planning and Resources Development Act—to the establishment of new health systems agencies (HSAs).[6,7]

In clinical nutrition and nursing, two effects of these changes, particularly, touch the dietitian and the nurse and involve the application of nutritional sciences to clinical practice. They both must reconcile the possible conflict between the *science* and the *art* of their professions and must function as members of the *health team*. This is true of other health team members as well.

The science and art of clinical care

Science is a body of systematic knowledge, facts, and principles that shows the operation of natural law. The rapid advances in scientific knowledge have provided clinicians with a stronger basis on which to build professional practice. *Art* is an exceptional ability to conduct any human activity. However, all practitioners must base their practice on sound scientific knowledge and must know and care about people and their needs. Scientific knowledge has little significance apart from application to human need. In each aspect of patient care the clinicians function as catalysts that bring scientific knowledge and human living together. They bring a particular knowledge and skill to bear on the patient's need at a particular point in his life. This role is shown diagrammatically in Fig. 1-1.

The health team approach

The health team approach has been devised as an attempt to meet some of the problems brought about by the rapid increase in population and the equally rapid expansion of scientific knowledge. It is based on a recognition that two groups of persons are directly affected by these developments—those in need of health care and those who are trained to give health care.

The rapidly increasing number of people needing care has brought tremendous pressure on community health resources. Physicians charged with the major responsibility of medical care have felt this pressure most. They have realized that the time is long past when they can be all things to all people. The modern physician is usually interested in the building of an effective health care team.

The rapid advance of science has brought an increasing complexity to health care. The cooperation of a team of specialists is required, who share their special knowledge and learn from each other for the welfare of the patient. Palmer and Thompson describe such an interdisciplinary team in action in the health care of children, in diagnosis as well as treatment.[8] The care of the total patient also requires a wide range of facilities. Even the most elaborate facilities, however, are useless unless they are available to the people whom the health team seeks to serve.

Unique position of the clinical dietitian and the nurse on the health team. Whether functioning in the hospital, the clinic, or the community, the clinical dietitian (the clinical nutrition specialist) and the nurse hold positions on the health team in a unique relation

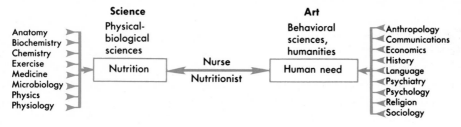

Fig. 1-1. The science and art of nutrition applied to human need.

to the patient. In certain respects they are closest to the patient and the family and have the opportunity to help determine many of the patient's needs, which include his basic nutritional requirements. They must coordinate services and often are the only ones who can help the patient understand and participate in his care. They have unparalleled opportunity to practice continuous patient-centered care that treats the whole person. In carrying out the other aspect of this role, it will frequently be the clinical dietitian or the nurse who reminds the entire health team that a person has emotional as well as physical needs, that he is part of a family whose members are also involved in his care, that he has an occupation, and that he lives in a specific community environment.

Such practitioners are concerned not merely with the *how* but also with the *why*. More pointedly still, they are concerned with the *who* and realize that their most therapeutic contribution is their genuine involvement and concern.

THE STUDY OF NUTRITION IN EDUCATION FOR THE HEALTH PROFESSIONS

In the light of the preceding discussion the question, "What place does knowledge of nutrition have in the practice of my profession?" can be considered.

The answer to the question must be sought in the context of the ideas about professional health practitioners that have been developed in this chapter. Food is fundamental to life and health, and a health care professional is concerned with helping each person under his or her care to achieve personal goals and to experience life and health to the fullest possible degree. In medical education, for example, certain nutrition concepts are increasingly viewed as essential in the education of the medical student.[9] The answer to the question lies in recognizing the evolving nature of the health care professions in a rapidly changing society. Since nutrition is an integral part of health care, the nutritionist is a key person who must be sensitive to current and future health needs and who must use these insights in setting professional directions.

The plan of study

Basic objective. The basic objective of this book is twofold. The objective is to provide sound, relevant background knowledge in the science of human nutrition and then to translate the scientific principles of nutrition into clear concepts with significant application to patient-centered care.

In this person-centered approach the science of nutrition is applied to individuals and their families in various situations and in the stress situation of illness.

Method. Four areas of nutrition in health care will be considered: (1) the scientific basis of nutrition, (2) nutrition as a part of community health, (3) the importance of nutrition in health care specialties, such as maternal-child health, geriatrics, psychiatry, and rehabilitation, and (4) the role of nutrition in clinical care.

Part I, Foundations of Nutrition, presents the fundamental principles of nutrition as they relate to human life and growth and emphasizes the scientific base of nutrition. In applying the scientific method to the study of human beings the whole must be considered first, and then each component part is studied in turn. This is the *analytical* method of scientific investigation. However, a human exists not in parts, but as a coordinated whole. The attempt is therefore made in each case to achieve a *synthesis,* which will relate each part to the whole. Emphasis will be placed on the fact that the unity of the whole is maintained by means of interrelationships between all the chemical elements and functions in the body.

In the spirit of mutual and open inquiry, Part I will be concerned with the basic nutrients (carbohydrates, fats, proteins), their nature, their fate and function in the body, and the regulatory roles of the accessory factors (vitamins and minerals). Part I will also be concerned with the way humans secure energy for their many life needs. In addition, the vital balance between water and electrolytes and the maintenance of the acid-base equilibrium will be discussed. Finally, the interrelationships in the overall process of digestion, absorption, and metabolism will be summarized.

Part II, Applied Nutrition in Community Health, applies the basic elements of nutritional science to persons as they live from day to day. It will deal with factors important in any life situation but will present facts that are particularly applicable to community health. Part II will be concerned with the reasons for and the dangers of food faddism. It will also be concerned with the community food supply and how it is protected and with cultural food patterns and the significant cohesive force they exert on community life. The cost of food and the wise use of the family food dollar, especially at low-income levels, will be considered. This part will also discuss ways of teaching nutrition in community settings, the need for family counseling, the use of dietary guides, and the basic nutritional deficiency diseases.

Part III, Nutrition in the Health Care Specialty, applies nutritional knowledge to the various specialty areas. The fundamental experience of birth and growth is the background for Chapter 17, Nutrition during Pregnancy and Lactation. This chapter considers the nutritional needs of the expectant mother and her newborn infant. Chapter 18, Nutrition for Growth and Development: Infancy, Childhood, and Adolescence, focuses on the nutritional needs of the growing child. In special needs, such as toxemias of pregnancy and deficiency diseases of childhood, modifications or emphases of diet therapy are correlated with the specific condition. Other sections of Part III are devoted to nutritional aspects of patient care in geriatrics, psychiatry, and rehabilitation.

Part IV, Nutrition in Clinical Care, applies basic nutritional science to the care of persons with specific diseases, on the premise that sound, optimal nutrition is a primary consideration in any illness and that therapeutic diets should modify an adequate diet only so far as is necessary to meet a specific condition. The introductory section deals with the study and care of the hospitalized patient and recognizes the stress that illness and hospitalization impose on him and the subsequent need for nutrition assessment as a basis for constant effective care planning. Other chapters deal with nutritional therapy in medical-surgical care with emphasis on the health teaching function of the health team members.

Tools for study

To aid and focus the overall study of nutrition and diet therapy, several learning devices will be used.

Concepts. Each idea is considered first from the point of view of basic principles, which are then applied to specific situations.

Terms. Words are important vehicles for communicating ideas. Many key words will be analyzed, and their derivations will be considered. To illustrate, the English word *concept* comes from a Latin root verb, *capere,* which means "to seize." The prefix *con-* is a derived form of the Latin word *cum,* meaning "with." When one combines the two parts, the literal meaning of concept is "to seize with," which means that one idea is "seized" and put "with" other ideas to construct a mental image of the whole idea. Diagrams will also be used in this book to further illustrate concepts. At the end of some chapters there will be a glossary of the key terms that have been introduced in the chapter. These do not simply contain dictionary definitions but have brief explanations of the concepts represented by the words. These glossaries should be useful tools for review.

Questions. When introducing basic material, salient questions will often be raised to stimulate the search for answers. A spirit of open inquiry is an important attitude to form in any scientific study. These questions will also serve as hooks on which to hang subsequent learning.

Clinical application. Abstract theory is of little practical value. It finds meaning only as it is applied to real situations. Throughout this study, emphasis will be placed on application of the nutritional science principles to specific clinical situations and individual needs. This book will look into the why of certain observations. The rationale for treatment and care will be considered in general terms and on an individual patient basis in various chapters under case studies.

General and specific references. As a stimulus to still further inquiry and reading, references are given at the end of each chapter. These include basic texts in the subject area and articles of related interest in journals, bulletins, pamphlets, and reviews. Also, at various points there will be boxed material entitled, To Probe Further. These offer additional material designed to take the curious student a step further with explanatory material or research on which theories are based.

Results of this approach to study of nutrition

An increasing awareness of the importance of nutrition programs is resulting from growing evidence of linkages between diet and disease and from the role nutrition may play in controlling the rising costs of medical care.[10] Indeed, the health care professions will be enriched as they outgrow their image of nutrition as a sterile, stereotyped, and often irrelevant set of diet lists and learn to take into consideration community needs and the fascinating subtleties of human relationships to food. The hospitalized patient, for example, looks forward to three events during each day — the physician's visit, the visit of loved ones, and the food tray. Hunger and its fulfillment must be placed in proper perspective as basic to vital,

patient-centered care. The health care professional must realize that food bears the imprint of culture and that it reflects a person's attitudes and the pattern of his social group. Nothing is more basic than food to an individual's physical existence and maintenance of health.

Recognizing the importance of food and nutrition will deepen and facilitate patient care. In such a personalized context, nutritional care can help to "humanize health care" and prevent "thinging" — the perception of persons as objects rather than as unique human beings.[11] It will help the health care practitioner (1) to think of patients as individual, unique human beings with specific needs, (2) to think of health care as a person-centered profession, and (3) to think of nutrition as a dynamic applied science that deals with both physical and psychosocial components. Nutrition as a science and an art not only is applicable to the patient on a special diet, but is a constant vital part of person-centered care for every patient.

REFERENCES
Specific

1. Paddock, W., and Paddock, P.: Famine—1975! America's decision: who will survive? Boston, 1967, Little, Brown and Co.
2. Mayer, J.: The dimensions of human hunger, Sci. Am. **235:**40, 1976.
3. Davis, K.: The world's population crisis. In Merton, R. K., and Nesbit, R. A., editors: Contemporary social problems, New York, 1966, Harcourt, Brace & World, Inc., p. 374.
4. Green, L. W.: Health promotion policy and the placement of responsibility for personal health care, Fam. Commun. Health, **2:**51, Nov., 1979.
5. Miike, L.: The future of new health practitioners, Fam. Commun. Health **2:**65, Nov., 1979.
6. Mott, P. D., Mott, A. T., Rudolph, J. M., et al.: Difficult issues in health planning, development, and review, Am. J. Public Health **66:**743, Aug., 1976.
7. United States Department of Health, Education, and Welfare: Health planning and resources development act of 1974, DHEW Pub. no. (HRA) 75-14015, Washington, D.C., 1975, U.S. Government Printing Office.
8. Palmer, S., and Thompson, R. T., Jr.: Nutrition: an integral component in the health care of children, J. Am. Diet. Assoc. **69:**138, 1976.

9. Gallagher, C. R., and Vivian, V. M.: Nutrition concepts essential in the education of the medical student, Am. J. Clin. Nutr. **32:**1330, June, 1979.
10. Quelch, J. A.: The resource allocation process in nutrition policy planning, Am. J. Clin. Nutr. **32:**1058, May, 1979.
11. Howard, J., et al.: Humanizing health care, Med. Care **15:**11, May, 1977.

General

American Dietetic Association: Position paper on the nutrition component of health services delivery systems, J. Am. Diet. Assoc. **58:**538-540, June, 1971.
American Public Health Association, Medical Care Section: Papers from Medical Sociology Section of the American Sociological Association, special studies: issues in promoting health, Med. Care, vol. 15 (special supplement), May, 1977.
Bates, B.: Doctor and nurse: changing roles and relations, N. Engl. J. Med. **283:**129, 1970.
Bray, G. A.: Nutrition in the Humphrey tradition, J. Am. Diet. Assoc. **75:**116-121, Aug., 1979.
Breslau, N., and Novack, A. H.: Public attitudes toward some changes in the division of labor in medicine, Med. Care **17:**859-867, Aug., 1979.
Chinn, P. L.: Child health maintenance: concepts in family-centered care, ed. 2, St. Louis, 1979, The C. V. Mosby Co.
Chou, M., and Harmon, D. P., Jr., editors: Critical food issues of the eighties, New York, 1979, Pergamon Press, Inc.
Collen, F. B., Madero, B., Soghikian, K., and Garfield, S. R.: Kaiser-Permanente experiment in ambulatory care, Am. J. Nurs. **71:**1371, 1971.
Corey, L., Epstein, M. F., and Saltman, S. E.: Medicine in a changing society, ed. 2, St. Louis, 1977, The C. V. Mosby Co.
Duval, M. K.: The challenge ahead, J. Am. Diet. Assoc. **60:**13-16, Jan., 1972.
Fox, J. G., editor: Controversial and legal issues, Fam. Commun. Health, vol. 2, Nov., 1979.
Garfield, S. R.: A new system of medical care delivery, Sci. Am. **222:**17, 1970.
Hamburg, D. A.: Disease prevention: the challenge of the future, Am. J. Public Health **69:**1026-1033, Oct., 1979.
Haug, M. R., and Lavin, B.: Public challenge of physician authority, Med. Care **17:**844-858, Aug., 1979.
Howard, J., Davis, F., Pope, C., and Ruzek, S.: Humanizing health care: the implications of technology, centralization, and self-care, Med. Care **15:**11-26, May, 1977.
Howard, J., and Strauss, A., editors: Humanizing health care, New York, 1975, John Wiley & Sons, Inc.
Kocher, R. E.: New dimensions for dietetics in today's health care, J. Am. Diet. Assoc. **60:**17-20, Jan., 1972.
Lee, P. R.: Nutrition policy—from neglect and uncertainty to debate and action, J. Am. Diet. Assoc. **72:**581-588, June, 1978.
Manocha, S. L.: Nutrition and our overpopulated planet, Springfield, Ill., 1975, Charles C Thomas, Publisher.
Moe, E. O., editor: Community assessment, Fam. Commun. Health, vol. 1, July, 1978.
Nutrition Subcommittee, Committee on Public Health of the New York Academy of Medicine: Recommendations concerning consultant dietitians in private practice, the colors of dietetics are raised on a medical flagship, Nutr. Today **14:**30-31, Sept./Oct., 1979.
Owen, A. L., and Owen, G. M.: Training public health nutritionists: competencies for complacency or future concerns, Am. J. Public Health **69:**1096, Nov., 1979.
Reinhardt, D. M., and Quinn, M. D., editors: Elements of family and community health, Fam. Commun. Health, vol. 1, April, 1978.
Shaw, S. H., and Miller, D.: Preventive medicine through nutrition: a model health care delivery system in San Diego County, J. Am. Diet. Assoc. **75:**49-51, July, 1979.
Simborg, D. W., Starfield, B. H., and Horn, S. D.: Physicians and non-physician health practitioners: the characteristics of their practices and relationships, Am. J. Public Health **68:**45-48, Jan., 1978.
Sims, L. S.: Identification and evaluation of competencies of public health nutritionists, Am. J. Public Health **69:**1099-1105, Nov., 1979.
Terris, M., Cornely, P. B., Daniels, H. C., and Kerr, L. E.: The case for a national health service, Am. J. Public Health **67:**1183-1185, Dec., 1977.
Turner, R. W.: Urgent care in the HMO, Med. Care **16:**361-371, May, 1978.
Vacek, P. M., Ashikaga, T., Mabry, J. H., and Brown, J. P.: A model for health care delivery with an illustration of its application, Med. Care **16:**547-559, July, 1978.
Williams, S. R., and Dickman, S. R., editors: Nutrition and health promotion, Fam. Commun. Health, vol. 1, Feb., 1979.
Winterfeldt, E. A.: Food and nutrition for the 1980's: moving ahead, J. Am. Diet. Assoc. **75:**115, Aug., 1979.

2 Carbohydrates

Over the ages, of all the basic nutrients that sustain man, carbohydrates have been of prime importance. Four factors have contributed to this primacy.

Availability. Carbohydrates comprise a large part of the world's available food supply. They are widely distributed in such easily grown plants as grains, vegetables, and fruits. In fact, in some countries these carbohydrate foods make up almost the entire diet of the people. Even in America, where a greater dietary variety is available, about 50% of the total caloric intake is in the form of carbohydrates. About 15% to 17% of the total diet's calories come from sugar—a per capita consumption of 36 to 45 kg (80 to 100 lb) per year.[1] Most of this American consumption has increased with a greater use of processed foods.[2,3] For nutritionists these have become disturbing trends.

Low cost. As a result of their wide distribution and supply, carbohydrate foods are relatively inexpensive. If the general income level of a people or an individual family lowers, the proportion of consumed carbohydrate foods rises. This becomes a concern for the health worker dealing with low-income families.

Ease of storage. Compared with other types of food, carbohydrate foods (grains and some fruits and vegetables) can be kept in dry storage for relatively long periods of time without spoilage. In many countries modern processing and packaging have extended the shelf life of carbohydrate products almost indefinitely. On the other hand, protein foods (such as meat and dairy products) must be kept under refrigeration.

Energy value. Because of the readily available glucose equivalent of carbohydrates, man depends on them for a main fuel source. The body rapidly oxidizes starches and sugars to yield carbon dioxide and water; this process is a major source of body heat and energy.

GENERAL AND CHEMICAL DEFINITIONS OF CARBOHYDRATES

General definition. For practical purposes in the discussion of dietetics, carbohydrates are starches and sugars. Plants are the main source of carbohydrate in the human diet. These food materials are produced by *photosynthesis* from carbon dioxide and water in the presence of sunlight and the plant's chlorophyll. The carbohydrate product is then stored in the various plant parts such as root, pod, seed, fruit, stem, or leaf. From animals, a lesser source, come carbohydrates in such forms as lactose (milk sugar) and fructose (the sugar in honey).

Chemical definition. Carbohydrates may be further defined according to their chemical elements—carbon, hydrogen, and oxygen. The hydrogen and oxygen occur in the same 2:1 ratio as that found in water (2 hydrogen atoms to 1 oxygen atom; H_2O), although the chemical joining differs from that in water. The name, ''carbo-hydrate,'' originally given to this group of food substances to indicate their basic chemical composition, fails to point out this different type of chemical joining.

The basic chemical structure of the simple sugars is a carbon chain, ranging from 3 to 7 carbon atoms, with the hydrogen and oxygen atoms attached singly and in alcohol or aldehyde groups. The most common carbon chain length is the 6-carbon chain—hexose. Of the hexoses, glucose ($C_6H_{12}O_6$), the most common simple sugar, serves as a good example of the structure (Fig. 2-1).

CLASSIFICATION OF CARBOHYDRATES
Monosaccharides

The simplest form of carbohydrate is the *monosaccharide,* often called simple sugar (Gr. *monos,* single or alone; L. *saccharum,* sugar). The monosaccharides are grouped according to the number of carbon atoms in their basic chain structure:

Trioses—3 carbons	Hexoses—6 carbons
Tetroses—4 carbons	Heptoses—7 carbons
Pentoses—5 carbons	

The *hexoses* are more important nutritionally and physiologically than all the others combined. The four monosaccharides in the hexose group are glucose, fructose, galactose, and mannose.

Glucose (also called dextrose because it is the *dextro*rotatory form of this molecule) is a moderately sweet sugar. It is found as preformed natural glucose in foods or is formed in the body from starch digestion. In human metabolism, all other types of sugar are converted by the body into glucose. Glucose is the form in which sugar circulates in the bloodstream and is oxidized to give energy. Sorbitol is a hexahydric alcohol derived from glucose and has the same caloric value as glucose. It is found in many fruits and vegetables, but is most commonly recognized as a sweetener in various dietetic products.

Fructose (also called levulose because it is

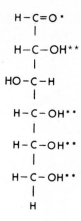

* Aldehyde group
** Alcohol group

Fig. 2-1. Chemical structure of d-glucose.

the *levo*rotatory form of the molecule) is the sugar found in fruits and honey. It is the sweetest of the simple sugars. In human metabolism it is converted to glucose for energy.

Galactose is not found free in foods but is produced from lactose (milk sugar) and is then changed to glucose for energy. The reaction is reversible, and during lactation glucose may be reconverted to galactose, since the lactose component in breast milk is produced from galactose.

Mannose, a relatively unimportant sugar in human nutrition, is not found free in foods but is derived from certain gums. Mannitol, an alcohol derived from mannose, is also used as a sweetener in dietetic products.

Disaccharides

Disaccharides (Gr. *di-,* twice, double) are more complex sugars made up of two monosaccharides. The three main disaccharides with their two component monosaccharides are

Sucrose = Glucose + Fructose

Lactose = Glucose + Galactose

Maltose = Glucose + Glucose

TO PROBE FURTHER

Monosaccharide combinations

Also of interest and importance in medicine and allied fields are combination forms of monosaccharide.

A *glycoside* is a monosaccharide plus a noncarbohydrate residue in the same molecule. Examples are the digitalis derivatives, which form drugs essential to cardiac therapy, and steroids, the adrenal hormones.

A *deoxy sugar* is a sugar with fewer oxygen than carbon atoms. An important and familiar example in physiology is *deoxyribose,* which occurs in nucleic acids such as *deoxyribonucleic acid* (DNA). *DNA* is the cellular substance that is believed to transmit genetic characteristics.

Amino sugars are sugars that contain an amino group (NH_2). An important example of their occurrence is in antibiotics such as the *mycin drugs.* The presence of these sugars is believed to give the antibiotic activity to such drugs.

In each of these disaccharides glucose is one of the two components.

Sucrose (common table sugar) is the most prevalent dietary disaccharide, contributing in today's changing food environment of increased processed foods about 65% of the total carbohydrate calories. It is found in many food sources, including cane and beet sugar, brown sugar, sorghum cane and molasses, maple syrup, pineapple, and carrot roots.

Lactose is the sugar in milk. It is formed in the body from glucose to supply the carbohydrate component of milk during lactation. It is the least sweet of the disaccharides, about one sixth as sweet as sucrose. It is often used in high-carbohydrate, high-calorie liquid feedings when the needed quantity of sucrose cannot be tolerated. When milk sours, as in the initial stages of cheese making, the lactose is changed to lactic acid and separates in the liquid whey from the remaining solid curd. The curd is then processed for cheese. Therefore, although milk has a relatively high-carbohydrate content (lactose), one of its main products—cheese—has none.

Maltose occurs in malt products and in germinating cereals. As such, it is a negligible dietary carbohydrate. However, it is important as an intermediate product of starch digestion.

Relative sweetness of the sugars. With sucrose as a base for comparison, given a value of 100, the general relative sweetness of the common sugars has been evaluated as follows:

Fructose	110 to 175
Sucrose	100
Glucose	75
Galactose	35 to 70
Lactose	15 to 30

Polysaccharides

Polysaccharides are even more complex carbohydrates, made up of many units of one monosaccharide.

Starch is the most significant polysaccharide in human nutrition. It is a compound made up of many branching glucose chains, hence it yields only glucose upon hydrolysis or digestion. Starch granules vary in size and shape according to the source (Fig. 2-2). Potato granules, for example, are relatively large, while rice granules are small.

Starch is by far the most important source of carbohydrate in most countries of the world. However, in recent years there has been a sharp

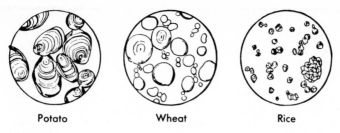

Potato   Wheat   Rice

Fig. 2-2. Starch granules of different sizes from different sources.

decline in starch use to about 25% of the total carbohydrate intake in the American diet. There is some indication currently, though, with an emphasis on use of whole grains, that the proportions of starch in the American diet may be increasing somewhat toward former levels. In other countries where it is the staple food substance, it makes up a higher proportion of the total diet. Major food sources include cereal grains, potatoes and other root vegetables, and legumes.

The cooking of starch not only improves flavor, but also softens and ruptures the starch cells, which facilitates enzymatic digestive processes. The reason starch mixtures thicken when cooked is that the amylopectin that encases the starch granules has a gel quality; this thickens in the same way that fruit pectin causes jelly to set.

Dextrins are polysaccharide compounds that are intermediate products of starch breakdown in the formation of maltose:

Starch + Water $\xrightarrow{\text{Ptyalin}}$ Soluble starch + Maltose

Soluble starch + Water $\xrightarrow{\text{Ptyalin}}$
Erythrodextrins + Maltose

Erythrodextrins + Water $\xrightarrow{\text{Ptyalin}}$
Achroodextrins + Maltose

Achroodextrins + Water $\xrightarrow{\text{Ptyalin}}$ Maltose

This breakdown is accomplished physiologically as a normal part of the body's digestion of starch (Starch → Dextrins → Maltose → Glucose), or commercially by a process of acid

hydrolysis. Dextrins form a soluble, gummy carbohydrate that is used commercially as mucilage for envelopes and postage stamps or as sizing for adhesive tape. Dextri-Maltose, an infant formula preparation, is a combination of dextrins and maltose.

Glycogen is often called animal starch. It is formed from glucose and is stored in relatively small amounts in the liver and in muscle tissue. (See Figs. 2-4, 2-5, 2-7, and 25-1.) Chief food sources therefore of stored glycogen would be animal foods—meat and seafood. Since glycogen is formed from glucose, it yields only glucose upon metabolism.

Inulin, a polysaccharide composed of fructose units, has little dietary significance. It is found only in a few common foods, such as onions, garlic, and artichokes. It is only partially digested, although further breakdown by bacteria may occur in the large intestine. Storage of inulin-containing foods also affects this carbohydrate. The fresh food may have much of its carbohydrate in this unavailable inulin form; however, upon storage much of the inulin may be converted to available sugar.

Although inulin is of small dietary significance, it is of interest and importance in medicine because it provides a test of renal function. Since inulin is filtered at the glomerulus, but neither secreted nor reabsorbed by the tubule, it can be used to measure glomerular filtration rate. This test is called the *inulin clearance test*.

The polysaccharide *cellulose* is but one of a larger group of nondigestible food substances collectively called "dietary fiber." Although all these substances are not carbohydrate, they are discussed here as a group to clarify the nutritional relationships among them and their general clinical significance.

DIETARY FIBER

In the past the common idea held about dietary fiber centered mainly on the basic notion that "bulk" or "roughage" in the diet was required as a normal laxative, or that it prevented so-called "autointoxication" of the body system caused by absorbed by-products of intestinal bacteria action. More recently, however, the information gap has narrowed. Current interest in dietary fiber has been stimulated by early observations and studies in Africa by the British physician Denis Burkitt[4,5,6] and by subsequent follow-up research by many other teams of investigators in different parts of the world. As a result a large body of epidemiologic evidence has grown linking modern low-fiber diets with various diseases. These data have been acclaimed by the popular press and picked up by food industries in products and advertising, often confusing the consumer and health practitioner alike.

Difficulties for the clinician in determining the more precise nutritional and clinical significance of fiber in the human diet have stemmed largely from problems of defining the variety of food substances involved, not all of which have the same properties, and from problems in accurately analyzing and measuring these substances in their variety of food sources. To help clarify these problems, consider the terms "dietary fiber" and "crude fiber" in defining fiber as to its types, respective physiologic properties and effects, nutritional and clinical applications, and practical dietary recommendations.

GENERAL DEFINITION. The word "fiber" is a diffuse term commonly applied to a variety of nondigestible carbohydrate and carbohydrate-related substances for which specific hydrolytic enzymes are lacking in the human digestive system. Confusion arises from the erroneous interchangeable use of the two terms "dietary fiber" and "crude fiber."

Dietary fiber is the total amount of naturally occurring material in foods, mostly plant sources, that is not digested.

Crude fiber is that material remaining after vigorous treatment of the food sources with acid and alkali in the laboratory. Thus it is derived from laboratory analysis and is the value given in most food value tables. These strong laboratory processes remove a good portion of the total dietary fiber that cannot withstand such treatment. Since the proportion of total dietary fiber and crude fiber varies widely among specific foods, depending on the fiber composition of a particular food, the fiber values given in food value tables have limited usefulness to the practitioner and must be used with qualification.

Types of fiber. Fiber may be classed as three general types according to structure and properties: cellulose, noncellulose polysaccharides, and the noncarbohydrate, lignin.

CELLULOSE. A major polysaccharide, cellulose is a carbohydrate of high molecular weight (100,000 to 2 million). This unbranched glucose polymer makes up the principal structural material in plant cell walls and provides most of the substance labeled "crude fiber." It is water insoluble but holds water and is thus bulk producing, reducing elevated intraluminal colon pressure.

NONCELLULOSE POLYSACCHARIDES. The noncellulose carbohydrates include hemicellulose, pectin, gums and mucilages, and algal substances.

Hemicelluloses are linear and branched chains of various saccharide units such as xylose and galactose, found in the cell wall of numerous plants. Hemicellulose holds water and is bulk producing, also contributing to reduced intraluminal colon pressure.

Pectins are polysaccharides composed mainly of methylated galacturonic acid units that form an intercellular cementing complex with protein in the structure of plant cell walls. This gellike structure absorbs water, slows gastric emptying time, and may bind bile acids.

Gums and mucilages are polysaccharides composed of galacturonic acid variously combined with units of mannose, rhamnose, arabinose, or xylose. They form base material for plant secretions or seeds. Their physical properties are similar to those of pectin: absorbing water, slowing gastric emptying time, and binding bile acids.

Algal substances are polysaccharides from algae and seaweeds composed of glucuronic acid with mannose, glucose, and xylose. These substances also have affinity for water, form bulk, slow gastric emptying time, and may bind bile acids.

LIGNIN. The only noncarbohydrate type of fiber, lignin is a polymer of phenyl propane units forming the woody part of plants. It acts as a cation exchange resin, combinging with bile acids to form insoluble compounds, thus preventing their absorption. This property is similar to that of the cholesterol-lowering drug, cholestyramine, an anion exchange resin.

Other related carbohydrate compounds that are not foods but occur in the body as structural or viscous secretory materials are mucopolysaccharides and mucoproteins. These materials include *keratosulfate* in nails, *dermatan sulfate* in skin, *chondroitin sulfate* in tissues such as cartilage, bone, skin, cornea, aorta and heart valves, *hyaluronic acid* in intercellular fluid material of joints and the vitreous humor of the eye, and *heparin* in the blood, an anticoagulant.

Physiologic effects. The physiologic properties of fiber produce various effects on the food mix consumed and its fate in the body.

Water absorption capacities of fiber contributing to its bulk-forming laxative effect influence the transit time of the food mass through the digestive tract and hence the rate of absorption of the various nutrients in the food mix. This action may have a smoothing effect, for example, on the rate of absorption of available glucose and subsequent blood glucose levels.

Binding effect of certain fiber such as the noncellulose materials may influence blood lipid levels through their capacity to bind bile salts and cholesterol and prevent their absorption. Some binding effects may be undesirable, however, such as those resulting from fiber materials that bind metals. For example, the phytate in wheat may absorb iron and zinc as well as calcium.

Relation to colon bacteria may have an effect on substances that are produced by these bacteria in the gastrointestinal tract. Some of the noncellulose fiber materials provide fermentation substrates for colon bacteria, producing volatile fatty acids and gas.

Satiety from food consumed may be enhanced by fiber, since it adds bulk to the food mix. Also, high-fiber foods usually take more time to eat. Both of these factors may help to control amount of food consumed, eating behaviors that contribute to management of obesity and diabetes.

Clinical significance. These physiologic effects of fiber have been the basis of much recent study concerning the possible clinical applications in disease prevention and control. This research has largely centered on the relation of fiber to gastrointestinal problems, cardiovascular disease, diabetes mellitus, and cancer.

GASTROINTESTINAL PROBLEMS. The relation of fiber to control of *constipation* is well established. Water absorption by the fiber softens and increases volume of the feces, causing the colon to contract and propel its contents faster. The fecal volume is also influenced by fiber's effect on increasing bacterial growth and bulk excreted, as well as colon flora production of volatile fatty acids, which stimulate fecal elimination. The bile acids that fiber transports to the colon may have similar cathartic effects. More recently, the role of fiber in diverticular disease has been established by investigators such as Plumley and Francis in England, who controlled symptoms of diverticulosis in their patients using a high-fiber diet.[7] Other researchers have found similar results.

CARDIOVASCULAR DISEASE. Fiber has been related to the control of blood lipids, especially cholesterol, through its binding effect, although results have been inconclusive.[8]

DIABETES MELLITUS. Studies relating fiber to control of blood glucose have demonstrated fiber's ability to lower hyperglycemia, probably through its effect on transit time and rate of nutrient absorption.[9,10]

CANCER. The role of fiber in colon cancer has been under investigation by a number of groups. Although these studies are inconclusive at this point, they are based on reasonable proposed mechanisms and have produced a large body of epidemiologic data pointing to such relationships.[11,12]

Clinical applications of the relation of fiber to these various medical problems are discussed in more detail in Part Four, Nutrition in Clinical Care.

Dietary recommendations. In the light of these physiologic and nutritional effects of fiber, what reasonable recommendation can a practitioner make about dietary fiber? Household surveys in recent years conducted by the U.S. Department of Agriculture have shown a decrease in fiber in the diet to about 4 g of crude fiber. Epidemiologic data seem to indicate correlation between incidence of disease, as indicated above, with low-residue or low-fiber diets. Extremes in use of crude fiber to as much as 25 g seems unwarranted in light of nutrient loss in some cases as in binding of iron, zinc, and calcium. A daily recommendation of about 6 to 8 g of crude fiber (total dietary fiber would be more) appears wise. This can be easily achieved through generous use of whole grains, vegetables, fruits, seeds, and nuts. Some added bran may be indicated, but indiscriminate use is not justified. More valid food values for total dietary fiber may be found in tables of selected foods provided by Southgate et al.[13]

FUNCTIONS OF CARBOHYDRATES IN THE BODY

Energy. The prime, overall function of carbohydrate in human nutrition is to provide energy. Although fat also is a fuel, it is primarily a storage form and the body may function without a dietary source of it. However, the body tissues require a constant dietary supply of carbohydrate to exist. The metabolic interrelationships involved are further discussed in this chapter in the section concerning the Krebs cycle (see pp. 27-30).

The amount of carbohydrate in the body is relatively small. A total of approximately 365 g is stored in the liver and the muscle tissues and is present in circulating blood sugar. The following shows the breakdown of carbohydrate storage in the body of a man weighing 70 kg (154 lb).

Liver glycogen	100 g
Muscle glycogen	245 g
Extracellular blood sugar	10 g
TOTAL	365 g
	(1,460 calories)

The 365 g of glucose provide energy sufficient for only about 13 hours of moderate activity. Carbohydrates must be ingested regularly and at moderately frequent intervals to meet the energy demands of the body.

Of the total carbohydrate ingested, however, three general factors affect the amount that will be available for use and the way the body will use it:

1. The state of the mucous membrane of the digestive tract and the time the carbohydrate is held in contact with this absorbing surface affect the availability of carbohydrates. Intestinal disease affecting the bowel lining or a hyperactive bowel

(which causes rapid passage of food materials) greatly decrease the proportion of the total ingested carbohydrate that will be used by the body.

2. Endocrine function is also important in carbohydrate availability. Several hormones play important roles in the use of carbohydrate. Among these are insulin and the several insulin antagonists such as hormones secreted by the pituitary gland, steroids secreted from the adrenal glands, glucagon secreted by the pancreas, and epinephrine secreted by the adrenal medulla. Imbalance among these various regulatory agents can greatly affect the body's use of carbohydrate.

3. Vitamins must be present in adequate amounts. Vitamins of the B complex especially are involved in the metabolism of carbohydrate. Thiamin, niacin, riboflavin, and others perform key functions in the enzyme systems for the oxidation of carbohydrate.

Special functions of carbohydrates in vital organs. In addition to their overall function as the body's main energy source, carbohydrates also serve special functions in certain vital organs.

LIVER. In the liver, carbohydrate not only is oxidized as fuel, but also serves two other important functions. First, it exerts a protective action by being present as glycogen and by participating in specific detoxifying metabolic pathways. For example, a glucose derivative, glucuronic acid, conjugates with certain toxic materials (drugs) to produce harmless forms for excretion.

Second, carbohydrate has a regulating influence on protein and fat metabolism. The presence of sufficient carbohydrate for energy demands prevents the channeling of too much protein for this purpose. This *protein-sparing action* of carbohydrate allows a major portion of protein to be used for its basic structural purpose of tissue building. The amount of carbohydrate present also determines how much fat will be broken down. Therefore it affects the formation and disposal rates of ketones. Ketones and intermediate products of fat metabolism, which normally are broken down to fatty acids. However, in extreme conditions (such as starvation or uncontrolled diabetes) in which carbohydrate is inadequate or inavailable, the ketones accumulate and produce a condition called ketosis or acidosis (see p. 30). The *antiketogenic effect* of carbohydrate prevents a damaging excess of ketone formation and accumulation.

HEART. Heart action is a life-sustaining muscular exercise. The glycogen in cardiac muscle is an important emergency source of contractile energy. In a damaged heart, poor glycogen stores or a low-carbohydrate intake may cause cardiac symptoms or angina.

CENTRAL NERVOUS SYSTEM. A constant amount of carbohydrate is necessary for the proper functioning of the central nervous system. Its regulatory center, the brain, contains no stored supply of glucose and is therefore especially dependent on a minute-to-minute supply of glucose from the blood. Sustained and profound hypoglycemic shock may cause irreversible brain damage. In all nerve tissue, carbohydrate is indispensable for functional integrity.

DIGESTION OF CARBOHYDRATES

The digestion of carbohydrate proceeds through the successive parts of the gastrointestinal tract, aided by both mechanical and chemical processes. The chemical processes involved are enzymatic in nature. An enzyme is a complex organic substance, protein in chemical nature, produced in a living cell and capable of causing certain chemical changes in other organic materials by acting as a catalyst. These processes are explained in greater detail in Chapter 5.

Mouth. Mastication breaks the food into fine particles and mixes it with the saliva. During this process a component enzyme of the saliva

Table 2-1. Summary of carbohydrate digestion

Organ	Enzyme	Action
Mouth	Ptyalin	Starch → Dextrins → Maltose
Stomach	None	(Above action continued to minor degree)
Small intestine	Pancreatic	
	Amylopsin	Starch → Dextrins → Maltose
	Intestinal	
	Sucrase	Sucrose → Glucose + Fructose
	Lactase	Lactose → Glucose + Galactose
	Maltase	Maltose → Glucose + Glucose

secreted by the parotid gland, a salivary amylase called *ptyalin,* acts on starch to begin its breakdown into dextrins and maltose.

Stomach. Mechanical digestion is continued in the stomach by successive wavelike contractions of the muscle fibers of the stomach wall. This action, peristalsis, further mixes food particles with gastric secretions to allow the chemical activity of digestion to take place more readily. The gastric juice contains no specific enzyme for the breakdown of carbohydrate, and hydrochloric acid (HCl) in the stomach counteracts the alkaline activity of ptyalin. Mechanical digestion continues to bring the carbohydrate to the pyloric valve as part of the food mass, now a thick, creamy *chyme,* ready for emptying into the duodenum, the first portion of the small intestine.

Small intestine. Peristalsis continues to aid digestion in the small intestine by mixing and moving the chyme along the length of the tube. Chemical digestion of carbohydrate is completed in the small intestine by enzymes from two sources: (1) The *pancreatic juice,* which enters the duodenum through the common bile duct, contains an amylase, *amylopsin,* which continues the breakdown of starch to maltose. (2) The *intestinal juice* contains three disaccharidases, *sucrase, lactase,* and *maltase,* which act on their respective disaccharides to

render the monosaccharides glucose, galactose, and fructose ready for absorption. Interestingly enough, these disaccharidases are almost exclusively *intracellular;* that is, they reside and carry on their activities within the cells of the mucosa (the inner layer of the intestinal wall). The digestion of disaccharides takes place not in the lumen of the intestine but within the intestinal mucosal cell.

A summary of the digestion of carbohydrate through these successive parts of the gastrointestinal tract is given in Table 2-1.

ABSORPTION OF CARBOHYDRATE INTO THE BLOODSTREAM

Carbohydrate is absorbed into the bloodstream as glucose, galactose, and fructose. The absorbing surface area of the small intestine is greatly enlarged by millions of villi, which are tiny, fingerlike projections of the mucous membrane. This large absorbing surface allows 90% of the digested food materials to be absorbed into the small intestine. Only water absorption remains to be accomplished in the large intestine.

By way of the capillaries of the villi, the simple sugars enter the portal circulation and are transported to the liver. Here the fructose and galactose are converted to glucose, and the glucose is in turn converted to glycogen for stor-

TO PROBE FURTHER
The process of carbohydrate absorption

The process by which glucose and other monosaccharides are absorbed across the epithelial cells of the intestine is complex and is another example of the specificity of the body's mechanisms. Classic research in the field of glucose absorption, synthesis to glycogen, and reconversion to glucose has been done by Drs. Carl and Gerty Cori* of Washington University School of Medicine. In 1947 they were awarded the Nobel Prize in medicine for their work.

Their studies seem to indicate that the common hexose sugars are absorbed at a fixed, fairly rapid rate, which is independent of their concentration in the intestinal lumen, even against an osmotic gradient. Simple diffusion would be dependent solely on the balance of osmotic forces on both sides of the cell wall. Therefore it is evident that a mechanism other than diffusion is also operating here.

Moreover, the Coris' data indicate that the rates of absorption of the different monosaccharides are not alike. Giving glucose an absorption rate of 100, the comparative rates for the other main simple sugars are 110 for galactose and 43 for fructose. The work of other researchers† concerning glucose jejunal absorption bears out this relative rate. There seems, then, to be a *specific selectivity* in the absorption of these monosaccharides.

Two mechanisms apparently are involved in sugar absorption: (1) *simple diffusion,* dependent on a greater sugar concentration within the intestinal lumen than in the mucosal cells and, in turn, in the blood plasma, and (2) *active transport* that requires energy, independent of the intestinal concentration (some sort of "pump"). This concept is further discussed in Chapter 10.

*Cori, C. F.: Mammalian carbohydrate metabolism, Physiol. Rev. **11**:143, 1931.
†Inglefinger, F. J.: Gastrointestinal absorption, Nutr. Today **2**:2, 1967.

age. The glycogen is reconverted to glucose as needed by the body.

Factors influencing absorption. The absorption of digested carbohydrate is influenced by four factors.

1. The rate at which the carbohydrate enters the small intestine affects its absorption. This rate of entry depends on the motility of the stomach and the control of the duodenal sphincter muscle, the pyloric valve.

2. The type of food mixture present influences the degree of competition for absorbing sites and available carrier transport systems.

3. Absorption is also influenced by the condition of intestinal membranes and the time carbohydrate is held in contact with these membranes. Any abnormality of the mucosal tissue (enteritis, celiac disease) or an abnormally rapid movement of the carbohydrate along the intestine (diarrhea) will hinder absorption.

4. Normal endocrine activity of the anterior pituitary and the related functioning of the thyroid is necessary for normal absorption. In addition, the adrenal cortex hormones regulate the body's sodium exchange, which indirectly influences the operation of the sodium pump.

METABOLISM OF CARBOHYDRATE

In this discussion and in those to follow concerning the other nutrients, a significant scientific principle will emerge. This principle may be stated as the *unity of the human organism*. The human organism is a whole made up of many parts and processes that possess unequaled specificity and flexibility. Intimate metabolic relationships exist among all the basic nutrients and metabolites, and it is impossible to understand any one of a human's metabolic processes without viewing it in relationship to the others that comprise the whole.

Metabolism is the sum of the physical and chemical processes in a living organism by which protoplasm, the basic substance of cells and tissues, is produced, maintained, or destroyed; and by which energy is made available for the functioning of the organism. A *metabolite* is a product of a specific metabolic process.

Three terms of medical importance that relate to blood sugar levels should be clearly understood by the practitioner, who will constantly encounter them in clinical work. *Normoglycemic* refers to blood sugar levels within the range of normal; *hypoglycemic* indicates blood sugar levels below the normal range; *hyperglycemic* means blood sugar levels above the normal range.

In cell nutrition the most important end product of the digestion of dietary carbohydrate is glucose, since fructose and galactose are eventually converted to glucose. The liver is the major site of the fascinating metabolic machinery that handles glucose, and much of the chemical activity takes place there. However, other tissues such as adipose fat tissue, muscle tissue, and renal tissue play important roles, and energy metabolism in general goes on in all cells.

The answers to four basic questions concerning carbohydrate metabolism are important to understand how the body handles glucose:

1. What are the sources from which glucose enters the blood?
2. What happens to glucose in the blood and tissues?
3. What hormones control the metabolism of glucose?
4. How is energy produced from glucose?

Sources of blood glucose

The sources of blood glucose are divided into carbohydrate and noncarbohydrate substances.

TO PROBE FURTHER
Sodium-potassium pump

An interesting mechanism believed to be operative in glucose absorption demonstrates the principle of *intimate metabolic interrelatedness of the nutrients*. It has been called the sodium-potassium pump, because it controls the ratio of sodium to potassium ion concentrations outside and inside the cell (Fig. 2-3).

Current evidence indicates that the entrance of glucose into intestinal wall cells and hence into the blood is sodium dependent. The work of Crane* has shown that a sodium deficiency inhibits glucose absorption. Moreover, when cells are incubated in a glucose-free environment, the pump is reversed: sodium and potassium leave the cell. When glucose is added, the pump reverts to its proper direction. This finely balanced homeostatic mechanism of active transport of glucose requires energy, which is supplied by metabolic processes within the cell.

*Crane, R. K.: Intestinal absorption of sugars, Physiol. Rev. **40**:89, 1960; Hypothesis for mechanism of intestinal active transport of sugars, Fed. Proc. **21**:891, 1962.

Carbohydrate sources. Carbohydrate sources include dietary carbohydrate, tissue glycogen, and products of intermediary carbohydrate metabolism.

Dietary carbohydrates are starches and sugars that are ingested, digested, and absorbed into the bloodstream. These form the major source of the body's glucose. *All* these carbohydrate food materials are converted into glucose.

Glycogen (also called glucogen) is stored in the liver and to a lesser extent in muscle tissue. It is the second main source of blood glucose. The hydrolysis of glycogen to form glucose is called *glycogenolysis* or *glycolysis.*

Products of intermediary carbohydrate metabolism include lactic acid and pyruvic acid. These products are formed by reversible reactions that may either proceed or return to their source material.

Noncarbohydrate sources. Protein and fat are the noncarbohydrate sources of glucose.

Certain *amino acids,* structural units of protein, are *glucogenic;* that is, they form glucose upon metabolic breakdown. After *deamination* (removal of the amino group, see p. 62), the remaining carbon chain forms the skeleton for glucose. This conversion process is catalyzed by adrenocortical steroids (such as cortisone). These steroids therefore have been called the S-hormones, or sugar-forming hormones. About 58% of the protein in a mixed diet is composed of glycogenic amino acids. Therefore it may be stated that more than half of the dietary protein, although it is consumed primarily for its tissue-building function, may ultimately be used for energy.

Fat is also converted into glucose. As will be seen later in greater detail in the discussion of fat metabolism (Chapter 3), after the breakdown of neutral fat into fatty acids and glycerol, the glycerol portion upon hydrolysis may be converted to glycogen in the liver and made available for glucose formation. Since glycerol comprises only about 10% of the fat, it normally contributes very little available glucose. However, under abnormal conditions of carbohydrate metabolism, as in diabetes mellitus, fat assumes a much more significant role in the complicating condition of ketosis.

The production of glucose from protein, fat, and the various intermediate carbohydrate metabolites is called *gluconeogenesis.*

Glucose in the blood and tissues

The body has several means of handling glucose. The blood sugar may be (1) burned for energy, (2) stored for reserve use, or (3) converted to other forms of nutrient. Together these uses of glucose serve to regulate the blood sugar to a normal range of 70 to 120 mg/dl.

The primary function of glucose is to supply energy according to the body's demands. Various metabolic pathways are used to accomplish this task in a highly efficient manner. The two main oxidative pathways, the Embden-Meyerhof glycolytic pathway and the Krebs cycle, together form one continuous pathway (see p. 29).

There are two major processes that convert glucose to storage forms. Glucose may be converted to glycogen and stored as such in the

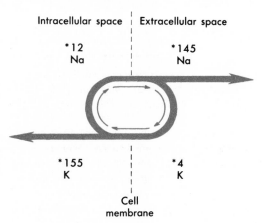

Fig. 2-3. Sodium-potassium pump. Active transport of ions across the cell membrane. (*Sodium and potassium concentration [meq/L] inside and outside the cell.)

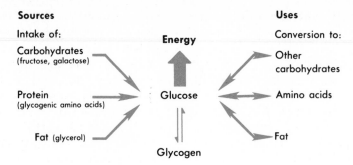

Fig. 2-4. Sources and uses of glucose.

liver and in muscle tissue. This conversion process is called *glycogenesis*. The capacity for this type of storage is limited. Only a small supply of glycogen is present at any one time, and it may be depleted rapidly. After energy demands have been fulfilled by oxidation of glucose and a limited amount has been stored for circulation and emergency reserves, any excess glucose is converted to fat and stored as adipose tissue. This process of conversion to fat is called *lipogenesis*. The capacity for this type of storage seems to be unlimited, to judge from the everyday observation of some human beings!

Some glucose is used in the production of various compounds that are important to the total functioning of the body. A relatively small amount of glucose goes into other carbohydrate compounds that have significant roles in overall body metabolism. Examples of these are

1. Ribose and deoxyribose, required for nucleic acids in the formation of DNA and RNA, which are believed to be key substances in genetic inheritance
2. Mannose, glucosamine, and galactosamine, required for mucopolysaccharides and glycoproteins, such as heparin and blood group materials responsible for the major blood types
3. Glucuronic acid, involved in various detoxification reactions by which the body excretes certain harmful substances

4. Galactose, required for glycolipids and for lactose during the lactation period

Certain amino acids that are synthesized in the body derive their carbon skeletons from glucose or its metabolites (see Chapter 4).

These sources and uses of glucose act as checks and balances to maintain the blood sugar within its normal range by adding sugar to the blood or removing it so that the body maintains a fairly constant internal environment that enables it to meet changing demands and stresses. This is but one more example of the remarkable *homeostatic* mechanisms of the body, built in to sustain life and promote health (Fig. 2-4).

Hormones that control metabolism of glucose

A number of hormones directly and indirectly influence the metabolism of glucose and regulate the blood sugar level according to the body's need. These hormones may be classified according to whether they lower or raise the blood sugar level.

Hormone that lowers the blood sugar level. *Insulin* is the only hormone that lowers the blood sugar. This hormone is perhaps more widely known than all the others. Insulin is produced by beta cells of the pancreas, which are specialized for this purpose. The beta cells form "islands" in the pancreatic tissue and are called the *islets of Langerhans*, named for the scientist Paul Langerhans, who as a young German medical student first discovered and studied them.

Insulin fosters *glycogenesis* by conversion of glucose to glycogen in the liver, where the glycogen is then stored.

Insulin also fosters *lipogenesis,* which is the formation of fat. Glucose is converted to fat for storage in adipose (fat depository) tissue. This conversion takes place mainly in the adipose tissue itself, but some glucose is converted to fat in the liver (see pp. 43-44).

Insulin increases *cell permeability to glucose* and allows glucose to pass from the extracellular fluids into the cells for oxidation to supply needed energy. The precise mechanism by which this is accomplished is not determined, but studies[14-17] indicate that a definite glucose-carrier system exists. Evidence demonstrates that in the presence of insulin, entry of sugar into certain cells is accelerated. Conversely, in the absence of insulin, sugar is prevented from entering. The cell wall presents a barrier to glucose, and an active transfer system is necessary to carry it into the cells. Insulin in some way acts on such a transfer system.

There is evidence that potassium as well as insulin is necessary for glucose entry into cells. When glucose enters the cell, potassium enters with it. Evidence for this association of potassium with glucose can be seen in the uptake of potassium in patients with diabetic acidosis who are treated with insulin. This makes potassium replacement an important part of treatment.

Apparently the cell's dependence on insulin for glucose entry differs in various tissues. For example, studies[18] indicate that glucose uptake is unaffected by the absence of insulin in the brain, red blood cells, intestinal mucosa, kidney tubules, and probably the liver. Tissues dependent on the presence of insulin for glucose uptake are skeletal muscle, adipose tissue, cardiac muscle, eye lens, the aqueous humor, leukocytes, and pituitary tissue.

Although some of the evidence may be inconclusive, insulin is also believed to influence *phosphorylation*. Phosphorylation is the initial and necessary phosphorus coupling step that allows glucose to enter the cell's metabolic pathway to produce energy. According to this theory[19,20] insulin acts on antagonists to the reaction to prevent them from inhibiting the action of *glucokinase* (glucokinase is the specific hexokinase needed to catalyze glucose phosphorylation).

Much evidence [21] exists that insulin promotes *protein synthesis*. However, this may be an indirect result of the increase in energy available for tissue building, which has been facilitated by glucose oxidation.

Hormones that raise the blood sugar level. A number of hormones effectively raise the blood sugar. These include glucagon, steroid hormones, epinephrine, the growth hormone, ACTH, and thyroxine.

Glucagon is also produced by the islets of Langerhans in the pancreas. However, it is produced in the alpha cells and has an effect opposite to that of insulin. Glucagon raises the blood sugar level by increasing hepatic *glycogenolysis,* the breakdown of liver glycogen to glucose. It probably does this by activating the hepatic enzyme catalyst for this conversion, phosphorylase. Glucagon may well be an important factor in maintaining the blood sugar level during starvation.

Somatostatin is a recently discovered hypothalamic hormone believed to operate through its suppression of the pancreatic hormones, insulin and glucagon. Thus this hormone also contributes to the maintenance of a normal blood sugar level. Somatostatin aids in the prevention of human diabetic ketoacidosis, providing evidence for an essential role of glucagon in the balance with insulin to sustain optimal blood glucose levels.[22,23] This breakthrough in diabetic and endocrinologic research provides further tools for management of diabetes.

The *steroid hormones* of the adrenal cortex raise the blood sugar level by stimulating *gluconeogenesis,* which releases glucose-forming carbon units from protein. The glucocorticoids influence glucagon secretion and plasma amino acid concentrations.[24] The steroids also act as insulin antagonists and block the sugar-lowering effect of insulin.

Epinephrine, which is secreted by the adrenal medulla, also raises the blood sugar level by stimulating *glycogenolysis.* Epinephrine is sometimes administered to diabetic patients in insulin shock to counteract severe hypoglycemia. Epinephrine causes a quick release of readily available glucose for immediate use. Apparently, epinephrine also influences the resynthesis and reactivation of phosphorylase in liver and muscle.

Growth hormone (GH), also called *somatotropin,* and *adrenocorticotropic hormone* *(ACTH)* are hormones secreted by the anterior pituitary gland. They raise the blood sugar level by acting as insulin antagonists.

The principal hormone secreted by the thyroid gland, *thyroxine,* has an elevating effect on blood sugar, probably because it influences the rate of insulin destruction, increases glucose absorption from the intestine, and liberates epinephrine.

Energy production from glucose

Once in the cell, glucose must undergo a series of reactions to produce energy for the body's varied demands. Two major pathways, which together form one continuous overall route, are most commonly used. By this route, glucose is broken down into the end products of carbon dioxide and water. Large amounts of energy are generated in the process of breakdown.

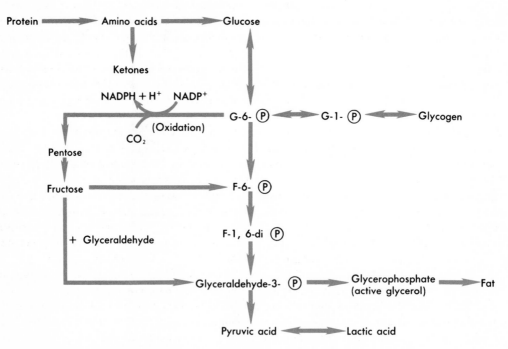

Fig. 2-5. The Embden-Meyerhof glycolytic pathway. F, fructose; G, glucose; P, phosphate; NADP, niacin adenine dinucleotide phosphate; NADPH, same as NADP, carrying H.

Embden-Meyerhof pathway. Through the Embden-Meyerhof pathway, the initial glycolytic pathway, glucose is converted to glycogen and glycogen to glucose. Glucose is also carried to pyruvic and lactic acids (Fig. 2-5). Several important steps along this pathway illustrate the principle of the metabolic interrelatedness of nutrients in human nutrition.

Initial phosphorylation is the first step in a series of reactions. This process adds phosphorus to glucose. The phosphorus traps the glucose in the cell and forms the compound glucose-6-phosphate, which begins the series of reactions that constitutes the Embden-Meyerhof pathway. Phosphate compounds are closely connected with the chemical energy bonds developed during the process of oxidation. An example is ATP (adenosine triphosphate), a compound with high energy bonds that "stores" the energy produced during glucose oxidation (p. 75). The phosphorylation reaction is catalyzed by the enzyme glucokinase, which is the glucose-specific hexokinase. This reaction is believed to be one of the key points at which insulin acts.

The reaction that forms *glycogen* is reversible. Glucose can be removed from the blood to be stored as glycogen, or glycogen can be broken down to form blood glucose.

Glyceraldehyde-3-phosphate provides the active form of glycerol needed for *lipogenesis* (the synthesis of fat from carbohydrate).

The formation of *pyruvic acid,* together with its product, *lactic acid,* ends the glycolytic pathway. The formation of pyruvic acid is important as a junction point because (1) pyruvic acid is the gateway to the final common pathway, the Krebs cycle, and (2) it provides the vital acetyl-CoA (active acetate), the metabolic step through which fatty acids (and in turn fat) are produced from glucose.

Cori cycle. Of interest also, especially in athletics, is the increased metabolism of glucose from muscle glycolysis to form lactic acid, which is then carried by the blood to the liver, where it is reconverted to glucose and returned as blood glucose to the muscles. Normally functioning muscle metabolism yields ATP for use as immediate fuel for muscle work, utilizing glucose, free fatty acids, and ketones as fuel. Basic fuels for resting muscles are fatty acids and ketones, which are converted to acetyl-CoA and enter the Krebs cycle for combustion. However, in actively contracting muscles, as in heavy sustained athletic events, additional glucose is called on to meet the greatly increased energy demand. This increased glucose is rapidly degraded by the glycolytic pathway to pyruvic acid, then in turn to lactic acid, with a consequent build-up of blood lactate in the process of its cycle to the liver for reconversion to blood glucose. It is this elevation of blood lactic acid in sustained strenuous exercise, as in long distance marathon running, for example, that causes a "pain threshold" to be reached. This metabolic cooperation between contracting skeletal muscle and the liver to support active muscle work is called the Cori cycle, named after the husband and wife team of scientists, Carl and Gerty Cori, who discovered and described its function. They were jointly awarded the Nobel Prize in medicine in 1947 for their work in carbohydrate metabolism.[25]

Krebs cycle. The Krebs cycle (also called citric acid cycle or tricarboxylic acid cycle) is the final common pathway that all nutrient metabolites involved in energy production finally enter in some form. It provides more than 90% of the body's energy (Fig. 2-6). Several reaction products along this pathway demonstrate the interrelatedness of the nutrients.

Several B-complex vitamins are involved in the formation of *acetyl*-CoA (active acetate). The compound itself contains pantothenic acid, which is one of the B vitamins. The formation of active acetate from pyruvic acid requires two other B vitamins, thiamin and lipoic acid, as coenzymes. The formation of active acetate is

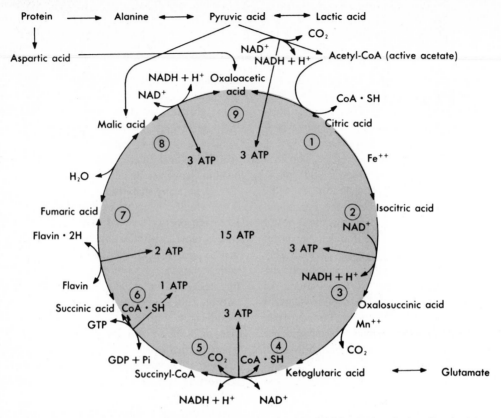

Fig. 2-6. The Krebs cycle. NAD, niacin adenine dinucleotide; NADP, niacin adenine dinucleotide phosphate; NADPH, same as NADP, carrying H; ATP, adenosine triphosphate.

TO PROBE FURTHER
Energy output from glucose oxidation*

The major route of carbohydrate oxidation—the Embden-Meyerhof glycolytic pathway together with the Krebs cycle—is a tremendously efficient producer of energy. It has been credited with an overall efficiency rate of 42%, which results from its ability to produce and store large amounts of energy, while relatively little energy is expended in "running the machine." According to engineering standards, this efficiency rate is above that of many man-made machines.

The energy produced in this route of glucose oxidation is trapped as chemical energy in phosphorus-containing compounds, such as ATP, which store the energy until it is needed. The body's energy supply is conserved rather than dissipated all at once (this point is further discussed in Chapter 5).

It has been calculated that the oxidation of 1 mole of glucose through this efficient system produces 38 high-energy phosphorus bonds—8 in the initial Embden-Meyerhof glycolytic pathway and 30 in the final common Krebs cycle. This is equivalent to an energy output of 288,800 calories!

*Harper, H. A.: Review of physiological chemistry, Los Altos, Calif., 1967, Lange Medical Publications, p. 228.

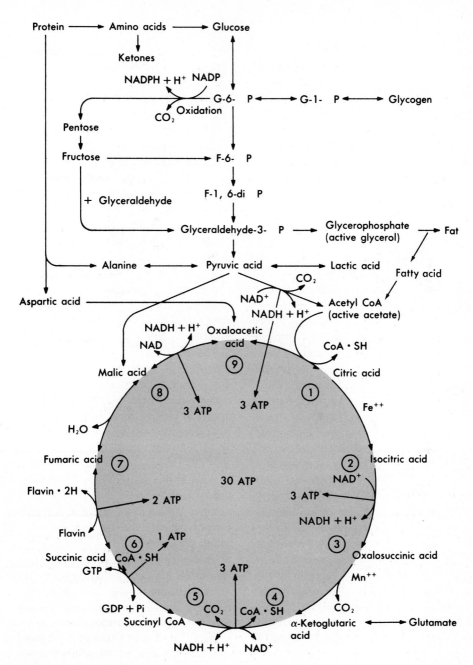

Fig. 2-7. Interrelationships between the two pathways for glucose oxidation—the Embden-Meyerhof pathway and the Krebs cycle.

a major junction point that integrates carbohydrate, fat, and protein metabolism, since acetyl-CoA can also be formed from fatty acids and certain amino acids.

Oxaloacetate (oxaloacetic acid) is formed from pyruvic acid as well as from certain amino acids. Active acetate reacts with oxaloacetate to form *citric acid*. Oxaloacetate is the carbohydrate fuel necessary to keep the process going, because with each complete cycle of reactions by which active acetate is broken down to produce carbon dioxide, water, and energy, another unit of oxaloacetate is produced, which begins the process again. If there is not adequate oxaloacetate from carbohydrate to maintain the cycle efficiently, active acetate from fat cannot be handled properly and is diverted to form ketone bodies. Under usual circumstances, ketones may be considered normal intermediates of fat metabolism. However, when the amount of glucose available is insufficient to perpetuate this process, fat is broken down so rapidly that it cannot be used for fuel. Without the necessary carbohydrate to handle the fat properly, the ketones accumulate, causing ketosis. These ketones are acids (acetoacetic acid, acetone, and β-hydroxybutyric acid), and their accumulation upsets the normal acid-base balance in the body, and acidosis results. Diabetic acidosis clearly demonstrates the interrelatedness of the nutrients and their metabolites. When glucose cannot be properly oxidized because insulin is lacking or unavailable, the oxaloacetate that is necessary to the maintenance of the Krebs cycle is not provided, and the active acetate from fat cannot be handled and instead is converted to ketones.

In summary, the Embden-Meyerhof pathway and the Krebs cycle serve several important metabolic functions:

1. They provide the body's major source of energy.
2. They provide glycogen formation and release.
3. They provide intermediates for fat formation (lipogenesis).
4. They provide intermediates for synthesis of some amino acids (protein synthesis).

The interrelationships between these pathways are shown in Fig. 2-7.

Alternate pathways. Alternate pathways open to glucose serve specific related functions.

The *pentose shunt* (also called the hexosemonophosphate shunt) of the Embden-Meyerhof pathway is a side channeling of glucose, and it serves a number of physiologic ends (see Fig. 2-5). It produces an important enzyme factor—NADPH (reduced niacin adenine dinucleotide phosphate)—essential in the synthesis of fatty acids. (NADPH is another example of the integration of a B vitamin, niacin, in glucose metabolism.) Insulin's role in lipogenesis may be that of stimulating the operation of this shunt pathway. NADPH is also involved as a cofactor in steroid synthesis, which makes the shunt active in the adrenal gland.

The *uronic acid pathway* is a side pathway that changes some of the glucose into glucuronic acid. Glucuronic acid in turn combines with certain toxic materials (such as some drugs) to remove them from the body, which is an important detoxifying function.

SUMMARY

What is the significance of this overall picture of carbohydrate metabolism for students of nutrition? What does all of this mean in the care of patients and the teaching of positive health principles? Certainly it is not important to remember all the details of metabolism—and only a few have been presented here. This sort of information is important to have only as reference knowledge. The complex and fascinating intricacies of body chemistry lie in the realm of the biochemist and the physiologist, whose imaginative research efforts have given the medical profession greater knowledge of the marvelous inner workings of the human body.

At least two basic concepts can be gained from this background knowledge: (1) the interrelatedness of nutrients and (2) the relation of the separate chemical reactions of the body to the total process of metabolism. There is an intimate metabolic interrelatedness between the basic nutrients and their metabolites. No one substance exists or operates along during metabolism. Rather, there is a tremendously significant interdependence among them all. From this fact, two practical conclusions may be drawn:

1. The emphasis in health teaching and in nutrition education should be on achieving a sound, balanced, normal nutritional basis for any dietary program.
2. It is entirely possible that some deficiency states may be iatrogenic, may have their origin in a fad, or may be caused by long-term, overzealous emphasis on one particular nutrient to the exclusion of other equally essential ones.

The general picture of carbohydrate metabolism can help one to understand more clearly how smaller segments, affecting a particular symptoms or condition, relate ultimately and intimately to the whole process of metabolism. Serious students will translate this information clearly and simply to individual patients. Because they perceive the relationship of the part to the whole, they will be able to help patients understand basic health needs and apply the treatment warranted by the specific situation.

GLOSSARY

disaccharides a class of compound sugars composed of two molecules of monosaccharide. The three common members are sucrose (table sugar), lactose (milk sugar), and maltose (grain sugar).

enzymes various complex organic substances produced by living cells that act independently of these cells. Enzymes are capable of producing certain chemical changes in other substances without themselves being changed in the process. Their action is therefore that of a catalyst. Digestive enzymes of the gastrointestinal secretions act on food substances to break them down into simpler compounds and greatly accelerate the speed of these chemical reactions. An enzyme is usually named according to the substance (substrate) on which it acts, with the common suffix *-ase; sucrase* is the specific enzyme for *sucrose* and breaks it down to glucose and fructose.

glucagon a hyperglycemic factor (HGF) secreted by the alpha cells of the pancreas, which stimulates glycogenolysis.

gluconeogenesis the formation of glucose from noncarbohydrate sources (protein or fat).

glycogen the polysaccharide of animal body (animal starch). It is formed in the body from glucose and stored in the liver and in muscle tissue.

glycogenesis the general term for formation of glycogen from glucose. It is usually used interchangeably with the term *glucogenesis*.

glycogenolysis the specific term for conversion of glycogen into glucose in the liver. Glycogenolysis is the chemical process of enzymatic hydrolysis or breakdown by which this conversion is accomplished.

glycolysis catabolism of carbohydrate (glucose and glycogen) by enzymes with release of energy and production of pyruvic acid or lactic acid.

hexoses a class of simple sugar (monosaccharides) that contain 6 carbon atoms ($C_6H_{12}O_6$). The most common members are glucose (dextrose), fructose (levulose), and galactose.

hormones various internally secreted substances from the endocrine organs, which are conveyed by the blood to another organ or tissue on which they act to stimulate increased functional activity or secretion. The tissue or substance acted on by a specific hormone is called its target organ or substance. For example, insulin, a hormone secreted by special cells of the pancreas (islets of Langerhans), acts to facilitate glucose metabolism.

metabolism the sum of all physical and chemical changes that take place within an organism, by which it maintains itself and produces energy for its functioning. Products of these various reactions are called *metabolites*. Interrelationships of substances in these processes are called *metabolic relationships*.

phosphorylation the combining of glucose with a phosphoric acid radical to produce glucose-6-phosphate as a first step in the cellular oxidation of glucose to produce energy. This reaction is catalyzed by the enzyme glucokinase, the specific hexokinase for this purpose.

photosynthesis the process by which plants containing chlorophyll are able to manufacture carbohydrates by combining carbon dioxide from the air and water from the soil. Sunlight is used as energy, and chlorophyll is a catalyst. The basic chemical reaction is

$$6CO_2 + 6H_2O + Energy \xrightarrow{\text{Chlorophyll}} C_6H_{12}O_6 + 6O_2$$

polysaccharides a class of complex carbohydrates composed of many monosaccharide units. The common members are starch, dextrins, dietary fiber, and glycogen.

portal an entryway, usually referring to the portal circulation of blood through the liver. Blood is brought into the liver by the portal vein and out by the hepatic vein.

REFERENCES
Specific

1. Stare, F. J., editor: Sugar in the diet of man, World Rev. Nutr. Diet **22:**237, 1975.
2. Page, L., and Friend, B.: Level of use of sugars in the U.S. In Sipple, H. L., and McNutt, K. W., editors: Sugars in nutrition, New York, 1974, Nutrition Foundation Academic Press.
3. Toscano, V. A.: Sugars and other carbohydrates. In White, P. L., Fletcher, D. C., and Ellis, M., editors: Nutrients in processed foods—fats, carbohydrates, Acton, Mass., 1975, Publishing Sciences Group Inc.
4. Burkitt, D. P., Walker, A. R. P., and Painter, N. S.: Effect of dietary fibre on stools and transit times, and its role in the causation of disease, Lancet **2:**1408, 1972.
5. Burkitt, D. P.: Epidemiology and etiology, J.A.M.A. **231:**517, 1975.
6. Burkitt, D. P.: Economic development—not all bonus, Nutr. Today **11:**6, Jan./Feb., 1976.
7. Plumley, P. F., and Francis, B.: Dietary management of diverticular disease, J. Am. Diet. Assoc. **63:**527, Nov., 1973.
8. Heaton, K. W.: Fiber, blood lipids, and heart disease, Am. J. Clin. Nutr. **29:**125, 1976.
9. Haber, G. B., Heaton, K. W., Murphy, D., et al.: Depletion and disruption of dietary fiber: effects on satiety, plasma glucose, and serum insulin, Lancet **2:**679, 1977.
10. Horwitz, D. L., and Miranda, P. M.: High-fiber diets in the treatment of diabetes mellitus, Ann. Intern. Med. **88:**482-486, 1978.
11. Modan, B., et al.: Low fiber intake as an etiologic factor in cancer of the colon, J. Natl. Cancer Inst. **55:**15, 1975.
12. Dales, L. G., Friedman, G. D., Ury, H. K., Grossman, S., and Williams, S. R.: A case-control study of relationships of diet and other traits to colorectal cancer in American blacks, Am. J. Epidemiol. **109:**132-144, Feb., 1979.
13. Southgate, D. A. T., Bailey, B., Collinson, E., et al.: A guide to calculating intakes of dietary fiber, J. Hum. Nutr. **30:**303, 1976.
14. Levine, R.: Concerning the mechanisms of insulin action, Diabetes **10:**421, 1961.
15. Levine, R., Goldstein, M. S., Huddleston, B., and Klein, S. P.: Action of insulin of "permeability" of cells to free hexoses, as studied by its effect on distribution of galactose, Am. J. Physiol. **163:**79, 1950.
16. Morgan, H. E., Regen, D. M., Henderson, M. J., Sawyer, T. K., and Park, C. R.: Regulation of glucose uptake in muscle. VI. Effects of hypophysectomy, adrenalectomy, growth hormone, hydrocortisone, and insulin on glucose transport and phosphorylation in the perfused rat heart, J. Biol. Chem. **236:**2162, 1961.
17. Morgan, H. E., Regen, D. M., and Park, C. R.: Identification of a mobile carrier-mediated sugar transport system in muscle, J. Biol. Chem. **239:**369, 1964.
18. Park, C. R., Johnson, L. H., Wright, J. H., Jr., and Batsel, H.: Effect of insulin on transport of several hexoses and pentoses into cells of muscle and brain, Am. J. Physiol. **191:**13, 1957.
19. Post, R. L., Morgan, H. E., and Park, C. R.: Regulation of glucose uptake in muscle. III. The interaction of membrane transport and phosphorylation in the control of glucose uptake, J. Biol. Chem. **236:**269, 1961.
20. Krahl, M. E.: The action of insulin on cells, New York, 1961, Academic Press, Inc.
21. Penhos, J. C., and Krahl, M. E.: Insulin stimulus of leucine incorporation into frog liver protein, Am. J. Physiol. **203:**687, 1962.
22. Gerich, J. E., Lorenzi, M., Bier, D. M., et al.: Prevention of human diabetic ketoacidosis by somatostatin: evidence for an essential role of glucagon, N. Engl. J. Med. **292:**985, 1975.
23. Maugh, T. H.: Diabetes: new hormones promise more effective therapy, Science **188:**920, 1975.
24. Wise, J. K., Hendler, R., and Felig, P.: Influence of glucocorticoids in glucagon secretion and plasma amino acid concentrations in man, J. Clin. Invest. **52:**2774, 1973.
25. Lehninger, A. L.: Short course in biochemistry, New York, 1973, Worth Publishers, Inc., p. 348.

General

Ackerman, L. V.: Some thoughts on food and cancer, Nutr. Today **7:**2, Jan./Feb., 1972.

Bogart, L. J., Briggs, G., and Calloway, D.: Nutrition and physical fitness, ed. 10, Philadelphia, 1974, W. B. Saunders Co.

Burkitt, D. P., and Trowell, H. C., editors: Refined carbohydrate foods and disease: some implications of dietary fibre, New York, 1975, Academic Press, Inc.

Davidson, S., Passmore, R., Brock, J., and Truswell, A.: Human nutrition and dietetics, New York, 1975, Langman, Inc.

Goodhart, R. S., and Shils, M. E., editors: Modern nutrition in health and disease, ed. 5, Philadelphia, 1973, Lea & Febiger.

Harper, H. A.: Review of physiological chemistry, ed. 15, Los Altos, Calif., 1975, Lange Medical Publications.

Howell, M. A.: Diet as an etiological factor in the development of cancers of the colon and rectum, J. Chronic Dis. **28:**67, 1975.

Jenkins, D. J. A., et al.: Effect of wheat fiber on blood lipids, fecal steroid excretion, and serum iron, Am. J. Clin. Nutr. **28:**1408, 1975.

Keihm, R. G., et al.: Beneficial effects of a high carbohydrate high fiber diet on hyperglycemic diabetic man, Am. J. Clin. Nutr. **29:**895, 1976.

Lehninger, A. L.: Short course in biochemistry, New York, 1973, Worth Publishers, Inc.

Mendeloff, A. I.: Dietary fiber and human health, N. Engl. J. Med. **297:**811, 1977.

Montgomery, R., Dryer, R. L., Conway, T. W., and Spector, A. A.: Biochemistry: a case-oriented approach, ed. 3, St. Louis, 1980, The C. V. Mosby Co.

Spiller, G. A., and Amen, R. H., editors: Fiber in human nutrition, New York, 1976, Plenum Publishing Corp.

Stefferud, A., editor: Food: the yearbook of agriculture, 1959, Washington, D.C., 1959, U.S. Department of Agriculture.

Trowell, H.: Definition of dietary fiber and hypotheses that it is a protective factor in certain diseases, Am. J. Clin. Nutr. **29:**417, 1976.

3 Fats

Since recorded history, and probably before, people have used fats to supply light and heat for shelter and to lubricate tools. They have even used fat for beautifying themselves.

The major use of fat, however, has been as food. There seems to be no set quantitative requirement of fat in human nutrition. People of many different cultures exist on widely various amounts of fat in their diets. For example, the fat intake of Japanese soldiers in wartime probably accounted for as little as 3% of their total calories, whereas the general Japanese population consumed from 6% to 10% of their total calories as fat.[1] About 40% of the total caloric intake of Americans is from this source, which is an excessive quantity according to some authorities. The Food and Nutrition Board of the National Research Council, the American Heart Association, and the American Medical Association recommend a decrease in proportion of dietary fat to no more than 30% of total calories, with 1% to 2% as the essential fatty acid, linoleic acid.[2] Other professional organizations, such as the Inter-Society Commission for Heart Disease Resources, have also added their appeal for a reduced intake of fats, especially animal fats and cholesterol.[3] Others have also advocated a "prudent diet" for controlled fat use.

GENERAL AND CHEMICAL DEFINITIONS OF FATS

General definition. Fats may be defined as a group of organic substances—fats, oils, waxes, and related compounds—that are greasy to the touch and insoluble in water but are soluble in alcohol or ether. Substances of this class are called *lipids* (Gr. *lipos,* fat). The food sources of fats are usually obvious to the consumer. The so-called visible fats include butter, margarine, oil, salad dressings, bacon, and cream. Egg yolk, meat fats, olives, avocado, and nuts are the so-called hidden fats.

Chemical definition. Fats may be defined according to their basic structural elements: carbon, hydrogen, and oxygen. Although these are the same elements that comprise the carbohydrates, in fat the relative hydrogen content is higher than in carbohydrate. Fats are actual or potential esters of fatty acids. (An *ester* is a compound of an alcohol and an acid.) These fatty acids are utilized in the metabolism of living organisms.

CLASSIFICATION OF FATS

The commonly used classification of fats suggested by Bloor and Deuel[4] divides fats into three main groups: simple lipids, compound lipids, and derived lipids.

Simple lipids. The simple lipids are neutral fats and waxes.

Neutral fats are esters of fatty acids with glycerol, in the ratio of three fatty acids to each glycerol base. They are therefore called *triglycerides* (Fig. 3-1).

Waxes are esters of fatty acids with straight-chain alcohols. Generally, these substances are more solid than fats. They have little importance in human nutrition, but are used more extensively in commercial products.

Compound lipids. Compound lipids are various combinations of neutral fat with other components. Three types of compound lipid are important in human nutrition: phospholipids, glycolipids, and lipoproteins.

Phospholipids are compounds of neutral fat, a phosphoric acid, and a nitrogenous base. The largest group of phospholipids, *lecithins,* contains glycerol, two fatty acids, phosphoric acid, and choline. Other important phospholipids are *cephalins* and *lipositols,* which are like the lecithins except that they contain other factors in place of choline.

Glycolipids are compounds of fatty acids that are combined with carbohydrates and nitrogen. Because they are found chiefly in brain tissue, these substances are also called *cerebrosides.*

Lipoproteins are compounds of various lipids with protein. Studies indicate that the intimate relation between plasma lipids and certain parts of the plasma proteins provides the main transport form of lipid substances in the bloodstream. These plasma lipoproteins contain cholesterol (free and esterified), phospholipids, neutral fat, unesterified (free) fatty acids, and traces of other related materials such as fat-soluble vitamins and the steroid hormones. Since fat is insoluble in water, lipids always travel in the blood bound with protein in varying ratios. The high or low density of the lipoprotein transport compounds is determined by their relative

ratios of fat and protein. The higher the protein ratio, the higher the density (see p. 607). This illustrates again the intimate interrelationships among the various nutrients and their interdependent nature.

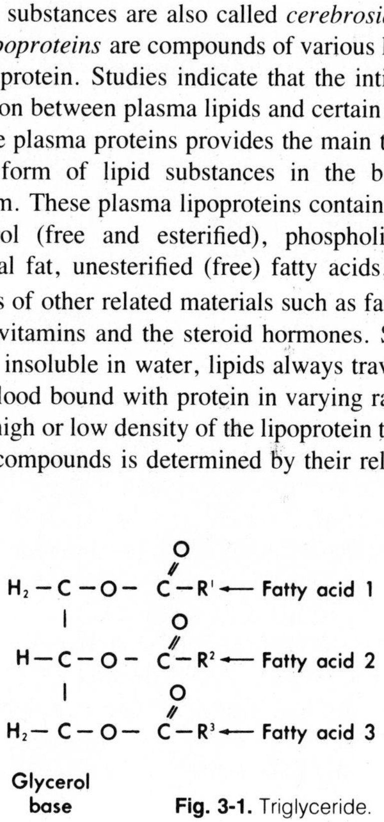

Derived lipids. Derived lipids are fat substances derived from simple and compound lipids by hydrolysis or enzymatic breakdown. Three important members of this group are fatty acids, glyercol, and steroids.

Fatty acids are the basic components of triglycerides (neutral fats), and they may be *saturated* or *unsaturated.*

Glycerol, the water-soluble component of triglycerides, is interconvertible with carbohydrate and therefore contributes to the total available glucose in the diet.

Steroids are a class of lipid substances that contain sterols, such as cholesterol and ergosterol (a precursor of vitamin D). Other important steroids are the bile salts, certain fat-soluble provitamins, and adrenal hormones.

FATTY ACIDS

Since fatty acids are the basic structural units of fats, a close study of them is important to an understanding of lipids. Terms applied to the fatty acids relate to their degree of chemical saturation or to their synthesis and function in the body.

Saturated and unsaturated fatty acids

The state of saturation or unsaturation of fatty acids is an important chemical characteristic. This state results from the ratio of hydrogen atoms to carbon atoms in the basic carbon chain that forms the individual fatty acid. In terms of chemical combining power, carbon has a *valence* of 4, meaning that *4* other atoms may attach themselves to positions on the carbon atom when various carbon compounds are formed. In a given fatty acid, if all of the available valence bonds of a basic carbon chain are filled with hydrogen, the fatty acid is said to be completely *saturated with hydrogen.* However,

Fig. 3-1. Triglyceride.

$$H—\overset{\displaystyle\overset{H}{|}}{\underset{\displaystyle\underset{H}{|}}{C}}—\overset{\displaystyle\overset{H}{|}}{\underset{\displaystyle\underset{H}{|}}{C}}—\overset{\displaystyle\overset{H}{|}}{\underset{\displaystyle\underset{H}{|}}{C}}—COOH$$

Saturated—butyric acid, as found in butter (4 carbons, no double bond)

$$H—\overset{\displaystyle\overset{H}{|}}{\underset{\displaystyle\underset{H}{|}}{C}}—(CH_2)_7—\overset{\displaystyle\overset{H}{|}}{C}=\overset{\displaystyle\overset{H}{|}}{C}—(CH_2)_7—COOH$$

Monounsaturated—oleic acid, component fatty acid in olive oil (18 carbons, 1 double bond)

$$H—\overset{\displaystyle\overset{H}{|}}{\underset{\displaystyle\underset{H}{|}}{C}}—(CH_2)_4—\overset{\displaystyle\overset{H}{|}}{C}=\overset{\displaystyle\overset{H}{|}}{C}—\overset{\displaystyle\overset{H}{|}}{\underset{\displaystyle\underset{H}{|}}{C}}—\overset{\displaystyle\overset{H}{|}}{C}=\overset{\displaystyle\overset{H}{|}}{C}—(CH_2)_7—COOH$$

Polyunsaturated—linoleic acid, found in various vegetable oils (18 carbons, 2 double bonds)

$$H—\overset{\displaystyle\overset{H}{|}}{\underset{\displaystyle\underset{H}{|}}{C}}—\overset{\displaystyle\overset{H}{|}}{\underset{\displaystyle\underset{H}{|}}{C}}—\overset{\displaystyle\overset{H}{|}}{C}=\overset{\displaystyle\overset{H}{|}}{C}—\overset{\displaystyle\overset{H}{|}}{\underset{\displaystyle\underset{H}{|}}{C}}—\overset{\displaystyle\overset{H}{|}}{C}=\overset{\displaystyle\overset{H}{|}}{C}—\overset{\displaystyle\overset{H}{|}}{\underset{\displaystyle\underset{H}{|}}{C}}—\overset{\displaystyle\overset{H}{|}}{C}=\overset{\displaystyle\overset{H}{|}}{C}—(CH_2)_7—COOH$$

Polyunsaturated—linolenic acid (18 carbons, 3 double bonds)

$$H—\overset{\displaystyle\overset{H}{|}}{\underset{\displaystyle\underset{H}{|}}{C}}—(CH_2)_4—\overset{\displaystyle\overset{H}{|}}{C}=\overset{\displaystyle\overset{H}{|}}{C}—\overset{\displaystyle\overset{H}{|}}{\underset{\displaystyle\underset{H}{|}}{C}}—\overset{\displaystyle\overset{H}{|}}{C}=\overset{\displaystyle\overset{H}{|}}{C}—\overset{\displaystyle\overset{H}{|}}{\underset{\displaystyle\underset{H}{|}}{C}}—\overset{\displaystyle\overset{H}{|}}{C}=\overset{\displaystyle\overset{H}{|}}{C}—\overset{\displaystyle\overset{H}{|}}{\underset{\displaystyle\underset{H}{|}}{C}}—\overset{\displaystyle\overset{H}{|}}{C}=\overset{\displaystyle\overset{H}{|}}{C}—(CH_2)_3—COOH$$

Polyunsaturated—arachidonic acid (20 carbons, 4 double bonds)

if at one point along the carbon chain there are 2 fewer hydrogen atoms, the 2 involved carbon atoms take up their 2 available valence bonds to make 1 mutual bond. When this newly created mutual bond is added to the already existing bond between them, a double bond between the 2 carbon atoms is created. If only 1 such double bond occurs along the carbon chain, the fatty acid is called a *monounsaturated* fatty acid. If 2 or more double bonds occur along the carbon chain of the fatty acid, it is called a *polyunsaturated* fatty acid. A comparison of the

basic structure of representative examples of each form of fatty acid is shown above.

Food fats. From the preceding facts, the concept of degrees of saturation and unsaturation of fatty acids can be derived. Fig. 3-2 shows the general saturated-unsaturated spectrum of food fats. One would expect the more saturated food fats to be the more solid, hard ones. Usually this is the case. The more saturated food fats have a higher melting point (solidification point). The fats on the saturated end of the spectrum are animal fats, and the fats toward

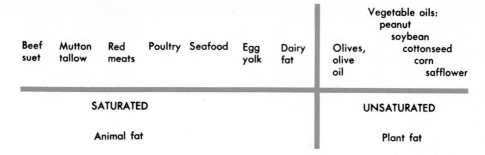

Fig. 3-2. Spectrum of food fats according to degree of saturation of component fatty acids.

the center of the spectrum become softer in texture. The fats on the unsaturated end of the spectrum are of plant origin and are usually free-flowing oils that do not solidify even at low temperatures.

Recent data are available concerning the comprehensive fatty acids in common food sources such as dairy products,[5,6] beef products,[7] eggs and egg products,[9] and pork products.[9]

Essential and nonessential fatty acids

The terms "essential" or "nonessential" when applied to fatty acid refer to the twofold physiologic fact: (1) a fatty acid is essential if its absence will create a specific deficiency disease. For example, a type of eczema in infants is caused by a lack of linoleic acid in the diet. (2) A fatty acid is essential if the body cannot manufacture it and must obtain it from the diet. Either or both of these things may be true of a specific fatty acid.

The three polyunsaturated fatty acids—linoleic acid, linolenic acid, and arachidonic acid—have for many years been called the essential fatty acids because they are essential for certain body functioning. Evidence also seemed to indicate that the body could not synthesize them. However, research[1,10] has since indicated that *linoleic acid* may be considered the one essential fatty acid for two reasons. Linolenic

acid has relatively little effect in relieving the skin lesions originally associated with a deficiency of the essential acids. Arachidonic acid can be synthesized by the body from linoleic acid and therefore does not have to be supplied as such in the diet.

These three fatty acids, especially linoleic acid, serve important functions in the body:

1. They strengthen capillary and cell membrane structure, which helps prevent an increase in skin permeability. A deficiency of linoleic acid leads to a breakdown in skin integrity with resulting eczematous skin lesions.
2. They combine with cholesterol to form cholesterol esters. They are also part of the phospholipid and lipoprotein complexes.
3. They lower serum cholesterol. Some investigators suggest that linoleic acid may play a key role in the transport and metabolism of cholesterol, although just what this role may be is not known at this time.
4. They prolong blood clotting time and increase fibrinolytic activity.

Although strong correlations have been shown to exist, the precise mechanism of the relationship between these fatty acids and the critical tissue change in coronary artery disease (atherosclerosis) has not been clearly determined.

The monounsaturated acid, oleic acid, is not

included as an essential acid because it can be readily synthesized in the tissues.

SOME COMMON CHEMICAL REACTIONS OF FATS

Certain common chemical reactions of fats have much dietary or commercial significance and should be clarified.

Hydrolysis. Hydrolysis is the process in which enzyme action by the lipases breaks down neutral fats in foods to their component fatty acids and glycerol (see section on Digestion of Fats, p. 39).

Saponification. Hydrolysis by an alkali breaks down fats into glycerol and the alkali salt of the fatty acids. The latter products are *soaps*. In certain abnormal states (for, example, sprue) the body produces soaps.

Hydrogenation. The process of hydrogenation introduces hydrogen into the available double bond linkages of unsaturated fats. Industrially, nickel is used as a catalyst. The process is also known as ''hardening.'' It has commercial value, as it converts liquid fats such as vegetable oils into a solid form for use as vegetable shortenings and margarines.

Rancidity. Rancidity is the result of chemical change in a fat caused by air exposure and age. The fat has an unpleasant odor and taste. Because oxygen in the air causes this chemical change, antioxidants are used in commercial food processing to prevent a fat from turning rancid.

FUNCTIONS OF FAT IN THE BODY

Fat serves two basic functions in the human body: (1) a primary metabolic function, to produce energy, and (2) a secondary mechanical or structural function, for example, the protection of vital organs.

Metabolic function. The primary function of fat in human nutrition is to supply the body's most concentrated source of energy. Fat has more than twice the fuel value concentration of either carbohydrate or protein. In colder climates and seasons therefore fat generally assumes a greater role in the diet to supply needed body heat.

Moreover, because of its concentration, high density, and low solubility, fat has value in the body as the storage form of energy. Carbohydrates and some proteins may also be converted to fat for storage as adipose fat tissue. The turnover of fats in adipose tissue is a dynamic, continuous process.

Mechanical or structural function. Fat provides a general padding for vital organs and nerves, which holds them in place and helps to absorb shocks. Further protection for the entire body is provided by the subcutaneous layer of fat, which insulates the body against rapid temperature changes or excessive heat loss.

Function of fat-related compounds. Other important functions of fat are those associated with fat-related compounds. Phospholipids, for example, are vital constituents of all cells. Brain and nerve tissues are especially rich in phospholipids. Unlike neutral fats, these compounds are water soluble and may therefore help facilitate the passage of neutral fats in and out of cells. Phospholipids probably also aid in the absorption of fats from the intestine. Cholesterol, another vital fat-related compound, is closely related chemically to the sex hormones and adrenal hormones.

DIGESTION OF FATS

Chemical digestion of fats takes place mainly in the small intestine; the general preparatory action occurs in the preceding parts of the gastrointestinal tract.

Mechanical digestion. Mechanical digestion of fats begins in the mouth. Mastication breaks the food up into fine particles and moistens it for passage into the stomach. In the stomach, peristalsis continues the mechanical mixing of fats with the stomach contents. No significant amount of enzyme specific for fats is present in the gastric secretions except a gastric lipase, tributyrinase, which acts on emusified butterfat.

As the main gastric enzymes act on specific nutrients, however, fat is separated from them and made more readily accessible to its own specific chemical breakdown in the small intestine.

Chemical digestion. It is not until fat reaches the small intestine that chemical digestion takes place. Agents from the *liver* and *gallbladder,* the *pancreas,* and the *small intestine* aid in this enzymatic breakdown of fats.

BILE SALTS FROM THE LIVER AND GALLBLADDER. The presence of fats in the duodenum stimulates the secretion of *cholecystokinin* from glands in the walls of the intestine. Cholecystokinin provides the stimulus for the contraction of the gallbladder, relaxation of the sphincter, and subsequent secretion of bile salts into the intestine via the common bile duct. Bile is produced in the liver and then is concentrated and stored in the gallbladder ready for use in the handling of fats. Its function is that of an emulsifier. Emulsification is an important first step in the preparation of fats for digestion by the enzymes. This emulsifying process has a twofold nature: (1) it breaks the fat into small particles or globules, which greatly enlarges the surface area available for action of the enzyme and (2) it serves to lower the surface tension of the finely dispersed and suspended fat globules, thus allowing greater ease of penetration of the enzymes. This is similar to the wetting action of detergents. The bile also provides an alkaline medium for the action of lipase.

ENZYMES FROM THE PANCREAS. The pancreatic juice contains an enzyme for fat and an enzyme for cholesterol. The pancreatic *lipase* that acts on fats is a powerful enzyme called *steapsin.* In a stepwise fashion, it breaks off one fatty acid at a time from the glycerol base of neutral fats. Thus one fatty acid and diglyceride, then another fatty acid and monoglyceride, are produced in turn. Each succeeding step of this breakdown is effected with increasing difficulty. In fact, separation of the final fatty acid from the remaining monoglyceride is such a slow process that less than one third of the total fat present actually reaches complete breakdown. The final products of fat digestion are fatty acids, diglycerides, monoglycerides, and glycerol (Table 3-1).

The formation of cholesterol esters by the combination of cholesterol and fatty acids is an important step in the preparation of free cholesterol for absorption by the bloodstream from the intestine. *Cholesterol esterase* is an enzyme of the pancreatic juice, which, along with bile salts, catalyzes this action.

ENZYME FROM THE SMALL INTESTINE. The small intestine secretes an enzyme in the intestinal juice called *lecithinase.* It acts on lecithin (a phospholipid) to break it down into its components of glycerol, fatty acids, phosphoric acid, and choline.

LARGE INTESTINE. Some remaining fat may be secreted into the large intestine and eliminated as fecal fat.

Table 3-1. Summary of triglyceride breakdown

Triglyceride	$+ H_2O \xrightarrow{\text{Lipase}}$ Diglyceride	$+$ 1 fatty acid
Diglyceride	$+ H_2O \xrightarrow{\text{Lipase}}$ Monoglyceride	$+$ 1 fatty acid
Monoglyceride	$+ H_2O \xrightarrow{\text{Lipase}}$ Glycerol	$+$ 1 fatty acid

Table 3-2. Summary of fat digestion

Organ	Enzyme	Activity
Mouth	None	Mechanical; mastication
Stomach	Gastric lipase (tributyrinase)	Emulsified butterfat, beginning breakdown Mechanical separation of fats as protein and starch digested out
Small intestine	Gallbladder Bile salts (emulsifier) Pancreatic	Emulsifies fats
	Lipase (steapsin)	Triglycerides to diglycerides and monoglycerides in turn, then fatty acids and glycerol
	Cholesterol esterase	Free cholesterol + Fatty acids to cholesterol esters
	Intestinal Lecithinase	Lecithin to glycerol, fatty acids, phosphoric acid, choline

A summary of fat digestion in the successive parts of the gastrointestinal tract is given in Table 3-2.

ABSORPTION OF FAT INTO THE BLOODSTREAM

Because of the increasing difficulty in breaking off the final fatty acid from original triglycerides, only about one third of the triglycerides are completely digested in the lumen of the small intestine. The major end products of fat digestion in the gastrointestinal tract are monoglycerides, some diglycerides, glycerol, and fatty acids.

The absorbing surface of the small intestine, with its millions of small villi, handles these products of fat digestion in various ways.

Initial fat absorption

Triglyceride products. Because it is water soluble, glycerol is easily absorbed into the portal blood system and carried to the liver.

The term "free" fatty acid is a misnomer, since all fats and fat products travel in the plasma bound with some small amount of protein. The term "free" here means *unesterified*. The unesterified fatty acids (UFA), short- and me-

dium-chain fatty acids, and medium-chain triglycerides may be absorbed directly into the portal vein and carried to the liver. For use in clinical conditions of impaired fat absorption, a medium-chain triglyceride preparation (MCT) is available in both oil and powder forms.[10]

The remaining monoglycerides, diglycerides, and long-chain fatty acids are less water soluble and require a wetting agent to facilitate their absorption. Bile salts perform this vital function and act as a ferry system to transport these products of fat digestion into the intestinal wall. With the monoglycerides and fatty acids, these bile acids form a micellar complex so fine that is is almost a clear solution, and the fat particles are about 1/100 the size of those that first entered the intestine. With the remaining unhydrolyzed triglycerides and diglycerides, bile forms an emulsion for absorption (Fig. 3-3).

Some electron microscopic observations suggest that the neutral fat complex may be absorbed by a process called *pinocytosis,* an engulfing of the globule directly by the cell membrane (see Fig. 9-3).

Absorption of fat-related products. *Cholesterol* may be taken in as such in the diet (exogenous cholesterol), or it may be synthe-

The efficiency of the enterohepatic circulation of bile salts demonstrates the body's amazing ability to conserve materials needed for its basic functions. These built-in conservation systems, because they maintain their own balance, are called *homeostatic mechanisms*. They are designed to sustain life in a relatively stable state of equilibrium between the multitude of interdependent elements and subsystems that comprise the human organism.

For example, of the 20 to 30 g of needed bile acids circulated daily in the body, only about 0.8 g is lost in the feces. Therefore only this small amount needs to be replaced daily by newly synthesized bile acids. After its tasks in digestion and absorption (emulsifying and transporting) are completed, the bile is separated from its fat complex, returned to the liver, and recirculated again and again (Fig. 3-4).

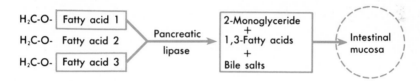

Fig. 3-3. Micellar complex of fats with bile salts for transport of fats into intestinal mucosa.

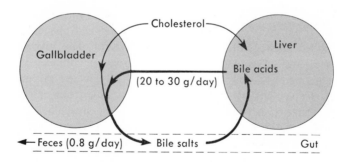

Fig. 3-4. Enterohepatic circulation of bile salts.

sized by the body (endogenous cholesterol). One of the major sites of cholesterol synthesis is intestinal tissue. Some cholesterol is absorbed with the aid of bile salts as free or unesterified cholesterol. Most of it, however, is esterified with fatty acids by the enzymatic action of cholesterol esterase and is absorbed as cholesterol esters.

The *phospholipids,* mainly lecithin, may also be taken in as such in the diet or synthesized in intestinal tissue. Some preformed dietary phospholipid, because of its *hydrophilic* nature (strong affinity for water), may be absorbed directly into portal blood. Other phospholipid synthesized in intestinal tissue becomes part of the lipoprotein complex (chylomicrons) that is

TO PROBE FURTHER
Chylomicrons

Following a meal, lipoprotein particles of fat, related fat products, and protein accumulate in the lymphatic vessels and the plasma. These particles are called *chylomicrons*. The term "chylomicrons" refers to their composition and size. These fat droplets contain mostly triglycerides but also small amounts of other fat products. Their approximate composition is

Triglycerides	81%
Cholesterol (free and esters)	9%
Phospholipids	7%
Free fatty acids	1%
Protein	2%

The chylomicrons disappear rather quickly from the plasma into various tissues for oxidation or storage. The efficient clearing factor is an enzyme, *lipoprotein lipase*, which begins its action in the plasma, but continues it mainly in the tissue by taking up the fat. It releases free (unesterified) fatty acids after their hydrolysis from depot fats. As one would expect, a large amount of the enzyme is present in adipose tissue, but none has been found in liver, where fat is not stored.

absorbed into the lymphatic system. It then passes into the portal blood circulation by way of the thoracic duct.

Subsequent steps in fat absorption carried out by the intestinal wall

A highly significant second stage of fat absorption takes place in the wall of the intestine. The mucosa does not act merely as passive tissue for a diffuse sort of entry and passage of fats. Rather, studies[12-14] have revealed it to be a dynamic metabolic tissue that is actively engaged in resynthesis of triglycerides and related fat products.

In the intestinal wall, bile salts are separated from the initial fatty acid complex absorbed from the intestinal lumen and are returned to the liver by way of the portal blood. In the liver the bile salts are then recirculated in the bile. This cycle, the *enterohepatic circulation of bile salts,* forms an efficient system for maintaining a constant supply as needed.

There is evidence[15] that an intestinal lipase (enteric lipase) exists within the cells of the intestine wall that continues the hydrolysis of the remaining triglycerides, diglycerides, and monoglycerides to fatty acids and glycerol. These fatty acids, together with those released from the initial bile salts–fatty acid complex, are activated and resynthesized with an activated glycerol. This glycerol is probably produced from the Embden-Meyerhof glycolytic pathway for glucose metabolism (see Chapter 2) and is not a new glycerol just produced by digestion. Resynthesized triglycerides are formed and are ready to be used by the tissues.

Final absorption and transport of fat

Through the metabolic action of the intestinal mucosa, final fat products are formed. These include fatty acids, phospholipids, free cholesterol, cholesterol esters, and triglycerides. This complex of materials is then bound with small amounts of protein to form a lipoprotein complex called *chylomicrons*. These chylomicrons penetrate the intercellular spaces of the intestinal mucosa and enter the abdominal lacteals. The chylomicrons can apparently cross

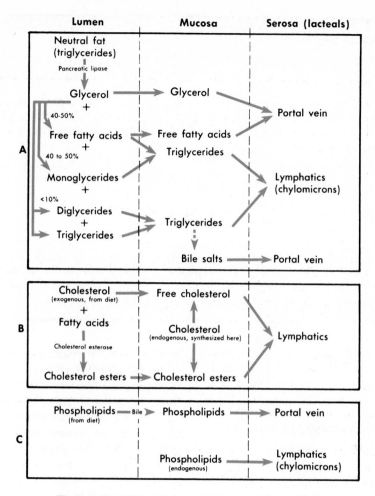

Fig. 3-5. Absorption of fat, cholesterol, and phospholipids.

the cell wall intact. These lipoprotein particles are transported through the lymphatic system to the thoracic duct, where they enter the blood through the left subclavian vein. The various stages in the overall process of fat absorption are summarized in Fig. 3-5.

METABOLISM OF FATS

Five factors work together to control the level of plasma lipids: (1) diet, (2) synthesis of fat in the tissues, (3) mobilization of fat from the depots, (4) the rate of oxidation in the various body tissues, and (5) deposition of fat in adipose tissue and the liver.

The main sites of utilization of lipids are adipose tissue and the liver. This basic interdependent relationship has been called the "liver-adipose tissue axis" (Fig. 3-6). Fat metabolism may be considered in terms of the fat-related activities of these two organ tissues. These metabolic activities in adipose and liver tissue are twofold: (1) *lipogenesis* (synthesis and deposit of fat) and (2) *lipolysis* (mobilization and oxidation of fat). Although these functions are

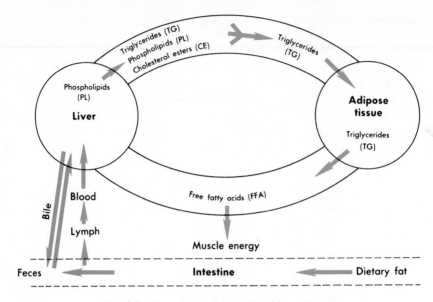

Fig. 3-6. Liver-adipose tissue axis of fat exchange.

considered separately here, they do not exist apart from each other; rather, they are constantly interbalanced to maintain blood lipid levels and to help supply energy needs.

Adipose tissue metabolism

Adipose tissue is by no means the static storage reserve of fat it was once thought to be. It is now known to be one of the most metabolically active body tissues. It maintains a constant turnover, depositing and mobilizing fat. In the body's total fat metabolism picture, endogenous as well as exogenous fat must be considered.

Fat synthesis and deposit. The most active site of lipogenesis in the human body is adipose tissue. Triglycerides are formed from fatty acids and glycerol. Two sources supply the needed fatty acids: (1) degraded neutral fat or dietary fat and (2) synthesized fatty acids from precursors such as carbohydrate and its metabolites (glucose, pyruvate, and active acetate). The synthesis of fatty acids from these precursors requires the presence of the niacin-containing coenzyme NADPH, which is produced by the

pentose shunt of the Embden-Meyerhof glycolytic pathway (see pp. 26-27). Tissues active in lipogenesis, such as adipose tissue and the lactating mammary glands, also have a very active shunt pathway. This helps to explain why glucose and insulin are necessary for lipogenesis. The required coenzyme, NADPH, is produced by glucose oxidation through this shunt.

The glycerol used in lipogenesis must be an activated form (it must contain phosphorus) rather than a newly released free glycerol. Since adipose tissue lacks the activating enzyme *glycerokinase,* active glycerol (α-glycerophosphate) must come from the glycolytic pathway of glucose metabolism (see p. 27).

These two factors of fat metabolism again demonstrate the closely interdependent relationships of the basic nutrients, fat and carbohydrate, and indicate that adipose tissue is in fact one of the major sites of insulin activity.

The synthesized fat is deposited in three major body sites: (1) subcutaneous connective tissue, (2) abdominal cavity, and (3) intermuscular connective tissue.

Fat mobilization and oxidation. Lipolysis also takes place in adipose tissue, since depot fat is constantly being mobilized by the body. The fat is again broken down into glycerol and fatty acids. The glycerol is released and subsequently converted in the liver to glycogen and is eventually oxidized as glucose. The free (unesterified) fatty acids released are transported to various cells as needed to be oxidized for energy. The turnover rate of these free fatty acids is high. They are the metabolically active forms of lipids. All tissues can oxidize them completely to carbon dioxide and water. They are even the preferred form of fuel for some tissues such as the myocardium.

Liver metabolism

In the overall balanced axis of fat metabolism, the liver also functions in lipogenesis and lipolysis.

Fat synthesis and deposit. The liver also synthesizes fatty acids and triglycerides, but to a lesser extent than that which occurs in adipose tissue. Unlike adipose tissue, however, the liver normally does not store deposits of fat. Such deposits produce a "fatty liver," an abnormal, pathologic state. Several conditions may contribute to the abnormal deposit of fat in the liver:

1. Excess mobilization of fat as in starvation or uncontrolled diabetes, which produces ketosis
2. Malnutrition, especially deficiencies in protein and key vitamins related to carbohydrate and fat metabolism
3. Alcoholism, which induces malnutrition
4. Hepatotoxins such as carbon tetrachloride, which injure liver tissue

Fat mobilization and oxidation. To prevent abnormal accumulation of fat in the liver certain *lipotropic* factors are active in this organ. By a process of *transmethylation* these lipotropic agents promote the production of lipoproteins, which transfer the fatty acids out of the liver.

A major example of such a lipotropic agent is choline, a component of the phospholipid lecithin. Choline, sometimes classified as a B-complex vitamin, is synthesized from methionine, an essential amino acid. The therapeutic effect of protein in early liver disease may derive in some measure from its lipotropic constituent amino acid, methionine.

A summary of fat metabolism is shown in Fig. 3-7 (see also Fig. 7-2).

The oxidation of fatty acids proceeds first through a gradual breakdown by 2-carbon fragments from the original carbon chain to form active acetate (acetyl-CoA) and shorter chain fatty acids. The active acetate then enters the Krebs cycle (see pp. 28-29) and is oxidized to form carbon dioxide and water.

The role of the liver in fat metabolism may be summarized as the synthesis of fatty acids from carbohydrate, the synthesis of cholesterol from 2-carbon acetate fragments, the synthesis of bile acids (the liver is the sole source of bile acids), and the synthesis of phospholipids and lipoproteins from protein sources. The liver also removes phospholipids, cholesterol, lipoprotein from plasma, and removes fatty acids from diet or deposit origin by degrading and oxidizing them when the body must call on fat as a major energy source. If oxidation is too rapid, excess ketones are formed.

Lipoproteins

It is clear therefore that lipoproteins provide the major vehicular form of fat in the blood serum. Elevation of these materials produces a clinical condition called *hyperlipoproteinemia* (see p. 607). Other terms used for this condition interchangeably are hyperlipidemia and hypertriglyceridemia. These lipoproteins are produced in two places: (1) the intestinal wall after initial absorption of dietary fat and (2) the liver.

The exogenous intestinal wall lipoproteins are called chylomicrons. They have the highest lipid content of all the lipoproteins, containing mostly triglycerides from the diet with a very small amount of protein as a carrier substance. The other major lipoproteins are endogenous, produced in the liver as transport fat to the tis-

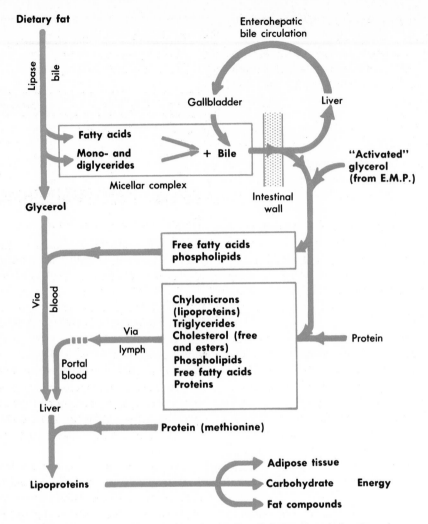

Fig. 3-7. Summary of fat metabolism. (EMP = Embden-Meyerhof pathway.)

sues for use in energy production and interchange with other metabolites. These are the prebeta, broad beta, beta, and alpha lipoproteins.

Thus the five types of lipoproteins in the blood may be grouped or classified according to their fat content and hence density, those with the highest fat content having the lowest density. These five groups of lipoproteins are, in order of lipid content:

1. Chylomicrons: lowest density, mostly tri-

glycerides (90%) with a small amount of protein, delivering dietary fat to cells (liver)

2. Prebeta lipoproteins: very low-density lipoproteins (VLDL), delivering endogenous triglycride to tissue cells

3. Broad beta lipoproteins: intermediate low-density lipoproteins (Int. LDL), continuing delivery of endogenous triglyceride to tissue cells

4. Beta lipoproteins: low-density lipopro-

teins (LDL), delivering cholesterol to the peripheral tissue cells

5. Alpha lipoproteins: high-density lipoproteins (HDL), transferring free cholesterol from the tissues to the liver for catabolism and excretion

Hormonal influences on fat metabolism

Since fat and carbohydrate metabolism are so closely interrelated, the same hormones that affect carbohydrate metabolism also affect fat metabolism.

1. Growth hormone (GH), adrenocorticotropic hormone (ACTH), and thyroid-stimulating hormone (TSH), which are all secreted by the pituitary gland, increase the release of free fatty acids from adipose tissue by imposing energy demands on the body.

2. Cortisone and hydrocortisone, which are secreted by the adrenal gland, cause the release of free fatty acids. Epinephrine and norepinephrine stimulate lipolysis, the breakdown of triglycerides.

3. The important lipogenic activity of insulin, which is secreted by the pancreas, has been described (pp. 25-26). Glucagon has an opposite effect by increasing the release of free fatty acids from adipose tissue.

4. Thyroxine, which is secreted by the thyroid gland, affects fat metabolism by stimulating adipose tissue release of free fatty acids. It also lowers blood cholesterol levels.

Effect of body temperature on fat metabolism

Lowering of body temperature stimulates the release of unesterified fatty acids. These fatty acids supply fuel to return the body temperature toward normal. Table 3-3 summarizes the factors that affect the rate of mobilization of free fatty acids from adipose tissue.

Table 3-3. Summary of factors affecting release of free fatty acids from adipose tissue

Increase release	Decrease release
Hormones	Insulin + Glucose
Diabetes	(lipogenesis)
Starvation (fasting)	Feeding
Cold	

Metabolism of cholesterol

Before the intestinal absorption of cholesterol can occur, bile and the pancreatic enzyme cholesterol esterase must be present. Cholesterol esterase catalyzes the esterification of cholesterol by fatty acids. By far the largest amount of cholesterol—80% to 90%—is absorbed in ester form.

The cholesterol esters and the small remaining amount of free cholesterol are then incorporated into the chylomicrons formed in the intestine wall and are transported by way of the lymph to the portal blood. The blood level of cholesterol is normally maintained at 150 to 300 mg/dl.

Although cholesterol may be synthesized by the liver as well as other tissues, alteration of dietary cholesterol does affect serum cholesterol more than was previously thought. Numerous studies indicate that diets reduced in cholesterol and saturated fat intake and increased in polyunsaturated fat *will* reduce serum cholesterol and other lipids and hence, presumably, the risk of coronary heart disease.[16,17] Radioactive-tagged cholesterol in the diet has been recovered in large quantities from atheromatous plaques.[18] Hence treatment for hypercholesterolemia or atherosclerosis may include a therapeutic restriction of cholesterol-rich foods. These foods include egg yolk, organ meats, shellfish, especially shrimp, and dairy fat.

Cholesterol is excreted by the liver in bile.

The liver therefore has a major cholesterol-regulating role, since it adds and removes cholesterol from the blood as needed.

GLOSSARY

cholecystokinin (Gr. *chole,* bile or gall; *kystis,* bladder; *kinein,* to move) a hormone that is secreted by the mucosa of the duodenum in response to the presence of fat. The cholecystokinin causes the gallbladder to contract. This contraction propels bile into the duodenum, where it is needed to emulsify the fat. The fat is thus prepared for digestion and absorption.

cholesterol a fat-related compound, a sterol ($C_{27}H_{45}OH$). It is a normal constituent of bile and a principal constituent of gallstones. In body metabolism, cholesterol is important as a precursor of various steroid hormones such as sex hormones and adrenal corticoids. It has been associated with atherosclerosis, a disease of blood vessels characterized by the formation of localized plaques within or beneath the intimal surface of the vessel wall. Cholesterol is one of the major components of these fatty plaques. Cholesterol can be synthesized by the liver. It is widely distributed in nature, especially in animal tissue such as glandular meats and egg yolk.

chyle the milklike contents of the lacteals and lymphatic vessels of the intestine. It consists principally of absorbed fats. Chyle is carried from the intestine by the lymphatic vessels to the cisterna chyli. The cisterna chyli (the cistern or receptacle of the chyle) is a dilated sac at the origin of the thoracic duct, which is the common trunk that receives all the lymphatic vessels. The cisterna chyli lies in the abdomen between the second lumbar vertebra and the aorta. It receives the lymph from the intestinal trunk, the right and left lumbar lymphatic trunks, and two descending lymphatic trunks. The chyle, after passing through the cisterna chyli, is carried upward into the chest through the thoracic duct and empties into the venous blood at the point where the left subclavian vein joins the left internal jugular vein.

chylomicrons (Gr. *chylos,* chyle; *mikros,* small) particles of fat appearing in the lymph and blood after a meal rich in fat. These particles are composed largely of triglycerides with lesser amounts of phospholipids, cholesterol, cholesterol esters, and protein. About two to three hours after a fat meal the chylomicrons cause lactescence (milkiness) in the blood plasma; this is termed *alimentary lipemia.*

emulsifier an agent that breaks down large fat globules to smaller, uniformly distributed particles. This action is accomplished in the intestine chiefly by the bile acids, which lower surface tension of the fat particles. Emulsification greatly increases the surface area of fat, facilitating contact with fat-digesting enzymes.

enterohepatic circulation (Gr. *enteron,* intestine; *hepar,* liver) the circulation of bile from the liver to the gallbladder, then into the intestine, from which it is absorbed and carried by the blood back to the liver to be returned to the circulation. This continual circulation efficiently conserves the bile. Of the 20 to 30 g of bile used daily by the body, only about 0.8 g is eliminated in the feces and must be replenished by the liver.

essential fatty acid (EFA) a fatty acid that is (1) necessary for body metabolism or function and (2) cannot be manufactured by the body and must therefore be supplied in the diet. The major essential fatty acid is linoleic acid ($C_{17}H_{31}COOH$). It is found principally in vegetable oils. Two other fatty acids usually classified as essential are linolenic acid and arachidonic acid.

ester a compound produced by the reaction between an acid and an alcohol with the elimination of a molecule of water. Esters are commonly lipids with characteristic fruity or flowery odors. Cholesterol esters are formed in the mucosal cells by combination with fatty acids, largely linoleic acid.

fatty acid the structural components of fats. See *glycerides.*

glycerides group name for fats, any of a group of esters obtained from glycerol by the replacement of one, two, or three hydroxyl (OH) groups with a fatty acid. Monoglycerides contain one fatty acid; diglycerides contain two fatty acids; triglycerides contain three fatty acids. Glycerides are the principal constituent of adipose tissue and are found in animal and vegetable fats and oils.

glycerol a colorless, odorless, syrupy, sweet liquid; a constituent of fats usually obtained by the hydrolysis of fats. Chemically, glycerol is an alcohol; it is esterified with fatty acids to produce fats.

hydrogenation the process of adding hydrogen to unsaturated fats to produce a solid, saturated fat. This process is used to produce vegetable shortening from vegetable oils.

hydrolysis the process by which a chemical compound is split into other compounds by taking up the elements of water. Common examples of hydrolysis are the reactions of digestion in which the nutrients are split into simpler compounds by the digestive enzymes; that is, the conversion of starch to maltose, of fat to fatty acids and glycerol, and so on.

hyperlipemia excess quantity of fats and fatty substances in the blood.

lecithin (Gr. *lekithos,* egg yolk) a yellow-brown fatty substance of the group called phospholipids. It occurs in animal and plant tissues and egg yolk. It is composed of units of choline, phosphoric acid, fatty acids, and glycerol. Commercial forms of lecithin, obtained chiefly from soybeans, corn, and egg yolk, are used in candies, foods, cosmetics, and inks. In the metabolism of fat in the liver, lecithin plays an important role. It provides an effective lipotropic factor, choline, which prevents the accumulation of abnormal quantities of fat.

linoleic acid the major essential fatty acid. It is polyunsaturated.

lipase (Gr. *lipos,* fat; *-ase,* the suffix for enzyme) any of a class of enzymes that break down fats. A small quantity of gastric lipase (lipase secreted by the gastric mucosa) acts on emulsified fats of cream and egg yolk. The major digestive lipase is pancreatic lipase, which acts on fats in the small intestine. Pancreatic lipase was formerly called *steapsin.* Enteric lipase acts within the mucosal cells.

lipids the group name for organic substances of fatty nature. The lipids include fats, oils, waxes, and related compounds.

lipogenesis the formation of fat.

lipolysis the breakdown of fat into its component fatty acids and glycerol.

lipoproteins compounds of fat with protein. The lipoproteins probably function as major carriers of lipids in the plasma, since most of the plasma fat is associated with them. Such a combination makes possible the transport of fatty substances in a predominantly aqueous medium such as plasma.

lipotropic factor (Gr. *lipos,* fat; *trope,* turning) an agent that has an affinity for lipids. It prevents or corrects an excess accumulation of fat in the liver. Choline is probably the most important of the lipotropic factors. Protein helps to prevent a fatty liver because it provides amino acids, such as methionine, that contribute to the synthesis of choline.

micellar bile-fat complex (L., *mica,* crumb, grain; *ella,* diminutive suffix) a micelle is a particle formed by an aggregate of molecules, a microscopic unit of protoplasm. In micellar bile-fat complex the particle is formed by the combination of bile salts with fat substances (fatty acids and glycerides) to achieve the absorption of fat across the intestinal mucosa.

phospholipids any of a class of fat-related substances that contain phosphorus, fatty acids, and a nitrogenous base. The phospholipids are essential elements in every cell, but seem to play a special role in the metabolism of fat within the liver.

saponification (L. *sapo,* soap; *facere,* to make) a characteristic reaction of fats and alkalis that produces soaps.

saturation (L. *saturare,* to fill) to cause to unite with the greatest possible amount of another substance through solution, chemical combination, or the like. A saturated fat, for example, is one in which the component fatty acids are filled with hydrogen atoms. A fatty acid is said to be saturated if all available chemical bonds of its carbon chain are filled with hydrogen. If one bond remains unfilled, it is a monounsaturated fatty acid. If two or more bonds remain unfilled, it is a polyunsaturated fatty

acid. Fats of animal sources are more saturated. Fats of plant sources are more unsaturated.

steroids any of a large group of fat-related organic compounds, including sterols, bile acids, sex hormones, hormones of the adrenal cortex, and D vitamins.

REFERENCES
Specific

1. Goodhart, R. S., and Shils, M. E., editors: Modern nutrition in health and disease, ed. 5, Philadelphia, 1973, Lea & Febiger.
2. Alfin-Slater, R. B.: Fats, essential fatty acids, and ascorbic acid, J. Am. Diet. Assoc. **64:**168-170, 1974.
3. Inter-Society Commission for Heart Disease Resources: Primary prevention of the atherosclerotic diseases, Circulation, vol. 42, Dec. 1970 (rev. April, 1972).
4. Deuel, H. J., Jr.: Lipids: their chemisty and biochemistry, vol. 1, Chemistry, New York, 1951, Interscience Publishers.
5. Posati, L., Kinsella, J., and Watt, B.: Comprehensive evaluation of fatty acids in foods. I. Dairy products, J. Am. Diet. Assoc. **66:**482-488, 1975.
6. Freeley, R., Criner, P., and Slover, H.: Major fatty acids and proximate composition of dairy products, J. Am. Diet. Assoc. **66:**140-146, 1975.
7. Anderson, B., Kinsella, J., and Watt, B.: Comprehensive evaluation of fatty acids in foods. II. Beef products, J. Am. Diet. Assoc. **67:**35-41, 1975.
8. Posati, L., Kinsella, J., and Watt, B.: Comprehensive evaluation of fatty acids in foods. III. Eggs and egg products, J. Am. Diet. Assoc. **67:**111-115, 1975.
9. Anderson, B. A.: Comprehensive evaluation of fatty acids in foods. VII. Pork products, J. Am. Diet. Assoc. **69:**44, 1976.
10. Mead, J. F.: The metabolism of the polyunsaturated fatty acids, Am. J. Clin. Nutr. **8:**55, 1960.
11. Harkins, R. W., and Sarett, H. P.: Medium-chain triglycerides, J.A.M.A. **203**(4):272, 1963.
12. Inglefinger, F. J.: Gastrointestinal absorption, Nutr. Today **2**(1):2, 1967.
13. Phelps, C. P., Rubin, C. E., and Luft, J. H.: Electron microscope techniques for studying absorption of fat in man, Gastroenterology **46:**134, 1964.
14. Porte, D., Jr., and Entenman, C.: Fatty acid metabolism in segments of rat intestine, Am. J. Physiol. **208:**607, 1965.
15. Guyton, A. C.: Textbook of medical physiology, Philadelphia, 1966, W. B. Saunders Co., p. 908.
16. Anderson, J., Grande, F., and Keys, A.: Cholesterol-lowering diets, J. Am. Diet. Assoc. **62:**133-142, 1973.
17. Hill, P., Reddy, B. S., and Wynder, E. L.: Effect of unsaturated fats and cholesterol on serum and fecal lipids, J. Am. Diet. Assoc. **75:**414, Oct., 1979.

18. Connor, W. E.: Dietary sterols: their relationship to atherosclerosis, J. Am. Diet. Assoc. **52:**202, 1968.

General

Albrink, M.: Triglyceridemia, J. Am. Diet. Assoc. **62:**626, 1973.

Atherosclerosis: The cholesterol connection, Science **194:** 711, 1976.

Brignoli, C. A., Kinsella, T. E., and Wahrauch, J. L.: Comprehensive evaluation of fatty acids in foods. V. Unhydrogenated fats and oils, J. Am. Diet. Assoc. **68:** 224, 1976.

Feeley, R. M., et al.: Cholesterol content of foods, J. Am. Diet. Assoc. **61:**134-148, 1972.

Food and Nutrition Board, Council of foods and nutrition, American Medical Association: Diet and coronary heart disease, Washington, D.C., 1972, National Academy of Sciences.

Fristrom, G. A., and Weikraugh, D. K.: Comprehensive evaluation of fatty acids in foods, J. Am. Diet. Assoc. **69:**517, 1976.

Goodhart, F. S., and Shils, M. E., editors: Modern nutrition in health and disease, ed. 5, Philadelphia, 1973, Lea & Febiger.

Hansen, A. W., et al.: Role of linoleic acid in infant nutrition, Pediatrics **31:**171, 1962.

Harper, H. A.: Review of physiological chemistry, ed. 15, Los Altos, Calif., 1975, Lange Medical Publications.

Institute of Shortening and Edible Oils, Inc.: Food fats and oils, ed. 4, Washington, D.C., 1974, The Institute.

Kolata, G. B.: Atherosclerotic plaques: competing theories guide research, Science **194:**592, 1976.

Kritchevsky, D.: Diet and cholesteremia, Lipids **12:**49, 1977.

Latner, A. L.: Cantarow and Trumper clinical biochemistry, ed. 7, Philadelphia, 1975, W. B. Saunders Co.

Lees, R. S., and Wilson, D. E.: The treatment of hyperlipidemia, N. Engl. J. Med. **248:**186, 1971.

Myant, N. B.: The influence of some dietary factors in cholesterol metabolism, Proc. Nutr. Soc. **34:**271, 1975.

Scott, L. W., et al.: Are low cholesterol diets expensive? J. Am. Diet. Assoc. **74:**558-561, May, 1979.

Truswell, A. S.: Diet and plasma lipids—a reappraisal, Am. J. Clin. Nutr. **31:**977, 1978.

Whyte, H. M., and Hevenstein, N.: A perspective view of dieting to lower the blood cholesterol, Am. J. Clin. Nutr. **29:**784, 1976.

Zilversmit, D. B.: Cholesterol index of foods, J. Am. Diet. Assoc. **74:**562-565, May, 1979.

4 Proteins

The Dutch chemist Gerardus Johannes Mulder first proposed the name *protein* in 1840 before much was known about these substances. The word *protein* comes from the Greek word *proteios,* meaning "primary, holding first place." Mulder applied the name well. Proteins make up the basic structure of all living cells and are an essential life-forming and life-sustaining ingredient of the diet of all animal organisms. The amount of protein in the diets of different cultures varies. In countries with adequate nutrition it contributes from 10% to 15% of the total calories. In the average American diet, protein contributes approximately 14% to 20% of the total calories, but there are increasing indications that our diet needs to be modified from our high consumption of animal protein with its attendant high ratio of animal fat.[1]

GENERAL AND CHEMICAL DEFINITIONS OF PROTEINS

General definition. Proteins may be defined as organic substances that upon hydrolysis or digestion yield their constituent unit building blocks—*amino acids*. Proteins are found in animal foods such as meat, milk, cheese, and eggs, and to a lesser extent in plant foods such as grains and legumes. Entirely free protein, such as albumin in egg white, is rare in nature. Usually protein is found in connection with fats and carbohydrates. For example, in the animal food sources protein is usually associated with fat (meat, milk, cheese, egg yolk). In plants, proteins are usually associated with carbohydrate (grains, legumes).

Chemical definition. A protein may be defined according to its basic elements. Like carbohydrate and fat, protein contains carbon, hydrogen, and oxygen. But protein is unique in that it also contains nitrogen (16% of its total composition; 6.25 g protein yields 1 g nitrogen upon metabolism) and often other elements such as sulfur.

The structure of protein is also different from that of either carbohydrate or fat. The proteins are much more complex compounds with high molecular weights, which range from a few thousand to a million or more. A given protein contains a specific number of specific amino acids linked in a sequence that is specific for that protein. It is this very *specificity* of protein structure in a definite amino acid sequence that gives various tissues their unique form, function, and character.

CLASSIFICATION OF PROTEINS
Chemical structure

More is yet to be learned about the composition of specific proteins, but the general structure and chemical nature of proteins provide a basis for the rather loose classifications of simple proteins, compound proteins, and derived proteins.

Simple proteins. Simple proteins contain only amino acids or their derivatives. A few common examples of simple proteins are

1. Albumin—lactalbumin in milk, serum albumin in blood
2. Globulin—ovoglobulin in egg, serum globulin in blood
3. Glutelin—gluten in wheat
4. Prolamin—zein in corn, gliadin in wheat
5. Albuminoid—collagen in supportive tissue, keratin in hair and skin, gelatin

Compound (conjugated) proteins. Compound proteins are compounds of simple proteins and some other nonprotein group. Examples include

1. Nucleoproteins (compounds of one or more proteins and nucleic acid)—purines, found in large amounts in glandular tissue
2. Glycoproteins and mucoproteins (compounds of a protein and carbohydrate)—mucin, found in secretions from mucous membranes
3. Phosphoproteins (compounds of a protein and a phosphorus-containing radical other than phospholipid or nucleic acid)—casein, found in milk
4. Chromoproteins (compounds of a protein and a chromophoric or pigmented group)—hemoglobin
5. Lipoproteins (compounds of a protein and a triglyceride or other lipid)—phospholipid or cholesterol
6. Metalloproteins (compounds of a protein and a metal such as copper or iron)—heme, the iron-binding portion of hemoglobin

Derived proteins. Derived proteins are fragments of various sizes. They are produced as large protein molecules initially and are progressively broken down during digestion. In order, from largest to smallest fragments of peptide chains, these derived proteins are proteoses, peptones, polypeptides, and peptides.

Function

Proteins may also be classified into seven broad categories according to their function in the body:

1. Structural proteins—collagen
2. Contractile proteins—muscle
3. Antibodies—gamma globulin
4. Blood proteins—albumin, fibrinogen, and hemoglobin
5. Hormones
6. Enzymes
7. Nutrient proteins—food sources of essential amino acids

AMINO ACIDS

Newer concepts of proteins interpret them in terms of their constituent amino acids. Students will need to recognize the names of these amino acids and know something of their nature, for they will be encountered in clinical practice. For example, in pediatrics one learns of *phenylketonuria,* a disease in children caused by the body's inability to properly handle the essential amino acid *phenylalanine.* Proteins also have a buffering effect for peptic ulcer patients because of the interesting *amphoteric* nature of amino acids.

Proteins should be viewed, then, in terms of their building blocks, amino acids. This chapter will look at the background of their discovery and at their unique dual structure.

History. Early in the 1800s, scientists recognized that proteins could be broken down (hydrolyzed) into a number of smaller structural units. Because these substances seemed to behave chemically with a dual nature—both acid and base—they were given the seemingly contradictory name *amino* (base) *acids.*

Glycine, the simplest amino acid, was identified in 1820; threonine was not identified until 1935. Since then, still other amino acids have been identified as metabolic products in the body. Much of the early work was contributed by Carl von Voit and his pupil Max Rubner in the late nineteenth century and by R. H. Chittenden in the early twentieth century. These basic studies were expanded and developed by Thomas B. Osborne and L. B. Mendel at Yale, W. C. Rose at the University of Illinois, and many others.

Classification of amino acids

Essential and nonessential amino acids. It was largely the brilliant work of Dr. Rose[2] that established an important differentiation among the amino acids. He termed amino acids "essential" or "nonessential." This grouping is based on two related factors: (1) whether the body can manufacture the particular amino acid and (2) whether the amino acid is essential for normal growth and development.

In his experiments, Rose used young rats. He first fed the rats on a known mixture of purified amino acids. Then, one at a time, he removed an amino acid from the mixture. If the rat continued to grow normally, he classified that amino acid as nonessential. If the rat ceased to grow normally or lost weight and died, he classified the amino acid as essential. It soon became apparent that in man, also, the protein requirement must be considered on the basis of the quality and not merely the quantity of the protein. It was obviously not only a matter of the total amount of protein needed but also of the specific amino acids needed. For example, gelatin alone is a rather worthless protein, for it lacks three essential amino acids—tryptophan, valine, and isoleucine—and has only small amounts of leucine.

On the basis of these distinctions in body dependence, eight amino acids have been demonstrated to be essential for adults. The approximately 12 remaining amino acids are nonessential or dispensable. The body can manufacture them, and thus they are not as necessary in the diet for normal growth and development. The following is a listing of the essential and nonessential amino acids.

Essential*	Nonessential*
Threonine	Glycine
Leucine	Alanine
Isoleucine	Aspartic acid
Valine	Glutamic acid

*Three other amino acids, cysteine, citrulline, and hydroxylysine, may be added to the nonessential list. Although not naturally occurring, they are nonetheless metabolically active in the body.

Essential	Nonessential
Lysine	Proline
Methionine	Hydroxyproline
Phenylalanine	Cystine
Tryptophan	Tyrosine
	Serine
	Arginine*
	Histidine*

Complete and incomplete proteins. According to the amounts of essential amino acids that given proteins in foods possess, proteins have been broadly classified as complete or incomplete. Complete proteins are those that contain all the essential amino acids in sufficient quantity and ratio to supply the body's needs. These proteins are of animal origin: meat, milk (cheese), and egg. Incomplete proteins are those deficient in one or more of the essential amino acids. They are of plant origin: grains, legumes, and nuts. In a mixed diet, animal and plant proteins supplement one another. Even a mixture of plant proteins may provide an adequate, balanced ratio of amino acids. The value of variety in the diet is therefore self-evident. The comparative nutritive quality of protein foods is discussed later in this chapter as the question of protein requirement is considered (pp. 66-67).

Basic structure of amino acids

Amphoteric nature. As indicated by its name, an amino acid has a chemical structure that combines both acid and base (amino) factors. This important chemical structure gives to amino acids a unique amphoteric nature (Gr. *amphoteros,* both). This dual nature can be seen in the fundamental pattern of an amino acid as shown in the diagrams above. The acid factor is the carboxyl group (COOH) and the base factor is the amino group (NH_2). A radical that is specific for the individual amino acid is grouped around a central carbon atom.

As a result of its dual nature, an amino acid in solution can *ionize* (dissociate or separate

*Arginine and histidine are necessary during growth but not during adulthood; they may be called "semiessential."

$$\text{Base (amino group)} \rightarrow \left(\begin{array}{c} H \\ | \\ H-N \end{array} \right) \begin{array}{c} \left(\begin{array}{c} O \\ \| \\ C-OH \end{array} \right) \leftarrow \text{Acid (carboxyl group)} \\ | \\ -C-H \\ | \\ (R) \leftarrow \text{Varying attached radical} \end{array}$$

Fundamental amino acid pattern

$$\begin{array}{c} COOH \\ | \\ NH_2-C-H \\ | \\ CH_3 \end{array}$$

Alanine (attached radical a methyl group)

$$\begin{array}{c} COOH \\ | \\ NH_2-C-H \\ | \\ H \end{array}$$

Glycine (attached radical a single hydrogen atom)

$$\begin{array}{c} COOH \\ | \\ NH_2-C-H \\ | \\ CH_2 \end{array}$$

Phenylalanine (attached radical a complex carbon ring structure)

into its constituent ions) to behave either as an acid or as a base, depending on the pH of the solution. This means that amino acids have a great *buffer* capacity, which is an important clinical characteristic. The interesting term commonly used for this unique phenomenon is "zwitterion." The term is taken from the German word *Zwitter,* meaning "hybrid," and the Greek word *ion,* meaning "wanderer." Amino acids behave like "hybrid wanderers," either acid or base, depending on the buffering need presented by the particular solution they are in.

Peptide linkage. This acid-base chemical nature of amino acids also enables them to join in the characteristic chain structure of proteins.

The amino group of one amino acid joins the carboxyl group of another. This characteristic chain structure of amino acids is called a peptide linkage. Long chains of amino acids linked in this manner are called *polypeptides* (Fig. 4-1).

Arrangement of peptide chains. Long polypeptide chains may be coiled or folded back on themselves in a spiral shape called a *helix.* They are held together in some instances by additional cross links of bonds involving sulfur and hydrogen. The helical shapes of these coils may be of two types: (1) *fibrous*—a protein that coils and unfolds on contraction and relaxation, such as myosin in muscle fiber, and (2) *globular*—a

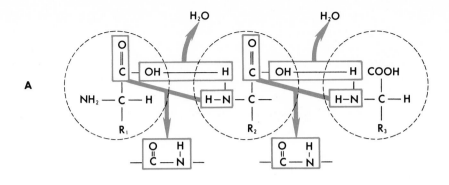

Fig. 4-1. Two stages in formation of peptide linkage by which amino acids are formed. **A,** Basic joining of the two amino acids, producing peptide bond and water. **B,** Polypeptide chain formed from numbers of specific amino acids linked in specific sequence. The different attached radicals (R_1, R_2 . . . R_{n-1}, R_n) determine the specific amino acids.

protein forming a dense compact coil, such as serum protein (albumin and globulin) and insulin.

The various component structures within the total structure of the protein molecule have been grouped according to increased complexity of arrangement. The *primary structure* is the basic polypeptide chain. The *secondary structure* is the helix with its coils linked to one another by crossbonds usually of hydrogen or sulfur. The *tertiary structure* is the characteristic arrangements of helixes that form specific layers on fibers of specific proteins.

FUNCTIONS OF PROTEIN

Growth and tissue maintenance. The primary function of dietary protein is the growth and maintenance of tissue. It does this by furnishing amino acids (of appropriate numbers and types) for efficient synthesis of specific cellular tissue proteins. In addition, protein supplies amino acids for other essential nitrogen-containing substances such as enzymes and hormones.

Specific physiologic roles of amino acids. All amino acids supplied by protein participate in growth and tissue maintenance, but some also perform other important physiologic and metabolic roles.

Methionine is a methylating agent that participates in the formation of such nonprotein cellular constiuents as choline. Methionine is also the precursor of the nonessential amino acid *cystine.*

Tryptophan is the precursor of the vitamin nicotinamide (niacin) and the precursor of the vasoconstrictor serotonin.

Phenylalanine is the precursor of the nonessential amino acid tyrosine. Together with tyrosine, phenylalanine leads to formation of the hormones thyroxine and epinephrine.

Energy. Protein also contributes to the body's overall energy metabolism. After removal of the nitrogenous portion of the constituent amino acid, the amino acid residue may be either *glycogenic* (capable of being converted to carbohydrate) or *ketogenic* (capable of being converted to fatty acids). Only leucine, phenylalanine, and tyrosine are fully ketogenic, and isoleucine is weakly so. The remaining amino acids are glycogenic. It has been estimated that on an average, 58% of the total dietary protein may become available as glucose and is oxidized as such to yield energy.

DIGESTION OF PROTEIN
Mechanical digestion

Mouth. Only mechanical breaking up of protein foods by mastication occurs in the mouth. Here the food particles are mixed with salivary secretions and pass as a semisolid mass into the stomach where the main chemical digestion of protein begins.

Chemical digestion

Stomach. Chemical digestion of protein begins in the stomach. In fact the stomach's chief digestive function in relation to all foods is the partial enzymatic breakdown of protein. Three agents contained in the gastric secretions participate in different ways in this beginning hydrolysis. These agents are pepsin, hydrochloric acid, and rennin.

Pepsin, the main gastric enzyme specific for proteins, is first produced as an inactive substance, *pepsinogen,* by a single layer of cells (the chief cells) in the mucosa of the stomach wall. Pepsinogen requires hydrochloric acid for activation to the enzyme pepsin. This active pepsin then begins breaking the peptide linkages of protein to produce *proteoses* and *peptones*. These are shorter chain polypeptides that are still rather large protein derivatives. If the protein were held in the stomach longer, pepsin could continue this breakdown until individual amino acids resulted. However, with normal gastric emptying time, only the beginning stage is completed by the action of pepsin.

Hydrochloric acid (HCl) is necessary to convert inactive pepsinogen to the active enzyme pepsin. Gastric hydrochloric acid is an important catalyst in gastric protein digestion. Clinical problems can be anticipated for patients who lack proper hydrochloric acid secretion.

Rennin is a gastric enzyme important in the infant's digestion of milk. Rennin and calcium act on the casein of milk to produce a curd. By coagulating milk, rennin prevents too rapid a passage from the stomach. In adults, however, rennin is apparently absent from the gastric secretions.

Small intestine. Protein digestion begins in the acid medium of the stomach and continues in the alkaline medium of the small intestine. A number of enzymes from both pancreatic and intestinal secretions take part.

PANCREATIC SECRETIONS. The protein-splitting enzyme *trypsin* is secreted first by the pancreas as an inactive substance called *trypsinogen*. Trypsinogen is activated to trypsin by the hormone *enterokinase,* which is produced by glands in the duodenal wall. This active enzyme trypsin acts on protein and proteoses and peptones carried over from the stomach to produce shorter chain polypeptides and dipeptides.

The pancreas also produces another protein-specific enzyme, *chymotrypsin,* preceded by its inactive precursor, *chymotrypsinogen*. Chymotrypsin is activated by the activated trypsin present. Chymotrypsin has the same protein-splitting action as trypsin and produces polypeptides and dipeptides. It also has more milk coagulating ability than trypsin.

Carboxypeptidase is one of a group of enzymes called peptidases. It is called carboxypeptidase because it attacks the end of the peptide chain where there is a free carboxyl (acid) group (COOH). It produces still simpler peptides and some free amino acids.

INTESTINAL SECRETIONS. Glands in the intestinal wall produce aminopeptidase and dipeptidase. There are two additional protein-splitting enzymes in the peptidase group.

Aminopeptidase attacks the amino (NH_2) linkages of the peptide chain. Through this cleavage action, Aminopeptidase produces

Table 4-1. Summary of protein digestion

| Organ | Enzyme | | | Digestive action |
	Inactive precursor	Activator	Active enzyme	
Mouth			None	Mechanical only
Stomach (acid)	Pepsinogen	Hydrochloric acid	Pepsin	Protein → Proteoses and peptones
			Rennin (infants) (calcium necessary for activity)	Casein → Coagulated curd
Intestine (alkaline) Pancreatic juice	Trypsinogen	Enterokinase	Trypsin	Protein, proteoses, peptones → Polypeptides, dipeptides
	Chymotrypsinogen	Active trypsin	Chymotrypsin	Proteoses, peptones → Polypeptides, dipeptides Also coagulates milk
			Carboxypeptidase	Polypeptides → Simpler peptides, dipeptides, amino acids
Intestinal juice			Aminopeptidase	Polypeptides → Peptides, dipeptides, amino acids
			Dipeptidase	Dipeptides → Amino acids

simpler short-chain peptides and free amino acids.

Dipeptidase is the final enzyme of the protein-splitting system. It acts on the remaining dipeptides to produce free amino acids.

By this system, the pancreatic and intestinal secretions break down the large complex proteins into progressively smaller peptides chains, and amino acids are split off from the ends of these chains. The end products of protein digestion (amino acids) are then ready for absorption by the intestinal mucosa.

A summary of protein digestion is outlined for review in Table 4-1.

ABSORPTION OF PROTEIN INTO THE BLOODSTREAM

The end products of protein digestion are water-soluble amino acids. These amino acids are absorbed rapidly from the small intestine directly into the portal blood system through the fine network of villous capillaries. Most of this amino acid absorption probably takes place in the proximal portion of the small intestine.

The mechanism of this absorptive transport is not completely known. Originally it was assumed that since amino acids are water soluble, all forms were absorbed through the intestinal wall by simple passive diffusion. However, studies[3,4] indicate that far more activity is involved. This process is currently believed to include several aspects.

Active transport system. An active and selective transport system is present, which is energy-dependent. The amino acids in their natural forms are transported by this active system; their isomers may be absorbed by free diffusion.

Vitamin B$_6$ cofactor. Vitamin B$_6$ (pyridoxine) in the form of pyridoxal phosphate appears to be intimately involved in the active transport of amino acids from the intestinal mucosa to the serosa. This vitamin also seems to play a role in the transport of amino acids into the cells for eventual metabolism. This relationship provides still another example of the concept of intimate interrelationships among the many nutrients and their metabolites in human nutrition.

Competition for absorption. Competition for absorption of the amino acids seems to exist. When a mixture of amino acids is fed to an organism, the quantitatively predominant amino acid may retard the absorption of the others. In the plasma, also, competition apparently exists among the circulating amino acids for entry into the cell.

Absorption of peptides and whole proteins. A few larger fragments of short-chain peptides may remain after digestion and be absorbed as such. This mucosal uptake of intact peptides is followed by hydrolysis within the absorbing cells to yield amino acids.[5] Even whole proteins are sometimes absorbed intact. These larger protein molecules apparently cannot be used in protein synthesis as can free amino acids, but they may play a part in the development of immunity and sensitivity. For example, antibodies in the mother's colostrum (the premilk breast secretion) are passed on to her nursing infant.

METABOLISM OF PROTEIN

In human nutrition the amino acids are the metabolic currency of protein. It is with the fate of these vital compounds that the metabolism of protein is ultimately concerned. The many metabolic processes involved in protein metabolism form a fascinating array of complex and intricately interwoven chemical activities. The metabolic activities of protein can be summarized under the three broad categories of *balance*, *building* tissue (anabolism), and *breakdown* of tissue (catabolism). These activities may be remembered as the "three B's" of protein metabolism.

Balance

Throughout the body many interdependent checks and balances exist. There is a constant ebb and flow of materials, a building up and breaking down of parts, and a depositing and mobilizing of constituents. Many body mechanisms maintain internal physiologic stability (equilibrium). The body has built-in controls that operate as coordinated responses of its parts of any situation that tends to disturb its normal condition or function. The resultant state of equilibrium is called *homeostasis,* and the various mechanisms designed to preserve it are called *homeostatic mechanisms*. This balance between body parts and functions is life sustaining.

Increasingly therefore as more and more is being learned about human nutrition and physiology, older ideas of a rigid body structure are giving way to a concept of dynamic equilibrium. All body constituents are in a constant state of flux, although some tissues are more actively engaged than others. This concept of dynamic equilibrium can be seen in carbohydrate and fat metabolism; however, it is especially striking in protein metabolism.

Protein turnover. Classic studies[6] with radioactive isotopes have clearly demonstrated that the body's protein tissues are continuously being broken down into amino acids and resynthesized. In such studies, when "labeled" amino acids are fed, they are rapidly incorporated into various body tissue proteins.

The rate of protein turnover varies in different tissues. It is highest in the intestinal mucosa, liver, pancreas, kidney, and plasma and lowest in muscle, brain, and skin tissue; there is almost no protein turnover in collagen tissue.

Endogenous body protein exists in a balance between two compartments—the tissue protein compartment and the plasma protein compartment. These endogenous stores are further balanced with exogenous dietary protein intake. Protein from one compartment may be drawn on to supply a need in the other. For example, during fasting, resources from the body protein stores may be used for tissue synthesis. But the interesting fact is that even when the intake of protein and other nutrients is adequate, the tissue proteins are still being constantly broken down and re-formed.

The adult body's state of stability, then, is the result of a balance between the rates of protein breakdown and resynthesis. In periods of growth, however, the synthesis rate is higher so that new tissue can be formed. In conditions of starvation and wasting diseases (and, more gradually, as in the aging process in the elderly) the rate of breakdown exceeds that of synthesis, and the body deteriorates.

Metabolic amino acid pool. Amino acids derived from endogenous tissue breakdown and amino acids from dietary protein both enter a common metabolic pool of amino acids. Thus a balance of amino acids is maintained to supply the body's total needs. Shifts and balances between tissue breakdown and dietary protein ensure the constant availability of a balanced

mixture of amino acids. From this amino acid pool, specific amino acids are supplied as needed for specific tissue protein synthesis and to make up body losses (Fig. 4-2).

Nitrogen balance. Nitrogen is also found in compounds other than amino acids. Nonprotein nitrogen is present in urea, uric acid, ammonia, creatine, creatinine, and other body tissues and fluids. *Total nitrogen balance* involves all these sources. The word balance refers to the balance between intake and output of a particular substance. The term *negative balance* is used to indicate that the output of a substance exceeds its intake. *Positive balance* is that state in which the intake of a given substance exceeds its output. Total nitrogen balance is the net result of all nitrogen gains and losses in all protein compartments, although it gives no picture of the shifts in distribution of nitrogen. For example, a tissue involved in a malignant neoplastic process may be robbing other tissues of nitrogen; yet this loss would not be reflected in total nitrogen balance. Nevertheless, the total nitrogen balance is a useful general measure of body equilibrium.

Nonprotein nitrogen plays a role in protein synthesis through its sparing effect on some

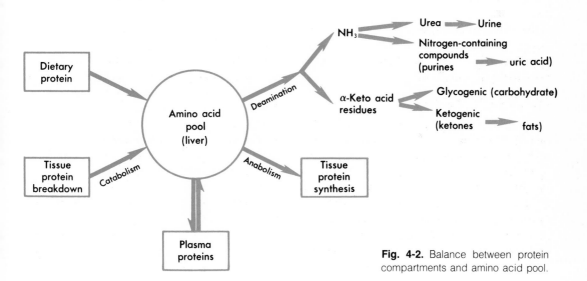

Fig. 4-2. Balance between protein compartments and amino acid pool.

amino acid requirements. By providing the amino group for transamination, it relieves the need for amino acid food sources to supply the nitrogen radical.

Building tissue (anabolism)

To maintain the vital balance in protein metabolism, amino acids have one of two possible fates in the body after absorption. They may be incorporated into tissue protein synthesis *(anabolism),* or they may be degraded or broken down into their constituent parts *(catabolism).* The products of protein catabolism are oxidized or excreted.

The building or synthesis of tissue protein is governed by a unique specificity with respect to the amino acid constituents that are required to produce a specific protein. This has been called the law of "all or none." All the necessary amino acids for a given protein must be present at the same time, or the protein will not be formed. Specific selection and supply of amino acids are mandatory.

Since the advent of the electron microscope, scientists have been able to study the intricate workings of cell metabolism and develop hypotheses concerning the process by which protein is synthesized by the living organism. To understand the process of protein synthesis one must consider both the basic substances governing the process and the basic steps or stages necessary to build the specific peptide chains. The following brief explanation of some of these processes is highly oversimplified from the point of view of the physical chemist, but it may be found convenient as a basis for conceptualization.

Substances that govern protein synthesis

DNA (deoxyribonucleic acid). DNA has been identified as the controlling mechanism by which genetic design is passed from generation to generation. It is the key material in the chromosomes of the cell nucleus. Each gene is probably composed of a complex nucleic acid molecule. DNA is a large double-chain *poly-*

mer (a compound of high molecular weight made up of many parts). It is composed of nitrogenous bases called nucleotides (purines, pyrimidines), a sugar (deoxyribose), and a phosphate group. DNA forms the basic pattern of the message code in each cell. This code or pattern determines what specific protein will be synthesized.

Messenger RNA (ribonucleic acid). RNA is formed by DNA in the cell nucleus and receives its own specific pattern imprint. (This relationship is similar to the way in which waffle batter receives the imprint of the waffle iron pressed against it.) RNA differs from DNA, however, in that it is only a single strand structure, it has a different sugar (ribose), and one of its nitrogen bases is a different compound. Once it is formed in the cell nucleus by the DNA, it carries the message pattern transferred to it by DNA to the cell cytoplasm. This type of RNA has been designated "messenger RNA." (Another type of RNA, "transfer RNA," is described below.) Out in the cell messenger RNA uses one of the membranous tubules of the endoplasmic reticulum as its working site. Here it attaches itself to the row of reticular granules (ribosomes) as an anchor point for its operations.

Ribosomes. Ribosomes are the small granules on the cell's network of endoplasmic reticulum. They are called *ribosomes* because they are minute bodies (Gr. *soma,* body) or spheres containing RNA (ribonucleic acid). The messenger RNA strand from the nucleus attaches itself to the ribosome and forms a template or mold to direct the lining up of amino acids in the exact sequence necessary to fit the master pattern for the desired protein. This is part of the marvelous *specificity* of protein synthesis at work.

Stages in the process of protein synthesis

Activated amino acids. For amino acids to be used in protein synthesis, they must first be activated. This means they must be energized to be capable of combining chemically with other substances. This is done in the cell's cytoplasm by an activating enzyme that is specific for each amino acid, plus an energizing phosphate compound—ATP (adenosine triphosphate) or AMP (adenosine monophosphate). The complex formed (Enzyme + AMP + Amino acid) produces an activated amino acid that is ready to go into its position in the protein molecule.

Transfer RNA. Many short-chain RNA molecules (transfer RNA) occur free in the cell's cytoplasmic fluid. There appear to be specific transfer RNA molecules for each amino acid used. Each transfer RNA molecule attaches itself to its specific amino acid partner and carries it to the strand of messenger RNA that is anchored on the ribosome. The amino acid slips perfectly into its correct slot. One beside another, the amino acids line up at their specific fitting sites along the grid of the ribosomal template as the messenger RNA is guided into place by the transfer RNA.

Peptide linkage. The activated amino acids, which have been lined up side by side in a precise sequence, are joined to each other by peptide linkages to form long polypeptide chains. This is the specific polypeptide chain of the protein originally designated by the pattern coded on the DNA in the cell nucleus. The newly formed polypeptide chain breaks free from the ribosome, and the transfer RNA molecules are freed from the messenger RNA template. The transfer RNA molecules are now available to perform the process all over again. These successive stages in protein synthesis are illustrated in Fig. 4-3.

Breaking down tissue (catabolism)

If a given amino acid is not used in tissue protein synthesis, it may be degraded or oxidized to yield energy. A nitrogenous group and a nonnitrogen residue result from catabolism of amino acids.

Nitrogenous group (NH₂). The first step in the metabolic breakdown of amino acids is

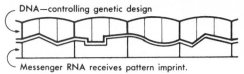

Stage 1:
Preparation in cell nucleus: DNA transfers specific protein pattern to messenger RNA

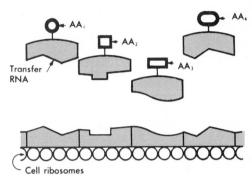

Stage 2:
Activated amino acids in cell cytoplasm attach to transfer RNA partner

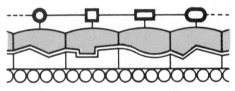

Stage 3:
Transfer RNA carries the active amino acids into position, and peptide linkage forms

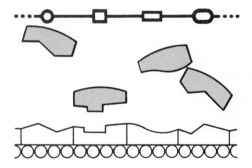

Stage 4:
Newly formed polypeptide chain breaks free; transfer RNA is released to repeat process

Fig. 4-3. Stages in protein synthesis.

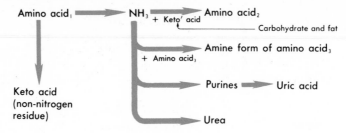

Fig. 4-4. Ways in which ammonia, derived from amino acid deamination, is disposed of by the body.

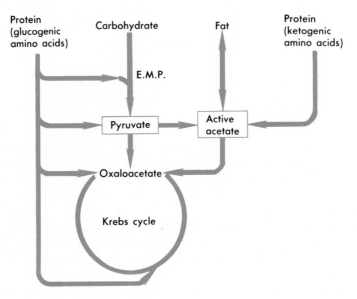

Fig. 4-5. Converging of glucogenic and ketogenic amino acids with carbohydrate and fat in the Embden-Meyerhof glycolytic pathway and the final common Krebs cycle for energy production.

the splitting off of the nitrogenous portion (the amino group, NH_2) by hydrolysis. This process, which takes place chiefly in the liver, is called *deamination*. The ammonia (NH_3) that is formed may be handled in several ways (Fig. 4-4).

1. Ammonia may be converted in the liver to urea and excreted by the kidney in the urine. The conversion is completed by a special urea cycle in the liver.
2. The ammonia may be used in production of purines and other nitrogen-containing compounds.

3. The ammonia may be combined with various carbohydrate derivatives of amino acid residues to form other amino acids. (Such amino acids would be nonessential because the body can manufacture them.) The process of transferring the amino group from an amino acid to a carbohydrate derivative or an amino acid residue is called *transamination*. The process is catalyzed by specific enzymes called *transaminases*. A vitamin B_6 derivative (pyridoxal phosphate) acts as a coenzyme. When tissue is damaged, trans-

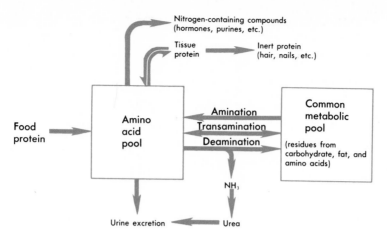

Fig. 4-6. Interrelationships between the amino acid pool and the common metabolic pool of residues from carbohydrates, fats, and amino acids.

aminases are released and their level in plasma rises.

4. Ammonia may be taken up by an amino acid to produce still another form of that acid, the *amine* form. This process is called *amination*. For example, a glutamic acid molecule may take up an NH_3 radical to form glutamine. The NH_3 radical may then be liberated from the glutamine molecule in distal tubules of kidney and excreted. These processes of amination and deamination provide an efficient way of removing a toxic substance (NH_3) from the body.

These four ways of processing ammonia furnish further illustrations of the body's constant metabolic interconversions between carbohydrate, protein, and fat.

Nonnitrogen residue. The nonnitrogen residue is called a *keto-acid*. The residue of a given amino acid is either glycogenic (leading to the formation of carbohydrate) or ketogenic (leading to the formation of fat). The ketogenic amino acids are phenylalanine, tyrosine, and leucine; isoleucine residue is also weakly ketogenic. The majority of the amino acids are glycogenic. Glycine, alanine, serine, threonine, valine, glutamic acid, aspartic acid, histidine, arginine, lysine, cystine, methionine, proline, and isoproline are all glycogenic. The glycogenic amino acid residues enter the Embden-Meyerhof glycolytic pathway at pyruvate (see Chapter 2) and the Krebs cycle at oxaloacetate and ketoglutarate. The ketogenic amino acid residues enter the same final oxidation pathways at active acetate (Fig. 4-5).

The intermediate metabolites from protein, carbohydrate, and fat enter a common metabolic pool. There is constant interplay between this pool and the amino acid pool (Fig. 4-6). Finally, metabolites from all three basic nutrients enter the Krebs cycle and produce the end products CO_2 and H_2O.

During a fasting period, glycogen stores are rapidly depleted; fat stores are then reduced more slowly. After the fat stores are diminished, the body, in its attempt to maintain itself, begins to break down tissue protein. It is for this reason that a diet sufficient in carbohydrate calories has a protein-sparing effect.

Hormonal influences on protein metabolism

The anabolism and catabolism of protein are regulated by certain hormones. Pituitary growth hormone (GH), androgens, insulin, and normal

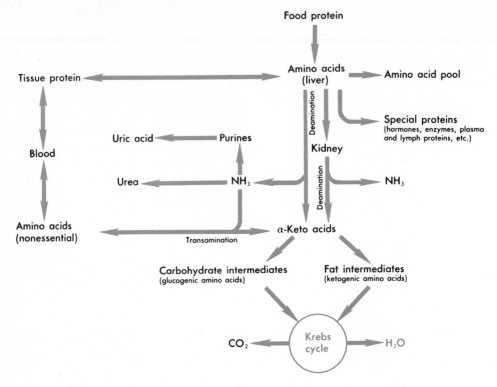

Fig. 4-7. Metabolic interrelationships between protein, carbohydrate, and fat.

amounts of thyroid hormone all have an anabolic effect.

Growth hormone stimulates body cells to retain protein and to maintain a positive nitrogen balance. It also allows greater protein tissue synthesis during growth periods. *Androgens* (gonadotropins), especially testosterone, stimulate tissue growth during puberty, chiefly in target reproductive organ tissue. *Insulin* is necessary for the protein synthesis effect of growth hormone and acts as an antagonist to the gluconeogenic effect of adrenocortical hormones. In normal amounts *thyroid hormone* works with growth hormone to stimulate protein synthesis.

Adrenal steroids and large amounts of thyroid hormone have a catabolic effect on protein metabolism. *Adrenal steroids* such as the glucocorticoids (cortisone, hydrocortisone) stimulate gluconeogenesis, deamination of amino acids, and conversion of the residue to glucose or glycogen. In this way, they act indirectly as protein catabolic agents.

Large doses of *thyroid hormone* stimulate excessive catabolism of muscle tissue. This effect is opposite to the anabolic action of the amounts normally secreted by the thyroid gland.

The summary of metabolic interrelationships among protein, carbohydrate, and fat given in Fig. 4-7 may be used for review.

PROTEIN REQUIREMENTS IN HUMAN NUTRITION
Factors that influence determination of protein requirements

Since protein is an essential nutrient, much study has been given to the question of how much protein the body actually requires. General requirements or recommendations for dietary protein intake have been developed on the basis of research pertaining to all age groups. A number of basic concepts influence (and confuse) one's understanding of the requirements of the various age groups.

Function of dietary protein. Because the primary purpose of furnishing protein in the diet is to supply amino acids in the quantity and kind necessary for growth and maintenance of tissue, the age and physical status of the individual should be taken into consideration when determining the amount required. Further, these amino acids must be supplied in an appropriate pattern for efficient synthesis of tissue protein and other nitrogen-containing substances. The nutritive value of a dietary protein is a measure of its ability to supply these needs. It can supply these needs, however, only if calorie needs are also met. Because protein's function is life sustaining, a deficiency in this dietary factor has a profound effect on various organs of the human body.

Metabolism of protein and amino acids. Knowing basic metabolic concepts is necessary to understand the body's protein requirement. The dynamic concept of protein compartments with an ebb and flow of nitrogen between tissue protein, dietary protein, and a common amino acid pool plays a role. Knowing the amount of protein reserves in the body is also necessary. Also, the concept of essential and nonessential amino acids aids in determining which specific amino acids the diet must supply. Moreover, the concept of the all or none law in protein synthesis aids in knowing which specific amino acids must be supplied at one time to produce a given tissue.

Nitrogen balance. The measure of net gain and loss of total nitrogen in all parts of the body gives a base for study of protein nutrition, although it gives no indication of internal shifts in distribution of nitrogen. An added difficulty is that this level is adaptive, and after a time the body adapts to a lower or higher level of nitrogen. Nitrogen balance alone is not enough to determine protein requirement.

In reference to nitrogen balance the nutritionist uses the term *biologic value* of a food source. This measure of the nutritive value of a given dietary protein refers to the percent of absorbed nitrogen that is retained by the body. However, some of the studies in this area are faulty. In some short-term observations, insufficient time is allowed for the organism to adapt to the diet change. In others, only a single tissue function is evaluated.

Digestibility factor. The degree to which a given protein is digested and absorbed will also influence the requirement for it. Absorption (digestibility) is affected by preparation and cooking and by the rate and completeness with which enzymes hydrolyze that specific protein.

Other factors affecting requirement. Other factors include the rate at which protein tissue is synthesized in the body at a given time and the nature and caloric value of the diet as a whole. The nature of the diet influences the quantitative protein requirement because of the protein-sparing effect of the carbohydrate and fat contained in the diet. The timing of meals, interestingly enough, plays a role also. Allowing time intervals between ingestion of protein foods apparently lowers the competition for absorption sites and enzymes. Other obvious factors affecting the body's need for protein are fever, disease processes, traumatic injury to tissues, and the postsurgical state.

Measure of protein requirements

A source of confusion in the determination of requirements is the unclear terminology applied to standards. General terms such as "minimum," "average," "adequate," and "optimum" are ambiguous. Does minimum mean the lowest adequate amount on record, the minimum requirement for the majority of the groups studied, or the minimum amount required to support growth? And how does one define optimum? Is it in terms of needed body reserves or of stress? How much is optimum? Actually the desirable size of body reserves has not been established, because it depends on a variety of circumstances.

An attempt to overcome this difficulty in terminology has brought into use the phrase, "recommended allowances." But this phrase also poses some problems. It is based on an excess margin of safety. However, the question of the rational size of such a margin must still be answered. One investigator, Rose,[1] has defined the optimum (safe) level as twice the minimal requirement.

Basic measures. Two basic measures of protein requirement must be considered: *quantity* and *quality*.

Protein quantity would establish the total protein requirement. The United States standard[7] has generally been set for adults at 0.8 g per kg (2.2 lb) of body weight. This amounts to about 56 g daily for a man weighing 70 kg (154 lb), and 44 g daily for a woman weighing 55 kg (120 lb). A total of 75 to 85 g daily is needed during pregnancy and lactation. The requirements for infants and children vary according to growth patterns (see Appendix M).

Since the value of a protein is dependent on its content of essential amino acids, in the final analysis the measure of protein requirement must be based on *quality,* that is, on the essential amino acid content.

Guidelines for protein needs, based on nitrogen balance studies[8-10] determining specific amino acid requirements, have been developed. One widely used guideline is the provisional amino acid pattern outlined by the Food and Agriculture Organization, a division of the World Health Organization (FAO/WHO) under the United Nations. This pattern is constructed according to the formula shown in Table 4-2. The amino acid that is required by the body in the smallest quantity is tryptophan. Tryptophan is therefore assigned the value of 1. Values for the other amino acids express the ratio between the body's tryptophan requirement and its need

for each other amino acid. On the basis of the provisional amino acid pattern, an ideal proportionality pattern of amino acids is constructed, against which the amino acid ratios in different foods may be measured. According to this method of study, egg and milk ranked highest as reference proteins against which to measure other foods (Fig. 4-8). Subsequent FAO/WHO protein standards, although somewhat lower than previous recommendations, continue to ensure a "safe level of intake" for healthy individuals in a population.[11]

A summary of the age group requirements of the essential amino acids, as determined by research balance studies, has been presented by the Food and Nutrition Board and is given in Table 4-3. These values probably represent minimal values for adults.

Protein quality in terms of essential amino acid content is of great practical significance in world health problems. In countries where the diet is limited to a few foods and protein is available in only one main plant food source, the protein intake could be made adequate by introducing other complementary plant proteins to make up the lacking amino acids.

Protein requirements in various vegetarian diets may be met by applying this same principle of combining complementary plant proteins to achieve the necessary balance of essential amino acids. Persons following such food patterns may be using one or more of the following four basic types of vegetarianism.

1. *Lacto-ovovegetarian diets:* All-vegetable diet supplemented with milk, cheese, and eggs. There would be no problem securing adequate protein with this combination.

2. *Lactovegetarian diets:* All-vegetable diet supplemented with only milk and cheese. Milk products add complete protein to this combination and enhance amino acid values.

3. *Pure vegetarian or vegan diets:* All-vegetable diet without any animal foods, dairy

Table 4-2. Food and Agriculture Organization* amino acid proportionality pattern for the adult based on essential amino acid requirements

Amino acid	Requirement (mg)	Proportionality pattern	Pattern simplified in common use†
Tryptophan	250	1.0	1.0
Threonine	500	2.0	2.0
Isoleucine	700	2.8	3.0
Lysine	800	3.2	3.0
Valine	900	3.6	3.0
Total sulfur amino acid	950	3.8	3.0
(methionine minimum)	(325)	(1.3)	
Leucine	1050	4.2	3.4
Total aromatic amino acid	1550	6.2	
(phenylalanine minimum)	(325)	(1.3)	2.0

*Food and Agriculture Organization: Protein requirements, FAO Nutritional Studies, No. 16, Rome, 1957 (adapted).
†Leverton, R. M.: Amino acids. In Stefferud, A., editor: Food, the yearbook of agriculture, 1959, Washington, D.C., 1959, U.S. Department of Agriculture.

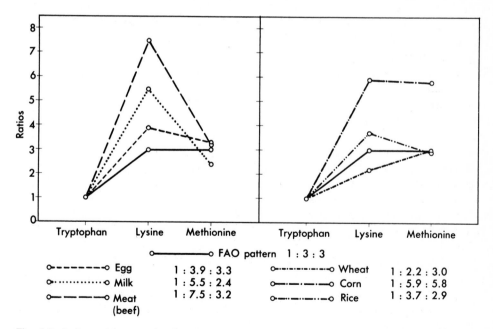

Fig. 4-8. Amino acid proportionality patterns of some animal and plant protein foods. Compare these with the amino acid pattern calculated by the Food and Agriculture Organization (FAO) to provide the daily adult requirements.

Table 4-3. Estimated amino acid requirements of humans*

Amino acid	Requirements (per kg body weight) mg/day			Amino acid pattern for high-quality proteins† (mg/g protein)
	Infant (3-6 mo)	Child (10-12 yr)	Adult	
Histidine (essential only for infants)	33	?	?	17
Tryptophan	19	4	3	11
Methionine (sulfur-containing amino acids including cystine)	45	22	10	26
Threonine	63	28	8	35
Isoleucine	80	28	12	42
Valine	89	25	14	48
Lysine	97	44	12	51
Leucine	128	42	16	70
Phenylalanine (aromatic amino acids including tyrosine)	132	22	16	73

*Food and Nutrition Board, National Research Council: Improvement of protein nutriture, Washington, D.C., 1974, National Academy of Sciences.
†Two grams per kilogram of body weight per day of protein of the quality listed in column four would meet the amino acid needs of the infant.

products, or eggs. More careful planning is required to achieve combinations providing the necessary amounts of the essential amino acids. A deficiency of B_{12} is a problem.

4. *Fruitarian diets:* Diet consisting of raw or dried fruits, nuts, honey, and olive oil. Potential inadequacy is greater here.

By using the reference table of amino acid values (Appendix B) for some representative vegetable protein foods, in comparison with the minimum adult amino acid requirements and the FAO proportionality pattern (Table 4-2), adequate and interesting diets may be planned. For example, some combinations of complementary food proteins may include the following:

Rice + Black-eyed peas (a southern United States dish called "Hopping John")

Whole wheat or bulgur + Soybeans + Sesame seeds (protein may be increased by the addition of yogurt)

Cornmeal + Kidney beans (a combination in many Mexican dishes, protein increased by the addition of cheese)

Soybeans + Peanuts + Brown rice + Bulgur wheat (an excellent sauce dish served over the rice and wheat)

Guidelines for such vegetable protein combinations and interesting recipes for preparing these foods have been developed and tested.[12]

Summary

This discussion of requirements is intended to help the student gain a sounder basis for teaching health to patients. The so-called protein requirements are not as rigid as they may appear when listed in National Research Council tables[4] (see Appendix M). Even the term "requirement" connotes an inflexible mandate, which simply is not the case.

The National Research Council's published standards for protein are intended to serve only as recommendations. They are designed to cover a wide range of need, and to provide a margin of safety to cover stress situations, they are approximately double the minimum allowances. They are not absolute, rigid requirements, but flexible *recommendations*. As such they can serve only as rough guides and should be adapted as needed to the individual patient.

There is a need for further research on proteins and amino acids. Better means of food analysis are needed to make food value tables more accurate and consistent. Further studies with animals are needed, as are studies with human subjects. Further research on protein deficiency diseases and field studies in areas of the world where protein malnutrition is prevalent are also needed.

Several general problems requiring further investigation have been identified by the National Research Council's Committee on Amino Acids:

1. What are the role, desirable level, and means of maintenance of the so-called protein reserves?
2. What is the specific role of protein in the development of resistance to and recovery from various stresses?
3. What is the effect of protein on longevity and the so-called degenerative diseases?
4. What are the possible effects of excessive protein and amino acids?

In applying basic knowledge of protein requirements to the individual patient, the student should always bear in mind that research along these and related lines is constantly modifying diet therapy. To cooperate intelligently with the health team, any health practitioner should maintain an open and inquiring mind toward news of these developments.

GLOSSARY

amination the taking up of an amino group (NH_2) by an amino acid to produce the *amine* form of that acid. This process is one means by which toxic nitrogenous products such as ammonia (NH_3) are removed from the system and made ready for excretion.

amino acid these compounds are the structural units of

protein. Out of a total of 20 or more, 10 are considered *essential*, or indispensable to life. (See *essential amino acid*.) The term "amino" represents the presence of the NH_2 group—a *base*. The unique chemical feature of the amino acids is that they contain *both* a base (NH_2, the amino group) and an acid (COOH, carboxyl group). Therefore they are capable of both acid and base reactions (amphoteric chemical nature). The various food proteins, when digested, yield their specific constituent amino acids. These amino acids are then available for use by the cells as the cells synthesize specific tissue proteins.

amphoteric (Gr. *amphoteros*, both) having properties of both an acid and a base and therefore able to function as either. Amino acids have this dual chemical nature because of their structure—they contain both an acid (carboxyl, COOH) and a base (amino, NH_2) group.

anabolism (Gr. *anabolē*, a building up) constructive metabolic processes that build up the body substances; the synthesis in living organisms of more complex substances from simpler ones. Anabolism *uses* energy; available energy generated by catabolic processes is taken up in forming the chemical bonds that unite the components of the increasingly complex molecules as they are developed in the anabolic processes. Anabolism is the opposite of catabolism.

catabolism (Gr. *katabolē*, a throwing down) the destructive phase of metabolism, the opposite of anabolism. Catabolism includes all the processes in which complex substances are progressively broken down into simpler ones. Catabolism usually involves the release of energy. Together, anabolism and catabolism constitute metabolism, which is the coordinated operation of anabolic and catabolic processes into a dynamic balance of energy and substance.

chymotrypsin a protein-splitting (proteolytic) enzyme produced by the pancreas that acts in the intestine. Together with trypsin, it reduces proteins to shorter chain polypeptides and dipeptides.

complete protein a protein that contains the essential amino acids in quantities sufficient for maintenance of the body and for a normal rate of growth. Such proteins are said to have a high biologic value. Egg, milk, cheese, and meat are complete protein foods.

deamination an initial step in the metabolic breakdown (catabolism) of amino acids in which the amino group (NH_2) is split off. Deamination takes place chiefly in the liver. The nitrogenous group thus formed (NH_3, ammonia) may be (1) converted to urea and excreted, (2) used in production of nitrogen-containing compounds such as purines, or (3) combined with carbohydrate derivatives or amino acid residues to form the amine form of that acid.

deoxyribonucleic acid (DNA) a complex, double-chain

protein of high molecular weight, which is the nucleic acid found in the chromosomes of the cell nucleus. It is believed to be the chemical basis of heredity and the carrier of genetic information for specific protein synthesis. DNA is composed of four nitrogenous bases (two purines, adenine and guanine; and two pyrimidines, thymine and cytosine), a sugar (deoxyribose), and phosphoric acid. A similar single-chain nucleic acid, ribonucleic acid (RNA, in which the sugar is ribose), also functions with DNA in protein synthesis in the cell.

essential amino acid an amino acid that is indispensable to life and growth and that the body cannot manufacture; it must be supplied in the diet. Eight amino acids are essential: threonine, leucine, isoleucine, valine, lysine, methionine, phenylalanine, and tryptophan.

homeostasis (Gr. *homio,* similar; *stasis,* a standing) a state of equilibrium of the body's internal environment.

keto-acid the amino acid residue after deamination. The glycogenic keto-acids are used to form carbohydrates. The ketogenic keto-acids are used to form fats.

nitrogen balance the difference between intake and output of nitrogen in the body. If intake is greater, a positive nitrogen balance exists. If output is greater, a negative nitrogen balance exists. For example, during growth when new tissue protein is being formed, nitrogen is retained for protein synthesis, and a state of positive nitrogen balance prevails.

nucleoprotein a conjugated protein found in cell nuclei that is formed from the combination of a protein with nucleic acid. Nucleoproteins are essential for cell division and reproduction. A common example of nucleoproteins is purines. Purines are found principally in meats, especially organ meats such as liver and heart.

pepsin the main gastric enzyme specific for proteins. Pepsin begins breaking large protein molecules into shorter chain polypeptides, proteoses, and peptones. Gastric hydrochloric acid is necessary to activate pepsin.

peptide linkage the characteristic joining of amino acids to form proteins. Such a chain of amino acids is termed a "peptide." Depending on its size, it may be a dipeptide fragment of protein digestion or a large polypeptide.

transamination the transfer of the amino group (NH_2) from an amino acid to a carbon residue to form another amino acid. The newly formed compound is classed a nonessential amino acid, since the body can synthesize it and is not dependent on the diet to supply it.

trypsin a protein splitting (proteolytic) enzyme secreted by the pancreas, that acts in the small intestine to reduce proteins to shorter chain polypeptides and dipeptides.

zwitterion (Ger. *Zwitter,* hybrid; Gr. *ion,* wandering) the term given to amino acids to describe the capacity, when ionized in a solution, to behave as either an acid or a base depending on the need of the solution in which they are present. This dual nature makes amino acids good buffer substances.

REFERENCES
Specific

1. Hegsted, D. M.: Protein needs and possible modifications of the American diet, J. Am. Diet. Assoc. **68:** 317, 1976.
2. Rose, W. C., et al.: The amino acid requirements of man, J. Biol. Chem. **217:**987, 1955.
3. Christensen, H. N., and Oxender, D. L.: Transport of amino acids into and across cells, Am. J. Clin. Nutr. **8:**131, 1960.
4. Sleisenger, M. H., and Kim, Y. S.: Protein digestion and absorption, N. Engl. J. Med. **300:**659, 1979.
5. Matthews, D. M., and Adibi, S. A.: Peptide absorption, Gastroenterology **71:**151, 1976.
6. Harper, H. A.: Review of physiological chemistry, ed. 11, Los Altos, Calif., 1967, Lange Medical Publications, p. 258.
7. Food and Nutrition Board: Recommended dietary allowances, 1979, ed. 9, Washington, D.C., 1980, National Academy of Sciences, National Research Council.
8. Calloway, D. H., and Margen, S.: Variation in endogenous nitrogen excretion and dietary nitrogen utilization as determinants of human protein requirements, J. Nutr. **101:**205-216, 1971.
9. Calloway, D. H., and Spector, H.: Nitrogen balance as related to caloric and protein intake in active young men, Am. J. Clin. Nutr. **2:**405-411, 1954.
10. Calloway, D. H., Odell, A., and Margen, S.: Sweat and miscellaneous nitrogen losses in human balance studies, J. Nutr. **101:**775-786, 1971.
11. FAO/WHO of the United Nations: Energy and protein requirements, WHO Tech. Rep. Ser. No. 522; FAO Nutr. Meet. Rep. Ser. No. 52, Geneva, 1973, The Organization.
12. Lappé, F. M.: Diet for a small planet, New York, 1971, Ballantine Books, Inc.

General

Adibi, S. A.: Intestinal phase of protein assimilation in man, Am. J. Clin. Nutr. **29:**205, 1976.

Broquist, H. P.: Amino acid metabolism, Nutr. Rev. **34:** 289, 1977.

Brown, H.: Protein nutrition, Springfield, Ill., 1974, Charles C Thomas, Publisher.

Chapra, J. G., Forbes, A. L., and Habicht, J. P.: Protein in the U.S. diet, J. Am. Diet. Assoc. **72:**253, 1978.

Food and Nutrition Board, National Research Council: Improvement of protein nutriture, Washington, D.C., 1974, National Academy of Sciences.

Food and Nutrition Board, National Research Council: Recommended dietary allowances, ed. 9, Washington, D.C., 1980, National Academy of Sciences.

Guyton, A. C.: Textbook of medical physiology, ed. 5, Philadelphia, 1976, W. B. Saunders Co.

Harper, H. A.: Review of physiological chemistry, ed. 15, Los Altos, Calif., 1975, Lange Medical Publications.

Harpstead, D. D.: High lysine corn, Sci. Am. **225:**34, Aug., 1971.

Hegsted, D. M.: Protein needs and possible modifications of the American diet, J. Am. Diet. Assoc. **68:**317, 1976.

Irwin, M. I., and Hegsted, D. M.: A conspectus of research on protein requirements of man, J. Nutr. **101:**385, 1971.

Latner, A. L.: Cantarow and Trumper clinical biochemistry, ed. 7, Philadelphia, 1975, W. B. Saunders Co.

Orr, M. L., and Watt, B. K.: Amino acid content of foods, home economics research report, no. 4, Washington, D.C., 1957, U.S. Department of Agriculture.

Payne, P. R.: Safe protein-calorie ratios in diets: the relative importance of protein and energy intake as causal factors in malnutrition, Am. J. Clin. Nutr. **28:**281, 1975.

Porter, J. W., and Rolls, B. A., editors: Proteins in human nutrition, New York, 1973, Academic Press, Inc.

VEGETARIANISM

Erhard, D.: Nutrition education for the ''now'' generation, J. Nutr. Educ. **2**(4):135, 1971.

Erhard, D.: The new vegetarians, Nutr. Today **8:**4, Nov.-Dec., 1973.

Dwyer, J. T., Kandel, R. F., Mayer, L., and Mayer, J.: The ''new'' vegetarians, J. Am. Diet. Assoc. **64:**376-382, 1974.

Dwyer, J. T., Mayer, L., Dowd, K., Kandel, R. F., and Mayer, J.: The ''new'' vegetarians: the natural high? J. Am. Diet. Assoc. **65:**529-536, 1974.

Hardinge, M. G., and Crooks, H.: Non-flesh dietaries. I. Historical background, J. Am. Diet. Assoc. **43**(6):545, 1963.

Hardinge, M. G., and Crooks, H.: Non-flesh dietaries. II. Scientific literature, J. Am. Diet. Assoc. **43**(6):550, 1963.

Hardinge, M. G., and Crooks, H.: Non-flesh dietaries. III. Adequate and inadequate, J. Am. Diet. Assoc. **45**(6):537, 1964.

Hardinge, M. G., Crooks, H., and Stare, F. J.: Nutritional studies of vegetarians. IV. Dietary fatty acids and serum cholesterol levels, J. Clin. Nutr. **10**(6):516, 1962.

Hardinge, M. G., Crooks, H., and Stare, F. J.: Nutritional studies of vegetarians. V. Proteins and essential amino acids, J. Am. Diet. Assoc. **48**(1):25, 1966.

Register, V. D., and Sonnenberg, L. M.: The vegetarian diet, J. Am. Diet. Assoc. **62:**253-261, 1973.

5 Energy metabolism

Energy is the basis of ongoing life. It is the power of an organism to do its work. Fundamental laws of physical existence ultimately revolve around the production of energy. The study of nutrition is concerned with the basic question of how the human body transforms the elements in its food into energy.

Several important interrelated concepts are involved in the study of energy metabolism. These deal with such basic questions as the following:

1. What are energy and metabolism?
2. How is energy measured?
3. How does the human body get its energy?
4. How is energy controlled in human metabolism?
5. How are basal and total energy needs determined?

DEFINITIONS OF ENERGY AND METABOLISM

The word *energy* comes from two Greek roots, *en* meaning "in" and *ergon* meaning "work." The Greeks put the two roots together to form *energon,* meaning "active." Hence energy is that force or power that enables the body to carry on life-sustaining activities. Death is the cessation of this activity. The word *metabolism* also comes from two roots, *meta* meaning "beyond" and *ballein* meaning "to throw." The greeks put these two roots together to form the noun *metabolē,* meaning "change." Metabolism is the total of all those chemical processes in the body by which substances initially in food are "thrown beyond themselves" to be changed into other substances. This very phrase gives the feel of the power involved in the processes that nurture and sustain life. *Energy metabolism* deals with the very real and dynamic concept underlying all life—*change.* It is these constant, multiple changes in the forms of physiologic constituents that produce energy.

MEASUREMENT OF ENERGY (CALORIES)

Since the body can perform work only as energy is released, and since all work takes the form of heat production, energy may be measured in terms of heat equivalents. Such a heat measure is the *calorie.* In nutritional and physiologic studies the unit of measure is the large calorie or kilocalorie, which is equal to 1,000 small calories. A kilocalorie is the amount of heat required to raise 1 kg of water 1° C. (The term "calorie" is used for the large calorie or kilocalorie in this text.)

The caloric values of various foods have been determined by the use of a metal instrument, which is called a bomb calorimeter because its shape resembles that of a bomb. A weighed amount of a food is placed into the core of the calorimeter, and the instrument is immersed in water. The food is then ignited by an electric spark in the presence of oxygen and burned. The increase in temperature of the surrounding water indicates the number of calories given off by the oxidation of the food.

The average caloric value of each of the three major nutrients is known as its respective *fuel factor*. One gram of carbohydrate yields 4 calories, 1 g of fat yields 9 calories, and 1 g of protein yields 4 calories.

In the metric system of measure the unit of energy is the *joule*. It was formally added to the Système International d'Unités (SI) in 1960 and adopted by the National Bureau of Standards in the United States in 1964. Nine tenths of the world is already on the metric system or is in the process of conversion. The joule was named for James Prescott Joule (1818-1889), an English physicist who discovered the first law of thermodynamics and invented an electro-magnetic engine. The letter J is used as the mathematical notation representing the 4.184×10^7 ergs needed to raise 1 g of water 1° C. Thus the conversion factor for changing kilocalories (kcal) to kilojoules (kJ) is 4.184: 1 kcal equals 4.184 kJ. For example, 55 calories would equal 230 J. The fuel factors expressed in joules would be carbohydrates, 17 J/g; protein, 17 J/g; fat, 38 J/g. Since the conversion product of diets in kilojoules is usually over 1,000, the notation MJ (megajoule: 1,000 kJ) is commonly used (see Table 5-2).

ENERGY IN THE HUMAN BODY

Energy cycle. It is clear that energy is not created. It exists in many forms and is constantly being transformed. In the human body, energy is available in four basic forms for life processes: *chemical, electrical, mechanical,* and *thermal*. It is constantly being cycled through these forms. In this perpetual cycle of energy the ultimate source of power is the sun with its vast reservoir of nuclear reactions. Through the process of photosynthesis, with water and carbon dioxide as raw materials, plants transform the sun's energy into food storage forms. In the body these food sources are converted to the basic energy unit of glucose, which is burned to

release energy. Water and carbon dioxide are the end products of this process of oxidation.

Transformation of energy—free and potential (Fig. 5-1). Metabolism is the process of converting chemical energy to other forms of energy for the body's work. This chemical energy is changed to *electrical energy* as in brain and nerve activity, *mechanical energy* as in muscle contraction, *thermal energy* as in regulation of body temperature, and to other types of *chemical energy* as in the synthesis of new compounds. In all these work activities of the body, heat is given off.

In human metabolism, as in any energy system, energy is always present as either *free* or *potential*. Free energy is the energy involved at any given moment in the performance of a task. It is unbound and in motion. Potential energy is the energy that is stored or bound in various chemical compounds and is available for conversion to free energy as needed. Energy stored in the sugar molecule is potential energy. When it is burned, free energy is released and work results. As work is done, energy in the form of heat is given off.

Whether the energy system is electrical, mechanical, thermal, or chemical, in the course of the many reactions that comprise its operation, free energy is decreased and the reservoir of potential energy is secondarily diminished. Therefore the system must be constantly refueled from some outside source. In the human energy system this source is food.

CONTROL OF ENERGY IN HUMAN METABOLISM

Controlled energy system—chemical bonding. The energy in any system may be uncontrolled and destructive as in an atomic bomb used for warfare, or it may be controlled and constructive as in an atomic reactor used for research and industry. In the human body also, the energy produced in its many chemical reactions, if "exploded" all at once, could be destructive. The mechanism by which energy

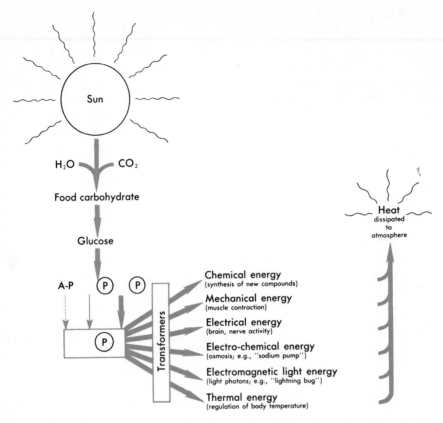

Fig. 5-1. Transformation of energy from its primary source (the sun) to various forms for biologic work by means of metabolic processes ("transformers").

is controlled in the human system is *chemical bonding*. The chemical bonds that hold the elements of the compounds together consist of energy. As long as that compound remains constant, energy is being exerted to maintain the atomic constellation that is characteristic for that molecule. It is in this sense that potential energy is stored in the compound. When the compound is broken into its parts, energy is released, and it becomes free energy. It is a characteristic of free energy that it immediately involves itself in the bonding of other atoms, which results either in a rearrangement of the atoms within the same compound or in new compounds.

The three types of chemical bonds by which energy is transferred in the body are *covalent bonds*, *hydrogen bonds*, and *phosphate bonds*.

COVALENT BOND. Valence refers to the chemical combining power of an element. A common example of covalent bonds are those shared between neighbor carbon atoms in the core of an organic compound:

$$-C-C-C-$$

HYDROGEN BOND. Hydrogen bonds are weaker bonds that attach hydrogen to various compounds. They are less rich in energy than covalent bonds. The very fact they can be broken easily gives them physiologic importance. They can alter molecular shapes as in protein molecules, and they can be transferred or passed readily from one substance to another.

HIGH-ENERGY PHOSPHATE BOND. Phosphate (PO_4) bonds (the bonds that attach the phosphate radical to a compound) play an important role in energy metabolism. Since the phosphate radical is highly labile, more energy is required to bind it than to bind carbon or most other radicals, and more free energy is released when the phosphate bond is broken. Many phosphate bonds are referred to as high-energy bonds. The sign $\sim$ is used to indicate them. An example of such a high-energy compound is adenosine triphosphate, commonly called ATP: $A - PO_4 \sim PO_4 \sim PO_4$.

Harper[1] has called ATP the "currency of the cell," which may be "cashed in" by the body for energy as needed to perform its work. Like storage batteries, these PO_4 bonds become the controlling force of any further energy needs.

Although more energy is required to bind the phosphate radical to any compound than is required to bind, for example, a carbon radical, there are some compounds in which the amount of energy required to bind the phosphate radical is relatively low. In such compounds the phosphate bond is called a low-energy phosphate bond.

Examples of low-energy phosphate bonds include those formed by the phosphorylation of glucose (glucose-6-phosphate, glucose-1-phosphate), which activates glucose for participation in cell metabolism. Later in the total process of oxidating glucose, high-energy phosphate bonds are formed.

Controlled reaction rates—enzymes, coenzymes, and hormones. The many chemical reactions that make up the finely developed energy systems in cell metabolism must also have controls. Some of the chemical reactions that break down proteins, for example, if left to themselves (as in sterile decomposition), would span several years. Such reactions must be accelerated, or else it might take years to get the needed energy from a meal. At the same time, they must be regulated so that too fast a reaction will not produce energy in a single explosion. Enzymes and coenzymes control biologic oxidation of the cells. The enzymes and coenzymes control numerous other biologic processes as well. The hormones also play a regulatory role in cell oxidation.

ENZYMES. David Green,[2] a noted enzymologist, once called enzymes "chemical keys of breath-taking eloquence." They are indeed just that! Life simply cannot go on without them.

The word enzyme comes from a Greek word meaning "in yeast." It was originally used because the first observations were of something in yeast that caused the fermentation of glucose to produce alcohol. All enzymes that have been isolated thus far are protein substances. They are produced in the cells, apparently under the control of specific genes. One specific gene is believed to control the making of one specific enzyme, and there are thousands of enzymes in each cell.

The substance on which a particular enzyme works is called its *substrate*. Enzymes possess a remarkable and highly significant degree of specificity for their special substrates; that is, a particular enzyme usually will act only on its own particular substrate. Like the interlocking pieces of a jigsaw puzzle, the specific shapes of enzyme and substrate must fit together perfectly, or the reaction will not take place. In this vital lock and key mode of action the enzyme and substrate first combine in a complex, then break apart and produce the new reaction products and the original unchanged enzyme.

Enzyme + Substrate → Enzyme-substrate complex

Activated enzyme-substrate complex →
Reaction products + Enzyme

While the substrate is locked in place with the enzyme, the enzyme places specific stress on it to break certain bonds and rearrange certain molecules. When unlocking occurs, dif-

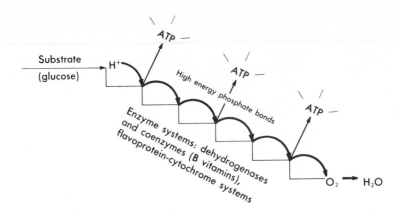

Fig. 5-2. The bouncing hydrogen ion—biologic oxidation in the cell to produce energy. Energy in the form of ATP (high-energy phosphate bonds) is produced through transfer of H^+ and electrons by means of enzyme systems (dehydrogenases and coenzymes, the B vitamins, and the flavoprotein-cytochrome systems). These enzyme chains are coupled with the glycolytic pathway and the Krebs cycle.

ferent reaction products are released, and the enzyme breaks away unchanged, ready to perform its remarkable feat over and over again. (Compare this action with that shown in Fig. 5-3.)

COENZYMES. The completion of reactions such as those involved in cellular oxidation to yield energy requires coenzymes. In respiratory chains for oxidation in the cells, oxygen was originally thought to enter into the process and to take part in the reactions. It is now known that energy is generated by a system of hydrogen ion transfer from product to product, with formation of high-energy phosphate compounds (ATP) along the way. The coenzymes act as a series of acceptors of the bouncing hydrogen ion until the hydrogen finally combines with oxygen to form water (Fig. 5-2).

Three such systems play a part in this hydrogen ion transfer to yield energy:

1. The *dehydrogenases*, with niacin as part of the coenzyme (Nicotinamide-adenine dinucleotide → Reduced nicotinamide-adenine dinucleotide [NAD → NADH]; Nicotinamide-adenine dinucleotide phosphate → Reduced nicotinamide-adenine dinucleotide phosphate [NADP → NADPH])

2. The *flavoprotein system*, containing riboflavin coenzymes

3. The *cytochrome system* (a "cousin" of hemoglobin), containing iron

An example of a dehydrogenase of clinical significance is *lactic dehydrogenase* (LDH), which catalyzes the change of lactic acid to pyruvic acid in muscle. When heart muscle is damaged, as in a myocardial infarction, the enzyme is released from the cells and accumulates in the blood. Hence a rise in the blood level of this enzyme is used as a diagnostic measure.

It may be helpful to think of the coenzyme as another substrate, for in receiving the material transferred the coenzyme is changed or reduced (Fig. 5-3).

Enzyme + Coenzyme + Substrate →
  Enzyme-coenzyme-substrate complex

Activated enzyme-coenzyme-substrate complex →
Reaction products + Reduced coenzyme + Enzyme

HORMONES. The word hormone comes from the Greek word *hormaein* meaning "set in mo-

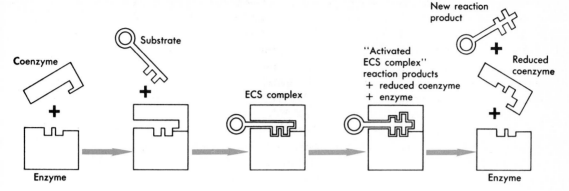

Fig. 5-3. Lock and key concept of the action of enzyme, coenzyme, and substrate to produce new reaction products.

tion'' or ''to spur on.'' Hormones are secretions of the endocrine glands, and they perform many regulatory functions in the body. In energy metabolism they act as chemical messengers to trigger or control enzyme action. For example, the rate of oxidative reactions in the tissues (the body's metabolic rate) is controlled by thyroxine from the thyroid gland, which in turn is controlled by the thyrotropic hormone from the anterior pituitary gland. Another familiar example is the controlling action of insulin from the pancreas on the rate of glucose utilization in the tissues. Steroid hormones also have the capacity to regulate the cell's ability to synthesize enzymes.

Types of metabolic reaction. The two types of reaction constantly going on in energy are anabolism and catabolism. Each requires energy; therefore each causes a decrease in free energy.

Anabolism is the synthesis of a more complex substance. Energy is required to generate this synthesis. The more complex the substance, the greater is its potential or bound energy.

Catabolism is the breakdown to simpler substances. This process releases free energy, but it also uses up some free energy for the breakdown. Therefore there is a constant energy deficit that must be supplied by food. When

food is not available, as in periods of fasting or starvation, the body draws for energy on its own stores:

1. Only a 12- to 48-hour reserve of glycogen exists in liver and muscle; this amount is quickly depleted.
2. Storage of energy (as protein) exists in limited amounts in the muscle mass, but in greater volume than glycogen stores.
3. The capacity for storage in the adipose tissue is virtually unlimited. This stored fat provides needed energy, but the supply varies from person to person and from circumstance to circumstance.

ENERGY METABOLISM—CALORIE REQUIREMENTS
Basal metabolism

Basal metabolism is a measure of the energy produced in the maintenance of the body at rest after a 12-hour fast. The basal metabolic rate (BMR) is the rate of internal chemical activity of resting tissue.

It is interesting to compare the contribution of various body tissues to the rate of basal metabolism. Certain small but vitally active tissues—brain, liver, gastrointestinal tract, heart, kidney—together make up less than 5% of the total body weight, yet they contribute about 60% of the total basal metabolic processes. Although resting muscle and adipose fat tissue are far larger in the mass, they contribute much less to the body's BMR.

Methods of measuring the BMR. Both direct and indirect methods of calorimetry have been used to measure the BMR. In direct methods a chamber large enough for a person to enter is used and his body's heat production is measured. Obviously such an instrument is large and costly and is therefore limited to research studies.

For clinical purposes the far more simple indirect calorimetry is sufficiently accurate. This method measures the exchange of gases in respiration while the subject is at rest; usually the calories are computed according to an average of the amount of oxygen consumed during two six-minute periods. In indirect calorimetry, metabolic rates are based on the *respiratory quotient* (RQ). This is the ratio between the volume of carbon dioxide given off and the volume of oxygen consumed:

$$\frac{\text{Volume } CO_2 \text{ produced}}{\text{Volume } O_2 \text{ consumed}} = RQ$$

It has been found that energy calculated in this manner is equivalent to the heat given off by the body. The BMR is calculated for a given person in terms of the number of calories given off per hour per square meter of body surface area, with corrections for age, sex, height, and weight. The results are then expressed in percent of variation above or below the normal number of calories per square meter of body surface area for a person of like height, weight, age, and sex. The ranges usually given as normal are -10% to $+10\%$, which includes about 75% of normal people, and -15% to $+15\%$, which includes about 95% of normal people.

When the BMR test is administered, certain conditions are necessary for accuracy.

1. The patient must have been in a fasting state (nothing by mouth, NPO) for the previous 12 hours. This assures that no digestive or absorptive activities are going on.
2. The patient must be in a relaxed state, both mental and physical. There should be a quiet atmosphere with at least a half hour of bed rest preceding the test.
3. The patient should be recumbent during the test.
4. The patient should be fully awake.
5. The room temperature should be 20° to 25° C (68° to 77° F).

Table 5-1. Energy expenditure per hour during different activities for a man weighing 70 kg*

Activity	Calories per hour	Activity	Calories per hour
Sleeping	65	Walking slowly (4.2 kmph, 2.6 mph)	200
Awake, lying still	77	Active exercise	290
Sitting at rest	100	Severe exercise	450
Standing relaxed	105	Swimming	500
Dressing and undressing	118	Running (8.8 kmph, 5.3 mph)	570
Sewing (tailoring)	135	Very severe exercise	600
Typewriting rapidly	140	Walking very fast (8.8 kmph, 5.3 mph)	650
Light exercise	170	Walking upstairs	1,110

*From Guyton, A. C.: Textbook of medical physiology, ed. 3, Philadelphia, 1966, W. B. Saunders Co., p. 980.

Factors that influence BMR. A number of factors influence the BMR and should be considered when interpreting results of tests.

1. Rates tend to be higher during growth periods. Generally the BMR slowly rises during the first five years of life, levels off, rises again just before and during puberty, and then declines into old age.
2. Surface area influence is relatively constant. Smaller persons of each sex tend to have a higher rate of metabolism per unit of surface area than larger persons.
3. Because of relative sex differences in body mass, women usually have a lower BMR than men.
4. The BMR rises during pregnancy be-

cause of increases in muscle mass of the uterus, size of mammary glands, fetal mass and placenta, cardiac work, and respiratory rate. This totals a 20% to 25% increase over the nonpregnant state, or about 300 calories.

5. The BMR also rises during the lactation period, because milk production utilizes energy. This is a large increase (about 60% or 1,000 calories) because breast milk has a value of 30 calories per ounce, and the average daily production is about 30 oz.
6. Fever increases the BMR about 7% for each .38° C (1° F) rise.
7. Although the effect of climate has been

Table 5-2. Daily energy requirements*

	Age (yr)	Weight kg	Weight lb	Height cm	Height in	Calories (kcal)	Joules (MJ)
Infants	0.0-0.5	6	13	60	24	kg × 115	kg × 0.48
	0.5-1.0	9	20	71	28	kg × 105	kg × 0.44
Children	1-3	13	29	90	35	1,300	5.5
	4-6	20	44	112	44	1,700	7.1
	7-10	28	62	132	52	2,400	10.1
Males	11-14	45	99	157	62	2,700	11.3
	15-18	66	145	176	69	2,800	11.8
	19-22	70	154	177	70	2,900	12.2
	23-50	70	154	178	70	2,700	11.3
	51-75	70	154	178	70	2,400	10.1
	76+	70	154	178	70	2,050	8.6
Females	11-14	46	101	157	62	2,200	9.2
	15-18	55	120	163	64	2,100	8.8
	19-22	55	120	163	64	2,100	8.8
	23-50	55	120	163	64	2,000	8.4
	51-75	55	120	163	64	1,800	7.6
	76+	55	120	163	64	1,600	6.7
Pregnant						+300	1.3
Lactating						+500	2.1

*Food and Nutrition Board, National Research Council, National Academy of Sciences: Recommended dietary allowances, ed. 9, Washington, D.C., 1980.

debated, most investigators indicate that the BMR rises in response to lower temperatures as a compensatory mechanism to maintain body temperature.

8. Small BMR differences have been recorded among people of different races. For example, the BMR of some Oriental individuals is lower than the rates of their Caucasian counterparts, and higher rates were noted in some Eskimos.

9. Diseases involving higher cellular activity (cancer, leukemia, polycythemia, certain anemias, cardiac failure, hypertension, dyspnea, emphysema) usually increase the BMR.

10. In starvation and malnutrition the BMR is usually lowered.

11. Thyroxine stimulates the BMR. The principal use of BMR testing in clinical practice is in the diagnosis of thyroid disease.

12. Obesity seems to have little effect on the BMR, although it may lower the rate somewhat.

Other influences on calorie requirements

Muscular work. Exercise is the other large factor that accounts for individual calorie requirements. The effects of various activities on energy metabolism have been measured by the oxygen consumption method (indirect calorimetry). Some representative calorie expenditures are given in Table 5-1.

Mental effort. Mental effort as in studying demands few if any calories. Feelings of fatigue following periods of study, for example, are due not to vast cerebral activity, but to various amounts of muscle tension involved.

Emotional state. Calories are expended during heightened emotional states because metabolic activity rises as muscle tension, restlessness, and agitated movements increase.

Diet. Food intake increases the expenditure of calories for digestion and absorption. Protein especially has a high specific dynamic action.

Total energy requirements

The total daily energy requirement of an individual is the number of calories necessary to replace daily basal metabolic loss plus loss from exercise and other activities.

These general calorie needs for various ages as indicated in the 1980 revisions of recommendations by the National Research Council are listed in Table 5-2.

GLOSSARY

adenosine triphosphate (ATP) a compound of adenosine (a nucleotide containing adenine and ribose) that has three phosphoric acid groups. ATP is a high-energy phosphate compound important in energy exchange for cellular activity. The splitting off of the terminal phosphate bond ($\sim PO_4$) of ATP to produce ADP (adenosine diphosphate) releases bound energy and transfers it to free energy, available for body work. The re-forming of ATP in cell oxidation again stores energy in the high-energy phosphate bonds for use as needed. They may be considered to act as biologic storage batteries that can be charged and discharged according to conditions in the cell.

basal metabolism (Gr. *basis*, base; *metabolē*, change) the amount of energy needed by the body for maintenance of life when the person is at digestive, physical, and emotional rest. The amount of oxygen consumed at rest is used as a measure of the basal energy requirements and is expressed as calories per square meter of body surface per hour. This basal metabolic rate (BMR) is reported as the percent of variation in the person above or below the normal number of calories required for a person of like height, weight, age, and sex.

calorie (L. *calor*, heat) a measure of heat. The *energy* required to do the work of the body is measured as the amount of *heat* produced by the body's work. The energy value of a food is expressed as the number of calories a specified portion of that food will yield when oxidized, either in the body or on being burned. Physicists use several different standard calories in investigative work. The calorie commonly used in metabolic studies and dietetic studies is the large calorie or kilocalorie, which is the amount of heat required to raise 1 kg of water 1° C.

calorimetry (L. *calor*, heat; Gr. *metron*, measure) the measurement of heat loss. An instrument for measuring heat output of the body or the energy value of foods is called a calorimeter.

chemical bonding the mutual attachment of various chemical elements to form chemical compounds. The chemical bonds that hold the elements of a compound together consist of stored potential energy. When the compound is broken up into its parts, free energy is released to do the body's work.

coenzyme (L. *co,* together; Gr. *en,* in; *zyme,* leaven) enzyme-activators required by some enzymes to produce their reactions. Coenzymes are diffusible, heat-stable substances of low molecular weight that combine with inactive proteins called *apoenzymes.* Each such combination of apoenzyme and coenzyme forms an active compound or a complete enzyme called a *holoenzyme.* A number of the B vitamins function as coenzymes in the energy-producing pathways in cell metabolism.

energy (Gr. *en,* in or with; *ergon,* work) the capacity of a system for doing work; available power. Energy is manifest in various forms — motion, position, light, heat, and sound. Energy is interchangeable among these various forms and is constantly being transformed and transferred among them.

enzyme a complex organic substance originating in living cells and capable of producing certain chemical changes in other organic substances by catalytic action. An enzyme is usually named for the substance on which it acts (its substrate) with the addition of the suffix -ase. For example, an enzyme that splits a protein may be called by the general name of proteinase. Enzymes are specific in their action; they will act only on a certain substance and no other. Some enzymes require coenzymes to make them active.

fuel factor the calorie value (energy potential) of food nutrients; that is, the number of calories 1 g of the nutrient yields when oxidized. The fuel factor for carbohydrate is 4; for protein, 4; and for fat, 9. These basic figures are used in computing diets and calorie values of foods.

hormone (Gr. *hormaein,* to spur on or to set in motion) a compound, produced in an endocrine organ (an organ of internal secretion; a ductless gland), secreted by the endocrine organ into the bloodstream, and transported by body fluids to a specific receptor or target organ whose function the hormone controls. Most hormones are complex proteins. They are usually active in minute quantities. In energy metabolism, a hormone does not supply energy, but acts as a chemical messenger, which triggers or controls enzyme action or synthesis.

joule energy unit in the metric system; 1 calorie = 4.184 J.

respiratory chain the series of chemical reactions in the cell's oxidation systems that transfer hydrogen ions or electrons to produce ATP (high-energy phosphate compounds). For example, the *riboflavin-cytochrome systems*

couple with the glucose oxidation pathways and Krebs cycle to produce such forms of energy.

respiratory quotient (RQ) the ratio between the volume of CO_2 produced and the volume of O_2 consumed:

$$\frac{CO_2}{O_2} = RQ$$

This ratio is used in indirect calorimetry as a basis for determining metabolic rates.

substrate the specific organic substance on which a particular enzyme acts.

REFERENCES
Specific

1. Harper, H. A.: Review of physiological chemistry, ed. 13, Los Altos, Calif., 1971, Lange Medical Publications, p. 480.
2. Cooley, D. J.: Enzymes: chemical keys to health and disease, Today's Health **39:**42, 1961.

General

Ames, S. R.: The joule-unit of energy, J. Am. Diet. Assoc. **57:**415, 1970.

Ball, E. G.: Energy metabolism, Reading, Mass., 1973, Addison-Wesley Publishing Co., Inc.

Bradfield, R. B., editor: Assessment of typical daily energy expenditure. Symposium, Am. J. Clin. Nutr. **24:**1109, 1971.

Bray, G. A., and Campfield, L. A.: Metabolic factors in the control of energy stores, Metabolism **24:**99, 1975.

Briggs, G. M., and Calloway, D. H.: Bogert's nutrition and physical fitness, ed. 10, Philadelphia, 1979, W. B. Saunders Co.

Calloway, D. H.: Recommended dietary allowances for protein and energy, J. Am. Diet. Assoc. **64:**157-162, 1974.

Carlson, L. D., and Hsieh, A. C. L.: Control of energy exchange, New York, 1970, Macmillan Publishing, Inc.

Davidson, S., Passmore, R., and Brock, J. F.: Human nutrition and dietetics, Baltimore, 1976, The Williams & Wilkins Co.

FAO/WHO of the United States: Energy and protein requirements, FAO nutrition meeting, Report No. 52; WHO Tech. Report No. 522, Geneva, 1973.

Food and Nutrition Board, National Research Council, National Academy of Sciences: Recommended dietary allowances, ed. 9, Washington, D.C., 1980.

Grande, F., and Keys, A.: Body weight, body composition, and calorie status. In Goodhart, R. S., and Shils, M. E., editors: Modern nutrition in health and disease, ed. 6, Philadelphia, 1980, Lea & Febiger.

Guyton, A. C.: Textbook of medical physiology, ed. 5, Philadelphia, 1976, W. B. Saunders Co.

Harper, A. E.: Remarks on the joule, J. Am. Diet. Assoc. **57:**416, 1970.

Harper, H. A.: Review of physiological chemistry, ed. 15, Los Altos, Calif., 1975, Lange Medical Publications.

Hegsted, D. M.: Energy needs and energy utilization, Nutr. Rev. **32:**33, 1974.

Konishi, F.: Exercise equivalents of foods, Carbondale, Ill., 1973, Southern Illinois University Press.

Konishi, F., and Harrison, S. L.: Body weight gain equivalents of selected foods, J. Am. Diet. Assoc. **70:**365, 1977.

Latner, A. L.: Cantarow and Trumper clinical biochemistry, ed. 7, Philadelphia, 1975, W. B. Saunders Co.

THE JOULE

Ames, S. R.: The joule—unit of energy. J. Am. Diet. Assoc. **57**(5):415, 1970.

Lord Ritchie-Calder: Conversion to the metric system, Sci. Am. **223**(1):17, 1970.

Moore, T.: The calorie versus the joule, J. Am. Diet. Assoc. **59**(4):327, 1971.

White, H. S.: SI—systeme international d'unites, J. Am. Diet. Assoc. **57**(5):418, 1970.

6 Vitamins: fat-soluble vitamins

INTRODUCTION

Probably no other group of nutritional elements has so captured interest and stimulated concern among biochemists, members of the health professions, and the general public as has the vitamin group. Over the past few decades the discoveries of the vitamins have formed a fascinating chapter in nutrition history. Numerous scientists have contributed to this unfolding story. Casimir Funk, a Polish chemist working at the Lister Institute in London in the early 1900s, with little financial means to carry on his experimental work, ordinarily fed his pigeons rice polishings that he swept up from the floor of a granary. That source of food supply was eventually closed to him, and he began to purchase rice that was whole-grain but polished. The pigeons soon developed a paralytic disease. Funk wondered whether the change of diet was related to the onset of the paralysis, and again fed the birds the waste polishings, and they recovered. Funk then sought some substance in the grain hulls that would account for the different response in the birds. In 1911 he discovered a nitrogen-containing material he thought was an amine. Because it was apparently vital to life, he called it *vitamine* ("vital-amine"). The final "e" was dropped later when other similarly vital substances turned out to be a variety of organic compounds. The name "vitamin" has been retained to designate compounds of this class.

One by one the list of vitamins has grown. Two characteristics mark a compound for assignment to the vitamin (or accessory factor) group: (1) it must be a vital organic dietary substance, which is neither a carbohydrate, fat, mineral, nor protein, but is necessary in very small quantities to the performance of particular metabolic functions or to the prevention of an associated deficiency disease, and (2) it cannot be manufactured by the body and therefore must be supplied in food.

Because of the intricacies of the human body, many such substances probably exist in addition to those already discovered. Those that have been discovered have probably been recognized because they exist in relatively small quantities in foods. Deficiencies are therefore more likely to occur, to be observed, and to be questioned.

The study of vitamins

Vitamins are usually grouped according to solubility. Although this distinction is sometimes an arbitrary one, it is still used for want of a better basis. The fat-soluble group includes vitamins A, D, E, and K. The water-soluble group includes vitamin C and the B-complex vitamins. This chapter will be concerned only with the fat-soluble group. The water-soluble vitamins will be considered in Chapter 7.

To clarify the current concepts concerning each known vitamin, this chapter and Chapter

7 will consider the answers to the following questions:

1. What is the nature of each vitamin?
2. How does the body handle each vitamin, and how is it absorbed into the bloodstream?
3. What is each vitamin's role in body functions?
4. What are the body's requirements for each vitamin?
5. What are the food sources for each vitamin?

VITAMIN A (RETINOL)

Chemical and physical nature of vitamin A

In 1917 E. V. McCollum and his co-workers at Johns Hopkins University in Baltimore demonstrated that an eye disease, xerophthalmia, was caused specifically by a lack of a fat-soluble substance. McCollum called this substance vitamin A.[1,2,3]

Chemically, vitamin A is a primary alcohol of high molecular weight ($C_{20}H_{29}OH$). Because it has a specific function in the retina of the eye, and because it is an alcohol, it has been given the name retinol. However, it is still commonly referred to by its letter name.

Vitamin A is soluble in fat and in ordinary fat solvents. Because it is insoluble in water, it is fairly stable in general cooking. It oxidizes readily, however, upon prolonged exposure to temperatures higher than those ordinarily used in cooking. Antioxidants, such as vitamin E, have been used with vitamin A to preserve it.

In its natural form, vitamin A is found only in animal sources and is usually associated with lipids. As an ester with fatty acids, it is deposited in such tissues as kidney, lung, fat depots, and especially liver. Since so limited an amount of vitamin A existed as such in these animal sources, investigators looked for a precursor in plants that the animals consumed. They believed that the animals must convert such a precursor in their bodies to vitamin A, and this proved to be the case.

Provitamin A (carotene). The ultimate source of all vitamin A is plants. The precursor of vitamin A (provitamin A) is a substance called carotene ($C_{40}H_{56}$), which is found in certain plant pigments. It is called carotene because it was first identified in the yellow pigment of carrots.

During the early study of these substances and their relation to vitamin A, confusion arose from the fact that the carotenes have such a deep, intense color, while pure vitamin A is colorless.

Several forms, α-, β-, and γ-carotene, have been found in deep yellow and green plants. Another form with similar properties, cryptoxanthin, has been found in yellow corn. Of these, β-carotene is the most significant to human nutrition and is the most common precursor of vitamin A. About two thirds of the vitamin A necessary in human nutrition is supplied by β-carotene.

Carotene occurs as crystals in plant cells. Cooking, by weakening the cell wall, helps to release these crystals, thus aiding their absorption in the intestine.

Vitamin A absorption

Substances that aid absorption. Vitamin A enters the body in two forms: as the preformed vitamin from animal sources and as carotene. Bile salts, pancreatic lipase, and fat aid in the absorption of vitamin A and carotene by the body.

BILE SALTS. Since oxygen easily destroys vitamin A, the natural antioxidant bile salts help to stabilize the vitamin. Therefore clinical conditions affecting the biliary system, such as obstruction of the bile ducts, infectious hepatitis, and cirrhosis of the liver, hinder vitamin A absorption. This is caused more by the rapid oxidation of the unprotected vitamin than by any primary defect in the absorptive process itself. Bile also aids in the absorption of vitamin A, as it does of other fat-related substances, since it serves as a vehicle of transport through the intestinal wall.

PANCREATIC LIPASE. The fat-splitting enzyme lipase is necessary for initial saponification or hydrolysis in the upper intestine of fat emulsions or oil solutions of the vitamin. This enzyme is not required for absorption of an aqueous dispersion form of the vitamin. Therefore in conditions where secretion of pancreatic lipase is curtailed, such as in cystic fibrosis, the aqueous dispersion form should be preferred.

FAT. The presence of some fat in the intestine, simultaneously absorbed, is apparently required for effective absorption of the vitamin. This seems to be more true of carotene than of vitamin A.

A warning must be given here about the non-food fat, mineral oil. This oil is not digested by the body, but goes through the gastrointestinal tract intact. If it is present in the intestine along with fat-soluble vitamins, such as vitamin A or carotene, it absorbs them and carries them out also. Therefore mineral oil should never be used with meals; nor should it be taken immediately before or after eating.

Carotene conversion and absorption. In the intestinal wall during absorption some of the carotene is converted to vitamin A. Animals vary greatly in their ability to make this conversion. The efficiency with which it is accomplished in man is not known, but it probably varies in different conditions. Thyroid hormone appears to stimulate this conversion. Some studies seem to indicate that conversion is impaired in uncontrolled severe diabetes and in lipoid nephrosis and that it is also affected by the amount and quality of protein in the diet. Normal whole blood levels of carotene range from 80 to 120 μg/dl. Serum levels are lower, about 40 to 60 μg/dl. When carotene levels exceed 250 μg/dl, as occasionally occurs with a large dietary intake, an interesting condition called xanthosis cutis develops. The skin takes on a deep yellow color that is particularly noticeable in the palms, ear lobes, and soles of the feet. It can be distinguished from jaundice because the sclerae or mucous membranes are not affected. It is harmless and fades in a few days after the quantity of ingested carotene is reduced.

Route of absorption and storage. The route of absorption of vitamin A and carotene is the same as that of fat. They enter the lymphatic system and are carried through the thoracic duct into the portal vein and then to the liver for storage and distribution. The liver is by far the most efficient storage organ. It contains about 90% of the total vitamin A in the body. This amount is sufficient to supply the body's needs for three to twelve months. Liver stores, as well as plasma levels, are reduced, however, during periods of infectious disease such as pneumonia and rheumatic fever. Studies also indicate that impaired storage of vitamin A as retinylesters, decreased hepatic synthesis, and release of retinol-binding protein occurs in liver disease such as cirrhosis leading to the vitamin A deficiency condition of night blindness.[4] At such times supplements of vitamin A may be indicated. Vitamin E may be given with the supplement to help prevent the rapid oxidation of vitamin A.

Influence of disease and age. Other conditions diminishing vitamin A absorption and utilization are intestinal diseases such as celiac disease, sprue, and colitis, which cause changes in the absorptive surface tissue of the mucosa. Age is also a factor in vitamin A absorption. In the newborn infant, especially the premature infant, absorption is poor. With advancing age the elderly person may experience increasing difficulties with absorption also.

Physiologic functions of vitamin A

Vitamin A has important functions in a number of human tissues. Its role in visual adaptation to light and dark has been well established, and studies indicate that it has a number of more generalized functions that influence epithelial tissue, growth, and development of teeth and endocrine function.

Vision. The ability of the eye to adapt to changes in light is dependent on the presence of a light-sensitive pigment, *rhodopsin* (commonly known as visual purple) in the rods of the retina. Rhodopsin is a conjugated protein; that is, it is made up of a protein attached to a nonprotein substance. The protein is *opsin;* the nonprotein part is a vitamin A compound called *retinene*.

When light hits the retina, rhodopsin is split into its two parts, opsin and retinene. In the dark the two components recombine to form visual purple again. Normally there is more than enough vitamin A in the pigment layer behind the rods and cones to ensure constant adjustments to variances in light. When the body is deficient in vitamin A, less retinene is available for formation of visual purple; the rods and cones become increasingly sensitive to light changes, which causes night blindness. This condition can usually be cured in a half hour or so by an injection of vitamin A, which is readily converted into retinene and then into visual purple.

The cones of the retina contain another pigment, visual violet, which influences color vision and the ability to see in bright light. Vitamin A is required as a component of this pigment also, but there is no evidence that vitamin A can cure color blindness.

$$\text{Rhodopsin (visual purple)} \underset{\text{Dark}}{\overset{\text{Light}}{\rightleftharpoons}}$$
(light-sensitive pigment)

$$\text{opsin + retinene} \rightleftharpoons \text{vitamin A}$$
(retinol)

Epithelial tissue. Vitamin A has a vital role in the formation and maintenance of healthy, functioning epithelial tissue, which forms the body's primary barrier to infections. The epithelium includes not only the skin but also the mucous membranes lining the ocular and oral cavities, and the gastrointestinal, respiratory, and genitourinary tracts.

This physiologic function of vitamin A in maintaining the integrity of epithelial tissue provides the basis for current research relating vitamin A to cancers of epithelial origin.[5] Syn-

thetic analogs of vitamin A, retinoids, are being developed as a "chemoprevention" approach in the treatment of common forms of these epithelial cancers. Such retinoids, with toxicity characteristics of vitamin A removed, could be used in larger doses than vitamin A.[6,7]

Without vitamin A the epithelial cells become dry and flat and gradually harden to form scales that slough off. This process is called *keratinization*. Keratin is a protein that forms dry, scalelike tissue such as nails and hair. When the body is deficient in vitamin A, many epithelial tissues may undergo keratinization.

1. In the eye the cornea dries and hardens. This condition, called *xerophthalmia*, may progress to blindness in extreme deficiency of vitamin A. The tear ducts dry, which robs the eye of its cleansing and lubricating means, and infection follows easily.

2. In the respiratory tract ciliated epithelium in the nasal passages dries, and the cilia are lost. A barrier to entry of infection is therefore removed. The salivary glands dry, and the mouth becomes dry and cracked, open to invading organisms.

3. In the gastrointestinal tract the secretory function of mucous membranes is diminished so that tissue sloughs off, which affects digestion and absorption.

4. In the genitourinary tract, as epithelial tissue breaks down, problems such as urinary tract infections, renal calculi, and vaginal infections become more common.

5. As the skill becomes dry and scaly, small pustules or a hardened, pigmented, papular eruption may appear around the hair follicles. This condition resulting from vitamin A deficiency is called *follicular hyperkeratosis* (Fig. 6-1).

Growth. It has been observed for some time that vitamin A deficiency is associated with retarded growth, but the mechanism is unknown. In man, nutritional deficiency usually involves multiple factors that make it difficult to isolate

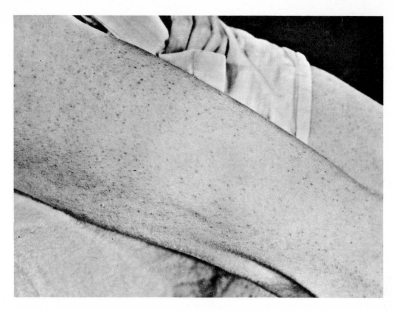

Fig. 6-1. Follicular hyperkeratosis caused by vitamin A deficiency. (From files of Therapeutic Notes, Parke, Davis & Co., Detroit, Mich.; courtesy Dr. Orson D. Bird.)

TO PROBE FURTHER
Clues to the growth puzzle

As is so often the case when there are no pat answers to puzzles in the functioning of the human body, clues may be found that point to possible solutions. Animal experiments in controlled laboratory situations have frequently provided the keys. Such is true concerning vitamin A's relation to growth.

Nitrogen uptake (necessary to protein synthesis) was found to be decreased in vitamin A deficiency in young, growing rats, but not in fully grown ones. This may suggest that vitamin A is required for growth of tissue but not for maintenance.*

In young animals deprived of vitamin A, bone growth slows, especially in the cranium and spine, while nerve tissue continues to grow. The result is ovrcrowding of the skull and spine, and mechanical compression damage to nerve tissue with paralysis and degeneration.

Mucopolysaccharides, the ground substance of collagenous tissue, are especially affected by vitamin A deficiency.

Protein synthesis is adversely affected by vitamin A deficiency.†

*Brown, E. F., and Morgan, A. F.: The effect of vitamin A deficiency upon the metabolism of the rat, J. Nutr. **35:**425, 1948.
†Roels, O. A.: Present knowledge of vitamin A, Nutr. Rev. **24:**129, 1966.

specific nutrient influences. For this reason, most studies of the effect of vitamin A on growth have been made in animals, where environment and variables can be controlled. Apparently vitamin A contributes in some essential way to the growth of skeletal and soft tissues, perhaps through an effect on protein synthesis, mitosis, or stability of cell membranes.

Teeth. Certain epithelial cells surrounding tooth buds in fetal gum tissue become specialized cup-shaped organs *(ameloblasts)* for forming the enamel structure of the developing tooth. Each cell carries out the fascinating task of producing and depositing minute prisms of enamel substance that eventually form the erupted tooth. Inadequate vitamin A produces faulty enamel-forming epithelial cells, which impairs the soundness of the tooth structure.

Endocrines. Studies with radioactive iodine have indicated that vitamin A deficiency reduces the rate of thyroxine formation. Also, goiter has been shown to occur more frequently in persons whose diet is deficient in vitamin A than in the general population.

Vitamin A requirement

The requirement for vitamin A is difficult to establish precisely because of the number of variables that modify the vitamin A needs. The amount stored in the liver, the form in which it is taken (as carotene or vitamin A), the medium in which taken (oil or aqueous disper-

Table 6-1. National Research Council recommended daily allowances for vitamin A

	Age (yr)	Retinol equivalents (µg RE)*	International units (IU)
Males and females	Birth-0.5	420	1,400
	0.5-1	400	2,000
	1-3	400	2,000
	4-6	500	2,500
	7-10	700	3,500
Males	11-14	1,000	5,000
	15-18	1,000	5,000
	19-22	1,000	5,000
	23-50	1,000	5,000
	51+	1,000	5,000
Females	11-14	800	4,000
	15-18	800	4,000
	19-22	800	4,000
	23-50	800	4,000
	51+	800	4,000
Pregnant		1,000	5,000
Lactating		1,200	6,000

*Assumed to be half as retinol and half as β-carotene, except for infants, when calculated from international units:

$$\frac{IU\ retinol}{3.33} + \frac{IU\ \beta\text{-carotene}}{10} = RE$$

sion), illness, and gastrointestinal defect all would have a bearing on the requirement.

National Research Council recommendations. To cover such variables, the recommendations of the National Research Council (NRC) allow a margin of safety above minimal needs (Table 6-1).

RETINOL EQUIVALENTS. Traditionally, vitamin A has been measured in international units (IU). One international unit is equivalent to the biologic activity* of 0.6 μg of pure β-carotene or 0.3 μg of retinol.

However, in 1967 an expert committee of the Food and Agriculture Organization, World Health Organization (FAO/WHO) decided to abandon the expression "vitamin A activity" in foods stated as international units and proposed instead that the biologic activity of vitamin A be stated as the equivalent of weight of retinol (vitamin A_1 alcohol) or "retinol equivalents."[8] Since then this change has been adopted by several countries including Great Britain.

As indicated in Table 6-1, the NRC's Food and Nutrition Board has also adopted the term "retinol equivalents" in its revised recommendations. This is a more accurate term than international units because intestinal absorption and conversion of provitamin A carotenoids are variable factors, and this variance is automatically included in the term "retinol equivalents." Also, because other countries and international agencies have adopted the term "retinol equivalents," a means is provided for clearer information exchange.

Since the proportions of vitamin A activity provided in the diet by preformed vitamin A and by precursor carotenoids may vary considerably, the use of retinol equivalents will provide a more accurate accounting of the total dietary intake. The following definitions and equivalencies agreed on internationally provide a basis for calculating conversions.

---

*The "biologic activity" of a vitamin is measured in rats according to its ability to forestall the development of a disease that is associated with deficiency of that specific vitamin.

DEFINITIONS. International units (IU) and retinol equivalents (RE) are defined as follows:

1 IU = 0.3 μg retinol (0.0003 mg)
1 IU = 0.6 μg β-carotene (0.0006 mg)

1 RE = 6 μg retinol
1 RE = 6 μg β-carotene
1 RE = 12 μg other provitamin A carotenoids
1 RE = 3.33 IU retinol
1 RE = 10 IU β-carotene

CONVERSION FORMULAS. On the basis of weight, β-carotene is one half as active as retinol, and on the basis of structure the other provitamin carotenoids are one fourth as active as retinol. Moreover, retinol is believed to be completely absorbed by the intestine, whereas the provitamin carotenoids are much less well utilized—an average absorption of about one third is assumed for man.[3] Therefore in overall activity, β-carotene is one sixth as active as retinol, and the other carotenoids are one twelfth as active. These differences in utilization provide the basis for the 1:6:12 relationship shown in the equivalencies above and the formulas below for calculating retinol equivalents from values of vitamin A, β-carotene, or other active carotenoids expressed either as international units or micrograms:

1. If retinol and β-carotene are given in micrograms:

$$\text{mg retinol} + \frac{\text{mg } \beta\text{-carotene}}{6} = \text{RE}$$

2. If both are given as international units:

$$\frac{\text{IU retinol}}{3.33} + \frac{\text{IU } \beta\text{-carotene}}{10} = \text{RE}$$

3. If β-carotene and other provitamin A carotenoids are given in micrograms:

$$\frac{\text{mg } \beta\text{-carotene}}{6} + \frac{\text{mg other carotenoids}}{12} = \text{RE}$$

Even though the current recommended allowances are given in retinol equivalents, complete transition to retinol equivalents from international units as a term of measuring vitamin A activity will await the listing of food composition in food value tables in terms of contents of retinol, β-carotene, and other provitamin A carotenoids separately on the basis of weight. In the interim, calculations may be made easily by using the conversion definitions and formulas, and recommended allowances will be given in both retinol equivalents and international units as in Table 6-1.

Hypervitaminosis A. Since the human liver has a great storage capacity for vitamin A and because megadoses of vitamin A have been erroneously administered by some persons, it is clearly possible to take potentially toxic amounts. Vitamins are substances that are required in small amounts. These small amounts are vital, but too much of some vitamins can be dangerous.

Hypervitaminosis A is manifested by joint pain, thickening of long bones, loss of hair, and jaundice. Such a case has been reported in an infant whose mother mistakenly gave vitamin A concentrate (dosage in *drops*) in amounts required for liver oil (dosage in *teaspoons*).[9] Other cases have also been reported.[19] Excess vitamin A may also cause liver injury with resulting portal hypertension and ascites.[11]

Food sources of vitamin A

There are few animal sources of preformed vitamin A. These include liver, kidney, cream, butter, and egg yolk. The major contributors are the yellow and green vegetable and fruit sources of carotene (carrots, sweet potatoes, squash, apricots, spinach, collards, broccoli, and cabbage). A number of commercial products may be fortified with vitamin A. Margarine, for example, is fortified with 15,000 IU of vitamin A per pound.

In summary, vitamin A deficiency may occur for three basic reasons:

1. Inadequate dietary intake
2. Poor absorption (lack of bile or defective absorbing surface)
3. Inadequate conversion of carotene (liver or intestinal disease)

VITAMIN D
Chemical and physical nature of vitamin D

A chemical characteristic of vitamin D, its resistance to oxidation, led to its discovery in 1922 by McCollum's group[1,2,3] at Johns Hopkins University. He eliminated vitamin A from a sample of cod liver oil by oxidation and named the undestroyed factor vitamin D. Vitamin D has since been identified as a group of sterols varying in potency. The crystalline form is white and odorless. All forms are soluble in fat and in organic solvents but not in water. They are heat stable and are not easily oxidized.

The two D vitamins most important in nutrition are D_2 and D_3. D_2 is formed by irradiating the provitamin D_2 (ergosterol) that is found in ergot and in yeast. The irradiated product is known as calciferol or viosterol.

Vitamin D_3 occurs in fish liver oils (and also in human skin). Provitamin D_3 (7-dehydrocholesterol) is converted to the active form by sunlight. However, the amount of vitamin D formed by the action of sunlight on skin is dependent on a number of variables, including length and intensity of exposure and color of skin. For example, heavily pigmented skin can prevent up to 95% of ultraviolet radiation from reaching the deeper layers of skin for adequate synthesis of vitamin D.

Vitamin D is unique among the vitamins in two respects. It occurs naturally in only a few common foods (mainly in fish oils and a little in egg and milk), and it can be formed in the body by exposure of the skin to ultraviolet rays either from the sun or from a lamp. Also, it has hormonelike functions closely interbalanced with the parathyroid hormone in calcium-phosphorus metabolism. Thus many scientists believe that is should be classed as a hormone rather than as a vitamin.[12,13]

Vitamin D absorption

Absorption of vitamin D accompanies that of calcium and phosphorus in the small intestine.

Since vitamin D is fat soluble, this absorption requires the presence of bile salts. Vitamin D, like vitamin A, is absorbed by mineral oil; therefore if mineral oil is taken, it should be ingested separately from food. Moreover, as with vitamin A, diseases such as celiac syndrome, sprue, and colitis hinder its absorption.

Synthesis of vitamin D in the skin. Synthesis in the skin upon exposure to sunlight is unique to vitamin D. Studies[14] have shown that perhaps synthesis occurs *on,* as well as *in,* the skin. After exposure to ultraviolet light, each subject's skin was washed, and the washings were found to have antirachitic properties. The skin washings from a control group not exposed to ultraviolet light had little potency.

After being produced on or in the skin, vitamin D is absorbed through the skin and carried to the liver and other organs for use. A somewhat lesser amount may be stored in the liver, compared with the liver's much larger capacity

for vitamin A storage. However, vitamin D is also stored in the body's fatty tissues, so that the toxicity potential with large intakes is a serious consideration. Vitamin D is excreted from the circulating blood by way of the bile.

Physiologic functions of vitamin D

Vitamin D in the body is predominantly associated with calcium and phosphorus. It influences the absorption of these minerals and their deposit in bone tissue. Here again is demonstrated a vital interdependency among the nutrients in the body's overall functioning.

Absorption of calcium and phosphorus. The primary action of vitamin D is to facilitate the absorption of calcium from the small intestine. This absorption appears to take place by active transport in the proximal segment of the small intestine and throughout the remainder of the intestine by passive diffusion. The absorption of phosphorus is apparently secondary.

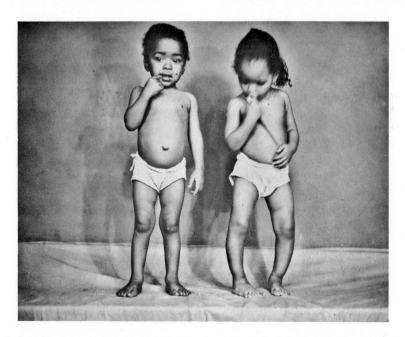

Fig. 6-2. Rachitic children. Note the knock-knees on the child on the left and the bowlegs on the child on the right. (From files of Therapeutic Notes, Parke, Davis & Co., Detroit, Mich.; courtesy Dr. Tom Spies and Dr. Orson D. Bird.)

Within the lumen of the intestine, calcium is bound to phosphorus as calcium phosphate. As calcium is removed from the intestine, uncombined phosphorus remains. Its absorption through the intestinal wall follows that of calcium. Vitamin D probably is responsible for the more rapid absorption of calcium; it makes the cell membranes more permeable to calcium, but not to phosphorus.

Calcification. After the absorption of calcium and phosphorus through the intestinal wall, vitamin D continues to work in partnership with calcium and phosphorus in the calcification aspect of bone formation. Tracer studies with radioactive isotopes have shown that vitamin D directly increases the rate of mineral accretion and resorption in bone, by which the tissue is built and maintained.

Renal phosphate clearance. Vitamin D also has an important effect on the kidney's handling of phosphates. When the body is deficient in vitamin D, as in rickets (a disease of bone formation, Fig. 6-2), the renal threshold for phosphate excretion is lowered thorugh the influence of parathyroid hormone, and the kidney excretes more phosphate than normal. Therapeutic doses of vitamin D raise the renal threshold by causing more tubular reabsorption, which conserves the plasma phosphate level. This renal mechanism gives another interesting example of the body's tenacious effort to adapt to the presence of disease and to maintain the integrity of the blood even at the expense of the tissue. The initial problem in rickets is lack of calcium due to absence of vitamin D. To preserve the vital balance between calcium and phosphorus in the blood, the kidney lowers its threshold point for phosphate and excretes more of it. If this adjustment were not made, the ratio of calcium to phosphorus would not be corrected, and tetany would result.

Citrate metabolism. Vitamin D also seems to play a role in citrate metabolism. Citrate is an important organic acid involved in many metabolic functions, including mobilization of minerals from bone tissue and removal of calcium from the blood. The removal of calcium results in an anticoagulant effect. This anticoagulant effect gives vitamin D a useful role in producing blood plasma and serum for medical use. In animal experiments, doses of vitamin D have produced increases in the citrate levels in many tissues such as bone, blood, kidney, heart, and the small intestine. Moreover, some investigators have even cured human rickets with citrate therapy alone. Orange juice given at the rate of 600 to 700 ml daily also proved effective therapy for rickets.

Knowledge about the physiologic role of vitamin D has been gained mainly through studies of its relation to rickets. More recent studies,[15] however, have indicated that this vitamin functions throughout the body in the movement of various divalent cations (for example, Mg^{++}). This is suggested by the wide dispersion of the vitamin in many systems and tissues.

Vitamin D requirement

Difficulties in establishing requirements for vitamin D arise from the limited number of food sources available and lack of knowledge of precise body needs. Also, the degree to which the body is able to produce vitamin D in response to irradiation is not precisely known. Thus a person's way of living determines the degree of exposure to sunlight and would therefore influence his individual need for additional vitamin D. A city dweller living in a high-rise apartment or in a tenement, and working indoors, needs more than a farmer who works out-of-doors all day. Elderly people or invalids who do not go out-of-doors have need for supplementary vitamin D. Growth demands in childhood, and in pregnancy and lactation, necessitate increased intake.

National research council recommendations. The NRC recommends 10 mg of cholecalciferol (400 IU) daily for children and for women during pregnancy and lactation. The daily recommendation for young adults is 7.5 mg and for older adults 5.0 mg. One international unit of vitamin D is equivalent to the biologic activity of 0.025 μg of pure crystalline vitamin D_3 (cholecalciferol).

Hypervitaminosis D. As with vitamin A, it is possible to ingest excess quantities of vitamin D, and so to produce toxicity. Thus excessive intakes of vitamin D are dangerous and should be avoided. The NRC reports that amounts of vitamin D above 50 μg cholecalciferol 2,000 IU per day (five times the recommended daily allowance) for prolonged periods have produced hypercalcemia in infants and nephrocalcinosis in infants and adults. It is clear that ingestion of vitamin D in excess of the recommended amounts provides no benefit and that large excesses are potentially harmful.[16,17] This is a special danger in infant feeding practices where fortified milk, fortified cereal, plus variable vitamin supplements are used. The infant needs only 10 μg or 400 IU daily, whereas the amount in all of the above items can easily total 100 μg (4,000 IU) or more. As vitamin D is now commonly added to many infant foods, it seems wise to reconsider the need for supplementation with vitamin D preparations.

Symptoms of vitamin D toxicity are calcification of soft tissue such as lungs and kidney, and bone fragility. Renal tissue is particularly prone to calcify; glomerular filtration is affected, and overall function is impaired.

Food sources of vitamin D

Few natural food sources of vitamin D exist. The two basic vitamins D_2 and D_3 occur only in yeast and fish liver oils. The main food sources are those to which crystalline vitamin D has been added or in which vitamin D has been produced by irradiation. Milk, because it is so commonly used, has proved to be the most practical carrier, and it is now a widespread commercial practice to standardize the added vitamin D content at 400 IU per quart. Milk is also a good companion for the vitamin because it provides calcium and phosphorus as well. Butter substitutes are also fortified.

VITAMIN E

Chemical and physical nature of vitamin E

Early vitamin research in animals led to observations that a certain factor was necessary for their reproduction. Between 1922 and 1924 the identification of this factor as an alcohol was reported.[18] Because of its function and chemical nature, it was named *tocopherol* (Gr. *tokos,* childbirth; *phero,* to bring, suffix *-ol,* alcohol). Tocopherol has come to be known as the antisterility vitamin, but it has been demonstrated to have this effect only in the rat and not in man—all specious advertising claims for its contribution to potency, virility, and the like notwithstanding! Pure vitamin E was finally isolated in 1936 from wheat germ oil. Its chemical structure was defined and its synthesis achieved in 1938.

A number of related compounds have since been discovered. In reality, vitamin E is a group of vitamins. Three of these, designated α-, β-, and γ-tocopherol, display the greatest biologic activity. Of these three, α-tocopherol is the most significant.

Vitamin E is a pale yellow oil, stable to acids but not to alkalis, and it is insoluble in water. It is also stable to heat. It oxidizes very slowly, which is one of its most important chemical characteristics.

Vitamin E absorption

Vitamin E is believed to be absorbed like the other fat-soluble vitamins through bile salts and fats. Storage takes place in different body tissues, but especially in adipose tissue.

Maternal transfer of vitamin E to the infant. The amount of vitamin E that crosses the placenta is apparently limited to immediate fetal needs. The amount transferred to the infant through mother's milk is apparently greater. Therefore vitamin E levels in breast-fed infants rise more rapidly than in bottle-fed infants. Vitamin E values in human colostrum range from 0.13 to 3.6 mg/100 ml, and in human milk from 0.10 to 0.48 mg/100 ml, with a mean of 0.24 mg/100 ml. This is about twice the value found in an infant feeding formula made of evaporated cow's milk diluted with an equal quantity of water, which can be compared to values found in other infant formulas.[19]

Physiologic functions of vitamin E in animals

The functions of vitamin E that have been determined up to this time are mainly those that have been demonstrated in laboratory animals and in animals important to commerce and industry. Even its role in animals gives it an important, although indirect, value to man. Such animals are of tremendous worth in research and in everyday life to supply food, clothing, and other human needs. A summary of these findings in animals may give some clues to the possible role of vitamin E in human nutrition.

Reproduction. Classic studies have established the role of vitamin E in the reproductive function of the rat (an animal widely used in nutrition research, from which some of the most important discoveries have come). In the female rat a deficiency of vitamin E causes poor placental implantation with consequent fetal resorption. In the male rat a deficiency of vitamin E causes testicular degeneration, with atrophy of spermatogenic tissue and consequent permanent sterility.

Muscle integrity. Vitamin E seems to be necessary for both the structure and function of smooth muscle, skeletal muscle, cardiac muscle, and vascular tissue. There is evidence that in a large number of animal species vitamin E deficiency causes muscular dystrophy. Affected muscles display various stages and forms of degeneration such as pallor, fragmentation of fibers, edema, nuclear breakdown, necrosis, calcification, fibrosis, and pigmentation. In some animals, cardiac muscle fibrosis leads to failure and death. Accelerated respiration with increased oxygen uptake is observed.

Liver integrity. Of interest are studies relating vitamin E to integrity of liver tissue. Massive liver necrosis in rats was made worse by vitamin E deficiency and improved by vitamin E treatment. The condition had been induced by a low-protein diet that was especially low in cystine, an amino acid that contains sulfur. If the diet was supplemented with cystine, vitamin E, and a compound called "factor 3" (a selenium compound), liver necrosis was prevented; if it had already occurred, it was reversed.[20]

Red blood cell integrity. Vitamin E is an effective antioxidant. Tests with strong oxidating agents such as hydrogen peroxide have indicated that the presence of vitamin E protects red blood cells against hemolysis. Vitamin E may preserve the integrity of the erythrocyte by inhibiting the action of the oxidase in hemoglobin on the unsaturated fatty acids of the cell membrane and may protect cellular unsaturated lipids from oxidative breakdown.

Coenzyme factor in tissue respiration. There is some evidence that vitamin E may function as a cofactor in various enzyme systems involved in cell respiration or in biosynthesis of cellular substances such as DNA. It is suggested that vitamin E may serve as an electron transfer agent in the cell's energy metabolism system (see p. 76).

Role of vitamin E in human nutrition

The preceding studies have been summarized to show how much must be learned about vitamin E in relation to its possible clinical applications. These studies suggest exciting directions for future research. Do these findings relate to human nutrition, and if so, in what ways? Although the specific role of vitamin E in human metabolism has not been clearly established, there are several possibilities.

Antioxidant agent. Already the antioxidant property of vitamin E is being made use of in commercial products to retard spoilage. Vitamin E is also added to therapeutic forms of vitamin A to protect the vitamin A from oxidizing before it is absorbed.

Anemias. The evidence concerning the role of vitamin E in erythrocyte protection has excited inquiry into possible relationships between this vitamin and blood dyscrasia. Several investigators have reported that plasma vitamin E levels are low in newborn infants and that erythrocytes tested in dilute hydrogen peroxide showed increased hemolysis. Malnourished infants with macrocytic anemia have responded to vitamin E therapy with a favorable hematologic response.[21] Also, infants fed formulas rich in polyunsaturated fatty acids and fortified with iron (an oxidant) appear to have an increased vitamin E requirement.[22]

Malabsorption and muscle defects. Cystic fibrosis of the pancreas causes steatorrhea. Patients with this disease have demonstrated low plasma vitamin E levels and increased erythrocyte hemolysis in the peroxide test. Muscle lesions similar to those seen in animal studies have been found postmortem in patients with cystic fibrosis.[23] Low plasma vitamin E levels and skeletal muscle lesions have also been reported in patients with kwashiorkor.

Relation to unsaturated fatty acid metabolism. Vitamin E may prove to have a definite correlation with protection of unsaturated fatty acids, especially linoleic acid, in the body. Studies seem to indicate that the vitamin E requirement can be directly correlated with the amount of polyunsaturated fatty acids in the diet.[24,25]

Polyunsaturated lipids, together with proteins and carbohydrates, constitute the principal structural components of living cells. Hence these lipids supply the material from which most of the membranous structures of the cells

are built. Polyunsaturated lipids are particularly useful in forming the endoplasmic reticulum in the cell, those rod-shaped structures that float about in the cell, and the mitochondria, which are the principal energy-producing sites in the cell. Therefore these lipids are needed in relatively large amounts for cell structure. Polyunsaturated lipids make up about 17% of the total fats in the American diet.

The aging process seems related to the role of lipids in cellular structure. The aging of our bodies is apparently influenced by the constant radiation bombardment we sustain from the atmosphere surrounding our planet. This radiation which occurs throughout life, causes gradual deterioration in the cell be penetrating the entire body and entering every cell, striking the polyunsaturated lipids present as a major structural component. If enough vitamin E is not present, the destructive process will proceed more rapidly, as these energetic rays strike the lipid molecules and cause complete oxidation. This lipid peroxidation (complete oxidation) is believed to be the mainspring of the aging process.[26,27]

Vitamin E requirement

Although the exact biochemical mechanism by which vitamin E functions in the body is still unknown, it is clearly an essential nutrient. Requirements vary with the amount of polyunsaturated fatty acids in the diet. In the revised dietary allowances published by the NRC in 1980, adult vitamin E needs are given in α-tocopherol equivalents (αTE) as 10 mg αTE for men and 8 mg αTE for women. Needs during childhood growth range from 3 to 8 mg αTE. (See Table 6-2.) These values are based on recent studies of American diets.[28] The stated recommendation is based on an estimate in the diet of 80% as α-tocopherol and 20% as other tocopherols with varying potencies. The current 1980 revisions state recommendations for vitamin E in terms of "α-tocopherol equivalents" to help eliminate confusion between interna-

Table 6-2. National Research Council recommended daily vitamin E allowances

	Age (yr)	Tocopherol equivalents (mg αTE)*
Males and females	Birth-0.5	3
	0.5-1	4
	1-3	5
	4-6	6
	7-10	7
Males	11-14	8
	15-18	10
	19-22	10
	23-50	10
	51+	10
Females	11-14	8
	15-18	8
	19-22	8
	23-50	8
	51+	8
Pregnant		+2
Lactating		+3

*Total vitamin E activity, estimated to be 80% as α-tocopherol and 20% as other tocopherols.

tional units and milligrams of the various forms of tocopherol.

Food sources of vitamin E

The richest sources of vitamin E are the vegetable oils. Curiously enough, these are also the richest sources of polyunsaturated fatty acids. Other food sources include milk, eggs, muscle meats, fish, cereals, and leafy vegetables.

VITAMIN K

Chemical and physical nature of vitamin K

In 1929 Henrik Dam, biochemist at the University of Copenhagen, discovered a hemor-

rhagic disease in chicks fed a fat-free diet. Later he determined that the absent factor responsible was a blood-clotting vitamin, which he called ''Koagulationsvitamin'' or vitamin K. In 1939 he succeeded in isolating and identifying the vitamin from alfalfa. In 1943 he was a recipient of the Nobel Prize for physiology and medicine in recognition of this brilliant work.

As with most of the vitamins, not one but several forms of vitamin K comprise a group of substances with similar biologic activity. There are three main K vitamins. Two occur in nature and are fat soluble: K_1 (phylloquinone or phytonadione), which was isolated from alfalfa by Dam; and K_2 (fanoquinone), which was isolated from putrefied sardine meal by other investigators.[1] Vitamin K_3 has been made synthetically and has wide clinical use. It is *menadione,* one of several vitamins that are synthetic products with similar structures and properties. A water-soluble form of menadione (its diphosphate ester) is available for clinical use in patients in whom a fat-soluble form would be less readily metabolized. Because vitamin K is sensitive to light and irradiation, it should be kept in dark bottles.

Vitamin K is synthesized by the normal intestinal bacteria so that an adequate supply is generally present. Since the intestine of a newborn infant is sterile at birth, however, the supply of vitamin K is inadequate until normal bacterial flora of the intestine develop about the third or fourth day of life.

Vitamin K absorption

The natural fat-soluble vitamins K_1 and K_2 require bile salts for absorption and therefore enter the metabolic system by way of the upper segment of the small intestine. They are absorbed with other fat-related products by way of the abdominal lacteals into the lymphatic system and then into portal blood and the liver. Vitamin K is apparently stored in small amounts, since considerable quantities are excreted after administration of therapeutic doses.

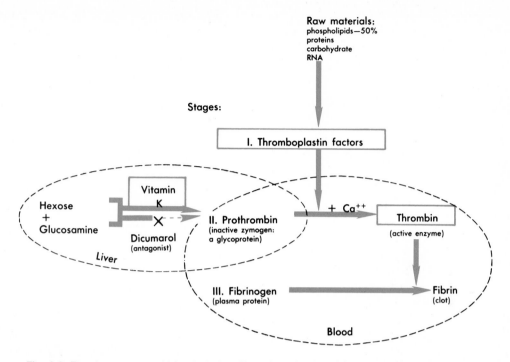

Fig. 6-3. The three stages of blood clotting. Note the role played by vitamin K in the production of prothrombin. Dicumarol, an anticlotting drug, acts as an antagonist (antimetabolite) to vitamin K and therefore inhibits the clotting mechanism at the start.

Physiologic functions of vitamin K

Blood clotting. The major function of vitamin K is to catalyze the synthesis of prothrombin by the liver (Fig. 6-3). Without vitamin K the whole vital process of blood clotting cannot be initiated. It acts as a catalyst, either as an enzyme or coenzyme. The mechanism for the production of prothrombin in the liver has recently been determined. It is now known that vitamin K participates in the chemical modification by carboxylation of the amino acid glutamine to produce the active form of prothrombin, which can then bind calcium, an essential element in blood clotting.[29,30] In the absence of functioning liver tissue, vitamin K cannot act. When liver damage has caused hypoprothrombinemia, and this in turn has led to hemorrhage, vitamin K is ineffective as a therapeutic agent.

Clinical applications. A number of clinical situations have important relationships with vitamin K.

OBSTETRICS. Since the intestinal tract of the newborn is sterile, the infant has no vitamin K during the first few days of life until normal bacterial flora develop. During this immediate postnatal period, hemorrhage may therefore occur. This condition is called hemorrhagic disease of the newborn. Vitamin K therapy may be given to the mother before delivery, but the effectiveness of placental transfer is debatable. Therefore a prophylactic dose of vitamin K is usually given to the infant soon after delivery.

Food sources of vitamin K

The items from which the natural vitamins K_1 and K_2 were originally extracted by Dam and others—alfalfa and putrefied sardine meal —are hardly human foods. However, vitamin

Table 6-3. Summary of fat-soluble vitamins

Vitamin	Physiologic functions	Results of deficiency	Requirement	Food sources
A (retinol)	Production of rhodopsin (visual purple)	Xerophthalmia	Adult male: 1,000 μg RE (5,000 IU) Adult female: 800 μg RE (4,000 IU) Pregnancy: 1,000 μg RE (5,000 IU) Lactation: 1,200 μg RE (6,000 IU) Children: 400 μg RE (2,000 IU) to 800 μg RE (4,000 IU)	Liver Cream, butter, whole milk Egg yolk
Provitamin A (carotene)	Formation and maintenance of epithelial tissue Toxic in large amounts	Night blindness Keratinization of epithelium Follicular hyperkeratosis Skin and mucous membrane infections Faulty tooth formation		Green and yellow vegetables Yellow fruits Fortified margarine
D (calciferol)	Absorption of calcium and phosphorus Calcification of bones Renal phosphate clearance Toxic in large amounts	Rickets Faulty bone growth Osteomalacia in adults	Adult: 5-10 μg cholecalciferol (200-400 IU) Pregnancy and lactation: 10-12.5 μg (400-500 IU) depending on age Children: 10 μg (400 IU)	Fish oils Fortified or irradiated milk
E (tocopherol)	Related to action of selenium Antioxidant with vitamin A and unsaturated fatty acids Hemopoiesis Reproduction (in animals)	Hemolysis of red blood cells; anemia Possible protection of unsaturated fatty acids Sterility (in rats)	Adult: 8-10 mg αTE Pregnancy and lactation: 10-11 mg αTE Children: 3-10 mg αTE	Vegetable oils
K (menadione)	Blood clotting, necessary for synthesis of prothrombin Possible coenzyme in oxidation phosphorylation Toxic in large amounts	Hemorrhagic disease of the newborn Bleeding tendencies in biliary disease or surgical procedures Deficiency in intestinal malabsorption (sprue, celiac disease, colitis) Prolonged antibiotic therapy Anticoagulant therapy (dicumarol counteracts)	Unknown	Green leafy vegetables Cheese Egg yolk Liver

K is also found in green leafy vegetables such as cabbage, spinach, kale, and cauliflower. Lesser amounts are found in tomatoes, cheese, egg yolk, and liver.

A summary of the fat-soluble vitamins is presented in Table 6-3 for review.

BILIARY DISEASE AND SURGERY. Any condition of the biliary tract affecting the flow of bile will prevent the proper absorption of vitamin K. Since vitamin K is a fat-soluble material, bile is necessary for its absorption. Bleeding tendencies would be enhanced in obstruction of the bile ducts, jaundice, gallbladder disease, hepatic injury, or liver disease. Water-soluble forms of vitamin K are available for therapeutic use. Parenteral use of menadione or oral administration of bile salts together with vitamin K may be indicated to counteract the delayed clotting.

Surgical procedures involving the biliary tract, such as operations on the common bile duct or removal of the gallbladder, usually necessitate vitamin K therapy to prevent excessive hemorrhage.

INTESTINAL DISEASE. Vitamin K deficiency is common in diseases such as celiac disease and sprue, which affect the absorbing mucosa of the small intestine, or other diarrheal diseases, such as ulcerative colitis, that cause rapid loss of intestinal contents. Intravenous administration of vitamin K may be indicated.

ANTIBIOTIC THERAPY. Prolonged use of antibiotics may adversely affect the normal bacterial flora of the intestine so that vitamin K deficiency occurs.

ANTICOAGULANT THERAPY. Use of heparin or bishydroxycoumarin (dicumarol) in anticoagulant therapy for coronary thrombosis or thrombophlebitis may counteract vitamin K. The molecular structure of dicumarol is similar to that of vitamin K, and it acts as an antimetabolite or antagonist to vitamin K because of the lock-and-key concept of enzyme action (see Fig. 5-3). Dicumarol almost fits into vitamin K's spot in the enzyme-substrate complex. It therefore gets in the way and prevents the nor-

mal reaction of vitamin K and prothrombin. This accounts for its anticoagulant action. In case of an overdose of the anticoagulants, vitamin K may be used as an antidote.

COENZYME ROLE. Recent studies suggest that vitamin K may have an additional metabolic function as an essential factor in oxidative phosphorylation (see pp. 27-28).

Vitamin K requirement

No requirement for vitamin K is stated, since a deficiency of vitamin K is unlikely except in the clinical situations indicated. An adequate amount is usually ensured because (1) the intestinal bacteria constantly synthesize a supply and (2) the amount the body needs is apparently small. The liver, however, must produce prothrombin if vitamin K is to be effective.

GLOSSARY

ameloblasts (Old Fr. *amel,* enamel; Gr. *blastos,* germ) special epithelial cells surrounding tooth buds in gum tissue, which form cup-shaped organs for producing the enamel structure of the developing teeth. Insufficient vitamin A causes faulty production of ameloblasts and it therefore impairs the soundness of the tooth structure.

antioxidant any substance that inhibits oxidation. Oxidation is a catabolic chemical process that breaks down or changes a substance by the introduction of oxygen. An antioxidant inhibits or slows such a deteriorating change. Vitamin E acts as an antioxidant in commercial products to retard spoilage.

carotene provitamin A. Carotene, which occurs in certain plant pigments, is the natural precursor that the animal body converts to vitamin A.

follicular hyperkeratosis a vitamin A deficiency condition in which the skin becomes dry and scaly and small pustules or hardened, pigmented, papular eruptions form around the hair follicles.

hypervitaminosis a toxic condition that results from intake of excess quantity of certain vitamins. The fat-soluble vitamins, especially A and D, have this distinct potential because they are stored by the body. The danger of toxicity does not hold for water-soluble vitamins, since the body eliminates any excess in the urine.

international units the measure traditionally used for vitamins A and D. The amount of the vitamin comprising a unit is determined by its biologic activity in rats; that is, the amount of the vitamin required to cure or prevent a disease that is associated with a deficiency of that specific vitamin.

keratinization (Gr. *keras, kerat,* horn) a process occurring in vitamin A deficiency states in which the epithelial cells either slough off or become dry and flattened, then gradually hardening and forming rough horny scales. This process may occur in the cornea, the respiratory tract, the gastrointestinal tract, the genitourinary tract, or the skin.

precursor (L. *praecursor,* forerunner) a substance that precedes and is converted into a second substance. For example, carotene is a natural substance in plant pigments that the body converts to vitamin A. Thus carotene is the precursor of vitamin A.

prothrombin (Gr. *pro,* before: *thrombos,* a clot) a protein (globulin) circulating in the plasma, essential to the clotting of blood. Prothrombin is produced by the liver. The process requires the presence of vitamin K.

retinol vitamin A; so named because of its chemical nature (an alcohol) and its function in the eye in the production of retinene, a necessary component of rhodopsin (visual purple).

retinol equivalents measure of vitamin A activity currently adopted by FAO/WHO and U.S. National Research Council's Food and Nutrition Board recommendations for vitamin A, replacing the term IU (international units). The measure accounts for dietary variances in preformed vitamin A (retinol) and its precursor, carotene. One RE (retinol equivalent) equals 3.33 IU or 1 μg retinol.

rickets a childhood disease that results from deficient deposition of calcium and phosphorus in developing cartilage and newly forming bone, producing abnormal bone shape and structure. Rickets is due primarily to vitamin D deficiency, which affects the absorption of calcium and phosphorus from the intestine, their deposition in bony tissue, and the reabsorption of phosphorus by the renal tubules.

tocopherol (Gr. *tokos,* childbirth; *pherein,* to bring) vitamin E; so named because of its association with reproduction in rats.

vitamin (L. *vita,* life; amine) any of a group of organic substances essential in small quantities to normal metabolism, found in minute amounts in natural foodstuffs; sometimes produced synthetically. Deficiencies of vitamins cause specific diseases and disorders.

REFERENCES
Specific

1. Kagan, B. M., and Goodhart, R. S.: The vitamins. In Wohl, M. G., and Goodhart, R. S., editors: Modern nutrition in health and disease, Philadelphia, 1964, Lea & Febiger.
2. McCollum, E. V.: Early experiences with vitamin A—a retrospect, Nutr. Rev. **10:**161, 1952.
3. Day, H. G., and E. V. McCollum: Doyen of nutrition science, Nutr. Rev. **37:**65, March, 1979.
4. Review: Cirrhosis, abnormal dark adaptation, and vitamin A, Nutr. Rev. **37:**73, March, 1979.
5. Basu, T. K.: Vitamin A and cancer of epithelial origin, J. Hum. Nutr. **33:**24, Feb., 1979.
6. Sparn, M. B., et al.: Prevention of chemical carcinogenesis by vitamin A and its synthetic analogs (retinoids), Fed. Proc. **35:**1332, May 1, 1976.
7. Review: Vitamin A, tumor initiation and tumor promotion, Nutr. Rev. **37:**153, May, 1979.
8. FAO/WHO of the United Nations: Requirements of vitamin A, thiamine, reboflavin, and niacin, FAO Nutr. Meet. Rep. Ser. No. 41; WHO Tech. Pre. Ser. No. 362, 1967.
9. Breslau, R. C.: Hypervitaminosis A; acute vitamin A toxicity, Arch. Pediatr. **74:**178, 1957.
10. Berger, S. S., and Raels, O. A.: Hypervitaminosis A, report of a case, Am. J. Clin. Nutr. **16:**265, 1965.
11. Russell, R. M., and Boyer, J. L.: Hepatic injury from chronic hypervitaminosis A resulting in portal hypertension and ascites, N. Engl. J. Med. **291:**435, 1974.
12. Loomis, W. F.: Rickets, Sci. Am. **223:**77, 1970.
13. DeLuca, H. F.: Vitamin D endocrinology, Am. Int. Med. **85:**367, 1976.
14. Kleiner, I. S., and Orten, J. M.: Biochemistry, ed. 7, St. Louis, 1966, The C. V. Mosby Co., p. 347.
15. Harper, H. A.: Physiological chemistry, ed. 11, Los Altos, Calif., 1971, Lange Medical Publications, pp. 67-68.
16. Food and Nutrition Board, National Research Council: Hazards of overdose of vitamin D, Am. J. Clin. Nutr. **28:**512, 1975.
17. Commentary: Hazards of overuse of vitamin D, J. Am. Diet. Assoc. **66:**453, May, 1975.
18. Gordon, H. H., and Nitowsky, J. M.: Vitamin E. In Wohl, M. G., and Goodhart, R. S., editors: Modern nutrition in health and disease, Philadelphia, 1964, Lea & Febiger, pp. 378-379.
19. Dicks-Bushnell, M. W., and Davis, K. C.: Vitamin E content of infant formulas and cereals, Am. J. Clin. Nutr. **20:**262, March, 1967.
20. Schwarz, K.: Factor 3, selenium, and vitamin E, Nutr. Rev. **18:**193, 1960.
21. Oski, F. A., and Barnes, L. A.: Vitamin E deficiency: a previously unrecognized cause of hemolytic anemia in the premature infant, J. Pediatr. **70:**211, 1967.
22. Williams, M. L., Shott, R. J., O'Neal, P. L., and Oski, F. A.: Role of dietary iron and fat on vitamin E deficiency anemia of infancy, N. Engl. J. Med. **292:**887, 1975.
23. Blane, W. A., Reid, J. D., and Andersen, D. H.: Avitaminosis E in cystic fibrosis of the pancreas, Pediatrics **22:**494, 1958.

24. Horwitt, M. K.: Vitamin E and lipid metabolism in man, Am. J. Clin. Nutr. **8:**451, 1961.

25. Horwitt, M. K., et al.: Vitamin E: a reexamination, Am. J. Clin. Nutr. **29:**569, 1976.

26. Tappel, A. L.: Where old age begins, Nutr. Today **2**(4):2, 1967.

27. Tappel, A. L.: Reactions of vitamin E, ubiquinol, and selenoamino acids and protection of oxidant-labile enzymes. In De Luca, H. F., and Suttie, J. W., editors: The fat soluble vitamins, Madison, Wis., 1970, University of Wisconsin Press.

28. Bieri, J. G., and Evarts, R. P.: Tocopherols and fatty acids in American diets, J. Am. Diet. Assoc. **62:**147, Feb., 1973.

29. Review: Vitamin K and the carboxylation of glutamyl residues in the formation of prothrombin, Nutr. Rev. **33:**25, 1975.

30. Fernlund, P., Stenflo, J., Roepstorff, P., and Thomsen, J.: Vitamin K and the biosynthesis of prothrombin, J. Biol. Chem. **250:**6125, 1975.

General

Bieri, J. G.: Fat-soluble vitamins in the eighth revision of the recommended dietary allowances, J. Am. Diet. Assoc. **64:**171, Feb., 1974.

Bieri, J. G., and Evarts, R. P.: Tocopherols and fatty acids in American diets, J. Am. Diet. Assoc. **62:**147, Feb., 1973.

Commentary: Who needs vitamin E? J. Am. Diet. Assoc. **64:**365, April, 1974.

Committee on Nutrition, American Academy of Pediatrics: The prophylactic requirement of toxicity of vitamin D, Pediatrics **35:**1022, 1965.

Elliott, R. A., and Dryer, R. L.: Hypervitaminosis A: report of a case in an adult, J.A.M.A. **161:**1157, 1956.

Food and Nutrition Board, National Research Council, National Academy of Sciences: Recommended dietary allowances, ed. 9, Washington, D.C., 1980.

Hegsted, D. M., editor: Present knowledge in nutrition, ed. 4, New York, 1976, The Nutrition Foundation.

Hodges, R. E.: Experimental vitamin A deficiency in human volunteers, summary of proceedings, workshop on biochemical and clinical criteria for determining human vitamin A nutriture, Washington, D.C., 1971, National Academy of Sciences.

Horwitt, M. K., editor: Symposium—vitamin E: biochemistry, nutritional requirements and clinical studies, Am. J. Clin. Nutr. **27:**939, 1974.

Jeghers, H., and Marraro, H.: Hypervitaminosis A: its broadening spectrum, Am. J. Clin. Nutr. **6:**335, 1958.

Johnson, B. C.: Dietary factors and vitamin K, Nutr. Rev. **22:**225, 1964.

McCollum, E. V.: Early experiences with vitamin A—a retrospect, Nutr. Rev. **10:**161, 1952.

McLaren, D. S., et al.: Xerophthalmia in Jordan, Am. J. Clin. Nutr. **17:**117, 1965.

McLaughlin, P. J., and Weibrauch, J. L.: Vitamin E content of foods, J. Am. Diet. Assoc. **75:**647, Dec., 1979.

Pereira, S. M., et al.: Vitamin A therapy in children with kwashiorkor, Am. J. Clin. Nutr. **20:**297, 1967.

Sebrell, W. H., Jr., and Harris, R. S., editors: The vitamins: chemistry, physiology, and pathology, vol. V, New York, 1972, Academic Press, Inc.

Udall, J. A.: Human sources and absorption of vitamin K in relation to anticoagulation stability, J.A.M.A. **194:**127, 1965.

Verner, J. V., Jr., et al.: Vitamin D intoxication: report of two cases treated with cortisone, Ann. Intern. Med. **48:**765, 1958.

Vietti, T. J., et al.: Observations on the prophylactic use of vitamin K in the newborn infant, J. Pediatr. **56:**343, 1960.

Vietti, T. J., et al.: Vitamin K prophylaxis in the newborn, J.A.M.A. **176:**791, 1961.

7 Vitamins: water-soluble vitamins

B-COMPLEX VITAMINS

The story of the B vitamins is a compelling one because it is the story of many people dying of a puzzling, age-old disease that other people observed and sought to cure. It was eventually learned that common, everyday food held the answer. The paralyzing disease beriberi had plagued the Orient for centuries and caused many men in many places to search for its solution. As early as 1882, a Japanese naval medical officer, Takaki, reported that he had cured beriberi in sailors of the Japanese navy by giving them less rice and more vegetables, barley, meat, and canned milk.

A few years later Christian Eijkman, a Dutch doctor at a prison in the Netherlands East Indies, observed the same type of paralysis in prison inmates and began to seek the answer through experiments with pigeons. Since he had little money for his research, he fed the pigeons scraps of the prison food, which was mostly polished rice. The same type of paralysis developed in the pigeons. When the unsympathetic prison director refused Eijkman permission to use the prison scraps, he was forced to buy some cheap natural (unmilled) rice to feed the birds. The dying birds revived and were soon well again. Eijkman experimented with numerous birds, and the same results followed. He could produce the disease and cure it simply by changing the diet! He reported his findings in 1897.

Eijkman's first theory was that the disease resulted from a poison in polished rice that was neutralized by an antidote in the hulls. Although this theory was wrong, his observation was an important clue. An associate of Eijkman, Dr. Grijns, offered another clue in 1901 with the idea that the disease was caused by something vital that was present in the polishings but was absent in the polished rice. In 1911, Casimir Funk isolated the vital nitrogen compound in the hulls, which he called a "vitamine" (see p. 83).

The international search gained momentum in the field and in the laboratory. A dedicated American, R. R. Williams, in the foreign service as chief chemist at the Philippine Bureau of Science from 1909 to 1916, applied these new findings and made tremendous strides in control and eradication of infantile beriberi by using extracts of rice polishings. In 1916, another American scientist then at the University of Wisconsin, E. V. McCollum, named the food factor "water-soluble B," because it was thought to be a single vitamin.

The widening search, however, proved that vitamin B was not a single substance, but about a dozen vitamin and vitamin-related factors. The B-complex family of vitamins is now recognized.

The B vitamins, originally believed to be important only in preventing the deficiency diseases that led to their discovery, have now been identified with many important metabolic functions. They serve as vital partners in many reactions as coenzymes in energy metabolism. Grouping them according to their function is therefore a useful step before the significance of each in relation to human nutrition is discussed.

Group I: Classic disease factors

1. Thiamin (vitamin B_1)—antiberiberi factor or antineruitic vitamin, called "aneurin" in Europe and some other areas; essential in carbohydrate metabolism
2. Riboflavin (vitamin B_2, formerly known as G)—essential in tissue respiration, hence in growth; and to the prevention of various skin disorders such as cheilosis (cracking at the corners of the mouth)
3. Niacin—nicotinic acid, originally called P-P factor (pellagra-preventing factor); a coenzyme essential to tissue oxidation and cell metabolism.

Group II: More recently discovered coenzyme factors

1. Pyridoxine (vitamin B_6)—essential coenzyme with amino acids; need for pyridoxine is increased in high-protein diets
2. Pantothenic acid—essential part of coenzyme A or active acetate (reread p. 27 to identify this pivotal key in the metabolism of carbohydrate, fat, and protein.)
3. Lipoic acid—coenzyme associated with thiamin in carbohydrate metabolism; a fatty acid, not a true vitamin
4. Biotin (formerly vitamin B_7 or H)—coenzyme in carbon dioxide fixation reactions in energy metabolism

Group III: Cell growth and blood-forming factors

1. Folic acid (formerly vitamin B_9 or B_{10})—a group of factors essential to the growth and reproduction of cells; associated with anemias because of their vital role in formation of red blood cells
2. Para-aminobenzoic acid (PABA)—part of folic acid molecule; sulfonamide antagonist; not a true vitamin
3. Cobalamin (vitamin B_{12})—red, cobalt-containing vitamin group; the antipernicious anemia factor; extrinsic factor (Castle)

Group IV: Other related nutrition factors (pseudovitamins)

1. Inositol—lipotropic agent in animal nutrition
2. Choline—essential metabolite, nerve mediator, lipotropic agent

CLASSIC DISEASE FACTORS
THIAMIN (B_1)

The search of many persons for the antiberiberi factor led eventually to a successful conclusion. In 1924 two Dutch workers in Java, Jansen and Donath, isolated and identified thiamin hydrochloride from rice polishings as the beriberi-preventive material. Subsequently, in 1935 the American workers, Williams and his associates,[1,2] finally synthesized thiamin, and the answer to the puzzle of beriberi was found. Its basic metabolic functions were essentially clarified during the 1930s.

Nature of thiamin

Thiamin hydrochloride is a white cystalline material sometimes described as having a nut-like and yeasty odor. It is water soluble and stable when dry, but is destroyed by alkalis. It is absorbed more readily in the acid medium of the proximal duodenum than in the lower duodenum where the acidity of the chyme is counteracted by alkaline intestinal secretions.

Thiamin is not stored in large quantities in the tissues. The tissue content is highly relative to heightened metabolic demand (fever, increased muscular activity, pregnancy, and lactation) or to composition of the diet. Carbohydrate increases the need for thiamin, while fat and protein spare thiamin. In addition, thiamin is constantly excreted in the urine.

Physiologic functions of thiamin

Coenzyme in carbohydrate metabolism. The manifestations of beriberi—polyneuritis, muscle weakness, and gastrointestinal disturbances—can be traced to physiologic problems related to the basic metabolic function of thiamin (see p. 104). When actively combined with phosphorus as thiamin pyrophosphate (TPP), thiamin plays a key role as a coenzyme in carbohydrate metabolism.

As stated in Chapter 5, enzymes act as *catalysts*. They not only speed up reactions that would otherwise be too slow, but also make possible the dynamic turnover of compounds without which life could not exist. Active partners in these processes are coenzymes.

For glucose oxidation, thiamin is such a coenzyme during decarboxylation and transketolation. *Decarboxylation* is the reaction in which pyruvate is converted to active acetate and carbon dioxide is removed. The enzyme is called *decarboxylase;* thiamin pyrophosphate acts as a *cocarboxylase*. This enables pyruvate to enter the Krebs cycle to produce vital energy. If there were no thiamin, there could be no energy (see p. 27).

In the hexose monophosphate shunt pathway for glucose oxidation, thiamin diphosphate (TDP) acts as a coenzyme in the important reaction that provides active glyceraldehyde. This is a key link providing activated glycerol for lipogenesis for the conversion of glucose to fat (see pp. 27-28). The process is called *transketolation* (keto-carrying), and the enzyme is a *transketolase*. Thiamin diphosphate is the key activator that provides the high energy phosphate bond. Ionized magnesium (Mg^{++}) is another cofactor present.

Clinical effects of thiamin deficiency

If thiamin is not present in sufficient amounts to provide the key energizing coenzyme factor in the cells, clinical effects will be reflected in the gastrointestinal system, the nervous system, and the cardiovascular system.

Gastrointestinal system. Various manifestations such as anorexia, indigestion, severe constipation, gastric atony, and deficient hydrochloric acid secretion may occur as a result of thiamin deficiency. As the cells of the smooth muscles and secretory glands are not able to receive sufficient energy from glucose, they cannot do their proper work in digestion to provide

still more glucose, and a vicious cycle ensues as deficiency continues.

Nervous system. The central nervous system is extremely dependent on glucose for energy to do its work. Without sufficient thiamin to help provide this need, neuronal activity is impaired, alertness and reflex responses are diminished, and general apathy and fatigue result. If thiamin deficiency continues, damage or degeneration of myelin sheaths of nerve fibers causes increasing nerve irritation, which produces pain and prickly or deadening sensations. Paralysis may gradually result if the process continues unchecked in a severe deficiency state.

Cardiovascular system. If the thiamin deficiency persists, the heart muscle weakens, and cardiac failure may result. Also, smooth muscle of the vascular system may be involved, causing peripheral vasodilation. As a result of the cardiac failure, peripheral edema may be observed in the extremities.

Thiamin requirement

The requirements for thiamin in human nutrition are usually stated in terms of the direct relation of thiamin to carbohydrate and energy metabolism, expressed as caloric intake. The studies of various investigators have indicated that the daily adult thiamin requirements are from 0.23 to 0.5 mg/1,000 calories. The National Research Council (NRC) 1980 allowances recommend 0.5 mg/1,000 calories, with a minimum of 1.0 mg for any intake between 1,000 and 2,000 calories. The correlations of thiamin with calories are shown in Table 7-1.

Clinical applications. Several important factors influence thiamin requirements and should be recognized in care of patients:

1. During growth periods of infancy, childhood, and especially adolescence, thiamin needs are increased.
2. Increased needs accompany gestation because of the increased metabolic rate characteristic of pregnancy and production of milk.
3. The larger the body and its tissue volume,

Table 7-1. National Research Council allowances for thiamin in relation to calories

	Age (yr)	Calories*	Thiamin (mg)
Males and	Birth-0.5	kg × 117	0.3
females	0.5-1	kg × 108	0.5
	1-3	1,300	0.7
	4-6	1,800	0.9
	7-10	2,400	1.2
Males	11-14	2,800	1.4
	15-18	3,000	1.4
	19-22	3,000	1.5
	23-50	2,700	1.4
	51+	2,400	1.2
Females	11-14	2,400	1.1
	15-18	2,100	1.1
	19-22	2,100	1.1
	23-50	2,000	1.0
	51+	1,800	1.0
Pregnant		+300	+0.4
Lactating		+500	+0.5

*Kilojoules (kJ) = 4.184 × kcal.

the greater its cellular energy requirements.

4. Fevers and infections increase cellular energy requirements, which also increase thiamin needs. Geriatric patients and those with chronic illness require particular attention to avoid deficiencies.

Food sources of thiamin

Good sources are lean pork, beef, liver, whole or enriched grains, and legumes. Eggs, fish, and a few vegetables are fair sources. Thiamin is less widely distributed in food than some of the other vitamins, such as A and C, and the quantities of thiamin in these foods are less than the naturally available quantities of vitamins A and C. Therefore a deficiency of thiamin is a distinct possibility in the average diet, especially when calories are markedly cur-

tailed, and in some highly inadequate special therapeutic diets.

Riboflavin (B$_2$)

Although as early as 1897 a London chemist named Blythe had observed a water-soluble pigment with peculiar yellow-green fluorescence in the milk whey, it was not until 1932 that riboflavin was actually discovered by workers in Germany.[3,4] The chemical group name, flavins (L. *flavus,* yellow), was given to the related compounds. Later, because the vitamin also contained the pentose sugar d-ribose, the term *riboflavin* was officially adopted.

Nature of riboflavin

Riboflavin is a yellow-green fluorescent pigment that forms yellowish brown needlelike crystals. It is water soluble and relatively stable to heat, but is easily destroyed by light and irradiation. It is stable in acid media and is not easily oxidized. However, it is sensitive to strong alkalis. Absorption seems to occur readily in the upper section of the small intestine and to be facilitated by combining with phosphorus in intestinal mucosa. Storage is relatively limited, although some amounts are found in liver and kidney. Day-to-day tissue turnover needs must be supplied by the diet. Urinary excretion varies according to intake and state of tissue depletion.

Physiologic functions of riboflavin

Coenzyme in protein metabolism. Just as thiamin is a partner in carbohydrate metabolism, riboflavin is a vital factor in protein metabolism. It, too, combines with phosphorus to form essential coenzymes in tissue respiration systems. The enzymes of which riboflavin is an important constituent are called *flavoproteins.* Two such riboflavin enzymes, flavin mononucleotide and flavin-adenine dinucleotide, operate at vital reaction points in the respiratory chains of cellular metabolism.

Flavin mononucleotide (FMN) is riboflavin phosphate activated with a high-energy phosphate bond. It is part of the enzyme systems that remove the amino group (NH_2) from certain amino acids. This process is called *deamination* (see Chapter 4 on protein metabolism).

Flavin-adenine dinucleotide (FAD) is a riboflavin enzyme that contains two high-energy phosphate bonds. It is a highly active form that operates in many reactions affecting amino acids, and carbohydrate. It helps in the deamination of glycine, an essential amino acid, and in the oxidizing of some of the lower fatty acids, such as butyric acid. It also acts in one of the systems of H^+ transfer in cellular oxidation (see Chapter 5). One such system is located in the Krebs cycle between succinic acid and fumaric acid (see Fig. 2-6 and Fig. 5-2).

Clinical effects of riboflavin deficiency

Manifestations of riboflavin deficiency center around tissue inflammation and breakdown.

1. Wound aggravation—even minor tissue injuries easily become aggravated and do not heal easily.
2. Mouth—cheilosis develops and the lips become swollen, crack easily, and characteristic cracks develop at the corners of the mouth.
3. Nose—cracks and irritation develop at nasal angles.
4. Tongue—the tongue becomes swollen and reddened (glossitis).
5. Eyes—extra blood vessels develop in the cornea (corneal vascularization), and the eyes burn, itch, and tear.
6. Skin—a scaly, greasy eruption may develop, especially in skin folds (seborrheic dermatitis).

Since nutritional deficiencies are usually multiple rather than single, riboflavin deficiencies seldom occur alone; they are especially likely to occur in conjunction with deficiencies of other B vitamins and protein.

Riboflavin requirement

The body's requirement for riboflavin is related to total caloric intake or energy needs and

Table 7-2. National Research Council allowances of riboflavin in relation to protein

	Age (yr)	Protein (g)	Riboflavin (mg)
Males and females	Birth-0.5	kg × 2.2	0.4
	0.5-1	kg × 2.0	0.6
	1-3	23	0.8
	4-6	30	1.0
	7-10	36	1.4
Males	11-14	44	1.6
	15-18	54	1.7
	19-22	54	1.7
	23-50	56	1.6
	51+	56	1.4
Females	11-14	44	1.3
	15-18	48	1.3
	19-22	46	1.3
	23-50	46	1.2
	51+	46	1.2
Pregnant		+30	+0.3
Lactating		+20	+0.5

to body size, metabolic rate, and rate of growth, all of which are related to protein intake. The lower the protein intake, the more riboflavin is excreted and lost. Studies indicate that tissue stores of riboflavin are not maintained when the dietary intake of this vitamin is less than 1.0 mg daily, and that 1.3 mg or more daily is necessary to maintain tissue reserves.

For practical purposes, the general 1980 NRC allowances for riboflavin have been stated as 0.6 mg/1,000 calories for all ages. The relation to protein intake is shown in Table 7-2.

Clinical applications. Attention should be given to certain risk groups or clinical situations in which riboflavin needs may be increased or where deficiencies are more likely to occur.

1. Cheap high-starch diets that are limited in protein foods such as milk, meat, and vegetables may be deficient in riboflavin.
2. Gastrointestinal disorders or chronic illness may result in a riboflavin deficiency

TO PROBE FURTHER
Niacin coenzymes and the "bouncing H⁺"

In the chain of agents that pass ionized hydrogen (H^+) and electrons along the distributing line to the waiting consumer, oxygen, two niacin compounds play key roles. This intricate network of systems within the cell provides energy precisely in the amounts necessary and at the time of need, which prevents waste and maintains orderly control (see Fig. 5-2).

These two niacin compounds are the following:

1. NAD (nicotinamide-adenine dinucleotide) coenzyme I; formerly called DPN (diphosphate nucleotide); the new term expresses the structure of the compound and is based on recognition of the important presence of the vitamin
2. NADP (nicotinamide-adenine dinucleotide phosphate) coenzyme II; formerly called TPN (triphosphate nucleotide)

In this oxidation system (the so-called respiratory chain) the niacin coenzymes often operate in partnership with thiamin and riboflavin coenzymes. For example, in the pivotal entry reaction of pyruvate into the Krebs final energy cycle, both niacin and thiamin coenzymes (NAD and TPP) are necessary. In the Krebs cycle itself, both niacin coenzymes (NAD and NADP) and riboflavin coenzymes (the flavoprotein system) operate together with cytochromes to generate bursts of energy (high-energy phosphate bonds at several different reaction points).

The total effect is similar to that of a generator. Energy is constantly produced and stored in "batteries" from which the body's cells may derive "current" when energy is needed. The carbon dioxide and water that are left at the end of these reactions are really by-products, but the controlling purpose of the entire series of reactions is to produce *energy*.

---

because food intake is affected by such disorders as anorexia, poor tolerance, or prolonged use of a too limited special diet. Disorders that affect absorption of nutrients can also cause riboflavin deficiency.

3. Wound healing, as in surgical procedures, trauma, and burns, increases the need for riboflavin because of the increased need for protein.
4. Periods of normal body stress such as growth periods, pregnancy, and lactation increase the need for riboflavin.

Food sources of riboflavin

The most important food source of riboflavin is milk. One of the pigments in milk, *lactoflavin,* is the milk form of riboflavin. Each quart of milk contains 2 mg of riboflavin, which is more than the daily requirement. Other good sources are the active organ meats (liver, kidney, and heart), and some vegetables contribute additional amounts. Cereals are poor sources unless they are enriched by commercial processing, which is now a common practice.

Since riboflavin is water soluble and destroyed by light, considerable loss can occur in open, excess-water cooking. Therefore covered containers and limited water are indicated.

Niacin (nicotinic acid)

Discovery of niacin. The discovery of niacin was the result of man's age-old struggle with disease. The disease associated with niacin deficiency is pellagra, which is characterized by a typical dermatitis and often has fatal effects on the nervous system (see p. 354). The unraveling of the mystery of pellagra forms a classic example of the interworking of talents and techniques from medicine, public health, epidemiology, nutrition, and nursing.

Observations of pellagra were first recorded in eighteenth century Spain and Italy where it was endemic in populations subsisting largely on corn. In the early 1900s Joseph Goldberger, a United States Public Health Service physician studying the problem of pellagra, worked in an orphanage in the rural southern United States. He noticed that although the majority of the children in the orphanage had pellagra in some degree, a few did not. He traced the absence of pellagra in the few to their pilfering of milk and meat from the orphanage's limited supply. His investigations established the relation of the disease to a certain food factor, which he called the P-P (pellagra preventive) factor or vitamin G. Casimir Funk in London isolated nicotinic acid from rice polishings in 1911, but did not recognize its disease-preventive significance. It was not until 1937 that Conrad Elvehjem,[5,6] a scientist at the University of Wisconsin, definitely associated the vitamin with pellagra by using it to cure the related disease, black tongue, in dogs.

Relation of niacin to tryptophan. As further study of the vitamin and pellagra continued, a new mystery developed concerning the relation of niacin to the essential amino acid, tryptophan. Again, curious observations were made. Why was pellagra rare in some population groups whose diets were actually low in niacin, whereas it was common in other groups whose diets were higher in niacin? And why did milk, which is low in niacin, have the ability to cure or prevent pellagra? Why was pellagra so common in groups subsisting on high-corn diets?[7]

At the University of Wisconsin, in 1945, Willard Krehl and his associates finally discovered that *tryptophan is a precursor of niacin.*[7,8,9] Here again was a vital link of a B vitamin with protein. Milk prevents pellagra because it is high in tryptophan. Almost exclusive use of corn contributes to pellagra because corn is low in tryptophan. Populations subsisting on diets low in niacin may never have pellagra because they happen to be also consuming adequate amounts of tryptophan. Gelatin is so poor a source of protein because it lacks tryptophan, whereas meat combines tryptophan and niacin.

This tryptophan-niacin relation led to the development of a unit of measure called *niacin equivalent (NE).* It was calculated that in a person with average physiologic needs, approximately 60 mg of tryptophan produces 1 mg of niacin. This amount of tryptophan was designated as a niacin equivalent. Dietary requirements are now usually given in terms of total milligrams of niacin and niacin equivalents.

Chemical nature of niacin

Two forms of niacin exist. Niacin (nicotinic acid) is easily converted to its amide form, *nicotinamide,* which is water soluble, stable to acid and heat, and forms a white powder when crystallized.

Physiologic functions of niacin

Coenzyme in tissue oxidation. Niacin is a partner with riboflavin in the cellular coenzyme systems that convert proteins and fats to glucose and that oxidize glucose to release controlled energy. In these systems the oxidation of glucose often takes place in the absence of free oxygen simply by the removal of hydrogen ions. These ions are passed down the line between the successively simpler compounds that comprise these systems to the eventual receiver, oxygen, and the end product is water. (See Chapter 5 on energy metabolism.)

Clinical effects of niacin deficiency

Since riboflavin and niacin have close interrelationships in cell metabolism, clinical manifestations of their deficiency closely parallel. Furthermore, if one of these two components is deficient, the other is usually deficient as well. General niacin deficiency is manifest as weakness, lassitude, anorexia, indigestion, and

Table 7-3. National Research Council niacin equivalent allowances in relation to calories and protein

	Age (yr)	Calories	Protein (g)	Niacin (mg NE)*
Males and females	Birth-0.5	kg × 115	kg × 2.2	6
	0.5-1	kg × 105	kg × 2.0	8
	1-3	1,300	23	9
	4-6	1,700	30	11
	7-10	2,400	34	16
Males	11-14	2,700	45	18
	15-18	3,800	56	18
	19-22	2,900	56	19
	23-50	2,700	56	18
	51+	2,400	56	16
Females	11-14	2,200	46	15
	15-18	2,100	46	14
	19-22	2,100	44	14
	23-50	2,000	44	13
	51+	1,800	44	13
Pregnant		+300	+30	+2
Lactating		+500	+20	+5

*On the average, 1 mg of niacin is derived from each 60 mg of dietary tryptophan.

various skin eruptions. More specific manifestations involve the skin and nervous system. Skin areas exposed to sunlight are especially affected, and they develop a dark, scaly dermatitis. If deficiency continues, the central nervous system becomes involved, and confusion, apathy, disorientation, and neuritis develop.

Niacin requirement

Studies with human requirements for niacin have indicated that the minimum for necessary tissue stores is about 9 mg/1,000 calories. Many factors affect requirement such as age and growth periods, pregnancy and lactation, illness, tissue trauma, body size, and physical activity. The 1980 NRC recommendations (6.6 mg/1,000 calories and not less than 13 niacin equivalents at intakes of less than 2,000 calories) are about 50% higher than minimum requirements to provide a safety margin to cover variances in individual need. These recommen-dations also allow for the contribution of tryptophan (in terms of niacin equivalents) from the dietary protein sources (Table 7-3).

Food sources of niacin

Meat is a major source of niacin. Peanuts, beans, and peas are also good sources. Enrichment makes good sources of all the grains; otherwise corn and rice are poor, because they are low in tryptophan. Oats are also low in niacin. Fruits and vegetables generally are poor sources.

MORE RECENTLY DISCOVERED COENZYME FACTORS
Pyridoxine (B₆)

Discovery of pyridoxine.[10,11] It was Joseph Goldberger, continuing his work with B vitamins, who suggested in 1926 that the group contained a factor that cured a particular dermatitis in rats. Because of this property, the factor was at first called *adermin* (or the rat-antidermatitis factor). In 1939 Harris synthesized the factor and noted that its chemical structure was distinguished by having a pyridine ring and so named it pyridoxine. In 1942 Snell's group isolated in animal tissue and synthesized the two companion products, pyridoxal and pyridoxamine. Umbreit and his group followed in 1945 with their report of coenzyme functions of the vitamin in its phosphate forms. The activity of another B vitamin in metabolic coenzyme reactions throughout the body was being clearly and systematically brought into view.

Chemical nature of pyridoxine

Three forms of vitamin B_6 occur in nature — pyridoxine, pyridoxal, and pyridoxamine. In the body all three forms undergo conversion to pyridoxal phosphate. By far the most potent and active forms in body metabolism are the phosphate derivatives of pyridoxal and pyridoxamine. The term *pyridoxine* or simply vitamin B_6 is used to designate the entire group, as well as one of its components.

Pyridoxine is a water-soluble, heat-stable vitamin that is sensitive to light and alkalis. It is absorbed in the upper portion of the small intestine and is found throughout the body tissues, which is evidence of its many essential metabolic activities. There is evidence that intestinal bacteria also produce this vitamin, but the full extent of this source and the degree to which it is utilized by the body are as yet undetermined.

Physiologic functions of pyridoxine

Coenzyme in protein metabolism. In its active phosphate forms (B_6-PO_4), pyridoxine is an active coenzyme factor in many types of reaction in amino acid metabolism:

1. Pyridoxine is active in decarboxylation. An example is the reaction that converts glutamic acid to γ-aminobutyric acid, a substance found in gray matter in the brain. Since aminobutyric acid affects central synaptic activity, it is a regulatory factor for the neurons. Also important to brain function is another such B_6-PO_4-dependent reaction involved in the conversion of tryptophan to serotonin. Serotonin, a potent vasoconstrictor, stimulates cerebral activity and brain metabolism.

2. Pyridoxine also aids in deamination. By removing the amino groups from amino acids, such as serine and threonine, B_6-PO_4 helps to render carbon residues available for energy.

3. In transamination reactions (transfer of amino groups), B_6-PO_4 acts as a coenzyme that splits off NH_2 and transfers it to a new carbon skeleton, which forms a new amino acid or other compound. This passage of the amino group from compound to compound is much like the hydrogen ion transfer systems in which thiamin, niacin, and riboflavin operate.

4. In transsulfuration (transfer of sulfur) B_6-PO_4 aids reactions of the sulfur-containing amino acids, as in the transfer of sulfur from methionine to another amino acid (serine) to form the derivative cysteine.

5. Pyridoxine is involved in nicotinic acid formation from tryptophan. Through its involvement in this reaction, B_6-PO_4 plays a role in niacin supply.

6. There is evidence that B_6-PO_4 is necessary for the incorporation of the amino acid glycine and succinate (a glucose metabolite in the Krebs cycle) into *heme,* the essential protein core of hemoglobin.

7. In amino acid absorption, B_6-PO_4 appears also to operate as part of an active transport system in the intestinal wall that aids in the absorption of amino acids and their entry into cells.

Coenzyme in carbohydrate and fat metabolism. To a lesser extent, B_6-PO_4 also plays a role in carbohydrate metabolism. By way of the transfer systems such as decarboxylation and transamination, metabolites are provided for energy-producing fuel in the Krebs cycle. B_6-PO_4 also participates in the conversion of the essential fatty acid, linoleic acid, to another fatty acid, arachidonic acid.

Clinical effects of pyridoxine deficiency

It is evident from such an impressive list of metabolic activities that pyridoxine may hold a key to a number of clinical problems.

Anemia. A hypochromic, microcytic anemia has been observed in several patients even in the presence of a high-serum iron level. A deficiency of pyridoxine was demonstrated by a tryptophan load test, and the anemia was subsequently cured by supplying the deficient vitamin.

Central nervous system disturbances. By virtue of its role in the formation of the two regulatory compounds in brain activity, serotonin and γ-aminobutyric acid, pyridoxine may have a place in control of related neurologic conditions. In infants deprived of the vitamin, there is increased hyperirritability that progresses to convulsive seizures. A classic object lesson occurred in the early 1950s when infants fed a commercial milk formula in which most of the pyridoxine content had inadvertently been destroyed by high-temperature autoclaving subsequently had convulsions. The seizures ceased soon after a B_6-supplemented formula was instituted.

Tuberculosis. Experience with isoniazid (isonicotinic acid hydrazide, INH), used as a chemotherapeutic agent for tuberculosis has shown it to be an antagonist for pyridoxine. By inhibiting the conversion of glutamic acid (the only amino acid the brain metabolizes), isoniazid has caused a side effect of neuritis in some patients. Treatment with large doses (50 to 100 mg daily) of pyridoxine prevents this effect.

Physiologic demands in pregnancy. Pyridoxine deficiencies during pregnancy have been demonstrated by tryptophan load tests and subsequently alleviated by supplementation with vitamin B_6. Fetal growth, in addition to creating greater maternal metabolic demands, increases the pyridoxine requirement. For some years vitamin B_6 has been used to treat the hyperemesis of pregnancy, but there is no real evidence to substantiate this practice.

Also, women on estrogen-progesterone oral contraceptives are reported to require additional vitamin B_6.[12] An abnormal state of tryptophan metabolism is indicated as a contributor to increased need.[13,14]

Pyridoxine requirement

For the first time in its 1968 recommendations, the NRC made a statement concerning pyridoxine needs. These recommended allowances were continued unchanged in the 1974 and 1980 revisions. Although exogenous pyridoxine is mandatory, the amount required is very small so that a deficiency is unlikely. Some of the vitamin is provided by bacterial synthesis in the intestine, but just how much is available from this source is not known. Since pyridoxine is involved in amino acid metabolism, the need for pyridoxine varies with dietary protein intake. It seems that for adults approximately 1 mg daily is minimal. However, the council has set a recommended allowance of 2 mg per day for adults to assure a safety margin for variances in individual need.

Food sources of pyridoxine

Pyridoxine is fairly widespread in foods, but many sources provide only very small amounts. Good sources include yeast, wheat and corn, liver and kidney, and other meats. There are limited amounts in milk, eggs, and vegetables.

Pantothenic acid
Nature of pantothenic acid

The presence of pantothenic acid in all forms of living things and the amount of it throughout body tissues account for the name given it by its discoverers. Pantothenic comes from the Greek word *pantothen,* which means "in every corner" or "from all sides." It is a white crystalline compound. Pantothenic acid was isolated and synthesized by R. J. Williams between 1938 and 1940.[15]

Intestinal bacteria synthesize considerable amounts of pantothenic acid. This, together with its widespread natural occurrence, makes deficiency unlikely. Deficiency states have been studied for the most part by inducing them in animals. Manifestations of deficiency are similar to those of other B vitamins. An additional manifestation, adrenal necrosis, has been observed in the deficient animals. This condition is related to the role of pantothenic acid in steroid synthesis.

Physiologic functions of pantothenic acid

Coenzyme role in metabolism. The coenzyme role of pantothenic acid is vital to overall body metabolism. In the metabolism of carbohydrate, active acetate (p. 27) is the point at which important reactions in a number of directions can involve carbohydrates, fats, and proteins. Pantothenic acid is an essential constituent of the enzyme CoA, which forms this key compound, and as such has extensive metabolic responsibility as an activating agent. The process of *acetylation* by the enzyme CoA is one of the prime chemical reactions of the body. Activation by pantothenic acid is necessary in the following reactions.

1. Activation of acetic acid to form active acetate enables the acetic acid derived from carbohydrate, fat, and amino acids to enter the Krebs cycle.
2. Activation of fatty acids provides for lipogenesis for oxidation of fat for energy or for production of intermediate products such as ketones.
3. Activation of amino acids allows them to combine in a number of synthesis reactions such as the formation of fat products

(ketogenic reactions) or the formation of carbohydrate products (glycogenic reactions).
4. Radioactive isoptope studies have shown that active acetate is a direct precursor of cholesterol.
5. Steroid hormones formed by the adrenal and sex glands are closely related to cholesterol and therefore to active acetate.
6. Activation of succinic acid from the Krebs cycle and glycine are necessary constituents of the first step in the formation of heme for hemoglobin synthesis.
7. Active acetate may combine with the sulfonamide drugs to facilitate their excretion.

Pantothenic acid requirement

The quantitative requirement for pantothenic acid in man has not been established, since deficiency is not likely. Studies with adults have shown that daily excretion rates range from 2.5 to 9.5 mg. The daily intake of pantothenic acid in an average American diet of from 2,500 to 3,000 calories is about 10 to 20 mg. Therefore a deficiency is not probable except perhaps under extreme metabolic stress.

Food sources of pantothenic acid

Sources of pantothenic acid are widespread. Yeast and metabolically active tissues such as liver and kidney are rich sources. Egg, especially the yolk, and skimmed milk contribute more. Fair additional sources include lean beef, milk, cheese, legumes, broccoli, kale, sweet potatoes, and yellow corn.

Lipoic acid
Nature of lipoic acid

The continuing study of thiamin as a coenzyme in carbohydrate metabolism revealed that this metabolic system required other coenzyme factors in addition to thiamin. One of these additional coenzymes, reported by Reed in 1951,[16] was discovered in work with lactic acid bacteria. On analysis, this new factor proved to be a fat-soluble acid and was named *lipoic acid* (Gr. *lipos,* fat). Subsequent study of its structure in natural sources proved it to be a *sulfur*-containing fatty acid ($LipS_2$, LSS). Although lipoic acid is not a true vitamin, because its coenzyme function is closely related to thiamin, it is classified here with the B-vitamin group.

Physiologic function of lipoic acid

Coenzyme role in metabolism. Lipoic acid is an essential coenzyme that functions with thiamin in the initial decarboxylation step of pyruvate (p. 27). Pyruvate, a key product in carbohydrate metabolism, is formed in the beginning pathway of glucose oxidation (Embden-Meyerhof glycolytic pathway, p. 26). This key reaction, oxidative decarboxylation, enables pyruvate ultimately to enter the Krebs cycle to produce energy. Lipoic acid, because it has two sulfur bonds of high-energy potential (LSS), combines with the active thiamin coenzyme with two high-energy phosphate bonds (thiamin pyrophosphate, TPP) to reduce pyruvate to active acetate, thereby sending it into the final energy cycle.

A review of Chapter 7 up to this point reveals not one, but *five* B vitamins are involved, together with ionized magnesium (Mg^{++}), in this one key reaction in energy metabolism—oxidative decarboxylation (Fig. 7-1).

This same type of team reaction occurs at a later point in the Krebs cycle. It is a striking illustration of that important general concept of the interdependent relationships among the various nutrients giving life to the organism. ''No man is an island,'' said the poet John Donne. Indeed, it seems that no nutrient is an island—even when it occurs in microorganisms!

Lipoic acid requirement

A quantitative requirement for lipoic acid in human nutrition has not been established. Only a minute amount appears to be needed for oxidative decarboxylation in microorganisms, and lipoic acid is widespread in active tissues. Further study may prove that this coenzyme is of even greater significance than is now known.

Food sources of lipoic acid

Lipoic acid is found in many biologic materials, including yeast and liver.

Biotin

Biotin, a member of the B-complex group of vitamins, has been called a ''micromicronutrient'' because such minute traces of it perform its metabolic task. Its potency is great. A natural deficiency is unknown.

Nature of biotin

Biotin is a water-soluble vitamin factor, and was first identified and synthesized from egg yolk in 1936 by German workers.[17] Previously, a curious syndrome characterized by eczema and paralysis had been observed in rats fed large amounts of raw egg white. This condition was counteracted by a factor in other foods such

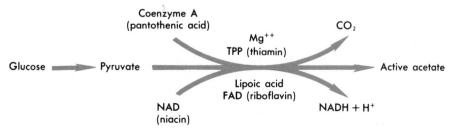

Fig. 7-1. Conversion of pyruvate to active acetate (acetyl CoA), illustrating the team action of five B vitamins and one mineral (magnesium).

as egg yolk. The corrective factor was subsequently identified as biotin, and the vitamin has been called the "anti-egg white injury" factor. Further study showed that the injurious substance in egg white, *avidin,* was a carbohydrate-containing protein, which apparently combines with biotin in the intestine and prevents its absorption. Biotin deficiency in human beings from such a cause is unlikely, unless one had an unusual taste for large amounts of raw eggs, but it has been known to occur.

Physiologic functions of biotin

Coenzyme role in metabolism. Biotin, even in very small amounts, appears to function as a coenzyme mainly in carboxylation and deamination.

CARBOXYLATION (CARBON DIOXIDE FIXATION, OR CARBON DIOXIDE ADDITION). Biotin serves as a coenzyme with active acetate in reactions that transfer carbon dioxide from one compound and fix it onto another. Examples of this combination of cofactors at work are

1. Initial steps in synthesis of some fatty acids
2. Conversion reactions involved in synthesis of some amino acids
3. Carbon dioxide fixation in forming purines

DEAMINATION. Biotin serves as a coenzyme with deaminases in splitting off the amino group from certain amino acids (aspartic acid, serine, threonine).

Biotin requirement

The human requirement for biotin has not been established in quantitative terms, since the amount needed for metabolism is so small. This coenzyme occurs in many natural foods and is apparently synthesized by intestinal bacteria.

Food sources of biotin

Examples of excellent food sources of biotin include egg yolk, liver, kidney, tomatoes, and yeast.

CELL GROWTH AND BLOOD-FORMING FACTORS
Folic acid (B_9)

The isolation and identification of folic acid are associated with laboratory studies of anemias and growth factors in animals. In 1938 Stokstad and Manning[18] described a growth factor for chicks, which they named vitamin U. Lately, in 1945, folic acid was obtained from liver and synthesized by Angier and Stokstad and their associates.[19] The vitamin was given the name *folic acid* (L. *folium,* leaf) or *folacin,* because a major source of its extraction was dark green leafy vegetables such as spinach. The reduced form of folic acid has since been discovered. It is *folinic acid,* first called *citrovorum factor* (CF) because it supplies an essential growth factor of *Lactobacillus citrovorum.*

Nature of folic acid

Folic acid is a conjugated substance made up of three acids, one of which is the amino acid glutamic acid. It is water soluble and forms yellow crystals. As with many of the B vitamins, folic acid is a group of related compounds that have similar actions in the body. It is absorbed throughout the small intestine. Apparently some amount is synthesized by intestinal bacteria.

Physiologic functions of folic acid

Coenzyme for single carbon transfer. The basic metabolic role of folic acid is to act as a necessary coenzyme in the important task of transferring single carbon (C_1) units for attachment in many interconversions. A number of key compounds are formed by these conversions.

1. *Purines* are part of a group of materials called *nucleoproteins,* which are essential constituents of all living cells. Because nucleoproteins are intimately related to the nuclear substance of the cells, they are involved in cell division and in the trans-

mission of inherited traits. It is clear, then, that any factor involved in the formation of nucleoproteins, such as folic acid, would play a vital role in cell growth and reproduction. Purines are therefore found in large quantity in tissues with very active cellular growth and reproduction, such as glandular tissue.

2. *Thymine* is an essential nucleoprotein material that forms a key part of DNA (deoxyribonucleic acid), the all-important material in the cell nucleus that is responsible for transmitting genetic characteristics (see p. 60). Folic acid participates in the reactions that synthesize thymine.

3. Folic acid performs its basic C_1-carrier role in the formation of heme, the iron-containing protein in *hemoglobin*. It is therefore not surprising that folic acid deficiencies would greatly affect blood cell formation.

Clinical applications

Anemias. Through continued study of *pernicious anemia,* it has been determined that other factors, not folic acid, are necessary to prevent this deficiency disease. Although the administration of folic acid results in blood cell regeneration in patients with pernicious anemia, its effect is not permanent; nor does it control the degenerative neurologic problems associated with the disease. Vitamin B_{12}, which was discovered after folic acid, proved to be the fully effective agent, both for blood regeneration and for the neurologic defect. The American Medical Association and the Food and Drug Administration have therefore recommended that no more than 0.4 mg of folic acid be included in nonprescription multivitamin preparations, as this would suffice for common needs, while at the same time it would not mask the development of pernicious anemia and prevent its diagnosis. A *nutritional megalaoblastic anemia* due to simple folic acid deficiency has been clearly described, however. A report of

seven cases[20] indicated low serum folic acid in the face of normal B_{12} levels and a rapid hematologic response to treatment with folic acid alone.

Some cases of *macrocytic anemia of pregancy* and *megaloblastic anemia of infancy* have been attributed to dietary folic acid deficiency (see p. 388). In one reported instance[21,22] a mother with macrocytic anemia and her 3-month-old nursing infant with megaloblastic anemia both responded to folic acid given to the mother alone.

Sprue. Folic acid has also been demonstrated to be effective in the treatment of sprue, a gastrointestinal disease characterized by intestinal lesions, malabsorption defects, diarrhea, macrocytic anemia, and general malnutrition. Response to folic acid has been excellent; both the blood-forming and gastrointestinal defects have been corrected.

Leukemia. A potent folic acid antagonist, *aminopterin,* has been used in the treatment of malignant neoplastic disease such as leukemia. An *antagonist* is a compound whose molecular configuration is almost, but not precisely, like that of a compound that is involved in a normal or abnormal metabolic process. An enzyme and its substrate (the ''key'') fits into particular sites on a molecule of the enzyme (the ''lock''). An antagonist is so similar in molecular structure to a specific enzyme that its molecule can compete with the molecule of that particular enzyme or coenzyme for the position of forming the lock. Once an antagonist molecule has got into the lock position, however, the slight dissimilarity between its configuration and that of the enzyme molecule prevents the key from fitting into it exactly, and the reaction will not proceed (see Fig. 5-3).

Folic acid is intimately involved in the normal synthesis of substances such as nucleic acid within the cell nucleus, which are responsible for cellular growth. Aminopterin, because it is an antagonist of folic acid, is able to block the rapid development of cells that is characteristic of malignant neoplastic disease. Unfortunately, although temporary remissions have been achieved with aminopterin, the leukemic cells seem to develop a resistance to the antagonist with continued use, and its effectiveness is overcome.

A closely related, more recently developed drug, methotrexate (amethopterin), is currently being used in cancer chemotherapy. Its major mechanism of action is to bind the enzyme dihydrofolate reductase and thus inhibit the C_1 fixing function of folic acid. The effect of this action is to prevent synthesis of DNA and purine in the cell.[23]

Folic acid requirement

Folic acid requirements were set for the first time by the NRC in its 1968 recommendations and continued in its 1980 allowances (Table 7-4). The average American diet contains about 0.6 mg of total folic acid activity (as measured by *Lactobacillus casei* assay). These recommended allowances cover variances in need and in the amount of available folic acid in foods. Note the increased requirement of folic acid during pregnancy and lactation. Stress, such as disease and growth, increases the requirement.

Food sources of folic acid

Liver, kidney, fresh green leafy vegetables, and asparagus are rich sources of folic acid. Fruit, milk, poultry, and eggs are relatively poor sources. Food values of folic acid for a variety of foods have been provided for reference use by the practitioner.[24,25,26]

Para-aminobenzoic acid (PABA)
Nature of para-aminobenzoic acid

Para-aminobenzoic acid is a structural unit of folic acid. Although it is not a true vitamin, PABA is sometimes listed as a separate factor because it is essential to the growth of certain microorganisms. However, its main role in human nutrition is secondary to that of folic acid; it is an essential component in folic acid formation.

Clinical application

In pharmaceutical levels, not as a vitamin, PABA has been reported to be effective in the treatment of some rickettsial diseases. The rickettsial diseases are disorders in man and animals caused by microscopically small parasites of the genus *Rickettsia*. They were named for their discoverer, Howard T. Ricketts, who was a pathologist at the American University of Chicago in the late 1800s and early 1900s. These minute organisms, which resemble small, rod-shaped bacterial cells, live in the intestinal tract of arthropods (mites, ticks, fleas, lice). When the arthropod bites a human being, the rickettsial parasite may be transmitted to the person's blood. It is capable of causing serious disease such as typhus or Rocky Mountain spotted fever.

The clinical use of PABA in attempts to combat rickettsial diseases is based on the concept

Table 7-4. National Research Council folic acid allowances

	Age (yr)	Folacin (μg)
Males and females	Birth-0.5	30
	0.5-1	45
	1-3	100
	4-6	200
	7-10	300
Males	11-14	400
	15-18	400
	19-22	400
	23-50	400
	51+	400
Females	11-14	400
	15-18	400
	19-22	400
	23-50	400
	51+	400
Pregnant		+400
Lactating		+400

of metabolic antagonism. PABA acts as an antagonist to a material essential to these organisms, para-oxybenzoic acid. The rickettsial organisms are killed because PABA blocks their essential metabolite.

Cobalamin (B_{12})

When folic acid was found to be lacking in full effectiveness as a specific agent in the control of pernicious anemia, the search continued for the remaining piece in the disease puzzle. In 1948 two groups of workers—one in America[27,28] and one in England[29]—crystallized a red compound from liver, which they numbered vitamin B_{12}. In the same year, it was clearly shown that this new vitamin could control both the blood-forming defect and the neurologic involvement in pernicious anemia.

Soon afterward a method of producing the vitamin through a process of fermentation with microorganisms was developed. This remains the main source of commercial supply.

Nature of cobalamin (vitamin B_{12})

Continued study of the vitamin's chemistry revealed its unique structure. B_{12} is the only vitamin that contains cobalt. It is a complex red crystalline compound of high molecular weight, with a single cobalt atom at its core ($C_{63}H_{90}O_{14}N_{14}PCo$). It has been given the generic name of *cobalamin*. It occurs as a protein complex in foods, so that its food sources are mostly of animal origin. The ultimate source, however, might be designated as microorganisms in the gastrointestinal tract of herbivorous animals. Such microorganisms are found in large amounts in the rumen (first stomach, containing cud) of cows. Apparently some synthesis occurs in the intestinal bacteria of man also, although the amount supplied from this source is not known.

Absorption of vitamin B_{12}. Absorption of vitamin B_{12} appears to take place in the ileum. It must be prepared for absorption, however, by two gastric secretions. It is the only human nutrient known to require exposure to stomach secretions before it can be absorbed. Hydrochloric acid in the stomach begins to split the B_{12} from its peptide bonds, and this splitting is continued by a group of enzymes in the intestine. The free B_{12} combines with *intrinsic factor*—a mucoprotein enzyme that is secreted by glands in the fundus and cardia of the stomach (although not in the pylorus). The combined material is conveyed to the ileum. In the presence of calcium, it remains for several hours attached to ileal receptors and is then carried by the blood to various organs where it is utilized or stored.

Storage of vitamin B_{12}. Vitamin B_{12} is stored in active body tissues. Organs holding the greatest amounts are the liver, kidney, heart, muscle, pancreas, testes, brain, blood, spleen, and bone marrow. Even these amounts are very minute, but because they are so vital, the body apparently holds tenaciously to its small supply. The stores are very slowly depleted. For example, a characteristic type of anemia, caused by loss of gastric secretions necessary for absorption of vitamin B_{12}, develops after surgical removal of the stomach. But this anemia does not become apparent until three to five years after the gastrectomy.

Physiologic function of vitamin B_{12}

Methylation in general metabolism. Vitamin B_{12} appears to have many metabolic interrelationships with the basic nutrients. It seems to be tied to protein metabolism, since the requirement for B_{12} increases as protein intake increases. Also, there is evidence that vitamin B_{12} is related to the utilization of fat and carbohydrate. The role of B_{12} in these various aspects of general metabolism seems to be associated with *methylation,* a process of forming or transferring key methyl groups (CH_3). In this role, B_{12} has been viewed as participating in the synthesis of nucleic acid and vital proteins in the cell. Coenzyme forms of B_{12} called *cobamides* have been found in tissue.

TO PROBE FURTHER

B$_{12}$ absorption defect in pernicious anemia*

Tracer studies with radioactive cobalt (Co$_{60}$) have given valuable additional information concerning the B$_{12}$ absorption defect in pernicious anemia. Since a single cobalt atom is the core structure of vitamin B$_{12}$, radioactive cobalt may be incorporated into the B$_{12}$ complex. The routine and activity of the vitamin can then be followed by various devices that detect the precise location of radioactivity in the body. The amount of radioactive substance necessary to label a compound so that it can be traced as it travels through the body is called a tracer dose.

A tracer dose of the vitamin is given by mouth, and the amount absorbed is determined by subtracting the quantity of radioactive substance that is excreted from the total amount of the tracer dose. After an interval, a second dose of radioactive B$_{12}$ is given, but on this occasion a dose of intrinsic factor is given at the same time. The amount absorbed is again calculated and compared with the amount that was absorbed when no intrinsic factor is given. Without intrinsic factor, only from 10% to 20% of the vitamin is absorbed.

The amount taken up by the liver after absorption has also been checked by counting radioactivity with instruments applied to the surface of the body over the liver.

*Shilling, R. F.: A new test for intrinsic factor activity, J. Lab. Clin. Med. **42:**946, 1953; Glass, G. B. J., et al.: Assay of intrinsic factor preparations: comparison of hepatic uptake of radioactive Co$_{60}$-B$_{12}$ with the hematopoietic response in pernicious anemia, J. Lab. Clin. Med. **46:**60, 1955.

Hematopoiesis. A well-established role of vitamin B$_{12}$ is its participation in the formation of red blood cells, and therefore in the control of pernicious anemia. It has been postulated that B$_{12}$ has an indirect effect on blood cell formation through activation of folic acid coenzymes. Within the developing red blood cell, activities that are dependent on folic acid are indirectly controlled by vitamin B$_{12}$. Perhaps this link with folic acid explains why folic acid may alleviate pernicious anemia only temporarily and why the folic acid must be supplemented by vitamin B$_{12}$ if the pernicious anemia is to be corrected over a long period.

Clinical applications

Pernicious anemia. The discovery of B$_{12}$ as a specific controlling factor in pernicious anemia was a great clinical breakthrough. Now a patient with this defect can be given from 15 to 30 μg of B$_{12}$ daily in intramuscular injections during a relapse and can be maintained afterward by an injection of about 30 μg every 30 days. This controls both the hematopoietic disorder and the degenerative effects on the nervous system.

Sprue. Like folic acid, vitamin B$_{12}$ has been effective in the treatment of the intestinal syndrome of sprue. However, it seems most effective when used in conjunction with folic acid. Therefore its role may be indirect in that it may facilitate the action of folic acid.

Vitamin B$_{12}$ requirement

The amount of exogenous vitamin B$_{12}$ needed for normal human metabolism appears to be very small. Reported minimum requirements have been from 0.6 to 1.2 μg per day, with a range upward to approximately 2.8 μg to allow adequately for individual variance. The ordinary diet easily provides this much and more. For example, 1 c of milk, one egg, and 4 oz of meat provide 2.4 μg.

In its 1980 revisions the NRC recommends a daily intake of 3.0 μg for adults. This amount allows a margin of safety to cover variance in individual need, absorption, and body stores.

Food sources of vitamin B₁₂

Vitamin B_{12} is supplied almost entirely by animal foods. The richest sources are liver and kidney, and lean meat, milk, egg, and cheese supply additional amounts.

Natural dietary deficiency is rare. The only reported manifestations of deficiency (general nervous symptoms, sore mouth and tongue, paresthesia, amenorrhea) have come from a group of true vegetarians, "Vegands," who live in Great Britain, and from other vegetarian groups in India and in the United States.

PSEUDOVITAMINS

Certain substances, although they are not true vitamins, are nonetheless related to vitamins in their activity and are usually classified with the B complex. These additional essential nutritional factors include inositol and choline. Lipoic acid and PABA, as indicated previously, may also be considered pseudovitamins.

Inositol
Nature of inositol

Inositol is a chemical compound found in meat extractives and is closely related in composition to glucose. It was first commonly called "muscle sugar" and given the name inositol from two Greek roots: *inos,* meaning sinews; and *-ose,* the suffix for sugars. It appeared to be an intermediary between aromatic substances and glucose.

Some years ago it was observed that certain patients' clinical records indicated a relationship between inositol and diabetes. Diabetic patients excreted larger amounts of inositol in the urine than did nondiabetics. It was not until much later, during the vitamin research of the 1940s, that the substance was used in animal experiments and a true deficiency state identified. In rats, early work showed that alopecia (baldness) of a particular type was found to be directly associated with inositol deficiency. A denuded area around the eyes gave the animals a curious speckled eye appearance. Although this relationship between inositol and alopecia in animals has been proved untrue, the initial belief that inositol was an essential nutritional factor led investigators to group it with the vitamins.

Phytic acid, found in grains, is a hexaphosphate ester of inositol. Phytic acid binds calcium in the intestine to form calcium phytate. It may therefore prove to be a cause of rickets.*

Inositol is stored largely in muscle tissue, particularly heart muscle and skeletal muscle. It is also stored in brain and eye tissue and in red blood cells. Apparently some is synthesized by intestinal bacteria.

Physiologic functions of inositol

No specific role of inositol in human nutrition has been established. Some evidence of a lipotropic effect (an affinity for fat, which enables some substances to decrease fat deposits in the liver) in animals led to its use in patients with cirrhosis. However, it failed to prove effective in reducing hepatic fat in such patients.

Inositol requirement

The requirement is unknown, since the role of inositol in human nutrition is undetermined.

---

*Notice the difference between the two words, "rickettsial" and "rickets." As explained in the section on PABA (p. 116), the term "rickettsial diseases" is based on the name of the discoverer of a group of microorganisms, Howard T. Ricketts. The term *rickets* is thought to have developed from an old English misspelling of the Greek word *rachitis.* The word rachitis is still a correct name for the group of diseases more familiarly known as rickets.

Food sources of inositol

Inositol is abundantly distributed in nature. It occurs in fruits, especially citrus fruits, in grains, nuts, and legumes. Animal sources include meat and milk.

Choline

Nature of choline

Choline is a second essential nutritional factor with vitaminlike activity and has long been known as a chemical compound. It was isolated from bile in 1862. It probably cannot be classified as a vitamin, since the body can manufacture choline and uses it in quantities larger than the small amounts that form part of the definition of the true vitamins (see p. 83). This biosynthesis of choline is established in animal experiments; it is not yet proved for man.

Choline deficiency states produced in animals include fatty liver and hemorrhagic kidney disease, but choline deficiency states have not been observed in man.

Choline is closely related to protein metabolism. Two essential amino acids are used by the animal body in the synthesis of choline.

Serine serves as a base, and methionine donates three methyl groups to complete it. Transferring these key single carbon groups to form vital products of metabolism is the important process of *transmethylation,* in which folic acid and vitamin B_{12} are coenzyme factors. Adequate dietary protein is therefore essential to supply building materials.

Choline is also a key component of two fat-related products. *Lecithin* is a phospholipid important in the metabolism of fat by the liver. *Sphingomyelin* is a phospholipid in brain and nerve tissue.

Physiologic functions of choline

Lipotropic agent. Choline seems to be an important lipotropic agent in hepatic fat metabolism. Lipotropic means "having an affinity for fat" (Gr. *lipos,* fat; *tropein,* to turn).

To prevent the accumulation of damaging amounts of fat in the liver, fat must be changed within the liver from storage forms to vehicular or transportation forms. Any substance that has an affinity for fat, and therefore attaches itself to fat in such a way that it changes the fat from

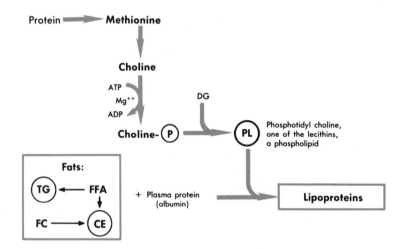

Fig. 7-2. Role of choline as a lipotropic agent in converting of fats to lipoproteins (transport form) for removal from the liver to adipose depots. Note that choline is produced from the essential amino acid methionine. (DG, diglyceride; TG, triglyceride; FFA, free fatty acid; FC, free cholesterol; CE, cholesterol ester; PL, phospholipid.)

a storage form into a transportation form, is called a lipotropic substance. The way in which choline acts in relation to hepatic fat has not been fully elucidated, but it is known that choline participates in phospholipid turnover. This turnover is the conversion of fatty acids to lipoproteins, the form in which they may be carried to the fat depots. This lipotropic role of choline may assume vital importance in liver disease such as hepatitis or cirrhosis. This important lipotropic role of choline is shown in Fig. 7-2.

Acetylcholine. Choline combines with active acetate to form acetylcholine, which reportedly functions as a mediator in nerve activity. There is some evidence that acetylcholine may have an influence on cell permeability.

Choline requirement

Dietary requirement for choline has not been stated. Materials required for its synthesis are choline precursors such as methionine.

Food sources of choline

Choline is widely distributed in foods, usually in association with proteins. Good sources include egg yolk, meat, cereals, and legumes. There is very little choline in fruits and vegetables.

A summary of the B vitamins and their roles in the body is given in Table 7-5.

VITAMIN C (ASCORBIC ACID)

Discovery of vitamin C. The fact that discovery is often the result of keen observation and asking why is illustrated in the history of the recognition of vitamin C and its association with the hemorrhagic disease scurvy (see p. 357). Documents describing the typical manifestations are as ancient as an Egyptian papyrus that dates from about 1500 BC. The Greek "father of medicine," Hippocrates, was concerned about scurvy. Crusaders of the thirteenth century observed the toll of the disease in their ranks. Jacques Cartier, exploring America in 1536, provided a clue to the cause of the

disease when he wrote in his log that he cured his dying men "almost overnight," simply by giving them a brew made from pine needles and bark. Officers of sailing vessels contributed further bits of information. In 1600 Captain Lancaster of the East India Company stated that he kept his crew hearty merely by the addition of a mandatory "three spoonfuls of lemon juice every morning." In 1753 the English naval surgeon, James Lind, concluded that the key must lie in a food factor in citrus fruit. The result was the official order for 1 oz of lemon or lime juice daily in every British sailor's food ration, and a name that stuck—"limies."

Thus the ground was laid for the research of the Norwegian scientists, Holst and Fröhlich, who in 1907 reproduced the disease in animals by feeding them a diet deficient in foods containing *ascorbic acid* (*a,* without; L. *scorbutus,* scurvy). In 1928 Szent-Györgyi, while working on cell oxidation in adrenal tissue, isolated a substance from the adrenals, and later from cabbage and from orange juice, which he believed to be a hexuronic acid derivative; he did not test it for antiscorbutic effect. In 1932 Charles Glen King[30] and W. A. Waugh, at the University of Pittsburgh, isolated and identified a hexuronic acid in lemon juice and demonstrated that it prevented or cured scurvy. The name ascorbic acid was given to this substance because of its antiscorbutic properties. The centuries-old scourge of scurvy had been defeated.[31]

Nature of vitamin C

Vitamin C is an odorless, white crystalline powder that is soluble in water but not in fat. It is an unstable, easily oxidized acid, and it can be destroyed by oxygen, alkalis, and high temperatures. It also reacts with the metallic ions of iron and copper.

A comparison of the chemical structure of vitamin C with glucose (Fig. 7-3) shows some striking similarities. Glucose is the natural precursor of vitamin C. Plants make the conversion

Table 7-5. Summary of B-complex vitamins

Vitamin	Physiologic functions	Clinical applications	Requirement	Food sources
Thiamin (B₁)	Coenzyme in carbohydrate metabolism: TPP—decarboxylation TDP—transketolation	Beriberi (deficiency) GI*: anorexia, gastric atony, indigestion, deficient hydrochloric acid CNS*: fatigue, apathy, neuritis, paralysis CV*: cardiac failure, peripheral vasodilation, and edema of extremities	0.5 mg/1,000 calories	Pork, beef, liver, whole or enriched grains, legumes
Riboflavin (B₂)	Coenzyme in protein of energy metabolism (flavoproteins) FMN (flavin mononucleotide) FAD (flavin-adenine dinucleotide)	Wound aggravation Cheilosis (cracks at corners of mouth) Glossitis Eye irritation; photophobia Seborrheic dermatitis	0.6 mg/1,000 calories	Milk, liver, enriched cereals
Niacin (nicotinic acid) (precursor —tryptophan)	Coenzyme in tissue oxidation to produce energy (ATP) NAD (nicotinamide-adenine dinucleotide) NADP (nicotinamide-adenine dinucleotide phosphate)	Pellagra (deficiency) Weakness, lassitude, anorexia Skin: scaly dermatitis CNS: neuritis, confusion	14-20 mg (NE)	Meat, peanuts, enriched grains
Pyridoxine (B₆)	Coenzyme in amino acid metabolism Decarboxylation Deamination Transamination Transsulfuration Niacin formation from tryptophan Heme formation Amino acid absorption	Anemia (hypochromic microcytic) CNS: hyperirritability, convulsions, neuritis Isoniazid is an antagonist for pyridoxine Pregnancy: anemia	2 mg	Wheat, corn, meat, liver
Pantothenic acid	Coenzyme in formation of active acetate (CoA)—acetylation	Contributes to: Lipogenesis Amino acid activation Formation of cholesterol		Liver, egg, skimmed milk

Vitamin	Physiologic function	Clinical significance	Requirement	Sources
		Formation of steroid hormones Formation of heme Excretion of drugs		
Lipoic acid (sulfur-containing fatty acid)	Coenzyme (with thiamin) in carbohydrate metabolism to reduce pyruvate to active acetate Oxidative decarboxylation	Undetermined (see thiamin)		Liver, yeast
Biotin	Coenzyme in decarboxylation (synthesis of fatty acids, amino acids, purines); deamination	Undetermined		Egg yolk, liver
Folic acid (B₉)	Coenzyme for single carbon transfer—purines, thymine, hemoglobin Transmethylation	Blood cell regeneration in pernicious anemia but not control of its neurologic problems Megaloblastic anemia Macrocytic anemia of pregnancy Sprue treatment Aminopterin is folic acid antagonist	400 μg Pregnancy: 800 μg Lactation: 800 μg	Liver, green leafy vegetables, asparagus
PABA (part of folic acid)		Treatment of rickettsial diseases Anemias (see folic acid)		Same as folic acid
Cobalamin (B₁₂)	Coenzyme in protein synthesis Formation of nucleic acid and cell proteins—red blood cells Transmethylation	Extrinsic factor in pernicious anemia—combines with intrinsic factor of gastric secretions for absorption; forms red blood cells (with folic acid) Sprue treatment (with folic acid)	3 μg	Liver, meat, milk, egg, cheese
Inositol	Lipotropic agent (?)	Undetermined		Citrus fruit, grains, meat, milk
Choline	Lipotropic agent Forms nerve mediator—acetylcholine	Fatty liver—hepatitis, cirrhosis (undetermined in human nutrition)		Meat, cereals, egg yolk

*GI = Gastrointestinal; CNS = Central nervous system; CV = Cardiovascular.

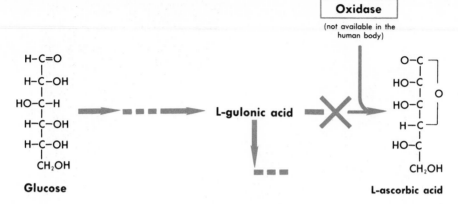

Fig. 7-3. Metabolic relation of glucose to ascorbic acid. In humans the absence of oxidase prevents this reaction, making the intake of preformed ascorbic acid in food necessary.

from glucose to produce the vitamin. Almost every animal species can also make ascorbic acid and, therefore do not require a food source for this vitamin. The exceptions include man, monkeys, guinea pigs, a rare Indian fruit bat, and the red-vented bulbul (a bird). These species lack the enzyme necessary to make the conversion from L-gulonic acid to ascorbic acid, and the material is diverted into other metabolites. Scurvy, then, in man in the final analysis can really be called a disease of distant genetic origin in the evolution of our species, an inherited metabolic error. A defect in carbohydrate metabolism results from the lack of an enzyme, which in turn results from the lack of a specific gene.

Metabolism of vitamin C. Vitamin C is easily absorbed from the small intestine.[32] Absorption is hindered by a lack of hydrochloric acid or by bleeding from the gastrointestinal tract. Vitamin C is not stored in single tissue depots, but is more generally distributed throughout body tissues. The amount of vitamin C in white blood cells is used as a general indicator of the degree of body tissue saturation. A small amount (from 1.0 to 1.2 mg/100 ml) circulates in blood plasma, and any excess is readily excreted. Excretion depends on the

quantity ingested and the state of tissue stores. Sufficient vitamin C for needs in early infancy is present in breast milk. Because cow's milk does not contain an adequate supply for the requirements of the human infant, formulas must be supplemented with ascorbic acid.

Physiologic functions of vitamin C

Intercellular cement substance. The well-established role of vitamin C in human nutrition concerns the provision of an intercellular cementing substance that is necessary to build supportive tissue. The presence of vitamin C is required to build and maintain bone matrix, cartilage, dentine, collagen, and connective tissue. Just how vitamin C functions in this process is not known, but when vitamin C is absent, the important ground substance does not develop into collagen. When vitamin C is given, formation of cartilaginous tissue follows quickly. *Collagen* is a protein substance that exists in many tissues of the body, such as the white fibers of connective tissue. The term is derived from two Greek words: *kolla,* glue; and *gennan,* to produce. Evidently vitamin C must help provide the glue.

Vascular tissue particularly is weakened without the cementing substance of vitamin C

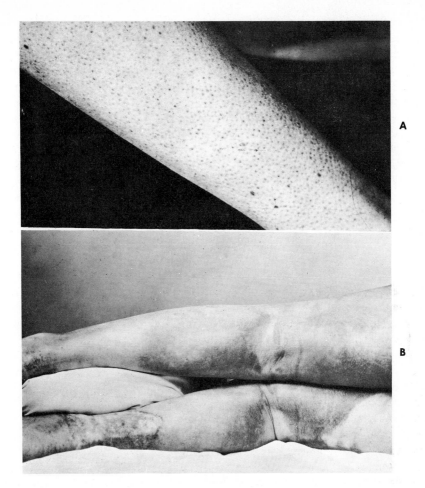

Fig. 7-4. A, Perifollicular hemorrhages of early scurvy. **B,** Ecchymosis of scurvy. (From Merck Report, May, 1956, Merck and Co., Inc., Rahway, N.J.)

to provide firm capillary walls. Therefore vitamin C deficiency states are characterized by fragile, easily ruptured capillaries with consequent diffuse tissue bleeding. Clinical conditions include easy bruising, pinpoint peripheral hemorrhages (Fig. 7-4), bone and joint hemorrhages, easy bone fracture, poor wound healing, and friable bleeding gums with loosened teeth (gingivitis).

General body metabolism. Continuing research is bringing to light facts that raise interesting questions and may indicate an even broader role in vitamin C in general body metabolism. The fact that there is a greater concentration of vitamin C in the more metabolically active tissues such as adrenal, brain, kidney, liver, pancreas, thymus and spleen, than in less active tissues, and that there is more vitamin C in a child's actively multiplying tissue than in adult tissue must mean there are vital interrelationships among vitamin C, protein, and cell metabolism processes.

In the formation of hemoglobin and maturation of red blood cells, vitamin C influences the removal of iron from ferritin (the protein-iron-phosphorus complex in which iron is stored), particularly in reticuloendothelial cells of the liver, spleen, and bone marrow. Because of this reaction more iron is made available in the body fluids. Vitamin C also influences the conversion in the liver of folic acid to a related compound, folinic acid. This is the citrovorum factor (p. 115) which has been used in the treatment of megaloblastic anemia.

A relationship of vitamin C to several amino acids may be indicated by certain observations made in the search for protein links:

1. Metabolism of phenylalanine and tyrosine is defective in premature infants who lack adequate vitamin C. In several reactions, tyrosine is not converted properly without vitamin C.
2. Vitamin C seems to participate in the synthesis of hydroxyproline from proline. This may be related to its role in collagen formation.

Large amounts of vitamin C are present in adrenal tissue; a dose of ACTH depletes the adrenal tissue of this substance.

Clinical applications

Wound healing. The significant role of vitamin C in cementing the ground substance of supportive tissue makes it an important agent in wound healing.[33] This has evident implications for vitamin C therapy in surgery, especially where extensive tissue regeneration is involved. For example, during the acute stage, a patient who has undergone mastectomy or a severe burn may need from 1 to 2 g daily of vitamin C, which is 10 times or more the usual daily allowance.

Fevers and infections. Infectious processes deplete tissue stores of vitamin C and necessitate additional intake. Apparently this is especially true of infection with bacteria. Optimum tissue stores of vitamin C help maintain resistance to infection.

Just how large a therapeutic dose may be re-

quired to maintain this prevention of infections is not known. There is much controversy concerning the effectiveness of massive doses of vitamin C in the prevention of the common cold. Although such large doses of vitamin C may have some pharmacologic or druglike effects, these are not related to the normal functioning of the vitamin at nutritional levels.[34] Vitamin C beyond the level at which tissue saturation is maintained is excreted in the urine. Hence with megadoses, one may only be producing an expensive urine rather than maintaining great therapeutic value. Fevers also deplete tissue stores of vitamin C as they accompany infectious processes and produce a catabolic effect on tissues.

Reaction to stress. Any body stress—injury, fracture, general illness, shock—calls on vitamin C tissue stores. This seems indicated by the large concentration of vitamin in adrenal tissue.[35]

Table 7-6. National Research Council allowances for vitamin C

	Age (yr)	Vitamin C (mg)
Males and females	Birth-0.5	35
	0.5-1	35
	1-3	45
	4-6	45
	7-10	45
Males	11-14	60
	15-18	60
	19-22	60
	23-50	60
	51+	60
Females	11-14	50
	15-18	60
	19-22	60
	23-50	60
	51+	60
Pregnant		+20
Lactating		+40

Growth periods. Additional vitamin C is needed during growth periods (infancy and childhood) and during pregnancy to supply demands for fetal growth and maternal tissues.

Vitamin C requirement

Difficulties in establishing requirements for vitamin C involve questions concerning individual tissue need, and whether minimum or optimum intakes are desired. Although studies indicate that a lower intake (from 20 to 30 mg daily) may suffice for the average adult, the NRC's revised 1980 allowances recommend 60 mg daily for optimum margins to cover variances in tissue demand (Table 7-6).

In considering vitamin C requirements, it seems wise to follow such logical recommendations as those of the NRC to provide safety ranges for optimum need. At the same time, it seems wise to avoid extravagant and wasteful excesses in the name of general good health when the situation does not demand therapeutic measures.

Food sources of vitamin C

Because of the ease with which vitamin C can be oxidized, the handling, preparation, cooking, and processing of any food source should be considered in evaluating its contribution of the vitamin. Well-known sources include citrus fruit and tomatoes. Less regarded, but good additional sources, include cabbage, sweet potatoes, white potatoes, and green and yellow vegetables. Other sources are seasonal, local, or regional foods such as berries, melons, chili peppers, green peppers, guavas, pineapple, chard, kale, turnip greens, broccoli, and asparagus.

A summary of vitamin C and its role in the body is given in Table 7-7.

BIOFLAVONOIDS
Nature of bioflavonoids

In the mid-1930s Szent-Györgyi and his co-workers[36] isolated a material from citrus rind that they called *citrin*. Their initial tests of it with scorbutic guinea pigs, reported in 1936, seemed to indicate that this new substance was effective, together with ascorbic acid, in decreasing capillary permeability and in curing scurvy. Therefore they named the substance "Permeabilitäts-Vitamin," or vitamin P.

Continued study proved that citrin was the flavanone hesperidin, which is one of a widely occurring group of natural pigments in flowers, fruits, grains, and vegetables. These substances were called *flavonoids* because of their basic yellow coloring (L. *flavus,* yellow). Some of these materials are naturally occurring yellow dyes.

Table 7-7. Summary of vitamin C (ascorbic acid)

Physiologic functions	Clinical applications	Requirement	Food sources

Intercellular cement substance:
  1. Collagen formation
  2. Firm capillary walls
General metabolism:
  1. Makes iron available for hemoglobin and maturation of red blood cells
  2. Influences conversion of folic acid to "citrovorum factor" (folinic acid)
	Scurvy (deficiency)
	Megaloblastic anemia
	Wound healing; tissue formation
	Fevers and infections
	Stress reactions
	Growth periods
		60 mg daily
		(adults)
			Citrus fruits
			Tomatoes
			Cabbage
			Potatoes
			Strawberries
			Melon
			Chili peppers

Nutritional significance of bioflavonoids

The early high hopes held for the flavonoids, however, did not materialize. Szent-Györgyi reported in 1938[28] that subsequent tests did not confirm the results of his earlier experiments, and similar work in other laboratories verified his conclusions. As a result, in 1950 the Joint Committee on Biochemical Nomenclature of the American Society of Biological Chemists and the American Institute of Nutrition recommended that the term "vitamin P" be discontinued. Since then the term "bioflavonoid" has been used instead, although the term "vitamin P" may still appear occasionally in the literature.

In the years since Szent-Györgyi's original work, numerous workers have studied the effects of the flavonoids (*citrin* from citrus rind and *rutin* from buckwheat) on capillary fragility, infections, the common cold, hypertension, and various hemorrhagic disorders. As yet, no therapeutic value has been demonstrated. Although the bioflavonoids may possess mild pharmacologic properties under certain conditions, they have no known nutritional functions, and cannot be considered essential nutrients.

GLOSSARY

antagonist a substance that counteracts the action of another substance. The antagonist prevents the normal action because its molecular structure is so like that of the first substance that it *almost* fits into the first substance's position in a metabolic process. It gets in the way and prevents the reaction from taking place.

beriberi (Sinhalese *beri,* weakness) a disease of the peripheral nerves caused by a deficiency of thiamin (vitamin B_1). It is characterized by pain (neuritis) and paralysis of the extremities, cardiovascular changes, and edema. Beriberi is common in the Orient where diets consist largely of milled rice with little protein.

bioflavonoids compounds that are widely distributed in nature as pigments in flowers, fruits, tree barks, vegetables, and grains. In the late 1930s, a bioflavonoid material found in the peel of citrus fruit (citrin) was thought to have antiscorbutic properties (decreasing capillary fragility) and was termed "Permeabilitäts-Vitamin," or "vitamin P." However, these results were refuted by later tests, and in 1950 the term "vitamin

P" was officially dropped. Since then the term "bioflavonoid" has replaced it. Continuing attempts to determine its role, if any, in capillary fragility, treatment of the common cold, and so on, have yielded no data that support any valid clinical role for the flavonoids.

biotin a B vitamin sometimes called the "anti-egg white injury" factor because it was discovered as the preventive substance for a curious eczema and paralysis observed in rats fed large amounts of raw egg white. In very small amounts, biotin appears to function as a coenzyme in metabolism during carboxylation and deamination reactions. It is found mainly in egg yolk.

cheilosis (Gr. *cheilos,* lips) a riboflavin deficiency condition in which the lips become swollen, crack easily, and characteristic cracks form at the corners of the mouth.

choline although not a true vitamin, choline is sometimes grouped with the B complex because it has vitaminlike activity related to animal growth. Choline has a vital role in nutrition as a lipotropic agent in the liver by preventing fat accumulation there. Choline is synthesized from the essential amino acid, methionine, and is a key component of the phospholipid lecithin. Choline also combines with active acetate to form the important compound acetylcholine, which mediates nerve activity.

citrovorum factor see *folinic acid.*

cobalamin (B_{12}) the B vitamin that controls pernicious anemia. B_{12} is the extrinsic factor, which combines with the intrinsic factor (a mucoprotein enzyme of the gastric secretions) to be absorbed and carried to various organs for use or storage. Many of its functions seem to be linked to those of folic acid, perhaps indicating that B_{12} may activate folic acid. B_{12} is a distinctive B vitamin. It is a large, complex compound of high molecular weight with a single red cobalt atom at its core. Its dietary sources are almost entirely animal foods—liver, lean meat, milk, egg, cheese. The only known natural dietary deficiency has been observed in true vegetarians.

collagen (Gr. *kolla,* glue; *gennan,* to produce) the protein in connective tissue and bones that helps give support, structure, and cohesiveness to the whole body. Collagen has a gelatinlike quality.

decarboxylation removal of the carboxyl group from certain chemical compounds to form other compounds. In the important decarboxylation of pyruvate to form active acetate (and hence its entrance into the Krebs cycle to produce energy) thiamin is part of the necessary coenzyme TPP. Thiamin is a vital key that unlocks and releases energy for action of muscles and nerves.

ferritin the protein-iron-phosphorus complex in which iron is stored, particularly in reticuloendothelial cells of the liver, spleen, and bone marrow. Vitamin C helps to make iron available for use by influencing its removal from the ferritin complex.

flavin-adenine dinucleotide (FAD) a riboflavin enzyme containing two high-energy phosphate bonds. It is a highly active coenzyme that operates in many reactions that affects amino acids, glucose, and fatty acids.

flavin mononucleotide (FMN) a riboflavin phosphate compound that acts as a coenzyme in the deamination of certain amino acids.

flavoproteins the enzymes of which riboflavin is an important constituent (FMN and FAD).

folic acid the B vitamin (B_9) discovered as a factor in the control of pernicious anemia. Folic acid only temporarily aids in regenerating the red blood cells in pernicious anemia and does not control the associated degenerative neurologic problems. Vitamin B_{12} has since been found to be the fully effective agent. A nutritional megaloblastic anemia due to folic acid deficiency has been clearly described, however, as well as a macrocytic anemia of pregnancy. Folic acid functions in metabolism as a coenzyme for transferring single carbon (C_1) units for attachment in many reactions. In this role, folic acid is a key substance in cell growth and reproduction through aiding in the formation of nucleoproteins and hemoglobin.

folinic acid a derivative of folic acid, which has been used in the treatment of megaloblastic anemia. Vitamin C influences this conversion of folic acid to folinic acid in the liver.

hematopoiesis (Gr. *haima*, blood; *poiein*, to form) the formation of blood.

inositol an intermediary compound between aromatic substances and glucose, classed in the B complex because it has vitaminlike activity. It seems to possess some lipotropic ability, but as yet its precise role in human nutrition is undetermined. Inositol occurs in grains, especially wheat, as an ester with phosphoric acid (phytin).

lactoflavin the form in which riboflavin occurs in milk.

lipoic acid a sulfur-containing fatty acid. Although it is not a true vitamin, lipoic acid is classed with the B vitamins because its coenzyme function is closely related to thiamin.

NAD (nicotinamide-adenine dinucleotide) a niacin compound with two high-energy phosphate bonds, which functions as an important coenzyme in tissue oxidation to release controlled energy.

NADP (nicotinamide-adenine dinucleotide phosphate) a niacin compound with three high-energy phosphate bonds, which acts as a vital coenzyme in the "respiratory chains" of tissue oxidation within the cell; controlled energy is made available by this reaction.

niacin a B vitamin, nicotinic acid, the lack of which produces pellagra. Important niacin compounds (NAD and NADP) function as key coenzymes in glucose oxidation. Niacin's relation to pellagra was discovered by Joseph Goldberger. Meat is a major source of niacin; also peanuts, enriched grains, and legumes. The essential amino acid, tryptophan, is a precursor of niacin.

niacin equivalent (NE) a unit of measure used for the amount of tryptophan (60 mg) that produces 1 mg of niacin in the body. Because tryptophan is a precursor of niacin and thus an additional source, dietary requirements for niacin are usually given in terms of total niacin and niacin equivalents.

PABA (para-aminobenzoic acid) although not a true vitamin, PABA is a structural component of folic acid. Its action as an essential cell growth factor is secondary to that of folic acid. Clinically, PABA has been used to treat some rickettsial diseases. It is effective because it acts as an antagonist to a material essential to the growth of the rickettsiae.

pantothenic acid (Gr. *pantothen*, from every side) a B vitamin found widely distributed in nature and occurring throughout body tissues. Pantothenic acid is an essential constituent of the enzyme CoA, which has extensive metabolic responsibility as an activating agent of a number of compounds in many tissues.

pellagra (L. *pelle*, skin; Gr. *agra*, seizure) a deficiency disease caused by a lack of niacin in the diet and an inadequate amount of protein containing the amino acid, tryptophan, a precursor of niacin. Pellagra is characterized by skin lesions that are aggravated by exposure to sunlight and by gastrointestinal, mucosal, neurologic, and mental symptoms. Four "D's" often associated with pellagra are dermatitis, diarrhea, dementia, and death.

pernicious anemia a chronic, macrocytic anemia occurring most commonly in Caucasians after age 40. It is caused by the absence of the intrinsic factor normally present in gastric juice. The intrinsic factor is necessary for the absorption of vitamin B_{12}, the extrinsic factor required for proper formation of red blood cells. Pernicious anemia is controlled by intramuscular injections of vitamin B_{12}.

pyridoxine (vitamin B_6) in its active phosphate form (B_6-PO_4), pyridoxine functions as an important coenzyme in many reactions in the metabolism of amino acids and to a lesser extent in the metabolism of glucose and fatty acids. Clinically, pyridoxine deficiency produces a hypochromic, microcytic anemia and disturbances of the central nervous system. Isoniazid (INH) used to treat tuberculosis, is a pyridoxine antagonist and produces side effects of pyridoxine deficiency. Large doses of pyridoxine prevent these side effects of neuritis.

riboflavin a B vitamin (B_2); a yellow-green pigment that contains ribose. B_2 is found mainly in milk as lactoflavin and also in leafy green vegetables and organ meats. Riboflavin forms coenzymes (FMN and FAD) important in the metabolism of amino acids, glucose, and fatty acids.

rickettsial diseases diseases in man and in animals caused by microscopic parasites of the genus *Rickettsia*. These are minute pathogenic organisms about midway in size between bacteria and viruses. They live in the intestinal tract of arthropods such as mites, ticks, fleas, and lice and are transmitted to humans by these biting insects. They cause such diseases as typhus and Rocky Mountain spotted fever.

scurvy a hemorrhagic disease caused by lack of vitamin C. Without vitamin C, the intercellular cement substance provided by this vitamin is missing; therefore capillary walls, bone matrix, cartilage, collagen, and connective tissue are not properly formed. As a result, diffuse tissue bleeding occurs, limbs and joints are painful and swollen, bones thicken due to subperiosteal hemorrhage, ecchymoses (large irregular discolored skin areas due to tissue hemorrhages) form, bones fracture easily, wounds do not heal well, gums are swollen and bleeding, and teeth loosen.

TDP (thiamin diphosphate) the activating coenzyme (acting with the enzyme *transketolase*) necessary for the transketolation reaction in the hexose monophosphate shunt (glucose oxidation) by which active glyceraldehyde is formed for lipogenesis (synthesis of fats).

thiamin a major B vitamin (B_1); essential for the normal metabolism of carbohydrates and fats. It acts as a coenzyme (TPP and TDP) in two key reactions: (1) decarboxylation by which active acetate is formed from pyruvate and (2) transketolation by which intermediate products are formed between carbohydrate and fat. A deficiency of thiamin hinders energy production and proper functioning of muscles and nerves. Muscle weakness and nerve irritation result, involving the gastrointestinal tract, the cardiovascular system, and the central nervous system. Extreme continued deficiency produces beriberi, paralysis, edema, and death. Thiamin is found in whole or enriched grains, meats, and legumes.

transketolation transfer of the first 2-carbon group

$$CH_2OH - \overset{\overset{\displaystyle O}{\|}}{C} - C -$$

($CH_2OH - C - C -$) from one sugar to another in the hexose monophosphate shunt (glucose oxidation pathway). This transfer produces active glyceraldehyde, a necessary component for synthesizing fats (triglycerides). The reaction requires thiamin diphosphate (TDP) as an activating coenzyme.

REFERENCES
Specific

1. Williams, R. R.: Toward the conquest of beriberi, Cambridge, Mass., 1961, Harvard University Press.
2. Williams, R. R.: Recollections of the "beriberi-preventing substance," Nutr. Rev. **11**:257, 1953.
3. Horwitt, M. K.: Thiamine, riboflavin, and niacin. In Wohl, M. G., and Goodhart, R. S., editors: Modern nutrition in health and disease, Philadelphia, 1964, Lea & Febiger, p. 385.
4. György, P.: Early experiences with riboflavin—a retrospect, Nutr. Rev. **12**:97, 1954.
5. Elvehjem, C. A.: Early experiences with niacin—a retrospect, Nutr. Rev. **11**:289, 1953.
6. Todhunter, E. N.: The story of nutrition. In Stefferud, A., editor: Food, the yearbook of agriculture, 1959, Washington, D.C., 1959, U.S. Department of Agriculture, p. 7.
7. Roe, D. A.: A plague of corn: the social history of pellagra, Ithaca, N.Y., 1973, Cornell University Press.
8. Goldsmith, G. A.: Niacin-tryptophan relationships in man and niacin requirements, Am. J. Clin. Nutr. **6**: 479, 1958.
9. Goldsmith, G. A., et al.: Efficiency of tryptophan as a niacin precursor in man, J. Nutr. **73**:172, 1961.
10. György, P.: The history of vitamin B_6, Am. J. Clin. Nutr. **4**:313, July-Aug., 1956.
11. Lepkovsky, S.: Early experiences of pyridoxine—a retrospect, Nutr. Rev. **12**:257, 1954.
12. Aly, H. E., Donald, E. A., and Simpson, M. H. W.: Oral contraceptives and vitamin B_6 metabolism, Am. J. Clin. Nutr. **24**:297, 1971.
13. Brin, M.: Abnormal tryptophan metabolism in pregnancy and with the contraceptive pill, Am. J. Clin. Nutr. **24**:704, 1971.
14. Lubby, A. L., Brin, M., Gordon, M., et al.: Vitamin B_6 metabolism in uses of oral contraceptive agents, Am. J. Clin. Nutr. **24**:684, 1971.
15. Williams, R. J.: Early experiences with pantothenic acid—a retrospect, Nutr. Rev. **12**:65, 1954.
16. Reed, L. J., et al.: Crystalline α-lipoic acid: a catalytic agent associated with pyruvate dehydrogenase, Science **114**:93, 1951.
17. Sydenstricker, V. P.: "Egg-white injury" in man and its cure with a biotin concentrate, J.A.M.A. **118**: 1199, 1942.
18. Viltner, R. W.: Folic acid. In Wohl, M. G., and Goodhart, R. S., editors: Modern nutrition in health and disease, Philadelphia, 1964, Lea & Febiger, p. 410.
19. Angier, R. B., Stokstad, E. L. R., et al.: The structure and synthesis of the liver *L. casei* factor, Science **103**: 667, 1946.
20. Unglaub, W. G., and Goldsmith, G. A.: Folic acid and vitamin B_{12} in medical practice, J.A.M.A. **161**:623, 1956.
21. Streiff, R. R., and Little, A. B.: Folic acid deficiency in pregnancy, N. Engl. J. Med. **276**:776, 1967.
22. Giles, C., and Shuttleworth, E.: Megaloblastic anemia of pregnancy and the puerperium, Lancet **7061**:1341, 1958.

23. Wong, R. I. H.: Practical drug therapy, Philadelphia, 1979, J. B. Lippincott Co., p. 606.
24. Butterfield, S., and Calloway, D. H.: Folacin in wheat and selected foods, J. Am. Diet. Assoc. **60:**310, 1972.
25. Streiff, R. R.: Folate levels in citrus and other juices, Am. J. Clin. Nutr. **24:**1390, 1971.
26. Thenen, S. W.: Food folate values, Am. J. Clin. Nutr. **28:**1341, 1975.
27. Rickes, E. L., et al.: Crystalline vitamin B$_{12}$, Science **107:**396, 1948.
28. West, R.: Activity of vitamin B$_{12}$ in Addisonian pernicious anemia, Science **107:**398, 1948.
29. Smith, E. L.: Purification of anti-pernicious anemia factors from liver, Nature **161:**638, 1948.
30. King, C. G.: Early experiences with ascorbic acid— a retrospect, Nutr. Rev. **12:**1, 1954.
31. Lorenz, A. J.: The conquest of scurvy, J. Am. Diet. Assoc. **30:**665, 1954.
32. Stevenson, N. R.: Active transport of L-ascorbic acid in the human ileum, Gastroenterology **67:**952, 1974.
33. Schwartz, F. W.: Ascorbic acid in wound healing—a review, J. Am. Diet. Assoc. **56:**497, 1979.
34. Anderson, T. W., Reid, D., and Beaton, G. H.: Vitamin C and the common cold: a double-blind trial, Can. Med. Assoc. J. **107:**503, 1972.
35. Hodges, R. E.: The effect of stress on ascorbic acid metabolism in man, Nutr. Today **5:**11, 1970.
36. Pearson, W. N.: Flavonoids in human nutrition and medicine, J.A.M.A. **164:**1675, 1957.

General

Abt, A. F., et al.: Vitamin C requirements of man re-examined, Am. J. Clin. Nutr. **12:**21, 1963.
Baber, S., and Srikantic, S. G.: Availability of folates from some foods, Am. J. Clin. Nutr. **29:**276, 1976.
Best, C. H., and Taylor, N. B., editors: The physiological basis of medical practice, ed. 8, Baltimore, 1966, The Williams & Wilkins Co.
Bridgers, W. F.: Present knowledge of biotin, Nutr. Rev. **25:**65, 1967.
Donald, E. A., et al.: Vitamin B$_6$ requirement of young adult women, Am. J. Clin. Nutr. **24:**1028, 1971.
Drapanas, T., et al.: Role of the ileum in the absorption of vitamin B$_{12}$ and intrinsic factor, J.A.M.A. **184:**337, 1963.
FAO/WHO of the United Nations: Requirements of vitamin A, thiamine, riboflavin, and niacin, FAO Nutr. Meet. Rep. Ser. No. 41; WHO Tech. Rep. Ser. No. 362, Rome, 1967.
Folic acid biochemistry and physiology in relation to the human nutrition requirement, Washington, D.C., 1977, National Academy of Sciences.
Food and Nutrition Board, National Research Council,

National Academy of Sciences: Recommended dietary allowances, Rev. 1980, Washington, D.C.
György, P.: Reminiscences on the discovery and significance of some of the B vitamins, J. Nutr. **91:**5, 1967.
Halstead, C. H.: The small intestine in vitamin B$_{12}$ and folate deficiency, Nutr. Rev. **33:**33, 1975.
Harper, H. A.: Review of physiological chemistry, ed. 15, Los Altos, Calif., 1975, Lange Medical Publications.
Hegsted, D. M., editor: Present knowledge in nutrition, ed. 4, New York, 1976, The Nutrition Foundation.
Hodges, R. E., et al.: Clinical manifestations of ascorbic acid deficiency in man, Am. J. Clin. Nutr. **24:**432, 1971.
Horwitt, M. K.: Nutritional requirements of man, with special reference to riboflavin, Am. J. Clin. Nutr. **18:** 458, 1966.
Hsu, J. M.: Effect of deficiencies of certain B vitamins and ascorbic acid on absorption of vitamin B$_{12}$, Am. J. Clin. Nutr. **12:**170, 1963.
Lopez, A., et al.: Influence of time and temperature on ascorbic acid stability, J. Am. Diet. Assoc. **50:**308, 1967.
McCollum, E. V.: The paths to the discovery of vitamins A and D, J. Nutr. **91:**11, 1967.
Noble, I.: Ascorbic acid and color of vegetables, J. Am. Diet. Assoc. **50:**304, 1967.
Reviews: The citrovorum factor, Nutr. Rev. **9:**24, 1951; Nutrition and metabolic bone disease in the elderly, Nutr. Rev. **25:**71, 1967; Riboflavin deficiency and anemia in man, Nutr. Rev. **23:**197, 1965; Vitamin B$_6$ component in various foods, Nutr. Rev. **23:**78, 1965.
Santini, R., et al.: The distribution of folic acid active compounds in individual foods, Am. J. Clin. Nutr. **14:**205, 1964.
Sherlock, P., and Rothschild, E. O.: Scurvy produced by a Zen macrobiotic diet, J.A.M.A. **199:**794, 1967.
Streiff, R. R., and Little, A. B.: Folic acid deficiency in pregnancy, N. Engl. J. Med. **276:**776, 1967.
Sydenstricker, V. P.: History of pellagra, its recognition as a disorder of nutrition and its conquest, Am. J. Clin. Nutr. **6:**409, 1958.
Unglaub, W. B., and Goldsmith, G. A.: Folic acid and vitamin B$_{12}$ in medical practice, J.A.M.A. **161:**623, 1956.
Viltner, R. W.: Vitamin B$_6$ in medical practice, J.A.M.A. **159:**1210, 1955.
Vitale, J. J.: Present knowledge of folacin, Nutr. Rev. **24:** 289, 1966.
Wachstein, M.: Evidence of abnormal vitamin B$_6$ metabolism in pregnancy and various disease states, Am. J. Clin. Nutr. **4:**369, 1956.
Wilson, T. H.: Intrinsic factor and B$_{12}$ absorption—a problem in cell physiology, Nutr. Rev. **23:**33, 1965.

8 The minerals

One remaining group of nutrients is essential to humans—the minerals. Minerals are inorganic elements widely distributed in nature, and many of them have vital roles in metabolism. Their metabolic roles are as varied as the minerals are themselves. These substances, which appear so inert in comparison with the complex, organic vitamin compounds, fulfill an impressive variety of metabolic functions. They are builders, activators, regulators, transmitters, and controllers. For example, ionized sodium and potassium exercise all-important control over shifts in the locale of body fluids; dynamic calcium and phosphorus provide structural body framework; oxygen-hungry iron gives a core to heme in hemoglobin; brilliant red cobalt is the atom at the core of vitamin B_{12}; and iodine is a necessary constituent of thyroxine. Far from being static, inert body materials, the minerals are active participants in the overall metabolic process.

The minerals found in the human body may be grouped according to whether they are present in large amounts (major minerals), are present in small amounts and have a known function (trace minerals), or are present in small amounts but their function is not understood. There are seven minerals in each of the first two groups and ten minerals in the third group. The major minerals contribute from 60% to 80% of all the inorganic material in the human body.

Group I: Major minerals

Calcium (Ca)
Phosphorus (P)
Magnesium (Mg)
Sodium (Na)
Potassium (K)
Chlorine (Cl)
Sulfur (S)

Group II: Trace minerals (known function)

Iron (Fe)
Copper (Cu)
Iodine (I)
Manganese (Mn)
Cobalt (Co)
Zinc (Zn)
Molybdenum (Mo)

Group III: Trace minerals (function unknown)

Fluorine (Fl)
Selenium (Se)
Aluminum (Al)
Boron (B)
Cadmium (Cd)
Chromium (Cr)
Nickel (Ni)
Tin (Sn)
Silicon (Si)
Vanadium (V)

Although the precise function of the trace minerals in group III is not altogether clear in human nutrition, new knowledge is constantly coming to light. Each of the minerals in groups I and II is known to act dynamically in human physiology. Each mineral will be considered separately. To trace the metabolic activity of each mineral, the answers to the following four questions will be considered:

1. How much of each mineral normally occurs in the body, and in what chemical form is it found?
2. What does each mineral do in the body; where and how does it act?
3. What is the clinical significance of each mineral, and what are some of its relationships to health and disease?
4. How much of each mineral is required in food, and what are the food sources of each mineral?

MAJOR MINERALS
Calcium
Occurrence in the body

Of all the minerals in the human body, calcium is present in by far the largest amounts.

It comprises about 1.5% to 2.0% of the total body weight. A person weighing 54 kg (120 lb) has about 0.9 kg (2 lb) of calcium in his body. Ninety-nine percent of this mineral is in skeletal tissue (bones and teeth) as deposits of the calcium salts dahllite or apatite. The ratio of calcium to phosphorus in the bone compartment is about 2:1.[1]

The remaining 1% of the total body calcium performs highly important metabolic tasks. This 1% occurs in the plasma and other body fluids.

The approximate distribution of calcium in plasma and interstitial fluids is indicated in Fig. 8-1. The normal serum calcium level is about 10 mg/dl of serum or 5 meq/L. The narrow normal range of 9 to 11 mg/dl indicates how strictly this level must be guarded and maintained. The main guardian of the serum calcium level is the parathyroid hormone, which will be discussed later in this chapter.

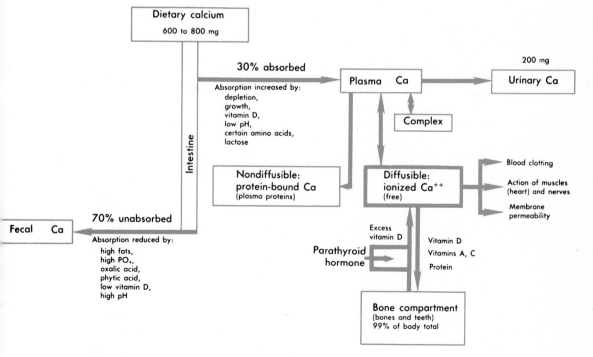

Fig. 8-1. Calcium metabolism. Note the relative distribution of calcium in the body.

The 1% of total body calcium that appears in the body fluids occurs in three forms: (1) nondiffusible, (2) diffusible, and (3) diffusible but a constituent of an organic complex. These three fractions are normally in equilibrium.

1. About half of the calcium in the plasma and other body fluids is bound with the plasma proteins, albumin and globulin. This is the nondiffusible fraction. Since the levels of plasma proteins vary, the size of this fraction also varies.
2. Diffusible calcium is ionized free calcium $(Ca++)$ and makes up the other half of the calcium in the plasma. It has the greatest physiologic effect of the three fractions. It exerts a profound influence on metabolism and function of bone, the nervous system, and the heart.
3. About 5% of the plasma calcium is diffusible but occurs as part of organic complexes such as citrate and other substances.

Metabolism of calcium

The metabolism of calcium, like that of any substance, may be considered in two broad aspects: (1) as a substance in its own right and (2) according to the physiologic function it performs in the body. It is taken for granted that calcium is important to the body, and inquiry is made into the ways in which the body maintains its calcium level. This leads directly to the concept of *homeostasis* (Gr. *homois,* unchanging; *stasis,* standing), which means to maintain a state of balance. Modern physiologists emphasize that every state of balance is maintained *dynamically* by constant interaction of the components that make up the whole. Calcium may also be looked at as a functioning component of the total body. Calcium is not only maintained by metabolic functions of the body, it contributes *to* the total metabolic interactions of the body and therefore has its own physiologic functions.

Homeostasis. Balance mechanisms are constantly at work to maintain the level of calcium in the circulating plasma within its narrow, normal range. The concepts that have emerged from physiologists' study of these mechanisms are basic to the understanding of the metabolism of many substances and are highly significant. As they apply to calcium, these homeostatic mechanisms involve four interrelated metabolic activities:

General metabolic concept	Application to calcium homeostasis
1. Maintenance of intestinal absorption-excretion balance	1. Intestinal adjustment of calcium absorption and excretion
2. Renal adjustment of excretion (the kidney threshold)	2. Renal adjustment of calcium excretion in the urine
3. Maintenance of a storage compartment	3. Maintenance of calcium stores in bone
4. Hormonal regulation	4. Parathyroid hormone control of calcium homeostasis

These mechanisms may be organized around two basic pairs of balances: (1) absorption-excretion balance and (2) deposition-mobilization balance.

Absorption-excretion balance

Absorption. From 10% to 30% of the calcium in an average diet is absorbed through the intestine. Absorption apparently takes place chiefly in the proximal intestinal tract (the duodenal area) where the pH tends to be lower than in the distal portion of the intestine because the acidity of the gastric juices has not yet been reduced. Calcium salts are relatively insoluble in a less acid medium. Vitamin D is necessary for the absorption of calcium through the intestinal mucosa. It appears to have some direct effect on the mucosa, which increases active transport of calcium across the membrane.

Calcium absorption is increased by greater body need, calcium ion concentration, carbohydrate and protein intake, and the acidity of the intestinal medium.

BODY NEED. During periods of greater body demand, such as growth or depletion states, more calcium is absorbed. For example, utilization of calcium is much more efficient in children of countries where the diet is low in calcium than in children studied in the United States, whose diets are high in calcium.

CALCIUM ION CONCENTRATION IN EXTRACELLULAR FLUID. Even a small change in the concentration of ionized calcium in the extracellular fluid is reflected in a several-fold rise in the rate of calcium absorption. The maintenance of ionized calcium concentration within this narrow range is controlled by the parathyroid hormone (see p. 136).

PROTEIN INTAKE. A greater percentage of calcium is absorbed when the diet is high in protein than when it is low in protein. This is probably due to the influence of the amino acids lysine, arginine, and serine on intestinal pH and on the formation of soluble calcium–amino acid complexes.

CARBOHYDRATE INTAKE. Lactose especially seems to enhance the absorption of calcium in the ileum, perhaps through action of the lactobacilli, to produce lactic acid, which lowers the pH. It is interesting that the only source of lactose is milk, which also contributes the major amount of calcium—a fortunate combination.

ACIDITY. Generally, lower pH favors solubility of calcium and consequently its absorption.

Factors that decrease calcium absorption include vitamin D deficiency, excess fat, the calcium to phosphorus ratio, the presence of oxalic or phytic acids, and the alkalinity of the intestinal medium.

VITAMIN D DEFICIENCY. If there is a deficiency in vitamin D, calcium cannot be absorbed into the bloodstream.

FATS. Excess fat in the diet or poor absorption of fats results in an excess of free fatty acids in the intestine. The fatty acids combine with free calcium to form insoluble calcium soaps—a process called *saponification*. These insoluble soaps are excreted, with consequent loss of the incorporated calcium.

CALCIUM TO PHOSPHORUS RATIO. The optimal *dietary ratio* of calcium to phosphorus is 1:1 in the diet of children and of women during the latter half of pregnancy and during lactation. Other adults require phosphorus in an amount one and one-half times the intake of calcium. If either mineral is taken in excess of this ratio, absorption of both is hindered, and excretion of the lesser mineral is increased. For example, excess phosphorus in relation to the amount of calcium in the intestine will result in the formation of more calcium phosphate, which binds the calcium and makes it unavailable for absorption.

The amounts of calcium and phosphorus in the serum are normally maintained in a definite relationship called the *serum calcium to phosphorus ratio*. This ratio is the product (solubility product) of calcium × phosphorus, expressed in milligrams of each mineral per 1 dl of serum. Since the serum level of calcium is normally 10 mg/dl, and that of phosphorus is normally 4 mg/dl in adults (5 mg/dl in children), the normal calcium to phosphorus ratios are $10 \times 4 = 40$ for adults and $10 \times 5 = 50$ for children. Briefly expressed, the ratios are $Ca:P = 40$ (adult) and $Ca:P = 50$ (child).

OXALIC ACID. Oxalic acid, a constituent of some foods, combines with calcium to produce calcium oxalate, a relatively insoluble compound, and thus prevents calcium absorption. The classic example is the unavailability of the calcium in spinach because of the oxalic acid also present in this leaf.

PHYTIC ACID. Phytic acid, found in the outer hulls of many cereal grains, especially wheat, also forms an insoluble compound with calcium —calcium phytate—which prevents the absorption of calcium.

ALKALINITY. Calcium is insoluble in an alkaline medium and therefore is poorly absorbed.

Excretion. The quantity of calcium excreted tends to balance the quantity absorbed.

Amounts ingested in excess of need and amounts remaining unabsorbed are excreted in the feces. From an average American diet, which contains ample amounts of this mineral, 70% to 90% of the total calcium ingested is so excreted. When calcium from food is plentiful, the body absorbs it less efficiently than when it is scarce.

When the calcium level in serum is high as a result of excess bone destruction or mobilization of calcium from any storage site, the excess calcium is excreted primarily in the urine. Ordinarily, however, about 99% of the ionized calcium filtered by the renal glomeruli is reabsorbed in the renal tubules.

Calcium is also excreted through the intestinal digestive secretions, especially the bile. The intestinal juices contain about 500 mg of calcium.

Deposition-mobilization balance

The second large homeostatic balance mechanism involves bone as a major site of calcium storage—the bone compartment of the total metabolic pool of calcium.* Formerly bone tissue was thought of as an inert site of static deposit of calcium for storage. It has been demonstrated that this is not true. Bone is a dynamic tissue, characterized by a constant turnover of calcium; balance results from an ongoing process of accretion and resorption. Circulating ionized calcium is constantly being deposited in bone, while the calcium stored in bone is perpetually mobilized and withdrawn. The calcium in the bone compartment appears to be divided into two portions. This division is not

a spatial separation; rather, there are two forms of calcium in bone that participate in this dynamic exchange at two different levels of activity. There is a more actively exchangeable reservoir of about 4 g in equilibrium with the free plasma ionized calcium, and there is a much larger, more stable calcium bone reserve which exchanges slowly. Parathyroid hormone and vitamin D influence this exchange of calcium.

Parathyroid hormone (PH). The parathyroid gland is particularly sensitive to changes in the circulating plasma level of free ionized calcium. When this level drops, the parathyroid releases its hormone, which acts in three ways to restore the normal calcium level: (1) it stimulates the intestinal mucosa to increase the absorption of calcium, (2) it mobilizes calcium rapidly from the bone compartment, and (3) it causes renal excretion of phosphate. These combined activities restore calcium and phosphorus to their correctly balanced ratio in the blood. Tetany* results from a decrease in the free ionized serum calcium; the action of parathyroid hormone prevents tetany (see also clinical application, p. 137).

Vitamin D. Vitamin D seems to play a role in the deposition of calcium in the bone matrix. Studies have shown that vitamin D has a direct effect on the calcification of bone tissue; however, its effect on calcium absorption from the intestine is much greater. The effect of parathyroid hormone is greater at the point of bone calcium mobilization.

Calcitonin. A third hormonal agent intimately involved in calcium metabolism is calcitonin, produced by special cells called C cells, in the thyroid gland.[2] Calcitonin prevents abnormal rises in serum calcium by decreasing the release of calcium from bone. Thus its ac-

---

*A metabolic pool is not to be thought of as a collection of a certain substance in any one place. When a physiologist talks about a metabolic pool, he is speaking of the total available reserves of a specific substance in the storage sites of the body. There may be one or several such sites. He frequently speaks of the "compartments" of this pool. The substances that are ascribed to pools are not necessarily liquids. For example, one speaks of a metabolic pool of calcium, 99% of which is in the bone compartment.

---

*Do not confuse *tetany* with *tetanus*. Although they come from the same Greek word *teinein* meaning "to stretch," they refer to very different syndromes. *Tetany* results from abnormal calcium metabolism; *tetanus* is an acute infectious disease.

tion counterbalances the action of parathyroid hormone to regulate serum calcium at normal levels in balance with bone calcium.

The cooperative action of these three factors, parathyroid hormone, vitamin D, and calcitonin, is a good example of synergistic* behavior of metabolic controls.

The overall relationship of the various factors involved in calcium absorption and metabolism may be visualized in Fig. 8-1.

Physiologic function of calcium

Bone and teeth formation. The physiologic function of 99% of the calcium in the body is to build and maintain skeletal tissue. This intricate and delicately balanced process is carried on by two types of cells. *Osteoblasts* continually form new bone matrix in which calcium phosphate is deposited and bone crystals develop. *Osteoclasts* continually balance this activity by absorbing bone tissue; they engulf (phagocytize) and digest minute bone crystals.

Calcium phosphate deposits are important to *tooth formation*. As the teeth develop, tooth-forming organs (ameloblasts) deposit calcium and other constituents; then mineral exchange continues, as in bone. This exchange occurs mainly in the dentine and cementum; very little occurs in the enamel.

Blood clotting. The remaining 1% of the body's calcium performs several vital physiologic functions. In blood clotting, calcium ions enhance bonding between fibrin molecules and give stability to the fibrin threads required for conversion of prothrombin to thrombin (see Fig. 6-3).

Muscle contraction and relaxation. Ionized serum calcium plays an important role in the initiation of muscle contraction. Each muscle fiber contains hundreds of small contractile units called *myofibrils,* which are composed of

the muscle protein filaments, *myosin* and *actin*. Alongside each myofibril is a fine system of tubes—the *tubular reticulum*. Calcium is firmly bound to this reticulum. When the signal for contraction comes, the calcium is suddenly released, ionized, and mobilized. The free calcium ions activate the chemical reaction between myosin and actin filaments that releases a large amount of energy from ATP and brings about contraction. The calcium ions are then immediately bound back on the reticulum, causing relaxation. Other elements, such as magnesium and potassium, are also involved in this process. The catalyzing actions of calcium ions on the muscle protein filaments, myosin and actin, which allows the sliding contraction between them to occur, is particularly vital in the contraction-relaxation cycle of the *heart muscle*.

Nerve transmission. Calcium is required for normal transmission of nerve impulses. Calcium ions in the extracellular fluid at the neuromuscular junction apparently cause the excitatory transmitting substance *acetylcholine* (see p. 121) to rupture through the separating membranes at the tips of the many nerve branches and excite the muscle fiber.

Cell wall permeability. Ionized calcium controls the passage of fluid through cell walls by affecting cell wall permeability. This is apparently the result of calcium's influence on the integrity of the intercellular cement substance.

Enzyme activation. Calcium ions are important activators of certain enzymes, such as adenosinetriphosphatase (ATPase), in the energy release for muscle contraction. They play a similar role with other enzymes, including lipase and some members of the protein-splitting enzyme system.

Clinical application

Tetany. A decrease in ionized serum calcium causes tetany, a state marked by severe, intermittent spastic contractions of the muscle and by muscular pain. It is manifested by a char-

---

*Synergism is the cooperative action of two or more factors, which in acting together produce a total effect greater than the sum of their separate effects. Many biologic and physiologic interactions provide examples of synergism.

acteristic carpopedal spasm of the muscles in the upper extremity, which causes flexion of wrist and thumb with extension of the fingers *(Trousseau's sign).*

Tetanylike responses may be caused by an increase in serum phosphorus fraction in the calcium to phosphorus ratio (p. 135), which causes a decrease in calcium level to maintain the solubility product of calcium × phosphorus. For example, a so-called milk tetany has been reported in newborn infants fed undiluted cow's milk. The ratio of phosphorus to calcium in cow's milk is greater than in human milk, and the kidneys of these infants could not clear this phosphate load. Phosphorus therefore accumulated in the serum. The rise in serum phosphorus caused a compensatory decrease in serum calcium; this in turn caused typical tetanic muscular spasms.

Occasional transient leg cramps of pregnancy have been attributed by some observers to a similar rise in phosphorus intake, if the gravid woman drinks in *excess* of the recommended amount of milk.

Rickets. As indicated in the discussion of vitamin D's relation to calcium and phosphorus in producing rickets (p. 91), when adequate calcium and phosphorus are not absorbed, proper bone formation cannot take place.

Renal calculi. The majority of renal stones are composed of calcium. A predisposing factor to the formation of renal calculi may be an increase in the amount of calcium that must be excreted in the urine as calcium is mobilized or withdrawn from the bone compartment. Immobilization of the body is one state that causes such resorption of calcium from bone stores into the blood. This has definite clinical implications. When a full body cast or some other orthopedic device immobilizes the body for a long period, dietary calcium intake should be adequate but should not exceed the usual daily allowances; if renal stones have already occurred, the amount of calcium in the diet should be somewhat reduced.

Hyperparathyroidism and hypoparathyroidism. Because calcium and phosphorus metabolism are so directly controlled by parathyroid hormone, conditions of the parathyroid gland that increase or decrease the secretion of its hormone will immediately be reflected in abnormal metabolism of these two minerals.

Dietary requirements of calcium

The National Research Council (NRC) recommended allowances (1980 revision) for calcium are 800 mg daily for men or women, increased to 1.2 g during pregnancy and lactation. Infants younger than 1 year should have 360 to 540 mg and children should have from 0.8 to 1.2 g daily.

Food sources of calcium

Dairy products supply the bulk of dietary calcium. One quart of milk contains about 1 g of calcium, and cheese contains a comparable amount. Secondary sources contribute much smaller quantities. These include egg yolk, green leafy vegetables, legumes, nuts, and whole grains. If the average American diet contained no dairy products, one would be hard pressed to account for more than about 300 mg of calcium.

Phosphorus

Phosphorus is closely associated with calcium in human nutrition. Both minerals occur in the same major food source—milk. Both function in the major task of bone building. Both are related to vitamin D in the absorption process. Both are regulated metabolically by parathyroid hormone. The two exist in the blood serum in definite ratio to one another.

Although phosphorus has been called the "metabolic twin" of calcium, it has some unique characteristics and functions. As the role of phosphorus in metabolism is considered here and the expected similarities to calcium are found, characteristics that distinguish it from calcium should also be looked for.

Occurrence in the body

Phosphorus makes up 0.8% to 1.1% of the total body weight. The body of a person weighing 54 kg (120 lb) contains about 0.54 kg (1.2 lb) of phosphorus. From 80% to 90% of this phosphorus is in the skeleton (including the teeth) compounded with calcium. The remaining 20% is, unlike calcium, uniquely distributed in every living cell, where it participates as an essential component in interrelationships with proteins, lipids, and carbohydrates to produce energy, to build and repair tissues, and to act as a buffer.

The serum phosphorus level normally ranges from 3.0 to 4.5 mg/dl in adults and is somewhat higher, 4 to 7 mg/dl in children. The higher range during growth years is a significant clue to its role in cell metabolism.

The total inorganic serum phosphorus exists in the form of the two balancing buffer anions: $HPO_4^=$ (phosphate), 2.1 meq/L; and $H_2PO_4^-$ (phosphoric acid), 0.26 meq/L. Other phosphorus in the body occurs as a constituent of organic compounds.

Absorption-excretion

The absorption of phosphorus is closely related to that of calcium. Equal amounts of the two minerals in the diet is an optimal ratio; excess of either causes increased fecal excretion of the other. Apparently phosphorus is more efficiently absorbed than calcium, as only 30% of the ingested phosphorus (bound to calcium) is excreted in the feces and about 70% is absorbed, compared with only 10% to 30% of dietary calcium that is absorbed.

The absorption of phosphorus is apparently secondary to that of calcium. Vitamin D enhances, but is not required for, the absorption of phosphorus. The direct action of vitamin D is on the absorption of calcium, and the absorption of phosphorus follows.

Since phosphorus occurs in food as a phosphate compound, mainly with calcium, the first step is the splitting off of phosphorus for absorption as the free mineral.

Factors similar to those that influence calcium absorption also affect phosphorus absorption. For example, an excess of calcium or

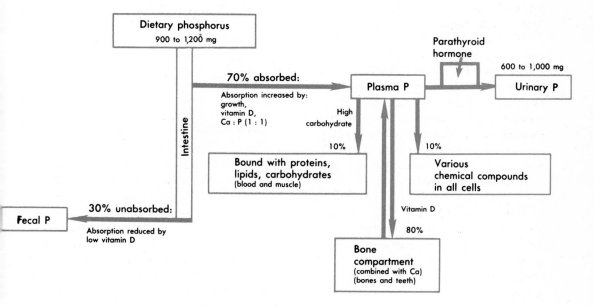

Fig. 8-2. Relative distribution and interchange of phosphorus in the body.

other material that may bind phosphorus in insoluble salts (such as aluminum or iron) will inhibit its absorption.

The kidneys provide the main excretory mechanism for regulation of the serum phosphorus level. The *renal threshold for phosphate* means that the amount of phosphate excreted by the kidney is relative to the serum phosphorus level. If the serum phosphorus level falls, the renal tubules return more phosphorus to the blood; if the serum phosphorus level rises, the renal tubules excrete more. When the diet lacks sufficient phosphorus, the renal tubules conserve phosphorus by returning it to the blood. By this means, normal serum phosphorus levels are maintained through the work of the kidney. The amount of phosphorus excreted in the urine of a person ingesting an average diet is from 0.6 to 1.0 g every 24 hours.

Metabolism of phosphate

Role of parathyroid hormone. The homeostatic mechanism by which the kidneys maintain the serum phosphorus level is controlled by the parathyroid hormone. This action is usually interdependent with calcium balance. When the serum phosphate level rises, the parathyroid hormone blocks renal tubular resorption of phosphorus so that more phosphorus is excreted in the urine. The serum phosphorus level and the calcium to phosphorus ratio are returned to normal.

The balance concept is also applicable to the equilibrium existing between the phosphorus in the bone compartment and in the circulating serum. These various balance relationships may be visualized in Fig. 8-2.

Physiologic functions of phosphorus

Eighty percent of body phosphorus contributes to mineralization of bones and teeth. As a component of calcium phosphate, it is constantly being deposited and reabsorbed in the dynamic process of bone formation.

Far out of proportion to the relatively small amount of the remainder, 20% of body phosphorus is intimately involved in overall human metabolism. Its vital role is indicated by its presence in every living cell. The various metabolic functions of phosphorus illustrate again the overarching concept of interrelatedness of the nutrients.

Absorption of glucose and glycerol. By the process of *phosphorylation,* phosphorus combines with glucose and glycerol (from fat) to promote the absorption of these substances from the intestine. Phosphorylation also promotes the renal tubular reabsorption of glucose, by which this sugar is conserved and returned to the blood.

Transport of fatty acids. By combination with fat as phospholipids, phosphorus helps to provide a vehicular form for fat.

Energy metabolism. Phosphorus is an essential part of such key cellular nucleoprotein substances as DNA and phosphatides, which also participate in the formation of numerous enzymes in the pathways for glucose oxidation and final energy production. These nucleoprotein substances are key power sources in the high-energy phosphate bonds of such compounds as ATP.

Buffer system. The phosphate buffer system of phosphoric acid and phosphate contributes additional control of acidotic and alkalotic states in the blood.

Clinical application

Situations involving physiologic changes in serum phosphorus level include growth and recovery from diabetic acidosis.

Growth. Growing children usually have high serum phosphate levels, probably resulting from high levels of growth hormone.

State of recovery from diabetic acidosis. Active carbohydrate absorption and metabolism use much phosphorus, depositing it with glycogen, thus causing temporary hypophosphatemia.

Changes in serum phosphorus level. Situations involving pathologic changes in serum phosphorus level include hypophosphatemia and hyperphosphatemia.

HYPOPHOSPHATEMIA. Intestinal diseases such as sprue and celiac disease in which phosphorus absorption is hindered, or bone disease such as rickets or osteomalacia in which the calcium to phosphorus balance is upset, are characterized by low serum phosphorus levels. The serum phosphorus level is also low in primary hyperparathyroidism, because the excess quantity of parathyroid hormone secreted results in excessive renal tubular excretion of phosphorus. Symptoms of hypophosphatemia include muscle weakness, because the muscle cells are deprived of phosphorus essential for energy metabolism.

HYPERPHOSPHATEMIA. Renal insufficiency or hypoparathyroidism causes excess accumulation of serum phosphate. As a result, the calcium side of the calcium to phosphorus ratio is low, which causes tetany.

Dietary requirement of phosphorus

During growth, pregnancy, and lactation, the ratio of phosphorus to calcium in the diet is ideally 1:1. In ordinary adult life, the intake of phosphorus is about one and one-half times that of calcium. In general, since these two minerals are found in the same food sources, if calcium needs are met, adequate phosphorus will be assured.

The NRC (1980 revision) recommends a phosphorus allowance equal to that for calcium for all ages except the young infant. For the infant the proportion of phosphorus is lower than calcium.

Food sources of phosphorus

Milk and milk products are the most significant sources of phosphorus, as they are for calcium. Because the role of phosphorus in cell metabolism assures the presence of phosphorus

in muscle cells, lean meats are also a good source.

Magnesium
Occurrence in the body

Magnesium, an essential nutrient, occurs in the body in appreciable quantities. There are about 25 g in an adult, and 70% of this is combined with calcium and phosphorus in the bone salts complex. The remaining 30% is distributed in various soft tissues and body fluids.

Plasma magnesium values range from 1.4 to 2.5 mg/dl. Unlike calcium, magnesium occurs predominantly in the red blood cells, and there is relatively little in the serum. About 80% of the blood magnesium is ionized and diffusible. The remainder is probably bound with serum protein, as is the nondiffusible calcium. It is also stored in bone. Muscle tissue contains more magnesium than calcium; blood contains more calcium than magnesium.

Absorption-excretion

In an average diet about 45% of ingested magnesium is absorbed, and 55% is excreted in the feces. Absorption apparently occurs in the upper small intestine; none appears to be absorbed in the colon. Urinary excretion is relatively low, since the kidney conserves magnesium efficiently. Aldosterone increases the renal clearance of magnesium, as it does that of potassium.

Factors that inhibit calcium absorption also hinder magnesium absorption. These include the presence of excess fat, phosphate, calcium, of alkalis. As with calcium, parathyroid hormone also increases magnesium absorption from the intestine. Vitamin D, however, apparently does not affect magnesium absorption.

Metabolic functions of magnesium

Ionized magnesium is essential to cellular metabolism of both carbohydrate and protein because it is a significant cation of the intracellular fluid. The following are the metabolic functions of magnesium.

1. In carbohydrate metabolism, ionized magnesium (Mg++) serves as an activator of many enzymes in the reactions of the initial Embden-Meyerhof glycolytic pathway for glucose oxidation (oxidative phosphorylation).
2. In protein metabolism, ionized magnesium is a coenzyme in protein synthesis in the cell ribosomes.
3. Magnesium is a constituent of molecules formed in the processes of growth and maintenance of tissues.
4. Magnesium is related to cortisone in the regulation of the blood phosphorus level.
5. Decreased ionized magnesium concentration causes vasodilation and inhibits smooth muscle action. Normally, ionized magnesium, like potassium, is concentrated in the intracellular fluid. Any changes in this concentration produce neuromuscular irritability. A tetanylike syndrome has been observed in animals fed a low-magnesium diet.

Clinical application

Gastrointestinal disorders. In prolonged diarrhea or vomiting or in diseases characterized by intestinal malabsorption, excessive amounts of magnesium may be lost. Fundamental to the treatment of such states is the restoration of the lost water by mouth or intravenously. Rehydration must be accompanied by adequate magnesium replacement; if it is not, the resulting low serum magnesium level may give rise to general neuromuscular irritability, manifested by tremor, spasm, and increased startle response to sound and touch.

Alcoholism. A tetanylike syndrome has been studied in persons with chronic alcoholism in whom magnesium deficiency has developed.

Serum cholesterol levels. Some recent study indicates a possible correlation of the serum magnesium level with the serum cholesterol level. As yet, this relationship is unclear.

Dietary requirement of magnesium

A natural magnesium deficiency in man is unlikely. Balance studies indicate that the average adult needs from 250 to 300 mg per day. The NRC (1980 revision) has set adult recommendations at 350 mg daily for men and 300 mg for women. Any deficiency would probably be long-term and cumulative and may have a role in chronic cardiovascular, neuromuscular, and renal diseases.

Food sources of magnesium

Magnesium is relatively widespread in nature. Its main sources include nuts, soybeans, cocoa, seafood, whole grains, dried beans, and peas.

Sodium
Occurrence in the body

Sodium, crucially important to many metabolic activities, is one of the more plentiful of the minerals in the body. Of the 120 mg (4 oz) or so in the body of a person weighing 70 kg (154 lb), about one third is present in the skeleton as inorganic bound material. The remaining two thirds are in the extracellular fluids. This extracellular ionized sodium (Na+) is largely distributed in plasma and in nerve and muscle tissue. Normal blood serum values range from 136 to 145 meq/L or from 310 to 340 mg/dl.

Absorption-excretion

Sodium is readily absorbed from the intestine, and normally only about 5% of all excreted sodium is lost in the feces. Larger amounts are passed by this route in such abnormal states as diarrhea. Ninety-five percent of the sodium that leaves the body is excreted in the urine. The renal control of sodium excretion is regulated largely by hormones of the adrenal gland, especially the powerful mineralocorticoid *aldosterone.* The aldosterone mechanism for sodium conservation is one of the major homeostatic controls of body sodium and hence of body water (see p. 188).

Metabolic functions of sodium

Fluid balance. Ionized sodium is the major cation of the extracellular fluid. Variations in the concentration of ionized sodium largely determine the shift of water by osmosis from one body area to another. These shifts of water from one part of the body to another are the means whereby substances in solution in the body water can circulate between the cells and the fluid that surrounds them. Such shifts also protect the body against large fluid losses. The role of sodium in the maintenance of fluid balance is discussed in Chapter 9 on water and electrolytes.

Acid-base balance. Through its association with chloride and bicarbonate ions, ionized sodium is an important factor in the regulation of the acid-base balance in the body.

Cell permeability. Cell permeability is affected by the sodium pump associated with glucose metabolism and cellular exchange of ionized sodium (see p. 23). By an active mode of transport of this type, sodium appears to be essential to the passage of such materials through cell walls.

Normal muscle irritability. Sodium ions play a large part in transmitting electro-chemical impulses along nerve and muscle membranes and therefore maintain normal muscle irritability or excitability. Potassium and sodium ions balance the response of nerves to stimulation, the travel of nerve impulses to muscles, and the resulting contraction of the muscle fibers.

Clinical application

Fluid-electrolyte and acid-base balance. Many clinical applications of these balance mechanisms, which are essential to health and to life itself, will be discussed in the next chapter. Suffice it to say here that perhaps no other

physiologic activity is so broad in scope or so profound in its effect on body systems (especially the cardiovascular, renal, and gastrointestinal systems) as the mechanisms by which the fluid-electrolyte and acid-base balances are maintained.

Muscle action. Abnormal serum levels of sodium may adversely affect the function of muscles, for example, the heart muscle. The consequences of serum sodium abnormalities on muscular function are, however, less profound than those of serum potassium abnormalities.

Dietary requirement of sodium

The specific dietary requirement for sodium is not stated. Apparently the body can function on a rather wide range of exogenous sodium through the operation of mechanisms designed to conserve or excrete this mineral. The amount of sodium in the average American diet (4 g of sodium in the average 10 g of table salt consumed daily) is about 10 times the quantity that the body requires for the maintenance of an adequate balance. An intake of about 5 g of table salt, or 2 g sodium (NaCl), has been recommended for adults. For those with a family history of hypertension, the recommended quantity in food is even less—from 1 to 2 g salt daily.

Food sources of sodium

Common salt, used in cooking and for seasoning, is the main dietary source of sodium. Other food sources include milk, meat, egg, and certain vegetables such as carrots, beets, spinach and other leafy greens, celery, artichokes, and asparagus.

Potassium
Occurrence in the body

Like sodium, potassium is a vital mineral element associated with physiologic fluid balance. This role will be discussed in greater detail in the next chapter.

Potassium is about twice as plentiful as sodium in the body. The body of an average man weighing 70 kg (154 lb) contains about 270 mg (9 oz, 4,000 meq) of potassium. By far the larger portion is found inside the cells; potassium is the major cation (K+) of the intracellular fluid (see p. 180). However, the relatively small amount in extracellular fluid has a significant effect on muscle activity, especially heart muscle. The normal blood serum values for potassium range from 3.5 to 5.0 meq/L, or 14 to 20 mg/dl. In comparison, the cell concentration is about 155 meq/L of cell water.

Absorption-excretion

Potassium ingested in food is easily absorbed from the small intestine. A considerable amount of potassium is also secreted into the intestine as a component of the digestive juices, but is later reabsorbed during the continuous cycle of gastrointestinal circulation of water and electrolytes. Little potassium is lost in the feces.

Urinary excretion is the principal route of loss. Since maintenance of serum potassium within the narrow, normal range is vital to heart muscle action and is an indicator of electrolyte balance, the kidney guards potassium carefully. The ability of the renal glomeruli and tubules to filter, reabsorb, secrete, and excrete potassium is so remarkable that the well-functioning kidney can maintain normal serum levels even in the face of relatively large injections of potassium. Changes in acid-base balance are reflected in compensatory changes in the amount of potassium excreted in the urine.

Hormones of the adrenal cortex, especially aldosterone, also influence potassium excretion. As a part of the aldosterone mechanism that conserves sodium, ionized potassium is excreted instead of ionized sodium, the two ions being exchanged for one another in the renal tubule (see p. 189).

Metabolic functions of potassium

Fluid-electrolyte balance. As the major cation of the intracellular fluid, ionized potassium functions in balance with the extracellular ionized sodium to maintain the normal osmotic pressures and water balance that maintain the integrity of the cellular fluid.

Acid-base balance. Ionized potassium also exerts an influence on acid-base balance through its operation with ionized sodium and ionized hydrogen.

Muscle activity. Ionized potassium plays a significant role in the activity of striated (skeletal and cardiac) muscle. As indicated, ionized potassium functions with ionized sodium and calcium to regulate neuromuscular excitability and stimulation, transmission of electrochemical impulses, and contraction of muscle fibers. This effect of ionized potassium is particularly notable in the action of heart muscle. Even small variations in serum potassium concentration are reflected in electrocardiographic changes. *Excess* serum potassium (hyperkalemia), a common and life-threatening complication of renal failure, severe dehydration, or shock, causes the heart to dilate and become flaccid, which slows its rate. Eventually, transmission of the electrochemical impulse that mediates the flow of the beat through the heart may be blocked between the atrium and the ventricles (atrioventricular block). An increase in serum potassium concentration to only two to three times the normal level may weaken cardiac contractions sufficiently to cause death.

Low serum potassium concentrations (hypokalemia) may cause muscle irritability and paralysis. The heart may develop gallop rhythm, tachycardia, and finally cardiac arrest.

Carbohydrate metabolism. When blood glucose is converted to glycogen for storage, potassium is stored with the glycogen. It has been calculated that for every 1 g of glycogen stored, 0.36 millimole (mmol) of potassium is also retained. When a patient in diabetic acidosis is treated by the administration of insulin and glucose, glycogen is rapidly produced and stored. The potassium that is to be stored with the glycogen is quickly withdrawn from the serum. The resulting hypokalemia may be fatal.

For this reason, the treatment of diabetic acidosis usually includes replacement of serum potassium.

Protein synthesis. Potassium is required for the storage of nitrogen as muscle protein. When muscle tissue is broken down, potassium is lost together with the nitrogen in muscle protein. Replacement therapy—the administration of amino acids to provide for resynthesis of muscle protein—should therefore also include potassium to ensure nitrogen retention.

Clinical application

As with sodium, variances in potassium levels have far-reaching clinical implications in fluid-electrolyte and acid-base balances. These are discussed in greater detail in Chapter 9. Other clinical situations related to potassium may be grouped under *elevated* or *decreased* serum potassium states.

Hyperkalemia (elevated serum potassium). Any condition that results in renal failure precludes the normal adjustment and clearance of ionized potassium. Serum potassium then rises to toxic levels. The too-rapid intravenous administration of potassium may also cause hyperkalemia. Hyperkalemia from either cause results in weakening of heart action, mental confusion, poor respiration (caused by weakening of the respiratory muscles), and numbness of extremities.

Hypokalemia (decreased serum potassium). Hypokalemia of dangerous degrees may be caused by a prolonged wasting disease with tissue destruction and malnutrition or by prolonged gastrointestinal loss of potassium as in diarrhea, vomiting, or gastric suction. The continuous use of diuretic drugs increases ionized potassium excretion and may leave the serum potassium level abnormally low. It is therefore recommended that the administration of such drugs be interrupted at intervals and that patients taking such agents receive potassium medication or use high potassium food sources for replacement.

Heart failure and subsequent depletion of ionized potassium in heart muscle makes the myocardial tissue more sensitive to digitalis toxicity and arrhythmia (irregular contractions). To prevent these complications of cardiac failure, potassium should be given, especially when potassium-depleting diuretics are used.

Diabetic acidosis, as indicated, requires replacement of potassium when insulin and glucose are given to offset the rapid withdrawal of potassium for incorporation with glycogen storage.

Dietary requirement of potassium

No dietary requirement is specified for potassium. The usual diet contains from 2 to 4 g daily, which seems ample for common need. No deficiency is likely, except in the clinical situations described in the preceding sections.

Food sources of potassium

Potassium is widely distributed in natural foods. Legumes, whole grains, certain fruits, leafy vegetables, and meats supply considerable amounts. Many other foods are supplementary sources.

Chlorine
Occurrence in the body

Chlorine occurs in the body as the chloride ion (Cl^-). It accounts for about 3% of the body's total mineral content. Ionized chlorine is the major anion of the extracellular fluid. The cerebrospinal fluid has the highest concentration of chloride (124 meq/L or 440 mg/dl). The normal range for plasma level is from 95 to 105 meq/L or 340 to 370 mg/dl. A relatively large amount of ionized chloride is found in the gastrointestinal secretions, especially as a component of gastric hydrochloric acid.

Absorption-excretion

Chloride is almost completely absorbed in the intestine with only a functional fecal loss. Excretion is accomplished chiefly through the kidney. Like sodium, chloride is a threshold substance. It is largely conserved by reabsorption in the renal tubules where it is returned to the circulating plasma. This reabsorption is enhanced by the adrenal hormone aldosterone. The reabsorption of chloride is secondary to aldosterone's control over the renal reabsorption of sodium.

Since ionized chloride is a major component of the gastrointestinal circulation, relatively large losses may occur in prolonged vomiting or diarrhea.

Metabolic functions of chlorine

Fluid-electrolyte balance. Together with ionized sodium, ionized chloride in the extracellular fluid helps to maintain water balance and to regulate osmotic pressure.

Acid-base balance. By participating in the chloride-bicarbonate shift mechanism, which operates between the plasma and the red blood cells, ionized chloride plays a special role in maintaining a constant pH in the blood. In response to changes in carbon dioxide tension in erythrocytes, ionized chloride goes into the red blood cell in exchange for HCO_3 (the chloride-bicarbonate shift). This provides constant bicarbonate buffering for the rapidly formed carbonic acid (H_2CO_3) from water and CO_3. These reactions are then reversed in the lungs as carbon dioxide is expired.

Gastric acidity. Chloride, secreted by the mucosa of the stomach as gastric hydrochloric acid, provides the necessary acid medium for digestion in the stomach and for the activation of enzymes (such as conversion of the pepsinogen to active pepsin for initial protein splitting).

Clinical application

Gastrointestinal disorders. As is true of sodium and potassium, large amounts of chloride may be lost during continued vomiting, diarrhea, or tube drainage, which would contribute the complications of hypochloremic alkalosis to the clinical state produced by dehydration. Prompt replacement of chloride is essential.

Alkalosis. Gastric secretions such as hydrochloric acid are low in sodium but high in chloride. When such secretions are lost, bicarbonate replaces the depleted chloride ions. A type of metabolic alkalosis called hypochloremic alkalosis results. Potassium deficiency is a frequent accompaniment.

Endocrine disorders. Cushing's disease, which is caused by hyperactivity of the adrenal cortex, or excessive quantities of ACTH or cortisone given as therapy may produce hypokalemia, and hypochloremic alkalosis may result.

Requirement and sources of chlorine

No quantitative statement of human requirement for chloride has been established. Almost the sole dietary source is as a partner to sodium in table salt (NaCl). When sodium intake is adequate, chloride will be amply supplied.

Sulfur
Occurrence in the body

Sulfur, an essential element, occurs in the body in a number of organic and inorganic forms. The inorganic forms of sulfur are the sulfates of sodium, potassium, and magnesium. Organic sulfur is divided into nonprotein sulfur and protein sulfur. Nonprotein organic sulfur includes sulfalipids and sulfatides. The following is a list of protein sulfurs.

1. Sulfur-containing amino acids—methionine and cystine
2. Glycoproteins—conjugates of sulfate and sulfuric acid with carbohydrate derivatives, such as chondroitin-sulfuric acid in cartilage, tendon, and bone matrix.
3. Detoxification products—conjugates such as phenol- and cresol-sulfuric acids, and indoxyl sulfate; some of these products are formed in part from bacterial putrefactive activity in the intestine
4. Other organic compounds such as heparin, insulin, thiamin, biotin, lipoic acid, and coenzyme A
5. Keratin—the protein of hair and skin

Sulfur occurs in some form throughout the body and is present in all cells, usually as an essential constituent of cell protein. The plasma sulfur level ranges from 0.7 to 1.5 meq/L.

Absorption-excretion

Inorganic sulfate is absorbed in the intestine as such and goes directly into the portal blood circulation. The sulfur-containing amino acids, methionine and cystine, are split off from protein during digestion and are also absorbed into the portal circulation. These two amino acids are the most important sources of sulfur in the body.

Sulfur is excreted by the urine. Since sulfur enters the body chiefly with protein, the amount excreted varies directly with the amount of protein ingested and with the extent of tissue protein breakdown.

Metabolic functions of sulfur

Maintenance of protein structure. Disulfide linkages (-S-S-) form an important secondary structure between parallel peptide chains to maintain the stability of proteins.

Activation of enzymes. Many enzymes depend on a free sulfhydryl group (-SH) to maintain their activity. Therefore sulfur participates in tissue respiration or biologic oxidation.

Energy metabolism. The sulfhydryl group also forms a high-energy sulfur bond similar to the high-energy phosphate bond (pp. 75-113). This is an important aspect of the metabolic activity of acetylcoenzyme A (CoA.SH) or active acetate.

Detoxification. Sulfur participates in several important detoxification reactions by which toxic materials are conjugated with active sulfate and converted to a nontoxic form and excreted in the urine.

Clinical application

Cystine renal calculi. A relatively rare hereditary defect in renal tubular reabsorption of the amino acid cystine causes excessive urinary excretion of cystine (cystinuria) and re-peated production of kidney stones formed of cystine crystals. They are yellowish in color because of the high sulfur content. A low-methionine diet is given to reduce the intake and synthesis of these sulfur-containing amino acids (see p. 658).

Requirement and sources of sulfur

No quantitative dietary requirement has been specified for sulfur. The major food sources are proteins containing methionine and cystine. Cystine may be synthesized in the body from its precursor methionine.

The major minerals are summarized in Table 8-1.

TRACE MINERALS WITH KNOWN FUNCTION

Seven essential minerals have been grouped as *trace elements* with known functions because they occur in the body in relatively small amounts—even minute amounts in most cases. Each, however, performs some vital function in human nutrition. These seven minerals are iron (Fe), copper (Cu), iodine (I), manganese (Mn), cobalt (Co), zinc (Zn), and molybdenum (Mo).

Iron
Occurrence in the body

The body contains about 45 mg of iron per kilogram of body weight. To calculate the amount of iron in the body, the formula 2.2 lb = 1 kg is used. A person weighing 55 kg (121 lb) would have about 2.5 g of iron.

This iron is distributed in the body in four main forms that point to its basic metabolic functions.

Transport iron. A very small amount of iron (from 0.05 to 0.18 mg/dl) is found in the plasma. This iron is being transferred from one point of use to another. While it is transferred, it is bound with one of the plasma β-globulins. The plasma protein that binds iron in this compound form and transports it is called *transferrin*.

Table 8-1. Summary of major minerals

Mineral	Metabolism	Physiologic functions	Clinical application	Requirement	Food sources
Calcium (Ca)	Absorption according to body need, aided by vitamin D; favored by protein, lactose, acidity; hindered by excess fats and binding agents (phosphates, oxalates, phytate) Excretion chiefly in feces, 70% to 90% of amount ingested Deposition-mobilization in bone compartment constant; deposition aided by vitamin D Parathyroid hormone controls absorption and mobilization	Bone formation Teeth Blood clotting Muscle contraction and relaxation Heart action Nerve transmission Cell wall permeability Enzyme activation (ATPase)	Tetany—decrease in ionized serum calcium Rickets Renal calculi Hyperparathyroidism Hypoparathyroidism	Adults: 0.8 g Pregnancy and lactation: 1.2 g Infants: 360-540 mg Children: 0.8-1.2 g	Milk Cheese Green leafy vegetables Whole grains Egg yolk Legumes, nuts
Phosphorus (P)	Absorption with calcium aided by vitamin D; hindered by excess binding agents (calcium, aluminum, iron) Excretion chiefly by kidney according to renal threshold blood level Parathyroid hormone controls renal excretion balance with blood level Deposition-mobilization in bone compartment constant	Bone formation Overall metabolism: Absorption of glucose and glycerol (phosphorylation) Transport of fatty acids Energy metabolism (enzymes, ATP) Buffer system	Growth Hypophosphatemia: Recovery state from diabetic acidosis Sprue, celiac disease (malabsorption) Bone diseases (upset Ca:P balance) Hyperphosphatemia: Renal insufficiency Hypoparathyroidism Tetany	Adults: 1½ times calcium intake Pregnancy and lactation: 1.2 g Infants: 240-400 mg Children: 0.8-1.2 g	Milk Cheese Meat Egg yolk Whole grains Legumes, nuts
Magnesium (Mg)	Absorption increased by parathyroid hormone, hindered by excess fat, phosphate, calcium Excretion regulated by kidney	In bones and teeth Activator and coenzyme in carbohydrate and protein metabolism Essential intracellular fluid (ICF) cation Muscle, nerve irritability	Tremor, spasm; low serum level following gastrointestinal losses	300-350 mg Deficiency in humans unlikely	Whole grains Nuts Meat Milk Legumes
Sodium (Na)	Readily absorbed Excretion chiefly by kidney, con-	Major extracellular fluid (ECF) cation	Fluid shifts and control Buffer system	About 0.5 g Diet usually has	Table salt (NaCl)

Mineral	Metabolism	Physiological functions	Clinical applications	Requirement	Food sources
	trolled by aldosterone, acid-base balance	Water balance; osmotic pressure Acid-base balance Cell permeability; absorption of glucose Muscle irritability; transmission of electrochemical impulse and resulting contraction	Losses in gastrointestinal disorders	more: 2-6 g	Milk Meat Egg Baking soda Baking powder Carrots, beets, spinach, celery
Potassium (K)	Secreted and reabsorbed in digestive juices Excretion guarded by kidney according to blood levels; increased by aldosterone	Major ICF cation Acid-base balance Regulates neuromuscular excitability and muscle contraction Glycogen formation Protein synthesis	Fluid shifts Losses in: Starvation Diabetic acidosis Adrenal tumors Heart action—low serum potassium (tachycardia, cardiac arrest) Treatment of diabetic acidosis (rapid glycogen production reduces serum potassium) Tissue catabolism—potassium loss	About 2-4 g Diet adequate in protein, calcium, and iron contains adequate potassium	Whole grains Meat Legumes Fruits Vegetables
Chlorine (Cl)	Absorbed readily Excretion controlled by kidney	Major ECF anion Acid-base balance—chloride-bicarbonate shift Water balance Gastric hydrochloric acid—digestion	Hypochloremic alkalosis in prolonged vomiting, diarrhea, tube drainage	About 0.5 g Diet usually has more:2-6 g	Table salt
Sulfur (S)	Absorbed as such and as constituent of sulfur-containing amino acid, methionine Excreted by kidney in relation to protein intake and tissue catabolism	Essential constituent of cell protein Activates enzymes High-energy sulfur bonds in energy metabolism Detoxification reactions	Cystine renal calculi Cystinuria	Diet adequate in protein contains adequate sulfur	Meat Egg Cheese Milk Nuts, legumes

Hemoglobin. About 75% of the body's iron is in hemoglobin. The greatest amount of the body's iron, about 70%, is found in red blood cells as a constituent of hemoglobin. Another 5% of the total body iron is a part of muscle hemoglobin—myoglobin.

Storage iron. About 20% of the total body iron is in various organs in storage form as the protein-iron compound *ferritin*. The main storage organs are the liver, spleen, and bone marrow.

Cellular tissue iron. The remaining 5% of total body iron is distributed throughout all cells as a major component of oxidative enzyme systems for production of energy.

Absorption-transport-storage-excretion

In the body, iron follows a unique system of interrelated absorption-transportation-storage-excretion. The system is unique in that the optimal levels of body iron are not maintained by urinary excretion as is the case with most plasma constituents. Rather, the mechanisms of control lie in an absorption-transportation-storage complex.

Absorption. Iron enters the body usually as ferric iron (Fe^{+++}) in food. It is reduced in the acid medium of the stomach to ferrous iron (Fe^{++}), the form necessary for absorption. Only about 10% to 30% of the ingested iron is absorbed, and this occurs mostly in the stomach and duodenum. The remaining 70% to 90% is eliminated in the feces.

Probably in a complex with amino acids, iron is carried into the mucosal cells of the intestine where it combines with a protein, *apoferritin,* to form ferritin. The factor that chiefly controls the absorption or rejection of ingested iron is the amount of ferritin already present in the intestinal mucosa. When all available apoferritin has been bound to iron to form ferritin, any additional iron that arrives at the binding site is rejected, then returned to the lumen of the intestine, and then passed on for excretion in the feces.

A number of factors influence the absorption of iron. Those that favor or facilitate absorption include the following:

1. The amount of reserve ferritin present in mucosal cells correlates with the body's need for iron. In deficiency states or in periods of extra demand as in growth or pregnancy, mucosal ferritin is lower, and more iron is absorbed. When tissue reserves are ample or saturated, iron is rejected and excreted.

2. Ascorbic acid (vitamin C) aids in absorption of iron by its reducing action and effect on acidity, changing dietary iron to the ferrous form in which it can be absorbed. Other metabolic reducing agents have similar effects.

3. The hydrochloric acid that is a normal constituent of gastric secretions provides the optimal acid medium for the preparation of iron for utilization.

4. An adequate amount of calcium helps to bind and remove agents such as phosphate and phytate, which if not removed would combine with iron and inhibit its absorption.

The following are factors that hinder iron absorption:

1. Phosphate, phytate, and oxalate are binding agents that remove iron from the body. Therefore a diet high in phosphate, phytate, or oxalate leads to a decrease in iron absorption.

2. Surgical removal of stomach tissue (gastrectomy) reduces the number of cells that secrete hydrochloric acid. The acid medium necessary for iron reduction is therefore not provided.

3. Severe infection hinders iron absorption.

4. Malabsorption syndromes or any disturbance that causes diarrhea or steatorrhea will hinder iron absorption.

Transport. Mucosal ferritin delivers ferrous iron to the portal blood system. The iron is converted back to the ferric state by oxidation. As ferric iron, it combines with a plasma β-globulin, *transferrin* (or siderophilin), to form

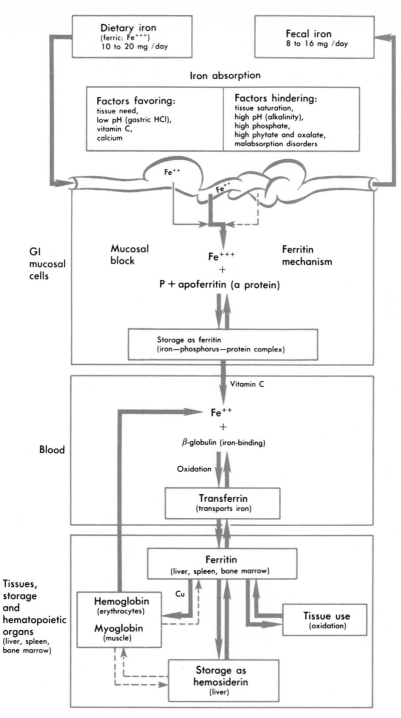

Fig. 8-3. Summary of iron metabolism, showing its absorption, transport, main use in hemoglobin formation, and its storage forms (ferritin and hemosiderin).

a ferric-protein complex, which is the plasma transport form of iron. Transferrin is from 30% to 40% saturated with iron, and the remaining 60% to 70% forms an unsaturated, unbound, latent reserve in the plasma for handling iron.

Storage. The plasma transferrin then conveys iron to the various body cells for storage and utilization. About 1 g is distributed throughout all the cells as an essential element in energy-producing enzyme systems. The main storage organs, however, are the liver, spleen, and bone marrow, which participate in the forming of red blood cells. In these sites the iron is stored as ferritin and as hemosiderin. Hemosiderin is a secondary, less soluble compound. It is a protein-bound ferric oxide with 35% iron. Hemosiderin formation increases as excess iron accumulates, such as during rapid destruction of red blood cells in hemolytic anemia. From these storage compounds, iron is mobilized for hemoglobin synthesis as needed. In the average adult, from 20 to 25 mg of iron is involved daily in hemoglobin synthesis. But the body avidly conserves the iron that it uses in the synthesis of hemoglobin. As red cells are destroyed after an average life span of about 120 days, approximately 90% of the iron that is released is conserved and is used over and over and over again. These iron absorption-storage mechanisms are diagrammed in Fig. 8-3. These relationships should be carefully compared.

Excretion. As indicated, since the main regulatory mechanism for control of iron levels is at the point of absorption, only very minute amounts are lost by excretion—about 0.5 to 1.0 mg daily. Average trace amounts excreted are 0.1 mg in the urine; 0.2 to 0.5 mg in feces; and 0.05 to 1.0 mg in sweat. In girls and women monthly menstrual losses are about 20 mg. From 400 to 900 mg of iron is lost during a usual pregnancy and delivery.

Metabolic functions of iron

Essentially, iron serves two major purposes in human metabolism.

Hemoglobin formation. Iron is the core of the heme molecule, the fundamental nonprotein conjugate of hemoglobin. Hemoglobin in the red blood cell is the oxygen transport unit of the blood that conveys oxygen to the cells for respiration and metabolism. Iron is also a constituent of a similar compound, myoglobin, in muscle tissue.

Cellular oxidation. Although in smaller amounts, iron also functions in the cells as a vital component of enzyme systems for oxidation of glucose to produce energy. In the Krebs cycle, for example, iron is a constituent of the *cytochrome* compounds, which are used in the oxidative chains producing high-energy ATP bonds (see p. 76).

Clinical application

Normal life cycle. During growth, the demand for positive iron balance is imperative. The newborn infant has at birth about a three to six months' supply of iron, which was stored in the liver during fetal development. Since milk does not supply iron, supplementary iron-rich foods must be added to prevent the classic milk anemia of young children. Iron is also needed during continued growth and to build up reserves for the physiologic stress of adolescence, especially the onset of menses in girls.

The woman's need for iron is increased during pregnancy to maintain the increased total number of red blood cells in an expanded circulating blood volume and to supply the iron for storage in the developing fetal liver. Finally, normal blood loss during delivery reduces iron stores.

Abnormal clinical situations. Because of the unique physiologic controls of the body's iron content, clinical abnormalities may result from either a deficiency or an excess of iron.

Deficiency of iron results in a hypochromic microcytic anemia. This lack of iron or inability to use it may result from one of several causes:

1. An inadequate supply of iron in the diet
   —*nutritional anemia*

2. Excessive blood iron loss—*hemorrhagic anemia*
3. Inability to form hemoglobin in the absence of other necessary factors such as vitamin B_{12}—*pernicious anemia* (p. 118)
4. Lack of gastric hydrochloric acid necessary to liberate iron for absorption—*postgastrectomy anemia*
5. The presence of inhibitors of iron absorption such as phosphate or phytate, or mucosal lesions that affect absorbing surface, leading to *malabsorption anemia*

Excessive amounts of iron may accumulate in the body because of the lack of an efficient excretory mechanism, and iron storage capacities may become saturated. This buildup of iron may result from one of several causes:

1. Excess iron intake or excess red blood cell destruction, as in malaria or hemolytic anemias (which release excess iron into the serum), produces a condition known as *hemosiderosis* (Gr. *hemo,* blood; *sidero,* iron). (An unusually high iron intake—about 200 mg per day—and resulting hemosiderosis have been reported among the Bantu natives of Africa. Their high-corn diet is low in phosphates to bind iron, and they cook their food in heavy iron pots. It seems that the continuous high-iron intake with little phosphate to hinder its absorption results in excessive liver storage and liver damage. This condition has been called Bantu siderosis.)
2. Excess intravenous iron or repeated transfusions may cause an accumulation of iron. This is associated with long-standing aplastic or hemolytic anemias with excess breakdown of red blood cells.
3. Hemochromatosis, a rare disease that occurs chiefly in males, is believed by some investigators to be genetically transmitted. Saturation of the body tissues with iron causes a bronze coloration, liver damage, and severe diabetes. A potent iron-chelating agent, *desferrioxamine,*

has been developed for use in treating such conditions. (The word *chelate* comes from the Greek word, *chele,* meaning claw. A chelating agent is a substance that can grasp and incorporate a metallic ion in its molecular structure, which binds it and removes the ion from a tissue or from the circulating blood.)

Dietary requirements of iron

The recommended allowances of the NRC (1980 revision) list a general daily adult dietary intake of 10 mg of iron for men and 18 mg for women during the childbearing years. This greater amount is needed to cover menstrual losses and the demands of pregnancy. It is doubtful that the woman's ordinary diet can supply this larger quantity of iron, and fortification with iron supplements is probably desirable. Infant allowances are 10 to 15 mg; recommendations for children are 15 mg for children ages 1 to 3, and 10 mg for children ages 3 to 12. The daily need is 18 mg for boys 12 to 18 and for girls from age 10 on through the reproductive years.

Iron needs vary with age and situations, and these allowances are designed to provide margins for safety.

Food sources of iron

Organ meats, especially liver, are by far the best sources of iron. Other food sources include meats, egg yolk, whole wheat, seafood, green leafy vegetables, nuts, and legumes.

Copper
Occurrence in the body

Broadly speaking, copper seems to behave in the body as a companion to iron. The two are metabolized in much the same way and share some functions.

The adult body contains from 100 to 150 mg of copper, distributed mainly in muscle, bone, the liver, heart, kidneys, and central nervous system. A small quantity is bound to plasma protein. The serum values are highly variable but range from 130 to 230 $\mu g/dl$. In the serum about 5% of the copper is bound with albumin, and about 95% is bound with a α-globulin as the copper-binding protein *ceruloplasmin*.

Absorption-transport-storage-excretion

Absorption. Copper is known to be absorbed in the proximal portion of the small intestine, although the mechanism for its absorption is not well understood.

Transport and storage. The absorbed copper is first taken up by the plasma albumin and probably is initially transported in this bound form. Within 24 hours, however, the copper is bound by an α-globulin to form ceruloplasmin. From 50% to 75% of the total body copper is stored in muscle mass and bones, with high concentrations in the liver, heart, kidneys, and central nervous system.

Excretion. The main route of excretion is the intestine. Some additional copper is lost in urine, sweat, and menstrual flow.

Metabolic functions of copper

Copper is associated with iron in several important metabolic functions:

1. Copper, like iron, is involved in the cytochrome oxidation system of tissue cells for energy production, as well as being a constituent of several other oxidative enzymes for amino acids.
2. Copper is essential, together with iron, in the formation of hemoglobin. A copper-containing protein, *erythrocuprein*, is in red blood cells.
3. Copper seems to promote absorption of iron from the gastrointestinal tract. Copper also appears to be involved in transporting iron from the tissues into the plasma.

In addition to these iron-related functions, copper is involved in two other areas of metabolism: (1) bone formation and (2) brain tissue formation and maintenance of myelin in the nervous system.

Clinical application

Deficiency states in man are unknown. However, low plasma copper levels *(hypocupremia)* due to urinary loss of ceruloplasmin have been observed in nephrosis. Sprue, because of malabsorption of copper, can also cause low plasma levels.

An excess accumulation of copper occurs in a rare inherited condition known as Wilson's disease, which is characterized by degenerative changes in brain tissue (basal ganglia) and in the liver. Large amounts of copper are absorbed, and storage is increased in the liver, brain, kidneys and cornea. A copper-chelate, penicillamine, is used to bind the excess copper and cause it to be excreted.

Requirement and food sources

Balance studies indicate that adults require about 2.5 mg of copper daily. Infants and children require about 0.05 mg/kg of body weight.

Copper is widely distributed in natural foods. The average daily diet contains from 2.5 to 5.0 mg. Therefore given a sufficient caloric intake, copper will be amply supplied.

Iodine

Occurrence in the body

Iodine is a trace element associated mainly with the thyroid gland. The total iodine in the body is from 20 to 50 mg. Approximately 50% is in the muscles, 20% in the thyroid gland, 10% in the skin, 6% in the skeleton. The remaining 14% is scattered in other endocrine tissue, in the central nervous system, and in plasma transport. By far the greatest iodine tissue concentration, however, is in the thyroid.

Absorption-excretion

Ingested iodine is absorbed in the small intestine as iodides. These are loosely bound with proteins and are conveyed by the blood to the thyroid gland. About one third of it is selectively absorbed by the thyroid cells and removed from circulation. The remaining two

TO PROBE FURTHER
The iodine pump and thyroxine formation

The cell membranes of the thyroid gland have a tremendous specific capacity to take up or trap iodides by an active transport mechanism. The concentration of iodides in these structures is normally about 25 times that of their concentration in the blood plasma. Highly active thyroid cells can accomplish an iodide concentration some 350 times that in blood.

Studies* with radioactive iodine (^{131}I) have traced the interesting interrelated role of iodine with protein in thyroxine formation. A neutral protein of large molecular weight, *thyroglobulin,* secreted into the thyroid follicle forms both the working base for synthesizing the hormone and the molecular storage complex for holding it until needed. This complex is called *colloid.* The amino acid tyrosine, a part of the thyroglobulin molecule, forms the base structure, which through successive stages of iodination, finally builds the hormone *thyroxine* (Fig. 8-4).

*Wolff, J.: Transport of iodide and other anions in the thyroid gland, Physiol. Rev. **44**:45, 1964.

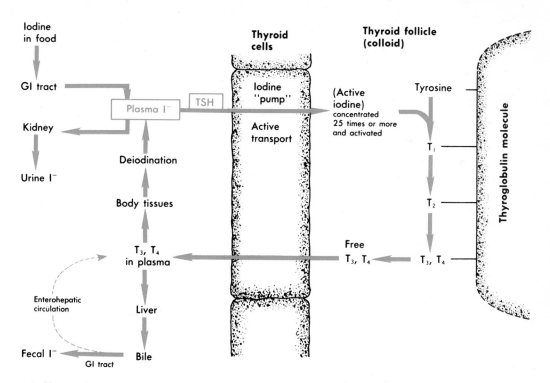

Fig. 8-4. Summary of iodine metabolism, showing active iodine pump in the thyroid cells and the synthesis of thyroxine in the colloid tissue of the thyroid follicles. (TSH, thyroid stimulating hormone; T_1, monoiodotyronine; T_2, diiodotyrosine; T_3, triiodothyronine; T_4, tetraiodothyronine.)

thirds is usually excreted in the urine within two to three days after ingestion. A pituitary hormone, TSH (thyroid-stimulating hormone or thyrotropic hormone), stimulates the uptake of iodine by the thyroid cells. The amount of TSH that is released by the pituitary is in turn governed by the level of thyroid hormone in the circulating blood. This circular or feedback mechanism normally maintains a healthy balance between supply and demand. Such a feedback mechanism is the characteristic pattern for governing all of the hormones from the several endocrine glands that are controlled by the pituitary (master) gland.

Metabolic function of iodine

Iodine participates in the synthesis of the thyroid hormone. This is the only known function of iodine in human metabolism. The thyroid hormone (thyroxine) in turn stimulates cell oxidation, apparently by increasing oxygen uptake and reaction rates of enzyme systems handling glucose. Therefore iodine indirectly exerts tremendous influence on overall body metabolism.

The free thyroxine with its associated iodine is secreted into the bloodstream and bound to plasma protein for transport to body cells as needed. This transport form of iodine is called serum *protein-bound iodine* (PBI). The serum level of PBI normally ranges from 4 to 8 μg/dl. After being used to stimulate oxidation in the cell, thyroxine is degraded in the liver, and the iodine is excreted in bile as inorganic iodine.

Clinical application

Thyroid function. Both hyperthyroidism and hypothyroidism affect the rate of iodine uptake and utilization. Endemic colloid goiter is a classic condition characterized by great enlargement of the thyroid gland. Endemic colloid goiter occurs in residents of areas where the water and soil (and therefore locally grown foods) contain little iodine. The thyroid gland that is starved for iodine cannot produce a nor-

mal quantity of thyroxine. The amount of thyroxine that is secreted into the bloodstream is therefore too low to shut off TSH secretion by the pituitary. The pituitary persists in putting out TSH, and these large quantities of TSH continue to stimulate the thyroid gland, calling on it to produce the thyroxine that it cannot supply. The only response that the iodine-starved gland can make is to increase the amount of thyroglobulin (colloid), which then accumulates in the thyroid follicles. Such a gland becomes increasingly engorged, and may attain a tremendous size, weighing 500 to 700 g (1 to 1½ lb) or more.

Tests for iodine metabolism

The *PBI test* measures the amount of iodine that is bound to thyroxine and in transit in the plasma. A small amount of free inorganic iodide may also be present. The normal range is from 4 to 8 μg/dl of serum. Values below 4 indicate hypothyroidism; those above 8 indicate hyperthyroidism. Unfortunately, false high readings may result from the presence in the system of other iodine compounds, such as certain iodine-containing radiopaque substances that may have been administered in conjunction with x-ray studies or iodine-containing therapeutic agents. Mercurial diuretics may cause false low readings.

Radioactive ^{131}I tests are tests that use radioactive iodine to measure the uptake and utilization of iodine by the thyroid gland.

The iodine cycle and dental caries. Prevention of dental caries has been attributed to the iodine cycle, which involves the salivary secretion of iodine. It is believed that increased saliva flow, by raising the concentration and secretion of iodine by the parotid and submaxillary glands, inhibits the formation of dental caries.

Requirement and food sources of iodine

Balance studies indicate that the adult needs to ingest from 100 to 200 μg of iodine daily and that the basal requirement is about 25 μg. The NRC (1980 revision) has recommended daily adult allowances of 140 μg for young men and 100 μg for young women. These needs normally decrease with age. The demand is increased during periods of accelerated growth such as adolescence and pregnancy.

Seafood provides a considerable amount of iodine; however, the quantity in natural sources varies broadly, depending on the iodine content of the soil. The average diet falls somewhat below the requirement. The commercial iodizing of table salt (1 mg to every 10 g of salt) provides the main dietary source of iodine.

Some question concerning the continued use of iodized salt has been raised on the basis of several current changes in our environment: (1) agricultural practices, especially in the diary industry, that increase the iodine content of milk products, (2) food technology, especially in the bread industry, where additive iodates in dough conditions may raise iodine content of a slice of bread to 250 μg, (3) use of iodine-containing drugs, and (4) increased absorption from polluted air. Also, ingestion of unusual iodine-rich items such as kelp and seaweed may contribute more. However, although the average consumption of iodine in the United States is five to ten times the recommended dietary allowance of the NRC's Food and Nutrition Board, an individual's iodine intake is highly variable and may be deficient, depending on geographic location and food supply, without the use of iodized salt. Therefore since moderately excessive iodine is relatively harmless and persons living in endemic goiter regions may be at risk, it is probably wise to continue using iodized salt as a precaution.[3]

Manganese
Occurrence in the body

In industry manganese is a metallic element used chiefly as an alloy in steel to give it toughness. In nutrition traces of manganese serve as essential activating agents that strengthen and stimulate a number of vital metabolic reactions.

Only about 10 mg of manganese is present in the adult body, chiefly in the liver and kidneys, with small amounts in other tissues such as the retina, bones, and salivary glands. Blood values are very low—4 to 20 μg/dl have been reported.

Absorption-excretion

Manganese, like iron, is poorly absorbed by the intestine; much is rejected by the intestine, and that which is rejected is eliminated directly in the feces. The small quantity that is absorbed in the small intestine, however, enters the bloodstream and is transported, loosely bound with protein, to the tissues for storage and utilization.

Excretion of manganese takes place almost entirely through the intestine. In addition to that which was rejected and eliminated directly, a small amount of the manganese that has been used by the tissues is ultimately carried to the bile, which returns it into the intestine, where this amount is excreted with other body wastes. Little or no manganese is excreted in the urine.

Metabolic functions of manganese

Studies of animals have clearly demonstrated the essential nature of manganese to a number of their metabolic functions. Although the participation of manganese has not been clearly shown in all of the parallel functions in human nutrition, studies with radioactive manganese (^{56}Mn) have shown that its active uptake sites are the cell mitochondria, in which the cell enzyme systems operate. Therefore it seems that the function of manganese in human nutrition may well be to participate in key coenzymes in these reactions. Some of these reactions include

1. *Urea formation*—activates an enzyme in the formation of urea; may help prevent ammonia toxicity
2. *Protein metabolism*—activates amino acid interconversions; activates peptidases for splitting specific amino acids such as leucine

3. *Carbohydrate metabolism*—activates several conversion reactions of the glycolytic pathway and Krebs cycle in glucose oxidation
4. *Fat metabolism*—activates the serum fat-clearing factor, lipoprotein lipase, and operates as a cofactor in the synthesis of long-chain fatty acids

Clinical application

Although many clinical evidences of manganese deficiency have been established in animals, none have been observed in humans. However, an industrial disease syndrome, representing *inhalation toxicity,* occurs in miners and other workers who undergo prolonged exposure to manganese dust. The excess manganese accumulates in the liver and central nervous system and eventually produces severe neuromuscular manifestations that resemble those of Parkinson's disease.

Requirement and food sources of manganese

Whether there is a specific human requirement of manganese is unknown. The average diet provides from 3 to 9 μg daily, which seems highly adequate.

The best food sources of manganese are of plant origin: cereal bran, soybeans, legumes, nuts, tea, and coffee. Animal foods are relatively poor sources.

Cobalt

Occurrence in the body

Cobalt occurs in only minute traces in the body tissues, and the main storage area is the liver. As an essential constituent of vitamin B_{12}, cobalt is largely associated with red blood cell formation. The normal blood level, representing the element in transit and in erythrocytes, is about 1 μg/dl.

Absorption-excretion

Variable amounts of cobalt are absorbed, and apparently quickly excreted in the urine.

Unabsorbed cobalt is lost in feces. The main form in which it is absorbed and used is as a constituent of vitamin B_{12}.

Metabolic function of cobalt

The basic function of cobalt in human nutrition that has been demonstrated is that of a constituent of vitamin B_{12}, an essential factor in the formation of red blood cells. The widespread distribution of cobalt in nature and its ready uptake by plants lead one to speculate about possible broader functions. As yet, however, such functions have not been established.

Clinical application

Deficiency of cobalt per se is well known to have deleterious effects in animals. In man a deficiency of cobalt is associated only with a deficiency of vitamin B_{12} and the consequent development of pernicious anemia (see p. 118).

Excess of cobalt has led to polycythemia, a condition characterized by the formation of an excess number of red blood cells that contain a relatively high concentration of hemoglobin.

Requirement and food sources of cobalt

The quantitative human requirement of cobalt is unknown, but is evidently minute. For example, as small an amount as 0.045 to 0.09 μg daily maintains bone marrow functions in patients with pernicious anemia.

Cobalt is widely distributed in nature; however, for man's chief need—as a constituent of vitamin B_{12}—cobalt is best obtained in the preformed vitamin, which is synthesized in animals by gastrointestinal bacteria.

Zinc

Occurrence in the body

Zinc occurs in the human body in amounts larger than those of other trace elements except iron. The body's total zinc content, from 1.3 to 2.3 g, is distributed in many tissues including the pancreas, liver, kidney, lung, muscles, bones, eye (cornea, iris, retina, and lens), endocrine glands, prostate secretions, and spermatozoa. The plasma zinc level is about 120 μg/dl.

Absorption-excretion

After zinc is absorbed in the small intestine it combines with plasma proteins for transport to the tissues. Isotope studies indicate that it first concentrates in the liver, pancreas, kidneys, and pituitary, then predominantly in red blood cells and bone, after which it appears to remain in circulation and use as long as from eight to twelve months.

Excretion of zinc is largely intestinal. Unabsorbed zinc is eliminated immediately. Zinc that has entered the blood and tissues is gradually excreted into the intestine in pancreatic and intestinal secretions, and a small amount is also excreted in the bile. Except in disease states, zinc is rarely excreted in the urine.

Metabolic functions of zinc

Enzyme constituent. Zinc functions mainly as an essential constituent of cell enzyme systems. It has its primary metabolic role as a component of various metalloenzymes, over 70 of which have been identified in various living systems.[4] Alkaline phosphatase, for example, is a zinc enzyme. Three other zinc enzymes may be used as examples: carbonic anhydrase, carboxypeptidase, and lactic dehydrogenase.

Zinc is an integral part of *carbonic anhydrase,* which acts as a carbon dioxide carrier, especially in red blood cells. It takes up carbon dioxide from cells, combines it with water to form carbonic acid (H_2CO_3), and then releases carbon dioxide from the capillaries into the alveoli of the lung. This enzyme also functions in the renal tubule cells in the maintenance of acid-base balance, in mucosal cells, and in glands of the body.

Zinc is a cofactor of the protein-splitting enzyme, *carboxypeptidase,* which removes the carboxyl group (COOH) from peptides to produce amino acids. Zinc therefore has a key role in protein digestion.

Zinc is a part of *lactic dehydrogenase.* This enzyme is essential for the interconversion of pyruvic acid and lactic acid in the glycolytic pathway for glucose oxidation. Thus zinc also plays a part in carbohydrate metabolism.

Two additional roles of zinc in metabolism are important, but their significance is less well understood.

Insulin. Zinc combines readily with insulin in the pancreas; zinc-insulin serves perhaps as the storage form of this hormone. The diabetic pancreas contains about half the normal amount of zinc.

Leukocytes. A considerable quantity of zinc bound to protein is present in leukocytes, although its function in white cells is unclear. Some investigators suggest that zinc affects the body's immune system through its essential role in the synthesis of nucleic acids and protein and is also needed for lymphocyte transformation.[5] Lymphoid tissue, which gives rise to lymphocytes, contains a large amount of zinc. All these factors support a cellular immunity role for zinc. The leukocytes of patients with leukemia contain about 10% less zinc than normal.

Clinical application

Hypogonadism and dwarfism from pronounced human zinc deficiency during growth periods have been found in some populations. Also, hypogeusia and hyposmia (impaired taste and smell acuity), which appear to be relatively widespread, are improved with increased zinc intake.

Wound healing is also related to zinc intake.[6] According to recent studies, zinc-deficient wounds seem to be common in the average hospital, and patients benefit from zinc supplementation. Some hospital diets, for example, reportedly contain only 11 mg/2,700 calories of zinc.[7] Certain bland diets probably contain even less. Zinc supplementation may be necessary in some cases. Older patients with poor appetites who subsist on marginal diets in the face of chronic wounds and illnesses may be particularly vulnerable.

A possible relation of zinc metabolism with liver disease has aroused the interest of investigators. In cirrhosis, serum zinc levels are low, urinary excretion is increased, and postmortem studies have revealed reduced zinc concentrations in the liver. It is speculated that the disease may increase the need for zinc, and therefore deficiency results from the usual intake.

Requirement and food sources of zinc

As with iron, an optimal intake of zinc in the United States population cannot be assumed. Thus for the first time in its 1974 revisions and continued in the 1980 standards, the NRC has established a recommendation for zinc in daily diets. For adults a standard allowance of 15 mg is given, with 10 mg indicated for children and 3 to 5 mg for infants.

The most vulnerable period of potential zinc deficiency is during times of rapid growth. For example, the newborn infant enters a phase of negative zinc balance in the first few months of life, returning to the initial (and adult) levels only at age 4. Thus it is important that infant formulas and foods contain enough zinc to meet recommended dietary allowances.

Another source of concern for optimal zinc intake lies with low-income diets and with the increased use of meat substitute items based on vegetable protein. Since the best food sources of zinc with the greatest availability are animal products rather than plants, a diet optimal in zinc may tend to be more expensive. A lower cost diet in which protein is obtained mainly from vegetable sources is likely to provide marginal amounts of zinc. Moreover, this problem may well be accentuated by the increasing production and consumption of meat analogs made from vegetable protein.

The best sources of zinc are seafood, meat, and eggs. Additional sources, although less available to the body, are legumes and whole grains. Food value tables for zinc content of a number of foods have been developed.[8] Adult needs for zinc can be met through the consistent use of a well-balanced diet, but it is more difficult when low-cost foods must be used. Therefore in the future it may be necessary to enrich certain staple foods with zinc.

Molybdenum
Occurrence in the body and function of molybdenum

Amounts of molybdenum in the body are very minute. This trace mineral is present in bound form as an integral part of various enzyme molecules and thus functions in facilitating the action of the specific enzyme involved. Examples of molybdenum-containing enzymes are xanthine oxidase and liver aldehyde oxidase.

In purine catabolism, xanthine oxidase catalyzes the oxidation of xanthine to uric acid. It has been isolated from milk and liver.

Liver aldehyde oxidase, a flavoprotein, catalyzes the oxidation of aldehydes to corresponding carboxylic acid.

Requirement and food sources of molybdenum

Food sources of molybdenum include legumes, whole grains, milk, leafy vegetables, and organ meats. There is no specific requirement given.

TRACE MINERALS WITH UNKNOWN FUNCTION

Several other minerals occur in trace amounts in the body, but their essential function is not clear. These include fluorine (Fl), selenium (Se), aluminum (Al), boron (B), cadmium (Cd), chromium (Cr), nickel (Ni), tin (Sn), silicon (Si), and vanadium (V).

Fluorine

The only relationship thus far established for fluorine in human metabolism is its association with dental health. Basic observations have centered around the results of an excess intake of fluorine and of a small intake.

Excess intake

Endemic dental fluorosis has been observed in communities where the natural fluorine content of the water supply is high. The largest known such region in the United States is the West Texas Panhandle. Apparently fluorine excesses act on teeth in the budding stage of formation, so that by the time they erupt their enamel is mottled, pitted, and discolored. Adults who habitually eat excessive quantities of fluoride may suffer from osteosclerosis. Osteosclerosis is abnormal density of the skeletal bone, which in some cases is so mild that it can barely be detected by x-ray film, but in other instances it is so severe as to be called crippling fluorosis.

Small intake

Dental caries has been demonstrated to be largely preventable by the addition of a small amount of fluorine to fluorine-poor drinking water or by the topical application of fluoride solutions to young developing teeth. Public health authorities advocate the fluoridation of public drinking water in the amount of one part per million in areas where the drinking water is low in fluoride content. The mechanism by which fluorine prevents dental caries is unknown.

Selenium

Interest in selenium has recently centered about the discovery of a potent, metabolically active, selenium-containing compound called "factor 3," which was observed to protect the liver against fatty infiltration and necrosis. This action of selenium is apparently related to that of vitamin E, since the two substances act synergistically in curing the hepatic disease and certain muscle disorders induced in animals.

Selenium functions as an essential constituent of glutathione (GSH) peroxidase, a major cellular antioxidant defense system. The activity of this system in human erythrocytes has been found to be correlated with the plasma vitamin E content.[9]

Aluminum

The amount of aluminum ingested in the average human diet ranges widely from about 10 mg to more than 100 mg daily. This element is found in many plant and animal foods. Despite this wide intake and distribution, no clear function in human nutrition has been established. A clue may be present in model systems studies of certain transaminase reactions with amino acids. The mechanism and significance of these reactions are not clear, however.

The total aluminum content of the adult human body is from 50 to 150 mg.

Boron

Minute traces of boron are found in body tissues, but no clues to its purpose have been discovered. Boron has been found to be essential for plant nutrition and growth, but experiments in animals have not demonstrated any evidences of deficiency after boron deprivation.

Cadmium

That traces of cadmium are present in body tissues has been known for some time. Not until 1960, however, was cadmium isolated as a definite component of a metal-containing protein. This protein, metallothionein, found in the renal cortex of the horse, contains cadmium, zinc, and sulfur. The significance of this cadmium-containing protein is not yet clear, but it points to the possibility that the mineral functions in some basic biologic system.

Chromium

Our bodies contain less than 6 mg of chromium. These minute traces of chromium present in the body were not recognized until analytic methods were developed that were sufficiently sensitive to detect them. There are about 20 parts of chromium in 1 billion parts of blood; however, certain cell proteins can achieve concentrations of chromium much higher than this. The greater concentration in cells has led to studies of chromium, which indicate a probable role in glucose metabolism. In animals made chromium-deficient by deprivation, fasting blood sugar levels were elevated and glycosuria followed. In humans, studies have shown the ability of chromium to raise abnormally low fasting blood sugar levels and to improve faulty uptake of sugar by body tissues. Physicians working in Jerusalem with refugee infants suffering from severe malnutrition and an inability to use sugar found that when small amounts of chromium were added to their diet, the infants made rapid recovery.

The work of Schwarz and Mertz has indicated that chromium functions as an active component of glucose tolerance factor (GTF). GTF is synthesized from inorganic chromium, niacin, and amino acids, probably in the liver or intestinal flora. It is released in response to increased blood insulin levels and potentiates the action of insulin in target tissues. Additional studies are being done to clarify these probable functions.[10]

The average daily human diet apparently contains from 80 to 100 μg of chromium, of which only 2 to 5 μg is absorbed. The absorbed chromium is stored in the tissues, from which it is released when glucose is ingested. It seems, however, that tissue levels are by no means consistent. Wide variances have been found in samples taken from different sites and at different times. Further study is needed to determine chromium's role in metabolism and its nutritional significance. In the meantime it is interesting to speculate concerning its possible link with chronic disease processes such as cardiovascular disorders and diabetes.

Nickel

Nickel has been established through animal studies to be an essential trace element, although additional study is needed to determine more specifically its role in human nutrition. It occurs in tissue as a metalloprotein, nickeloplasmin, and appears to be associated with thyroid hormone and RNA in the cell. A deficiency of nickel in animals has been related to low-ered oxygen uptake, increased plasma lipids, changes in liver tissue, impaired reproduction, sparse rough hair, and lethargy. Possible clinical relationships in humans may be in plasma lipid levels, in cirrhosis of the liver, and in chronic uremia. There is a relatively high concentration of nickel in sweat—49 μg/L. Human dietary needs for nickel have been estimated to be under 0.6 μg daily. It occurs mainly in plant foods, especially grains and vegetables, with little in animal food sources.

Tin

Trace amounts of tin occur in many tissues and dietary items. Until recently, it has been considered more an "environmental contaminant" than the essential trace mineral it is now known to be. Its chemical properties suggest that it may contribute to the tertiary structure of proteins (see p. 55) and also participate in certain oxidation-reduction reactions in the cell's enzyme systems, such as with the flavine enzymes (see p. 76). Daily dietary needs have been estimated to be under 1 mg. It is found in food sources such as meats and other animal products, whole grains, legumes, vegetables, and fruits, especially in acidic juices canned in tin.

Silicon

Animals deprived of silicon evidence depressed growth, pallor of mucous membranes, and skeletal alterations and deformities, especially of the skull. These skeletal changes apparently involve the cartilage matrix, and it is postulated that silicon may function as an essential agent in developing crosslinking in structure and resilience of connective tissue. It has been shown to be essential for bone calcification. The daily dietary need for humans is unknown. It is found in all plant foods, especially whole grains.

Vanadium

Studies have shown vanadium to be an essential element for higher animals, related to tooth

Table 8-2. Summary of trace minerals

Mineral	Metabolism	Physiologic functions	Clinical application	Requirement	Food source
Iron (Fe)	Absorption according to body need controlled by mucosal block—ferritin mechanism; aided by vitamin C, gastric hydrochloric acid Transport—transferrin Storage—ferritin, hemosiderin Excretion from tissue in minute quantities; body conserves and reuses	Hemoglobin formation Cellular oxidation (cytochrome system producing ATP)	Growth (milk anemia) Pregnancy demands Deficiency—anemia Excess—hemosiderosis; hemochromatosis	Men: 10 mg Women: 18 mg Pregnancy: 18+ mg Lactation: 18 mg Children: 10-18 mg	Liver Meats Egg yolk Whole grains Enriched bread and cereal Dark green vegetables Legumes, nuts
Copper (Cu)	Transported bound to an α-globulin as ceruloplasmin Stored in muscle, bone, liver, heart, kidney, and central nervous system	Associated with iron in Enzyme systems Hemoglobin synthesis Absorption and transport of iron Involved in bone formation and maintenance of brain tissue and myelin sheath in nervous system	Hypocupremia: Nephrosis Malabsorption Wilson's disease—excess copper storage	2-2.5 mg Diet provides 2-5 mg	Liver Meat Seafood Whole grains Legumes, nuts Cocoa Raisins Food cooked in copper utensils
Iodine (I)	Absorbed as iodides, taken up by thyroid gland under control of thyroid-stimulating hormone (TSH) Excretion by kidney	Synthesis of thyroxine, the thyroid hormone, which regulates cell oxidation	Deficiency—endemic colloid goiter; cretinism	Men: 140 μg Women: 100 μg Infants: 35-45 μg Children: 60-140 μg	Iodized salt Seafood
Manganese (Mn)	Absorption limited Excretion mainly by intestine	Activates reactions in Urea formation Protein metabolism Glucose oxidation Lipoprotein clearance and synthesis of fatty acids	No clinical deficiency observed in humans Inhalation toxicity in miners	2.5-7 mg (estimated) Diet provides 3-9 μg	Cereals, whole grain Soybeans Legumes, nuts Tea, coffee Vegetables Fruits

Continued.

Table 8-2. Summary of trace minerals—cont'd

Mineral	Metabolism	Physiologic functions	Clinical application	Requirement	Food source
Cobalt (Co)	Absorbed chiefly as constituent of vitamin B_{12}	Constituent of vitamin B_{12} essential factor in red blood cell formation	Deficiency associated with deficiency of vitamin B_{12}—pernicious anemia	Unknown	Supplied by preformed vitamin B_{12}
Zinc (Zn)	Transported with plasma proteins Excretion largely intestinal Stored in liver, muscle, bone, and organs	Essential enzyme constituent: Carbonic anhydrase Carboxypeptidase Lactic dehydrogenase Combined with insulin for storage of the hormone	Possible relation to liver disease Wound healing Taste and smell acuity Retarded sexual and physical development	Adults: 15 mg Children: 10 mg Infants: 3-5 mg	Widely distributed Liver Seafood, especially oysters Eggs Milk Whole grains
Molybdenum (Mo)	Minute traces in the body	Constituent of specific enzymes involved in Purine conversion to uric acid Aldehyde oxidation		450-500 μg (estimated)	Organ meats Milk Whole grains Leafy vegetables Legumes
Fluorine (Fl)	Deposited in bones and teeth Excreted in urine	Associated with dental health	Small amount prevents dental caries Excess causes endemic dental fluorosis	1-3 mg (estimated)	Water (1 ppm. Fl)
Selenium (Se)	Active as cofactor in cell oxidation enzyme systems	Associated with fat metabolism	Constituent of "factor 3," which acts with vitamin E to prevent fatty liver	Under 100 μg (estimated)	Seafoods Meats Whole grains

Mineral		Function		Amount (estimated)	Food sources
Chromium (Cr)	Improves faulty uptake of glucose by body tissues	Associated with glucose metabolism; raises abnormally low fasting blood sugar levels	Infants unable to metabolize sugar, and adult diabetics show definite improvement when small amounts of chromium added to diet. Possible link with cardiovascular disorders and diabetes	20-50 μg (estimated)	Animal proteins, especially meats (except fish). Whole grains
Nickel (Ni)	Binding by phytate reduces intestinal absorption	Constituent of the protein nickeloplasmin. Associated with thyroid hormone. High in RNA	Plasma levels decreased in cirrhosis and chronic uremia	Under 0.6 μg (estimated)	Whole grains, Legumes, Vegetables, Fruits
Tin (Sn)		Structural element in protein synthesis. Associated with cell enzyme systems in energy metabolism	Wound healing, Tissue growth	Under 1 mg (estimated)	Meats, Whole grains, Legumes, Vegetables, Fruits, Acid juices canned in tin
Silicon (Si)		Essential agent in formation of bone, cartilage, connective tissue	Bone calcification and healing	Unknown	All plant foods
Vanadium (V)		High in teeth; may have role in bone and tooth formation	Possible relation to lipid metabolism, blood lipid levels	0.1-0.3 mg (estimated)	Grains, breads, Root vegetables, Nuts, Vegetable oils

and bone development. It also appears to have a role in lipid metabolism, as deficiency states have been related to lowered cholesterol levels. Additional study is needed to determine vanadium function and requirements in man, but adequate vanadium nutrition should not be taken for granted. It is found widely distributed in primary foods such as grains, root vegetables, nuts, and vegetable oils. The daily need in human nutrition has been estimated to be about 0.1 to 0.3 mg.

Some of the trace minerals are summarized in Table 8-2.

GLOSSARY

anemia blood condition characterized by decrease in number of circulating red blood cells, hemoglobin, or both. Anemias may be caused by lack of dietary iron intake, hemorrhage, lack of other substances necessary to form hemoglobin (vitamin B_{12}), lack of factors necessary for absorption of iron (hydrochloric acid), or intestinal diseases affecting absorbing surface.

apoferritin (Gr. *apo,* from away, separation; L. *ferr,* iron) protein base in intestinal mucosa cells, which will bind with iron (from food) to form ferritin, the storage form of iron.

bone compartment the body's total content of skeletal tissue. The bone compartment contains 99% of the body's total metabolic calcium pool.

calcitonin a quick-acting hormone secreted by the parathyroids in response to hypercalcemia, which acts to induce hypocalcemia. A similar substance from the thyroid gland, thyrocalcitonin, also lowers calcium levels. These substances are believed to participate in the feedback mechanism that controls and maintains stable blood calcium levels.

calcium to phosphorus ratio (Ca:P ratio) since calcium and phosphorus are intimately related in metabolism, two ratios between them are significant. (1) The dietary calcium to phosphorus ratio affects absorption of these minerals; a 1:1 ratio is ideal for growth, pregnancy, and lactation periods. Otherwise, for adults a 1:1½ ratio of calcium to phosphorus is required. (2) The serum calcium to phosphorus ratio is the solubility product of the two minerals in the serum. An increase in one mineral causes a decrease in the other to maintain a constant product of the two. The normal serum level of calcium is 10 mg/dl; of phosphorus, 4 mg/dl in adults (5 mg in children). Thus the normal serum calcium to phosphorus ratio for adults is 40 (10×4), and for children 50 (10×5).

calculus (L. pebble; plural, calculi) any abnormal accretion within the body of material that forms a "stone." Calculi are usually composed of mineral salts. The most commonly formed renal calculi are composed of calcium salts.

chelate (Gr. *chele,* claw) a chemical compound capable of grasping and incorporating a metallic ion into its molecular structure. By binding the metal, the chelate removes it from a tissue or from the circulating blood. For example, *desferrioxamine* is a chelating agent developed by chemists for the treatment of hemochromatosis, a disease in which excess iron is stored in body tissue. The desferrioxamine removes iron from the tissues and transports it to excretion sites.

chloride-bicarbonate shift the exchange of bicarbonate for chloride in red blood cells. To provide constant bicarbonate buffering for the rapidly forming carbonic acid from water and carbon dioxide ($H_2O + CO_2$), chloride replaces bicarbonate in the cell, which allows bicarbonate to participate in the carbonic acid-base bicarbonate buffer system. In the lungs, as carbon dioxide is expired, the reaction forming carbonic acid is reversed, and bicarbonate is not needed, so the shift changes.

cystinuria a condition caused by a rare hereditary defect. It is characterized by excessive urinary excretion of cystine (a sulfur-containing amino acid). In this disease, cystine crystals often accumulate and form characteristic, small, smooth, yellow kidney stones—cystine renal calculi.

feedback mechanism the mechanism that regulates production and secretion by an endocrine gland (A_g) of its hormone (A_h), which stimulates another endocrine gland (T_g; the *target gland*) to produce its hormone (T_h). As T_g produces sufficient T_h to supply the body's needs, the blood level of T_h rises. This rise in the blood level of T_h signals A_g to stop secreting A_h. The blood level of A_h then gradually falls. T_g recognizes this as its signal to produce more A_h. The rise in A_h tells T_g to increase its production of T_h. Example: the anterior pituitary-thyroid interaction. Here A_g is the anterior pituitary gland; T_g is the thyroid gland. The anterior pituitary secretes thyroid-stimulating hormone (TSH). TSH stimulates the thyroid to secrete thyroxine. When the blood level of thyroxine reaches optimum, the anterior pituitary ceases to secrete TSH. The thyroid thereupon stops secreting thyroxine, and the blood level of thyroxine falls. When it falls below the level needed by the body, the anterior pituitary responds to this low blood level of thyroxine by again liberating TSH into the bloodstream.

ferritin the protein-iron compounds in which iron is stored in the tissues—the storage form of iron in the body. The so-called ferritin mechanism in the mucosal cells of the stomach and small intestine regulates iron absorption.

When the ferritin protein compound is satured with iron, no more iron is absorbed.

fluoridation the process by which fluorine is added to a substance. Proper fluoridation of public water supplies in areas where the fluorine content is naturally low has been demonstrated to control the incidence of dental caries.

goiter (L. *guttur,* throat) endemic colloid goiter is an enlargement of the thyroid gland caused by lack of sufficient available iodine to produce the thyroid hormone, thyroxine.

hemochromatosis (Gr. *haima,* blood; *chroma,* color) a disturbance of iron metabolism in which excessive iron storage causes a bronze discoloration of skin and viscera, liver and pancreas damage, and diabetes (bronzed diabetes). The condition is believed to be genetically transmitted by a defect occurring chiefly in males.

hemoglobin (Gr. *haima,* blood; L. *globus,* globe) the protein that gives the color to red blood cells. Hemoglobin is a conjugated protein composed of an iron-containing pigment called heme and a simple protein, globin. Hemoglobin is the oxygen carrier of the blood and combines with oxygen to form oxyhemoglobin.

hemosiderin (Gr. *haima,* blood; *sideros,* iron) an insoluble iron oxide–protein compound in which iron is stored in the liver if the amount of iron in the blood exceeds the storage capacity of ferritin. Such accumulation of excess iron occurs in diseases that are accompanied by rapid destruction of red blood cells (malaria, hemolytic anemia).

hemosiderosis a condition in which large amounts of the iron storage compound hemosiderin are deposited, especially in the liver and spleen. Hemosiderosis may occur as the result of excessive breakdown of red blood cells in diseases such as malaria and hemolytic anemia, or after multiple blood transfusions.

hyperkalemia excessive amounts of potassium (K) in blood plasma. Hyperkalemia is a serious complication of renal failure, severe dehydration, or shock; it causes the heart to dilate, and the heart rate is slowed by weakened contractions. Potassium plays a vital role with ionized sodium and calcium (Na^+ and Ca^+) in regulating neuromuscular stimulation, transmission of electrochemical impulses (such as those that mediate the flow of the beat through the heart), and contraction of muscle fibers.

hyperphosphatemia high serum phosphorus. Hyperphosphatemia may be caused by renal insufficiency because the kidney cannot excrete phosphorus adequately or by hypoparathyroidism, which causes an insufficient secretion of parathyroid hormone, which regulates the renal excretion of phosphorus. When serum phosphorus rises, serum calcium falls, causing tetany.

hypochloremic alkalosis excessive loss of gastric secretion (hydrochloric acid) results in loss of chlorides, and bicarbonate replaces the depleted chloride ions. Hypochloremic alkalosis (a type of metabolic alkalosis) results. Such gastrointestinal disorders as excessive vomiting may lead to hypochloremic alkalosis. Therefore prompt replacement of chloride is essential.

hypocupremia low serum copper level. Hypocupremia may be caused by urinary loss of *ceruloplasmin* (the copper-binding protein of the plasma) in nephrosis or by malabsorption of copper in sprue.

hypokalemia low blood potassium. Hypokalemia is a serious complication of severe diarrhea, for example, in which large amounts of potassium are lost in intestinal secretions. Hypokalemia may also result from rapid glycogenesis during the recovery phase of diabetic acidosis. Replacement therapy in both instances should involve added potassium.

hypophosphatemia low serum phosphorus. Hypophosphatemia may be caused by decreased absorption of phosphorus as in intestinal diseases (sprue, celiac disease), by an upset serum calcium to phosphorus ratio as in bone disease (rickets, osteomalacia), or by excess secretion of parathyroid hormone with resulting excessive renal excretion of phosphorus, as in primary hyperparathyroidism.

ionized calcium (Ca^{++}) free, diffusible form of calcium in the blood and other body fluids. Although free ionized calcium makes up a very small amount of the total body calcium (1%), it exerts a profound influence on the function of bone, the heart, and the nervous system. (The remaining 99% of the total body calcium is deposited as calcium salts in bone tissue.)

myofibrils (Gr. *myo,* muscle; L. *fibrilla,* small fiber) the contractile element in muscle tissue, a tiny fiber running parallel to the cellular long axis. Calcium ions activate the chemical reaction between the constituent muscle protein filaments, myosin and actin, which releases a burst of energy from ATP bonds and brings about contraction of the myofibril units in the muscle.

myoglobin muscle protein (globin) that contains iron (also called *myohemoglobin*).

osteoblasts (Gr. *osteo,* bone; *blastos,* germ) bone-forming cells.

osteoclasts (Gr. *osteo,* bone; *klan,* to break) giant, multinuclear cells found in depressions on bone surfaces, which cause resorption of bone tissue and the formation of canals.

parathyroid hormone (PH) hormone of parathyroid gland, which controls calcium and phosphorus metabolism in three ways: (1) it stimulates the intestinal mucosa to increase calcium absorption, (2) it mobilizes calcium rapidly from bone, and (3) it causes renal excretion of phosphate. All of these responses act together as needed to regulate the circulating amounts of calcium and phosphorus to maintain them within normal levels.

PBI protein-bound iodine. The PBI test is used to measure thyroid activity by determining the amount of iodine that is bound to thyroxine and in transit in the plasma.

polycythemia a condition characterized by the presence of excess red blood cells that contain a high concentration of hemoglobin. There are several types of polycythemia. One type may be caused by an excess of cobalt. Cobalt is the core of vitamin B_{12}, which is an essential factor in red blood cell formation.

radioactive ^{131}I tests tests of thyroid function using a radioactive isotope of iodine, ^{131}I. After the test dose is administered, the uptake and utilization of iodine by the thyroid gland is measured by tracing the ^{131}I.

sulfhydryl group the -SH radical that forms high-energy sulfur bonds in chemical compounds. These are similar to the high-energy bonds formed by phosphates in compounds such as ATP. In such compounds sulfur participates in important tissue respiration (oxidation) reactions.

synergism (Gr. *syn,* with or together; *ergon,* work) the joint action of separate agents in which the total effect of their combined action is greater than the sum of their separate actions. Each agent potentiates the action of the other.

tetany a disorder caused by abnormal calcium metabolism. Severe, intermittent, tonic contractions of the extremities and muscular pain occur, which are usually caused by lowered blood calcium levels. A characteristic diagnostic sign is the inward muscular spasm of the wrist called Trousseau's sign.

thyroid-stimulating hormone (TSH) a hormone secreted by the anterior pituitary gland that regulates uptake of iodine and synthesis of thyroxine by the thyroid gland.

thyroxine the iodine-containing hormone produced by the thyroid gland.

transferrin an iron-binding protein complex, a serum β-globulin; the transport form of iron in the body.

Wilson's disease a rare hereditary disease of abnormal copper metabolism. Large amounts of copper are absorbed by, and accumulate in, the liver, brain, kidneys, and cornea. The disease produces degenerative changes in brain and liver tissue. A copper-chelate, *penicillamine,* is used to bind the excess copper and excrete it.

REFERENCES
Specific

1. Hegsted, D. N.: Calcium. In Goodhart, R. S., and Shils, M., editors: Modern nutrition in health and disease, ed. 5, Philadelphia, 1973, Lea & Febiger, p. 268.
2. Rasmussen, H., and Pechet, M.: Calcitonin, Sci. Am. **223:**42, 1970.
3. Cullen, R. W., and Oace, S. N.: Iodine; current status, J. Nutr. Educ. **8:**101, 1976.
4. Solomans, N. W.: On the assessment of zinc and copper nutriture in man, Am. J. Clin. Nutr. **32:**856, April, 1979.
5. Alford, R. H.: Metal cation requirements for phytohemagglutinin-induced transformation of human peripheral blood lymphocytes, J. Immunol. **104:**698, March, 1970.
6. Pories, W. J., et al.: Metabolic factors affecting zinc metabolism in the surgical patients. In Prasad, A. S., editor: Trace elements in human health and disease, vol. 1, New York, 1976, Academic Press, Inc., p. 115.
7. Food and Nutrition Board, National Research Council, National Academy of Sciences: Zinc in human nutrition, Washington, D.C., 1971.
8. Murphy, E. W., Willis, B. W., and Watt, B. K.: Provisional tables on the zinc content of foods, J. Am. Diet. Assoc. **66:**345, 1975.
9. Chow, C. K.: Nutritional influence on cellular antioxidant defense systems, Am. J. Clin. Nutr. **32:**1066, May, 1979.
10. Mertz, W.: Effects and metabolism of glucose tolerance factor, Nutr. Rev. **33:**129, 1975.

General
GENERAL MINERAL

Burch, R. E., and Sullivan, J. F., editors: Trace elements, Med. Clin. North Am. vol. 60, 1976.

Food and Nutrition Board, National Research Council, National Academy of Sciences: Recommended dietary allowances, ed. 9, Washington, D.C., 1980.

Goodhart, R. E., and Shils, M., editors: Modern nutrition in health and disease, ed. 6, Philadelphia, 1980, Lea & Febiger.

Hegsted, M., editor: Present knowledge of nutrition, New York, 1976, The Nutrition Foundation.

Maugh, T. H.: Trace elements: a growing appreciation of their effects in man, Science **181:**253, 1973.

Mertz, W., and Cornatzer, W. E., editors: Newer trace elements in nutrition, New York, 1971, Marcel Dekker, Inc.

Prasad, A. S., and Oberleus, D., editors: Trace elements in health and disease, vol. 1 and 2, New York, 1976, Academic Press, Inc.

Underwood, E. H.: Trace elements in human and animal nutrition, ed. 3, New York, 1971, Academic Press, Inc.

World Health Organization: Trace elements in human nutrition, WHO Technical Report Series No. 532, Geneva, 1973.

CALCIUM AND PHOSPHORUS

Hegsted, D. M.: Nutrition, bone, and calcified tissue, J. Am. Diet. Assoc. **50:**105, 1967.

Holemans, K. C., and Meyer, B. J.: A quantitative relationship between the absorption of calcium and phosphorus, Am. J. Clin. Nutr. **12:**30, 1963.

Johansen, E.: Nutrition, diet, and calcium metabolism in dental health, Am. J. Public Health **50:**1089, 1960.

Lutwak, L.: Osteoporosis—a mineral deficiency disease? J. Am. Diet. Assoc. **44:**173, 1964.

Margen, S., Chu, J. Y., Kaufmann, N. A., et al.: Studies in calcium metabolism. I. The calciuretic effect of dietary protein, Am. J. Clin. Nutr. **27:**584, June, 1974.

Review: Dietary phosphorus, PTH, and bone resorption, Nutr. Rev. **31:**124, 1973.

Wiels, M. R.: Intestinal absorption of calcium, Lancet **1:**820, 1973.

MAGNESIUM

Anast, C. S., et al.: Evidence for parathyroid failure in magnesium deficiency, Science **77:**606, 1972.

Briscoe, A. M., and Ragan, C.: Effect of magnesium or calcium metabolism in man, Am. J. Clin. Nutr. **19:**296, 1966.

Caddell, J. L.: Studies in protein-calorie malnutrition. II. A double-blind clinical trial to assess magnesium therapy, N. Engl. J. Med. **276:**535, 1967.

Caddell, J. L., and Goddard, D. R.: Studies in protein-calorie malnutrition. I. Chemical evidence for magnesium deficiency, N. Engl. J. Med. **276:**533, 1967.

Friedman, R., et al.: Primary hypomagnesemia with secondary hypocalcemia in an infant, Lancet **1:**687, 1967.

Kahil, M. E., et al.: Magnesium deficiency and carbohydrate metabolism, Diabetes **15:**734, 1966.

Review: Magnesium deficiency, Nutr. Rev. **30:**335, 1962.

Seelig, M. S.: The requirement of magnesium by the normal adult, Am. J. Clin. Nutr. **14:**342, 1964.

Shils, M. E.: Magnesium deficiency and parathyroid hormone levels in man, Am. J. Clin. Nutr. **28:**421, 1975.

Wacker, W. E. C.: Magnesium metabolism, J. Am. Diet. Assoc. **44:**362, 1964.

FLUORIDE

Ast, D. B., and Schlesinger, E. R.: The conclusion of a ten-year study of water fluoridation, Am. J. Public Health **46:**265, 1956.

Bernstein, D. S., et al.: Prevalence of osteoporosis in high- and low-fluoride areas in North Dakota, J.A.M.A. **197:**499, 1966.

Kramer, L., Osis, D., Wiatrowski, E., et al.: Dietary fluoride in different areas in the United States, Am. J. Clin. Nutr. **27:**590, June, 1974.

Report: Fluoride protects against bone loss, J.A.M.A. **200:**31, 1967.

Waldbott, G. L.: Fluoride in food, Am. J. Clin. Nutr. **12:**455, 1963.

World Health Organization: Fluorides in human health, Geneva, 1970.

IRON

Cook, J. D., and Finch, C. A.: Iron nutrition, West. J. Med. **122:**474, 1975.

Cook, J. D., et al.: Serum ferritin as a measure of iron stores in normal subjects, Am. J. Clin. Nutr. **27:**681, 1974.

Dietary iron controversy: Nutr. Today **7:**2, 1972.

Finch, C. A.: Iron balance in man, Nutr. Rev. **23:**129, 1965.

Finch, C. A., and Monsen, E. R.: Iron nutrition and the fortification of food with iron, J.A.M.A. **219:**1462, 1972.

Frieden, E.: The ferrous to ferric cycles in iron metabolism, Nutr. Rev. **31:**41-44, 1973.

Hallberg, L., Harwerth, H. C., and Vannotti, A., editors: Iron deficiency pathogenesis, clinical aspects, New York, 1970, Academic Press, Inc.

Jacobs, A., and Norwood, M.: Iron in biochemistry and medicine, New York, 1974, Academic Press, Inc.

Review: Iron deficiency anemia, Nutr. Rev. **20:**164, 1962.

Review: Iron storage in bone marrow, Nutr. Rev. **21:**99, 1963.

COPPER

Al Rashid, R. A., and Spangler, J.: Neonatal copper deficiency, N. Engl. J. Med. **285:**841, 1971.

Ashkenazi, A., et al.: The syndrome of neonatal copper deficiency, Pediatrics **52:**525, 1973.

Cartwright, G. E.: The questions of copper deficiency in man, Am. J. Clin. Nutr. **15:**94, 1964.

Cartwright, G. E., and Wintrobe, M. M.: Copper metabolism in normal subjects, Am. J. Clin. Nutr. **14:**224, 1964.

Cordano, A., and Graham, G. G.: Copper deficiency complicating chronic intestinal malabsorption, Pediatrics **38:**596, 1966.

Danks, D. M., Campbell, P. E., Stevens, B. J., et al.: Menkes' kinky hair syndrome. An inherited defect in copper absorption with widespread effects, Pediatrics **50:**188, Aug., 1972.

Holtzman, N. A.: Menkes' kinky hair syndrome: a genetic disease involving copper, Fed. Proc. **35:**2276, 1976.

Hook, L., and Brandt, I. K.: Copper content of some low-copper foods, J. Am. Diet. Assoc. **49:**202, 1966.

Pennington, J. T., and Calloway, D. H.: Copper content of foods, factors affecting reported values, J. Am. Diet. Assoc. **63:**143, 1977.

Report: Preventing Wilson's disease sequelae (abnormal copper metabolism), J.A.M.A. **200:**41, 1967.

Solomons, N. W.: On the assessment of zinc and copper, Am. J. Clin. Nutr. **32:**856, April, 1979.

Vilter, R. W., Bozian, R. C., Hess, E. V., et al.: Manifestations of copper deficiency in a patient with systemic sclerosis on intravenous hyperalimentation, N. Engl. J. Med. **291:**188, July 25, 1974.

Wolf, W. R., Holden, J., and Greene, F. E.: Dietary intakes of zinc and copper from self-selected diets, Fed. Proc. **36**:1175, 1977.

SODIUM AND POTASSIUM

American Academy of Pediatrics, Committee on Nutrition: Salt intake and eating patterns of infants and children in relation to blood pressure, Pediatrics **53**:115, 1974.

Cooper, G. R., and Heap, B.: Sodium ion in drinking water. II. Importance, problems, and potential applications of sodium-iron-restricted therapy, J. Am. Diet. Assoc. **50**:37, 1967.

Dahl, L. K.: Salt, fat and hypertension, Nutr. Rev. **18**:97, 1960.

Dahl, L. K.: Salt and hypertension, Am. J. Clin. Nutr. **24**:231, 1972.

Gros, G., Weller, J. M., and Hoobler, W. W.: Relationship of sodium and potassium intake to blood pressure, Am. J. Clin. Nutr. **24**:605, 1971.

Krehl, W. A.: The potassium depletion syndrome, Nutr. Today **1**:20, 1966.

Krehl, W. A.: Sodium, a most extraordinary dietary essential, Nutr. Today **1**:16, 1966.

Parijs, J., Joossens, J. V., Van der Linden, L., et al.: Moderate sodium restriction and diuretics in the treatment of hypertension, Am. Heart J. **85**:22, Jan., 1973.

Review: Salt in the infant's diet, Nutr. Rev. **25**:82, 1967.

Seftel, H. C., and Kew, M. C.: Early and intensive potassium replacement in diabetic acidosis, Diabetes **15**:694, 1966.

White, J. M., Wingo, J. G., Alligood, L. M., et al.: Sodium ion in drinking water. I. Properties, analysis and occurrence, J. Am. Diet. Assoc. **50**:32, Jan., 1967.

TRACE ELEMENTS

Carlisle, E. M.: A relationship between silicon, glycosaminoglycon, and collagen formation, Fed. Proc. **33**:704, 1974.

Carlisle, E. M.: Silicon in the osteoblast, the bone-forming cell, Fed. Proc. **34**:927, 1975.

Glinsmann, W. H., Feldman, F. J., and Mertz, W.: Plasma chromium after glucose administration, Science **152**:1243, May 27, 1966.

Hambridge, K. M.: Chromium nutrition in man, Am. J. Clin. Nutr. **27**:505, 1974.

Hopkins, L. L., Jr., and Mohr, H. E.: Vanadium as an essential nutrient, Fed. Proc. **33**:1773, 1974.

Lang, V. M., et al.: Manganese metabolism in college men consuming vegetarian diets, J. Nutr. **85**:132, 1965.

Mayer, J.: Trace elements: pinning down the facts, Fam. Health, **7**:43, May, 1975.

Mertz, W., and Cornatzer, W. E., editors: The newer trace elements in nutrition, New York, 1971, Dekker Publishing Co.

Mertz, W., et al.: Present knowledge of the role of chromium, Fed. Proc. **33**:2275, 1974.

Milne, D. B.: Trace mineral intake of enlisted military personnel, J. Am. Diet. Assoc. **76**:41, Jan., 1980.

National Research Council, National Academy of Sciences: Manganese, Washington, D.C., 1973.

Neilsen, F. H., and Sandstead, H. H.: Are nickel, vanadium, silicon, fluorine, and tin essential to man? A review, Am. J. Clin. Nutr. **27**:515, 1974.

Schroeder, H. A.: Cadmium as a factor in hypertension, J. Chronic Dis. **18**:647, 1965.

Schroeder, H. A.: Essential trace elements in man: molybdenum, J. Chronic Dis. **23**:481, 1970.

Schroeder, H. A., Nason, A. P., and Tipton, I. H.: Chromium deficiency as a factor in atherosclerosis, J. Chronic Dis. **23**:123, Aug., 1970.

Schwartz, K.: Recent dietary trace element research, exemplified by tin, fluorine, and silicon, Fed. Proc. **33**:1748, 1974.

Underwood, E. H.: Trace elements in human and animal nutrition, ed. 3, New York, 1971, Academic Press, Inc.

Vought, R. L., and Landon, W. T.: Dietary sources of iodine, Am. J. Clin Nutr. **14**:186, 1964.

ZINC

Food and Nutrition Board, National Research Council, National Academy of Sciences: Zinc in human nutrition, Washington, D.C., 1971.

Haeflein, K. A., and Rasmussen, A. I.: Zinc content of selected foods, J. Am. Diet. Assoc. **70**:610, 1977.

Halstead, J. A., Smith, J. C., Jr., and Irwin, M. E.: A conspectus of research on zinc requirements of man, J. Nutr. **104**:345, 1974.

Hambridge, K. M., et al.: Low levels of zinc in hari, anorexia, poor growth, and hypogeusia in children, Pediatr. Res. **6**:868, 1972.

Henkin, R. I., Schechter, P. J., Hoge, R., et al.: Idiopathic hypogeusia with dysgeusia, hyposmia, and dysosmia. A new syndrome, J.A.M.A. **217**:434, July 26, 1971.

Henzel, J. H., DeWeese, M. S., and Lichti, E. L.: Zinc concentrations within healing wounds. Significance of zincuria on availability and requirements during tissue repair, Arch. Surg. **100**:349, 1970.

Jacob, R. A., Sandstead, H. H., Solomons, N. W., Rieger, C., and Rothberg, R.: Zinc status and vitamin A transport in cystic fibrosis, Am. J. Clin. Nutr. **31**:638, April, 1978.

Kay, R. G., Tasman-Jones, C., Pybus, J., et al.: A syndrome of acute zinc deficiency during total parenteral alimentation in man, Ann. Surg. **183**:331, April, 1976.

Klevay, L. M.: Coronary heart disease: the zinc/copper hypothesis, Am. J. Clin. Nutr. **28**:764, 1975.

Nelder, K. H., and Hambridge, K. M.: Zinc therapy of

acrodermatitis enteropathica, N. Engl. J. Med. **292:**879, 1975.

Pories, W. J., Henzel, J. H., Rob, C. G., et al.: Acceleration of wound healing in man with zinc sulfate given by mouth, Lancet **1:**121, Jan., 1967.

Pories, W. J., Strain, W. H., Hsu, J. M., and Woolsey, R. L., editors: Clinical applications of zinc metabolism, Springfield, Ill., 1974, Charles C Thomas, Publisher.

Prasad, A. S.: Zinc metabolism, Springfield, Ill., 1966, Charles C Thomas, Publisher.

Prasad, A. S.: Nutritional metabolic role of zinc, Fed. Proc. **26:**172, 1967.

Sandstead, H. H.: Zinc nutrition in the United States, Am. J. Clin. Nutr. **26:**1251, 1973.

Sandstead, H. H., Prasad, A. S., Schulert, A. R., et al.: Human zinc deficiency, endocrine manifestations and response to treatment, Am. J. Clin. Nutr. **20:**422, May, 1967.

Solomons, N. W.: On the assessment of zinc and copper nutriture in man, Am. J. Clin. Nutr. **32:**856, April, 1979.

Solomons, N. W., Rosenberg, I. H., and Sandstead, H. H.: Zinc nutrition in celiac sprue, Am. J. Clin. Nutr. **29:**371, 1976.

Swanson, C. A., and King, J. C.: Human zinc nutrition, J. Nutr. Ed. **11:**181, Oct.-Dec., 1979.

Tucker, S. B., Schroeter, A. L., Brown, P. W., Jr., et al.: Acquired zinc deficiency. Cutaneous manifestations typical of acrodermatitis enteropathica, J.A.M.A. **235:**2399, May 31, 1976.

9

Water and electrolytes

Water is the one nutrient most vital to a human being's existence. A human can survive far longer without food than without water. Only air is a more constant need. Fulfilling the body's need for a continuous supply of water and maintaining the body's water composition are major economic, nutritional, and physiologic tasks.

Several basic concepts are essential to the understanding of the uses of water in the human body. First, there is the idea of a unified whole. A human is one continuous body of water. The "sea within" is held in shape by a protective envelope of skin. Water diffuses freely to all parts and is controlled only by the water's own chemical potential. In this warm, fluid, chemical environment, life processes are sustained. Second, there is the concept of compartments of water within the whole. These compartments are separated by membranes. The quantities of water contained in each compartment are balanced by forces that maintain an equilibrium along the parts. Third, basic to an understanding of these balancing forces, there is the concept of particles (charged electrolytes and other solutes) in the water solution. It is the concentration and distribution of these particles that determine internal shifts and balances in body water.

Involved throughout is the unifying concept of homeostasis. The body has a tremendous resilience through its capacity to employ nu-

merous, finely balanced homeostatic mechanisms that protect its vital fluid supply. To relate these various parts to the whole, the following questions should be considered carefully:

1. Where is the water in the body and how is it distributed?
2. What is the overall balance between intake and output of water?
3. What forces control the distribution of water?
4. What is the role of the gastrointestinal tract in water distribution and use?
5. What is the role of the kidney with respect to body water?
6. How do hormones influence water balance?

BODY WATER AND ITS DISTRIBUTION

The body of a man has been found by various investigators to be from 55% to 65% water; that of a woman is from 50% to 55% water. The higher water content in men is generally because of the greater muscle mass. (Striated muscle contains more water than any body tissue other than blood). The remaining 40% of a man's weight is about 18% protein and related substances, 15% fat, and 7% minerals.

The body water performs three functions that are essential to life: (1) it helps give structure and form to the body through the turgor it provides for tissue, (2) it gives the aqueous environment that is necessary for cell metabolism, and (3) it provides the means for maintaining a stable body temperature.

The body water may be thought of as the total water outside the cells plus the total water inside the cells. These two quantities of water have been called compartments of body water: (1) the *extracellular fluid compartment* (ECF) is made up of all the water outside the cells and (2) the *intracellular fluid compartment* (ICF) is made up of all the water inside the cells.

Extracellular fluid compartment (ECF)

The collective water outside the cells makes up about 20% of the total body weight. Approximately one fourth of this (5% of body weight) is contained in the blood plasma. The remaining three fourths (15% of body weight) is made up of water surrounding the cells, water in dense tissue, and water in transit secretions. *Plasma* includes the total extracellular fluid within the heart and blood vessels. The *interstitial fluid*

and lymph include the fluid environment in which the cells are bathed; it provides a transfer medium for materials entering and leaving the cells. *Fluid in dense tissue* includes water in dense connective tissue, cartilage, and bone. *Fluid in transit* includes transcellular water in cerebrospinal fluid and in secretions such as those of the salivary glands, thyroid gland, liver, pancreas, gallbladder, gastrointestinal tract, gonads, various mucous membranes, skin, kidneys, and eye spaces.

Intracellular fluid compartment (ICF)

The total water inside the body cells amounts to about twice that outside the cells. This is not surprising, since the cell is the basic unit of structure of the entire body, and the cells are the sites of the vast basic metabolic activity of the body. The intracellular fluid compartment makes up about 40% of the total body weight.

These relative total amounts of body water in the different compartments are compared in Fig. 9-1.

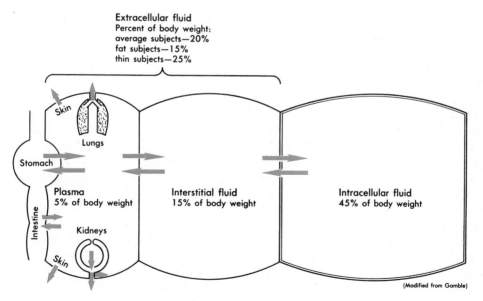

Fig. 9-1. Body fluid compartments. Note the relative total quantities of water in the intracellular compartment and in the extracellular compartment.

OVERALL WATER BALANCE: INTAKE AND OUTPUT

The average adult metabolizes from 2½ to 3 L of water per day in a constant turnover balanced between intake and output. Normally, water enters and leaves the body by various routes, controlled by such basic mechanisms as *thirst* and *hormonal control of renal excretion.* Control centers that regulate water intake through operation of the thirst mechanisms are located in the brain and in the hypothalamus.[1] Thirst is a distinct physical sensation and a conscious demand for water caused by (1) extracellular dehydration, (2) low cardiac output or hemorrhage, (3) intracellular dehydration, and (4) dryness of the mouth. The hormonal regulation of renal excretion is under the control of the antidiuretic hormone (ADH; also called vasopressin), which is secreted by the pituitary gland. These mechanisms of dehydration and hormone control will be discussed later. First, the routes of water intake and water output will be compared.

Water intake

Water enters the body in three main forms: (1) as preformed water in liquids, (2) as preformed water in foods, and (3) as a product of oxidation.

Preformed water in liquids. Water and other beverages are the main source of ingested fluid. From 1,200 to 1,500 ml of liquid is ingested daily in this form.

Preformed water in foods. Foods vary with respect to their water content from those with a large amount, such as tomatoes, oranges, and watermelon, to those that contain little water, such as dried fruit and legumes. The water ingested in foods that are eaten (rather than as liquid that is drunk) contributes from 700 to 1,000 ml daily.

Water of oxidation. When nutrients are burned or oxidized in the body, one of the end products is water. The amount of metabolic water produced varies with different nutrients.

For example, 100 g of fat produces 107 g of water; 100 g of carbohydrate produces 55 g of water, and 100 g of protein produces 41 g of water. On the whole, from 200 to 300 ml of water is contributed daily from the body's metabolic activity. This brings the daily water intake from 2,100 to 2,800 ml.

Water output

Water leaves the body through the kidneys, the skin, the lungs, or the feces.

Kidneys. The kidneys of an adult normally excrete from 1 to 2 L of urine daily. The water in this total amount is made up of two portions, the obligatory water excretion and the facultative water excretion. *Obligatory water excretion* is the amount of water that the kidney is "obligated" to excrete to rid the body of its daily load of urinary solutes. Since about 15 ml of water is required to dissolve 1 g of solute, the quantity of obligatory water excretion depends on how large a load of metabolic end products (solutes such as urea and other metabolites) is seeking excretion and also on the concentrating power of the kidney. The average obligatory water excretion of an adult is approximately 900 ml daily. *Facultative water excretion* occurs in addition to obligatory water loss. An additional 500 ml, more or less, may be excreted according to fluctuating body need and the renal tubular reabsorption rate.

Skin. About 350 ml of water is lost daily through the skin by diffusion. Because a person is unaware of this loss, it is called *insensible water loss.* An additional 100 ml may be lost in normal perspiration. Heavier sweating caused by heat or increased activity may cause the loss of 250 ml of water, more or less, according to body need. Therefore under usual circumstances, from 450 to 700 ml of water is lost daily through the skin. Excessive sweating or loss of skin as in extensive burns further increases the water output.

Lungs. An insensible water loss of about 350 ml occurs daily through normal respiration

Table 9-1. Approximate daily adult intake and output of water

	Intake (replacement) ml per day		Output (loss)	
			Obligatory (insensible) ml per day	Additional (according to need) ml per day
Preformed		Lungs	350	
Liquids	1,200-1,500	Skin		
In foods	700-1,000	Diffusion	350	
Metabolism (oxidation	200- 300	Sweat	100	±250
of food)		Kidneys	900	±500
		Feces	150	
TOTAL	2,100-2,800	TOTAL	1,850	750
(approx. 2,600 ml per day)		(approx. 2,600 ml per day)		

vapor. This amount varies with climate, being least in hot, humid weather and greatest in very cold temperatures.

Feces. A small amount of water, from 150 to 200 ml, is usually lost daily through intestinal elimination. In abnormal conditions, such as diarrhea or dysentery, much greater losses will occur.

On the average, daily water output from the adult body totals about 2,600 ml. This comparative intake and output balance is summarized in Table 9-1.

FORCES INFLUENCING WATER DISTRIBUTION

Forces that influence and control the distribution of water in the body revolve around two factors: (1) the *solutes* (particles in solution in body water) and (2) the *membranes* that separate the water compartments.

Solutes

Three types of solutes influence internal shifts and balances of body water. These are electrolytes, plasma proteins, and organic compounds of small molecular size.

Electrolytes. Certain inorganic compounds (usually an acid, an alkali, or a salt) partly dis-

sociate into their constituent ions when they are dissolved in water. An *ion* is an atom or a group of atoms that carries an electrical charge. This charge may be *positive,* because the atom has *lost* one of the negatively charged electrons that orbit around its nucleus, or *negative,* because the atom has *gained* a negatively charged orbiting electron. The word *ion,* which is derived from the Greek word meaning "wanderer," emphasizes that such an atom wanders freely in a solution, dissociated from the compound of which it was a part. A compound that dissociates into ions when in solution is called an *electrolyte* (Gr. *electron,* amber + *lytos,* a solution). This term refers to the fact that a solution containing one of these substances can transmit an electric current. If an electric current is passed through a volume of water in which an electrolyte is dissolved, the ions that dissociate themselves from the electrolyte migrate toward the pole that carries the electric charge opposite to the electric charge of that particular ion; the positively charged ions cluster around the negative pole, and the negatively charged ions migrate to the positive pole. The two forms of ions are cations and anions. A *cation* is an ion that carries a positive charge (Na^+, K^+, Ca^{++}, Mg^{++}); an *anion* is an ion that carries a negative charge (Cl$^-$, HCO$_3^-$, HPO$_4^=$, SO$_4^=$). Electrolytes constitute a major force controlling fluid balances within the body (see also pp. 177-178).

Plasma proteins. Plasma proteins are organic substances of large molecular size, mainly albumin and globulin, which influence the shift of water from one compartment to another. They are called colloids (Gr. *kolla,* glue) and form *colloidal solutions.* Such a solution is a mixture of large, gelatinous particles or molecules that do not readily pass through separating membranes. Therefore they normally remain in the blood vessels where they exert a *colloidal osmotic pressure* (COP), which maintains the integrity of the blood volume in the vascular compartment.

Organic compounds of small molecular size. Organic compounds of small molecular size include such substances as glucose, urea, and amino acids. Because of their small size, they diffuse freely and therefore affect water balances only if they occur in unusually large amounts. For example, the large amount of glucose in the urine of a patient with uncontrolled diabetes causes an abnormal osmotic diuresis or excess water output.

Separating membranes

Two basic types of separating membranes are involved in the movements of water and solutes within the body. These are the capillary wall and the cell wall. The capillary wall is a relatively free or rapid membrane, across which electrolytes pass readily. The cell wall is a slow membrane and is more difficult to penetrate. It is composed essentially of a lipid matrix, covered on either surface by a layer of protein. The metabolic processes within the cell usually govern the passage of electrolytes (and therefore water) across this barrier.

Mechanisms for movement of water and solutes across membranes

According to the type of membrane and the number of particles in the involved solution, water and solutes move across membranes by one or more of five mechanisms: osmosis, diffusion, active transport, filtration, or pinocytosis.

Osmosis. The word osmosis comes from the Greek word *osmos* meaning ''to push'' or ''to thrust.'' Osmosis is the process by which water molecules pass through a semipermeable membrane separating two solutions. The molecules pass from the more dilute solution (water concentration is *higher,* the solute concentration is *lower*) to the more dense solution (water concentration is *lower,* the solute concentration is *higher*). Osmotic pressure is created by the difference in molecular pressure on either side of the membrane. The process may be thought of as a thrusting force in which water molecules, relatively unimpeded by the presence of many solute particles, push through the membrane more freely than the molecules that are laden with solute. It may also be thought of as a pulling force exerted by the denser solution, in which the burden of solute particles hinders the movement of the water molecules. As a consequence, the solution that is laden with solutes draws to itself a greater number of water molecules to enhance its mobility. Whether osmosis is thought of as a pushing or a pulling force, it tends to equalize the concentration of solutes and the fluid pressure on each side of a membrane. As it does so, it effectively controls the movement of water from place to place in the body.

Diffusion. The word diffusion comes from the Latin word *diffundere,* meaning ''to spread'' or ''to pour forth.'' It is the process by which particles in solution spread throughout the solution and across separating membranes, from the place of highest solute concentration to all spaces of lesser solute concentration. It may be simple passive diffusion or it may be carrier mediated (see p. 214). The movements of molecules in osmosis and diffusion are compared in Fig. 9-2.

Active transport. Many times a significant movement of substances across a membrane

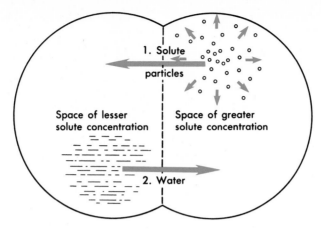

Fig. 9-2. Movement of molecules, water, and solutes by osmosis and diffusion.

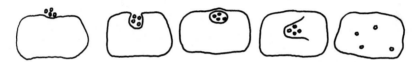

Fig. 9-3. Pinocytosis—engulfing of large molecules by the cell.

is accomplished even against the usual pressure gradient. This may be compared to a person swimming upstream or walking uphill against gravity's pull. Obviously such movement against pressure requires energy. In the case of substances moving across membranes in the body, the requisite energy comes from metabolism in the cells. Usually some vehicle or mechanism of transport is needed in addition. An example of such active transport is the operation of the sodium pump by which glucose is absorbed from the intestinal lumen and into individual cells (see Fig. 2-3). Other molecules such as amino acids and fatty acids enter and leave cells by a similar means of active transport.

Filtration. Fluid is forced or filtered through membranes when there is a difference in pressure on the two sides. For example, filtration occurs across the capillary walls because the hydrostatic pressure within the capillary is greater than that in the surrounding interstitial fluid area. Small molecules pass with the fluid out of the capillary lumen, but the large molecules of plasma protein remain. These pressures are diagrammed in Fig. 9-5.

Pinocytosis. Proteins and fats sometimes enter cells by the interesting process of pinocytosis (see Fig. 9-3). The word means "cell drinking." It does not mean the cell itself is engulfed; rather, as these large molecules becomes attached to the cell's outer surface, the cell membrane forms a pocket and encircles them. This creates an invagination or incupping on the cell surface, from which the engulfed material is eventually released into the cell cytoplasm. Apparently this is the mechanism by which fat, for example, is absorbed from the small intestine (see Fig. 3-5).

ELECTROLYTES

Because the electrolytes play such a prominent role in the control of water balance in the body, it will be well to discuss them in greater detail. They may be considered in four important aspects: (1) *measurement* of electrolytes in body fluids, (2) electrolyte *composition* of body fluids, (3) electrolyte *balance* within fluid compartments, and (4) electrolyte *control of body hydration.*

Measurement of electrolytes in body fluids

The chemical activity of a solution is determined by the concentration of electrolytes (charged solutes) in a given volume of the solution. Concentration is a function of volume, since the degree of concentration indicates the number of particles or charges in a unit volume. It is the *number* of particles in a solution, not the *weights* of the various particles, that is the important factor in determining chemical combining power. Electrolytes are dynamically active chemicals; the ions that are released when the electrolyte enters into solution carry charges of electrical energy, and each particle contributes chemical combining power to the whole according to its *valence,* not its weight. Therefore electrolytes are measured according to the total number of particles in solution rather than total weight.

The unit of measure commonly used is an *equivalent,* with hydrogen as a reference point. One equivalent of a substance is equal to the combining power of 1 g of hydrogen. Since small amounts are usually in question, most physiologic measurements are expressed in terms of *milliequivalents.* One milliequivalent (meq) is equal to the chemical combining power of 1 mg of hydrogen. The term "milliequivalent" refers to the *number of ions* (cations and anions) in solution, as determined by their concentration in a given volume. This measure is expressed as the number of milliequivalents per liter (meq/L).

The relation of milliequivalents to milligrams of an ionized substance in solution may be determined in the following manner: Equivalents of an ionized substance in solution are calculated in terms of the molecular weight and valance of that substance. One equivalent (eq) is 1 mole (mol; the gram-molecular weight of the substance, that is, the molecular weight of the substance in grams) divided by its valence. The milliequivalent is one one-thousandth of an equivalent. Thus

$$1 \text{ eq Na}^+ = \frac{23 \text{ g (mol wt of sodium)}}{1} = 23 \text{ g}$$
$$1 \text{ meq Na}^+ = 23 \text{ mg}$$

$$1 \text{ eq Ca}^{++} = \frac{40 \text{ g (mol wt of calcium)}}{2} = 20 \text{ g}$$
$$1 \text{ meq Ca}^{++} = 20 \text{ mg}$$

Thus the milliequivalents per liter equals the milligrams per liter divided by the equivalent weight. Equivalent weight equals gram molecular weight (atomic weight) divided by valence.

Electrolyte composition of body fluids

Electrolytes are distributed in the body water compartments in a definite pattern, which has great physiologic significance. This distribution pattern (the pattern of relative positions and concentrations) provides the overall regulation of water shifts and balances as well as the basis of respective tissue functions.

The comparative profiles of electrolyte distribution are shown in Fig. 9-4. Several electrolyte characteristics of each major fluid compartment are important to note and remember.

Extracellular fluid (ECF). Ionized sodium (Na^+) is the main cation in extracellular fluid. Sodium provides about 90% of the total base concentration (or about 45% of the total electrolyte concentration) in the body water outside the cells. Its concentration here is much greater than inside the cells. The sodium in the extracellular fluid provides the primary osmotic force that maintains the water volume necessary for the cell environment. The amounts of the other cations (K^+, Ca^{++}, Mg^{++}) in the extracellular fluid are relatively small.

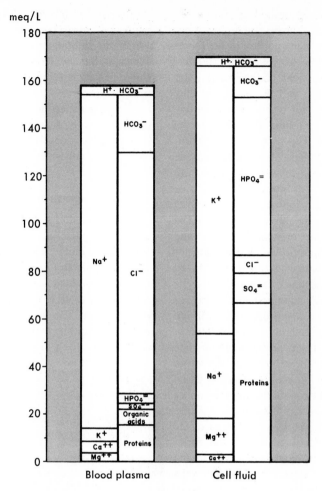

Fig. 9-4. Electrolyte distribution in extracellular fluid and in intracellular fluid. (From Gamble, J. L.: Chemical anatomy, physiology and pathology of extracellular fluid, Cambridge, Mass., 1954, Harvard University Press.)

Ionized chlorine (Cl^-) is the main anion in extracellular fluid. Chloride provides the main balancing anion in the extracellular fluid. It is present in particularly high concentration in gastric secretions as a constituent of hydrochloric acid and in interstitial lymph.

The extracellular fluid also contains the variable anion bicarbonate (HCO_3^-), the fixed anions phosphate ($HPO_4^=$), sulfate ($SO_4^=$), and protein, together with various organic acids (such as lactic acid and pyruvic acid). A fixed anion

is one that is not destroyed by the metabolic processes, for example, Cl^-, $HPO_4^=$, and $SO_4^=$. Because they are not destroyed metabolically, the fixed anions are excreted in the urine. A variable or unfixed anion is one that is converted during metabolism to other chemical forms; for example, bicarbonate is converted to carbon dioxide and water, which are used in various metabolic processes. Organic anions are similarly converted and used. The variable ions do not have to be excreted in the urine, since they do not cause the kidney to perform work in selecting them for passage in the urine.

Protein is in the plasma portion of the extracellular fluid. If the electrolyte profiles of interstitial and plasma portions of the extracellular fluid are compared, it will be noted that they are the same, except for one important difference. The extracellular fluid protein is in the plasma portion only. These are the plasma proteins present in the blood vessels that provide the colloidal osmotic pressure necessary to maintain the integrity of blood volume.

Intracellular fluid. Ionized potassium (K^+) is the main cation in the intracellular fluid. The relative concentrations of ionized sodium and potassium in the intracellular fluid are the reverse of those in the extracellular fluid. Ionized potassium is concentrated within the cells where it provides a major osmotic force for maintaining the necessary water volume inside the cell. Most of the cellular potassium is free. However, a significant amount—about one third—is bound with the cell protein. Therefore when cell protein is broken down, as in tissue oxidation of extensive tissue destruction, more potassium is freed and influences fluid shifts.

Phosphate ($HPO_4^=$) is the main anion in the intracellular fluid. Because of the significant role of phosphate in cell metabolism in the various energy-producing chains and pathways for glucose oxidation, a much greater concentration of this anion is found inside the cells than outside.

The quantity of protein in the cell fluid is three or four times greater than that in the extracellular plasma. Again, this is not surprising because of the greater protoplasmic mass in tissue cells and the important work of protein synthesis constantly going on in each cell. Together with phosphate, then, protein constitutes a major cellular anion.

Electrolyte balance within fluid compartments

Biochemical and electrophysical laws demand that in a stable solution the number of positively charged particles must equal the number of negatively charged particles. In other words, the solution must be electrically neutral. When shifts and losses occur, compensating shifts and gains follow to maintain electroneutrality.

Such a balance does indeed exist in body fluids, as can be seen by adding up the respective concentrations of cations and anions in each fluid compartment expressed in meq (see Table 9-2).

Electrolyte control of body hydration

As indicated, ionized sodium is the chief cation of extracellular fluid, and ionized potassium is the chief cation of intracellular fluid. These two electrolytes, with the others present in smaller amounts, exercise control over the amount of water to be retained in any given compartment. The usual bases for these shifts in water from one compartment to another are changes occurring in the *extracellular* concen-

Table 9-2. Balance of cation and anion concentrations in extracellular fluid (ECF) and intracellular fluid (ICF), which maintains electroneutrality within each compartment

		ECF (meq/L)	ICF (meq/L)
Cation	Na^+	142	35
	K^+	5	123
	Ca^{++}	5	15
	Mg^{++}	3	2
	TOTAL	155	175
Anion	Cl^-	104	5
	$HPO_4^=$	2	80
	$SO_4^=$	1	10
	Org. acids	5	
	Protein	16	70
	HCO_3^-	27	10
	TOTAL	155	175

trations of these electrolytes. The terms *hypertonic dehydration* and *hypotonic dehydration* refer to the electrolyte concentration of the water *outside* the cell, which in turn causes a shift of water into or out of the cell.

Hypertonic dehydration. In the extracellular fluid, when water loss exceeds electrolyte loss, the extracellular fluid becomes hypertonic to the intracellular fluid (the osmotic pressure of the extracellular fluid is higher than that of the intracellular fluid). The imbalance in osmotic pressures causes water to shift from the cell into the extracellular fluid spaces. This situation could occur from either excess water loss or water restriction. Clinical manifestations include severe thirst, hot, dry body (especially the tongue), vomiting, disorientation, and scanty and concentrated urine.

Hypotonic dehydration. When large amounts of water are added to the extracellular fluid without the addition of sufficient electrolytes to maintain the normal density of the solutions, the extracellular fluid becomes hypotonic to the intracellular fluid. This type of imbalance in osmotic pressures causes a compensatory shift of water from the extracellular fluid into the cell. The result is a dangerous shrinking of the extracellular fluid, especially the blood volume. Renal blood flow is impaired, and swelling of cells (cellular edema) occurs. This serious situation could result either from overzealous hydration of patients (giving too much plain water without accompanying electrolytes) or from losses of both water and electrolytes and replacement with water only. Clinical manifestations include progressive weakness without thirst or decreased urine output. Also, the hematocrit reading and the red blood cell count are elevated because of concentration of the blood.

Influence of protein on internal fluid shifts

Protein influences the internal shifting of body water in three areas. These are the water exchange across capillary walls, water exchange across cell walls, and lymph drainage of tissue water.

Water exchange across capillary walls. The plasma proteins exert a tremendous colloidal osmotic pressure within the capillaries, which pulls fluid and solutes from the interstitial spaces into the blood. This maintains the necessary plasma volume. About 70% of this total colloidal osmotic pressure comes from the albumin, which is present in a greater quantity than any other plasma protein; the remaining 30% is from the presence of globulins and fibrinogen. Because the molecules of the plasma proteins are for the most part too large to pass through the capillary wall, they exert a constant osmotic pull on the interstitial fluid. However, this osmotic pull is balanced by an opposite outward thrust (hydrostatic pressure) of the blood within the capillary. This blood pressure tends to push fluid *out* of the capillary lumen into the interstitial fluid. Throughout the length of the capillary—from the end at which it emerges from the arteriole to the end at which it merges into the venule—these two forces play against one another in an intricate and subtle opposition that produces an exquisite balance. At the arteriole end of the capillary, the hydrostatic pressure predominates just enough to filter some water and solutes (including salts and a small amount of protein) out into the tissue fluids. By the time the blood has reached the venous end of the capillary, it has lost so much water that the relative osmotic pull of the plasma proteins within its lumen has risen considerably. Meanwhile, the opposing hydrostatic outward thrust has diminished because the fluid is just that much farther from the heart, which sent it on its way. The balance topples to the other side; water and solutes are drawn through the wall of the capillary into its lumen.

The statement of this equilibrium of pressures was first proposed in 1895 by E. H. Starling, and is now called *Starling's law of the capillaries,* or the *capillary fluid shift mechanism.* This equilibrium is one of the body's most important homeostatic mechanisms to

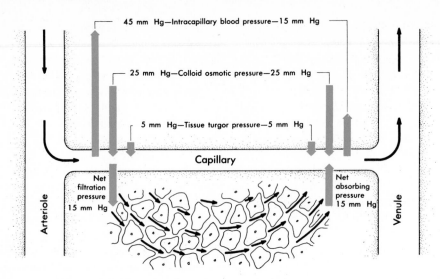

Fig. 9-5. The fluid shift mechanism. Note the balance of pressures that controls the flow of fluid.

maintain fluid balance. The diagram illustrating this fluid shift (Fig. 9-5) should be studied carefully.

The blood enters the capillary from the arteriole under a hydrostatic pressure from the heartbeat of about 45 mm Hg, which is the intracapillary blood pressure. Working against this pressure is the colloidal osmotic pressure of the protein molecules (approximately 25 mm Hg) and a small amount of resisting tissue turgor of the capillary wall (approximately 5 mm Hg). If the total of these resistant pressures (30 mm Hg) is subtracted from the blood pressure of 45 mm Hg, a net filtration pressure at the arteriole end of the capillary is 15 mm Hg. Under this thrust, the water with its small amount of diffusible solutes (glucose, amino acids) goes out into the interstitial spaces to bathe the cells.

As the capillary flow continues to the venule end, the protein molecules that are too large to pass through the capillary wall accumulate and maintain the colloidal osmotic pressure at about 25 mm Hg; but the blood pressure (from the cardiac impulse) has diminished to about 15 mm Hg. The balances are now reversed; the colloidal osmotic pressure exceeds the blood pressure, a net absorbing pressure of 15 mm Hg now prevails, and water is drawn back into the vascular compartment. The constant operation of this mechanism maintains the plasma volume and provides the transfer fluid environment to serve the cell's needs.

Water exchange across cell walls. In much the same way that the plasma proteins provide colloidal osmotic pressure that helps to maintain the integrity of the extracellular fluids, the cell protein (protoplasm) helps to provide the osmotic pressure that maintains the integrity of the intracellular fluid. Added to the osmotic pressure from the cell protein is the osmotic pressure provided by the intracellular ionized potassium. Balanced against the total intracellular pressure from these two sources is the osmotic pressure outside the cell, which is maintained by ionized sodium. As a result of the balance between the intracellular and the extracellular osmotic pressures, water and nutrients flow in, and water and metabolic wastes flow out through the cell membrane.

Lymph drainage of tissue water. Protein in the lymphatic fluid provides a further means of removing excess water from the tissue spaces. During periods of relative inactivity of tissue, the capillaries are adequate to drain away the water that remains after exchanges. In an active organ, however, such as a contracting muscle, more water is produced. Here, the lymphatic vessels help to carry off the excess water, averting the accumulation of fluid (edema) in the interstitial spaces. The severe leg edema seen in elephantiasis is a result of the cutting-off of this lymph circulation. A parasitic worm lodges in the lymph vessel and obstructs it, these fluids accumulate, and the leg swells.

ROLE OF THE GASTROINTESTINAL TRACT

In considering total fluid and electrolyte balance in the body, it is easy to lose sight of the vast importance of the gastrointestinal secretions in maintaining that balance. Water from the plasma, containing ions in patterns that vary according to numerous factors, is converted by the appropriate sections of the gastrointestinal tract into digestive secretions. These secretions, which are produced daily, function progressively throughout the alimentary system in the processes of digestion and absorption. They circulate constantly between plasma and secreting cells. Finally, in the distal portion of the intestine, most of the water and electrolytes are reabsorbed into the plasma to circulate again.

These fluids should be considered according to the sheer magnitude of the gastrointestinal secretions and the serious results of fluid loss from the upper or the lower portion of the gastrointestinal tract.

Magnitude of the gastrointestinal secretions. Seldom realized are the enormous quantities of water and electrolytes secreted daily into the gastrointestinal tract. As indicated in Table 9-3, the total amount of fluid participating in the gastrointestinal circulation has been

Table 9-3. Approximate total volume of digestive secretions produced in 24 hours by adult of average size*

Saliva	1,500 ml
Gastric	2,500
Bile	500
Pancreatic	700
Intestinal	3,000
TOTAL	8,200 ml

*From Gamble, J. L.: Chemical anatomy, physiology and pathology of extracellular fluid, ed. 6, Cambridge, Mass., 1954, Harvard University Press.

Table 9-4. Approximate concentration of certain electrolytes in digestive fluids (meq/L)

	Na$^+$	K$^+$	Cl$^-$	HCO$_3^-$
Saliva	10	25	10	15
Gastric	40	10	145	0
Pancreatic	140	5	40	110
Jejunal	135	5	110	30
Bile	140	10	110	40

variously estimated at 7,500 to 10,000 ml daily. The distribution of this total volume in the various secretions should be noted.

Because of the large quantities of fluid that are returned into the plasma, only from 100 to 150 ml of water is left for fecal elimination.

The approximate total volume of the gastrointestinal secretions is 8,200 ml, while the total blood volume in the average sized adult is only 3,500 ml. The blood volume is less than half that of the gastrointestinal fluids. It is no wonder, then, that imbalances in gastrointestinal circulation, if allowed to go uncorrected, rapidly lead to serious consequences.

In addition, surprisingly large amounts of key cations and anions are present in the gastrointestinal tract. Table 9-4 shows the distribution of these electrolytes.

If the relative ionized potassium values of the various gastrointestinal secretions are compared, the *total* quantity of gastric ionized potassium is two to five times that of the blood serum. In the rest of the gastrointestinal tract, ionized potassium concentration is equal to that of the extracellular fluid. Also, there are large amounts of ionized sodium in the gastrointestinal fluids. These total approximately 1,000 meq per day, which is about one third of the total body sodium. An adequate diet supplies sufficient amounts of these two cations—from 75 to 100 meq (3 to 4 g) of potassium and from 130 to 250 meq (8 to 15 g) of salt.

The gastrointestinal fluids are held in *isotonicity* (equality of osmotic pressure due to ion equilibrium) with the extracellular fluid compartment. When water is drunk without solutes or accompanying food, electrolytes and salts enter the intestine from the extracellular fluid. If a hypertonic solution or food is ingested, additional water is drawn into the intestine from the extracellular fluid. In each instance, water and electrolytes are shifted from compartment to compartment to maintain solutions in the alimentary tract isotonic with the extracellular fluid. This law of isotonicity has many clinical implications. For example, what would happen if a patient on gastric suction drank water, or if a patient being maintained by tube feeding were given his formula too rapidly at too concentrated a dilution? In the first case, the water would cause the stomach to produce more secretions containing electrolytes; the electrolytes would in turn be lost in the suctioning. The plasma, from which the electrolytes are supplied, would be gradually depleted of them and unable to supply these essential nutrients to tissue cells. In the second case, the hypertonic solution being given by tube would cause a shift of water into the intestine, which would rapidly shrink the vascular volume of the extracellular fluid.

Upper and lower gastrointestinal losses. It is not surprising, because of the large amounts of water and electrolytes involved, that loss of gastrointestinal secretions is the most common cause of clinical fluid and electrolyte problems. The biochemical problem differs according to whether the upper or the lower portion of the alimentary tract is involved. For example, in persistent vomiting, much fluid and hydrochloric acid are eliminated, and dehydration, a potassium deficit, and alkalosis result. In prolonged diarrhea, large amounts of water, sodium, chlorine, and bicarbonate are lost. As sodium losses continue, sodium is shifted from the plasma and interstitial fluid to replace it, and potassium then moves out of the cells to replace the extracellular sodium. The loss of potassium is compounded by the triggering of the aldosterone mechanism, a hormonal device for conservation of sodium, and more potassium is eliminated in the process (Fig. 9-8).

ROLE OF THE KIDNEYS

The major responsibility for regulating the water and electrolyte balance in the body falls to the kidney. This marvelous organ is central to the successful operation of many other organs and tissues. In his delightful book, *From Fish to Philosopher,* Homer Smith places the kidney in a primary position in the body's hierarchy of parts. He states:

It is no exaggeration to say that the composition of the body fluids is determined not by what the mouth takes in but by what the kidneys keep: they are the master chemists of our internal environment. . . . Recognizing that we have the kind of internal environment we have because we have the kind of kidneys that we have, we must acknowledge that our kidneys constitute the major foundation of our physiological freedom. Only because they work the way they do has it become possible for us to have bones, muscles, glands, and brains. Superficially, it might be said that the function of the kidneys is to make urine; but in a more considered view one can say that the kidneys make the stuff of philosophy itself.[2]

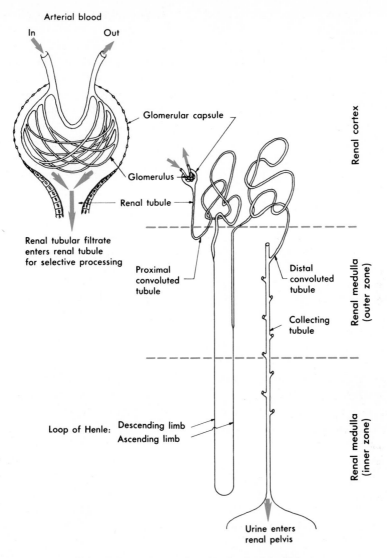

Arterial blood

In   Out

Glomerular capsule

Glomerulus

Renal tubule

Renal tubular filtrate
enters renal tubule
for selective processing

Proximal
convoluted
tubule

Distal
convoluted
tubule

Collecting
tubule

Loop of Henle: Descending limb
Ascending limb

Urine enters
renal pelvis

Renal cortex

Renal medulla
(outer zone)

Renal medulla
(inner zone)

Fig. 9-6. The nephron—functional unit of the kidney.

The basic anatomy and physiology of the kidney should be reviewed carefully in terms of water and electrolyte balance. The kidney's functional unit, the *nephron,* is particularly well adapted in structure for this vital regulatory role (Fig. 9-6). There are two significant aspects of this role: (1) the nepron's basic functions, for which it is uniquely structured and (2) the hormonal homeostatic mechanisms involved in renal control of water and electrolyte conservation and excretion.

Functions of the nephron

In the cortex of each kidney there are about 1 million minute, finely structured functioning units called nephrons. The tremendous capacity of these units to select, reject, conserve, and eliminate is demonstrated over and over again as they cleanse the blood 15 to 18 times every day. Filtration, tubular reabsorption, and secretion are the three basic functions involved in this overall control process.

Filtration. Filtration has been defined (p. 177) as one of the ways in which water and certain solutes move across capillary walls as the result of pressure differences on either side. Because the intracapillary fluid pressure is greater than the interstitial fluid pressure, water and small, freely diffusible molecules pass out of the capillary through its wall into the surrounding interstitial fluid and thence into the absorbing capsule of the renal tubule. In the nephron, several structures are especially adapted to facilitate this initial filtration process. These structures are the arterioles and the cells in the walls of the glomerulus and the capsule.

AFFERENT AND EFFERENT ARTERIOLES. The head of the nephron consists of a cuplike structure called Bowman's capsule, which holds the glomerulus (a tuft of branching capillaries). The afferent (entering) arteriole is relatively large. As it breaks up into its many branching capillaries it offers a narrowing stream bed, which effectively slows down the renal blood flow to promote filtration. The loops of the capillary tuft join again to form a single vessel, the efferent (leaving) arteriole, which is of smaller diameter than the afferent arteriole. This offers resistance to flow and produces additional backward pressure to favor filtration.

Further control is added by the ability of the uniquely muscular afferent and efferent arterioles to constrict or dilate independently of one another, according to blood pressure requirements. For example, when the blood pressure is lower, the afferent arteriole may dilate and the efferent arteriole constrict to provide

---

TO PROBE FURTHER
Renal reabsorption of sodium by the countercurrent system

The reabsorption of sodium is continuously carried on in the nephron as one of its most significant tasks in reclaiming this vital electrolyte. The reabsorption of sodium occurs between the two limbs of the loop of Henle, and is believed to involve a *countercurrent system* of active transport. This countercurrent theory, advanced by Wirz* and now widely held, contributes a significant step in the knowledge of renal function and physiology. As the fluid that has passed through the proximal convoluted tubule flows through the portion of the loop of Henle that descends into the inner zone of the renal medulla, much of its water passes out into the interstitial fluid, while the sodium moves on into the ascending limb of the loop of Henle. From this site, the sodium is actively transported out of the ascending limb into the interstitial fluid of the medulla, then back into the descending limb by means of a series of sodium pumps. The result is a progressive increase in sodium concentration (and therefore in the osmolarity) of the fluid in all structures from the inner to outer portion of the renal medulla. The net effect is to conserve water and concentrate the urine in the distal collecting duct as it passes through this hyperosmolar section of the medulla on its way to the renal pelvis. The total system that controls levels of osmolarity has come to be known as the *countercurrent multiplier of concentration*. These relationships are shown in Fig. 9-7.

*Wirz, H.: Kidney, water, and electrolyte metabolism, Annu. Rev. Physiol. **23**:577, 1961.

additional pressure favoring filtration. If the blood pressure is high, this reaction may be reversed.

CELLS IN WALLS OF GLOMERULUS AND CAPSULE. The glomerulus and the receiving tubular capsule are lined with long, thin, flat cells especially structured to provide optimal filtration and absorbing surfaces. Resistance to flow is therefore minimized, and filtration occurs readily.

Tubular reabsorption. After water and filterable solutes are filtered from the blood via the glomerulus into the receiving capsule, they pass in turn through the three portions of the tubule in which selective reabsorption takes place. These areas are the proximal tubule, the loop of Henle, and the distal tubule. It is in these areas that the nephron carries on its highly selective process of reabsorbing needed materials and rejecting others for eventual elimination. In this process, the nephrons perform several tasks. They control the amount of water in the body and the electrolyte level, they excrete various electrolytes as waste products, and they excrete excess metabolic materials.

AMOUNT OF WATER IN THE BODY. By varying the amount of water retained or eliminated, the nephrons effectively control and guard the total fluid volume. This control is largely regulated in turn by certain hormones, such as the antidiuretic hormone (ADH, vasopressin) from the posterior pituitary (neurohypophysis). Indirect control is also exerted by aldosterone from the adrenals. These two important homeostatic mechanisms are discussed on pp. 188-189. As the result of the renal tubular control of hydration, 99% of the water filtered is recovered and returned into the bloodstream to be reused.

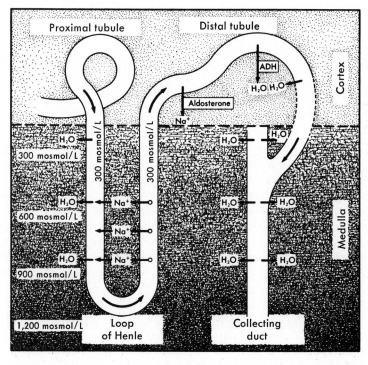

Fig. 9-7. Countercurrent system of sodium (Na) and water exchange operating between the two limbs of the loop of Henle.

LEVELS OF ELECTROLYTES IN THE BODY. The nephrons also have the task of maintaining various electrolyte blood levels within normal ranges. The integrity of the concentration of certain electrolytes, especially of sodium and potassium, is necessary for delicate fluid-electrolyte and acid-base balances throughout the body. The control of sodium concentration illustrates the adaptation of the nephron's structure and function to the maintenance of the proper supply of electrolytes. Two interesting mechanisms are involved. One is the aldosterone mechanism, which is periodically triggered by a threatened loss of sodium. The other is a continuous, active transport process that involves a countercurrent system against the usual osmotic pressure gradient. This system makes use of the sodium pump.

EXCRETION OF VARIOUS METABOLITES AS WASTE PRODUCTS. The waste products excreted by the nephrons include such materials as urea and excess ketones, which the nephrons selectively reject and discard, thus preventing their harmful accumulation in the blood.

EXCRETION OF EXCESS METABOLIC MATERIALS. The nephrons excrete harmful excess loads of otherwise beneficial metabolic materials. Glucose, for example, is a beneficial product of the metabolism of carbohydrates. Normally, it is not excreted but is conserved for use. However, in uncontrolled diabetes, the glucose accumulates in the blood to harmful levels, and the kidney then begins to excrete these excesses.

Secretion. A third major function of the kidney involved in control of fluid and electrolytes, especially as related to acid-base balance, is secretion. Control of acidity is affected by secretion of hydrogen ions and ammonia from the blood. This function is further detailed in the general discussion of acid-base balance on p. 193.

Hormonal control of water and electrolyte balance

The two hormonal mechanisms designed to guard the body's water and electrolytes and to maintain their state of equilibrium are the antidiuretic hormone (ADH) mechanism and the aldosterone mechanism. These mechanisms function to protect the integrity of the blood volume and to maintain adequate circulation despite real or threatened deprivation of water or sodium.

ADH mechanism. The antidiuretic hormone secreted by the posterior lobe of the pituitary gland acts mainly in the distal collecting tubule. It stimulates the reabsorption of water according to body need. Excess secretion of the hormone may be triggered by a real or apparent loss of body water. The actual loss of body water, as in hemorrhage, engages the ADH mechanism in an effort to conserve water. In certain situations, such as congestive heart failure, the body water is not actually diminished but is shifted from the circulating plasma into the interstitial extracellular fluid spaces by the diminished action of the heart. Included in this general reduction of plasma flow to all organs is reduction of plasma flow to the kidney. The kidney interprets this diminished plasma flow to mean that the body is deprived of water, and the ADH mechanism is set in motion in an effort to conserve water for the total body.

The mechanism by which ADH is released from the pituitary is believed to be mediated by changes of the osmotic pressure in the plasma that bathes the hypothalamus. It is further believed that in the hypothalamus there are pressure-sensitive centers called *osmoreceptors* (volume receptors). Their precise location within the hypothalamus is not known. Various stress reactions inducing shock stimulate release of the hormone to guard water and electrolytes.

Aldosterone mechanism. A second important hormone that governs the renal control of water and electrolyte balance is the aldosterone mechanism. This mechanism is primarily a sodium-conserving device, but in carrying out this function it also exerts a secondary control over the diuresis of water. Therefore it essen-

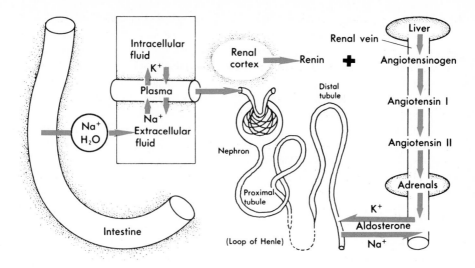

Fig. 9-8. The aldosterone mechanism that conserves sodium in exchange for potassium and causes increased reabsorption of water.

tially restores the volume of extracellular fluid and of circulating blood in times of stress and threatened loss. The operation of the aldosterone mechanism involves a specific cycle of events (Fig. 9-8):

1. When sodium intake is decreased, or sodium is lost, or body fluid volume is contracted, the renal cortex forms the enzyme *renin* and secretes it into the blood via the renal vein. In the blood, renin acts on its specific substrate from the liver, *angiotensinogen,* to form *angiotensin I,* which in turn is converted to *angiotensin II*. Angiotensin II is an active pressor substance that increases the force of the heartbeat, constricts the arterioles, and diminishes renal blood flow.

2. Angiotensin II stimulates secretion of aldosterone by the adrenals. Aldosterone then causes retention and reabsorption of sodium and therefore of water; improved renal circulation follows. A secondary result of aldosterone activity is a potassium loss in the tubular ion exchange for sodium.

3. Aldosterone is operative chiefly in the distal renal tubule. It can increase reabsorption up

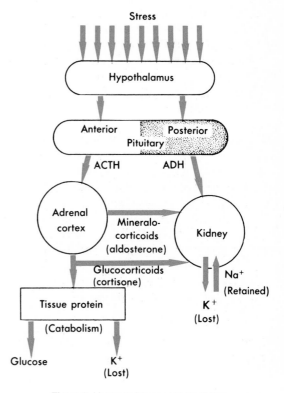

Fig. 9-9. Hormonal response to stress.

to 98% as in shock because of lowered blood volume. Shock shrinks the total fluid compartment; less fluid therefore circulates through the kidneys, and reabsorption of greater quantity is needed to supply the deficit.

Aldosterone release may also be stimulated by ACTH, a hormone secreted by the anterior pituitary in response to body stress. Both ADH and aldosterone mechanisms may be activated by stress situations such as bodily injury or surgery. The relationship of these hormones to stress is illustrated in Fig. 9-9.

Clinical applications

Many applications of these fluid and electrolyte balance principles may be discovered in daily clinical practice. The following are questions concerning clinical situations that should be reviewed carefully to try to work out the chain of successive events that produce serious water and electrolyte imbalances. The linear diagrams of these triggering chains are given at the end of this chapter on pp. 196-199.

1. What accounts for the edema of starvation?
2. Why would cellular dehydration result from drinking sea water?
3. Why does potassium depletion occur in prolonged diarrhea?
4. Why would oliguria occur, and why is there a danger of potassium depletion following surgery?
5. What is the danger of trying to hydrate a patient (one with diarrhea, for example) with plain water?
6. Why should patients on gastric suction not be allowed to have water in liquid or solid form?
7. Which is preferable for a gastric lavage— plain water or isotonic saline solution? Why?
8. Why are salt tablets supplied for men working at the open hearth in a steel mill? What is the danger of satisfying their thirst only with water?

Additional clinical applications center around postgastrectomy and other surgical problems, edema in congestive heart failure, ascites in advanced liver disease, and renal disease such as the nephrotic syndrome. These specific situations are discussed in greater detail in Part IV, Nutrition in Clinical Care.

Other clinical applications concern lack of the controlling hormone ADH. Lesions in the hypothalamus or pituitary stalk cause ADH production to cease, producing the disease *diabetes insipidus*. Without the water reabsorbing hormone, ADH, large quantities of dilute urine are excreted daily. The volume may be from 5 to 30 L per day. The disease is controlled by subcutaneous administration of posterior pituitary extract or by nasal instillation of the extract.

ACID-BASE BUFFER SYSTEM

Water and electrolytes are involved in a second area that has broad physiologic implications—the *acid-base buffer system*. This system is essential to the maintenance of an optimal acid-base balance throughout the body. To understand the physiologic buffer systems, the answers to the following questions will be considered:

1. What is the difference between an acid and a base?
2. What is a buffer?
3. What ratio should exist between acids and bases if the buffer system is to successfully offset changes in the ionized hydrogen concentration in the extracellular fluid?
4. What role do the kidney and lung play in maintaining the acid-base balance in the extracellular fluid?
5. What are acidosis and alkalosis?

Definitions of acid and base

A substance is *more or less* acid, according to the degree of its concentration of ionized hydrogen. Its degree of acidity is expressed in terms of pH. The symbol pH is derived from a mathematical term. It is the negative logarithm expressed as an exponential *p*ower of the *Hy*drogen ion concentration. If the pH of a solution is 5.0, its hydrogen ion concentration is 10^{-5}. The hydrogen ion concentration in pure water is 10^{-7}; therefore the pH of pure water is 7.0. A pH of 7.0 is the neutral point between an acid and an alkaline (base). Substances with a pH *lower* than 7.0 are *acid*. (Since the pH is the *negative* logarithm, the higher the hydrogen ion concentration, the lower the pH.) Substances with a pH above 7.0 are *alkaline*.

Acids. An acid may be defined as a compound that has enough hydrogen ions to give some away. When in aqueous solution, an acid releases hydrogen ions. The following are some examples of acids and their donation of ionized hydrogen when in aqueous solution:

$$H_2CO_3 \rightarrow H^+ + HCO_3^-$$
$$HCl \rightarrow H^+ + Cl^-$$
$$H_2SO_4 \rightarrow 2H^+ + SO_4^=$$
$$H_3PO_4 \rightarrow 2H^+ + HPO_4^=$$

Bases. A base possesses *few* hydrogen ions. It therefore takes up ionized hydrogen. The following are examples of bases:

$$OH^- + H^+ \rightarrow H_2O$$
$$HCO_3^- + H^+ \rightarrow H_2CO_3$$
$$OH^- + H_2CO_3 \rightarrow H_2O + HCO_3^-$$

Buffers

The word *buffer* comes from a Middle English root meaning "to protect from blows." In the seventeenth century it referred to a coat of armor. In chemistry, a buffer is a mixture of acidic and alkaline components, which protects a solution against wide variations in its pH, even when strong bases or acids are added to it. A solution containing such a protective mixture is called a *buffered solution*. A buffer protects the acid-base balance of a solution by rapidly offsetting changes in its ionized hydrogen concentration. It works by protecting against either added acid or base.

Protection against added acid. If a strong acid is added to a buffered solution, the base partner of the acid-base buffer reacts with the added acid to form a weaker acid. The acidity of the total solution is effectively lowered toward (or to) the starting point. Formula 9-1 shows the reaction when hydrochloric acid is added to a buffered solution. The H^+ donated by the hydrochloric acid is taken up by the bicarbonate to form a weaker acid.

Protection against added base. If a strong base is added to a buffered solution, the acid partner of the buffer donates ionized hydrogen, which combines with the intruder to form a weaker base, and restores the pH to the starting point. Formula 9-2 shows the reaction that occurs if sodium hydroxide is added to a buffered solution.

The human body contains many buffered solutions, including those that involve hemoglobin, oxyhemoglobin, protein, and the disodium hydrogen phosphate–sodium dihydrogen phosphate $(Na_2HPO_4–NaH_2PO_4)$ system. Its main buffer system is the relatively weak carbonic acid–sodium bicarbonate $(H_2CO_3–NaHCO_3)$ system. The body selects this as its principal buffer system for two reasons: (1) the raw materials for the production of carbonic acid $(CO_2 + H_2O = H_2CO_3)$ are readily avail-

(strong acid)		(base-buffer)		(weaker acid)		(salt)	
HCl	+	$NaHCO_3$	$\rightarrow$	H_2CO_3	+	NaCl	**(9-1)**
hydrochloric acid		sodium bicarbonate		carbonic acid		table salt	

(strong base)		(acid-buffer)		(weaker base)		(water)	
NaOH	+	H_2CO_3	$\rightarrow$	$NaHCO_3$	+	H_2O	**(9-2)**
sodium hydroxide		carbonic acid		sodium bicarbonate		water	

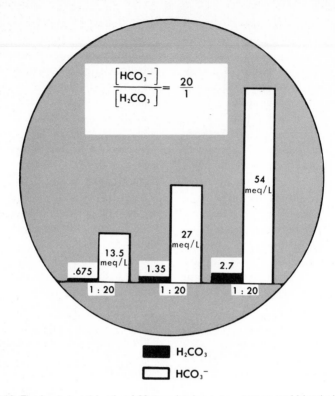

$$\frac{\left[HCO_3^-\right]}{\left[H_2CO_3\right]} = \frac{20}{1}$$

54 meq/L

27 meq/L

13.5 meq/L

.675   1.35   2.7

1 : 20   1 : 20   1 : 20

■ H_2CO_3

☐ HCO_3^-

Fig. 9-10. The base to acid ratio of 20:1 maintains a constant normal blood pH of 7.4.

able and (2) the lungs and kidneys can easily adjust to ratio alterations between carbonic acid and the base bicarbonate, sodium bicarbonate.

Buffer system ratio in the extracellular fluid. The normal pH of the extracellular fluid is 7.4, with a normal range from 7.35 to 7.45. Maintenance of the pH within this narrow range is necessary to sustain the life of cells. The carbonic acid–sodium bicarbonate buffer system is able to make an effective contribution to the stabilization of the extracellular fluid at this pH because the base bicarbonate partner in this buffer system is about 20 times as abundant as the carbonic acid. This 20:1 base to acid ratio is normally maintained even though the absolute amounts may fluctuate during compensation periods from the normal concentrations of 27 meq/L of base bicarbonate and 1.35 meq/L of carbonic acid. As long as the 20:1

ratio is maintained, the extracellular fluid acid-base balance is held constant (Fig. 9-10).

Roles of the lungs and kidneys

The lungs and kidneys guard the body's acid-base balance by regulating the supply of components of the carbonic acid–sodium bicarbonate buffer system. According to the body's immediate need, each of these two organs conserves or releases substances that are essential to the production of either base or acid. This permits the buffer system to perpetuate the necessary 20:1 base to acid ratio.

Lungs. The lungs ultimately control the body's supply of carbonic acid. Carbonic acid is formed from carbon dioxide and water:

$$CO_2 + H_2O \rightarrow H_2CO_3$$

Changes in rate and depth of breathing alter the

amounts of carbon dioxide that enter the body, which effectively controls the level of carbonic acid in blood and tissues. When the blood level of sodium bicarbonate goes down, the lungs expel excess carbon dioxide; this decreases the quantity of raw material available for the production of carbonic acid, and the ratio of base to acid in the buffer system is restored to 20:1.

Kidneys. The kidneys maintain the base bicarbonate component of this buffer system. In the renal tubule, hydrogen ions are secreted; in an ion exchange with hydrogen, sodium is recaptured and returned to the bloodstream. The sodium is combined with HCO_3^- to form sodium bicarbonate ($NaHCO_3$).

The kidney also conserves base by eliminating extra hydrogen ions through the production and excretion of ammonia (NH_4):

$$NH_3 + H^+ \rightarrow NH_4$$
$$\updownarrow$$
$$\text{from}$$
$$\text{deamination}$$
$$\text{of amino acids}$$

ACIDOSIS AND ALKALOSIS

The key concept that has enabled investigators to understand the clinical states of acidosis and alkalosis is ionized hydrogen *concentration*. It was not possible to develop adequate therapy for these states as long as they were thought of merely as conditions in which the blood was ''more acid'' or ''more alkaline.'' *In acidosis, the ionized hydrogen concentration is above normal. In alkalosis, ionized hydrogen concentration is below normal.* Either of these abnormal states initiates compensatory responses of the buffer system, lungs, and kidneys, which cause body fluids to accept, to release, or to excrete ionized hydrogen. Increases and decreases in ionized hydrogen concentration are therefore modified so that the pH is not significantly changed from its normal range of 7.35 to 7.45. Failure of either the lungs or the kidneys to carry out their functions results in acidosis or alkalosis. If the failure is predominantly related to the pulmonary system, the clinical result is called respiratory acidosis or respiratory alkalosis. If the failure is chiefly related to the renal system, the resultant clinical state is called metabolic acidosis or metabolic alkalosis.

Respiratory acidosis

Cause. Diseases that interfere with normal breathing impede the release of carbon dioxide from the lungs. The retained carbon dioxide combines with water and forms carbonic acid. The carbonic acid level may rise to twice normal. In addition, the carbon dioxide combining power in the serum is increased by the presence of the carbon dioxide that was retained by the lungs.

Pulmonary compensation. The lung attempts to increase ventilation to expel excess carbon dioxide. It is often prevented from doing so by the same pulmonary disease that initiated the retention of carbon dioxide.

Renal compensation. Two compensatory responses take place in the kidney. First, increased ionized hydrogen is secreted by the renal tubule and exchanged for sodium; the sodium is combined with HCO_3^- to form sodium bicarbonate ($NaHCO_3$) and is returned to the bloodstream. This elevates the base bicarbonate component in this buffer system. Second, increased quantities of ammonia are formed so that more ionized hydrogen is excreted.

Clinical examples. The exchange of oxygen and carbon dioxide occurs at the alveolocapillary membrane. A variety of diseases that affect the lung involve this membrane and therefore contribute to the development of respiratory acidosis. These include emphysema, bronchiectasis, asthma, pulmonary edema, bronchial pneumonia, and congestive heart failure. A similar effect may follow administration of inhalation anesthesia to a patient whose pulmonary function is marginal or weak. Respiratory acidosis may also occur because of paralysis of respiratory muscles as in poliomyelitis.

Respiratory alkalosis

Cause. The primary cause of respiratory alkalosis is excess carbon dioxide output, which in turn is caused by hyperventilation. The decrease in available carbon dioxide lowers the production of carbonic acid, and the ionized hydrogen concentration therefore falls (pH rises). In addition, because less carbon dioxide is available, carbon dioxide combining power is diminished.

Pulmonary compensation. The lung cannot initiate efforts to compensate for respiratory alkalosis, as it is directly involved in the cause; however, the decreased carbonic acid level in the extracellular fluid tends to gradually depress respiration.

Renal compensation. The major task of compensation falls to the kidneys where tubular ionized hydrogen formation is suppressed so that sodium bicarbonate is excreted. Ammonia formation is also diminished so that further sodium is excreted.

Clinical examples. Common causes of respiratory alkalosis are the hyperventilation syndrome (brought about by hysteria or acute anxiety); hyperpnea (labored breathing) in response to hot weather, high altitude, or fever; or excessive breathing forced on a patient by a poorly adjusted mechanical respirator. Respiratory alkalosis may also result from overstimulation of the respiratory center in the brain; this may be brought about by salicylate (aspirin) poisoning (a frequent occurrence in children) or by meningitis or encephalitis.

Metabolic acidosis

Cause. In certain metabolic disorders the blood may contain an excess of specific metabolic organic acids (ketones, lactic acid). Part of the bicarbonate in the buffer system is displaced by these acids, and the ionized hydrogen concentration rises.

Pulmonary compensation. To reduce the carbonic acid level, the lungs attempt to expel carbon dioxide by deep, pauseless breathing (air hunger or Kussmaul breathing). Kussmaul breathing is characteristic of diabetic acidosis, for example.

Renal compensation. The renal tubule increases its secretion of hydrogen ions, which are exchanged for sodium. The sodium is returned to the blood as sodium bicarbonate. Ammonia production rises, taking up ionized hydrogen and excreting it in the urine.

Clinical examples. It is interesting to trace (as in Fig. 25-2) the chain of events, for example, that characterizes states of fluid and electrolyte imbalance in diabetic acidosis. These potentially disastrous consequences are brought about because, in these situations, the body cannot properly metabolize blood glucose and turns for its energy to the catabolism of protein and fat.

A similar metabolic situation prevails in starvation when the body turns to its own body stores of protein and fat to supply its needs. In states of accelerated metabolism, such as thyrotoxicosis when increased metabolic demand rapidly depletes carbohydrate stores, the body burns protein stores, producing ketosis. Gastrointestinal problems may also produce metabolic acidosis. For example, although initial vomiting may cause metabolic alkalosis because of loss of gastric hydrochloric acid, prolonged vomiting frequently causes metabolic acidosis as the inability to eat results in decreased carbohydrate intake, glycogen depletion, burning of body protein and fat, and finally ketosis. Severe diarrhea may induce acidosis because large amounts of bicarbonate (HCO_3^-) and sodium (Na^+), as components of intestinal contents, are swept away. Chronic and acute renal diseases may contribute to metabolic acidosis as the kidney becomes unable to compensate in the face of excess ionized hydrogen concentrations.

Metabolic alkalosis

Cause. Metabolic alkalosis is characterized by a fall in ionized hydrogen concentration (rise in pH) caused primarily by an increase in bicarbonate. Such an excess of bicarbonate may be caused by excretion or loss of large amounts of ionized hydrogen, by excessive intake of bicarbonate, or by decrease in potassium stores: as ionized hydrogen and sodium move into the cell to replace lost potassium, the extracellular fluid concentration of ionized hydrogen is reduced.

Pulmonary compensation. The decreased ionized hydrogen concentration (increased pH) gradually suppresses ventilation; the lungs tend to conserve carbon dioxide, which increases the production of carbonic acid.

Renal compensation. The renal tubule suppresses secretion of ionized hydrogen, which allows sodium bicarbonate to be excreted rather than reabsorbed. Ammonia production is re-

duced so that more base is excreted. The excretion of various acid metabolites is also reduced.

Clinical examples. Loss of ionized hydrogen and chlorine, as in initial vomiting, induces metabolic alkalosis. The same ions are lost in excessive gastric suction or when the proximal intestine is obstructed, as by pyloric stenosis. Conditions that involve potassium depletion also induce alkalosis, as ionized hydrogen and sodium move into the cells to replace lost potassium. This reduces the extracellular fluid hydrogen concentration. Such conditions include lack of potassium intake, gastrointestinal loss of potassium, or ACTH (adrenocorticotropic hormone) therapy. (ACTH induces renal tubular reabsorption of sodium in an ion exchange for potassium, and therefore potassium

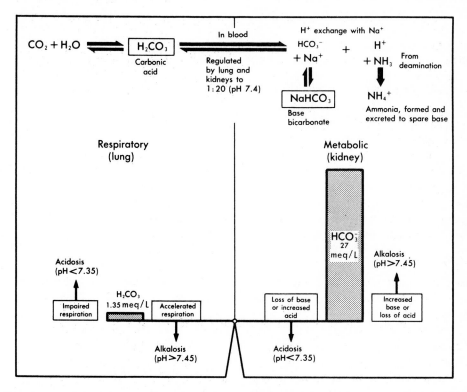

Fig. 9-11. Carbonic acid to sodium (base) bicarbonate buffer system. Note the types of clinical situations that lead to respiratory acidosis and alkalosis and to metabolic acidosis and alkalosis.

is excreted.) Excess intake of alkali powders or sodium bicarbonate, as in long-term ulcer therapy, may also contribute to alkalosis.

In all states of acid-base imbalance, two basic rules of treatment apply. First, the primary cause of the acidosis or alkalosis is treated. Second, efforts are made to aid the various compensatory responses of the lungs and kidneys. Each of these therapeutic attempts calls for careful and continuous adjustment. The summary diagram (Fig. 9-11) of the acid-base buffer system involving all four clinical situations (respiratory acidosis and alkalosis, metabolic acidosis and alkalosis) should be reviewed.

GLOSSARY

acid (L. *acidus*, sour) a substance that is sour to taste and neutralizes base substances. Acids are essentially ionized hydrogen donors—in solution they provide H ions.

acidosis a disturbance in acid-base balance in which there is a reduction of the alkali reserve. Acidosis may be caused by an accumulation of acids (as in diabetic acidosis) or by an excess loss of bicarbonate (as in renal disease).

active transport the movement of solutes in solution (for example, products of digestion such as glucose) across a membrane *against* the usual pressure gradient. Movement against pressure requires energy, which is supplied by the cell. Sometimes an additional transporting substance is required such as the sodium pump for absorbing glucose and the intrinsic factor (IF) for absorbing vitamin B_{12}.

ADH antidiuretic hormone, secreted by the posterior pituitary gland in response to body stress. It acts on the renal tubules (chiefly the distal tubule) to cause reabsorption of water. The ADH mechanism is the body's primary water-conserving mechanism and is therefore essential to life; see also *vasopressin*.

aldosterone potent hormone of the cortex of the adrenal glands, which acts on the distal renal tubule to cause reabsorption of sodium in an ion exchange with potassium. The aldosterone mechanism is essentially a sodium-conserving mechanism, but indirectly conserves water also as water reabsorption follows the sodium reabsorption.

alkalosis a disturbance in acid-base balance in which there is a reduction of the acid partner in the buffer system, or an increase in the base. In either case, the necessary 20:1 ratio between base and acid is upset by an increase in the relative amount of base.

Answers to questions on p. 190.

1

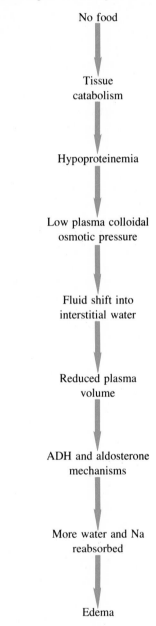

No food

Tissue catabolism

Hypoproteinemia

Low plasma colloidal osmotic pressure

Fluid shift into interstitial water

Reduced plasma volume

ADH and aldosterone mechanisms

More water and Na reabsorbed

Edema

2

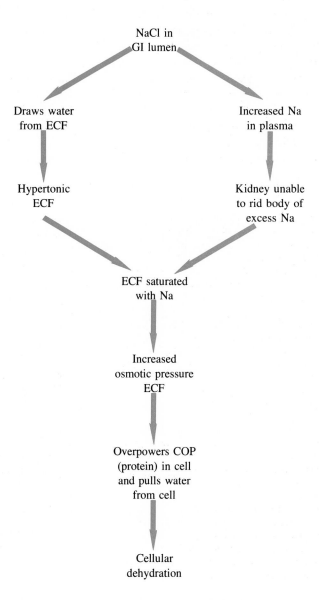

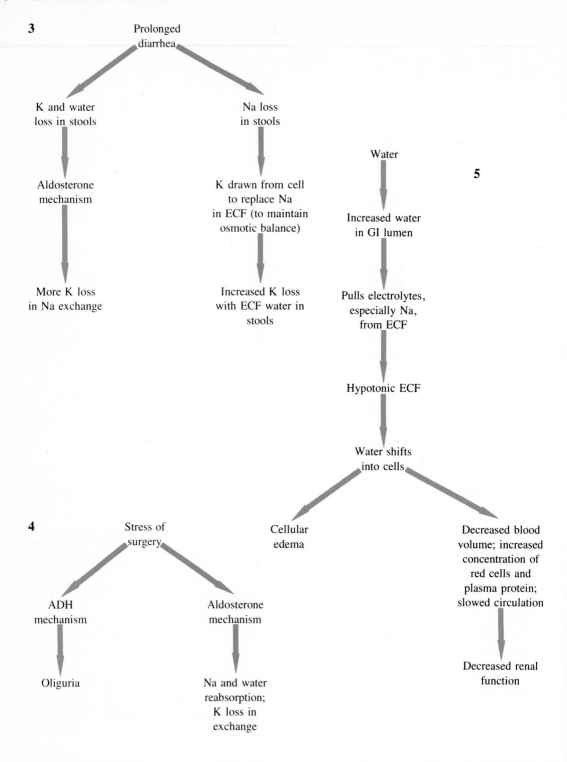

3 Prolonged diarrhea

K and water loss in stools

Aldosterone mechanism

More K loss in Na exchange

Na loss in stools

K drawn from cell to replace Na in ECF (to maintain osmotic balance)

Increased K loss with ECF water in stools

Water

Increased water in GI lumen

Pulls electrolytes, especially Na, from ECF

Hypotonic ECF

Water shifts into cells

5

Cellular edema

Decreased blood volume; increased concentration of red cells and plasma protein; slowed circulation

Decreased renal function

4 Stress of surgery

ADH mechanism

Oliguria

Aldosterone mechanism

Na and water reabsorption; K loss in exchange

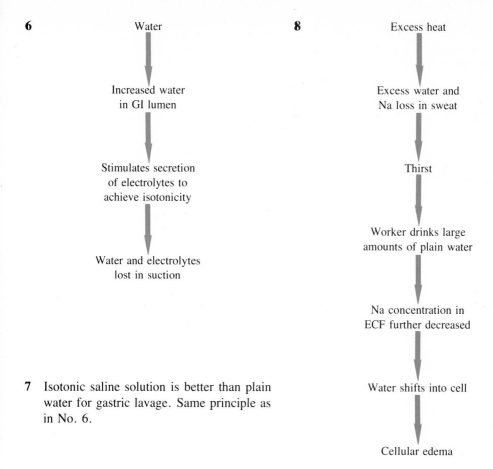

6

Water
↓
Increased water
in GI lumen
↓
Stimulates secretion
of electrolytes to
achieve isotonicity
↓
Water and electrolytes
lost in suction

8

Excess heat
↓
Excess water and
Na loss in sweat
↓
Thirst
↓
Worker drinks large
amounts of plain water
↓
Na concentration in
ECF further decreased
↓
Water shifts into cell
↓
Cellular edema

7 Isotonic saline solution is better than plain water for gastric lavage. Same principle as in No. 6.

angiotensin (Gr. *angeion,* vessel; L. *tensio,* stretching, pressure) a pressor substance produced in the body by interaction of the enzyme renin, produced by the renal cortex, and a serum globulin fraction, angiotensinogen, produced by the liver. Successive products are formed by the interaction—angiotensin I and II. Angiotensin II is the active pressure substance that increases arterial muscle tone and triggers the production of aldosterone by the adrenal gland. Angiotensin I and II therefore are key products in the cycle of the aldosterone mechanism.

anion an ion that carries a negative electrical charge.

base a chemical substance that is capable of neutralizing acid by accepting hydrogen ions from the acid. A synonymous term is *alkali*.

base bicarbonate in the term "base bicarbonate" the word "base" refers to *any* base that might be combined with bicarbonate. In the main buffer system of the human body, this base is sodium bicarbonate.

buffer a mixture of acidic and alkaline components, which, when added to a solution, is able to protect the solution against wide variations in its pH even when strong acids and bases are added to it. If an acid is added, the alkaline partner reacts with it to counteract its acidic effect. If a base is added, the acid partner reacts with it to counteract its alkalizing effect. A solution to which a buffer has been added is called a buffered solution.

capillary fluid shift mechanism the process that controls the movement of water and small molecules in solution (electrolytes, nutrients) between the blood in the capillary and the surrounding interstitial area. Filtration of water and solutes out of the capillary at the arteriole end and reabsorption at the venule end are accomplished by shifts in balance between the intracapillary hydrostatic blood pressure and the colloidal osmotic pressure exerted by the plasma proteins.

carbonic acid (H_2CO_3) the acid partner in the carbonic acid–base bicarbonate buffer system in the body.

cation an ion that carries a positive electrical charge.

colloidal osmotic pressure (COP) pressure produced by the protein molecules in the plasma and in the cell. Because proteins are large molecules, they do not pass through the separating membranes of the capillary cell walls. Thus they remain within their respective compartments, exerting a constant osmotic pull that protects vital plasma and cell fluid volumes in these compartments.

compartment the collective quantity of material in a given type of tissue space in the body. For example, in speaking of body water, the physiologist calls all the water in the body that is outside of cells the extracellular fluid compartment (ECF). In like manner, he calls all the water in the body that is inside of cells the intracellular fluid compartment (ICF).

diffusion (L. *diffundere*, to spread or to pour forth) the process by which particles in solution spread throughout the solution and across separating membranes from the place of highest solute concentration to all surrounding spaces of lessert solute concentration.

electrolyte (Gr. *electron*, amber [which emits electricity if it is rubbed] + *lytos*, soluble) a chemical compound, which in solution dissociates by releasing ions. (An ion is an atomic particle that carries a positive or a negative electrical charge.) The process of dissociating into ions is termed ionization.

filtration (Medieval L. *filtrum*, felt used to strain liquids) passage of a fluid through a semipermeable membrane (a membrane permeable to water and small solutes, but not to large molecules) as a result of a difference in pressures on the two sides of the membrane. For example, the net filtration pressure in the capillaries is the difference between the outward-pushing hydrostatic force of the blood pressure and the opposing inward-pulling force of the colloidal osmotic pressure exerted by the plasma proteins retained in the capillary.

hydrostatic pressure the pressure exerted by a liquid on the surfaces of the walls that contain it. Such pressure is equal in the direction of all containing walls. In body fluid balance, hydrostatic pressure usually refers to the blood pressure, which, together with the plasma proteins, maintains fluid circulation and volume in the blood vessels.

hypertonic dehydration loss of water from the cell as a result of hypertonicity (excess solutes, hence greater osmotic pressure) of the surrounding extracellular fluid.

hypotonic dehydration increase of water in the cell (cellular edema) at the expense of extracellular fluid, as a result of hypotonicity (decreased solutes, hence diminished osmotic pressure) of the extracellular fluid surrounding the cell. A dangerous shrinking of the extracellular fluid (especially blood) volume follows.

interstitial (L. *interstitium*, standing between) spaces or interstices between the essential parts of an organ that comprise its tissue. For example, interstitial fluid is the fluid that occupies the spaces between the cells of a body tissue. This interstitial fluid is freely exchanged and in balance with the vascular fluid (fluid in blood and lymph vessels) that services the tissue area.

ion (Gr. *ion*, to wander) a molecular constituent of one or more atoms that is a free-wandering particle in solution. An ion carries a positive or a negative electrical charge. Ions carrying positive charges are called cations; those carrying negative charges are called anions.

isotonic (Gr. *isos*, equal; *tonos*, tone, tension) having the same tension or pressure. Two given solutions are isotonic if they have the same osmotic pressure and therefore balance each other. For example, the law of isotonicity operates between the gastrointestinal fluids and the surrounding extracellular fluid. Shifts of water and electrolytes in and out of the gastrointestinal lumen are controlled to maintain this state of isotonicity.

milliequivalent the unit of measure used for electrolytes in a solution. It is based on the number of ions (cations and anions) in solution, as determined by their concentration in a given volume, not the weights of the various particles. The term refers to the chemical combining power of the solution and is expressed as the number of milliequivalents per liter (meq/L).

nephron (Gr. *nephros*, kidney) the structural and functional unit of the kidney. The nephron includes the renal corpuscle (glomerulus), the proximal convoluted tubule, the loop of Henle, the distal convoluted tubule, and the collecting tubule (which empties the urine into the renal medulla). The urine passes into the papilla and then to the pelvis of the kidney. Urine is formed by filtration of blood in the glomerulus and by the selective reabsorption and secretion of solutes by cells that comprise the walls of the renal tubules. There are approximately 1 million nephrons in each kidney.

osmosis (Gr. *osmos*, a thrusting) the passage of a solvent such as water through a membrane that separates solutions of different concentrations. The water passes through the membrane from the area of lower concentration of solute to that of higher concentration of solute, which tends to equalize the concentrations of the two solutions. The rate of osmosis depends on (1) the difference in osmotic pressures of the two solutions, (2) the permeability of the membrane, and (3) the electric potential across the membrane.

pH symbol used in chemistry to express the degree of acidity or alkalinity (the concentration of H^+) of a solution. It is mathematically based on the negative logarithm expressed as an exponential power (pH = *power of Hydrogen ion concentration*). Therefore the acidity of a solution varies inversely with the figure expressing it—the smaller the pH number, the greater the degree of acidity. A neutral solution (pure water) has a pH of 7.0. Solutions with a lower pH are acid; those with a higher pH are alkaline. The blood buffer system maintains the blood at a pH of 7.4.

pinocytosis (Gr. *pinein*, to drink; *kytos*, cell) the absorption of large molecules (products of digestions such as fat substances) by engulfing them directly into the cell cytoplasm.

renin (properly pronounced rēnin) This word is often mispronounced rĕnin. It may then be confused with *rennin,* an enzyme from a calf's stomach used to sour milk to make cheese or puddings. A protein substance formed in the renal cortex, which, in response to blood pressure changes, is secreted to act as an enzyme on its specific substrate, angiotensinogen, to form angiotensin I and II. Angiotensin II is a powerful vasoconstrictor. Angiotensin II also stimulates the adrenal glands to produce aldosterone, which causes reabsorption of sodium by the distal renal tubule, thus holding water and maintaining the plasma volume.

solute a dissolved substance; particles in solution.

valence (L. *valens,* powerful) the power of an element or a radical to combine with (or to replace) other elements or radicals. Atoms of various elements combine in definite proportions. The valence number of an element is the number of atoms of hydrogen with which one atom of the element can combine.

vasopressin (ADH) a hormone secreted by the anterior pituitary gland, which acts on the distal renal tubule, causing the reabsorption of water. The result is diminished urinary output, hence the term *antid*iuretic *h*ormone (ADH).

REFERENCES
Specific

1. Anderson, B.: Thirst and brain control of water balance, Am. Sci. **57**:408, 1971.
2. Smith, H. W.: From fish to philosopher, New York, 1961, Doubleday & Co., Inc.

General

Beck, L. H., and Goldberg, M.: Diuretic therapy, Primary Care **1**:165, 1974.

Best, C. H., and Taylor, N. B.: The physiological basis of medical practice, ed. 8, Baltimore, 1966, The Williams & Wilkins Co.

Bland, J. H.: Clinical metabolism of body water and electrolytes, Philadelphia, 1963, W. B. Saunders Co.

Boedeker, E. C., and Danber, J. H.: Manual of medical therapeutics, ed. 21, Boston, 1974, Little, Brown and Co.

Camien, M. N., Simmons, D. H., and Gonick, H. C.: A critical reappraisal of acid-base balance, Am. J. Clin. Nutr. **22**:786, June, 1969.

Cannon, W. B.: The wisdom of the body, New York, 1932, W. W. Norton & Co., Inc.

Collins, R. D.: Illustrated manual of fluid and electrolyte disorders, Philadelphia, 1976, J. B. Lippincott Co.

Earley, L. E., and Dougherty, R. M.: Sodium metabolism, N. Engl. J. Med. **28**:72, 1969.

Fichman, M. P., Vorherr, H., Kleeman, C. R., et al.: Diuretic-induced hyponoturemia, Ann. Intern. Med. **75**:853, Dec., 1971.

Filley, G. F.: Acid-base and blood gas regulation, Philadelphia, 1971, Lea & Febiger.

Gamble, J. L.: Chemical anatomy, physiology and pathology of extracellular fluid, ed. 6, Cambridge, Mass., 1954, Harvard University Press.

Goldberger, E.: A primer of water, electrolyte and acid-base syndromes, ed. 4, Philadelphia, 1970, Lea & Febiger.

Goodhart, R. S., and Shils, M. E., editors: Modern nutrition in health and disease, ed. 4, Philadelphia, 1973, Lea & Febiger.

Gozansky, D. M., and Hermon, R. H.: Water and sodium retention in the fasted and refed human, Am. J. Clin. Nutr. **24**:869, 1971.

Guyton, A. C.: Textbook of medical physiology, ed. 5, Philadelphia, 1976, W. B. Saunders Co.

Harper, H. A.: Review of physiological chemistry, ed. 15, Los Altos, Calif., 1975, Lange Medical Publications.

Kleeman, C. R., and Fichman, M. P.: The clinical physiology of water metabolism, N. Engl. J. Med. **277**:1300, 1967.

Krehl, W. A.: The potassium depletion syndrome, Nutr. Today **1**:20, 1966.

Krehl, W. A.: Sodium: a most extraordinary dietary essential, Nutr. Today **1**:16, 1966.

Latner, A. L.: Cantarow and Trumper clinical biochemistry, ed. 7, Philadelphia, 1975, W. B. Saunders Co.

Mason, E. E.: Fluid, electrolyte, and nutrient therapy in surgery, Philadelphia, 1974, Lea & Febiger.

Maxwell, M. H., and Kleeman, C. R.: Clinical disorders of fluid and electrolyte metabolism, ed. 2, New York, 1972, McGraw-Hill Book Co.

Robinson, J. R.: Water, the indispensable nutrient, Nutr. Today **5**:16, 1970.

Rocchio, M. A., and Randall, H. T.: Wound kinetics; water and electrolyte changes from zero to sixty days in clean wounds, Am. J. Surg. **121**:460, 1971.

Stroot, V. R., Lee, C. A., and Schaper, C. A.: Fluids and electrolytes; a practical approach, Philadelphia, 1975, F. A. Davis Co.

Taylor, W. H.: Fluid therapy and disorders of electrolyte balance, Oxford, 1980, Blackwell Scientific Publications.

Wilson, R. F.: Fluids, electrolytes and metabolism, Springfield, Ill., 1973, Charles C Thomas, Publisher.

Wintrobe, M. M., et al.: Harrison's principles of internal medicine, ed. 7, New York, 1974, McGraw-Hill Book Co.

10 Digestion, absorption, and metabolism

Thus far in this study, each of the fundamental nutritional components has been examined separately, and each has been considered with respect to its particular role in human nutrition. At the same time that the components have been separated to consider them in detail, the all-important concept of *the interrelatedness of the nutrients* has been emphasized. This has been largely a biochemical study, although it has certainly not been exclusively biochemical, since such matters as the clinical significance of each nutrient and its availability in foods have also been considered. In addition, other aspects have been considered that must be understood if the individual is to receive the correct balance of needed nutrients.

In this chapter the body's use of nutriment will be looked at in still another way—from the point of view of the anatomy and physiology of the organs that digest and absorb nutrients. Once the body receives nutrients, how does it go about converting them into forms it can use? The physiologic process can be separated into components and can be understood only as one recognizes that it consists of three events: digestion, absorption, and metabolism. Again, however, because the process of analysis is a necessity for the human mind, each of these phases will be considered separately, even though analysis as such does not characterize nature. All the while that these three processes are being studied separately, they are functioning as a digestion-absorption-metabolism continuum—*a dynamic unit.*

The question of why this intricate complex of biochemical and physiologic activities is necessary may be asked at this point. Two reasons are apparent. First, food as it naturally occurs (and as man consumes it) is not a single component, but is a mixture of substances. If these substances are to be induced to release their energy for use, they must be separated into their components so that each component may be handled by the body as a separate unit. Second, because in most instances the still simpler chemical units that make up their nutrient components are still unavailable to the body, some additional means of changing their form must follow. The intermediate units must be broken down, simplified, regrouped, and rerouted. This exceedingly complex chemical work must take place because a human being is the most highly organized and intricately balanced of all organisms, whose life is developed and sustained in an internal chemical environment. This view of the human body as an integrated physiochemical organism is basic to an understanding of human nutrition.

To achieve this picture of the digestion-absorption-metabolism process as a whole, the general principles related to each phase should be noted. The student should then be able to follow the fate of food components as they travel together through the successive parts of the gastrointestinal tract and into the body cells.

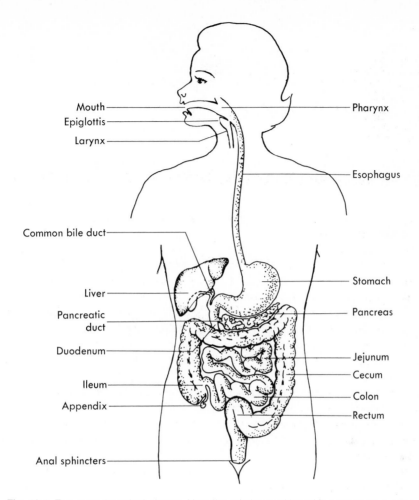

Fig. 10-1. The gastrointestinal system. Note the relative position of the successive parts.

For reference, these respective components of the gastrointestinal tract and their relative position in the overall system should be carefully reviewed (Fig. 10-1).

DIGESTION
Basic principles of digestion

Digestion achieves the initial preparation of food for use by the body. Two basic types of action are involved: (1) mechanical or muscular activity, which produces gastrointestinal motility and (2) chemical or enzymatic activity, which results from gastrointestinal secretions. The cells and glands of the gastrointestinal tract also secrete mucus and water and electrolytes.

Gastrointestinal motility. Mechanical digestion takes place through a number of neuromuscular, self-regulatory processes. These actions work together to move the food components along the alimentary tract at a rate that is optimal for digestion and absorption of nutrients.

Four types of muscle in the stomach and intestine contribute to this motility: (1) a layer of

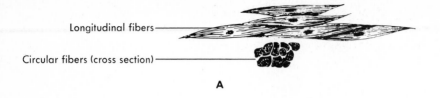

Longitudinal fibers

Circular fibers (cross section)

A

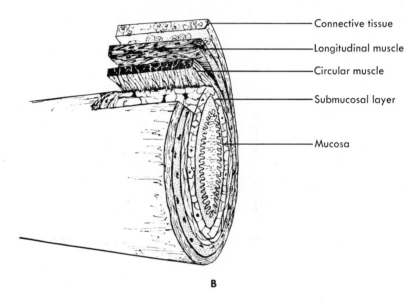

Connective tissue

Longitudinal muscle

Circular muscle

Submucosal layer

Mucosa

B

Fig. 10-2. Layers of smooth muscle in the intestinal wall. **A,** Microscopic appearance of muscle tissue. **B,** Arrangement of layers of muscle.

circular, contractile rings that break up, mix, and churn the food particles, (2) longitudinal muscles that help to propel the food mass along, (3) sphincter muscles that act as valves (the pyloric, ileocecal, and anal valves) to control passage of material to the next segment of the intestine, and (4) a thin, mucosal layer of smooth muscle that can raise intestinal folds to increase the absorbing surface. The interaction of these four types of muscles produces two general types of movement: (1) a general muscle tone or tonic contraction, which ensures continuous passage and valve control and (2)

periodic, rhythmic contractions, which mix and propel the food mass. These alternating muscular contractions and relaxations that force the contents forward are known by the term *peristalsis*. The layers of smooth muscle making up the gastrointestinal wall are shown in Fig. 10-2.

Specific nerves regulate these muscular actions. A complex, interrelated network of nerves within the gastrointestinal wall, the *intramural nerve plexus,* extends from the esophagus to the anus. The intramural nerve plexus controls muscle tone of the gastrointes-

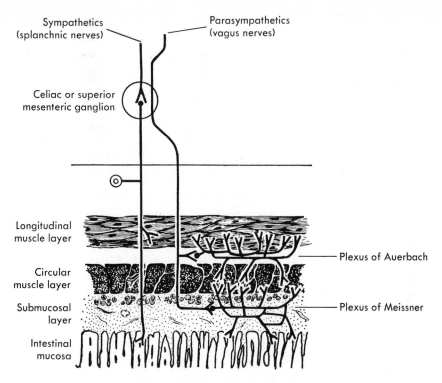

Sympathetics
(splanchnic nerves)

Parasympathetics
(vagus nerves)

Celiac or superior
mesenteric ganglion

Longitudinal
muscle layer

Plexus of Auerbach

Circular
muscle layer

Submucosal
layer

Plexus of Meissner

Intestinal
mucosa

Fig. 10-3. Innervation of the intestine, showing the plexus of Auerbach and the plexus of Meissner.

tinal wall, regulates the rate and intensity of periodic muscle contractions, and coordinates the various movements (Fig. 10-3).

Gastrointestinal secretions. Food is digested chemically by the action of a number of secretions. Generally, these secretions are of four types:

1. Enzymes—specific in kind and quantity for the degradation of a given nutrient
2. Hydrochloric acid and buffer ions—to produce the pH necessary for the activity of given enzymes
3. Mucus—for lubrication and protection of the gastrointestinal tract
4. Water and electrolytes—in quantities sufficient to carry or circulate the organic substances

There are several kinds of cells and glands that produce these secretions. There are single mucous cells on the epithelial surface called *goblet cells,* which act alone. In the small intestine there are *multicellular tubular glands,* such as the simple pits lined with goblet mucous cells (crypts of Lieberkühn). Enzymes and hydrochloric acid are secreted by the deeper branched *gastric glands.* In addition, there are complicated *glands outside the gastrointestinal tract,* such as the salivary glands, the pancreas, and the liver. These secrete enzymes and bile from organized secretory cell structures called *acini,* which feed into ducts that empty into the gastrointestinal lumen. The secretory action of these various special cells or glands may be stimulated locally by the presence of food, by sensory nerve stimuli, or by hormones specific for certain foods.

Digestion in the mouth and esophagus

Mechanical digestion. Mastication (biting and chewing) begins the breaking up of food into smaller particles. The teeth and other oral structures are particularly suited for this function. The incisors cut; the molars grind. Tremendous force is supplied by the jaw muscles —25 kg (55 lb) of muscular pressure is applied through incisors, and 91 kg (200 lb) is applied through the molars. Mastication makes it possible for an enlarged surface area of food to constantly be exposed to enzyme action, and the fineness of the food particles eases the continued passage of material through the gastrointestinal tract.

Swallowing of the mixed mass of food particles and its passage down the esophagus are accomplished by peristaltic waves controlled by nerve reflexes. In the usual upright eating position, gravity aids this movement down the esophagus. However, for a bed patient in a prone position, it is more difficult. At the point of entry into the stomach, the gastroesophageal constrictor muscle relaxes to allow food to enter, then constricts again to prevent regurgitation of stomach contents up into the esophagus. (When regurgitation does occur, through failure of this mechanism, the patient feels it as "heartburn.") Clinical conditions such as cardiospasm, caused by failure of the constrictor muscle to relax properly, or hiatus hernia (protrusion of the stomach into the thorax through an abnormal opening in the diaphragm, which allows food to be held in the outpouched area) hinder normal food passage at this point.

Chemical or secretory digestion. Three pairs of salivary glands—parotid, submaxillary,

---

TO PROBE FURTHER

"Executive monkeys"

Interesting data concerning the relationship of emotional states to gastric hypersecretion and the development of peptic ulcer disease were obtained from the now classic experiments of Brady* and his associates performed on monkeys.

In the first experiment an electrical shock was applied to the animals' feet. The animals were taught that, by pressing a level at regular intervals, they could avoid this shock. After a long period of such testing, the animals incurred gastric hypersecretion, excessive acid rise, and resulting duodenal ulcers with perforation.

In the second experiment two monkeys were placed together in a test situation like the first. Each was supplied with a lever to press. This time, however, the lever for monkey A did not control the shock. The lever of monkey B, if pressed on schedule, prevented the shock to both. Monkey A soon learned that he had no control over his situation and incurred no gastric hypersecretion. But monkey B—the "executive" who had to make the decisions for both of them—did incur gastric hypersecretion.

Although complicating factors in the experiments make simple cause-and-effect conclusions impossible, the observations raise interesting speculation. They may suggest that the greater the controlling power one has over the lives and fortunes of others, the worse off he is physically. And perhaps if we consider the "executive syndrome" repeatedly observed in the driving "organization man in the gray flannel suit" of our industrial age, we may conclude that not all monkeys are in cages. Or is it that we build cages for ourselves of another sort?

*Brady, J. V.: Ulcers in "executive monkeys," Sci. Am. **199**:95, 1958.

and sublingual—secrete a serous material containing *ptyalin,* an enzyme specific for starches and a mucous material that lubricates and binds the food particles. These salivary secretions amount to 1,000 to 1,500 ml per day. They usually are only slightly acid (pH about 6.8). However, they may range around neutrality (pH from 6.0 to 7.0). Stimuli such as sight, smell, taste, and touch—and even the thought of likes or dislikes in foods—greatly influence these secretions.

Because food remains in the mouth only a short time, starch digestion by ptyalin is relatively unimportant, since it is terminated by the more acid medium of the stomach. Secretions of mucous glands that line the esophagus aid in swallowing and movement of the food mass toward the stomach.

Digestion in the stomach

Mechanical digestion. The major parts of the stomach are shown in Fig. 10-4. Muscles in the stomach wall provide three basic motor functions of the stomach: storage, mixing, and slow, controlled emptying. As the food mass enters the stomach it lies against the stomach walls, which can stretch outward to store as much as 1 L. Gradually, local tonic muscle waves increase their kneading and mixing action as the mass of food and secretions moves on toward the region of the pyloric antrum at the distal end of the stomach. Here, waves of peristaltic contractions reduce the mass to a semifluid chyme. Finally, with each peristaltic wave, small amounts of chyme are forced through the pyloric valve. This pyloric pump controls the emptying of the stomach contents into the duodenum by constrictive action of the sphincter muscle (the pyloric valve) and by controlling the rate of propulsive peristaltic activity in the antrum. This control releases the acid chyme slowly enough so that it can be buffered by the alkaline intestinal secretions.

Chemical or secretory digestion. About 2,000 ml of gastric secretion are produced daily. Two basic types of gland in the stomach wall—the gastric and pyloric glands—secrete materials that act on specific nutrients.

GASTRIC GLAND SECRETION. Gastric glands are located in the upper portion of the stomach and the wall of the body and fundus. They secrete enzymes, hydrochloric acid, and some mucus.

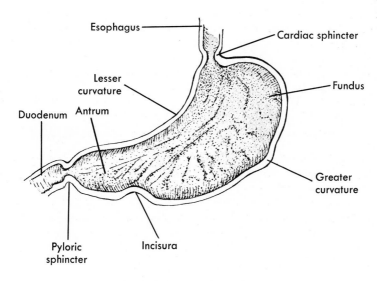

Fig. 10-4. Major parts of the stomach.

These gastric glands are tubular and are lined with secreting cells.

The *chief cells* (also called the *adelomorphous cells*) secrete pepsinogen, which is activated by previously formed pepsin and hydrochloric acid to form the active enzyme pepsin. A highly acid medium (pH approximately 2.0) is required for this enzyme activation. Pepsin begins the enzymatic breakdown of proteins to smaller polypeptides. The *parietal cells* secrete the necessary hydrochloric acid. *Mucous cells* secrete mucus, which helps to protect the gastric mucosa and to give body and cohesiveness to the food mass. Other enzyme-secreting cells produce small amounts of a specific gastric lipase, tributyrinase, which acts on the tributyrin in butterfat; this is a relatively minor activity.

The *pyloric glands* secrete additional thin mucus. Surface *goblet cells* produce a thicker, more viscous mucus, which coats and protects the stomach wall. When irritation occurs, a still greater quantity of mucus is produced.

Stimuli for all of these secretions are twofold.

1. Nerve stimulus is produced in response to sensation, to food taken in, and to emotions. For example, in response to anger and hostility, secretions increase. Fear and depression decrease secretions and inhibit blood flow and motility as well.

2. Hormonal stimulus is produced in response to the entrance of food into the stomach. Certain stimulants, especially coffee, alcohol, and meat extractives cause the release of *gastrin* from mucosal glands in the antrum, which in turn stimulates the parietal cells to secrete more hydrochloric acid. When the pH reaches 2.0, a feedback mechanism stops secretion of the hormone to prevent excess acid formation. Another hormone, *enterogastrone,* produced by glands in the duodenal mucosa, counteracts excessive gastric activity by inhibiting acid and pepsin secretion and gastric motility.

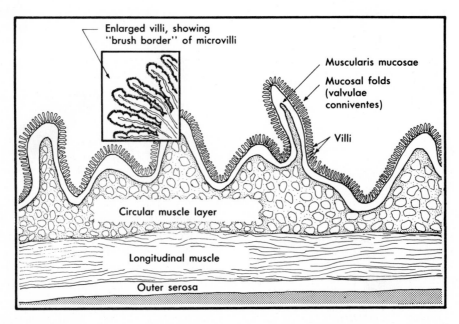

Fig. 10-5. Intestinal wall. Note the arrangement of muscle layers and the structures of the mucosa that increase the surface area for absorption—mucosal folds, villi, and microvilli.

Digestion in the small intestine

Up to this point, the digestion of food consumed has been mainly mechanical, delivering to the small intestine a semifluid chyme made up of fine food particles mixed with watery secretions. Chemical digestion has thus far been limited. Starch was slightly attacked by ptyalin in the mouth, but this action was quickly terminated by stomach acid. The breakdown of complex proteins to polypeptides has been barely begun in the stomach by the action of pepsin; but even this is not vital, since a full enzyme system for the digestion of proteins is available in the small intestine. Therefore the major task of digestion (and of absorption that

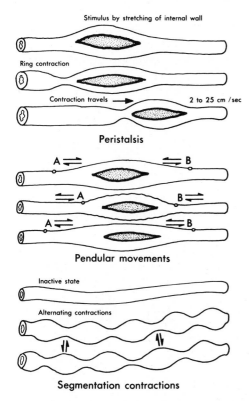

Fig. 10-6. Types of movement produced by muscles of the intestine: peristaltic waves from contraction of deep circular muscle, pendular movements from small local muscles, and segmentation rings formed by alternate contraction and relaxation of circular muscle.

follows) occurs in the small intestine. Its structural parts, its synchronized movements, and its array of enzymes are highly developed for this all-important final task of mechanical and chemical digestion.

Mechanical digestion. The structural arrangement of the intestinal wall is shown in the diagrammatic section in Fig. 10-5.

Finely coordinated intestinal motility is achieved by the three basic layers of muscle: (1) the thin layer of smooth muscle in the mucosa (muscularis mucosa) with fibers extending up into the villi, (2) the circular muscle layer, and (3) the longitudinal muscle next to the outer serosa. Under the control of the nerve plexus, of the wall stretch pressure from food present, or of the hormonal stimuli, these muscles produce several types of movement that aid mechanical digestion (see Fig. 10-6):

1. Segmentation rings from alternate contractions of circular muscle progressively chop the food mass into successive boluses. This action constantly mixes the food materials with secretions.
2. Longitudinal rotation by the long muscle running the length of the intestine rolls the slowly moving food mass in a spiral motion, mixing it and exposing new surfaces for absorption.
3. Pendular movements from small local muscle contractions sweep back and forth and stir chyme at the mucosal surface.
4. Peristaltic waves, produced by the contraction of deep circular muscle, propel the food mass slowly forward. The intensity of the waves may be increased by food intake or by the presence of irritants. In some cases this causes long, sweeping waves over the entire length of the intestine.
5. Motions of the villi also aid mechanical digestion. Alternating contractions and extensions of mucosal muscle fibers constantly agitate the mucosal surface. This action stirs and mixes chyme that is in contact with the intestinal wall and ex-

poses additional nutrient material for absorption. A specific hormone, *villikinin,* is released from the upper intestinal mucosa when it is bathed by chyme entering from the proximal gastrointestinal tract. Villikinin stimulates these contractions, which in turn constantly shorten and lengthen the intestinal villi.

Chemical or secretory digestion. Since the major burden of chemical digestion falls on the small intestine, this portion of the alimentary tract secretes a large number of enzymes, each of which is specific for one of the fundamental types of nutrient. These important specific enzymes are secreted from the intestinal glands and the pancreas.

A. Intestinal glands in the mucosa (crypts of Lieberkühn)
   1. Fat—intestinal lipase converts fat to glycerides and fatty acids
   2. Protein
      a. Enterokinase converts the inactive precursor trypsinogen to active trypsin.
      b. Amino peptidase removes from polypeptides the terminal amino acids that contain a free amino

(NH_4) group by attacking the peptide bond.
      c. Dipeptidase converts dipeptides to amino acids.
      d. Nucleosidase converts nucleosides to a purine or a pyrimidine base, and pentose sugar.
   3. Carbohydrate—disaccharidases (maltase, lactase, sucrase) convert maltose, lactose, and sucrose to their constituent monosaccharides (glucose, fructose, and galactose).
B. Pancreas
   1. Fat—pancreatic lipase converts fats to glycerides and fatty acids
   2. Protein
      a. Trypsin causes initial breakdown of proteins and polypeptides to smaller polypeptides. It also activates chymotrypsinogen to chymotrypsin.
      b. Chymotrypsin breaks down proteins and polypeptides to smaller polypeptides.
      c. Carboxypeptidase removes carboxyl (COOH) terminal amino acid from polypeptidases.

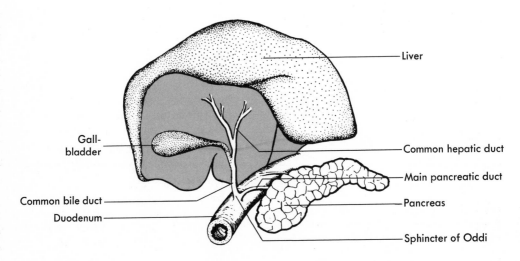

Fig. 10-7. Organs of the biliary system and the pancreatic ducts.

Table 10-1. Summary of digestive processes

Nutrient	Mouth	Stomach	Small intestine
Carbohydrate	Starch $\xrightarrow{Ptyalin}$ Dextrins		**Pancreas** Starch $\xrightarrow{Amylase}$ (Disaccharides) Maltose and sucrose **Intestine** Lactose $\xrightarrow{Lactase}$ (Monosaccharides) Glucose and galactose Sucrose $\xrightarrow{Sucrase}$ Glucose and fructose Maltose $\xrightarrow{Maltase}$ Glucose and glucose
Protein		Protein $\xrightarrow[Hydrochloric\ acid]{Pepsin}$ Polypeptides	**Pancreas** Proteins, Polypeptides $\xrightarrow{Trypsin}$ Dipeptides Proteins, Polypeptides $\xrightarrow{Chymotrypsin}$ Dipeptides Polypeptides, Dipeptides $\xrightarrow{Carboxypeptidase}$ Amino acids **Intestine** Polypeptides, Dipeptides $\xrightarrow{Aminopeptidase}$ Amino acids Dipeptides $\xrightarrow{Dipeptidase}$ Amino acids
Fat		Tributyrin $\xrightarrow{Tributyrinase}$ Glycerol Fatty acids (butterfat)	**Pancreas** Fats $\xrightarrow{Lipase}$ Glycerol Glycerides (di-, mono-) Fatty acids **Intestine** Fats $\xrightarrow{Lipase}$ Glycerol Glycerides (di, mono-) Fatty acids **Liver and gallbladder** Fats $\xrightarrow{Bile}$ Emulsified fat

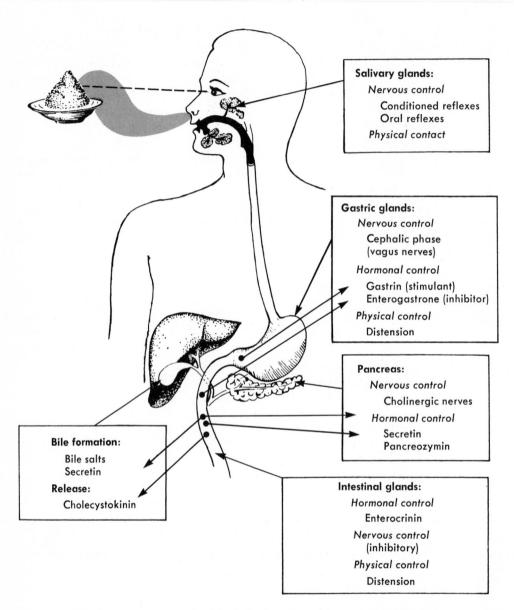

Fig. 10-8. Summary of factors influencing secretions of the gastrointestinal glands.

d. Nucleases convert nucleic acids (RNA and DNA) to nucleotides.

3. Carbohydrate—pancreatic amylase converts starch to disaccharides.

MUCOUS GLANDS. In addition to enzymes, large quantities of mucus are secreted by intestinal glands (Brunner's glands) located immediately inside the duodenum. This secretion protects the mucosa from irritation and digestion by the highly acid gastric juices, which enter the intestine at this point. Emotions inhibit these mucous secretions and are an important factor in the production of duodenal ulcers. Additional mucous cells on the mucosal surface or in intestinal glands continue to secrete mucus as they are touched by the food mass to provide lubrication and protection of tissues. The combined secretions of the mucous glands of the intestine and pancreas total about 4,200 ml daily (3,000 ml from intestinal glands and 1,200 ml from the pancreas).

HORMONAL STIMULUS FOR SECRETIONS. The hormone *secretin,* produced by the mucosa of the upper part of the small intestine, stimulates the pancreatic secretions and regulates their pH so that they are maintained at the alkalinity that is necessary to stop the acidic enzyme activity of chyme entering from the stomach. The unprotected intestinal mucosa alone could not withstand this high degree of acidity. The resultant alkalinity of the medium also provides the pH (8.0) that is optimal for pancreatic enzyme activity.

BILE. Another important aid to digestion and absorption in the small intestine is bile, since it is an emulsifying agent for fats. Bile is produced by the liver, and is concentrated and stored by the gallbladder. When fat enters the duodenum, the hormone *cholecystokinin* is secreted by intestinal mucosa glands and stimulates the gallbladder to contract and release bile. From 600 to 700 ml of bile is produced daily and provides for the repeated circulation of bile salts in the enterohepatic circulation (see Fig. 3-4). The interbalanced system of gastrointestinal hormones, including secretin and cholecystokinin, constitutes a vital regulatory network maintaining specific secretory and motor action throughout the tract.[1]

The organs of the biliary system and the pancreatic ducts are illustrated in Fig. 10-7. A summary of these digestive processes is given in Table 10-1. Many factors influence the various secretions of the gastrointestinal tract. Control by hormone, by nerves, and by physical contact is summarized in Fig. 10-8.

ABSORPTION

After digestion of the food nutrients is complete, the simplified end products are ready to

Table 10-2. Daily absorption volume in human gastrointestinal system

	Intake (L)	Intestinal absorption (L)	Elimination (L)
Food ingested	1.5		
Gastrointestinal secretions	8.5		
TOTAL	10.0		
Fluid absorbed in small intestine		9.5	
Fluid absorbed in large intestine		0.4	
TOTAL		9.9	
Feces			0.1

be absorbed. These end products include monosaccharides such as glucose, fructose, and galactose from carbohydrates, fatty acids and glyceride from fats, and amino acids from proteins. Some small peptides can apparently be absorbed intact and hydrolyzed to amino acids within the mucosal absorptive cells, a process that plays an important role in facilitating the absorption of protein digestion products.[2] Also liberated are vitamins and minerals. Finally, with a water base for solution and transport, plus necessary electrolytes, the total fluid food mass forms the material that is involved in a constant, life-sustaining, gastrointestinal circulation.

The absorptive powers of the gastrointestinal circulation may be visualized in terms of the total fluid volume handled daily (Table 10-2).

Small intestine

Surface structures. Viewed from the outside, the serosa of the intestine appears smooth. But the inner mucosal surface is different. There are three types of convolutions and projections that are progressively smaller in size. These mucosal folds, villi, and microvilli increase the inner surface area some 600 times over that of the outer serosa! These special structures of the mucosal surface of the small intestine, plus the contracted length of the live organ (630 to 660 cm [21 to 22 ft]), combine to produce a tremendously large absorbing surface. The remarkable potential of the luminal surface of the small intestine is a total absorbing surface area as large or larger than half a basketball court!

Fig. 10-5 should be referred to again to compare the three structures that enlarge the absorptive surface of the luminal serosa.

MUCOSAL FOLDS. Easily seen by the naked eye are heaped-up folds along the mucosa surface, like so many hills and valleys in a mountain range.

VILLI. Closer examination by light microscope reveals small, fingerlike projections, the villi, covering these convoluted folds of mucosa. These villi further increase the area of the exposed surface. To receive the absorbed nutrients, each villus has an ample vascular network that involves venous and arterial capillaries and central *lacteals*. Lacteal is the special name given to a lymphatic vessel in the small intestine. It is like any other lymphatic vessel in structure and function. It receives this special name because the chyle that fills it during digestion looks like milk.

MICROVILLI. An electron microscope focused on the surface of a single villus brings to view extremely numerous minute surface projections. This vast array of microvilli covering the edge of each villus is called the "brush border," because they look like bristles on a brush. At the base of the brush border is the basement membrane.

All three of these mucosal surface structures function as a unit for the absorption of nutrients. Although the small intestine is popularly thought of as the lowly "gut," it is actually one of the most highly developed, exquisitely fashioned, specialized tissues in the human body!

Mechanism of absorption. Absorption is accomplished by the small intestine by means of a number of processes, including passive diffusion, active ferrying, energy-driven transport, and penetration by engulfment.

PASSIVE DIFFUSION (OSMOSIS) THROUGH EPITHELIAL MEMBRANE PORES. Where no opposing pressure exists, molecules small enough to pass through the capillary membranes diffuse easily into the capillaries of the villi, in the direction of pressure flow, in quantities that represent their concentration or electrochemical gradient. For example, electrolytes diffuse in and out of the intestinal lumen as electrochemical need demands, and water molecules flow back and forth as osmotic pressures vary (p. 177).

CARRIER-MEDIATED DIFFUSION. Ferry systems carry molecules across the epithelial cells and basement membrane of microvilli into the capillary circulation of villi. Molecules too large to traverse membrane pores must be helped through the barrier of the cell wall. If the pressure gradient is from greater to lesser, a molecule of another nutrient combines with the large molecule to help carry the large molecule through the barrier.

For example, the stomach secretes the highly specialized ferry called intrinsic factor (IF), which is required to carry the very large molecule of vitamin B_{12} out of the intestinal lumen into the circulating blood. If the stomach fails to secrete IF, the large vitamin B_{12} molecule lacks the ferrying molecule and cannot enter the blood. Lacking vitamin B_{12}, the red blood cells cannot mature normally, and pernicious anemia results (p. 118).

ENERGY-DEPENDENT ACTIVE TRANSPORT. Even against a pressure gradient, nutrient molecules must cross the intestinal epithelial membrane to feed hungry tissue cells. Such work requires extra machinery and energy. This need is supplied by a mechanism that physiologists have come to call a pump,* which continuously picks up the waiting molecules and carries them across the membrane. Energy to operate the pump is supplied from the cell's metabolism. The sodium pump, which transports glucose molecules, it an example of this fascinating mechanism (see Fig. 2-3).

ENGULFING (PINOCYTOSIS). Some even larger macromolecules require still another means of reaching the tissue circulation outposts in the villi. In these instances, epithelial cells of the villi act like amebae or leukocytes and ingest

---

*The use of the word *pump* for this type of mechanism may be confusing at first. It must be remembered that what makes a pump *pump* is the *threat of vacuum*. A pump pulls material from one place to another by the exercise of negative pressure. The pump is able to suck material from one place to another because the new site *cannot endure the absence of material*. It is from this characteristic that biochemists and physiologists have adopted the name *pump*. The avidity of the empty site for something to fill its space provides the power to move the molecules across membranes. A biochemical ''pumping mechanism'' is one that works by pulling a fresh molecule in to fill a place that has been emptied by the removal of a molecule that was formerly present.

---

foreign particles. A small portion of the edge of the cell, on coming in contact with the material to be transported, dips inward (invaginates), engulfs the particle, and opens to swallow the particle into the interior of the cell. The particle is conveyed through the cytoplasm to the opposite side of the epithelial cell that borders on the capillary lumen. Here the particle is discharged into the intracapillary blood. Occasionally whole proteins are absorbed by pinocytosis. This mechanism is probably also involved in the absorption of neutral fat droplets (chylomicrons) and their transportation into the lacteals of the villi (see Fig. 9-3).

Routes of absorption. After their absorption by any of these processes, each of the nutrient components from carbohydrates and proteins enters the portal blood system and travels to the body tissues. Only fat is unique in its route. After enzymatic processing in the cells of the intestinal lumen, the fat is largely converted into esterified lipids. These molecules are small enough to pass between the cells of the intestinal mucosa and into the lymph vessels in the center of the villi. From these, they flow into the larger lymph vessels of the mesentery and finally enter the common portal blood flow at the thoracic duct. Exceptions are the medium- and short-chain fatty acids, which are absorbed directly into villi blood circulation. However, most commonly consumed fats are made up of long-chain fatty acids, which travel the lacteal route.

Large intestine (colon)

The main absorption task remaining for the large intestine is that of taking up water. However, related factors are involved, such as the absorption of sodium and other minerals, absorption of some vitamins and amino acids, the action of intestinal bacteria, the collection of nondigestible residue, and the formation and elimination of feces.

Water absorption. Within a 24-hour period, about 500 ml of remaining isotonic chyme leaves the ileum (the last portion of the small intestine) and enters the cecum (the pouch at the start of the large intestine). The *ileocecal valve* exerts important control over passage of the semiliquid chyme. Normally the valve remains closed. With each peristaltic wave, however, it relaxes briefly to allow a small amount of chyme to squirt into the cecum. This control mechanism holds the food mass in the small intestine long enough to ensure adequate digestion and absorption of vital nutrients. Such timing is necessary because no digestive enzymes are secreted by the colon.

The chyme continues to move slowly through the large intestine, aided by mucus secretion from glands in the colon and by muscle contractions. Segmentation contractions mix the residue mass and aid absorption by exposing more of the mass to the mucosa. Long muscles produce peristaltic waves to propel the mass forward. The major portion of the water in the chyme (from 350 to 400 ml) is absorbed in the proximal half of the colon; only from 100 to 150 ml remains to form and aid in elimination of the feces.

Studies with test meals[3] indicate that the food residue mass moves through the large intestine at a gradually slowing pace. Usually the test meal, having traversed the 630 to 660 cm (21 to 22 ft) of small intestine, starts to enter the cecum about four hours after it is consumed. About eight hours later it reaches the sigmoid colon, having traveled through the large intestine for a distance of about 90 cm (3 ft)! In the sigmoid colon, the mass descends still more slowly toward the anus. Even 72 hours after the meals has been eaten, as much as 25% of it may still remain in the rectum!

Mineral absorption. Electrolytes, principally sodium, are transported into the bloodstream from the colon. From 20% to 70% of ingested calcium is eliminated in the feces, as is from 80% to 85% of ingested iron, a considerable amount of phosphates, and some carbonate.

Bacterial action—vitamin absorption. Bacteria in the colon are closely associated with a number of vitamins. At birth the colon is sterile, but very shortly thereafter intestinal bacterial flora is well established. The adult colon contains large numbers of bacteria, the predominant species being *Escherichia coli*. Great masses of the bacteria are passed in the stool. The colon bacteria synthesize vitamin K and some vitamins of the B complex (especially biotin and folic acid), which are absorbed from the colon in sufficient amounts to meet the daily requirement.

Although vitamin B_{12} (cyanocobalamin) is also synthesized by intestinal bacteria, it is not absorbed from the large intestine. What factor, secreted by the gastric mucosa, necessary for B_{12} absorption, and present in the small intestine, is not present in the large intestine? (See p. 118.) Since the large intestine lacks this cofactor, the vitamin cannot be transported through the wall of the colon and is eliminated in the feces.

Other bacterial action. Intestinal bacteria also affect the color and odor of the stool. The brown color represents bile pigments, which are formed by the colon bacteria from bilirubin. Thus in conditions where bile flow is hindered, the stools may become clay-colored or white. The characteristic odor results from amines, especially indole and skatole, formed by bacterial enzymes from amino acids.

Gas, or flatus, formed in the large intestine contains hydrogen sulfide or methane produced by the bacteria. Gas formation, however, is attributable not so much to specific foods per se as to the state of the body that receives them. Many foods have been labeled gas formers, but in reality such classifications have little or no scientific basis.[4]

Residue. Since humans, unlike herbivorous animals and some insects such as the termite, have no microorganisms or enzymes to break down cellulose, this plant product remains after digestion and absorption as residue. Cellulose contributes important bulk to the diet and helps form the feces. Cellulose and several other

Table 10-3. Intestinal absorption of some major nutrients

Nutrient	Form	Means of absorption	Control agent or required cofactor	Route
Carbohydrate	Monosaccharides (glucose and galactose)	Competitive Selective Active transport via sodium pump	— — Sodium	Blood
Protein	Amino acids	Selective	—	Blood
	Some dipeptides	Carrier transport systems	Pyridoxine (pyridoxal phosphate)	Blood
	Whole protein (rare)	Pinocytosis	—	Blood
Fat	Fatty acids	Fatty acid-bile complex (micelles)	Bile	Lymph
	Glycerides (mono-, di-)		—	Lymph
	Few triglycerides (neutral fat)	Pinocytosis	—	Lymph
Vitamins	B_{12}	Carrier transport	Intrinsic factor (IF)	Blood
	A	Bile complex	Bile	Blood
	K	Bile complex	Bile	From large intestine to blood
Minerals	Sodium	Active transport via sodium pump	—	Blood
	Calcium	Active transport	Vitamin D	Blood
	Iron	Active transport	Ferritin mechanism	Blood (as transferritin)
Water	Water	Osmosis	—	Blood, lymph, interstitial fluid

groups of nondigestible substances comprise the total dietary fiber consumed. This important group of materials is discussed in detail in Chapter 2 (p. 16). The feces contain about 75% water and 25% solids. The solids include fiber, bacteria, inorganic matter (mostly calcium and phosphates), a small amount of fat and its derivatives, some mucus, and sloughed-off mucosal cells.

Some major features of nutrient absorption in the intestines are summarized in Table 10-3.

METABOLISM

The various absorbed nutrient components, including water and electrolytes, are carried to the cells as raw materials to produce a myriad of substances needed by the body to sustain life. Metabolism encompasses the total, con-

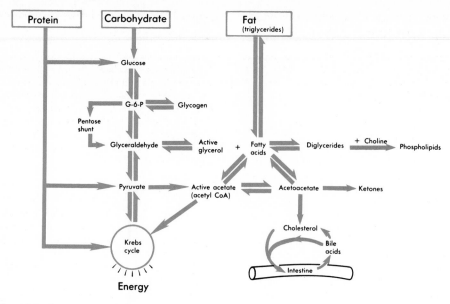

Fig. 10-9. Summary diagram of metabolism of the nutrients. Note metabolic interrelationships of carbohydrate, protein, and fat.

tinuous complex of chemical changes that determine the final use of the individual nutrients.

Purposes. Each of these chemical processes is purposeful, and all are interdependent. The processes are designed to fill two essential needs: (1) to produce energy and (2) to maintain a dynamic equilibrium between the building-up or breaking-down of tissue. The controlling agents in the cells are the cellular enzymes, their coenzymes (many of which are B vitamins), other cofactors, and hormones.

Interrelationships. The main features of cell metabolism of the fundamental nutrients and of some vitamins and minerals are summarized in Fig. 10-9. This summary diagram should be studied carefully. Here some of the important relationships between individual components that work together to comprise the whole can be visualized. All in all, it is an exciting biochemical system. By it, the human body works to develop, sustain, and protect its most precious possession—life itself.

GLOSSARY

absorption (L. *ab,* away + *sorbere,* to suck in) the process by which digested food materials pass through the epithelial cells of the alimentary canal (mainly of the small intestine) into the blood or lymph. A number of variables influence absorption—the chemical nature of the nutrient, the cell membrane, and electrochemical pressure differences between the solutions in the intestinal lumen and in the mucosal cells. Therefore different absorptive mechanisms may be used—simple osmosis or passive diffusion, energy-dependent active transport, or direct amebalike engulfing (pinocytosis).

acini (L. *acinus,* grape) groups of secretory cells in glands such as the salivary glands, the pancreas, and the liver. These organized clusters of cells are called acini because their shape resembles that of a bunch of grapes. Their secretions of enzymes and bile feed into ducts that empty into the gastrointestinal lumen.

Brunner's glands mucus-secreting glands in the duodenum, that provide mucus to protect the mucosa from irritation and erosion by the strongly acid gastric juices entering from the stomach. Emotional tension and stress inhibit these mucous secretions—a large factor in duodenal ulcer formation.

chief cells special cells in the lining of the tubular gastric glands, which secrete pepsinogen. Previously formed pepsin and hydrochloric acid in the stomach convert the inactive pepsinogen to the active enzyme pepsin, which begins the breakdown of protein to polypeptides.

crypts of Lieberkühn (Gr. *kryptein,* to hide) tubular glands of the intestine that secrete intestinal juice. These special secretory organs open between the bases of the villi. Their walls are lined with special cells that secrete digestive enzymes, water, and electrolytes.

digestion (L. *dis,* apart + *genere,* to carry; *digerere,* to separate, arrange, dissolve, digest) the process by which food is broken down chemically in the gastrointestinal tract through the action of secretions containing specific enzymes. Digestion separates complex food structures into their simpler parts, which are the chemicals needed by the body to sustain life.

enterogastrone a hormone produced by glands in the duodenal mucosa, which counteracts excessive gastric activity by inhibiting acid and pepsin secretion and gastric motility.

gastrin a hormone secreted by mucosal cells in the antrum of the stomach that stimulates the parietal cells to produce hydrochloric acid. Gastrin is released in response to entry of stimulants (especially coffee, alcohol, meat extractives) into the stomach. When the gastric pH reaches 2.0, a feedback mechanism cuts off gastrin secretion and prevents excess acid formation.

goblet cells special single secretory cells on the mucosal surface that produce mucus. Mucin droplets accumulate in the cell, causing it to swell. The free surface finally ruptures and liberates the mucus. This mucus coats and protects the mucosa.

intramural nerve plexus (L. *intra,* within; *murus,* wall; *plexus,* a braid) a network of interwoven nerve structures within a particular organ. The action of smooth muscle layers comprising the gastrointestinal wall is controlled by such a network of nerve fibers. The interlacing of short nerve fibers in the muscle layers forms the *plexus of Auerbach;* in the submucosal layer, a similar network forms the *plexus of Meissner.* Together these systems regulate the alternating muscular contractions and relaxations that produce the synchronized waves of motion along the gastrointestinal tract.

microvilli minute surface projections that cover the edge of each intestinal villus. They are visible only through the electron microscope. This vast array of microvilli on each villus is called the brush border. The microvilli add a tremendous surface area for absorption.

mucus a viscid fluid secreted by mucous membranes and glands, consisting mainly of mucin (a glycoprotein), inorganic salts, and water. Mucus serves to lubricate and protect the gastrointestinal mucosa and to help move the food mass along the digestive tract.

parietal cells (L. *paries,* wall) cells of the gastric glands in the fundus of the stomach that produce hydrochloric acid.

secretin a hormone produced in the mucous membrane of the duodenum in response to the entrance of the acid contents of the stomach into the duodenum. Secretin in turn stimulates the flow of pancreatic juice, providing needed enzymes and the proper alkalinity for their action.

villikinin a hormone produced by glands in the upper intestinal mucosa in response to presence of chyme entering the intestine. Villikinin stimulates alternating contractions and extensions of the villi. This motion of the villi constantly agitates the mucosal surface, which stirs and mixes the chyme and exposes additional nutrient material for absorption.

REFERENCES
Specific

1. Rayford, P. L., Miller T. A., and Thompson, J. C.: Secretin, cholecystokinin, and newer gastrointestinal hormones, N. Engl. J. Med. **294**(20):1093, **294**(21):1157, 1976.
2. Matthews, D. M., and Adibi, S. A.: Peptide absorption, Gastroenterology **71**:151, 1976.
3. Menguy, R.: Motor function of the alimentary tract, Annu. Rev. Physiol. **26**:227, 1964.
4. Report: Joint Committee of the American Dietetic Association and the American Medical Association: diet as related to gastrointestinal function, J. Am. Diet. Assoc. **38**:425, 1961.

General

Bogert, L. J., Briggs, G., and Calloway, D.: Nutrition and physical fitness, ed. 10, Philadelphia, 1979, W. B. Saunders Co.

Brown, J. C.: "Enterogastrone" and other new gut peptides, Med. Clin. North Am. **58**:1374, Nov., 1974.

Gangl, A., and Ockner, R. K.: Intestinal metabolism of lipids and lipoproteins, Gastroenterology **68**:167, Jan., 1975.

Ganong, E. F.: Review of medical physiology, ed. 7, Los Altos, Calif., 1975, Lange Medical Publications.

Goodhart, R. S., and Shils, M. E., editors: Modern nutrition in health and disease, ed. 6, Philadelphia, 1980, Lea & Febiger.

Guyton, A. C.: Function of the human body, ed. 4, Philadelphia, 1974, W. B. Saunders Co.

Guyton, A. C.: Textbook of medical physiology, ed. 5, Philadelphia, 1976, W. B. Saunders Co.

Harper, H. A.: Review of physiological chemistry, ed. 15, Los Altos, Calif., 1975, Lange Medical Publications.

Ingelfinger, F. J.: Gastrointestinal absorption, Nutr. Today **2**:2, 1967.

Ingelfinger, F. J.: Gastric function, Nutr. Today **6**:2-11, Sept.-Oct., 1971.

Ingelfinger, F. J.: How to swallow, and belch and cope with heartburn, Nutr. Today **8**:4, Jan.-Feb., 1973.

Latner, A. L.: Cantarow and Trumper clinical biochemistry, ed. 7, Philadelphia, 1975, W. B. Saunders Co.

Lehninger, A. L.: Biochemistry, ed. 2, New York, 1975, Worth Publishers, Inc.

Levitt, M. D., and Bond, J. H.: Volume, composition and source of intestinal gas, Gastroenterology **59:**921, Dec., 1970.

Liebow, C.: Enteropancreatic circulation of digestive enzymes, Science **189:**472, 1975.

Luckey, T. D.: The villus in chemostat man, Am. J. Clin. Nutr. **25:**1266, 1974.

Pike, R. L., and Brown, M. L.: Nutrition: an integrated approach, ed. 2, New York, 1975, John Wiley & Sons, Inc.

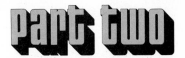

APPLIED NUTRITION IN COMMUNITY HEALTH

Community health care presents the alert and skilled pracitioner with a unique opportunity—indeed, even a responsibility—to apply knowledge of the science of human nutrition to help meet human need.

These scientific principles are not applied abstractly in a vacuum. They have meaning only in terms of *people*—people in families, people in communities, people in various work situations, people in financial distress, people with housing problems, people with deeply ingrained habits and customs, people with differing religious and cultural backgrounds— young people, old people, fat, thin, ill, well, discouraged, happy, clean, not so clean, educated, and illiterate people. There are many kinds of people in many places with many needs. Each person is a human being with unique dignity and pride and worth.

Therefore knowledge alone is not enough. Human compassion and concern are needed as well as practical guides, insights, appreciations, and skills to apply knowledge in a useful and helpful manner. The chapters in this study unit will help to provide a background on which health practitioners will be able to draw as they try to fill these human needs.

First, because some efforts to help people are hindered by their food fads or by their belief in false claims about foods, the chapter on Food Misinformation compares myths and magic to scientific facts.

Second, to guard against diseases that are spread by improper handling of food and to confront serious questions concerning the increasing use of food additives, the chapter on Protecting the Food Supply describes the problem and suggests ways of guarding food throughout its journey from producer to consumer.

Third, because cultural forces so strongly influence the meanings of food and its use in the family, the chapter on Cultural, Social, and Psychologic Influences on Food Habits provides a frame of reference for work with individual families.

Fourth, because knowing and doing are two different things, and because money spent for food is a large part of any family budget, the chapters on Nutrition Education and Family Diet Counseling—Food Needs and Costs offer tools and techniques and methods and materials for the effective delivery of sound nutrition guidance and education.

Finally, because in some pockets of extreme poverty in communities in the United States or in less developed countries the added factor of gross deficiency diseases may be encountered, the chapter on such conditions briefly pictures the classic examples of malnutrition.

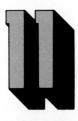

Food misinformation

Every year millions of dollars are spent by zealously health-conscious Americans as they respond to the claims of self-styled "scientists" who offer panaceas for ills. The panacea may be a pill, pellet, book, lecture, special food, or food supplement. Often message is couched in garbled, pseudoscientific jargon, which seems to the unwary to indicate knowledge. But the pitch is usually the same—a glibly worded advertisement that appeals more to the emotion than to the intellect. The result is an immense "health food" industry. Surrounding that industry are satellite personalities who capitalize on the insatiable anxiety of people about their health through lectures and publications full of half-truths or outright error.

At one time or other, and with great frequency in some communities, the worker in the health profession will confront these barriers to sound health teaching. Health practitioners need to know the nature and extent of food faddism, to understand why it exists, and to have a clear concept of the harm it may do. They need to be able to identify, among the people they serve, the risk groups who may be particularly vulnerable to the bogus authority of the food fad salesman. They will want to determine effective countermeasures to enticing misstatements made.

The first step is to understand the problem of food misinformation as objectively as possible. The term "as objectively as possible" is used because if all persons are entirely honest, they will probably acknowledge that there is some vestige of superstition about foods lying deep within them. Perhaps most people gullibly accept certain myths because they (like primitive peoples) secretly suspect there is something magical in nearly every kind of food. We must scrutinize our own beliefs and the beliefs of others and ask some fundamental questions:

1. What is a food fad or food myth?
2. What are some examples of these fallacies? How do they hold up in the light of nutritional science?
3. What harm is there in fads?
4. Why do faddists and quacks exist?
5. Who is especially vulnerable?
6. What can be done to prevent fallacies about nutrition from harming patients?

DEFINITIONS

Food fads. The word "fad" is a shortened form of an old word, *faddle* (it is retained today in the phrase "fiddle-faddle"), meaning "to play with." A fad is something one "plays with" for awhile. A fad is any popular fashion or pursuit, without substantial basis, that is followed enthusiastically. Most fads are short-lived; but some persist, and a few eventually become incorporated into a society's customs or mores.

Food fads are scientifically unsubstantiated beliefs about certain foods, which may persist for a time in a given community or society. Some may be perfectly harmless. Others have more serious implications concerning the health and welfare of their followers.

Food faddist. A food faddist is one who follows such food customs for a time. Usually he does so with exaggerated fervor as do some enthusiasts for molasses, wheat germ, yogurt, and so on. He may be an individual faddist, whose practice may have its basis in an acute or chronic psychologic problem. Or the faddist may be a member of a group that has accepted some rigid, stereotyped dietary practice in the belief that it will improve health or cure disease.

Food myths. The word *myth* comes from the Greek word *mythos* meaning "story" or "fable." The Greeks applied it to the vast array of stories that accumulated through the centuries about their gods and goddesses—their mythology. A myth is a traditional legend without a determinable basis of fact; it is an invented story, idea, or concept. Food myths are unproved stories or beliefs about food that are accepted uncritically, or are used to justify one's own desires, interests, or practices.

Over the years many myths have developed around foods. Current myths that have been identified by the U.S. Food and Drug Administration (FDA) center on food and disease. To a large extent, they represent a reactionary response to advances in scientific agriculture and food technology (see p. 258).

Quack. The word *quack,* as used in this sense, has an interesting history. It is a shortened form of "quacksalver," a term invented centuries ago by the Dutch, to describe the pseudophysician or pseudoprofessor who sold worthless salves, "magic" elixirs, and cure-all tonics. He proclaimed his wares, like a barker, in a patter that skeptical people compared to the quacking of a duck. The quacksalver made much loud noise but had no real medical ability or knowledge.

In medicine, nutrition, and allied fields, a quack is a fraudulent pretender who claims to have skill, knowledge, or qualifications he does not possess. His motive is usually money. By a cruel hoax, he feeds on the physical and emotional needs of people. The food quack exists because food faddists exist.

The food quack can usually be recognized by four aspects basic to his method of operation:

1. He uses the direct sales approach to promote the sale of his special food products. Although he may start by appealing to the gullible in a comparatively mild way, eventually his lectures, writings, and special products are foisted on the unwary at extravagant prices. The buyer of such products becomes persuaded that he should ignore the advice of the reputable physician and nutritionist in favor of self-diagnosis and treatment.
2. The quack makes exaggerated claims. He promises that his treatment will cure or prevent all diseases.
3. The quack warns his customers against American agriculture and established food distributors; he creates distrust in all scientific technology.
4. He uses emotionally convincing double-talk, which is full of half-truths and misinterpretations. Often he quotes out of context leading medical and nutritional authorities to support his claims. He is usually a charming person, with a flair for words and a clever wit.

Food misinformation. To misinform is to give false or misleading information. Food misinformation is a statement about food that is not based on or is not in agreement with scientific evidence. False information may have arisen out of a traditional fallacy, or it may represent a belief in magic or folklore. It may be built on outright lies, more subtle half-truths, innuendos, and inferences that are the stock-in-trade of the ingenious quack.

Scientific nutritional concepts. Opposed to food misinformation is the body of nutritional concepts that have been built on scientific evidence. Although concern for food safety and wholesomeness clearly existed long before the advent of the scientific method, it is on a sound basis of scientific knowledge and approach that wise food choices can best be made and misinformation can be recognized as such.[1] Scientifically sound concepts are the result of persistent research and testing over many decades. They represent organized, tested knowledge. The scientific or problem-solving method, here as in all other branches of modern learning, involves four steps:

1. Recognizing that a problem exists, identifying the problem, and determining some desirable goals in relation to it

2. Gathering all possible pertinent data, background knowledge, and principles, and on the basis of this information forming a hypothesis (an educated guess) about the solution to the problem

3. Testing this hypothesis under controlled conditions, which entails isolating the pertinent variables and studying one variable at a time; usually a large number of cases must be observed in detail before valid results accrue

4. Evaluating these test results, and if the hypothesis seems to be borne out, applying the results to a much larger population, while continuing to observe critically for errors that may become apparent only with time and broad application over a wide range of circumstances

Whenever one is confronted with questionable food information from a quack or a faddist, it is highly legitimate to ask, "What is your evidence?"

MYTHS AND FADS VS. SCIENTIFIC FACT
Basic food myths

It is an intriguing test of one's own beliefs to notice how some sample myths appear in the light of facts that have been amassed by scientific observers. Four basic food myths, which occur in many different disguises, have been identified by the American Medical Association (AMA) and the FDA. Each myth is compared with scientifically tested facts.

Myth: All disease is the result of faulty diet. The proponents of this myth contend that certain chemical imbalances in the body are the cause of disease and that these imbalances are the direct result of improper or inadequate diet. Since it is impossible for the average person to eat an adequate diet, according to the myth, he must supplement it with whatever product is being sold at the time. The product in question usually contains a long list of ingredients, including those labeled as "mysterious substances as yet unknown to nutritional scientists."

Here, for example, is the colorful "line" of one such food supplement salesman, as tape-recorded by an investigator employed by the FDA: "You eat food to make blood. You send down junk, your body will be junk. Your body will wind up in the junk pile. You send down vital elements that are needed, you're okay. Whenever you get your body normalized, you won't have no condition. You can't even take a cold. I don't care how you're exposed to freezing temperature, wet feet and cold feet, you'll never take it if you get your blood stream up to par."[2] And, of course, according to the salesman, the only way to "get your blood stream up to par" was to take large numbers of the special pills he was selling.

FACT. Disease is caused by many sorts of variation from normal states, such as inherited defects, and by any of a host of agents such as microorganisms and parasites. A large number of these causes of disease have no specific etiologic relationship to nutrients.

The few classic nutritional deficiency diseases, such as scurvy, rickets, pellagra, kwashiorkor, and a small number of others, have been well studied by medical science. They are still a major health problem in some impoverished parts of the world, including sections of the

United States (see p. 342). In such areas the problem is usually one of a complex web of factors including politics, economics, social alienation, education, or rejection of middle-class health values—not food availability alone.

Myth: Soil depletion causes malnutrition. People who believe this myth argue that the soil has lost its vitality from long overuse and that crops grown on it are deficient in nutrients.

FACT. Both scientists and farmers have repeatedly observed that if a soil lacks minerals and other materials necessary for plant growth, the plant simply will not grow. Poor soil affects only the *quantity* of food grown on it, not the *quality*. Extensive, controlled tests indicate these two facts:

1. Fertilizing the soil significantly increases the yield, not the nutritive content, of the food grown on it.[3]
2. The kind of fertilizer used—commercial chemical mix or organic manure—makes no difference in the food's nutritional composition.[4]

American agriculture has worked to meet two advancing pressures: (1) a rapidly growing population—demographers predict there will be approximately 400 million people by the year 2000—and (2) an even more rapidly shrinking amount of farmland as cities and suburbs spread over soil once used to grow food. The purpose that dominates agrarian research and the development of chemical fertilizers is to increase the yield of available land.

Myth: Food processing destroys the nutritive value of food. Many food supplement exponents insist that all processed food is inadequate or harmful, even labeling canned and frozen food as well as pasteurized milk as worthless or inferior because processing has removed the natural vitamins and minerals. They even lament that cooking causes further nutritive loss and advocate the use of raw foods, often liquefied in a blender. Some promote the sale of special cookware (at inflated prices), claiming that certain utensils, especially aluminum, slowly poison the body.

FACT. Three false premises in this myth are refuted by scientific observations:

First, consumers need to use discrimination in selection of so-called processed foods. It is true that many nutritionally empty "junk" foods do exist in the marketplace, and valid questions are raised concerning the rapidly changing food environment. However, many good products exist also that may add nutrition to the diet.

Modern food processing methods are scientifically developed and highly controlled to preserve or restore nutritional values in foods. For example, processing times, temperatures, and quality are rigidly controlled in the canning and freezing of vegetables and fruit to preserve the nutrients that are present. Enrichment of grain products restores much of their major natural vitamin and mineral content. United States food enrichment laws in general have been a primary factor in almost eliminating from the American population deficiency diseases that were once prevalent. A clinical case of ordinary vitamin D–deficiency rickets, for example, is now hard to find, largely because milk has been fortified for some years with 400 IU of vitamin D (10 μg cholecalciferol) per quart. Food enrichment regulations must undergo constant study so that current practice can be coordinated with developing scientific knowledge. One result of such continuing study is the body of FDA regulations concerning vitamin and mineral additions to foods (see p. 259). There is need, however, for still more rigorous study to meet the pressures generated by the rapidly changing food environment and socioeconomic problems. Better labeling regulations for processed foods is a step toward better consumer awareness and selection of food items.

Second, the nutritive qualities of vitamins and minerals as they occur naturally in foods do not differ from those that are synthetically produced in a laboratory and added to food. Categorically and unequivocally, *a vitamin is a vitamin.*

Third, aluminum is a trace element in the

human body and widespread in nature. There is no evidence to indicate that these trace amounts are harmful or that the amounts that may be ingested in food that has been cooked in an aluminum utensil significantly increases the total amount in the body. Extensive use of aluminum cookware, even in quantity cookery in governmental and industrial food service installations, has produced none of the harmful effects claimed by promoters of this myth. Statements by the American Cancer Society, the U.S. Public Health Service, and the AMA's Council on Foods and Nutrition declare that there is absolutely no scientific basis for such a claim.

Myth: The United States population suffers from widespread subclinical deficiencies requiring supplements of vitamins and minerals. Many times in advertisement one hears or reads about "that tired feeling" or "tired blood" or vague aches and pains, for which the advertiser has blamed dietary deficiencies. The very vagueness of this myth makes it difficult to refute. It is particularly appealing to the anxious person who constantly worries about his health and who fears that there must be something wrong with him, which the physicians simply have not been able to detect. Such a person accepts the claims of the vitamin or tonic salesman and purchases his product, perhaps because it provides the emotional support he needs. The vitamin is his placebo.

FACT. The word *subclinical* is a general, nonspecific term given to conditions for which there are no observable symptoms. It can be used in almost any context, depending on the purposes of the user. It is therefore rather meaningless in itself, and if used by an irresponsible person it may be misleading. Moreover, every normal person occasionally experiences such vague feelings of fatigue due to any of a variety of life situations. Should such feelings persist, however, the person should consult a qualified physician for competent examination and individually indicated treatment. In fact, excessive intake of some fat-soluble vitamins such as A

and D may have toxic effects. Also, adverse interrelationships may exist between other vitamins; for example, an excessive intake of vitamin C has been found to destroy vitamin B_{12}.[5] Supplementary vitamins and minerals will be prescribed only if they are needed by the patient. A sound, normal diet including a variety of foods will supply ample amounts of the essential nutrients.

Fallacious claims by food faddists

Types of claims. Food faddists make exaggerated claims for certain types of food. These claims fall into four basic classifications:

1. Certain foods will cure specific conditions.
2. Certain foods are harmful and should be omitted from the diet.
3. Special food combinations are very effective as reducing diets and have special therapeutic effects.
4. Only "natural foods" can meet body needs and prevent disease.

Basic error. If the above claims are examined carefully, the reader will notice that each one focuses on foods per se, not on the chemical components in them—the nutrients—which are the actual physiologic agents of life and health. *It is the nutrients, not specific foods as such, that have specific functions in the body.* Each of these nutrients may be found in a number of different foods. *People require specific nutrients, never specific foods.*

Examples of food fads. A number of food fads have flourished from time to time. The following are a few examples and the fallacies they represent.

1. Milk and fish form a harmful combination and should never be eaten together.

FACT. Both milk and fish are excellent foods, alone or together. Only if either milk or fish is contaminated or spoiled by improper handling or lack of refrigeration may difficulty be encountered.

2. Pasteurized milk is a "dead milk" and should be replaced by raw milk.

FACT. The process of pasteurization may destroy a small amount of vitamin C. But the quantity of vitamin C in cow's milk is so small that it makes no significant contribution to the human diet, and its destruction by pasteurization is therefore not important. Control of microorganisms by pasteurization and the prevention of the spread of disease by this means far outweigh any imagined dietary loss.

3. Citrus fruits such as oranges and lemons make the body acid or produce "acid stomach."

FACT. Hydrochloric acid, secreted by the parietal cells in gastric mucosal glands, forms the normally acid medium of the stomach. Citrus fruits have no influence on this secretion. As they undergo metabolism by the body, almost all fruits form an alkaline, not an acid, residue.

4. Onion and garlic will cure a cold; or will purify the blood.

FACT. No such powers are inherent in either food—unless, of course, copious use of such pungent partners so isolate him socially as to free him from viral contagion! Extension of the superstition that garlic has an effect on the blood is the basis on which the quack is able to sell "garlic pills" to cure high blood pressure.

5. Yogurt, blackstrap molasses, honey, and other such "wonder foods" assure good health.

FACT. Yogurt is merely a fermented, cultured form of milk; it has no mysterious additional properties. It costs more than plain milk. Blackstrap molasses is a syrup formed in the process of refining sugar. It contains vitamins and minerals; but so do many, many other foods in more common use. Honey is simply a form of sugar (fructose). Some have claimed any number of unfounded curative properties for honey combined with vinegar.

6. Oysters, olives, lean meat, and raw eggs enhance sexual potency and fertility.

FACT. Perhaps the notion that there is a connection between lean meat and potency had its origin in the primitive belief that eating certain foods gave the consumer the characteristics of the thing eaten. Hence, lean meat (animal flesh) was supposed to arouse animal passions. Such folklore has no basis in fact. There is no food that has any effect on sexual potency.

7. Grape juice, tomato juice, red wine, and beets are strong blood builders.

FACT. The main nutrients necessary to the production of red blood cells are protein and iron, neither of which these foods supply. Presumably, this superstition arises from the color of these foods; they, like blood, are red.

8. Fish, celery, and nutmeg are good brain foods; raw beef juice is good nerve food.

FACT. No food as such builds any specific tissue. Again it is the specific nutrients in foods that are required for the building of specific tissue. Nervous tissue, including brain tissue, is built and repaired from amino acids contained in protein, and protein is, of course, found in many foods.

9. Gelatin in large amounts builds strong fingernails.

FACT. Gelatin is an incomplete protein, which alone builds nothing. Nail formation is influenced by many other factors such as general body nutrition, disease, environment, and local nail care.

10. Seaweed or kelp products are important dietary supplements that prevent serious iodine deficiency.

FACT. Although there is some current question concerning the general environmental changes in iodine sources,[6,7] the small amount of iodine needed by the body is usually supplied in iodized table salt, which is commonly used in the American diet, and in seafood. To spend money on seaweed because it provides additional iodine is unnecessary.

11. Special food combinations are highly effective as reducing diets. Examples of such odd combinations are bananas and skimmed milk, lamb chops and pineapple, steak and spinach, or just eggs and more eggs.

FACT. A weight reduction program is successful only when calorie intake is smaller than caloric output (energy expenditure). For optimal nutrition during such a program, the diet must contain a wisely balanced group of nutrients. These faddish reducing combinations do not.

12. Special foods influence pregnancy and lactation by marking the child, by tainting breast milk, or by increasing milk production. Examples of such taboos and unfounded notions about the need for special foods are

a. Strawberry birth marks on infants are caused by strawberries eaten by the mother during her pregnancy.
b. Cravings for specific foods or for clay or cornstarch indicate physical needs of the gestating woman.
c. Beer increases lactation.
d. Foods such as cabbage, chocolate, and onions taint breast milk and produce gastrointestinal upsets in the nursing infant.

FACT. It is not specific foods that are needed for optimal maternal nutrition, although increased amounts of specific nutrients may be required. No food can mark the developing fetus. No food taints breast milk. The lactating mother does not need beer, although she may well need to increase her total daily fluid intake. Each of the beliefs listed here is unfounded.

DANGERS OF FOOD FADS

Why should the health worker be concerned about food faddism and food quackery? What harm may they do? Essentially, food fads involve four basic dangers, which concern all members of the health professions.

Dangers to health. Responsibility for care of one's health is fundamental. However, self-diagnosis and self-treatment can be dangerous. When such action is based on questionable sources, the dangers are multiplied. By following such a course, a person with a real illness may fail to secure proper medical care. Many anxious patients who have cancer, diabetes, or arthritis have been misled by quacks who fraudulently claimed that they had a cure for these diseases, and these patients have postponed effective therapy.

Money spent needlessly. Some of the foods and supplements used by faddists are harmless; but many are expensive. All money spent for useless food is wasted. When dollars are scarce, the family may neglect to buy foods that will fill its basic needs to purchase a "guaranteed cure."

Lack of knowledge of scientific progress. Misinformation spread by charlatans hinders the development of our society along lines that have been opened by scientific progress. The supersititions that are perpetuated by quacks counteract sound health teaching in the minds of many persons.

Distrust of food market. There is an increased current need for intelligent concern and rational problem-solving approaches to meet nutritional needs within our rapidly changing food enviornment. A wise course is to purchase a majority of one's foods among those "closer to the source"—having minimal processing, with a few carefully selected processed items for specific uses. However, blanket, erroneous teaching concerning food and health breeds public suspicion and complete distrust of the common food market and of food technology and agriculture in general. Many food products make possible the multitude and variety of standard quality food items. Each food product must be evaluated on its own merits in terms of individual consumer needs—nutrient contribution, esthetic values, and cost.

REASONS FOR EXISTENCE OF FOOD FADDISM

In the face of unprecedent advances in the knowledge available to scientists, why should some consumers use unsound and wasteful practices? Several reasons may be considered. They relate to both group culture pressures and individual human needs. These reasons include the rapid scientific and technologic advances, the population increase, the growth of the American economy, the communications media, individual social and emotional needs, and lack of general health education.

Scientific advances. The very rapidity of technical advance in itself has contributed to the problem. As medical knowledge has increased, most acute diseases have come under control.

Everyone is familiar with the statement: *During the first half of this century there was a dramatic increase in human longevity.* This has been stated many, many times. Do people feel its impact? Do people who live in the second half of the twentieth century sense the profound change that the promise of longevity has made in the human psyche?

The statement has more meaning when it is realized that the change was not so much a lengthening of the life span of those individuals who survived the acute diseases of childhood and the dangers of childbirth as it was a remarkable rise in the *total number of persons who lived to reach old age.* Today most people take it for granted that the average man and woman can reasonably expect to live to the age of 70. Yet this is the most exciting news that has ever come out of humankind's endeavors. This one fact created in the peoples of developed countries, within a single generation, a new attitude toward life; people *expect* to live.

A woman, if she plans to marry, does not carry in the back of her mind a haunting dread of the possibility that she may die if she has a child. If a woman is pregnant, she does not have to grope about for ways of facing a haunting terror that her baby will probably die before his or her fifth birthday. With the exception of persons with specific genetically transmitted diseases, such fears as these hardly enter the consciousness of healthy-minded young people today. Yet, a single example of what life was like in all former centuries, even for well-off professional people, shows how different their expectations were. It gives a gauge by

which the change in human attitudes can be measured that has resulted from the conquering of acute disease and of the high rate of deaths in childbirth. The composer Johann Sebastian Bach, who even in his own day was famous and successful and who came from vigorous stock, had 20 children from his two wives. His first wife died young, after bearing the first seven children. Of those 20 children, only 10 survived their infancy, and this infant death rate was not unusual. The effect that the nearness of death had on people's thoughts and feelings will become clear after considering how often and how deeply this man, who was the respected friend of princes, knew grief.

The mastery in the twentieth century of most of the diseases that killed mothers and young children pushed the thought of death far into the background of the average person's consciousness. Taking its place has been an eager determination to live. An American today looks for ways to ensure that he will get his full share of happiness while he is alive and that he will live out his full measure of years.

Americans are fully aware through the popular press that this change has come about through the application of scientific principles to biologic problems. They therefore look to science to give them still more of this good thing, life. Unfortunately the alterations has been so swift that public education has not had time to catch up. Even young persons whose total education has been within the scientific era do not always apply scientific principles to all phases of their lives. Persons educated before World War II or those who attend schools where teaching is less than optimal are sometimes unable to perceive the relationship between the glittering achievements of science and the sober step-by-step work of physiology, pathology, and calculus. Without having gone through those painstaking steps, thousands have felt themselves to be emotionally converted to science as they might be converted to a belief in magic if they saw proof that it worked. Such enthusiasts are easily duped by any hoax that masquerades in pseudoscientific jargon and that offers glib explanations that sound as though they are scientific. Thus faith in the results of science is distorted into gullibility toward pseudoscience.

Such converts turn toward pseudomedicine for quack cures. And they turn toward the propaganda of the food faddist for the same reason—there is a real basis for believing that nutrition is related to health. New knowledge of nutrition has yielded undeniable evidence of the role of proper diet in disease prevention and in the maintenance of sound health. What the food quack does *not* mention is that nutrition is a relatively infant science. More reliable information about food and its production, composition, and functions in maintaining health has been discovered within the past few decades than was established in all humankind's previous history. But the true scientist is far from ready to make the glib assertions and the broad promises of the quack.

Food technology advances. Together with the increased knowledge of nutritional science has come a revolution in food technology. The American food supply has become almost transformed by new methods of food preservation, processing, distribution, packaging, and transportation. The food quack points to these new processes with suspicion. He knows and uses the psychologic basis for building a wall of distrust in that which is new and unfamiliar.

The human mind maintains its stability by means of an equilibrium between eagerness for the new and distrust of the unfamiliar. Professional workers respect this equilibrium. The same sort of balancing activity goes on in the minds of physicians as they assess the value of a new drug. Interest is aroused by the claims of the manufacturer, by the reasonable way in which the pharmacologic chemist has worked out a respectable hypothesis, by the convenience of a new form of administration, by attractive packaging, which tends to help patients

accept the treatment. But trained skepticism is also aroused. Is the new agent effective? Is it safe? Physicians have been taught the tests to apply in making an informed judgment as to when to take advantage of the new and when to rely on the old.

Less well-trained persons often do not know. Many intelligent people are unfavorably impressed or are calmly unimpressed by gaudy packaging and extravagant claims. The trouble starts when this healthy conservatism is outbalanced by superstitions clinging to the old, for one reason only—simply because it is familiar.

The notion that people in those mythical ''good old days'' enjoyed better food and better nutritional health than people do today is nonsense. Rates of death and disease were far higher then, and the average chance of living out the full human life span was much less. The present food supply presents a broad spectrum of food forms—some wise selections and some poor buys. Today's consumer can no longer afford to be unknowledgeable, but basic research in food technology has enabled the *prudent* shopper in the community food market to procure good food of high quality for family health and enjoyment.

Population increases. Population explosions the world over have focused attention on the amounts of food that will be needed to sustain the increasing numbers of people. The pressure to develop more and better means of food production and distribution has led to revolutionary changes in agriculture. It has been necessary to increase the efficiency of agricultural workers through new techniques and to increase the yield of farmland by the intelligent, careful, and economical use of chemicals. These developments are an example of the application of technologic advance to the fulfillment of pressing human need.

American economic growth. Oddly enough, America's great economic growth has also contributed to food faddism. By and large, food faddism with its many special foods and gadgets is a costly practice, one that only a relatively affluent society can maintain. Today's worker has more money than any worker in history. Automation has given him more leisure time in which to seek new interests; those who are so inclined will spend much of this time in seeking foods that will fill some imagined need. And there are some persons who feel that to require a special food is to prove that one has a higher status than ordinary people. Appeals to each of these peculiarities have been used by clever promoters to enhance their products.

Mass communication media. Through television, radio, and public press, a health-conscious culture has been developed in the United States. Public awareness of medical advances, of nutrition's role in health, and of food technology has created a general desire for more information. This very desire for information provides a fertile soil for the growth of faddism. Some of the statements of faddists are honest errors of misguided zeal. Some statements made by quacks are deliberately deceptive.

Social and emotional needs. Very real contribution to food faddism arises from the social and emotional needs of people.[8] Food has emotional value for the average person. Everyone knows this from personal experience. People today live in a world of many pressures. This era has been called the age of anxiety. Sometimes these anxieties are converted into an exaggerated concern for health, and attachment to certain food practices may result.

In human societies, especially where scarcity of food is not a problem, food assumes significance far beyond fulfillment of hunger as a basic drive. Eating toether symbolizes social acceptance, friendliness, cultural identification, prestige, and position. Eating with one's peers, and the exclusion of those who do not rank with the peer group, may even be a form of weapon. Foods are used as bribes or rewards. From infancy, foods mean love, comfort, pleasure, and protection. In the anxious adult, these associations may form the basis of compulsive drives to overeat. Faddism appeals to such human emotional values and drives. Quackery makes direct capital of them.

Lack of general health education. In many instances, faddism has grown because nurses, nutritionists, and physicians have failed to communicate sound information about relationships between food and health. Sometimes health workers have not been sufficiently person centered to appreciate the emotional value of foods. Sometimes, by being rigidly fact centered, they have repelled rather than appealed to those persons who are vulnerable to fads. Although the information given must be scientifically grounded, the importance of a balance between intellect and emotion must not be ignored. Professional medical persons often are depicted as sterile, cold personalities, perhaps more concerned with maintaining their own professional status than with meeting the needs of people. If this image is contrasted with the warmly sympathetic, soothing tones of the pseudoprofessional food quack, it is no wonder that many frightened or anxious persons reject the first and accept the latter.

Groups vulnerable to food faddism

Food fads appeal especially to certain groups of people with particular needs and concerns. Among these are the middle aged, the elderly, the adolescent, the obese, and people whose living depends on their physical appearance.

Fear of the changes that come about as youth and potency wane leads many middle-aged persons to grasp at exaggerated claims that some purchasable product will restore their vigor.

When in pain and discomfort, perhaps facing chronic illness, the elderly patient may respond to the hope that the food quack holds out for a sure cure. Desperately ill and lonely people are an easy prey for a cruel hoax.

Figure-conscious girls and muscle-minded boys frequently respond to advertisements that glowingly depict a crash program for attaining the perfect body. Young people, particularly those who are lonely, but also many who have exaggerated ideas of glamour, hope to achieve peer group acceptance by these means.

One of the most disturbing health problems in America today is obesity. It is often frustrating to treat. Obese persons, faced with a bewildering barrage of propaganda advocating diets, pills, candies, wafers, and devices, are likely to succumb to fads.

People in the public eye—entertainers and athletes—are often prey to those who make false claims that certain foods, drugs, or dietary combinations will enable them to retain the physical appearance and strength on which their careers depend.

These groups are vulnerable for obvious reasons. There seems to be no segment of the population, however, that is completely free from food faddism's appeal. Particularly in metropolitan areas, large groups of faddists present a constant array of misinformation that hinders the efforts of the members of the legitimate health professions to raise the community standards in nutrition.

ANSWERS TO THE PROBLEM

What is the answer to the problems associated with food faddism, misinformation, and outright quackery? What can workers in the health professions do? What *should* they do? At least six courses of action merit consideration:

1. Members of the health professions must assess their own attitudes and habits. They cannot teach another until they have first examined their own position. Instruction based on personal conviction, practice, and enthusiasm will achieve far more than teaching that says, in effect, "Do as I say, not as I do."

2. Sound facts must be obtained from reliable sources. Two types of background knowledge are vital. (1) Health workers must have facts that will accurately controvert specific items of misinformation and that will clearly explain why a certain product is worthless, harmful, inflated in price, or cannot have the effects claimed for it. One must have facts about people involved in a given instance of fraud or in a specific kind of fraud. One must avoid making broad generalizations or vague charges; effective counteraction is necessarily based on knowledge of the adversary. (2) Health workers must also have facts concerning human nutritional physiology and about the scientific approach to the solution of health problems. Health workers must have facts about food technology, agricultural methods, and other related data, since these facts are tools. To have them at their command, health workers must keep up with relevant research and be alert to scientific discoveries and to the constant developments in the practices of applied science.

3. Health workers must recognize the basic human needs involved in nutrition. They must observe in themselves and others how psychologic and cultural factors affect food habits. One cannot effectively combat false information without considering the emotional needs that are symbolically fulfilled by foods, by the eating of food, and by the rituals with which everyone surrounds the eating of food. In planning a program of nutritional education for a group or for a single patient, these emotional needs must be respected. Everyone has them. They are part of life. The power that foods and eating rituals possess for filling those needs should be welcomed. The power should be used intelligently and worked into a health worker's program. Foods should not be disparaged as a mere "crutch." Even when there is reason to believe that the patient is using food as a crutch for an ailing emotional adjustment, the value to him of such an adjustment must be considered. A wise teacher has put it well. "We must avoid 'breaking crutches' without offering alternative support." This should be remembered particularly when a patient falls within one of the categories that is especially vulnerable to food faddism.

4. Health workers must be alert to community opportunities and resources. Any opportunity that arises with a community should be

taken to present sound health information to groups or individuals, formally and informally. Workers should know what community resources are available, such as a local or state university agricultural extension service, volunteer health agencies, clinic and hospital facilities, federal, state, county, and city public health departments, and professional health organizations. Workshops, conferences, meetings, classes, clinics, demonstration projects, displays, exhibits, bulletins, newsletters, and many other channels are excellent devices for promoting sound nutritional concepts. Skill in communication is essential to success in using these devices. Clarity in speech and writing is all important. Monotony should be avoided, and workers should possess a well-disciplined imagination. Without this, the message will not convince.

5. Young people should be taught to think scientifically. While very young, children may be introduced to the problem-solving approach to everyday situations. Children are naturally curious. A child often seeks evidence to support statements with which he is confronted. Far too often the system of education fails to develop this spirit of inquiry. Children can learn early that it is valuable to ask legitimate questions such as, what do you mean, how do you know, and what is your evidence.

6. Health workers should know the work of responsible authorities and support them in their direct dealing with quacks. The FDA is charged with the legal responsibility for controlling the quality and safety of all food and drug products marketed in this country, but it needs the vigilance of consumers to help fulfill so large a task. Every worker in the health professions should know of this organization and its work and should relay to it information about illegal food handling or food quackery.

Other governmental, professional, and private organizations provide additional resources for consumer education. The Federal Trade Commission exerts control of consumer products. The U.S. Department of Agriculture maintains a broad program of research, regulation, and education. The Agricultural Extension Service extend this department's work into communities. A group of scientists form the Food and Nutrition Board of the National Research Council (NRC), which studies human nutrient requirements and recommends standards and guidelines.

On a worldwide basis, the Food and Agriculture Organization and the World Health Organization, divisions of the United Nations, help to raise living standards, attach the problem of insufficient food for the world's increasing population, and contribute to general nutritional health. Two other United Nations agencies, UNESCO and UNICEF, also work in the area of world nutrition.

Professional organizations, such as the American Public Health Association, the Food and Nutrition Council of the AMA, the Society for Nutrition Education, and the American Dietetic Association, provide additional educational resources through their printed materials and local group activities.

An important private foundation, The Nutrition Foundation, Inc., provides service through research, publication, and education.

CASE STUDY 1
A young family trying to cope

Sarah Brown, age 20, and her husband Charles, age 21, live in a small flat in a low-rent district of the city with their three young children—a boy of 3, a girl 18 months old, and their new baby, 6 weeks old. Sarah has gained more weight, so that now she weighs 93 kg (205 lb). Already she feels old and unattractive. She has always been rather dependent on her mother and, lately, on her husband. But now she seems less and less able to cope.

Charles works in a gas station during the day and sometimes gets extra mechanic work at night, but still he can barely make enough to meet expenses. There are many unpaid bills. The friction between Charles and Sarah has increased, and Charles is absenting himself increasingly from home.

Recently, about the time that Sarah came home from the county hospital with the new baby, Sarah's mother, Mrs. Miller, aged 50, came to live with the Brown family. She had been living alone, but now because her arthritis was worse and had begun to cripple her more she could no longer work or care for herself. There seemed to be no other place to go but to her daughter's home.

A district public health nurse in the county, Miss Jordan, was visiting Sarah and her new baby for a 6-week checkup. When Miss Jordan arrived at the apartment, she found Sarah distraught and in tears. Charles, she said, had gone off to work that morning angrily saying that he might not return until she grew up and learned how to manage things better. Sarah was wearing an old housecoat, and her hair was uncombed. She held a formula bottle in her hand, seemingly not knowing quite what to do with it. The apartment was crowded and cluttered. Dishes filled the small kitchen sink, and every available space seemed taken up with used utensils. The two older children were thin and fretful, hitting at each other over a toy both wanted, pulling at their mother's housecoat for her attention.

Although it was midmorning, the children had had no breakfast. The baby was in a crib in a corner of the room, crying, waiting for the bottle Sarah was trying to fix to feed her. Sarah's mother was lying on the couch; the crutches she had to use to walk with were close by.

Miss Jordan offered to feed the baby, for which Sarah seemed grateful. After the feeding Miss Jordan weighed the baby and found that she was not gaining weight as she should. Sarah said that none of the formula seemed to agree with the baby, and she was constantly spitting it up.

At this point a knock sounded at the door. It was Mrs. Bryant, who lived in the flat above the Brown family. She was older than Sarah, about 45, a loud and dominant-appearing woman. She was bringing a bottle of some food supplement to Sarah, for which Sarah, after searching and finally finding her purse, gave her a $10 bill. All the while Sarah was searching for her purse, Mrs. Bryant enthusiastically told Miss Jordan about her special health food products.

"This is a special high-protein food supplement. It isn't sold through stores but only through special agents like me who know its real worth. You know, all this processed food you buy in the markets is worthless. There's no food value left in it. It's no wonder everybody's half sick. It's all caused by bad diet. But this supplement will make up the difference. It's a natural food substance, organically grown. It's the very thing Sarah needs to get her strength back and to help her lose weight. As for the children," she continued, "it's just what they need, too, to put some meat on their bones."

Then Mrs. Bryant turned to Sarah's mother and patted her arm. "You poor dear. As soon as you start using this, too, a double dose daily for a while, your arthritis will be cured."

As she was leaving, Mrs. Bryant said to Miss Jordan, "You look a little peaked yourself. You could use some, too. Here, let me leave this leaflet with you that tells all about it."

After Mrs. Bryant left, Sarah explained that Charles' anger that morning resulted from her buying the expensive special food supplement when their family budget was so tight.

Continued.

CASE STUDY 1
A young family trying to cope—cont'd

After talking briefly with Sarah and her mother, Miss Jordan made definite arrangements to return the following week. As she drove away from the apartment building, she was thinking about her observations and the problems she had encountered in the Brown family. Already she had decided that when she returned to the district public health office she would consult with the nutritionist and leave the food supplement pamphlet with her to investigate. She also decided to speak with the psychiatric nursing consultant and a social worker in the social service department.

Questions to guide your inquiry

1. Imagine you are the nutritionist or the nurse. What important questions come to your mind from your observations?
2. What problems do you identify? What are Sarah Brown's needs? What are her husband's needs?
3. What solutions can you propose? How would you involve other health department persons in your solutions or plan of action?
4. Consider each of the children. What growth and development needs—physical, psychosocial, as well as nutritional—does each child present? What food and feeding practices are related? (See age group needs in Chapter 18.)
5. What solutions can you propose to meet each child's needs?
6. What are Mrs. Miller's needs? How is nutritional therapy related to arthritis?
7. Why is this family vulnerable to the ''health food'' sales pressures of the neighbor, Mrs. Bryant?
8. What food myths or misinformation did you find?
9. What dangers are involved in such food fads or quackery?
10. Why does food faddism exist?
11. What can health workers do about the problems of food faddism?
12. What other questions have been raised in your mind from your analysis, to this point, of this family situation?
13. What additional information would you need to work with this family? What possible sources or means would you use to obtain it?

REFERENCES
Specific

1. Day, H. G.: Food safety—then and now, J. Am. Diet. Assoc. **69:**229, Sept., 1976.
2. Bell, J. N.: Let 'em eat hay, Today's Health, Sept., 1958.
3. Maynard, L. A.: Effect of fertilizers on the nutritional value of foods, J.A.M.A. **161:**1478, 1956.
4. Beeson, K. C.: Effects of fertilizers on nutrition quality of crops and health of animals and man, Plant Food J. **5:**7, 1951.
5. Herbert, V.: Destruction of vitamin B_{12} by ascorbic acid, J.A.M.A. **230:**241, 1974.
6. Kidd, P. S., Trowbridge, F. L., Goldsby, J. B., and

Nichaman, M. Z.: Sources of dietary iodine, J. Am. Diet. Assoc. **65:**420, Oct., 1974.
7. Cullen, R. W., and Oace, S. M.: Iodine: current status, J. Nutr. Educ. **8:**101, 1976.
8. Schaefer, R., and Yetley, E. A.: Social psychology of food faddism, J. Am. Diet. Assoc. **66:**129, Feb., 1975.

General

Bruch, H.: The allure of food cults and nutrition quackery, J. Am. Diet. Assoc. **57:**316, Oct., 1970.
Deutsch, R. M.: The new nuts among the berries, Palo Alto, Calif., 1977, Bull Publishing Co.
Henderson, L. M.: Programs to combat nutritional quackery, J. Am. Diet. Assoc. **64:**372, April, 1974.

Jalso, S. B., Burns, M. M., and Rivers, J. M.: Nutritional beliefs and practices, J. Am. Diet. Assoc. **47:** 263, Oct., 1965.

New, P. K., and Priest, R. P.: Food and thought: a sociologic study of food cultists, J. Am. Diet. Assoc. **51:**13, July, 1967.

Nutrition misinformation and food faddism, Nutr. Rev. **32**(suppl. 1), July, 1974.

Rhee, K. S., and Stubbs, A. C.: Health food users in two Texas cities, J. Am. Diet. Assoc. **68:**542, June, 1976.

Shifflett, P. A.: Folklore and food habits, J. Am. Diet. Assoc. **68:**347, April, 1976.

12 Protecting the food supply

America's abundant (although sometimes maldistributed) food supply is the result of an increasing application of scientific knowledge to a vast heritage of fertile acres. However, wise ways to use, develop, and more equitably distribute our food supply must be found.

The rapid growth of the population is increasing the demand for food at the same time that it is reducing the available farming land. Every year, hundreds of thousands of acres of rich farm soil are sacrificed to the spread of cities and suburbs. The agricultural sections are pushed farther away from the consumers who are crowded into the cities, where virtually no food can be grown. This means that foods must be hauled greater distances than ever before. It is one more factor that poses a problem of food preservation. But there are many additional reasons why there is never freedom from the threat of food spoilage and waste, or from disease carried by food either by microorganisms and parasites, or by the poisons used to combat them. Therefore to maintain this abundant harvest and ensure its safety and high quality, safeguards within the agricultural, the chemical, and the food industries are imperative.

In considering ways of protecting the food supply, knowledge of five factors is important: (1) food- and water-borne disease agents, (2) food additives, (3) protection of food during handling from farm to table, (4) means of food preservation, and (5) control agencies to ensure food safety and quality. This study should be focused on the following questions:

1. What agents of disease may be spread by food?
2. How is food guarded during production from spoilage and harmful agents?
3. How is food preserved for continuing use?
4. What agencies control food safety and quality?

Human ecology and nutrition. Many advances have been made in hygiene, sanitation, and preventive medicine in the struggle to protect human beings from the pathogenic organisms that are constantly present in the environment and are transmitted by contaminated food and water. Epidemiologic studies of the classic triad of host, agent, and environment and the interactions among them have led to valuable knowledge of how to control the environment and make it more healthful. All of these problems are by no means solved. Even scientific advances sometimes create new difficulties. Everyone is cognizant of advancing environmental pollution and radioactivity that are by-products of technical achievements. The study of a human's relation to his environment—human ecology—has arisen out of his awareness of pressing needs. Constant vigilance is necessary to control the diseases that result when that relationship is disturbed.

FOOD- AND WATER-BORNE DISEASE AGENTS

The agents of disease carried by food and water may be classified in three main categories: (1) pathogenic organisms, which carry disease to humans, usually by the fecal-oral route through contaminated food and water or through unsanitary food handling, (2) natural poisons in certain plants and animals, and (3) man-made chemical contaminants.

Pathogenic organisms

The organisms pathogenic to humans that are transmitted through food or water are parasites, bacteria, viruses, and fungi.

Parasites

A number of protozoa and helminths inhabit a human's intestinal tract. The term *helminth* means "worm," but medical workers usually use it to indicate pathogenic worms. Two types of worm are of serious concern in conjunction with food: (1) *nematodes,* or roundworms, of which the trichina worm found in pork is an example, and (2) *cestodes,* or flatworms, such as the common tapeworms of beef and pork.

Trichina worm *(Trichinella spiralis).* The trichina worm is transmitted through unsanitary garbage eaten by hogs. The larvae become embedded in the pork muscle. If a person eats such infested meat, the organism grows and multiplies in his intestinal tract, then moves into muscle tissue and causes fever and intense pain. In some fatal cases of trichinosis, millions of encysted larvae have been found in the muscle tissue at the time of autopsy. Two measures are imperative to prevent trichinosis: (1) Underdone pork should never be eaten. It should be cooked thoroughly until the meat is all white and no pink color remains. (2) Hog food sources must be controlled. Garbage must be cooked before it is fed to hogs. Since 1952 laws in all states have banned the feeding of uncooked garbage to swine. As a result, cases of trichinosis are now rare in the United States.

However, a recent outbreak on a cruise ship, traced to a meat grinder being used for pork and beef preparation, indicates the need for constant vigilance.

Tapeworms. The beef tapeworm, *Taenia saginata,* and the pork tapeworm, *Taenia solium,* are transmitted by the fecal-oral route, usually in the form of mature eggs in segments of the worm. These cysts are eaten by cattle in sewage-polluted pastures or by hogs in polluted garbage. The larvae develop in the animal's intestine, then encyst in the muscle. If a human eats the infected meat raw or rare, the adult tapeworm matures in his intestine and continues its reproductive cycle. Important controls are prevention of sewage pollution of pastures, sanitary hog-raising operations, and avoidance of eating rare beef and underdone pork.

Amebae. Although numerous harmless amebae normally inhabit a human's intestinal tract, some are highly pathogenic. The most widely known pathogenic species is that which causes amebic dysentery—*Entamoeba histolytica* (Gr. *ent,* inside; *histo,* tissue; *lytic,* dissolving). The name indicates its mode of attack. The organisms are ingested as cysts in contaminated food or water. In the intestine the cysts grow into adult forms which produce tissue-destroying enzymes that enable the organism to burrow into the intestinal lining and cause ulcers. Occasionally such embedding may be deep enough to produce intestinal rupture, and the patient may die of resulting peritonitis. The amebae may also enter the intestinal lymph vessels and blood vessels and travel to liver, lungs, brain, and other organs, where they may localize and form large, destructive abscesses.

Transmission is entirely by the human fecal-oral route. A human is the reservoir, the carrier, and the passer. Fecal contamination of food and water is caused by soiled, unwashed hands and by flies. Carriers who are food handlers contaminate food and utensils. Leaking sewers may pollute water supplies. Control obviously centers on strict sanitation measures and personal hygiene.

Bacteria

Two terms that relate to bacterial sources of food-borne disease need to be distinguished. These terms are food infection and food poisoning.

Food infections (bacterial). Food infections result from the ingestion in food of large amounts of viable bacteria that multiply inside the host (humans) and cause infectious disease. Each specific disease is caused by a specific organism. Because incubation and multiplication of the bacteria take time, symptoms of food infection develop relatively slowly, usually 12 to 24 hours or more after the infected food has been eaten.

SALMONELLOSIS. The typhoid and paratyphoid bacilli, which infect humans, belong collectively to the genus *Salmonella*. They produce various infections (salmonellosis) of the intestinal tract. Some bacilli such as the typhoid bacillus, also invade the blood and cause general infection. The genus is named for the American bacteriologist and veterinarian, Daniel E. Salmon, who in 1885 first isolated from a pig a species of the organisms that infects animals. Humans are sometimes involved indirectly in the animal infection chain by eating infected meat or meat products (pork and poultry). However, the types of *Salmonella* that are chiefly responsible for human disease are *S. typhi* and *S. paratyphi*. They are largely restricted to humans, and they spread either directly or indirectly from person to person.

Salmonellae are rod-shaped bacteria that resist cold and survive for long periods in soil, ice, water, milk, and foods. Since they do not form spores, they are easily killed by being boiled for five minutes or by pasteurization. Drying and direct sunlight also kill them. The organisms grow easily in simple, common foods such as milk, custards, egg dishes, salad dressings, and sandwich fillings. Seafoods from polluted waters may also be a source of infection.

Immunization practices and regulations controlling the sanitation of community water and food supplies have reduced the incidence of typhoid fever to rare outbreaks. However, paratyphoid organisms continue to frequently infect food. As is true of most species that cause enteric infections, transmission of the several *Salmonella* species that cause paratyphoid fever (enteric fever) is by the oral-fecal route, through careless, unsanitary handling of foods and utensils. One carrier may infect a large number of persons at one meal by preparing a dish ahead of time and leaving it in a warm room for several hours, which would incubate the bacilli. The resultant cases of gastroenteritis may vary in intensity from mild diarrhea to severe attacks.

Authorities warn that salmonellosis appears to be increasing in America.[2] This poses an ominous health hazard requiring more rigid control.

SHIGELLOSIS. Bacillary dysentery (shigellosis) is caused by rod-shaped bacteria of the genus *Shigella*. The organism is named for the Japanese physician, Kiyoshi Shiga, who was the first to discover a species of the organism during an epidemic in Japan in 1898. Shigellosis is usually confined to the large intestine and may vary from mild transient intestinal disturbance (as is most common in adults) to fatal dysentery (as occurs more often in young children).

The *Shigella* organisms grow easily in foods, especially in milk, which is a common vehicle of transmission to infants and children. The boiling of food and water or the pasteurization of milk kills the organisms; but the food or milk may easily be reinfected subsequently through unsanitary handling by a carrier. The several species that may cause shigellosis are spread in much the same way as are those that produce salmonellosis—by feces, fingers, flies, milk, and food and by articles handled by unsanitary carriers.

CHOLERA. Chiefly an Asiatic disease, cholera is caused by *Vibrio cholerae* (also called *V. comma*), an organism that resembles *Salmonella* in many respects. It also is a nonspored bacillus that may be easily killed by boiling, pasteurization, and disinfectants. Transmission is from person to person in the same manner as that of *Salmonella*. Attacks of cholera are usually more severe than attacks of salmonellosis; diarrhea, prostration, and emaciation often proceed rapidly to death unless treatment is given in time.

Food- and water-borne epidemics are common in Asiatic countries. In the nineteenth century, five such epidemics originating in Asia swept through western countries and killed millions of persons. Some of these epidemics even reached the United States. It is only because of the alertness of public health agencies and continuous environmental sanitation that most countries of Europe and America are free of cholera today.

BRUCELLOSIS. Milk from infected cows or goats may transmit the cocobacilli that cause brucellosis (undulant fever). The genus *Brucella* was named for Sir David Bruce, a British-Australian physician who, working in Malta in 1887, discovered the organisms in goats and in British soldiers who had drunk the goats' milk. The disease in humans is characterized by intermittent fever that recurs daily over a period that may vary from days to years, with general malaise and aching and stiffness of the back and joints. In mild forms it may be regarded as "intestinal flu."

Brucella organisms may be transmitted in the milk of goats or cows or through cuts or scratches on the skin of persons who work with infected animals. Thus butchers, slaughterhouse workers, stock raisers, and veterinarians are particularly exposed. The disease is pre-

vented by using only pasteurized milk and other dairy products and by avoiding contact with infected animals.

LEPTOSPIROSIS. (Gr. *leptos,* thin [literally, stripped]; L. *spira,* coil.) The genus *Leptospira* is so named because it is the smallest and most delicately formed of the spirochetes (spiral-shaped bacteria). The organisms are transmitted to humans mainly in polluted water—by drinking it or by swimming or wading in it and acquiring the organisms through cuts or scratches on the skin. Infected animals that may pollute streams include dogs, cattle, swine, mules, rats, and many wild animals. The disease in humans, characterized by high fever and intense, hemorrhagic jaundice and hepatitis, was originally called Weil's disease, after Adolf Weil, a German physician. It is common among persons who work in foul, watery places such as trenches in wartime, poorly built mines, sewers, rice fields, and the like where urine-polluted water and rats abound. It may also occur, however, in persons who do not enter such situations but who ingest food or water that has been polluted, usually by rats.

Careful storage of foods in the home, general cleanliness in housekeeping, and constant control of rats are obvious measures for the prevention of leptospirosis.

TULAREMIA. The bacterial genus *Pasteurella,* named for Louis Pasteur, includes one species that occasionally causes food-borne disease in humans. The organism is *P. tularensis,* named for Tulare County in California where it was first observed. The disease is commonly called tularemia. It is popularly known as rabbit fever, because it is frequently transmitted to rabbit hunters, trappers, and handlers (market men and housewives) from wild rabbits that have been infected by ticks, fleas, lice, or other insects that carry the microorganism. Such an infectious disease of animals, usually transmitted by arthropods, is called a *zoonosis.* A human may accidentally enter the animal-insect-animal transmission cycle. Tularemia resembles plague, although it is much milder. It is characterized by focal ulcers at the site of infection, recurrent fever, prostration, myalgia, and headache.

Restrictions against the sale of wild rabbits have sharply reduced the incidence of tularemia. Caution should be exercised in eating rabbits of wild or unknown origin.

ESCHERICHIA COLI INFECTIONS. Several *Escherichia coli* species normally inhabit the human gastrointestinal tract in enormous numbers. The bacterial genus *Escherichia* was named for a German physician, T. Escherichia, who first studied them. *Escherichia* are widely distributed in nature. The species that normally inhabits the human colon receives the name *E. coli* from its location in humans. Ordinarily *E. coli* cause their host no difficulty; but certain strains produce enteritis, especially in infants. Babies' formulas prepared under unsanitary conditions are the usual route of infection.

CLOSTRIDIUM PERFRINGENS FOOD INFECTION. *Clostridium perfringens,* the bacterium that causes gas gangrene when it infects deep wounds, is also capable in certain circumstances of inducing gastrointestinal illness. Rarely is the illness fatal, and then only in elderly, debilitated patients. Its symptoms are usually mild—diarrhea, acute abdominal cramping, nausea, and headache. Most patients recover in 24 hours or at most within a few days.

The *C. perfringens* spores are in soil, water, dust, refuse—everywhere. They are resistant to drying, heat, cold, chlorination, and irradiation. Some heat-resistant strains can survive in boiling water for more than six hours. In cold storage tests, some spores survived at least six months in frozen raw beef.

The organism multiplies in cooked meat and meat dishes held for extended periods at warming temperatures or at room temperature. A number of outbreaks of clostridia infection from food eaten in restaurants, college dining rooms, and school cafeterias have been reported. In each case, cooked meat was improperly handled in preparation and refrigeration. Control rests principally on careful preparation and adequate cooking of meats, prompt service, and immediate refrigeration at sufficiently low temperatures.

Food poisonings (bacterial toxins). Food poisoning is caused by the ingestion of bacterial toxins that have been produced in the food by the growth of specific kinds of bacteria before the food is eaten. The powerful toxin is ingested directly, and symptoms of food poisoning therefore develop rapidly, usually within one to six hours after the food is eaten.

STAPHYLOCOCCAL FOOD POISONING. Several organisms in this group, including *bacillus cereus,* are responsible for causing food poisoning.[3] However, of the bacterial food poisonings observed in the United States, staphylococcal food poisoning is by far the most common. Powerful preformed toxins in the contaminated food produce illness within one to six hours after ingestion. The manifestations appear suddenly. There is severe cramping and abdominal pain with nausea, vomiting, and diarrhea, usually accompanied by sweating, headache, and fever. There may be prostration and shock. Recovery is fairly rapid, however, and the symptoms subside within 24 hours. The amount of toxin ingested and the susceptibility of the individual eating it determine the degree of severity.

The source of contamination is usually a locus of staphylococcal infection on the hand of a worker preparing the food. Often it is only a minor infection, considered harmless or even unnoticed by the food handler. Custard or cream-filled bakery goods are particularly effective culture beds for staphylococci and are common carriers of the toxins formed during their growth. Other foods that often support the development of staphylococci are processed meats, ham, tongue, cheese, ice cream, potato salad, sauces, chicken and ham salads, and combination dishes such as spaghetti and casseroles. The toxin causes no change from the normal appearance, odor, or taste of the food, so the victim is not warned.

A careful food history is necessary to determine the source of the poisoning. If possible, portions of the food are obtained for bacterial examination. Few bacteria may be found, for heating kills these organisms but does not destroy the toxin they produce.

Prevention of staphylococcal food poisoning rests upon enforcement of three practices:

1. Strict observance by food handlers of the rules of hygiene
2. Careful and immediate refrigeration of all perishable foods
3. Reheating foods only immediately before serving; not allowing them to stand long periods at room temperature

Education of food handlers, an ongoing activity of many public health departments, is vital to the prevention of food poisoning incidents in the community.

BOTULISM. Serious, often fatal food poisoning results from ingestion in food of the toxin produced by the bacteria *Clostridium botulinum.* Depending on the dose of toxin taken and individual response, the illness may vary from mild discomfort to death within 24 hours. Mortality rates are high. Nausea, vomiting, weakness, and dizziness are initial complaints. Progressively, the toxin irritates motor nerve cells and blocks transmission of neural impulses at the nerve terminals (myoneural junction); gradual paralysis follows. Sudden respiratory paralysis with airway obstruction is the major cause of death.

C. botulinum spores are widespread in soil throughout the world. These spores may be carried on harvested food to the canning process. Like all clostridia, this species is anaerobic (develops in the absence of air) or nearly so. The relatively anaerobic environment in the can and canning temperatures (above 27° C [80° F]) provide good conditions for toxin production. The development of high standards in the commercial canning industry has eliminated this source of botulism, but a few cases still result each year from the eating of carelessly home-canned foods. Since boiling for 10 minutes destroys the toxin (not the spore), all home-canned food, no matter how well preserved it is considered to be, should be boiled *at least* 10 minutes before eating.

Viruses

Illnesses produced by viral contamination of food are few in comparison with those pro-

---

TO PROBE FURTHER
"Ptomaine poisoning"—a misnomer

A misnomer is a misapplied name or designation. It is an error in naming a person or thing. Such an error has crept into common usage as a term used by laymen for food poisoning—the use of the word *ptomaine.* There is no such thing as "ptomaine poisoning" in humans.

The word ptomaine comes from the Greek word *ptoma,* meaning "dead body." Ptomaines are members of a large class of basic nitrogenous substances, some of them highly poisonous, which are produced during putrefaction of animal or plant protein. They are easily detectable by the deteriorated appearance of the material almost to a liquid state and by the powerful, obnoxious odor they produce. Food in such a condition is hardly human fare!

The word ptomaine is therefore erroneously used when it is applied to other common food infections or poisonings, such as salmonellosis or staphylococcal intoxication.

TO PROBE FURTHER
Alimentary toxic aleukia (ATA)

An extreme example of food poisoning caused by mycotoxins occurred in grain-producing areas of the Soviet Union during World War II.* Because of the wartime shortage of farm workers, large crops of grain had to remain in the fields during the winter snows. Alternate freezing and thawing in the early spring produced excellent conditions for growth of soil fungi on the grain. As a result, the grain became highly toxic to animals and human beings and produced a syndrome of profound bone marrow suppression and decrease in white blood cells (aleukia). Large numbers of persons became ill, and many deaths resulted. Incidents such as this have stimulated new research concerning mold toxins in foods.† Undoubtedly others will be discovered.

*Jaffee, A. Z.: Toxin production in cereal fungi causing toxic alimentary aleukia in man. In Wogan, G. N., editor: Mycotoxins in foodstuffs, Cambridge, 1965, Massachusetts Institute of Technology Press, p. 77.
†Wogan, G. N.: Current research on toxic food contaminants, J. Am. Diet. Assoc. **49:**95, 1966.

---

duced by bacterial contamination of food. These include upper respiratory infections and viral infectious hepatitis.

Common upper respiratory infections. Persons infected with viruses that produce diseases of the upper respiratory tract such as colds and influenza often transmit these illnesses through foods. They may, with soiled hands, handle unwrapped foods in stores or cafeterias; or they may sneeze or cough over them.

Viral infectious hepatitis (virus A). Acute viral hepatitis, an inflammatory disease of the liver, is caused by either of two strains of virus: virus A causes infectious hepatitis (IH), virus B causes serum hepatitis (SH). Virus B has been found only in blood and is transmitted only by parenteral inoculation (intravenous transfusion of infected blood or injection with a contaminated needle). Virus A is usually transmitted by the fecal-oral route common to food- and water-borne diseases. Explosive epidemics have occurred in towns, schools, and other communities after fecal contamination of water, milk, or food. Shellfish contaminated by living in polluted water have been a source of several outbreaks. Continuous vigilance in maintaining community controls of water, milk, and food supplies and stringent personal hygiene and sanitary practices by food handlers are essential to the prevention of infectious hepatitis.

Fungus toxins (mycotoxins)

Crop damage by molds has long been an economic problem. Only recently, however, has it been demonstrated that foods may be contaminated by toxins that are produced by molds (fungi). Such toxins are called mycotoxins (Gr. *myco,* fungus; L. *toxicum,* poison). Several toxins formed by fungi have been studied.

Aflatoxins. First found in peanut meal fed to poultry, aflatoxins were extracted and found to be produced by strains of *Aspergillus flavus,* a common storage mold.[4] The name aflatoxins comes from the abbreviation *A. flavus.* Isolation and identification of four aflatoxins was accomplished in 1963. Apparently the toxins are produced immediately after harvesting and early in the storage period. Rapid drying, improved storage conditions, and possible use of fungicides would be important control measures.

Natural food poisons

Naturally occurring toxicants in foods are ubiquitous. In general, though, they do not present hazards to health in the average diet of normal healthy individuals because concentrations are usually low, the toxicities are not additive, or neutralizing interactions occur.[5,6]

However, certain plants and animals contain poisonous substances that do occasionally cause human illness or death. Most of these toxic substances are poisonous alkaloids, such as strychnine, atropine, scopolamine, and solanine. For unknown reasons some organisms are toxic at one season of the year and not at others; some plants produce toxic substances at one point in their growth cycle and not at others. Humans have been cognizant for centuries of some of these toxic plants and animals; others have been recognized, and their toxins isolated, only recently. A few examples of these organisms that are poisonous as food are listed in the following sections.

Poisonous plants

Cottonseed. A toxic pigment, *gossypol,* contained in cottonseed, has created problems in preparing protein-rich food supplements for use in combating protein malnutrition throughout the world. Procedures for removing the toxin from cottonseed meal during processing have been devised, and efforts are being made to develop strains of the plant that do not contain gossypol.

Soybeans. A trypsin inhibitor in *raw* soybeans is responsible for a toxic substance contained in them. Fortunately this substance is destroyed by heat and is therefore easily inactivated by cooking.

Cycad nuts. Plants of the genus *Cycas,* common in tropical and subtropical areas, are intermediate in appearance between ferns and palms. Many species have a thick, unbranched, columnar trunk bearing a crown of large, leathery, pinnate leaves. The nuts are sometimes eaten in times of extreme need, as during famine; they were investigated in Guam as a possible cause of a disease of the nervous system, *amyotrophic lateral sclerosis* (ALS), observed in persons who had eaten them. In 1960 they were found to contain the active toxin *cycasin,* which was isolated and chemically identified. The toxin is now removed from the nuts by a washing process before they are eaten.

Potatoes. The green part of sprouting white potatoes contains sufficient amount of the toxic substance solanine to cause gastroenteritis, jaundice, and prostration. Solanine is a poisonous, narcotic alkaloid. Usually it is removed with the peel before the potato is cooked.

Mushrooms. Certain species of mushroom belong to the poisonous genus *Amanita.* Wild mushrooms should be strictly avoided as food. A number of edible species of mushrooms are grown commercially.

Rhubarb leaves. The large amount of oxalic acid contained in rhubarb leaves causes illness. These leaves should not be used as leafy greens for cooking and eating. Edible leafy greens are spinach, chard, mustard, turnip, and a few others.

Fava bean. *Favism* is the name given to a severe form of hemolytic anemia produced by the ingestion (or by the inhalation of pollen) of fava beans *(Vicia faba)* in persons sensitive to them. This sensitivity is caused by a genetically controlled deficiency of the enzyme glucose-6-phosphate dehydrogenase in the shunt pathway (see hexose monophosphate shunt, p. 30) for glucose oxidation normally found in the red blood cell. This genetic trait was first observed in certain members of the Mediterranean (Sicilian and Sardinian) and African populations, and has more recently been noted in about 10% of blacks in the United States. The same genetic trait provides some protection against falciparum malaria. It is a good example of an evolutionary genetic adaptation of a population group to a disease process. Susceptible individuals also react to antimalaria drugs such as primaquine phosphate and to the analgesic phenacetin in the same way they react to fava beans.

Wild plants. Hemlock, wild parsnip, monkshood, foxglove, and deadly nightshade are a few of the many wild plants known to be poisonous. Occasionally they are mistaken for harmless plants they resemble and are inadvertently eaten.

Poisonous animals

Puffer fish. The puffer fish (family Tetraodontidae) is so named because it is capable of inflating its body with water or air until it forms a globe. It has a gland containing a powerful neurotoxin, *tetraodontoxin,* which causes death soon after ingestion. Nonetheless, the puffer fish is considered a delicacy in the Orient, and chefs take pride in their ability to remove the gland with great care before cooking the fish. This game of chance brings death from tetraodontoxin poisoning to a number of persons each year whose chefs' knives slipped!

Clams and mussels. During the summer months, certain species of clam and mussel in waters along the Pacific Coast from Alaska to California feed on marine organisms, plankton, which infect the fish and produce a toxic alkaloid similar to strychnine. At this season the eating of these fish can be fatal.

Herring. At different seasons in various locations, herring apparently become poisonous as human food. Poisonings have been observed from herring caught in the waters around Cuba and Tahiti from May to October and in waters around the New Hebrides Islands in the South Pacific from April to July. Just what accounts for these seasonal changes is not known.

Barracuda. Observations have been made of seasonal poisoning from barracuda. In Florida, in the spring and summer of 1954, four outbreaks of poisoning were traced to the eating of barracuda.

Food spoilage

Food-borne disease and economic waste may also be caused by general food spoilage.

Food may deteriorate or become contaminated by chemical or physical changes, by microbial growth, or by contact with insects or rodents.

Chemical spoilage. Chemical spoilage may be due to oxidation. Fats may become rancid, and fruits may be discolored. Hydrogen gas formation in canned foods may cause cans to swell. Enzymatic activity causes color changes and a haylike flavor in old frozen vegetables.

Physical spoilage. Physical spoilage may be manifested as granulation, as in honey or ice cream. (While granulation does not spoil honey in the sense that it becomes harmful as food, this change in its appearance and texture makes it unacceptable to many customers.) Sunlight destroys the riboflavin content of milk.

Microbial spoilage. Microbial spoilage may be caused by bacteria, yeasts, or molds. Souring of milk, contamination of cooked food that has been held too long before eating, mold growth on bread, and rotting of fruits and vegetables may present problems of disease control and economic loss.

Animal and insect spoilage. Food storage problems are constantly presented by insects and rodents. Hairs, droppings, fragments of insects, and disease organisms may be deposited. Rigorous vector control programs are attempted by public officials, but in some areas the problem may exceed the community resources to combat it adequately.

Radioactivity in foods

Many communities are concerned with the extent of food contamination by radioactive fallout. Peacetime uses of atomic energy release small amounts of radioactive materials into the environment. The benefits that may be gained by the use of atomic energy, in contrast to its biologic risk and cost, demand more careful scientific and philosophic study.

Vegetation may be contaminated directly or through the soil, and animals, especially cattle, can become contaminated both directly and through their forage and water. Humans, in turn, ingest radioactivity in milk (strontium-90) and meat and their products.

Monitoring systems reveal that present radiation levels are far below those permissible in the human life span. Radioactivity in foods is checked extensively and continuously by the Federal Drug Administration (FDA), the Public Health Service, and the Atomic Energy Commission. Their current findings do not seem to warrant government action or changes in habits of buying or preparing foods.

FOOD ADDITIVES (man-made chemicals)

A number of chemicals have been developed by the agricultural and food processing industries to increase and preserve food. They have rapidly changed the character of America's present food supply and its environment in a complex "feeding web," which has increasingly raised issues in nutritional ecology.[7] As a result, some critics voice concerns in the public press as consumers become increasingly aware of the rapid changes food processing has brought to our overall food environment.[8] They wonder if the chemist more than the farmer determines the American diet. In any event, knowledge of these food processes is important to the consumer and to the health practitioner as a basis for making wise food choices and providing prudent counseling.

These man-made chemicals may be intentional or incidental (adventitious) additives.

Intentional food additives

In the past three decades chemicals intentionally added to foods have to an increasing degree become components of the food supply. The present variety of marketed items would be impossible without them.

The use of additives has been a major factor in the rapid evolution of the corner grocery store into the supermarket. The change that has swept the food marketing system during the last 25 years is rooted in a deeper social revolution and in scientific advance. Among the reasons

for development and use of food additives are the following:

1. Because of the unprecedented population growth, more food must be produced. However, this greater quantity must be produced on less land, and it is more important than ever before that food be preserved and protected from waste and spoilage.

2. New and widely publicized discoveries have increased the food purchaser's awareness of nutritional needs and have impressed him with the importance to health of a well-balanced diet. Specific foods are enriched or fortified to help supply these needs.

3. There is an increased desire for variety in foods and creativity in cooking. Foods from local and distant places provide great variety in choice. New types of foods change cooking procedures in the average American kitchen.

4. The increasing complexity of family life and the number of working wives and mothers have created a desire for convenience foods that require little preparation time.

5. People generally want safe, quality food. Wholesome food is an increasing concern of individuals and families. Most Americans are becoming more aware that their health depends on an adequate supply of fresh or properly preserved foods. Efforts of the consumer to purchase quality food are backed by laws governing food production, processing (including the use of intentional additives), and sale. However, the rapidly changing food environment requires constant reevaluation of these laws to ensure their adequacy to meet needs.

Purposes served by food additives

Intentional additives may be grouped according to the purpose they serve in a particular food.

Addition of specific nutrients. Certain foods have proved to be good carriers for factors essential to sound nutrition. To other foods, nutrients have been added to replace those removed in processing. Examples include the addition of iodine to salt, ascorbic acid to many fruit juices, vitamin D to milk, vitamin A to margarine, and the B vitamins (thiamin, niacin, and riboflavin) and iron to cereal products. As a result of enrichment, controlled in many instances by enrichment laws, deficiency diseases such as goiter and pellagra have largely been eliminated from the American population. The enrichment of bread and cornmeal has helped to control pellagra in the southern United States. The addition of vitamin D to milk has reduced the incidence of rickets in this country.

Production of uniform sensory properties. The esthetic value of food is enhanced by such sensory properties as color, flavor, aroma, texture, and general appearance. For many persons, otherwise nutritious foods may be unappealing in appearance, taste, aroma, or texture and may often go uneaten. In their natural state, samples of a given food may vary widely in color and flavor according to the season or locality in which they are harvested or to the species. Natural and synthetic flavoring agents, colorings, preservatives, and texturing materials have been added by food processors to give increased appeal and characteristic uniformity to common food products.

An example of color control is the addition of bleaching agents to processed flour. Small quantities of natural pigments in freshly milled wheat flour give it a yellowish color, which many persons find less attractive than pure white. Such flour also lacks the qualities necessary to make the elastic stable dough necessary for making bread of the texture that seems to be preferred by many Americans. Natural aging and ripening permit the development of these characteristics, and for years long aging was the only way millers and bakers could make desired products. Natural aging, however, was time consuming, costly, and wasteful. Deterioration and infestation from insects and rodents took a great toll. About 1915, a process for bleaching flours was discovered, and a little later a method for accelerating its maturation was found. Today bleaching and maturing agents produce uniform products for immediate use. Without these agents, cakes, breads, and cake mixes as they are known today could not exist.

Standardization of functional properties. A number of additives enhance and standardize the functional properties of given foods. In this class are emulsifiers, stabilizers, moisture retainers, thickeners, binders, dough conditioners, anticaking agents, jelling agents, and others. Many of the common processed foods would be impossible or far more difficult to prepare without such additives.

Preservation of food. Many agents are added to food to help maintain it long past the peak of harvest time or the time of processing. Salt and certain curing agents preserve meat and make possible a variety of meat products. Antioxidants prevent discoloration of fruits and rancidity of fats. Antimycotic agents, such as mold inhibitors, and bacterial control agents, such as "rope" inhibitors, preserve bread and other baked products. Sequestrants (L. *sequester,* a depository) set apart, in an inactive form, trace substances in food that would otherwise interfere with its processing. For example, in fats, sequestrants combine with trace minerals such as iron and copper and prevent their catalytic action, which would hasten oxidation— the cause of rancidity in fats. Sequestrants also inactivate certain minerals in the water that is used in making soft drinks. This prevents turbidity caused by the minerals settling out during processing.

Control of acidity or alkalinity. The acidity or alkalinity of foods often affects their flavor, texture, and the cooked product. Various acids, alkalis, buffers, and neutralizing agents are used in processed foods to achieve the desired balance or flavor. For example, acids contribute flavor to candy and help prevent a grainy texture. The flavor of many soft drinks is modified by the addition of acid. Acids and alkalis constitute leavening agents such as baking powder. In making butter, alkali is added to sour

Table 12-1. Some examples of intentional food additives

Function	Chemical compound	Common food uses
Acids, alkalis, buffers	Sodium bicarbonate	Baking powder
	Tartaric acid	Fruit sherbets
		Cheese spreads
Antibiotics	Chlortetracycline	Dip for dressed poultry
Anticaking agents	Aluminum calcium silicate	Table salt
Antimycotics	Calcium propionate	Bread
	Sodium propionate	Bread
	Sorbic acid	Cheese
Antioxidants	Butylated hydroxyanisole (BHA)	Fats
	Butylated hydroxytoluene (BHT)	Fats
Bleaching agents	Benzoyl peroxide	Wheat flour
	Chlorine dioxide	
	Oxides of nitrogen	
Color preservative	Sodium benzoate	Green peas
		Maraschino cherries
Coloring agents	Annotto	Butter, margarine
	Carotene	
Emulsifiers	Lecithin	Bakery goods
	Monoglycerides and digylcerides	Dairy products
	Propylene glycol alginate	Confections
Flavoring agents	Amyl acetate	Soft drinks
	Benzaldehyde	Bakery goods
	Methyl salicylate	Candy; ice cream
	Essential oils; natural extractives	
	Monosodium glutamate	Canned meats
Nonnutritive sweeteners	Saccharin, calcium, and sodium cyclamates	Diet packed canned fruit Low-calorie soft drinks
Nutrient supplements	Potassium iodide	Iodized salt
	Vitamin C	Fruit juices
	Vitamin D	Milk
	Vitamin A	Margarine
	B vitamins, iron	Bread and cereal
Sequestrants	Sodium citrate	Dairy products
	Calcium pyrophosphoric acid	
Stabilizers and thickeners	Pectin	Jellies
	Vegetable gums (carob bean, carrageenan, guar)	Dairy desserts and chocolate milk Confections
	Gelatin	"Low-calorie" salad dressings
	Agar-agar	
Yeast foods and dough conditioners	Ammonium chloride	Bread, rolls
	Calcium sulfate	
	Calcium phosphate	

cream so that it will churn properly and yield a satisfactory flavor.

Some common examples of intentional food additives are listed in Table 12-1.

Problems in control of food additives

Although food additives have served many useful purposes in the development of the modern food industry, problems have accrued along with these gains. These problems are of increasing concern to consumers and producers.

Food Additives Amendment and Delaney Clause. The Food Additives Amendment of the Federal Food, Drug, and Cosmetic Act of 1938 was passed on September 6, 1958. This amendment, which took effect on March 6, 1960, completely altered the U.S. government's method of regulating the use of additives in food. The law provided for the first time that no additive could be used in food unless the FDA after a careful review of the test data, agreed that the compound was safe at the intended levels of use. An exception was made for all additives in use at that time, which, because of years of widespread use without deleterious effects reported, were "generally recognized as safe" (GRAS) by experts in the field. This approach was a compromise between giving blanket approval to all additives then in use or banning all untested food additives until several years of laboratory safety studies could be conducted.

The Delaney Clause was attached in the final hours of congressional debate on the legislation. This clause to the Food Additives Amendment states that "no additive shall be deemed safe if it is found to induce cancer when ingested by man or animal, or if it is found after tests which are appropriate for the evaluation of the safety of food additives, to induce cancer in man or animal." It was under this clause, for example, that cyclamates were banned in 1969.[9] Saccharin is now under the threat of a similar fate, and new alternative sweeteners are being sought.[10,11]

GRAS list. The result of the Food Additives Amendment has been to establish what is now known as the GRAS list, that large number of food additives "generally recognized as safe" but not having undergone rigid testing requirements. This list includes several thousand food additives, including salt, sugar, baking powder, spices, flavorings, vitamins, minerals, preservatives, emulsifiers, and nonnutritive sweeteners. Some of them are restricted to uses in certain foods and at certain levels, but most are limited only to their "intended use" and to "good manufacturing practice."

Problems, however, exist with the GRAS list. First, there is an uncertainty as to how many GRAS items there are, and no single compilation of them exists. Quoted statements concerning the number range from approximately six hundred to several thousand. FDA officials themselves are uncertain about how many GRAS items there are. Second, in the years since the GRAS list was formulated, two developments have had direct bearing on the soundness of the original GRAS concept. (1) We have become much more sophisticated about toxicity testing, and we have recognized the inadequacy of relying on a lack of reported human adverse effect as the sole measure of safety. (2) We have also seen the demands of modern technology increase the uses of certain GRAS items well beyond the exposure patterns considered in the original development of the GRAS list. In short, the total food environment has changed radically, creating new problems.

As a result, the U.S. government has directed the FDA to reevaluate all the items on the GRAS list for safety. However, this poses an almost impossible task with present allocations of funds and manpower to accomplish the directive. Herein lies the basis of our present dilemma; food additives are facing increasing public scrutiny.

Incidental (adventitious) food additives

The chemicals used in American agriculture have made possible the advances in food production that are required to meet the demands of a growing population. Today's farmer uses chemicals to control a wide variety of destructive insects, to kill weeds, to control plant diseases, to stop fruit from dropping prematurely, to make leaves drop so that harvesting will be easier, to make seeds sprout, to keep seeds from rotting before they sprout, and for many other purposes related to increased yield and improved marketing qualities.

Pesticide residues in food

Another source of increasing concern to farm workers, consumers, and the general public is the effect of current levels at which agricultural chemicals are used to increase needed food production practices that have led to our present "pesticide dilemma."[12] The use of these agricultural chemicals brings hazard as well as gain. Recognition of the necessity for control led to the initial Federal Food, Drug, and Cosmetic Act of 1938, which established procedures for setting "safe" (a difficult determination at best when human health and life are involved) limits (tolerances) on the amount of pesticide residues permitted on crops. An effort was made by Congress to establish more workable and realistic controls through the 1958 Food Additives Amendment, which gave the FDA greater responsibility and authority for controlling chemical residues in food. Today the FDA directs a pesticide control program in two phases: (1) requirement for initial approval and (2) continued surveillance.

Initial approval of a chemical for use. Any chemical for which an agricultural use is planned is subjected by the manufacturer to several years of development and controlled testing before it is submitted to the FDA to be approved for use. The FDA, if it grants its approval, also sets the tolerances under which the chemical must be used. A tolerance is granted only on definite proof, by pharmacologic tests, that the residues are safe at levels greatly exceeding those remaining on the food. An effort is made to set the tolerance amount at the lowest level that will accomplish the agricultural purpose, even if it is thought that larger amounts would still be safe.

Enforcement through continued surveillance. The FDA seeks to enforce the laws governing use of pesticides in three ways: through public education, sampling of field produce, and market basket studies.

PUBLIC EDUCATION. FDA inspectors and laboratory scientists keep in constant touch with producers, growers, county agents, insect control specialists, pesticide dealers, and agriculture stations. They try to learn the nature of pest problems in various localities throughout the United States. They observe which pesticides are being recommended and used in different localities and what violations may be most likely. All known violations are acted on immediately.

OBJECTIVE SAMPLING OF FIELD PRODUCE. In all states crops are periodically sampled at random and inspected at producing, shipping, and destination points. A large number of samples are taken to ensure reliable results. Tests are sometimes conducted on the spot in mobile trailer laboratories. If excessive residues of harmful chemicals are found, the goods are seized and, if necessary, destroyed. Although as a result of this sampling program most growers are careful to comply with directions and laws governing the use of pesticides, complete enforcement is difficult and problems may occur in various locations from human error or lack of concern.

MARKET BASKET STUDIES. In 1961, annual surveys of pesticide residues in the total diet of persons living in the United States were begun as an additional check on the chemical safety of food consumed. Since a 19-year-old man eats more than almost any other American, he was selected as the reference person. Each year in five regions and 30 cities of the United States, a list of the food that would be eaten by a 19-year-old man over a two-week period is made out by nutritionists. All food on the list is purchased in local markets and prepared for the table. After the prepared food has been grouped into 12 classes to facilitate analysis, the foods of each group are homogenized, and a composite sample is examined by highly sensitive laboratory tests for a number of pesticide residues. The test results are compared with the daily intake levels jointly set as acceptable by the United Nations Food and Agriculture Organization and the World Health Organization Expert Committee. These studies have indicated that the amounts of pesticide residue in foods as consumed are below the currently acceptable levels. This information supplements the data from field sampling.

FOOD PROTECTION FROM FARM TO TABLE

From producer to consumer, modern devices and practices are applied to protect food and to ensure its quality and safety. However, despite these assurances the "pesticide dilemma" is a real presence. In a carefully researched *National Geographic* article, Boraiko graphically illustrates the reality of the public problem facing scientists, farmers, and government alike.[12] Much activity is involved in providing consumers with the variety of foods that are available today.

Crop control and protection. Before a specific crop is sown, the seed is selected from the improved strains that are constantly being developed and tested in agricultural research units. While the crop is growing, it is protected from damage by numerous insect, plant disease, and weed control measures. The U.S. Department of Agriculture operates an alert plant disease forecasting program, similar to the weather forecasts supplied by the Weather Bureau, so that farmers can plan for crop protection.

Harvesting. The eating quality of many foods depends on their being harvested rapidly at the right moment in their development. Quality also depends on getting them immediately from the field to the processor. Mechanization has speeded most harvesting processes. For example, large machines move through lettuce fields and, in one complex operation, harvest the lettuce, wrap each head individually in film, and box it. It is then ready to be picked up by a side truck and transported to the wholesale market under refrigeration.

Transportation. Modern refrigeration design and equipment in trucks, trailers, and railroad cars have reduced losses of fresh produce. For overseas shipment, refrigerated trailer vans ("fishybacks") are driven to dockside, and the entire trailer van container is lifted aboard ship and carried to its destination as a unit. Opening of the van and handling of its contents during transfers en route are eliminated. For example, Florida grapefruit arrives at Swiss markets intact and in excellent condition. Better loading patterns and newer fiberboard boxes have also prevented much bruising and damaging during transportation.

Milk and meat protection. Because milk and meat are particularly susceptible to contamination by harmful microorganisms, special laws govern their production and marketing.

MILK PRODUCTION. The modern dairy industry is founded on many years of experience and research, which have built dependable safeguards into milk processing to ensure high quality. Rigidly enforced government ordinances regulate the handling of milk from farm to consumer.

Disease in milk-producing cows is eradicated by veterinary programs under government control. For example, bovine tuberculosis, brucellosis, and mastitis are quickly eliminated by constant, sensitive testing and vaccination and by the isolation and treatment of affected cows. Personnel and equipment involved in care and milking of the animals and in the handling of the milk are required to pass rigid health and sanitation inspections.

Cows are usually milked by machines, which pipe the milk to storage tanks without exposure to contaminating dust and insects. In these refrigerated tanks, the milk is cooled quickly to about 3° C (38° F) and held at that temperature throughout a brief storage period and while it is being transported in refrigerated tank trucks to the dairy.

At the processing plant the milk is first subjected to a vacuum treatment which removes objectionable flavors that may have resulted from certain grasses or from wild onions, for example, that have been eaten by the cow. Next it is pasteurized by any of several legal heat treatments. For example, the milk can be held at 63° C (145° F) for 30 minutes or at 72° C (161° F) for 15 seconds. Pasteurization destroys disease-producing organisms that might be present in the milk and also kills bacteria that could grow during storage under refrigeration. It renders milk and milk products not only safe for consumption but also less likely to spoil during storage and marketing.

Homogenization is usually associated with pasteurization. By homogenization the fat globules are reduced in size and evenly dispersed so that the cream does not separate from the milk. Vitamin D is added to compensate for the lack of this vitamin in milk. The standard supplement is 400 IU (10 μg cholecalciferol) per quart. Finally, the milk is packaged and kept refrigerated until it is delivered to the consumer. At each step the production, processing, marketing, and delivery of milk are constantly regulated and supervised by law enforcement agencies. These include at the federal level the U.S. Public Health Service, the U.S. Department of Agriculture, and the FDA; at the state level the state departments of health and agriculture; and at the local level city and county governments.

MEAT PRODUCTION. The circular purple stamp placed on meat and poultry that have passed government inspection is the consumer's guarantee of a safe, wholesome product. Under the Meat Inspection Act of 1906 and the Poultry Products Inspection Act of 1957 the Consumer and Marketing Service of the U.S. Department of Agriculture controls the commercial marketing of meat and poultry. Qualified inspectors scrutinize meat production and marketing in

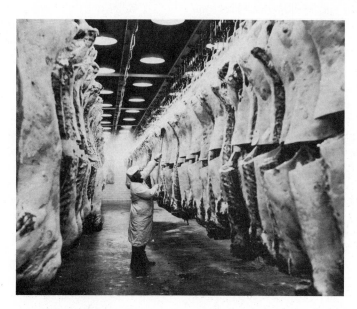

Fig. 12-1. Meat inspection and grading. A U.S. Department of Agriculture meat grader marks the quality grade on beef carcasses at an Omaha, Nebraska, packing plant. (USDA photograph.)

every detail. They are concerned with sanitation of the processing plant, inspection of animals at the stockyard before slaughter, immediate examination of the carcass and internal organs, and inspection during meat processing, curing, canning, and smoking. They also regulate disposal of condemned material, the marking and labeling of products, and inspection of imported meat (Fig. 12-1). There is need, however, for better labeling instructions for consumers to prevent disease from improper handling of the meat after initial inspection. At present no such labeling requirements exist.

Storage. Tremendous amounts of food are stored each year for consumption by market animals and by the population of our country and for shipping overseas. Well-built storage facilities are constantly checked for temperature and humidity. Effort is made to protect the stored food from harm by insects, fungi, mold, bacteria, and rodents through the application of control measures.

Marketing. Safeguards applied in most supermarkets continue to protect food for the consumer. Temperature and humidity controls keep the food in optimal condition until it is purchased. Programs for inspection of perishables are designed to maintain high standards. Problems exist in many communities, however, because of insufficient funds and inspection personnel to vigorously carry out the programs to enforce existing codes. There are specific codes for regulating the handling and temperature of frozen foods, for rotating shelf goods to maintain the freshness of canned and packaged foods, and for sanitary handling and facilities to ensure cleanliness.

Home care. The final steps in the protection of food for the family are the responsibility of the consumers. Unless they handle the products intelligently, the industry's efforts to supply them with safe, high-quality food are wasted. They should first select foods of the best quality they can afford, either from the market or from the farm. Alert consumers will purchase sound,

fresh produce and will look for reliable grades in processed food, reading labels carefully. At home they will store foods promptly under proper conditions of space, ventilation, and refrigeration and will use each within the recommended storage periods. Finally, they will prepare and serve the food and will care for leftovers by methods that protect their natural goodness and food value and that avert spoilage. Ultimately a large part of the power to effect change and regulate food production and marketing lies with the consumer. With the present and increasing complexity of the food environment and changing food forms and channels, the consumer can no longer afford to be apathetic or unknowledgeable.

FOOD PRESERVATION

To keep seasonal excess quantities for later use, to enable foods to withstand transportation to distant places, and to protect them from spoilage and contamination, various methods of food preservation have been developed.

Drying

Perhaps the oldest known method of preserving food is drying. Removing most of the moisture from highly perishable fruits and vegetables, for example, halts the growth of bacteria contained in them and extends the period in which they are edible. Drying is a *bacteriostatic* method of preservation. Fresh grapes rot quickly. But for many centuries, grapes have been preserved by making them into raisins by a method that is essentially unchanged even today. The fruit is laid out on open racks and dried in the sun. Since primitive times, people have preserved meat and fish by drying and have added smoking, salting, and curing to the process.

Newer forms of dried foods include such items as skimmed milk and eggs. Impetus was given the exploration of drying processes by the successful development of field rations used by soldiers in World War II and by the obvious convenience of such products both to the consumer and to the marketer. Properly dried foods lose none of their nutrients, are light to handle, occupy far less storage space than fresh foods, and are exceedingly simple to prepare. In this busy era and in homes with limited storage space, these are important advantages. An entire new branch of the food industry has been developed to prepare and market an array of instant foods—potatoes, tea, coffee, fruit juice, sauces, soups, and substitutes for coffee cream. The list of such items grows daily.

Canning

Canning is a *bactericidal* method of food preservation. It destroys bacteria with heat. The history of the canning process is a story of human response to the pressure of crisis and of human persistent ingenuity in finding a solution.

In the late 1700s France was burdened by wars with England, Prussia, Austria, and Spain and with revolution at home. By 1795 more French soldiers were dying from malnutrition and scurvy than from bullets. In desperation the five-man French Directory offered a prize of 12,000 francs to the patriot who could find a way to preserve food long enough so that it could be transported to the front. An obscure French citizen, Nicolas Appert, took the offer seriously. Until then he had drifted in and out of a number of jobs involving food and drink. He had been chef, pickler, preserver, candymaker, winemaker, brewer, and distiller. In response to this challenge, he began to work in earnest. For 14 years he experimented with methods and materials. In 1810 he succeeded in preventing food from spoiling by packing it in an airtight container. He was awarded the prize by the French Minister of the Interior. In 1811 Appert published an account of his method, *L'art de conserver, pendant plusieurs années, toutes les substances animales et végétales* (The Art of Preserving for Several Years All Animal and Vegetable Substances). Appert knew from long

trial and error that heat applied to food sealed in an airtight container prevented spoilage. But he did not know why. It was not until 1857 that another Frenchman, Louis Pasteur, demonstrated chemically that spoilage was caused by microorganisms, which Appert's canning method destroyed. Although Appert did not know that microorganisms existed, he stated the two essentials that have long been proved valid and are still followed: (1) complete cleanliness in the process and (2) a permanent seal on the container to exclude air.

From France, Appert's method immediately spread to England, where in 1810 Peter Durand developed and patented a container made of iron and tin. The word canister, from the Greek word *kanastron,* meaning "basket of reeds," was being used in England for the reed baskets that held tea, coffee, spices, or fruit. Durand called his crude container a metal canister.

In 1819, canning reached America. William Underwood in Boston began using cumbersome glass jars with sealed cork stoppers; in 1839 he substituted the metal canisters. His workmen shortened the word to "can," and the slang term shortly became accepted as the official name. It has remained to label a giant modern food industry.

Modern "tin" cans are not actually made of tin. They are thin sheets of specially prepared steel, coated with tin by dipping or electroplating. Today's canning plant, with its sanitary, automated production line and sophisticated quality controls, is a far cry from Appert's crude beginnings. But the hermetically sealed container, filled under sanitary conditions and sterilized by heat, still preserves food by destroying microorganisms.

Freezing

Although ancient tribes living in cold climates no doubt learned that meat and fish could be held in frozen form for long periods, quick freezing came into being only in the 1920s when Clarence Birdseye first applied rapid freezing methods to fish for commercial purposes. In 1927 the process was extended to vegetables, and the frozen food industry began to grow. Frozen precooked food was first offered for sale in the late 1940s. Today more than 700 frozen items are found in supermarkets and more are yet to come.

Freezing destroys many microorganisms and inhibits the growth of others. Because frozen foods are not sterile, they must be handled as perishables from the time they are processed until they are eaten. The moment they are thawed, bacteria begin to multiply. This is no problem with such frozen foods as vegetables and meats, which are cooked in the same way as fresh foods. However, precooked frozen foods are exposed to greater hazards of contamination during processing so that it is necessary to take extra precautions at all stages of preparation. The two factors that have proved important in the control of microorganisms and in the maintenance of high quality in the frozen product are time and temperature. Rapid, sanitary food preparation followed immediately by quick freezing controls bacterial growth and prevents damage to the cell walls, which would break down the texture. Quick freezing is made possible by the use of liquid nitrogen ($-160°$ C [$-320°$ F]) or fluidized-bed freezers. After the initial quick freezing, it is imperative that the food be stored at a low temperature and used before expiration of the recommended storage time. Most frozen food should be held at $-18°$ C ($0°$ F) or lower; $-23°$ C ($-10°$ F) is better.

Newer methods of food preservation

Two methods that represent attempts to combine the best features of freezing and drying and one method that is based on the pharmacologic destruction of microorganisms are already in commercial use; a fourth, irradiation, is in an advanced phase of practical application but is still being extensively tested.

Freeze-drying. Piece-form foods such as fruits and seafoods are kept frozen while they dry in a vacuum. This retains the original size and shape of the food but greatly reduces its weight. A freeze-dried strawberry is the same size as the fresh strawberry, but weighs only one sixteenth as much. This lightness is an advantage in handling and transportation. Because vacuum drying by piece is a costly method of water removal, it is usually restricted to high-cost foods such as meats and seafoods or to special military situations. At the present stage, piece-form foods processed by this technique are less excellent in taste and meet with less acceptance than do quick-frozen or canned foods. Other nonfood items such as coffee are now freeze-dried for the convenience of quick preparation.

Dehydrofreezing. Fruits and vegetables are first dehydrated to about 50% of their original weight and volume, but not until their quality is impaired, then frozen. The quality of dehydrofrozen foods is usually equal to that of foods processed by the standard quick-freezing methods. They have the advantages of lighter weight and less bulk, and therefore they cost less to package, freeze, store, and ship. Foods that have been satisfactorily dehydrofrozen include potatoes, carrots, peas, apples, apricots, berries, and cherries. They are used chiefly in commercially prepared combinations, as vegetables in soup or fruits in pies.

Use of antibiotics. In 1955 and 1956 the FDA approved the use of chlortetracycline and oxytetracycline for the preservation of raw poultry. Tolerance levels were established in 1959 for chlortetracycline in preserving certain kinds of raw fish and shellfish. Since about 10% of the population of the United States are sensitive to various drugs, the addition of antibiotics to foods must be carefully controlled. Only small amounts of the antibiotic may be employed. Residues in tissues are destroyed in cooking. Used under specified conditions, these antibiotics significantly increase retention of quality in fresh poultry and fish during storage.

A food-grade antibiotic (from 10 to 20 ppm.)

is added to the ice-slush that chills cleaned and dressed poultry carcasses. Usually the poultry remains in this solution from one to two hours and then is drained and packaged for shipment to retailers. Antibiotics are a constituent of preservative dips for fresh fish fillets, of refrigerated brines in which dressed whole fish are held in fishing vessels, and in ice used to refrigerate fish during transport, processing, and marketing. The feed of agricultural animals is supplemented with antibiotics to stimulate growth and to treat disease. Many crop sprays contain antibiotics. When properly used in any of these ways, antibiotics have not been shown to constitute a hazard to human health.

IRRADIATION. Although the process of ionizing radiation has not developed as yet as an acceptable method of food preservation, it has been used experimentally during the past few years to determine its effectiveness and safety. It was first approved by the FDA in 1963 for use on canned bacon and bulk wheat, largely on the basis of extensive test data submitted by the U.S. Army Quartermaster Research Organization and others. Gamma radiation was used to kill insect life in bulk wheat; the electron beam was used to sterilize bacon. Irradiation under approved processes does *not* cause the food to become radioactive or to retain radioactivity that may have lingered in it from previous exposure.

Radiation, in its simplest terms, means the sending of energy from a source to an absorbing substance. Heat and sunlight are forms of radiation. In relation to radiation of food, however, the term is most often used to refer to the sending of electromagnetic X rays or gamma rays, both of which have a shorter wavelength than heat or light rays. These rays are used together with electrons, given off by a radioactive isotope or other radioactive subtance. The use of X rays, gamma rays, or electrons on food kills bacteria, inactivates some enzymes, and destroys insects. Cobalt 60 has been used as a source of gamma radiation. When used in food processing, the radioactive

isotope is sealed in a container that allows only the gamma rays to penetrate and radiate. Electron beams are best secured from man-made generators that accelerate electrons by high-voltage electrical fields.

Aside from high costs, there are two problems in developing a practical food irradiation process. First the radiation changes the characteristics of the food. Radiation high enough to completely sterilize food sometimes causes undesirable changes in flavor, appearance, and texture. Cooked meats, normally brown or gray, turn pink, lettuce wilts, egg whites thin, and baked products are reduced in volume. Second, there is the problem of safety. Thorough study, however, has now resulted in techniques that render safe levels and kinds of irradiation. Controlled gamma rays, such as from cobalt 60, do not produce radioactive elements in foods.

Although not yet applied on a commercial scale, irradiation may be used extensively for food preservation in the future. It may be employed not only to sterilize certain foods (4,500,000 rads destroys *C. botulinum,* the most resistant spoilage bacterium) to give them an indefinite shelf life, but also in smaller quantities (100,000 to 500,000 rads) to control other forms of spoilage. Such smaller doses of irradiation combined with refrigeration may greatly increase the preservation and storage life of perishables.

CONTROL AGENCIES TO PROTECT FOOD SAFETY AND QUALITY

A number of government and private agencies and professional organizations are charged with various responsibilities toward ensuring the safety and high quality of food. Among them are the organizations introduced in the previous chapter (p. 225) in relation to their work concerning food misinformation.

Foremost among concerned groups in the U.S. Department of Health and Human Services are the FDA and the Public Health Service; in the U.S. Department of Agriculture there are the Agricultural Research Service and the Consumer and Marketing Service. Also acting to protect the consumer are the Federal Trade Commission and the National Bureau of Standards.

Food and Drug Administration

The broad work of the FDA serves as an example of the U.S. government's effort to protect and control the food supply. In essence, the FDA is a law enforcement agency charged by Congress to ensure, among other things, that the food supply is safe, pure, and wholesome. It seeks to carry out its responsibility through scientific research and public education as well as by surveillance and enforcement. However, our rapidly changing environment and the problems it presents pose increasing problems.

Food standards. Section 401 of the Federal Food, Drug, and Cosmetic Act was designed "to promote honesty and fair dealing in the interest of Consumers." It directed the secretary of the Department of Health, Education, and Welfare (now the Department of Health and Human Services) to establish, for any food deemed necessary, regulations governing definition and standard of identity, reasonable standard of quality, and standards of fill of container. The food label must indicate these standards and must tell what is in the package. It must not be false or *misleading* in any particular.

STANDARDS OF IDENTITY. Reference standards have been established for a number of common foods such as jams, jellies, macaroni, noodles, mayonnaise, salad dressing, catsup, and cheese. A ratio of ingredients (or percentage of constituents) is established as specifically identifying that food item, and any food bearing that name on the label and sold as such must have been prepared exactly by that standard.[13] On such identified foods there is no requirement to list the ingredients, since they are named in the standard. For many less common foods, no standards of identity have been established, and the label must list all of the ingredients *in the order of their predominance* in the food.

Single copies of the complete text of these standards may be obtained without charge from the FDA.

STANDARDS OF QUALITY. For a number of canned fruits and vegetables, minimum standards have been set concerning such properties as tenderness, color, and freedom from defects. If such a fruit or vegetable is safe for human consumption but does not meet these standards, its label must carry a specific statement of the characteristic in which it is defective; for example, "broken parts," "excessive peel," or other indication.

STANDARDS OF FILL OF CONTAINER. For many foods, standards of fill have been established to protect the consumer against slack fillings. These are especially necessary for products that settle after filling, such as cereals, or for products that consist of a number of pieces packed in a liquid such as fruit cocktail. The legal standards ensure that no air, water, or space is sold as food and that the container fits the food.

STANDARDS FOR ENRICHED PRODUCTS. Standards are set for enrichment of flour, cereals, margarine, and other foods with specific quantities of vitamins and minerals. Any such product labeled "enriched" or "fortified" must contain precisely the specified amount of added nutrients.

Food labeling. Reports of inadequate nutrition in the U.S. population have accumulated, and public pressures have been generated during the past decade by the White House Conference on Food, Nutrition, and Health.[14-16] Also, consumer advocates have voiced needs for reexamination of control agencies and regulations.[17-19] These reports have triggered a reassessment of the FDA's program of food standards and labeling. As a result, new guidelines for the nutritional quality and labeling of process foods are being developed and tested.[20-22]

Over the next few months and years, food labels are going to take on a new look with more ingredient listing, nutrient accounting,

TO PROBE FURTHER
Early FDA regulations: "truth in packaging" laws

The Fair Packaging and Labeling Act. A law enacted in 1966, which took effect in July, 1967, initiated the procedures for bringing into being regulations requiring fuller and more prominent information on the labels of packaged foods. After initial publication of these proposed regulations and consideration of written comments and objections that were subsequently filed, the provisions were adopted in September, 1967.

Four basic regulations concerning label information have been specified*:

1. A statement of the food's identity must appear on the principal display panel in bold type.
2. The name and address of the manufacturer, packer, and distributor must be conspicuously stated.
3. A statement of the net contents must appear in concise standard measure. No qualifying terms, such as "giant quart," or "jumbo pound," may appear.
4. A statement listing ingredients, when required, must appear in type of legible size on a single panel of the label. The common names of the ingredients must appear in decreasing order of predominance.

Dietary foods regulations. The regulations also involve proposals for special diet foods, with particular reference to vitamin and mineral supplementation and low-calorie foods.† These proposals became effective upon completion of hearings and amendments in early 1969.

1. Vitamins and minerals:
   a. The following statement is proposed for use on all vitamin and mineral supplements: "Vitamins and minerals are supplied in abundant amounts by the foods we eat. The Food and Nutrition Board of the National Research Council recommends that dietary needs be satisfied by foods. Except for persons with special medical needs, there is not scientific basis for recommending routine use of dietary supplements."
   b. It is proposed that the National Research Council's recommended dietary allowances replace the outmoded, misleading, and frequently abused concept of "minimum daily requirement."
   c. It is proposed that eight classes of food that may be fortified with vitamins and minerals be stated and that the specific elements and amounts that may be used in these foods be clearly stipulated. These food groups are (1) pastes (macaroni products), (2) whole milk (fluid and powdered) for drinking, (3) fluid skimmed milk and fluid low fat milk for drinking, (4) fruit juices and drinks, (5) fruit products for infants, (6) processed cereals, (7) salt, and (8) formulas for infant feeding.
   d. It is proposed that extravagant, deceptive promotion of "shotgun" multivitamin and mineral supplements that serve no dietary need be prohibited. It is also proposed that specific required and optional elements and their amounts be indicated. In multivitamin products six ingredients are to be required (vitamin A, vitamin D, ascorbic acid, thiamin, riboflavin, niacin or niacinamide), and five others are to be optional (vitamin E, vitamin B_6, folic acid, pantothenic acid, vitamin B_{12}). In mineral supplements calcium and iron are to be required; phosphorus, magnesium, copper, and iodine are to be optional.
2. Low-calorie foods:
   a. It is proposed that use of the term "low calorie" on labels be restricted to those foods that contain 15 or fewer calories per serving.
   b. It is proposed that use of the term "lower in calories" be limited to those foods that contain at least 50% fewer calories than their ordinary food counterpart. Such comparison of calories in equivalent servings is to be clearly stated on the label. Any nonnutritive ingredients, such as artificial sweeteners or added bulk, are to be declared.

*Friedelson, I.: Fair packaging: synopsis of food packaging and labeling regulations, FDA Papers **1:**21, 1967.
†FDA proposes major overhaul of dietary food regulations, FDA report on enforcement and compliance, FDA, U.S. Dept. of Health, Education, and Welfare, Washington, D.C., July, 1966, p. 3.

and open dating.[23] In this age of consumerism there is increasing interest in food and nutrition and greater concern with food costs. Labels on foods will have to tell consumers what is in the food they buy and what its general freshness and quality is. To this end, new nutrient labeling regulations are being developed and put into practice to guide consumers.[24-27] Tools for its use are being developed.[28] This increased nutrient analysis of food products will also influence revised food value tables.[29]

Safe use of food additives. The many intentional food additives that make possible our wide variety of food products must first be approved for use by the FDA. The bureau frequently checks currently sold products to make certain that processors are following the rules that ensure the safety of the product. Problems, however, exist with the GRAS list of food additives (see p. 250).

Safe limits for pesticide residues in food. The amount of chemical residue from sprays and dusts applied to crops that may safely remain on food is carefully set as a tolerance limit by FDA scientists. FDA field inspectors check food shipments to see that these limits are observed. Market basket tests assure that food as consumed by the day-to-day buyer does not contain pesticide residues in excess of tolerance.

Nutritional misinformation. The FDA wages a continual campaign against food quackery and misinformation. Thousands of persons spend millions of dollars yearly on food supplements they do not need, some of which may be harmful. In the previous chapter on Food Misinformation this problem is discussed in detail.

Interstate food shipments and food imports. FDA officials constantly inspect food establishments and processing plants to see that standards of sanitation, food safety, and quality are maintained. Samples of foods shipped from one state to another are examined for purity and quality. Food imported from other countries is checked to see that it complies with U.S. law.

Check on food contamination in disasters. In cooperation with local and state officials, the FDA inspects food that has been damaged by flood, hurricane, fire, or other disaster and assists in the removal of contaminated items from the market.

Education of consumers. The Division of Consumer Education of the FDA carries on an active program of consumer protection through education and public information. Many excellent materials are prepared and distributed to individuals and student and community groups. Consumer specialists work through all FDA district offices.

Scientific research. As a basis for all its activities, in a world of burgeoning technology, the FDA scientists constantly seek to provide a

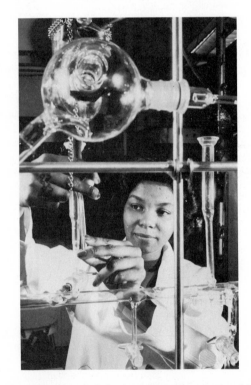

Fig. 12-2. Research in food chemistry. A chemist in the U.S. Department of Agriculture's Agricultural Research Service makes an adjustment on a molecular still used in a project to aid in the manufacture of dry milk. (USDA photograph.)

background of evaluation through their own research (Fig. 12-2). That they discharge this responsibility in a notable manner was formally recognized in 1956 by the presentation to them of the Lasker Award, with the statement that the FDA is "both a scientific institution and a federal law enforcement agency."

The declared intent of the persons in charge of the FDA is that food safety must be interpreted not only in the traditional sense that food must be free from danger, but also in the more positive sense that its nutritional value must be clear. Certainly it is reasonable for consumers to insist that additives introducing possible hazard without adding any benefits to food—for example, the use of sodium nitrate in baby foods, which has no value whatsoever for the baby and may be harmful—must be avoided.[30] Wise leaders in government and in the food industry will heed such real concerns.

To this end the FDA has asked the National Academy of Sciences to develop nutritional guidelines for certain food products, including formulated main dishes, new foods such as meat analogs, foods important as groups having high malnutrition risks, fruit juices and drinks, and snack foods. This is a broad jump from the former regulatory philosophy of years past and should go far toward meeting changing needs in these changing times.

CASE STUDY 2
A community food poisoning incident

John and Eva Wesson, a middle-aged couple, agreed that their lodge dinner had been the best they had ever had, especially the dessert ~~was good~~—custard-filled cream puffs, John's favorite. John had eaten two of them, despite Eva's protests at the time. Maybe that was why he began to feel ill shortly after they arrived home. Eva's stomach felt a little upset too, so John and Eva both took some antacid pills, thinking their "stomach ache" was from eating more rich food than they were accustomed to having. They went to bed early.

By 11 PM, however, Eva woke up alarmed. John was vomiting and having diarrhea and increasingly severe stomach cramps. He complained of headache. His pajamas were wet with sweat. He had a fever and appeared to be in shock. Eva herself began to have similar pains and symptoms, although not as severe as John's.

The phone rang. It was one of their friends who had also been at the lodge dinner. She and her husband were also experiencing the same reactions.

Now Eva was really frightened; John had recently begun to have some heart trouble, and she thought this attack was related. By now he was prostrate, unable to move. Eva immediately called their doctor, who arranged for John to be taken to the hospital. After treatment in the emergency room for shock, followed by observational care and rest the following day, John's symptoms had subsided, and he was allowed to go home. The doctor advised them to eat lightly for a few days and get more rest, and he said in the meantime he would investigate the cause. They learned during the next few days that almost all their lodge friends who had been at the dinner had had an experience similar to theirs.

The doctor contacted the public health department to report the incident. His was one of several similar calls, a public health officer said, and the department was already investigating.

The following week the officer returned the doctor's call to report his findings. The cream puffs served that evening by the restaurant had been purchased from a local bakery. At the bakery the health officials had located a worker with an infected cut on his little finger; a small thing, the worker said. He couldn't understand what all the fuss was about.

The health officials also located the delivery truck driver, who had started out at midmorning to make his rounds and take the cream puffs to the restaurant. On questioning the driver, however, they learned that the truck had "broken down" during the afternoon deliveries before he reached the restaurant. He said he remembered because he had been irritated by a three-hour wait at the garage while the truck was being fixed. But he still got the order to the restaurant in time for the dinner, he said, so what was the problem?

At the restaurant the chef said that everyone was so busy with the dinner that when the cream puffs finally arrived, no one had time to give much notice to them. They had decided there was no point in putting the cream puffs in the refrigerator at the time, since they were to be served in a very short while.

When John and Eva's doctor called them afterward to report the story, John and Eva decided they would not eat at that restaurant again. Besides, by then John had lost his taste for cream puffs.

CASE STUDY 2
A community food poisoning incident—cont'd

Questions to guide your inquiry

1. Why is control of a community's food supply an important responsibility of the health department?
2. What disease agents may be carried by food or water?
3. What was the agent causing John and Eva's illness? Was this a food infection or a food poisoning? How do you know?

   While the investigation was going on and before John and Eva learned the real cause of their illness, John thought it must have been caused by "those things farmers and food processers put into food these days. I've been reading about those things in the paper. It's a wonder we're not sick all the time."

4. What substances did John mean? Can you give some examples?
5. Why are these materials used for growing and processing food?
6. What controls do we have for their use?
7. What are some ways in which food is protected from its point of production to our tables?
8. How can food be preserved for later use?
9. What agency controls food safety and quality? How does it go about this important work? What are food standards? What are the current labeling regulations for food products?

REFERENCES
Specific

1. Most, H.: Current concepts in parasitology: trichinosis, N. Engl. J. Med. **298:**1178, May 25, 1978.
2. Goddard, J. L.: Incident at Selby Junior High, Nutr. Today **2**(3):2, 1967.
3. Terranova, W., and Blake, P. A.: Bacillus cereus food poisoning, N. Engl. J. Med. **298:**143, Jan. 19, 1978.
4. Ashcroft, R.: In Goldblatt, L., editor: Aflatoxin; scientific background, control, and implications, New York, 1969, Academic Press, Inc., p. 237.
5. Food and Nutrition Board, Committee on Food Protection, National Research Council: Toxicants occurring naturally in foods, ed. 2, Washington, D.C., 1973, National Academy of Sciences.
6. Coon, J. M.: Natural toxicants in food, J. Am. Diet. Assoc. **67:**213, Sept., 1975.
7. Gussow, J. D.: The feeding web: issues in nutritional ecology, Palo Alto, Calif., 1978, Bull Publishing Co.
8. Serrin, W.: Let them eat junk, Saturday Rev., Feb. 2, 1980, p. 17.
9. Wiegand, R. G.: Cyclamate. In Sweeteners: issues and uncertainties, Washington, D.C., 1975, National Academy of Sciences.
10. Food and Drug Administration: Saccharin and its salts, proposed rule and hearings, Federal Register **42:** 19996, April 15, 1977.
11. Wightman, N.: Saccharin—are there alternatives? J. Nutr. Educ. **9:**106, July-Sept., 1977.
12. Boraiko, A. A.: The pesticide dilemma, National Geographic **157:**145, Feb., 1980.
13. Report: Standard of identity, Nutr. Rev. **32:**29, 1974.
14. Enloe, C. H.: Hitched to everything in the universe, Nutr. Today **4**(4):2 1969-70.
15. Stare, F. J., and Choate, R. B.: Responses to the White House Conference, Nutr. Today **5**(1):13, 1970.
16. Shaefer, A. E., and Johnson, O. C.: Are we well fed? . . . the search for the answer, Nutr. Today **4**(1):2, 1969.
17. Turner, J.: The chemical feast, New York, 1970, Grossman Publishing Co.
18. Stokes, R. C.: The Consumer Research Institute's nutrient labeling research program, Food Drug Cosmet. Law J. **27:**249, 1972.
19. Lenahan, R. J., et al.: Consumer reaction to nutritional labels on food products, J. Consumer Affairs **7:**1, 1973.
20. Breeling, J. L.: Nutritional guidelines, J. Am. Diet. Assoc. **59:**102, Aug., 1971.
21. Cooke, J. A.: Nutritional guidelines and the labeling of foods, J. Am. Diet. Assoc. **59:**99, Aug., 1971.
22. Food labeling: goals, shortcomings, and proposed changes, U.S. General Accounting Office, MWD-75-19, Washington, D.C., 1975.
23. Ross, M. L.: What's happening to food labeling? J. Am. Diet. Assoc. **64:**262, March, 1974.
24. Federal Register **38:**2124, Jan. 19, 1973, **38:**6950, March 14, 1973.
25. LaChance, P. A.: A commentary on the new F.D.A. nutrition labeling regulations, Nutr. Today **8:**18-23, Jan.-Feb., 1973.
26. McGill, M.: Nutrition labeling, Fam. Health **6:**35-37, Nov., 1974.
27. Johnson, O. C.: The Food and Drug Administration and labeling, J. Am. Diet. Assoc. **64:**471, May, 1974.
28. Peterkin, B., Nichols, J., and Cromwell, C.: Nutrient labeling: tools for its use, U.S. Dept. of Agriculture, A18 No. 382, Washington, D.C., 1975.
29. Watt, B. K., Gebhardt, S. E., Murphy, E. W., et al.: Food value tables for the 70's, J. Am. Diet. Assoc. **64:**257, March, 1974.
30. Jacobson, M. F.: Eater's digest, the consumer's factbook of food additives, New York, 1972, Doubleday & Co., Inc.

General

Agar, E. A., and Dolman, C. E.: Type E botulism, J.A.M.A. **187:**538, 1964.

Beacham, L. M.: Food standards, F.D.A. Papers **1**(6):4, 1967.

Bird, K.: Freeze-dried foods, Marketing Research Report No. 617, U.S. Dept. of Agriculture, Washington, D.C., 1963.

Black, H., et al.: The Berkeley co-op food book, Palo Alto, Calif., 1980, Bull Publishing Co.

Brooke, M. M.: Epidemiology of amebiasis in the United States, J.A.M.A. **188:**519, 1964.

Call, D. L.: The changing food market—nutrition in a revolution, J. Am. Diet. Assoc. **60:**384, May, 1972.

Clydesdale, F. M.: Nutritional realities—where does technology fit? J. Am. Diet. Assoc. **74:**17, Jan., 1979.

Crosby, W. H., et al.: The experts debate the added enrichment of bread and flour with iron, Nutr. Today **7**(2):2, 1972.

Day, H. G.: Food safety—then and now, J. Am. Diet. Assoc. **69:**229, Sept., 1976.

Despaul, J. E.: Food poisoning microorganisms—a study of characteristics and methods of detection with particular emphasis on *Clostridium perfringens,* Washington, D.C., 1964, U.S. Government Printing Office.

Despaul, J. E.: The gangrene organism: a food poisoning agent, J. Am. Diet. Assoc. **49:**185, Sept., 1966.

Eadie, G. A., Molner, J. G., Solomon, R. J., et al.: Type E botulism, J.A.M.A. **187:**496, Feb. 15, 1964.

Evans, T. E.: Madison Avenue vs. the medical establishment, Nutr. Today **12:**41, Sept.-Oct., 1977.

Food labeling regulations (summary from Federal Register, Jan. 19, 1973), Nutr. Today **8:**14, Jan.-Feb., 1973.

Food and Nutrition Board Food Protection Committee, National Research Council: Selected publications. Chemicals used in food processing, Pub. 1274, 1965; An evaluation of public health hazards from the microbiological contamination of foods, Pub. 1195, 1964; Food packaging materials—their composition and uses, **645,** 1958; Radionuclides in foods **988,** 1962.

Friedelson, I.: Fair packaging: synopsis of food packaging and labeling regulations, FDA Papers 1(8):21, 1967.

Fritz, J. H.: The milk and food program of the Food and Drug Administration, Am. J. Public Health **62:**414, March, 1972.

Furia, T. D., editor: Handbook of food additives, ed. 2, Cleveland, 1972, CRC Press.

Graham, D. M., and Hertzler, A. A.: Why enrich or fortify foods? J. Nutr. Educ. **9:**166, Oct.-Dec., 1977.

Grant, J. D.: Nutritional guidelines and labeling, J. Am. Diet. Assoc. **60:**381, May, 1972.

Gussow, J.: Counternutritional message of TV ads aimed at children, J. Nutr. Educ. 4(2):48, 1972.

Hartley, H. L.: Vox populi, Nutr. Today 7(2):28, 1972.

Hodges, R. E.: The toxicity of pesticides and their residues in food, Nutr. Rev. 23:225, 1965.

Hickey, R. J., and Cleland, R. G.: Hazardous food additives: nitrite and saliva? N. Engl. J. Med. **298:**1036, May 4, 1978.

Jacobson, M. F.: Eater's digest, the consumer's factbook of food additives, New York, 1972, Doubleday & Co., Inc.

Kramer, A.: Benefits and risks of color additives, Food Technology **32:**65, Aug., 1978.

Lovell, R. T., and Flick, G. T.: Irradiation of gulf coast area strawberries, Food Technology 20:99, 1966.

Milstead, K. L.: Science works through law to protect consumers, J. Am. Diet. Assoc. **48:**187, March, 1966.

Most. H.: Trichinellosis in the United States, J.A.M.A. **193:**871, 1965.

National Academy of Sciences, Subcommittee on Food Technology: Technology of fortification of foods. Workshop poceedings, Washington, D.C., 1975.

Norman, C.: New food regulations make strange bedfellows, Nutr. Today **8:**26, Sept.-Oct., 1973.

Ostrander, J., Martinsen, C., McCullough, J., et al.: Egg substitutes: use and preference—with and without nutritional information, J. Am. Diet. Assoc. **70:**267, March, 1977.

Patterson, M. I., and Marble, B.: Dietetic foods, Am. J. Clin. Nutr. **16:**440, May, 1965.

Protecting our food: yearbook of agriculture, 1966, Washington, D.C., 1966, U.S. Government Printing Office.

Report: Nutritional claims for food, Berkeley, Calif., 1976, Soc. Nutr. Educ.

Robinson, H. E., and Urbain, W. M.: Radiation preservation of foods, J.A.M.A. **174:**1310, 1960.

Roe, R. S.: Pesticide regulatory activities of the Food and Drug Administration, Am. J. Public Health **55**(pt. 2):36, 1965.

Schwartzberg, L., George, C., and Phillips, M. C.: Issues in food advertising—the nutrition educator's viewpoint, J. Nutr. Educ. **9:**60, April-June, 1977.

Sharon, G. S.: Of (iron) pots and pans, Nutr. Today **7**(2):34, 1972.

Stalvey, R. M.: Legislation by litigation, Nutr. Today **7**(2):26, 1972.

Strong, D. H., Weiss, K. F., and Higgins, L. W.: Survival of *Clostridium perfringens* in starch pastes, J. Am. Diet. Assoc. **49:**191, Sept., 1966.

Stumpf, S. E.: Social aspects of benefit/risk analysis of the food supply, Food Technology **32:**68, Aug., 1978.

Thatcher, F. S.: Food-borne bacterial toxins, Can. Med. Assoc. J. **94:**582, 1966.

Vermeersch, J. A., and Swenerton, H.: Consumer responses to nutrition claims in food advertisements, J. Nutr. Educ. **11:**22, Jan.-March, 1979.

Ward, G. M., Johnson, J. E., and Wilson, D. W.: Deposition of fallout cesium-137 on forage and transfer to milk, Public Health Rep. **81:**639, 1966.

Ward, J. C.: The functions of the Federal Insecticide, Fungicide, and Rodenticide Act in the United States, Am. J. Public Health **55**(suppl.):27, July, 1965.

13 Cultural, social, and psychologic influences on food habits

In public health work, as in other aspects of their professional activities, nutritionists, physicians, nurses, and other health workers are confronted constantly with the fundamental question of why people eat what they eat. The health professions are concerned with the nutritional needs of persons and families in communities. They know that food is necessary to sustain life and health. But they also recognize that people eat for many reasons other than physical sustenance and that they seldom eat to supply their bodies with the good nutrition that a health worker may propose. Food has many meanings, and a person's food habits are intimately tied up with his whole way of life.

Important as a sound knowledge of the science of human nutrition is, it is not enough to provide the health workers with the means of carrying out their function in relation to persons. That is only the beginning. Unless this knowledge is applied realistically to persons in their unique life situations with their particular cultural conditioning, the health worker does not help them. Indeed the health worker may even create barriers and problems rather than help find solutions.

Consider the example of the public health nurse working with a family whose income is relatively limited and who is faced with several health problems involving inadequate nutrition. The nurse knows the necessity of an adequate and safe food supply, knows food values and nutrients and their functions in the body, and can outline a well-balanced family meal pattern that will assure all these nutritional essentials. The nurse proceeds with great enthusiasm to accomplish this for the mother by telling her and her family to eat "three good, square meals a day," which *everyone* should have for health.

But must everyone have three meals a day? Why not two meals a day or five or six? Why orange juice and egg only for breakfast? Why meat only for dinner? Why dinner only in the evening? Perhaps this particular family has different eating habits. Failing to recognize or explore this family's cultural variation in spite of good intentions, the nurse may have unconsciously confused *biologic necessity* which the meal plan surely does not represent, with *cultural patterning,* which the meal plan does represent—the pattern of *the nurse's own* cultural background. Perhaps the nurse persists in a plan against the family's resistance. The nurse remains unperceptive to the family's uniqueness and continues to project his or her own cultural values. When *the nurse's* plan for the family fails, the nurse is likely to label them "uncooperative" and so describe them in a report, still unaware that the problem is his or her own, not the family's.

Perhaps this is an extreme and unlikely example. But it is just such failures to find the means of helping that have made it necessary for there to be greater awareness on the part of the health care professions of the human factors that operate in a human being's repsonse to health and illness.

Traditionally medical care has been based on the physical and biologic sciences. A knowledge of these is essential, of course, if one is to understand disease and care for persons who are ill. However, complexity is increasing from two points of view. Throughout the world, societies are becoming more complex with the intermingling of cultures and exchange of health workers across cultural boundaries. The study of disease processes and the growing concept of preventive medicine prove increasingly the need to understand the social and cultural aspects of human behavior and especially to analyze human responses to health care.

This need is strikingly evident in the area of nutrition and is of increasing interest and concern to nutritionists and other health professionals. If they are thoughtful, if they know their patients' basic nutritional needs or deficiencies, yet observe differences in ways of eating and the strong emotional responses to proposed changes in habits, they ask themselves questions. Why do people eat what they eat? Why do they choose one food and reject another? What accounts for the total complex of behaviors that constitute food habits?

Food habits, like other forms of human behavior, are the result of many personal, cultural, social, and psychologic influences. Studies in the behavioral sciences—anthropology, sociology, and psychology—have contributed much insight concerning the bases of these habits. Perhaps all persons tend to be somewhat ethnocentric—centered in their own culture—so that they view their own way as the best or right way. Habits of another who differs are looked on as foreign or wrong or superstitious or stupid. If people are honest enough to recognize their own biases, many of the misconceptions that prevent understanding other people can be cleared away. Such misconceptions

hinder the health worker's ability to give patients sensitive, constructive care.

There is an increasing awareness of the need for a closer working relationship between nutrition and behavioral science. This need has been the focus recently in several programs on prevention and control of health problems sponsored by the National Heart, Lung, and Blood Institute (NHLBI) of the National Institutes of Health (NIH), U.S. Department of Health, Education, and Welfare (now the Department of Health and Human Services).[1] Several working papers have developed from their Science to Practitioner Project that help nutrition practitioners apply principles from behavioral science in their work. Two areas of behavioral science applied to nutrition in this project are behavior modification[3] and social psychology.[4] Both reports provide helpful background for the practitioner, emphasizing self-responsibility of the patient, influence of environment on food behaviors, and manageable realistic goals for dietary change.

In the last analysis it is the cultural, social, and psychologic factors in the individual patient that will prove most influential in personal nutritional behavior. In each patient these factors are interwoven into a behavioral complex. To study them, each will be looked at separately.

CULTURAL INFLUENCES
Concept of culture

A century-old definition by E. B. Taylor describes culture as "that complex whole which includes knowledge, belief, art, law, morals, custom, and any other capabilities and habits acquired by man as a member of society." Modern anthropologists have enlarged the definition of culture to include the entire way of life of a people. Margaret Mead stated that culture involves not only the more obvious and historical aspect of a person's communal life (his language, religion, politics, technology, and so on), but also all the little habits of everyday living such as preparing and serving food and caring for children, feeding them, and lulling them to sleep. Often the most significant thing that can be known about a culture is what it takes for granted in daily life.

These many facets of a person's culture are *learned*. Gradually as the child grows up within a given society, the slow process of conscious and unconscious learning of values, attitudes, habits, and practices takes place through the conscious and unconscious influence of parents, teachers, and other enculturating agents of that society. Whatever is invented, transmitted, and perpetuated—socially acquired knowledge and habits—persons learn as part of their culture. These become internalized and entrenched.

Function of culture

The culture of people develops over a long period, partly as the result of *adaptation to the environment*. The environment may be harsh and hostile, and the way of life developed by a people is what has enabled them to survive. Sometimes the changing of these habits by an outsider who does not understand these adaptations may upset this balance with nature. Such change will then do more harm than good. This has been the case when some health workers have tried to impose Western culture and habits on people in other parts of the world, without prior study and appreciation of established customs. Programs have failed for this reason.

The culture of a people also develops as a means of *interpreting common (and sometimes terrifying) life experiences,* such as birth, death, illness, disease, sex, and phenomena of nature. Rituals, taboos, totems, habits, and practices develop to explain, placate, or protect and to establish human and environmental relationships. A certain poisonous plant, for example, may have become taboo as a food because the tribal ancestors observed that it caused death.

Food in a culture

Food habits are among the oldest and most entrenched aspects of many cultures. They exert deep influence on the behavior of the people. The cultural background determines what shall be eaten as well as when and how it shall be eaten. There is, of course, considerable variation; and both rational and irrational and beneficial and injurious customs are found in every part of the world. Nevertheless, by and large, food habits are based on food availability, economics, or symbolism. Included among these influential factors are the geography of the land, the agriculture practiced by the people, their economy and market practices, and their history and traditions.

Cultural determination of what food is. Items considered to be food in one culture may be regarded with disgust or may actually cause illness in the persons of another culture. In America milk is valued as a basic food; in many other cultures it is rejected with revulsion as an animal mucous discharge. In the Philippines the Ifugao tribesmen of northern Luzon are famous for adapting their steep mountain terrain to the production of rice by forming multiple, narrow, terraced, dry rice fields in which they grow a major portion of this staple food (an example of overcoming geographic barriers to food production). They are also known for their enjoyment of other dietary items that they prize, such as dragonflies and locusts, which they boil, dry, and grind into a powder. Crickets, flying and red ants, beetles, and water bugs are fried in lard.

The use of the staple item, bread, is another example. Many a diet-obsessed American rejects bread. In a Greek home bread is the main food. It is *the* meal. All other foods are considered accompaniments to bread and are eaten between bites of bread. So strong is the place of bread in the diet throughout much of the Middle East that in Egypt wives have been divorced because they seldom provided fresh bread for their husbands.

Religious aspects of culture also control food rejection and use. Pork is unacceptable as food for a Moslem or an orthodox Jew; any meat is unacceptable for the Seventh Day Adventist; the strict Hindu or Buddhist eats no meat, and even the liberal Hindu may not eat beef. In his youth, Mahatma Gandhi is said to have intellectually agreed that beef was a good food for human use and he therefore ate some. But his Hindu culture and rejection of beef was so deeply ingrained and internalized that the food made him violently ill.

Appetite for specific foods. Foods acceptable for one meal may be rejected for another meal. For example, the main breakfast food in a Greek home may be bread and cheese; in Europe, a sweet roll; in America, ham and eggs. Inhabitants of different regions within a country also vary in their choices. In America the Westerner would probably have fried potatoes at breakfast with his ham and eggs; the Southerner would consider potatoes a dinner food and have grits (a porridge made with coarsely ground white corn) for breakfast instead; the New Englander is fond of pie for breakfast.

How and where food is eaten. In a highly urban, industrialized society such as America, in which value is placed on action, speed, and productivity, lunch for the working person may be a quick snack he or she eats while standing at a lunch counter. Even the form of food is geared for quick eating—fruit in juice form and meat in a sandwich. To the Spanish or Latin American merchant such a lunch is unthinkable. His less tensely paced culture allows him to close his shop for two hours in the middle of the day while he enjoys a leisurely meal and siesta at home with his family.

Appropriate occasion for specific foods. The force of dietary patterning is seen in the Thanksgiving turkey, the Easter ham, and until recently (and still for strict observers) the Friday fish. Times of religious observance, such as Lent, call for specific food patterns. Food becomes an integral part of transmitting and teaching many aspects of one's particular culture.

Symbolism of food in a culture

Within every culture there are certain foods that are deeply imbued with symbolic meaning.

These symbols are related to major life experiences from birth through death, to religion, to politics, and to general social organization. (In the following examples many foreign food names are mentioned. These terms are explained in the section of this chapter on Cultural Food Patterns.)

Major life experiences. The birth of a child is observed in many cultures by a meal that symbolizes a general celebration of the beginning of life. It is an occasion for feasting or, in some cultures, for offering special foods to one or more deities. Soon after birth a baptism or dedication ceremony may be followed by a special family meal. Birthdays are celebrated with special foods—in modern America, with a cake decorated with candles. Stages of the young person's development are often observed by special food uses. At a coming-of-age ceremony such as the bar mitzvah for Jewish boys at the age of 13, honey cake and wine, canapes, strudel, knishes, and pirogen are generally served. Puberty rites in other cultures often involve the eating of special foods. Graduation ceremonies marking levels of attainment in educational, occupational, religious, or social life may require special feasting or, in some cultures or instances, fasting.

Weddings are especially surrounded with symbolic foods. The bride's cake and the wedding reception are common in Western culture. Family feasting often lasts for several days in other cultures where it is the eating of special foods together that seals the marriage pact.

Pregnancy is attended by many food symbols, taboos, and practices. Certain foods may be avoided in the belief that they will mark the infant. Certain foods may be denied the pregnant woman in the belief that she will contaminate the food supply. For example, in the Zulu tribe of South Africa the pregnant woman may not go near the cattle enclosure or drink any milk from the cows because of the belief that she will exert an evil influence on the prized herd. In rural southern United States and some other areas, pica (the eating of clay or of starch) is sometimes practiced by pregnant women who profess strong cravings for it.

In many cultures the death of a member of the group involves food use symbolizing the fact that each individual life has its end. In one group, food may be buried with the body to sustain the departed on his journey to the hereafter. In another group, food may be the main expression of sympathy, sorrow, or support for the bereaved, and many offerings of food are brought to the home by neighbors. A special funeral supper may be a part of the mourning prescribed in still another group.

Religion. Food symbolism plays a large role in most religions of the world. From early times ceremonies and religious rites surrounded acts pertaining to fertility and the harvest seasons. Food gathering, preparing, and serving followed specific customs and commemorated special events of religious significance. Many of these customs remain.

Among the Jewish people a number of special feast or fast days commemorate significant events in their history (Table 13-1) and are a means of teaching cherished beliefs and traditions to the children. The Jewish New Year, Rosh Hashanah, occurs in September or October and begins the Hebrew calendar of holidays. At this time it is customary to serve apple slices dipped in honey, signifying the yearning for a sweet and happy year. Carrots in some form are served to signify the wish for pros-

Table 13-1. Jewish holidays and associated foods

Holiday	Month	Event	Traditional foods
Rosh Hashanah (New Year)	September or October	Beginning of Jewish New Year (Tishri 1)	Honey, honey cake, carrot tzimmes
Yom Kippur	September or October	Day of Atonement	Fast day (total)
Sukkoth	October	Feast of Booths, Harvest festival; symbolizes booths in which Israelites lived on flight from Egypt and wilderness wanderings	Kreplach or holishkes (chopped meat wrapped in cabbage leaves) Strudel
Chanukah	December	Feast of Lights; celebrates heroic battle of the Maccabees for Jewish independence (165 BC) Home festival with candles	Grated potato latkes, potato kugel
Chamise Oser b'Sh'vat	January	Festival of the Trees (Arbor Day); blossoming time of trees in Palestine	Bokser (St. John's Bread) fruits, nuts, raisins, cakes
Purim	March	Feast of Esther; celebrates downfall of Haman and deliverance of Hebrews by influence of Queen Esther to King Xerxes of Persia	Hamantaschen (three-cornered pastry), apples, nuts, raisins
Passover (Pesach)	April	Festival of Freedom; celebrates escape of Israelites from Egyptian slavery	Seder meal; matzoth and matzoth dishes, wine, nuts
Shevuoth	May	Feast of Weeks (Pentecost); celebrates the day Moses received Ten Commandments on Mt. Sinai	Cheese blintzes, cheese kreplach, dairy foods

perity in the coming year. A carrot tzimmes is usually served. Perhaps the two most significant holidays that follow in the Jewish calendar are Yom Kippur (Day of Atonement), the high holy day of fast, which comes in September or October; and Passover (Pesach), which occurs in April. On the evening before the fast day, Yom Kippur, no highly spiced or seasoned foods are served. At the end of the fast, the *Kiddush* (the blessing over wine) is observed, followed by a special meal of Sabbath dishes such as stuffed herring (gefüllte fish), noodle soup, poultry, vegetables, salad, fruit, and strudel.

Observance of Passover, usually celebrated for eight days in April, commemorates the liberation of the Israelites from Egyptian bondage. This feast has come to play an important role in the democratic struggle for human dignity for many peoples of the world, to strengthen conviction that justice and freedom for all persons may yet prevail on the earth. The holiday begins with a highly symbolic family meal on the evening before the Passover—the Seder, at which each food eaten signifies a specific aspect of the historical deliverance.

Among the Moslem people, a month of fast-

TO PROBE FURTHER
The Seder, beginning of the Jewish Passover

On the eve of Passover Week, perhaps the most beloved of all the Jewish festivals, a special ceremonial meal is held in Jewish homes to commemorate the deliverance of the Israelites from Egyptian bondage. This symbolic meal is called the Seder, which means ''order''; the word refers to the prescribed order of the Passover service. Each item of the table setting and each food used has special significance.

Candles—ancient symbol of enlightenment or human consciousness growing out of prehuman darkness

Ke'arah—the seder plate containing the symbolic objects used for the ceremony

Betzah—roasted egg, symbol of an offering; the shape, without beginning or end, signifies eternal redemption and liberation of all humankind

Zeroa—roasted lamb or chicken bone, symbol of the paschal lamb, sacrificed the night of Passover in the Temple

Morar—bitter herb (grated horseradish), symbol of the bitter life of the Hebrews in bondage

Karpas—green vegetable (parsley, lettuce, or watercress) dipped in a dish of salt water and eaten as a relish; symbolizes the manner of leisurely eating enjoyed by free men in olden times

Kharoses—mixture of chopped nuts, apples, cinnamon, and wine; symbol of the mortar and clay used by the ancient Israelites in making bricks when they toiled under Pharaoh

Three matzoth—(1) bread of poverty eaten by the afflicted Israelites, (2) symbol of haste in which Israelites fled from Egypt—the dough had not leavened because they could not tarry, (3) symbol of ancient ceremonial custom, The Feast of Unleavened Bread

Arba Kosos—wine goblet for each person, from which four cups of wine are drunk, symbolizing the four expressions in the Bible relating to redemption

Cup of Elijah—extra goblet left for Elijah, the herald of the messianic era

Hard-cooked eggs and salt water are passed to each person at the feast as an entrée to the main meal, symbolic of mourning for the destruction of the Temple. The eggs also symbolize Life, the perpetuation of existence.

TO PROBE FURTHER

Id al-Fitr, the post-Ramadan festival

Traditionally in Moslem countries at the conclusion of Ramadan, Islam's holy month of prayer and fasting, wealthy merchants and princes hold public feasts for the needy. This is the festival of Id al-Fitr.

Over the years many delicacies have been served to symbolize the joy of return from fasting and the heightened sense of unity, brotherhood, charity that the fasting experience has brought to the people. Among the foods served are chicken or veal, sautéed with eggplant and onions, then simmered slowly in pomegranate juice and spiced with tumeric and cardamon seeds. The highlight of the meal usually is kharuf mahshi, a whole lamb (symbol of sacrifice) stuffed with a rich dressing made of dried fruits, cracked wheat, pine nuts, almonds, onions, and seasoned with ginger and coriander. The stuffed lamb is baked in hot ashes for many hours so that it is tender enough to be pulled apart and eaten with the fingers.

At the conclusion of the meal, rich pastries and candies are served. These may be flavored with spices or flower petals. Some of the sweets are taken home and savored as long as possible as a reminder of the festival.

---

ing is observed during Ramadan[5] (the ninth month of the Islamic lunar calendar, thus rotating through all seasons). The fourth pillar of Islam is fasting. "O ye who believe! Fasting is prescribed to you as it was prescribed to those before you, that ye may ward off evil," commands the Koran. Ramadan was chosen for the sacred fast because it is the month in which Mohammed received the first of the revelations that were subsequently compiled to form the Koran and also the month in which his followers first drove their enemies from Mecca in AD 624.

During the month of Ramadan, Mohammedans all over the world observe rigid daily fasting, taking no food or drink from dawn to sunset. Nights, however, are often spent in gay feasting. First, an appetizer is taken, such as dates or a refreshing drink. A popular modern beverage is a sherbetlike liquid made from dried apricots, called qamar-al-deen ("moon of religion"). After this appetizer, the family enjoys an "evening breakfast," the iftar. At the end of Ramadan a feast lasting up to three days climaxes the observance. Special dishes

mark this joyous occasion. There are delicacies such as thin pancakes dipped in powdered sugar, savory buns, and dried fruits.

Among the Christian people of the world, there is prescribed the six-week fast period of Lent that precedes Easter. There is a special light-meal pattern and abstinence from meat in symbolic preparation of the spirit to observe the holy season of Easter, which commemorates the death and resurrection of Christ. Throughout the year the Communion meal (the Lord's Supper, the sacrament of the Mass) involves symbolic use of foods. Bread is taken as the body of Christ, broken and offered for men, and wine is taken as the blood of Christ, shed in sacrificial redemption for men. For the Christian, the simple line of the Lord's Prayer, "Give us this day our daily bread," the saying of grace at mealtimes, and the offering of thanks at harvest time all relate food to faith.

Many of the religious rituals associated over the years with the preparation and use of food result not only from symbolic meaning but also from wisdom regarding possible contamination and spread of disease. For example, the Jains, members of an ascetic religious sect founded in India in the sixth century by a Hindu reformer as a revolt against the caste system, eat their meals before sunset to avoid the possibility of insect pollution in their food. They avoid root vegetables because such foods carry on their skins organisms that proliferate in the earth.

Politics. Food use has had political significance in history as well as religious significance. In India the fasts of Gandhi wielded tremendous political power, which contributed enormously to that country's achieving independence from Great Britain. The Boston Tea Party was concerned with important interrelationships among food, economics, and a budding nation's political views. Tea was considered to be an almost essential commodity by the American colonists, and English taxes on tea stimulated the politics of American independence.

SOCIAL INFLUENCES
Concept of social organization

Sociology may be defined in simplest terms as the study of group life. It is concerned with human group behavior, the numerous activities, processes, and structures by which social life goes on. Through the discipline and methods of sociology, human behavior is understood in terms of social phenomena. Such fields and problems as social change, urbanism, rural life, the family, the community, race relations, crime, and delinquency are studied.

This broad behavioral science has many implications for nutrition. Two aspects of social organization that concern health care professionals are class structure and value systems.

Class structure. The structure of a society is largely formed by groupings according to such factors as economic status, education, residence, occupation, or family. Within a given society many of these groups exist, whose values and habits vary. These subgroups within a larger culture are called subcultures. They may be established on the basis of region, religion,

age, sex, social class, occupation, or political party. Within these subgroups there may be still smaller groupings with distinguishing attitudes, values, and habits—the community juvenile gang, the college fraternity, the industrial executives, the army officers, the families in a given neighborhood, or the physicians in a hospital hierarchy. A person may be a member of several subcultural groups, each of which influences his values, attitudes, and habits.

Social class, especially, influences value systems, responses and behavior patterns. Social classes may be considered as comprising those persons having similar community status, responsibilities, and privileges. In America social classes are less distinct and rigid than in some countries. For example, class barriers clearly separate the aristocrat from the commoner in Great Britain, and a severe caste system characterizes the Hindu population of India. Nonetheless, social classes are present in America and do influence behavior. One classic study of an American urban community reported the presence of six social layers.[6] Perhaps this is a fair sample and may roughly serve as a model, although current social change is effecting some lessening of these distinctions:

1. Upper-upper class—old-line community aristocrats
2. Lower-upper class—the newly rich of the community
3. Upper-middle class—professional persons, business owners, executives
4. Lower-middle class—tradesmen, white collar workers, some highly skilled workers
5. Upper-lower class—skilled and semi-skilled workers
6. Lower-lower class—laborers, some unassimilated foreign groups

These class lines are often blurred, and movement from class to class occurs. Essentially the distinctions are based on the related factors of income, occupation, education, and residence.

A later study at Yale University[7] identified five classes in the community of New Haven, Connecticut. This stratification may have been typical of similar U.S. cities of 250,000 population at that time. Using an index of social position based on area of residence, occupation, and education (including a sampling of income and behavior patterns regarding books and periodicals read, radio and television programs heard and viewed, and organization and club memberships), the researchers found the comparative results shown in Table 13-2.

The democratic and equalitarian philosophy of American society and the humanitarian ideals on which members of the health professions have been nurtured combine to make the reality of class differences difficult to accept. Yet the differences do exist, and they probably influence the approach to patients, relationships with them, and the outcome of those relationships more than the health care worker may be aware or care to admit.

Value systems. Another important aspect of a society's social organization is its value system, which develops as a result of its history and heritage. Values held in America, for example, stem largely from its relatively recent pioneer history. The majority of American settlers were from rigidly Puritan backgrounds. Their highest values were placed on industry, self-denial and self-control, work, willpower, cleanliness, honesty, responsibility, and initiative. These values became intensified because the survival of the settlers often depended on the exercise of these characteristics. Pleasure and entertainment were considered to have secondary value at best, and in most instances they were held by the settlers who lived through the most difficult pioneer periods to be unworthy or even evil.

Table 13-2. American urban social class structure*

Class	Occupation	Residence	Education	Social life	Population (%)
1	Inherited wealth; business and professional leaders	"The best"	College graduation; famous private schools	Private clubs; family cliques; exclusive organizations	3
2	High managerial positions; professions; live well but no great wealth	"Better" residential areas	College graduation; graduate professional study	Family; church; clubs; community and professional organizations	9
3	Small businessmen; office and sales workers; skilled workers	"Good" residential areas	High school graduation; business school; 1 to 2 yr college	Family; low-prestige churches; lodges	20
4	Semiskilled factory industrial workers	Scattered	Older members: elementary school Young adults: high school	Family; neighborhood; labor unions; public places	50
5	Semiskilled factory hands and unskilled laborers	Tenements, cold-water flats	Lower grades of elementary school	Family; flat; street; neighborhood; social agencies	18

*Hollingshead, A. B., and Redlich, F. C.: Social class and mental illness, New York, 1958, John Wiley & Sons, Inc.

Jurgen Ruesch[8] has identified four basic premises on which the present American value system is based: *equality, sociality, success,* and *change*. All of these values influence attitudes toward health care and food habits. The placement of a high value on equality leads health workers to establish standards of quality health care for all people. The high respect accorded to sociality builds peer group pressures and status-seeking within social groups. Foods may be accepted because they are high-status foods or rejected because they are low-prestige foods. The esteem in which success is held often leads persons to measure life in terms of competitive superlatives. They want to set the best table, to provide the most abundant supply of food for the family, and to have the biggest eater and the fattest baby of any in the neighborhood. The value that is placed on change leads families or individuals to seek constant variety in their diets, to be geared for action, and to seek quick-cooking, conveniently prepared foods. In response to such market demands, food technologists are producing an increasing array of food products each year.

Food and social factors

The food habits of people in any setting are highly socialized. These habits perform significant social functions, some of which may not always be evident to the persons who have such habits.

Social relationships. Food is a symbol of sociability, warmth, friendliness, and social acceptance. The breaking of bread together binds a group. From the earliest Christian era, such custom enriched fellowship and became the symbol of the Communion meal. "And they, continuing daily with one accord, breaking bread from house to house, did eat their meat with gladness and singleness of heart" (Acts 2:46).

Similar use of food for binding fellowship is seen in the honor reception, the wedding breakfast, the political party banquet, and the serving of food to visitors. Very early socialization was observed once in a young child who offered his little friend his "sucking thumb" for awhile! From the first hours of life, eating is not a solitary experience. It is a matter of two people—a feeding adult and an eating newborn.

An extreme example of the social function of food is seen in the practice of the mountain Arapesh, a Papuan people of New Guinea. With great effort, sometimes in groups of six families, they clear small plots for gardens, often at long distances from their homes. They raise animals for food, and they hunt game. But none of this is ever for themselves! Each person gives the product of his labors to other members of the group, frequently traveling great distances over mountain trails to do so. The worst thing an Arapesh man can do is keep some of his produce for himself. The entire process of food production, gathering, and consumption is a means of social warmth and intercourse. By American standards this practice might be called highly inefficient and even irrational, for about one third of the tribe's time is spent in traveling the difficult terrain for the purpose of feeding others. But for these warm, happy people it is a source of group fellowship and strength. And which of these basic values is more important?

Persons involved in social relationships. People tend to accept food more readily from those persons viewed as friends or allies. People most enjoy eating with those persons to whom they feel close. New foods from persons who seem congenial are acceptable. Advice about food is accepted from persons who are considered to be authorities and with whom is felt a warm relationship. For example, some people are more willing to take such counsel from the family physician than from the more remote nutritionist. People tend to distrust food given to them by strangers and outsiders. Emotional feelings about people are transferred to their food. The more alien the authority figure, the more he is considered to be unconcerned, and it is more likely that his food suggestions will be considered as outlandish or perhaps even harmful.

Maternal role. Food is symbolic of motherliness. In the family the early feeding process is the vehicle of much conscious and unconscious learning between mother and child. The mother teaches what is acceptable as food, when to eat, how much to eat, and why it is eaten. Many mothers are unaware that they impart their own likes and dislikes to their children. Yet how often statements about food are prefaced with the words, ''My mother always . . .''!

A mother's self-esteem is deeply involved in feeding her family. She feels it necessary to be confident that she has done the right thing for them as a mother. Depending on her education, she decides who is an authority to advise her about child feeding. If she is relatively unsophisticated and has little education, she is likely to view her own mother and her neighbors as her best guides. If she has somewhat more education, she perhaps accepts more readily the advertising of business concerns as the greatest authority. Mothers with middle-class or better education place most faith in a professional medical authority. Under the stress of emergency, however, most mothers of all educational levels are likely to turn to the recognized health professional for advice about food for a sick infant.

Status foods. Status is often sought in terms of food. A person may build a reputation as a gourmet. To accomplish this he may eat and become an expert with respect to exotic foods (which he secretly may not enjoy), simply as a means of gaining prestige among his peers. (Compare the enthusiast for opera who attends every first-night performance and knows who designed every high fashion gown worn by the women in the audience, but is ignorant of what opera is being performed or what artists are singing lead roles.) High-prestige foods such as roasts or steaks are usually served for dinner when guests are invited, and lower prestige foods such as hamburger or liver are rarely served. For some social groups, forms of bread vary in status. White bread is preferred to dark bread. In some social groups, purchased bread has higher status than homemade biscuits; in others, the reverse is true.

Food in family relationships. Eating together as a family group builds closeness and family solidarity. Food habits that are most closely associated with family sentiments are the most tenacious throughout life. The role of each family member is most clearly illustrated to the child as the family eats together. Long into adulthood, certain foods trigger a flood of childhood memories, and these foods are valued for reasons totally apart from any nutritional value.

Certain meals have more family significance than others. In America breakfast and lunch may be rather impersonally served and eaten by various family members at individual times. Dinner is more family-centered and its pattern is more complex. Its foods are often more symbolic. Changes in one's food habits or the introduction of new foods may tend to be more acceptable at breakfast or lunch than at dinner. Strong religious factors associated with food also tend to have their origin and reinforcement within the family meal circle.

Economic factors. People tend to eat foods that are readily available to them and that they can afford. Family income, community sources of food, and market conditions influence food habits and ultimate food choices.

Social problems and food habits

Among the many effects of rapid social change, with the uprooting and displacing of persons and families, are changes in the food habits of millions of persons.

Poverty. In large urban centers, growing numbers of persons who are members of minority groups live in slums, where they are unassimilated and often disregarded by the mainstream of a sophisticated, affluent society. They are unprepared for earning a living in industry's automated age and are often frightened, insecure, and lonely. Many persons from such nearby places as Puerto Rico, Cuba, and Mexico or from some areas of the United States such as the rural South have made their way to the cities where they hoped to find a new life. Instead, they sometimes find obstacles that they cannot surmount and live a marginal existence at best. Inadequate housing is attended by problems related to cooking, refrigeration, storage, and sanitation. Malnutrition, broken spirits, and hostility often result.

Family disintegration. Abject poverty for some workers and increased affluence for others has resulted from industrialization and changing urban-surburban living patterns. These newly emerging patterns appear to have contributed to changes in family patterns and values. An increasing number of families seldom gather for meals; in such families the reinforcement of group unity and stability that was formerly felt from eating together is lost. Children who are left to shift for themselves incur erratic eating habits and tend to fill their stomachs with a diet that is nutritionally inadequate. The increased number of teenage marriages, often between young people with limited means of support and little knowledge of food preparation or of child feeding, may lead to poor food choices and poor eating habits.

Alcoholism. Alcoholism is frequently associated with poor nutrition. Both the addict and his family may be adversely affected. If the wage earner is addicted, he or she may spend a great portion of the family's small income for alcohol; inadequate funds remain for feeding the family. The alcoholic who does not deprive others of food frequently damages his own health by obtaining in alcohol the mere calories requisite for direct energy expenditure. He neglects to eat a proper diet that would supply the many other nutrients his body needs, and malnutrition results.

PSYCHOLOGIC INFLUENCES
Social psychology—understanding dietary patterns

Social psychology is the most recent of the behavioral sciences. It began in the last part of the nineteenth century and combines concepts from psychology and sociology. This discipline is concerned with social interaction in terms of its effect on individual behavior and with the social influences and determining factors of individual perception, motivation, and action. How does a particular individual perceive a given situation? What basic needs motivate his action and response? What social factors surround his particular action? Social psychologists are particularly interested in the effect of culture on personality, the socialization of the child, differences in individuals and groups, group dynamics, group attitudes and opinions, and leadership. The detailed individual case study is much used as a social psychology research method.

The science and methods of social psychology have made important contributions to nutrition, medicine, nursing, and allied health care, especially to problems of human behavior under stress. Intensive study has been made of the psychosocial aspects of physical disability, aging, obesity, problems attending surgical procedures such as mastectomy, gastrectomy, and colostomy, and those related to chronic diseases such as peptic ulcer.

It must be borne in mind by the health worker, for example, that deep psychologic connotations lead to exceedingly sensitive areas in the individual's total structure as a person capable of meeting life and carrying out responsibilities. Knowing that such connections exist, persons planning health care will need to use this knowledge to avoid mistakes and to better understand the depth of the roots of the problems that will be encountered. However, they will also recognize the limits beyond which it would be unwise to probe. Foods as symbols may lead the psychiatrist to discoveries the primary care practitioner should be aware of in general and can refer as needed to the specialist.

Food and psychologic factors

Individual behavior patterns including those related to eating are the result of many interrelated psychosocial influences and factors. Factors that are particularly pertinent to the shaping of food habits are motivation and perception.

Motivation. People are not the same the world over. People of differing cultures are not motivated by the same needs and goals. Even primary biologic drives, such as hunger and sex, are modified in their interpretation, expression, and fulfillment by many cultural, social, and personal influences. The kinds of food sought, prized, or accepted by one individual at one time and place may be violently rejected by another individual living in different circumstances. In the person existing in a state of basic hunger or semistarvation, food is his whole perception and motivation. Such a person thinks, talks, and dreams about food. Under less severe circumstances, however, the concern for food may be on a relatively abstract level and may involve symbolism that is associated with other levels of need.

Maslow[9] has developed a useful concept of a hierarchy of human needs, wants, and strivings. He indicates that only as each level of need is met is the individual able to progress to the next level of experiences and awareness. He described five levels that operate in turn, each building on the prior ones:

1. Basic physiologic needs—hunger, thirst
2. Safety needs—physical comfort, security, protection
3. Love, affection, ''belongingness'' needs —giving and receiving affection
4. Self-esteem, status, recognition needs— sense of self-worth, strength, self-confidence, capability, adequacy
5. Self-actualization—self-fulfillment, creative growth

Although these levels overlap and vary with time and circumstance, Maslow's concept of such hierarchy can help the health care worker to understand patient needs and to plan health care accordingly.

Perception. Perception is the process of adding meaning to what is taken in through the senses. It is perception that enables people to create a relatively stable environment out of an otherwise chaotic assortment of sensory impressions. Perception also limits understanding. Each phenomenon that the outer world offers is perceived through social and personal lenses. In every experience of a person's life, what is perceived is a blend of three factors: (1) the external reality, (2) the message of the stimulus that is conveyed by the nervous system to the integrative centers where thinking and evaluation go on, and (3) the interpretation that each person puts on each datum of experience. A host of subjective elements such as hunger, thirst, hate, fear, self-interest, values, and temperament influence response to the phenomena that are presented by the outer world. Those responses are called behavior.

The philosopher Justus Buchler[10] has suggested the term *pro*ception as being more accurate. By proception, Buchler means all one's past relations to one's world, one's accumulated experience, and the future toward which this very personal past and present propel each one of us. The individual acquires this direction from native temperament, culture, cumulative habit, situation, and emotional character. In short, proception is the total process of relevant behavior from input to act. The procept opens and closes the gate to the percept.

This concept relates significantly to health education. Allport[11] states that health workers are selected, well-educated specialized persons who tend to be intellectualizers, abstract thinkers, and less emotionally dependent than uneducated persons are on the surrounding environment. But the people for whose health they assume certain responsibilities usually do not think abstractly, particularly under the stress of illness, anxiety, and pain. The responses of such persons to attempts at health education may vary from overreaction to repression. The patient who is repressing response to the health worker's efforts may seem to be turning a deaf ear to the message. However, if the health worker concludes that the patient is deliberately excluding the message, *the health worker's* perception is at fault. The patient wants to know and understand. Deep within all people is a basic desire for meaning. Every person searches for meaning in all personal life experiences including illness, suffering, and death. It is an important part of the health worker's task to shape instructions to the patient's perception and to be sensitive to the individual patient at any particular stage of development. Health workers must respect patients as unique beings if they are to help them find the answers in their search for meaning.

It is this dimension that makes a health professional's work profound. Health workers cannot impose on patients mechanical routines of sanitation, hygiene, and nutrition born of their own antiseptic cultural values. Patients will not carry them out if they are presented in this way. The health worker must look *at* his or her own spectacles and not just *through* them. At the same time the health worker must also look *at* and *through* the spectacles of the patient. This takes skill, and the health worker must care enough to work at it. Only after attaining a higher level of perception will he or she realize that glib answers fail. In the last analysis, persons learn because they sense an urgent need to know. They learn because their curiosity is aroused. They learn by exploring, making mistakes and correcting them, testing, and verifying. *All of these things individuals must do for themselves.* This is true of everyone's learning. It is true of the learning health workers desire for their patients. The process cannot be changed or shortened or avoided.

Diet and behavior—psychodietetics

Emotional responses to food stem from many sources. The practices and relationships that surrounded one's early infant feeding experiences build lasting emotional responses. Cultural and family conditioning, and religious and economic factors all mold the adult's behavior with respect to food.

Food feeds the psyche as well as the body. Several areas of psychologic significance give symbolic meaning to foods.

Milk. Of all commonly used foods, milk is perhaps imbued with more psychologic meaning than any other. To many persons milk symbolizes security and comfort. This is especially likely to be true if the individual's early relationships with the mother figure were satisfactory. At the same time, milk may mean dependence and helplessness, particularly in periods of stress. For example, ulcer patients may prefer prolonged treatment of milk every few hours because they find in such a routine a socially accepted form of symbolic regression. In fact, the ulcer itself may in part stem from an inner dependent-independent conflict and a fear of success.

Sex-related attitudes. Certain foods, such as meat and bread, carry masculine meanings. They connote the paternal role of hunter, provider, and acceptor. These notions about meat have been traced by anthropologists to the beliefs of primitive tribes. Meat was (and still is in many cultures) considered the only food that would make a warrior strong and courageous. A plethora of traditions about the magic power of meat and blood is known to anthropologists. Warriors are forbidden to eat any food but meat. In certain cultures a youth to be initiated into the warrior group may have to drink tiger's blood or eat bear's meat or eat the flesh of a sacred animal. Some of this ancient tradition has been handed down to modern times in every culture. In some cultures it has been modified by the wish of the group to eradicate ferocity; therefore eating meat is forbidden. In America the tradition that strong men eat meat has been fostered until modern times by frontier history. The survival of the pioneers depended on their physical energy, strength, activity, and aggression. Meat has been the center of the meal, both in terms of menu planning and money expended. In modern industrial America it remains the main concern of many wives that they have strong husbands and active children. Although they may know that eggs are nutritionally equal to meat (actually better in ideal amino acid combination), eggs never quite make the grade as a meat substitute. They are offered only as a last resort. The homemaker's attitude toward a given food market may be based on the quality of meat it sells.

Vegetables and fruits carry feminine meanings. They connote the maternal role of the one who feeds and gives. This symbolic concept also has a fascinating anthropologic history. When early human beings first settled down after a purely nomadic and hunting existence to an agricultural life, it was women who tilled the fields, while men continued to hunt and fight. The supremacy of the man is bound up with his belief in the "feminine weakness" represented by "mere" fruits and vegetables. The less educated (and the less psychologically developed) a man is, the more likely he is to scorn fruits and vegetables on emotional grounds—although he usually is totally unaware of the reason for his preference and attributes it simply to the taste of the food itself.

Fruits are most feminine in meaning. The apple for the teacher, the gift basket, grapes, and peaches and cream symbolize love, beauty, sexuality, esteem, and luxury. The reproductive notion is basic in the word fruition, the bearing of fruit. Vegetables carry ideas related to even more primitive and earthy aspects of femininity—vegetate, vegetation. Fruits and vegetables are seasonal, ripe, brightly colored, and pleasantly shaped.

Age. Milk and strained foods, sometimes necessary components of a therapeutic diet for the adult, are considered infant foods and may be rejected, particularly by the person who is uncertain that he has genuinely attained adult status. Such a person may be of any chronologic age.

In the latency period the child's food horizon widens. As he leaves home for school, he encounters new foods and is given greater freedom of choice. He also compares his family's food to that of his peers and begins to learn the social status of foods. Certain foods, such as peanut butter, become labeled as children's food and are promoted as such by advertisers.

During adolescence, the tenacious struggle for selfhood ensues. Not only clothes, late hours, driving, and dating, but also foods become battlegrounds between the generations. The teenager periodically adopts food fads, exhibits intense likes and dislikes, and displays enormous appetite. His obsession with his body image is basically a sexual problem. It may take the form of muscle-building foods for boys or figure-control diets for girls.

Adulthood brings certain ideas of food privileges. Foods such as olives, shrimp, and gourmet dishes may be considered adult. Drinks such as coffee, tea, or alcohol are reserved in most groups for adults.

Reward foods. Sweets are often used to bribe children; they are given as rewards for good behavior and are withheld for bad behavior. This pattern may carry over into adulthood. In a moment of self-pity a person may think, "Life has deprived me of my fair reward; therefore I shall eat chocolate cream pie." Sometimes unusual foods, special ways of preparation, or rare delicacies become symbolic rewards or punishment.

Illness. Illness is a period of psychologic repercussion. During illness, some degree of regression usually manifests itself. The patient may become picky and finicky about his food and make frequent special demands. Poor appetite may compound the feeding problem. The patient, more than the well person, needs to be involved in the selection of his food. The same person who when well cares little about the style of food service may as a patient find that his appetite is surprisingly dependent on esthetic appeal in preparation and service.

CULTURAL FOOD PATTERNS

A number of different cultural food patterns are represented in American community life. Many have contributed characteristic dishes or modes of cooking to American eating habits, and in turn many of the food habits of these subcultures have been Americanized. Traditional foods tend to be used more consistently by the older members of the families, while the members of younger generations may use such foods only on special occasions or holidays. Nonetheless, these traditional food patterns have strong meanings and serve to bind families and cultural communities in close fellowship. A few representative cultural food patterns are given here. The unique characteristics of each should be noted. It should be remembered that among persons of all cultures individual tastes vary, geographic patterns within a country vary, and economic factors make for wide differences as does the educational level.

Jewish food pattern

Adherence to Jewish dietary food laws varies among the three basic groups within Judaism: Orthodox—strict observance: Conservative—nominal observance; and Reform—less ceremonial emphasis and minimum observance of the general dietary laws. This body of laws is called the rules of kashruth,[12] and food selected and prepared accordingly is called kosher food. Both words come from the Hebrew word *kasher,* meaning "right" or "fit." The basis of these laws is primarily self-purification and a means of service to God, although they probably also had some hygienic or ethical foundation in their inception. Most of these rules relate to ordinances given to the ancient Hebrews as recorded in the Old Testament books of the law (Leviticus and Deuteronomy) and to the Jewish traditions accumulated through the ensuing centuries. These were collected and interpreted in the Talmud, a body of laws set down in the fourth to sixth centuries BC.

Since the original Hebrew religion was centered in practices of animal sacrifice, and the blood had special ritual significance, the present dietary laws apply specifically to the selection, slaughter, preparation, and service of meat, to the combining of meat and milk, to fish, and to eggs.

Food restrictions

1. The only meat allowed is the meat of cloven hoofed quadrupeds that chew a cud (cattle, sheep, goat, deer), and only the forequarters may be used. The hind quarter may be eaten only if the Sinew of Jacob (hip sinew of the thigh) is removed (Leviticus 11:1-8; Deuteronomy 14:3-8; Genesis 32:33).

2. Chicken, turkey, goose, pheasant, and duck may be eaten (Leviticus 11:13-19).

3. Ritual slaughter follows rigid rules based on minimal pain to the animal and maximal blood drainage. This process of preparing kosher meat involves several steps. The meat is soaked in water in a special vessel. It is then rinsed and thoroughly salted with coarse salt. It is placed on a perforated board tilted to permit blood to flow off, and the meat is left to stand for an hour. After it has drained thoroughly it is washed three times before being used in cooking.

4. No blood may be eaten as food in any form, as blood is considered synonymous with life (Genesis 9:4; Leviticus 3:17, and 17:10-14; Deuteronomy 12:23-27).

5. No combining of meat and milk is allowed. This prohibition is based on the oft-repeated Old Testament command, "Thou shalt not seethe a kid in its mother's milk" (Exodus 23:19, 34:26; Deuteronomy 14:21). Milk or milk food (cheese, ice cream) may be eaten just before a meal, but not for six hours after eating a meal that contains meat. In the Orthodox Jewish home it is customary to maintain two sets of dishes, one for serving meat meals and the other for serving dairy meals.

6. Only those fish with fins and scales are allowed; no shellfish or eels may be eaten (Leviti-

cus 11:9-12; Deuteronomy 14:9-10). Fish of the type permitted may be eaten with either dairy or meat meals.

7. No egg that contains a blood spot may be eaten. Eggs may be taken with either dairy or meat meals.

8. There are no special restrictions on fruits, vegetables, or cereals.

Foods for special occasions

Many of the traditional Jewish foods are related to the different festivals of the Jewish calendar. These holidays and associated foods are summarized in Table 13-1.

Special Sabbath dishes. In Orthodox Jewish homes no food is prepared on the Sabbath, which begins at sundown on Friday and ends when the first star becomes visible Saturday evening. Foods are prepared on Friday and held for use on the Sabbath. A long-honored custom is that of inviting a guest (an orach) to share the Sabbath meals as a remembrance of the Biblical injunction, ''For you were strangers in the land of Egypt'' (Exodus 22:21). A few of the special Sabbath dishes follow:

1. Challah—a special loaf of white bread shaped as a twist or a beehive coil; used at the beginning of the meal after the Kiddush (the blessing over wine)
2. Gefüllte (gelfilte) fish (Ger. ''stuffed fish'')—first course of the Sabbath eve meal; fish fillet, chopped, seasoned, and stuffed back into the skin or minced and rolled into balls
3. Cholent (chulent, or shalet)—a one-dish meal of meat and vegetables, usually beef, potatoes, dried beans, onion, and chicken fat
4. Kugel—a sweet pudding seasoned with spices, raisins, and almonds
5. Tzimmes—carrot pudding made as a main dish with white and sweet potatoes, beef, and onion; may also be a sweet carrot pudding made with honey and spices; prunes may be used instead of carrots

Other representative foods

1. Bagel—a doughnut-shaped hard yeast roll
2. Blintzes—thin filled and rolled pancakes
3. Borsht (borsch)—soup of meat stock, beaten egg or sour cream with beets, cabbage, or spinach; served hot or cold
4. Bubke—coffee cake
5. Farfel—grated noodle dough or crumbled matzoth, used in soup
6. Kasha—buckwheat groats (hulled kernels), used as a cooked cereal or as a potato substitute with gravy
7. Knaidlach or kloese—dumplings, served with chicken soup
8. Knishes—pastry filled with ground meat
9. Latkes—pancakes (potato *latkes* especially popular)
10. Lox—smoked, salted salmon
11. Lukshen—noodles
12. Matzo—flat, unleavened bread
13. Strudel—thin pastry filled with fruit and nuts and rolled, then baked

Greek food pattern

In the close-knit, traditionally organized life of the Greek family, food and the ceremonial aspects of meals constitute primary values. In many Greek homes the meal is a family ritual. A blessing is said or sung, and hospitality is extended to guests. Everyday meals are simple, but holiday meals are the occasion for serving a great variety of delicacies. Bread is always the center of every meal, indeed it is *the* meal, with other foods considered accompaniments to it. Bread is eaten between bites of other food. During religious holidays such as Lent there are fast days of meat-free meals with large use of vegetables.

Food groups

Milk. A relatively small amount of milk is used as a beverage by adults who usually take this food in the form of yogurt. Children drink hot boiled milk sweetened with sugar. Cheese is a favorite food; varieties include feta, a special white cheese made from sheep's milk and preserved in brine, and two hard, salty cheeses, caceri and cephalotyri.

Meat. Lamb is the favored meat. Little beef but some pork and chicken are taken. Frequent use is made of organ meats and fresh fish. Eggs are sometimes taken as a main dish, but not at breakfast. Some characteristic meat dishes include

1. Kreas souvlas—barbecued lamb; brizoles —broiled lamb or pork chops; yiouvarlakia—meat balls and rice with egg-lemon sauce or tomato sauce
2. Mousaka—alternate layers of fried potato, eggplant or squash, cheese, cooked ground meat in spiced tomato sauce covered with thin pastry and baked
3. Ketta vrasti—boiled chicken, eaten hot or cold
4. Psari scharas—broiled fish with olive oil and lemon sauce seasoned with chopped parsley and mustard
5. Psari plake—baked fish with tomatoes, onions, parsley, and olive oil

Vegetables. Vegetables are usually cooked until very soft and are seasoned with meat broth or tomato with onions, olive oil, and parsley. Vegetables are often the main dish. Large amounts of many varieties are eaten. Fresh vegetables are preferred. A combination salad of thinly cut raw vegetables and feta cheese with a simple dressing of olive oil and vinegar or lemon juice is used often. Many legumes (beans, peas, lentils, and chick peas) are eaten; often a meal is made of cooked dried beans served with olives and pickles. Characteristic vegetable dishes include

1. Yiachni—chopped onion browned in olive oil, vegetable added with tomato and seasonings, simmered until soft
2. Dolmathes—meat and rice mixture rolled in cabbage or vine leaves, steamed, served with egg sauce
3. Paragemista—stuffed vegetables such as eggplant, zucchini, green peppers, tomatoes
4. Tiganita—fried vegetables served with garlic or tomato sauce
5. Fasolia yiachni—dried beans cooked with tomatoes and onions

Fruits. Large amounts of fruit are eaten. Peeled raw fruit is an everyday dessert.

Bread and cereals. Bread made of plain wheat flour, water, salt, and yeast is an indispensable part of every meal. It is preferred plain without a spread of butter, jam, or jelly. Dark breads are used by some families. Wheat products such as noodles, macaroni, and spaghetti may be used plain or with meat and tomato sauce. Rice is commonly used. The following are some characteristic cereal dishes:

1. Pilafi—rice to which, after it has been browned in butter, broth or water is added, and simmered until the liquid is absorbed
2. Tyropetta and spanacopetta—cheese pie and spinach pie; thin layers of pastry brushed with olive oil alternating with layers of cheese and egg mixture or cheese and spinach
3. Pastitsio—alternating layers of noodles, macaroni, or spaghetti with tomato sauce containing meat and spices and cheese, covered with thick white sauce, bread crumbs, more cheese, and baked
4. Macaronia me kima—macaroni with meat-tomato sauce
5. Kritharaki—cooked cereal made of flour and water; formed into grains shaped like rice added to cooked meat

Desserts. Desserts other than raw fruit are usually served on special occasions such as holiday meals. Some of these characteristic dishes include

1. Tsoureki—an Easter holiday bread similar to coffee cake, shaped in a braid and glazed with fruit and nuts
2. Baklavas—many layers of very thin pastry brushed with butter and sprinkled with

nuts, sugar, and spices, cut in diamond shapes and baked, served with honey or syrup

3. Loukoumathes—batter of plain flour, yeast, water, dropped in deep fat and fried, served with honey and cinnamon
4. Melomacarona—short dough (flour, oil, orange juice, soda, sugar) filled with mixture of nuts, sugar, and spices, sealed and baked, dipped in syrup and sprinkled with nuts
5. Risogalo—rice custard sprinkled with cinnamon

Italian food pattern

The sharing of food and companionship is an important part of the Italian pattern of life. Meals are associated with much warmth and fellowship, and special occasions are marked by the sharing of food with families and friends. Leisurely meals are customary, with a light breakfast, the large main meal in the middle of the day, and a small evening meal. Bread and pasta are the basic Italian foods. On religious fast days, such as Fridays, Lent, and the period of Advent before Christmas, pasta is prepared with meatless sauces or with fish.

Food groups

Milk. Milk is seldom used alone as a beverage. Frequently it is consumed with coffee in a mixture of about half coffee and half milk. Cheese, however, is a favorite food. Parmesan and Romano are hard grating cheese used in cooking; ricotta and mozzarella are two soft Italian cheeses used in cooking or with bread.

Meat. Chicken baked with oil or in tomato sauce is used often. Beef and veal are used as meatballs, meat loaf, cutlets, stews, roasts, and chops. Roasted or fried Italian pork sausage is common. A number of Italian cold cuts are famous—salami, mortadella (bologna-type sausage), coppa (peppered sausage), and prosciutto (Italian cured ham). Many kinds of fish are used. Fresh fish are preferred, but some canned fish such as tuna, sardines, anchovies, and special salted codfish are used also. Some characteristic meat dishes are pollo alla cacciatora (chicken browned in olive oil, then simmered in wine and tomato sauce), scaloppina di vitello (thin, floured strips of veal browned in olive oil and simmered in sauce flavored with wine and herbs), Italian meatballs with spaghetti, and baccala (dried salted codfish, soaked several days, browned in olive oil, and simmered with tomato sauce and herbs).

Vegetables. Favorite vegetables include zucchini and other squash, broccoli, spinach, eggplant, escarole and other salad greens, green beans, peppers, and tomatoes. Tomatoes are used in sauces either whole or as paste, or they are pureed. Vegetables are usually cooked in water, drained, and seasoned with olive oil or with oil and vinegar. A combination salad of greens such as escarole, chicory, lettuce, endive, and romaine, seasoned with a simple dressing of olive oil, vinegar, garlic, salt, and pepper is called insalata.

Fruits. Fresh fruit in season is taken as dessert.

Bread and cereals. Bread is present at every Italian meal as a highly regarded principal food. It is made in loaves of many shapes. Each is characteristic of a different Italian province. All Italian breads are made of wheat flour and are white, crusty, and substantial. Some rice and corn meal are used in special dishes. For example, risotto ala Milanese is a dish made of rice cooked in broth with saffron, Parmesan cheese, onion, and mushrooms. Polenta is a thick, yellow cornmeal mush sometimes made into a casserole with sausage, tomato sauce, and cheese.

A basic item in the Italian food pattern is pasta. This term is used for all of the wheat products made into various shapes and forms such as spaghetti, macaroni, and egg noodles. Pasta is served in many ways. Spaghetti is commonly used with a characteristic tomato sauce and cheese or with added meatballs or fish. Special dishes of pasta of various kinds filled with meat mixtures are served on holidays—

ravioli, lasagna, manicotti, tortellini, and cannelloni. A dry red or white wine is usually served also.

Soups. Thick soups often serve as the main food for lighter meals. Minestrone is made with vegetables, ceci (chick peas), and pasta. Pasta e fagioli is a substantial bean soup.

Seasonings and basic cooking method. Herbs and spices characteristically used in Italian dishes include oregano, rosemary, basil, saffron, parsley, and nutmeg. Garlic is used often, as are wine, olive oil, tomato puree, salt pork, and cheese. The basic processes of Italian cooking of main dishes are the initial browning of the seasonings in olive oil, adding meat or fish for browning also, then covering with wine, tomato sauce, or broth and simmering slowly on low heat for several hours.

Puerto Rican food pattern

Indigenous tropical vegetables and fruits form the base of the Puerto Rican food pattern. Almost everyone eats the main food, viandas (compare the English word ''viands''), which are starchy vegetables and fruits such as plantain and green banana. The two other staples of the diet are rice and beans. Milk, meat, yellow and green vegetables, and other fruits are used in limited quantities.

Food groups

Viandas. The many kinds of vianda eaten every day include piche verde (green banana), platano verde (green plantain), plantano maduro (ripe plantain), batata blanca (white sweet potato), batata amarilla (yellow sweet potato), name blanco (white yam), panapen (breadfruit), yautia (tanier), and yuca (cassava). Viandas are cooked in many ways. Usually codfish and onion are added, and if income permits, some avocado and hardboiled eggs are also added. This dish is called serenata. A Puerto Rican soup containing vianda and meat is called sancocho.

Rice. A large proportion of the daily calories is obtained from rice. Most Puerto Ricans eat about 7 oz daily. The rice is usually cooked in salted water and seasoned with lard (arroz blanco—white rice). Other dishes prepared with rice include arroz con habichuelas, rice stewed with beans and sofrito (a sauce of tomatoes, green pepper, onion, garlic, salt pork, lard, herbs); arroz con pollo, rice with chicken, seasoned with olives, red peppers, and sofrito; arroz con dulce, a dessert made with rice, sugar, and spices; and asopao, a thick soup of chicken and rice.

Other cereal grains. Some wheat is used in the form of bread, noodles, and spaghetti. Oatmeal and cornmeal mush may be added if income permits.

Beans. Legumes used include chick peas, navy beans, red kidney beans (preferred), and dried peas. Usually they are boiled until tender and cooked with sofrito.

Milk. Low-income groups can afford little milk. Most of that which is taken is boiled and used with coffee (café con leche). Some cocoa and chocolate are used in the same way.

Meat. Most Puerto Rican families cannot afford meat, although pork and chicken are used when income allows. The only animal protein the majority can buy is dried codfish.

Vegetables and fruits. Small amounts of other vegetables are used by the Puerto Rican people. Many tropical fruits are available. Puerto Rico is the home of the acerola, the tiny, sour West Indian cherry that looks like a miniature apple and has the highest quantity of ascorbic acid known to be contained in any food (about 1,000 mg/100 g). Other fruits include oranges, pineapples, grapefruits, papayas, and mangos.

Meal pattern

In most homes a typical day's food would include coffee with milk for breakfast, a large plate of viandas with codfish for lunch, and rice, beans, and viandas for dinner. If income permits, egg or oatmeal may be added to the breakfast, some meat to dinner, and some fruit may be taken between meals. This simple daily diet is in contrast with a holiday meal such as that enjoyed at Christmastime—whole pig roasted on a spit (lechon asado), blood sausage, green bananas or plantains cooked in the ashes, rice, pasteles (plantain dough filled with chopped pork, sofrito, olives, raisins, and boiled peas), rice pudding, and wine, beer, or brandy.

An effort is being made by the U.S. government to improve the diet of the Puerto Rican people by listing the basic foods everyone eats (rice, beans, viandas, codfish, lard, sugar, coffee) and suggesting things that need to be added, such as milk in the form of goat's milk or dry milk, meat and egg, yellow and green vegetables, and fresh native fruit.

Mexican food pattern

A blending of the food habits of the Spanish settlers and native Indian tribes formed the basis for the present food patterns of the people of Mexican heritage who now live in the United States (chiefly in the Southwest). Three foods are fundamental to this pattern—dried beans, chili peppers, and corn. Variations and additions may be found in different localities or among those Mexicans of different income levels.

Food groups

Milk. Very little milk is used. A small amount of evaporated milk may be purchased for babies.

Meat. Because of its cost, little meat is taken. Beef or chicken may be eaten two or three times a week. Eggs also are used only occasionally, and fish rarely.

Vegetables. Corn (fresh or canned) and chili peppers are the main vegetables. Chicos is steamed green corn dried on the cob. Pasole is similar to whole grain hominy (lime-treated, hulled whole kernels), Chili peppers provide a good source of vitamin C. They are usually dried and ground into a powder. Pinto beans or calice beans are used daily. They may be reheated by frying (refried beans), or they may

be cooked with beef, garlic, and chile peppers (chili con carne).

Fruits. Depending on availability and cost, oranges, apples, bananas, and canned peaches are used.

Bread and cereals. For centuries corn has been the basic grain used as bread and cereal by the Mexican people. Masa (dough) is made from dried corn, which has been heated, soaked in limewater, washed, and ground wet to form a mass with a consistency of putty. This dough is formed into thin, unleavened cakes and baked on a hot griddle to make the typical tortilla. Wheat is now replacing corn for making tortillas. Unless the wheat flour is enriched, the calcium that is a dietetically important constituent of the lime-treated corn is lost to the Mexican diet. Cornmeal gruel, or atole, is served with hot milk. Rice cooked in milk may be used as a dessert. Oatmeal, a popular breakfast cereal, is eaten by those who can afford it.

Beverage. Large amounts of coffee are used. In many families coffee is given to young children.

Seasonings. Chili pepper, onion, and garlic are used most frequently. Occasionally other herbs may be added. Lard is the basic fat.

Chinese food pattern

Traditional Chinese cooking is based on three principles: (1) the natural flavors must be enhanced, (2) the texture and color must be maintained, and (3) undesired qualities of foods must be masked or modified. Like the French, Chinese cooks feel that refrigeration lessens natural flavors. They select the freshest possible foods, hold them the shortest possible time, then cook them quickly at a high temperature in small amounts of liquid or fat. By these means natural flavor, color, and texture are preserved. Vegetables are cooked just before serving so that they are still crisp and flavorful when eaten. The only sauce that may be served with them is a thin, translucent one, perhaps made with cornstarch. A thick gravy is never used. To mask some flavors or textures or to enhance others, foods that have been dried, salted, pickled, spiced, candied, or canned may be added as garnishes or relishes.

Food groups

Milk. Very little milk and limited amounts of cheese are used.

Meat. Pork, lamb, chicken, duck, fish, and shellfish are used in many ways. Eggs and soybeans (soybean curd and milk) add to the protein content of the Chinese diet. Some characteristic dishes include egg roll, a thin dough spread with meat and vegetable filling, rolled and fried in deep fat; egg foo yung, an omelet of egg, chopped chicken, mushrooms, scallions, celery, and bean sprouts; and sweet and sour pork, pork cubes fried, then simmered in a sweet-sour sauce of brown sugar, vinegar, and other seasonings. Chow mein is an American invention. It is a mixture of meat, celery, and bean sprouts served over rice or noodles and seasoned with soy sauce.

Vegetables. Cooked by the characteristic method described, vegetables such as cabbage, cucumbers, snow peas, melons, squash, greens, mushrooms, bean sprouts, and sweet potatoes are made into many fine dishes.

Fruits. Usually fruits are eaten fresh, without addition; but pineapple and a few others are sometimes used in combination dishes.

Bread and cereals. Rice is the staple grain used at most meals.

Beverage. The traditional beverage is unsweetened green tea.

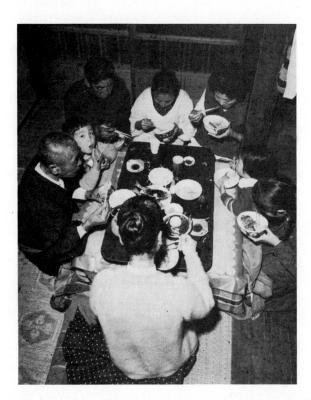

Fig. 13-1. Japanese family at dinner. The evening meal consists of rice, vegetables, pickles, and seafood. Sometimes chicken is prepared. The favorite dish is sashimi, pieces of raw fish dipped in soy sauce. (WHO photograph by T. Takahara.)

Seasonings. Soy sauce is a basic seasoning. Almonds, ginger, and sesame seeds are also used. The most frequently used cooking fats are lard and peanut oil.

Japanese food pattern

Japanese food patterns are in some ways similar to Chinese. Rice is a basic constituent of the diet, tea is the main beverage, and soy sauce is used for seasoning. However, there are some characteristic differences. The Japanese diet contains more seafood, especially raw fish. A number of taboos prohibit certain food combinations or the use of certain foods in specific localities or at specific times. Some of these taboos are associated with religious practices such as ancestor veneration.

Food groups

Milk. Little milk or cheese is used. Some evaporated or dried milk may be added in cooking or given to babies.

Meat. On the Japanese islands, where no city is far from the ocean, the main animal protein source is seafood. Many varieties of fish and shellfish are served, such as raw squid or octopus. Other unusual saltwater fare are eels, abalone, globefish (puffer fish); more familiar to the Westerner are crab, shrimp, mackerel, carp, and salmon. Families living inland, especially, may also eat rabbit, chicken, and occasionally beef or lamb. Eggs are a source of additional protein.

Vegetables. Japanese menus include many vegetables, usually steamed and served with soy sauce. Pickled vegetables are also well liked.

Fruits. Fresh fruit is eaten in season. A tray of fruit is a regular course of the main meal.

Bread and cereals. While rice is the staple grain, some corn, barley, and oats are served, and white wheat bread is coming into increasing use in Japanese cities.

Meal sequence

A specific sequence of courses is followed at most meals (Fig. 13-1). A dinner is served in this order: green tea, unsweetened; some appetizer such as soy or red bean cake, a raw fish (sashimi) or radish relish (komono); broiled fish or omelet; vegetables with soy sauce; plain steamed rice; herb relish; fruits in season; a broth base soup (shirumise); and perhaps more unsweetened green tea. Typical dishes include tempura (batter fried shrimp) and aborakge (fried soybean curd). Sukiyaki is as American as chow mein. It is a mixture of sautéed beef and vegetables served with soy sauce. Soybean oil is the main cooking fat.

CASE STUDY 3
The generation gap in a Jewish family

Abe Goldstein, aged 68, was a lonely man. Ever since his wife, Ruth, died suddenly last spring, the house seemed so quiet. When the children were growing up at home, they always had some of their young friends around. During those years he was teaching, too, and his students came by frequently to discuss problems.

There had always been a guest to share the Sabbath meal, which Ruth had prepared on Friday. After the *Kiddush* and wine they broke bread together, the special coiled white loaf, challah. Then came the gefüllte fish in sharply seasoned little balls, followed by hearty bowls of cholent, and finally the sweet tzimmes with honey and spices.

Even now the thought caused Abe, lying alone in his hospital room, to run his tongue over his lips. But instead of honey, the taste in his mouth now seemed bitter. Since his retirement no one seemed to need him any more, and without Ruth nothing mattered. The older children were married and lived too far away to visit often. Now there was only the youngest son, Benjamin, at home. At 18 Benjamin seemed so tall, almost grown, but his ways were so different. These days he was rarely at home, and when he was, there seemed to be little that they shared. With Passover coming soon, Abe had hoped he and his son could invite some friends for the Seder meal just as the family used to do in the old days. But when he suggested it, Benjamin only replied, ''Oh, that's old-fashioned stuff, and besides, I don't think any of my friends would care about it.''

It was the following week that Abe had collapsed as he was leaving the synagogue. His friend, Joseph Goldberg, had taken him to the hospital, where he felt more alone than ever. The doctor had said he was all right, though, and could go home the next day. This was just a little warning, the doctor said, but with his heart condition he would have to take it easy, rest more, and eat more nourishing food to regain some weight. Abe's thin, sparse frame seemed almost bony.

But in the hospital the food was so foreign. With his orthodox Jewish practices, he had eaten very little. The nutritionist, however, seemed particularly concerned, and said she would come in later to discuss his diet with him. With this thought Abe lay his head back on the pillow and began to relax a bit. ''Maybe she can help me,'' he thought.

Questions to guide your inquiry

 1. What meanings does food have for Abe Goldstein?
 2. What is the basis for the Jewish dietary laws?
 3. What food restrictions need to be remembered in helping Abe with his diet?
 4. What is the Seder meal? How are foods used in this meal as symbols?
 5. What psychologic factors were influencing Abe's present eating habits? What social factors?
 6. What are the nutritional needs of a man Abe's age?
 7. Why may a person in Abe's situation develop malnutrition?
 8. In what general ways will culture influence food habits? Give some examples.
 9. What is food symbolism? Give some examples of such meanings related to food.
10. What social factors influence food habits?
11. Give some examples of the present American value system and its influence over attitudes toward food.
12. What social problems cause changing food habits and contribute to nutritional problems?
13. What are some psychologic factors that influence food habits?
14. Why is perception—both the patient's and the practitioner's—such an important factor in health education?
15. What are some psychologic meanings that we will attach to some of our common foods?

REFERENCES
Specific

1. Barlow, D. H., and Tillotson, J. L.: Behavioral science and nutrition: a new perspective, J. Am. Diet. Assoc. **72:**368, April, 1978.
2. Tillotson, J. L., editor: Proceedings of the Nutrition-Behavior Research Conference, DHEW Pub. No. (NIH) 76-978, 1975.
3. Mahoney, M. J., and Caggiula, A. W.: Applying behavioral methods of nutrition counseling, J. Am. Diet. Assoc. **72:**372, April, 1978.
4. Evans, R. I., and Hall, Y.: Social-psychologic perspective in motivating changes in eating behavior, J. Am. Diet. Assoc. **72:**378, April, 1978.
5. Sakr, A. H.: Fasting in Islam, J. Am. Diet. Assoc. **67:**17, July, 1975.
6. Warner, W. L., and Lunt, P. S.: The social life of a modern community, New Haven, Conn., 1941, Yale University Press.
7. Hollingshead, A. B., and Redlich, F. C.: Social class and mental illness, New York, 1958, John Wiley & Sons.
8. Ruesch, J., and Bateson, G.: Communication: the social matrix of psychiatry, New York, 1951, W. W. Norton & Co., Inc., pp. 94-134.
9. Maslow, A. H.: Motivation and personality, New York, 1954, Harper & Bros.
   (See also Maslow's Toward a psychology of being, Princeton, N.J., 1962, D. Van Nostrand Co.)
10. Buchler, J.: Nature and judgment, New York, 1955, Columbia University Press.
11. Allport, G. W.: Perception and public health. In Katz, A. H., and Felton, J. S., editors: Health and the community, New York, 1965, The Free Press.
12. Natow, A. B., Heslin, J., and Reven, B. C.: Kashruth in a dietetics curriculum: integrating the Jewish dietary laws into a dietetics program, J. Am. Diet. Assoc. **67:**13, July, 1975.

General

American Dietetic Association: Cultural food patterns in the U.S.A., Chicago, 1976.
Cardenas, J., Gibbs, C. E., and Young, E. A.: Nutritional beliefs and practices in primigravid Mexican-American women, J. Am. Diet Assoc. **69:**262, 1976.
Chang, B.: Some dietary beliefs in Chinese folk culture, J. Am. Diet. Assoc. **65:**436, 1974.
Cosper, B. A., and Wakefield, L. M.: Food choices of women: personal, attitudinal, and motivational factors, J. Am. Diet. Assoc. **66:**152, 1975.
Fathauer, G. H.: Food habits—an anthropologist's view, J. Am. Diet. Assoc. **37:**335, 1960.
Gifft, H. H., Washbon, M. B., and Harrison, G. G.: Nutrition, behavior, and change, Englewood Cliffs, N.J., 1972, Prentice-Hall, Inc.
Grivetti, L. E., and Panghorn, R. M.: Origin of selected Old Testament dietary prohibitions, J. Am. Diet. Assoc. **65:**634, Dec., 1974.
Heller, C. A.: The diet of some Alaskan Eskimos and Indians, J. Am. Diet. Assoc. **45:**425, 1964.
Judd, J. E.: Century-old dietary taboos in the 20th century Japan, J. Am. Diet. Assoc. **33:**489, 1957.
Kaufman, M.: Adapting therapeutic diets to Jewish food customs, Am. J. Clin. Nutr. **5:**676, 1957.
Longman, D. P.: Working with Pueblo Indians in New Mexico, J. Am. Diet. Assoc. **47:**470, 1965.
Lowenberg, M. E., and Lucas, B. L.: Feeding families and children—1776 to 1976, J. Am. Diet. Assoc. **68:**207, 1976.
Lowenberg, M. E., et al.: Food and man, ed. 2, New York, 1974, John Wiley & Sons.
Manning, M. L.: The psychodynamics of dietetics, Nurs. Outlook **13:**57, 1965.
Mayer, J.: The nutritional status of American Negroes, Nutr. Rev. **23:**161, 1965.
Mead, M.: Dietary patterns and food habits, J. Am. Diet. Assoc. **19:**1, 1943.
Mead, M.: Cultural patterning of nutritionally relevant behavior, J. Am. Diet. Assoc. **25:**677, 1949.
Reaburn, J. A., Krondi, M., and Lau, D.: Social determinants in food selection, J. Am. Diet. Assoc. **74:**637, June, 1979.
Schwartz, N. E.: Nutritional knowledge, attitudes, and practices of high school graduates, J. Am. Diet. Assoc. **66:**28, 1975.
Valassi, K. V.: Food habits of Greek Americans, Am. J. Clin. Nutr. **11:**240, 1962.
Zifferblatt, S. M., Wilber, C. S., and Pinsky, J. L.: Understanding food habits, J. Am. Diet. Assoc. **76:**9, Jan., 1980.

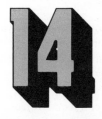

Nutrition education

In the previous chapter the question of why people eat what they eat was explored. This question is fundamental to understanding people's food habits. Cultural, social, and psychologic factors shape the patterns of attitudes, beliefs, and values that govern food habits of groups and individuals.

The second question fundamental to success as effective health professionals is *How can insights contributed by the behavioral sciences be used to improve family and community nutrition?* What principles must guide health education work with individuals, families, and communities? How can these principles be applied in practical ways so that people can be reached and helped to meet their health needs through improved food habits? What methods, approaches, and materials may be most effective?

In the search for answers there are four aspects of nutrition education and applied community nutrition that should be considered: (1) the relationship of cultural forces to changes in food habits, (2) the teaching-learning process, (3) health teaching in patient care, and (4) community nutrition education. Throughout all of these ramifications of the problem, one underlying concept is essential. The health workers themselves must become imbued with a concept of *change* if their efforts are to succeed. Life—always a dynamic process—and learning—which is manifested in terms of changed behavior—are in essence based on the principle of change. Biologically and educationally, to be static is to be dead. To be alive is to be willing to change. The more people are to change in ways that lead to improvement for themselves and others, the more they are alive.

CULTURAL FORCES AND FOOD HABIT CHANGE

Many examples could be cited to demonstrate the power of social and cultural forces in determining food habit behavior. Three classic studies clearly illustrate the far-reaching implications of these forces in efforts to reach people needing health care. Two of these studies were in other cultures; one was made in an American community. Experiences of workers in a health center serving a Zulu community in the Republic of South Africa and those of workers in a child welfare clinic in West Bengal, India, reveal the strong and intimate relationships that exist between cultural forces and health practices, hence the necessity for health personnel to know and understand such forces. Kurt Lewin's important wartime study of food habits in a midwestern U.S. community defined the social and economic forces that channel food from source to consumer and identified the various "gatekeepers" who control those channels.

A health program among South African Zulus

John Cassel's[1] study of health habits in a community of Zulu tribesmen in southwestern Natal, South Africa, underscored two principles important to health education: (1) The more central and strongly integrated segments of a culture, especially those closely related to moral codes governing interpersonal conduct, resist change. Other segments made up of persons who are less deeply concerned with such codes are more open to change. (2) The health team that works *in* —not apart from—the community and that integrates health education and disease prevention activities with curative aspects of health practice can produce desirable changes in the beliefs of persons and can alter their habits in ways that will improve health and general living standards.

In 1940 when the Polela Health Centre organized its first multidiscipline teams, each consisting of a family physician, a family nurse, and a health educator, health conditions in the African community described in this report were extremely poor. Infant and crude mortality rates were high. Eighty percent of the people bore marks of malnutrition, and epidemics were common. After only 10 years of operation the health program's results were evident. The infant mortality rate had been greatly reduced by the improved nutritional state of the babies, the incidence of pellagra and kwashiorkor had fallen from 12 or more cases a week to fewer than 12 a year, and epidemics of infectious diseases were better controlled.

Reeducation for better nutrition. Since severe malnutrition was the major health problem, the Health Centre based its program on reeducation for better nutrition. The first step was a detailed survey of existing dietary habits, and analysis of factors behind these habits, and a study of current attitudes and beliefs about food. The team learned that the tribe subsisted on a monotonous diet that was composed principally of maize (corn), with some dried beans, little or no milk, occasional potatoes or pumpkins in season, and large quantities of beer brewed from millet (sorghum). Factors that contributed to malnutrition were eroded soil, extreme poverty (money was earned by migrant

labor in distant cities), traditional ideas about foods, ignorance of food values and of the body's needs for food, inefficient use of available resources, and cooking methods that destroyed much of the nutritional value of food.

After analysis had led the team to a clear understanding of the community's needs, the workers approached the problem of changing the ingrained food habits of the people. They began with activities aimed at creating awareness of needs and increasing interest in possible dietary changes. Informal group discussions in the Zulu language were held in key homes. Other homes throughout the community were visited periodically. Subjects discussed were food values, ideas about digestion, fetal nutrition, how the body is nourished, comparison of the people's poor diet with the better diet of their ancestors, and available but unused food resources. The members of the community agreed on three changes: (1) the addition of vegetables, to be grown in home gardens, (2) the addition of eggs, by overcoming negative but not strongly entrenched economic and cultural notions concerning the bad effects of this food, and (3) the addition of milk from the tribe's prized herds of cattle.

General results of the program. Under the impetus of continued group discussions, demonstrations, and instructions, the first two of these aims were accomplished with little difficulty. To induce these people to take milk in any form, including curd or cheese, proved to be a far more complex problem. According to their ancient and deep-seated religious belief, the link between a man and his ancestors was his cattle. The members of the tribe strove to maintain their cattle at all costs, even though the size of the herd exceeded food and pasture resources. Only by doing so could a man retain the goodwill of his ancestors; and only his ancestors' beneficence could ward off misfortune, ill health, and harm. Cattle were also prized as an index of wealth and as payment of the bride price necessary to obtain a wife and to seal the marriage contract. Only the kin group of the male head of a household could use milk from his cattle. Since a menstruating or pregnant woman had power to bewitch the cattle, milk was excluded from the diet of all girls past puberty. A double prohibition fell on a married woman. She was a woman, and she lived in her husband's family as a "foreigner" to his kin group, to his ancestors, and hence to his cattle and their milk. This was, of course, particularly unfortunate for the married woman during her childbearing years, when nutritional demands are especially pronounced.

It was soon evident that factual knowledge about the nutritional value of milk, especially for pregnant and lactating mothers who were a major health concern, could not change so deep a system of cultural and religious beliefs. Another way had to be found. The need was met ingeniously by the introduction of powdered milk! This the people readily accepted, calling it "meal" or "powder" and consuming it in large quantities.

Numerous social and economic problems remained to be solved at longer range. Methods of agriculture and stockraising needed to be improved, and there were other difficulties beyond the scope of the health program. But the inclusion in the diet of more vegetables, eggs, and milk was a beginning, and its value was reflected in improved maternal and child health.

This experience serves to emphasize that health conditions in a community do not exist in isolation. They are bound up in a network of economic, political, ecologic, and cultural factors and must be approached in such a context.

A health program among West Bengal Indians

In 1947 the province of Bengal, which had been developed in northeast India while that country was under British rule, was divided between India and East Pakistan. West Bengal, whose population was largely Hindu, became a part of India; East Bengal, largley Moslem, was absorbed into the newly created, divided country of Pakistan. The personal experience of D. B. Jelliffe[2] in a rural welfare clinic in West Bengal reinforces the need to know the cultural pattern of a community in relation to foods and illness and to work within this cultural pattern to find effective ways of meeting health needs. In describing his experience, Jelliffe emphasized three important principles of health education: (1) People will accept new knowledge about health and nutrition only to the extent that the new information can be amalgamated into existing patterns of custom and belief. (2) Cross-cultural exchanges are mutually beneficial. People of less highly industrialized cultures can learn from health workers, but the health workers also can learn much from other cultures that will enrich their own. (3) Interest in individuals of other cultures and appreciation of the personal and social functions they perform build rapport between health workers and the families they seek to serve. Unless rapport exists between these two groups of persons, all efforts to educate are wasted.

Cultural influences. Most of the women who brought their children to the West Bengal clinic were illiterate villagers of a low socioeconomic class. They practiced the Hindu religion. The Hindu is taught that foods are to be classified in two ways. First, there is the all-important distinction between *amish* (vegetarian) and *niramish* (nonvegetarian) nutrients. Second, these mothers followed closely the ancient Indian classification of foods as *garam* (hot) and *thanda* (cold). The classification into garam and thanda is based on properties believed to be inherent in certain foods, which enable them to exert specific influences on the body. Combinations of garam and thanda foods are believed to be especially harmful. Traditional Hindu medicine classifies illnesses also into those that are garam and thanda and restricts the patient's diet accordingly. During a garam illness, one may not eat garam food, because to do so would intensify the disease; during a thanda sickness, the patient must eat no thanda food. Eggs, meat, milk, honey, and sugar are garam foods; lemon, orange, rice water, acid buttermilk, and curd (yogurt) are thanda foods.

The health workers of Jelliffe's group had to use ingenuity to integrate their treatment into this system of beliefs. In treating an upper respiratory infection the physician might want the child to increase his fluid intake and to receive ascorbic acid in the form of water and orange juice, and he might want to prescribe rice as an easily digested source of energy. But that diet would be unacceptable to the mother, because both this illness and these foods are regarded as thanda. Knowing this, the physician advised that she put a little honey in the water and juice and that she cook the rice in milk. Since honey and milk are garam, they will neutralize the thanda of the other foods. This the mother readily accepted, and so the health needs of the child were met.

A similar difficulty arose in prescribing for children recovering from diarrhea. Even when the child could tolerate milk, the mother did not want to give it, because both milk and diarrhea are classified as garam. Some of the Hindus avoided milk so persistently that they incurred kwashiorkor or another protein deficiency disease. Aware of these traditions, the physician would prescribe a low-residue rice gruel and a pectin-containing apple sherbet— both thanda foods. Dilute acid buttermilk, a thanda food, was also a good choice on two accounts. Medically it was well tolerated and contained needed protein, and culturally it was acceptable.

Principles of approach. Throughout this effort, the health workers in the West Bengal clinic made use of a threefold approach: (1) They made an intensive study of the cultural practices related to health. (2) They carried out an *unprejudiced* analysis of these practices in the light of the scientific principles on which modern western medical care is based and in consideration of local conditions. (3) They encouraged those traditional practices that were beneficial, did not interfere with those that were harmless, and sought to overcome the harmful practices by means of persuasion and demonstration. Where it was medically important to introduce a treatment that was unacceptable on cultural grounds, they devised ways of neutralizing it or of presenting the essential aspect of the treatment in a culturally acceptable form.

Food behavior among midwestern U.S. homemakers

A widely known study of food habits in America was conducted by a field staff at the Child Welfare Research Station of the State University of Iowa in 1942 under the direction of Kurt Lewin.[3] This study has given important insights into the forces that influence food habits in America and has provided a basis for the development of more effective methods of changing those habits. Combining the approaches of cultural anthropology and the quantitative methods of psychology, Lewin studied five population groups: Caucasian Americans of three income levels and two subcultural groups, Czech and black. He interviewed homemakers to determine factors behind family food behavior. To evaluate the efficacy of methods that might be used in attempts to change food habits, he compared the responses to lectures and to group discussions.

His results led him to two conclusions: (1) Food reaches the family table from its point of origin through a series of channels. These channels are controlled at various points by "gatekeepers." The flow of food through these channels depends on the ideas about food and the values of these "gatekeepers." (2) Changes in food habits come about more readily as a result of group discussion and decision than in response to lecture and request. It will be worthwhile to look more closely into Lewin's findings.

Channel theory

Food channels. From production point to consumer, food moves through a series of channels. A channel is a single step in the complex process of food delivery. It may refer to as simple a step as delivery of a head of lettuce from the kitchen garden to the family table. It may refer to home canning or home cooking. The channel may also be one of the many routes through which a food may be bought—a market, a wayside stand, a home delivery service. Again, a channel may be the preparation of food for sale by baking, by freezing, or by cooking and serving in a restaurant. It may be the holding of quantities of food at storage points (refrigeration plants, freezers, and warehouses).

Gatekeepers. Each of these channels is governed by a "gatekeeper," who in turn is controlled both by psychologic and cultural forces and by nonpsychologic forces.

PSYCHOLOGIC AND CULTURAL FORCES. Each gatekeeper—farmer, wholesale food dealer, storekeeper, homemaker, or other person who controls one of the channels through which food is delivered from field to table—is more or less consciously influenced by tradition, childhood memories related to specific foods, taste preference, religious or other taboos, and beliefs or knowledge about the value or danger of specific items. Some of these psychologic forces operate through the culture as a whole (such as having turkey at Thanksgiving). Others are individual matters (Mrs. Black does not like olives). Important among psychologic forces are resistance (Mr. Blue refuses to eat sweets because his physician has warned him against them) and conflict. (Miss Green wonders whether to serve filet mignon when her boss comes to dinner—will he think she should show her appreciation by this special treat or will he decide that if she can afford this she does not need another raise?)

NONPSYCHOLOGIC FORCES. The gatekeepers of the food channels are also responsive to such objective pressures as the ability to raise certain foods in certain soils or under certain weather conditions, available means of transportation, the chance to buy a certain food (as a restaurant features fruits in season, a baker runs a "special" of fresh blueberry pie, or a butcher advertises a bargain in spring lamb), and available money (Miss Green counts her dimes and decides to do miracles with beef à la stroganof; a year later, married to the chief junior executive, she serves the filet with truffles).

Main gatekeeper. Although family patterns and roles are changing, historically the most significant gatekeeper in the food channel system is the mother in the home. Often it is she who determines what food is served and in what condition it is delivered to the plate. It is she who selects, from among the many reasons that are presented to her for choosing this or that item, the set of reasons that for her are decisive. *The personal values of the main gatekeeper* are, in the last analysis, the key to the food habits of a family.

Regardless of which member in the family assumes the role, the main gatekeeper determines *what is food* for the family: what is food for breakfast, food for lunch at home, food for lunch at school or work, food for family dinner, food for Sunday dinner, and food for guests, for summer, for winter, for the sick child, and for the growing boy and girl. Within the main gatekeeper's personal system, a specific item (meat, milk, potato, salad, bread, egg, or pie) plays various roles in relation to various family members and in accordance with the meal pattern. If a conflict arises between the cost of food and the meaning of food, the main gatekeeper's decision may vary according to the response to the pressure considered most important.

Methods of changing food habits. Many methods have been and are being used to bring about desired changes in the food habits of the American people. The approaches range from individual depth therapy, as with a disturbed child, to propaganda campaigns carried on through the mass media—radio, television, newspapers, magazines, billboards, and other advertising devices. Lewin was interested in detecting the most effective means by which health workers could reach and persuade people to improve their nutritional patterns. He therefore focused on the approaches that would retain the impact of personal, face-to-face meeting, while conserving the time of the health worker. These techniques were midway between individual instruction and mass methods and involved two types of group meeting—lecture-request and discussion-decision.

To test the relative effectiveness of these two group methods in bringing about a change in food habit, it was decided to attempt the introduction of a rather widely rejected type of food: organ meats, such as kidneys, heart, and brains. A pair of groups were selected as the target from each of the three broad socioeconomic classes: low, middle, and high. One group of each pair was approached by the lec-

ture-request method; the other group was approached by the discussion-decision method.

LECTURE-REQUEST GROUPS. In attempting to induce the desired food habit change in the lecture-request groups, the nutritionist sought to establish motive by pointing out the relationships between nutrition and general health and by emphasizing high food values and economic advantages in these particular meats. By using detailed explanations and charts and other devices, the nutritionist told of various ways of cooking the organ meats to overcome aversions to odor, texture, appearance, and flavor. The nutritionist concluded by handing out recipes and requesting the group members to try them during the week.

DISCUSSION-DECISION GROUPS. In trying to persuade the members of the discussion-decision groups from each socioeconomic level, the nutritionist opened each meeting with a brief introductory statement. The nutritionist acknowledged the difficulties involved in changing food

---

Table 14-1. Change of food habits in members of groups according to method used and economic level of participants*

Socioeconomic level	Group decision				Lecture			
	Low	Middle	High	Total	Low	Middle	High	Total
Number of participants	17	16	13	46	13	15	13	41
Percent of persons serving one or more of the three meats	35	69	54	52	15	13	0	10
Percent of persons serving a meat they had *hardly* ever served before	20	53	54	44	0	8	0	3
Percent of persons serving a meat they had *never* served before	13	36	50	32	0	8	0	3
Total percent of persons serving one or more of the new meats who had never used any of the three meats prior to the experiment				29†				0‡

*Lewin, K.: Forces behind food habits and methods of change. In The problem of changing food habits, Washington, D.C., 1943, National Academy of Sciences, National Research Council
†Out of a total number of 14 participants who had never before used any of the meats.
‡Out of a total number of 11 participants who had never before used any of the meats.

habits and frankly said that she hoped to gain the group's cooperation. The nutritionist then withdrew from the discussion, and the members of the group took it up. Step by step they identified the problem more completely until they as a group acknowledged that it was necessary to do something about it. This led to exploration of the reasons for rejection of these particular foods. The question was then stated by the members of the group: "How can we overcome these objections?"

At this point the group turned to the nutritionist and asked for her expert help. The nutritionist now gave the same information that she had given to the lecture-request groups, but in a different manner and in a much more condensed form, and distributed recipes. The group decided by vote to try the meats during the following week.

RESULTS. A comparison of the results shown in Table 14-1 clearly indicates the greater effectiveness of the discussion-decision method. Perhaps the most telling contrast is that between the responses of those group members who had never before tried any of these foods. Twenty-nine percent of such participants in the discussion groups used one or more of the meats in family meals for the first time after the experience described; *not one member of the lecture group tried the meats for the first time.*

Principles for successful nutritional education

Such studies and field work, both in other cultures and in America, teach important principles with which health workers can improve their work in nutrition and in health education.

Knowledge of people. Health workers need to have an intimate knowledge of the people's beliefs, attitudes, values, behavior, and extent of knowledge before they attempt to introduce changes or new practices. Habits are never developed in a vacuum. All people in every culture have *some* knowledge of nutrition. If the health worker assumes that they know nothing simply because their concepts differ, the worker shall only arouse their resistance to the information that he or she has to convey.

Understanding reasons for habits. All beliefs and practices, no matter how strange they may appear, serve psychologic and social functions. If health workers hope to communicate effectively with others, they will find their path remarkably smoothed and their results strikingly better if they analyze the habits that people have. The habits should be evaluated objectively, and the overall pattern or system into which the customs and beliefs fit should be determined.

Identification of customs that need to be changed. Many practices, even though they may differ from the health worker's, are beneficial and should be encouraged. Some may be harmless and need not be disturbed. Others are harmful. To overcome the harmful ones successfully, a sympathetic approach is necessary. Techniques of persuasion will have to be developed, and points must be proved by demonstration. It is useful to integrate good nutritional practices with existing habits wherever ways can be found to do it.

Meeting individual needs. A flexible attitude that is sensitive to the needs of individuals in specific situations at specific times allows health workers to be effective. They cannot be effective if they are bound by rigid ideas. Changes cannot be brought about in others if the health workers cling blindly to a few methods and materials that were learned at a specific time, in a specific set of circumstances, as though they were universal laws. Health workers can most successfully free others if they themselves are free to adjust, adapt, and tailor. There is always more than one way to do something; health workers should work with open systems.

Self-knowledge. It is an exciting adventure for a person to study the degree to which he is culturebound. Each person has, perhaps without realizing it, a culturally determined system of values. Success is unlikely for the person who unconsciously attempts to impose his system on the behavior of others. It is possible that genuine introspection on the part of health workers may lead to some major reorientation in certain areas of their own philosophy.

Involvement of key people. The leadership patterns in the community should be studied. Ways to enlist the cooperation and guidance of key individuals and families should be sought.

Main gatekeeper of the food channels. As stated previously, the wife and mother in the home is usually the main gatekeeper who ultimately determines the food habits of her family. Wives and mothers, by virtue of their feeling of responsibility for the health of the family, are probably the most open and educable members of population groups. It is also most important from the health worker's point of view that these women be reached, since they are the persons who are mainly responsible for the nutrition of children and for the development of the food habits of persons as they grow from infancy to adulthood.

Involvement of people. Group discussions, by creating awareness of needs, help to motivate persons to action. Group decisions, because they reflect the finding of solutions by the persons themselves usually represent a sense of identification with that solution. This sense of identification is most helpful in producing long-term results.

Communication skills. To often people are unaware that they are speaking in a way that their hearers either misunderstand or fail to understand. Those trying to teach are then puzzled at their listeners' lack of response or at their misinterpretation. Health workers are almost sure to make this kind of error if they are not sensitive to the hearer's frame of reference and to the associated ideas that arise out of his background. The health worker needs to seek a common meeting ground, to perceive the situation as his hearer sees it, to think in the hearer's idioms, and to understand the meanings that words and actions have for the hearers. Sometimes health workers have had little or no training in educational principles or techniques.

Lacking the awareness that is developed by such training, they are prone to suppose that the methods by which they were taught—lectures and demonstrations—will suffice for others. Perhaps they need to forget the textbook practices in order to look honestly and sympathetically at the situation before them.

Evaluation of results. At the end of an episode in which the health worker has tried to effect a change in the behavior of others, it is often useful simply to ask: what happened, was the teaching realistic, was it necessary, did it work, and did it meet the need? Questions such as these help the health worker to appraise immediate results and to anticipate long-range effects. They may well be necessary to maintain perspective and direction.

TEACHING-LEARNING PROCESS

There is far more to learning than merely dispensing information, yet the myth prevails in health education that if enough information is provided, harmful health practices will be changed.[4] Bruner, a leading educator, underscores the dynamic nature of learning and teaching: "Knowing is a process, not a product."[5]

Definition of learning. Learning means *change*. There is a vast difference between a person who has *learned* and a person who has only been *informed*. Learning must ultimately be measured in terms of changed behavior. To be valid, education must focus not on the teacher, nor on the content, but on the *learner*. The teacher's primary responsbility is not to teach facts but to educate persons. The teacher's major task is to create situations in which the person can learn, succeed, and develop self-direction and self-motivation.

Aspects of human personality involved in learning

The teaching-learning process involves three fundamental aspects of human personality—cognition, emotion, and will.

Cognition. Cognition is the thought process itself by which information is grasped. Cognitions shape, and are shaped by, the terms in which the mind thinks about a given body of facts. The thought process usually starts with a diffuse sensation. This is followed by a more focused perception that leads to the construction of a concept and to identification of specific principles involved. The total process of cognition provides the background knowledge that is the basis for reasoning and analysis. The learner senses the contribution of cognition to the learning process as, "I know how to do it."

Emotion. In each individual, specific feelings and responses are associated with given items of knowledge and with given situations. These emotions reflect the desires raised and the needs aroused. Emotions provide impetus. They create the tensions that spur a person to act. When he feels unfulfillment, lack, or need, he wants to do something about it. If the teacher understands the learner's emotions, the teacher can direct the impetus in ways that will forward the learning process. The learner senses the contribution of emotion to the learning process as, "I want to do it."

Will. The will to act arises from the conviction that the knowledge discovered can fill the felt need and relieve the sense of tension. The will focuses our determination to act on the knowledge received, to change an attitude, a value, a thought, or a pattern of behavior. The learner senses the contribution of the will to the learning process as, "I will do it."

Principles of learning

Basic principles of learning, focused on the learner, are individuality, contact, listening, participation, need fulfillment, and appraisal.

Individuality. Learning can only be individual. Each person in the final analysis must learn for himself, according to his need, in his way, in his time, and for his purpose. To teach, the teacher must discover who the learner is. To do this the teacher must ask questions that make clear the relationship of the learner to the problem under consideration.

Contact. Learning starts from a point of contact between prior experience and knowledge, an overlap of the new with the familiar. To teach a person, the teacher must know what the individual already knows and to what past experience the present situation can be related. The process of learning must start at that point. It is the teacher, not the learner, who must find and identify this point of contact. A teacher is very likely to fail to reach and teach the individual if it is merely *assumed* that the learner is at a given point of experience and knowledge. The teacher must search for the areas of association that are present in the individual learner. The teacher must then relate teaching to that point of contact.

Listening. Because learning is individual and because it is a process that must move from a point of contact that reflects the learner's present knowledge to a desired outcome, it must involve listening—the *teacher's* listening! (Certainly the learner must listen also, but teaching him to listen is part of the teacher's task.) The most mature teacher is the most expert listener. The listening of a fine teacher is the kind of client-centered activity that Rogers[6] has called creative listening. Listening should be a skilled effort to understand a person and his situation from *his* perspective. Such listening is by no means passive. It is active concentration, an alert attempt to view the situation as the patient is experiencing it. The active listener is sensitive not merely to the words the learner is speaking but also to the *meaning* the learner is consciously and unconsciously communicating. There is much subsurface significance to communication. It is conveyed in tone, gesture, posture of the whole body and each of its parts, the context in which words are used, and even silences. Indeed these aspects of the communication are often the most significant.

Participation. Since learning is an active process through which behavior changes, the learner must become personally involved. He must participate actively. One means of securing participation is through *planned feedback*. Feedback may take several forms. One method is to ask questions that require more than a yes or a no answer. The question should elicit statements that will reveal the learner's degree of understanding and motivation. Another feedback method is to use return demonstrations by the learner under the guidance of the teacher. These usually take the form of brief periods in which procedures are practiced or skills discussed. Such guided practice develops ability, self-confidence, and security, and it enables the learner to clarify his grasp of the principles involved. The third feedback method is for the learner to try the new learning outside the teacher-directed situation in the circumstances of his own life. Such trials are alternated with return visits in which the learner reviews his experiences with the teacher; the teacher answers, or helps him to answer, the questions raised and provides continued support and reinforcement.

Need fulfillment. People learn only what they feel will be useful to them. They retain only what they believe they need or shall need. The more immediately persons can put new learning to use, the more readily they grasp it. The more it satisfies their immediate goals, the more effective the learning will be. Only the intelligent and the mature put forth the effort to learn for long-term goals.

Appraisal. If teachers accept the premise that learning means changed behavior, they must appraise the learner's progress toward the determined goal. They must, at appropriate intervals, take stock of the changes that the learner has made in outlook, attitude, and action toward the specific goal in health education. What is the learner *doing?* Careful, sympathetic questioning may reveal blocks to learning. These may be cognitive (misunderstandings that are hindering the learner's progress), or they may be emotional (points of negative feelings). They may also be volitional. The learner may understand (more or less) what is to be done and emotionally think that it would be a fine idea to do it, but lack the firm will to achieve.

In addition to speeding the learning process, such person-centered concern will reveal to the health worker personal progress as a teacher. It will show the health worker whether he or she is communicating successfully, making contact, and making the best choices of method. It will recall to the health worker principles that may have been glossed over. It may reveal to him or her significant clues to the learner's behavior, which may have been missed entirely. In the final analysis the measure of success in teaching lies not in the number of facts transferred, but in the *change for the better that has been initiated in persons.*

HEALTH TEACHING IN PATIENT CARE

From the preceding discussion of how learning takes place, it is abundantly clear that if health teaching is to be valid, it must be patient centered. Health teachers must focus on the *learner.* To translate this principle into action, the role of the health worker in teaching patients about nutrition should be considered.

Definitions. First, what does *not* constitute nutrition teaching—or any health teaching—should be considered. The term "health teaching" is often misused grammatically and mechanically: "Go down to Mrs. Smith's room before she leaves and health teach her about her diet." Or, "Has anyone given Mr. Jones some health teaching for his ulcer?" This attitude toward health teaching is analogous to applying a dressing with no knowledge of what might be festering beneath the surface or administering a drug with no knowledge of what reaction might occur.

Learning is the *continuing* process of interaction between a person and his environment that leads him to *changed behavior.* Along the way at certain points of individual and group need, this interaction is aided by helping vehicles—persons equipped with knowledge, skill, and personality to provide tools and direction according to need. These persons are called *teachers.* It is the function and the responsibility of the teacher to challenge and help motivate, to provide an atmosphere conducive to learning, to create specific learning situations, and to help provide resources as indicated. All this is done with one objective—that the learner may learn *for himself*. In the health field, practitioners are such helping vehicles.

To help keep this larger view in mind perhaps the broader term *health education* is better than health teaching. Health education implies the overall teaching-learning concept of the educative process.

Health education may be defined as the involvement of persons in their own health care and the creation of a general climate and specific situations in which persons may participate in decisions and activities concerning their health. Valid health education is based on the accurate statement of related facts that have been demonstrated scientifically and on the application of these facts to the protection, maintenance, and improvement of health by the patient himself or by those responsible for his well-being.

Clinician-teacher

Health education cannot be separated from the total nutritional care function. It is caring and sharing. The key word that characterizes an alert and sensitive clinician-teacher is *awareness*.

1. Awareness of the patient's uniqueness; being sensitive to cultural, social, personal, and physical needs
2. Awareness of the dynamic nature of knowledge; having a sound basis of scientific background principles, but being flexible and open to current concepts
3. Awareness of self; understanding that feelings influence the ability to perceive the needs of others; knowing the healing value of genuine care and concern for other persons
4. Awareness of the specific skills necessary

TO PROBE FURTHER
Basic nutrition concepts*

1. Nutrition is the food you eat and how the body uses it. We eat food to live, to grow, to keep healthy and well, and to get energy for work and play.
2. Food is made up of different nutrients needed for growth and health.
   a. All nutrients needed by the body are available through food.
   b. Many kinds and combinations of food can lead to a well-balanced diet.
   c. No food, by itself, has all the nutrients needed for full growth and health.
   d. Each nutrient has specific uses in the body.
   e. Most nutrients do their best work in the body when teamed with other nutrients.
3. All persons, throughout life, have need for the same nutrients, but in varying amounts.
   a. The amounts of nutrients needed are influenced by age, sex, size, activity, and the state of health.
   b. Suggestions for the kinds and amounts of food needed are made by trained scientists.
4. The way food is handled influences the amount of nutrients in food, its safety, appearance, and taste.
   a. Handling means everything that happens to food while it is being grown, processed, stored, and prepared for eating.

*Interagency Committee on Nutrition Education (ICNE), Agricultural Research Service, U.S. Dept. of Agriculture, Nutr. Program News, Sept.-Oct., 1964.

for communicating and relating to others; identifying and learning these skills, and continuing to improve them throughout professional life (these skills include listening, perceiving, verbalizing, clarifying, analyzing, encouraging, enlarging, supporting, and sharing information) Each of these characteristics of the sensitive teacher stems from an underlying awareness that all human beings need recognition, a sense of self-worth and a feeling that they belong. They need assurance that they are making progress and confidence that they can succeed. The sensitive teacher tries to foster and nuture the fulfillment of these needs.

Content of health teaching

Because the clinician-teacher is not merely purveying information but is educating persons, he or she derives the content of health teaching from the two sources of specific needs of persons and scientific knowledge. The specific needs of persons may arise from illness (care of a patient with a particular disease), preventing illness (positive health care), or daily living problems (concerns about physical needs and human relationships). The teacher also needs an organized body of scientific knowledge relative to these needs of persons. These scientific principles are learned from the biologic sciences, the social sciences, and the humanities. They are the tools of the educated, caring health worker.

Basic nutrition concepts. An example of a simple statement of basic concepts for use in health education is the outline of basic nutrition concepts developed by the Interagency Committee on Nutrition Education (ICNE), first published in 1964 by the Agricultural Research Service, U.S. Department of Agriculture (see above). Since this statement's appearance, various nutrition agencies have used it as a basis for in-service training of public health nurses and for teaching elementary school teachers to integrate nutrition activities into social studies

and health programs. It has been used in workshops with physical education and home economics teachers, health educators, and agricultural extension workers in counseling individuals who require dietary modification for the control of disease and for countless other purposes.

Mutual activity in health teaching

In dynamic, purposive health teaching, the clinician-teacher and the patient-learner share responsibility for the outcome. Each has something to give to the teaching-learning process.

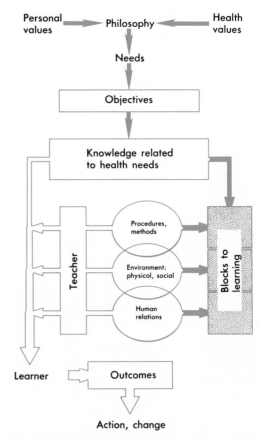

Fig. 14-1. The role of the clinician-teacher as a helping vehicle or channel in the teaching-learning process of health education.

The clinician gives special knowledge and skills. The patient gives unique personal experience with the particular problem at hand. Together they explore the problem and consider alternative plans for solution. Ultimately the patient must choose a plan and must carry out the plan of his choice by appropriately modifying his health behavior.

Role of the clinician-teacher. Throughout the interview, the practitioner is attempting to see the patient's world as he sees it and to help him achieve increased insight and ability to cope with his individual situation more adequately and comfortably. For example, the primary care practitioner acts as a helper to bridge the distance between the *health objective* (based on the patient's needs and philosophy) and the *outcome* (the desired change in health behavior). To do this the practitioner helps the patient to understand the facts he needs to know and in so doing will often have to work through blocks that exist because of a variety of factors. These factors include the patient's environment (his educational level, economic resources, social conditioning, cultural habituation) and methods used by the persons around him. His own or his wife's cooking methods, the necessity of eating lunch in a company cafeteria or bringing a lunch from home may be factors. Patients who regularly eat in a boarding school, campus dining room, boarding house, or restaurant need special consideration. There are many other human relations involved. This vital "facilitator" function in the teaching-learning process may be visualized in Fig. 14-1.

COMMUNITY NUTRITION EDUCATION
Changing concepts in community health care

The rapid changes that are occurring in population and family patterns and in medical and allied scientific knowledge bring with them inevitable changes in society that directly involve the teaching of nutrition to patients. These changes are reflected in shifting emphases in medical care itself. Until very recent years, stress was almost exclusively placed on the cure or amelioration of disease by surgery and drugs. While advances in these areas continue to be made with great rapidity, there is also an increasing tendency to blend curative practices with disease-preventive, health-oriented primary care. Generally a more sophisticated, affluent society knows more, has more, and asks more than a simple culture. People seek more involvement in their own health care. As the population increases, the greater numbers of people also demand more efficient approaches. Attempts to meet these demands have taken many forms, including group medical practice by specialists, clustering of medical facilities, and health insurance plans. There has been pronounced change in the role of the community hospital. It is rapidly emerging as the community health center of the future. Within its environs, nutrition education is becoming recognized by professional workers and by the community at large as an essential aspect of education for total health.

Concept of the community health center

Curative and preventive health systems. Although the concept of the community health center as a focus for the coordination of curative and preventive health care is not fully formed, it is developing as a result of social pressures and correlated trends in American medicine. Increasingly leaders in medicine and hospital administration voice these changes in direction.[7] Project studies and pilot programs are indicating the needs, and as a result the gap between the curative and preventive health systems is closing. These reports indicate that the curative system (largely the professional practitioners and the hospitals) is doing more work in home care programs, in coordinated activities with chronic disease hospitals and nursing homes, in health care financing, and in areawide hospital planning. The preventive system (largely public health departments and other government agencies and programs) is organizing its services for the delivery of general health care, care of the chronically ill, rehabilitation work and overall community health planning (especially centered in families of high-risk, low-income population groups), and broad community health screening programs.

Coordination of the two health systems. The great need felt by leaders in the health care field is for increased functional coordination between the two health systems. In some situations this coordination may be a blending of the community hospital and the local health department, and it may include parts of the local welfare agency. In other situations, services of the two systems could be coordinated in activities such as home care programs, outpatient clinic services, and broad public community education programs. Such coordination would prevent much costly and inefficient overlapping and fragmentation, such as now exist in many communities. Fresh vision in planning and in program development would give needed vitality and human dignity to pressing community health needs.

Community health education center

Among community health centers being developed in this country is the health education center formed by a group of physicians in Oakland, California, the Permanente Medical Group, in conjunction with their affiliated community health facilities, the Kaiser Foundation Health Plan and Hospitals. A directing staff that serves as a model health team (physician, nurse, nutritionist and health educator) coordinates and administers a long-range program of health education. Expanded facilities, centrally located, provide space for individual staff offices and counseling rooms, small conference rooms for discussion groups, and a larger auditorium for meetings, conferences, workshops, and lectures. A library, an exhibit theater, and individual teaching machine booths are available. A long-standing activity of the medical group, its comprehensive multiphasic health screening program, has been expanded and involves extensive data processing equipment. These data provide a broad basis for continuing research in limitless numbers of health problems. The multiphasic health screening program is a fundamental part of the expanded health education program. Numerous primary care programs similar to the Kaiser model have developed in other parts of the country.

Methods and approaches in the community health center

The community health center provides varied opportunities for health education and care through its facilities and personnel.

Health team. The coordinated health team approach underlies the basic program of a community health center. Under the guidance of the physician, specialists in various areas of health care work together with the patients to explore needs and provide services for family-centered health care.

METHODS. The methods used include individual counseling, small discussion groups, classes, use of libraries and exhibits, and self-teaching devices.

INDIVIDUAL COUNSELING. Either by appointment or in the open clinic according to need, individuals may have personal conferences with members of the health team, such as physician, psychologist, nutritionist (Fig. 14-2), nurse, or social worker. Instruction may be given concerning some aspect of health care as the need for such instructions becomes apparent. Dietary modification is high on the list of probabilities for such instruction. Team conferences, under the direction of the family internist and pediatrician, are held in which workers in relevant disciplines explore and coordinate plans for family health care.

SMALL DISCUSSION-DECISION GROUPS. Studies such as those of Lewin demonstrate that per-

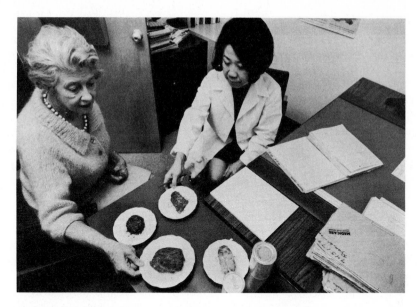

Fig. 14-2. The clinic dietitian reviews nutritional needs with a patient. She discusses dietary modifications based on a sound food plan adapted to individual requirements and desires.

sons are more likely to carry out a decision if they have participated in the forming of it than if the decision has been made for them by others. Small discussion-decision groups provide opportunity for persons to explore needs, to obtain information about health care, to learn whether alternatives are open to them, and to gain motivation and support for action. Such discussion-decision groups are proving effective instruments for the education of persons with common health problems. Patients with diabetes, obesity, heart disease, or peptic ulcer or persons wanting to improve their health by stopping the smoking habit have found positive direction and emotional reinforcement through discussion-decision sessions. Well persons with common health interests, such as parents of young children, expectant parents, teenagers, or older persons, have taken a lively interest in learning and sharing in these ways.

CLASSES. More structured classes in subjects related to various health needs also provide needed information in such areas as prenatal care, natural childbirth, infant and child care, and family planning. Other classes may be provided for persons with heart disease, diabetes, peptic ulcer, renal disease, genetic disease, and other chronic or long-term problems. Classes in broad areas of health interest may be planned as needed. These may be in areas such as family meal planning and marketing, preventive family health care through wise use of available comprehensive health plans and group medical practice, human relations, or current medical research in a wide variety of areas. The possibilities are as broad as the need in the individual community.

For effective teaching in such classes, the health worker will need to plan carefully. The teaching plan will include sound research and other preparation and plans for the creation of a learning situation, for the guidance of learning activities, and for helping each person who attends to apply the material to his individual situation so that he may translate what he learns into action. Various teaching aids may be planned, prepared, secured, and arranged. Equipment and classroom facilities will need to be checked. During the class the pace at which material is presented, flexibility, and group involvement will be significant factors. After the completion of each class and at the end of the series, a follow-up evaluation in the light of the stated objectives will be essential as the basis for planning future classes or series of classes.

LIBRARY AND EXHIBITS. Health education materials, books, pamphlets, leaflets, models, pictures, and charts in an organized health library under the care of a qualified librarian provide rich learning resources as a part of a community health center. An exhibit area where displays of visual and graphic materials related to various aspects of health care may be presented is another highly effective means of health education.

SELF-TEACHING DEVICES. Booths may be provided with individually operated devices such as teaching machines and recorded audiovisual materials. Persons may use these as desired to obtain new information or to review certain health care principles and practices.

Community health resources

In various forms in many types of communities, other health agencies and organizations provide opportunities and resources for community health education.

Government agencies. Public health departments conduct many service and educational activities on the local, state, and national levels. Public health nutritionists help survey community nutrition needs, plan nutrition components of community health programs (Fig. 14-3), and provide training, consultation, and teaching materials for public health workers in other specialties such as nursing and sanitation. Public health nurses work with families through various health services, help organize and conduct clinics, and teach community health classes. Other government health agencies working in specific community projects include those formed in response to the Eco-

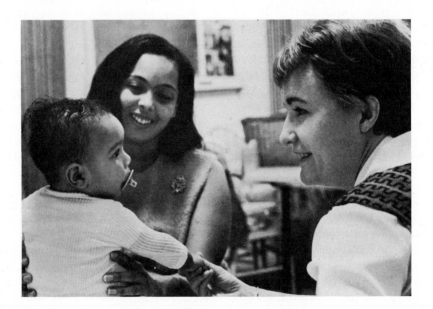

Fig. 14-3. Public health nutritionist discussing infant feeding with a young mother at a community child health conference.

nomic Opportunity Act, such as Vista (Volunteers in Service to America) and other groups operating in poverty areas, the Indian Health Program, and the School Lunch Program.

Volunteer agencies. A host of volunteer health agencies, such as the American Heart Association, American Diabetes Association, and the American Cancer Society, provide educational opportunities and materials through their local chapters. In some larger urban areas, nutrition committees have classes taught by local nutritionists, nurses and physicians. These are sometimes arranged through cooperation with the local adult evening school. There are nutrition consultation and diet counseling services provided by a staff nutritionist with educational materials developed and printed by community physicians and health workers. There are also professional workshops on specific health problems. Volunteer nutritionists and nurses also work with local chapters of the American Diabetes Association in their annual diabetes detection drives, and they teach classes in the local adult evening and extension schools.

Specific health-interest clubs. Local chapters of organizations formed for the study and dissemination of information related to specific health problems offer support and a sharing of information to persons having such needs. These groups include ones such as the Ileostomy and Colostomy Clubs, TOPS (Take Off Pounds Sensibly), and Weight Watchers. Community health workers are often invited to speak at meetings of the members.

School, church, civic, and fraternal groups. A number of lay organizations conduct health-related activities for groups of persons having special needs. An example is the excellent ''Meals-on-Wheels'' program conducted in some cities by volunteers who prepare and deliver hot meals to persons in need of such service. These are usually patients referred by the physician of the community. They are for the most part persons who are chronically ill or who are undergoing rehabilitation and are often elderly and alone. In rooming houses and apartment districts food is delivered by couriers on a regular schedule for a nominal fee. Often this courier is the only person who visits the patient for days at a time; he or she is awaited eagerly each day and brings more than food into the patient's life.

Professional groups. A particularly important group of nutrition educators is found in the Society for Nutrition Education with offices in Berkeley, California.* A National Nutrition Education Clearing House is maintained with a library of materials representing a wide spectrum of sound educational media. A number of educational listings and guides are published and available. A quarterly *Journal of Nutrition Education* is also published.

Other local professional organizations—medical, nursing, dietetics—provide health education in a number of ways. They sponsor workshops, participate in mass communication through such media as radio and television, and issue staff-written articles for publication in newspapers and magazines. A unique activity of the American Dietetics Association, for example, is the ''Dial-a-Dietitian'' program that has been established in many urban areas. Through a telephone-answering service, persons may make inquiries about food and nutrition; dietitians return the calls and give information or clarify a confused point.

Food industry groups. A number of food industries sponsor research, provide nutrition educaton materials, and underwrite community nutrition projects. Among these organizations are the National Dairy Council and its affiliated state groups and the National Livestock and Meat Board.

County interagency nutrition councils. In many counties a nutrition council whose members represent the various nutrition agencies in

---

*Society for Nutrition Education, 2140 Shattuck Ave., Suite 1110, Berkeley, Calif. 94704.

the community coordinates the work of all of the represented groups. These nutrition councils plan and sponsor community health activities such as projects and workshops that may be carried out through the local high schools. They also develop adult conferences on nutrition and issue teaching materials.

Information concerning nutrition education work in a community may be obtained by writing or telephoning one of the following sources:

1. Agricultural Extension Service, usually located in the state university
2. Home advisors or home economists in district agricultural extension offices

---

TO PROBE FURTHER
Teaching plan for group instruction

I. Preparation
  A. Research the subject and make a careful study. Prepare an outline and finally reduce the kernel of the material to one sentence.
  B. Make out a teaching plan.
    1. *Aim.* Define the patient-learning goals. Make sure that this goal (a) relates to this patient's needs so that he can identify with it, (b) suggests teaching procedure, and (c) is a realistic one that you can attain within the class period.
    2. *Approach.* Create a learning situation that will (a) secure attention and interest, (b) stimulate learning readiness, (c) be relevant and lead into the class topic, and (d) raise pertinent questions.
    3. *Answers.* Guide learning experiences and activities so that they (a) secure group involvement, (b) lead to the organization of concepts, (c) provide an opportunity to explore background and alternative answers, (d) provide resource material for analysis and discussion, and (e) allow for continuous feedback by a variety of methods.
    4. *Application.* To help each patient to apply the proffered material to his own needs (a) summarize key points, (b) bring the group to a decision concerning a plan of action, if indicated, and (c) enable each patient to ask specifically, "What does this mean to me?"—and to perceive the answer with clarity.
    5. *Assignment.* To secure carry-over into life situations (a) obtain any further needed information from sources in the community and (b) if the program involves a series of classes, propose possible feedback for the next class.
  C. Prepare and check out all aids and equipment ahead of time.
II. Presentation
  A. Arrange in advance for the room, chairs, speaker's desk, displays, materials, and equipment necessary.
  B. Carry out the teaching plan.
    1. *Timing.* Begin and end on time, and pace the material for balance and interest.
    2. *Group involvement.* Maintain a relaxed and permissive atmosphere. Be flexible and allow for an adjustment of the original plan as the situation warrants. Use resource people as needed.
III. Purpose fulfilled?
  A. Evaluate class results in light of its objective.
  B. Plan follow-up activity.

3. Registered dietitians in local hospitals
4. Clinical and community nutritionists in private practice
5. Public health nutritionists in local health departments or clinics
6. Nutrition instructors in high schools, colleges, and nursing schools
7. Volunteer health agency office, the local chapter of the American Heart Association or of the American Diabetes Association

Tests of the success of teaching about nutrition

Because health teaching involves dynamic interaction between teacher and learner, health workers who would educate patients about nutrition and health will at frequent intervals reassess their own developing comprehension of the dynamics of human behavior, of growth and development, and of learning. They will evaluate from time to time their own growth in recognizing the needs and perceptions of persons and their increased sensitiveness to others. Such appraisals will help to equip them with realistic self-understanding. (How do health workers see themselves—as an "authority figure who knows best," or as a "helping vehicle of learning" who is present when needed to guide a person's own learning?) In testing one's own success as an educator in the special field of nutrition, the health worker will use the techniques of self-appraisal that have become standbys in other aspects of health care. These are the methods developed by such students of human interactions as Carl Rogers,[6] Abraham Maslow,[8] and Thomas Weiss.[9] The health worker will want to reread the findings and recommendations of these and other authorities and consider them afresh in their application to the complex field of nutrition and the teaching of nutrition to patients and to community groups.

Key questions. To further this self-analysis,

each health care worker should ask himself or herself the following key questions:

1. *Do I listen when the patient talks?* Do I listen to the patient's words? Have I become alert to the difference between "Certainly!" and "Yes, I think so . . ."? Am I sure *this* patient knows the difference between whole milk, low-fat milk, and fat-free milk? Does he know the difference between "a little sugar" and a heaping teaspoonful of sugar to a half cup of coffee? If the patient does not speak English fluently, am I sure, from his own words, that he is certain of the information I have given him? Do I listen to the patient's inflections? Do I notice the fall of the voice that conveys reluctance, doubt, lack of faith in the therapy recommended, indifference, discouragement, revulsion, or hostility? These emotions, if not offset by stronger and more valid considerations, will negate all carefully constructed reasoning once the patient has left the environment of the health center.

2. *Does the patient understand what I am saying?* Are the words and phrases that I use related to his experience so that he may identify with them and build on them?

3. *Do I respect the necessity for cultural harmony?* Does my teaching conflict in any way with the patient's cultural values and conditioning? Since I know that such conflict will result in lack of confidence and probably in rejection or confusion, do I have the imagination to find ways to integrate my knowledge with this patient's conditioning?

4. *Am I comfortable with silences that allow the patient to think through a thought raised?* Do I allow the patient to translate our conversation into his own thinking at his own pace? Do I respect the slow thinker? Am I patient with the person who has a mind of his own and will not change it until he sees convincing cause? Am I easily fooled by the fast thinker, who seems to agree so readily with my suggestions (but who will ignore them)? Do I rec-

ognize the various qualities of silence of each of these types of person? Do I have the poise that allows the person to go through the behind-scenes events that take place in that silence? Do I *value* the silence, because of these events —knowing that until he has gone through that inner process he cannot reach a meaningful decision?

5. *Do I accept without approval or disapproval what the patient says?* Have I set aside my judgmental tendencies, left behind my infantile wish to praise or blame? Do I see evidence for the maturity and freedom of my own approach in the frankness with which patients are able to discuss with me their cravings, their aversions, or their boredom?

6. *Do I keep the conversation patient-centered? Do I allow him to set the direction of discussion about himself?* Do I conserve the patient's energy and time (and my own time,

---

TO PROBE FURTHER

The problem-solving method in nutrition education

Increasingly efforts of leaders in the health professions to develop a unique body of theory have been based on the method of problem-solving. The problem-solving method is a stepwise organization of concepts and activities directed toward the solution of specific problems. One of its essentials is the requirement for clear definitions at each step before attempting the next phase of solution. To apply the problem-solving method to nutrition education, a definition of the function of nursing, for example may be helpful.

The function of nursing* is to provide for a person undergoing illness, medical treatment, or the formulation of a plan for medical care, such help as he may require for the fulfillment of his needs, while encouraging him to optimum self-care. *Nursing practice* based on this premise (clearly distinguished from medical care) must revolve around three further factors:

1. Identified patient needs—*the nursing diagnosis*
2. The plan of action, derived through consideration of needs, goals, and possible actions by patient and nurse together—*the nursing care plan*
3. Mutual exploration of results—*nursing evaluation*

Within this same framework, *nutritional care practice* may also be planned by the nutritionist around three factors: (1) nutritional diagnosis, (2) nutritional care plan, and (3) nutritional care evaluation. A useful outline for a problem-solving approach to the education of patients about nutrition may be as follows:

Identified need	What is the specific nutrition problem in this patient?
Goal	What is the specific nutrition goal for this patient?
Background knowledge	What scientific principles are applicable to this need and goal?
Plan	What plan of nutrition improvement is organized (with the patient's participation) to meet this need and to reach this goal?
Results	What happened? Did the plan enable the patient to reach his goal? Was the goal reached completely, partially, or not al all? (If work remains to be done, the problem-solving activity is begun again with new definitions of the need and goal.)

*Orlando, I. J.: The dynamic nurse-patient relationship, New York, 1961, G. P. Putnam's Sons.

too, for which I am responsible to others) by concentrating on the business at hand—the health of this patient?

7. *Do I reflect, without interpretation, key words and phrases expressed by the patient?* (This technique, which is highly developed by the psychologic counselor, is useful to the health educator insofar as it helps him to understand *precisely* what the patient is telling him. The patient who says, "I eat two eggs a day," may be relating a simple fact; or he may be telling the health educator that he has no intention of eating eggs and that he wants to stop discussing that subject once and for all. The obese woman who declares, "I *never* eat sweets," will make this assertion with increasing passion if she feels that she is being probed for a confession of dietary sin. The health educator who calmly restates, without interpretation, those statements he or she suspects of masking an emotion-loaded situation is sometimes able to help the patient face the truth by dispelling fear or anger.)

8. *Am I genuinely interested?* Do I show my interest? Do I indicate my concern by looking directly at the patient, by my facial expression, nod of head, and tone of voice?

9. *Has my teaching been practical?* Will my suggestions prove workable for this patient in his special situation? Does he have the resources to carry out such a plan?

10. *Has my teaching been important?* Does this teaching really matter to the patient's health? If he makes the changes agreed upon, will they really make a difference in the outcome?

11. *If other persons are present and I must discuss the patient with them, do I keep all communication directed to and through him?*

12. *At the end of the interview, do I leave the door open to further reflection and exploration as needed?*

Health workers must evaluate nutrition teaching by applying these 12 tests to each program that is planned and, in retrospect, to daily work with individuals and groups. If you are dissatisfied with your rating, reevaluate your approach. The therapy for failure on any point can be summarized in a simple formula: *Explore more closely with the patient the patient's real needs.*

CASE STUDY 4
A Mexican-American family's struggle in a new country

As she drove toward the poorer section of town, Mrs. Parker, a skilled and concerned nutritionist, thought of Rosa Torres and her little family, struggling to make their way against many difficulties. Rosa and Manuel Torres had come to the valley with the migrant farm workers from Mexico the year before, but because Rosa had wanted to make a settled home, they had remained here. Somehow, Manuel had made the necessary arrangements, had gotten a job in a warehouse, and was taking night classes in English at the local high school. Their two girls, 6 and 8 years old, were in school and had soon learned to speak English. Rosa, however, seldom went out because she was self-conscious about her inability to speak English.

Six months ago the Torreses had had a third child, a boy. Manuel was overjoyed. Nothing was too good for the son he had so long wanted. During the last two or three months of Rosa's pregnancy she had been under close observation because of increasing edema, excessive weight gain, and elevated blood pressure. However, she had not returned to the clinic afterward for follow-up care of herself and the baby.

Mrs. Parker had continued to make visits to the home to observe Rosa and the baby. The child seemed to thrive under Rosa and Manuel's care—in fact, too much so. To them, the larger a baby was, the healthier he was. So they pushed him to drink more of his rich milk formula and constantly fed him extra crackers and cereal. Now he had folds of fat on his chubby body and was so overweight he was beginning to have some difficulty breathing. Rosa was still overweight herself, becoming increasingly fatigued and finding it difficult to carry her son about or care for him.

Mrs. Parker stopped her car in front of the house where the Torreses lived in a small, three-room basement apartment. She wondered as she picked up her bag and walked down the alley between the houses toward the back entrance just how she could best help Rosa and Manuel in their effort to make a home in this new and different community and to meet the health needs of their growing family.

Questions to guide your inquiry

1. What health problems can you identify in the Torres family?
2. What factors have helped create the baby's excessive weight? What health problems does it pose?
3. What communication barriers may exist in reaching Rosa Torres? How might Mrs. Parker plan to overcome them?
4. How could Mrs. Parker evaluate the children's nutritional needs?
5. What plan of approach do you think Mrs. Parker might use to help Rosa and Manuel perceive the baby's situation and to motivate them to alter their food behavior toward him?
6. What diet modifications would you suggest for the baby? For Rosa? How would you teach these modifications to Rosa and Manuel?
7. How do you think Rosa and Manuel would accept this teaching?
8. What food-buying problems might exist? What solutions would you suggest?
9. Describe the food pattern in Mexican-American culture. What nutritional problems might it pose?

REFERENCES
Specific

1. Cassel, J.: A comprehensive health program among South African Zulus. In Paul, B. D., editor: Health, culture and community, New York, 1955, Russell Sage Foundation, pp. 15-41.
2. Jelliffe, D. B.: Cultural variation and the practical pediatrician, J. Pediatr. **49:**661, 1956.
3. Lewin, K.: Forces behind food habits and methods of change. In The problem of changing food habits, Washington, D.C., 1943, National Academy of Sciences, National Research Council, pp. 35-65.
4. Evans, R. I., and Hall, Y.: Social-psychologic perspective in motivating change in eating behavior, J.A.D.A. **72:**378, April, 1978.
5. Bruner, J. S.: Toward a theory of instruction, Boston, 1966, Harvard University Press, p. 72.
6. Rogers, C.: Freedom to learn, Columbus, Ohio, 1969, Charles E. Merrill Publishing Co.
7. Clark, H. T., Jr.: Shaping the hospital for its future role, Hospitals **40:**50, 1966.
8. Maslow, A.: The farther reaches of human nature, New York, 1971, Viking Press.
9. Weiss, T. M., Moran, E. V., and Cattle, E.: Education for adaptation and survival, San Francisco, 1975, International Society for General Semantics.

General

Anderson, J. V., and Cines, B.: Teaching behavior modification to nutrition students, J. Nutr. Educ. **11:**39, Jan.-March, 1979.

Bois, J. S.: The art of awareness, ed. 2, Dubuque, Iowa, 1973, William C. Brown Co., Publishers.

Cave, W. M., and Chesler, M. A.: Sociology of education, New York, 1974, Macmillan Publishing Co., Inc.

Chidester, F. H.: Programmed instruction: past, present, and future, J. Am. Diet. Assoc. **51:**413, 1967.

Coleman, J. C., and Hammer, C. L.: Contemporary psychology and effective behavior, Glenview, Ill., 1974, Scott, Foresman and Co.

Craig, D. G.: Guiding the change process in people, J. Am. Diet. Assoc. **58:**22, Jan., 1971.

DeCecco, J. P., and Crawford, W. R.: The psychology of learning and instruction, ed. 2, Englewood Cliffs, N.J., 1974, Prentice-Hall, Inc.

Fabun, D.: The dynamics of change, Englewood Cliffs, N.J., 1967, Prentice-Hall, Inc.

Forest, R. P.: What everyone should know about semantics, a scriptographic booklet, Greenfield, Mass., 1967, Channing L. Bete Co.

Gagne, R. M.: The conditions of learning, ed. 2, New York, 1970, Holt, Rinehart and Winston, Inc.

Garrett, A.: Interviewing: its principles and methods, New York, 1942, Family Service Association of America.

Ginther, J. R.: Educational diagnosis of patients, J. Am. Diet. Assoc. **59**(6):560, 1971.

Glock, M. D.: Guiding learning, New York, 1971, John Wiley & Sons, Inc.

Gnagey, W. J., Chesebro, P. A., and Johnson, J. J.: Learning environments, New York, 1972, Holt, Rinehart and Winston, Inc.

Guthrie, H. A.: Is education not enough? J. Nutr. Educ. **10:**57, April-June, 1978.

Juhas, L.: Nutrition education in day care programs, J. Am. Diet. Assoc. **63:**134, Aug., 1973.

Klausmeier, H. J., and Ripple, R. E.: Learning and human abilities, ed. 3, New York, 1971, Harper & Row, Publishers.

Kolasa, K., et al.: Home-based learning—implications for nutrition educators, J. Nutr. Educ. **11:**19, Jan.-March, 1979.

Leverton, R. M.: What is nutrition education? J. Am. Diet. Assoc. **64:**17, Jan., 1974.

Mager, R. F.: Preparing instructional objectives, Palo Alto, Calif., 1962, Fearon Publishers.

Mager, R. F.: Developing vocational instruction, Palo Alto, Calif., 1967, Fearon Publishers.

Mager, R. F.: Developing attitudes toward learning, Palo Alto, Calif., 1968, Fearon Publishers.

Marino, M. A.: Developing and testing a programmed instruction unit on PKU, J. Am. Diet. Assoc. **76:**29, Jan., 1980.

Marshall, W. H.: Educational directions, J. Am. Diet. Assoc. **58**(6):509, 1971.

Mead, M.: The dietitian as a member of the therapeutic team, J. Am. Diet. Assoc. **21:**424, 1945.

Mead, M.: Food habits research: problems of the 1960's, Washington, D.C., 1964, National Academy of Sciences, National Research Council, Pub. No. 1225.

Mead, M.: Culture and commitment, New York, 1970, Natural History Press.

Mico, P. R., and Ross, H. S.: Health education and behavioral science, Oakland, Calif., 1975, Third Party Associates, Inc.

Myers, M. L.: The ambulatory clinic in community and public health nutrition, J. Am. Diet. Assoc. **59:**48, 1971.

Paulson, B. K., and Beneke, W. M.: Long-term results from a weight loss program, J. Nutr. Educ. **11:**42, Jan.-March, 1979.

Richmond, F. W.: The role of the federal government in nutrition education, J. Nutr. Educ. **9:**150, Oct.-Dec., 1977.

Rogers, C.: Freedom to learn, Columbus, Ohio, 1969, Charles E. Merrill Publishing Co.

Slowie, L. A.: Patient learning—segments from case histories, J. Am. Diet. Assoc. **59**(6):563, 1971.

Somers, A. R.: Health care in transition: directions for the future, Chicago, 1971, Hospital Research and Educational Trust.

Talmage, H., Hughes, M., and Eash, M. J.: The role of evaluation in nutrition education, J. Nutr. Educ. **10:**169, 1978.

Toffler, A.: Future shock, New York, 1970, Random House.

U.S. Dept. of Health, Education, and Welfare: A white paper: toward a comprehensive health policy for the 1970's, Washington, D.C., 1971, U.S. Government Printing Office.

Vargas, J. S.: Teaching as changing behavior, J. Am. Diet. Assoc. **58**(6):512, 1971.

Wagner, M. G., Huyck, M. C., and Hinkle, M. M.: Evaluation of the Dial-a-Dietitian Program. I. Program organization. II. Impact on the community, J. Am. Diet. Assoc. **47:**381, Nov., 1965.

Wilson, J., Roheck, M., and Michael, W.: Psychological foundations of learning and teaching, New York, 1974, McGraw-Hill Book Co.

Zifferblatt, S. M., and Wilbur, C. S.: Dietary counseling: some realistic expectations and guidelines, J. Am. Diet. Assoc. **70:**591, 1977.

15 Family diet counseling—food needs and costs

The public health worker frequently needs to apply the basic principles of health teaching in family diet counseling. The term "counseling" is appropriate here, for if the nutritionist or the nurse works with the family in the light of counseling principles, various members will be led to explore their own situation, to determine their own needs, and to find methods of meeting those needs that are best suited to their life situation and tastes.

TYPES OF FAMILIES REQUIRING COUNSELING

The families that need counsel fall into two large categories, the well family and the family that requires therapeutic modifications.

The well family. The well family is one in which no member is acutely or chronically ill from any disease that specifically requires modification of the diet as therapy. Obviously there may be problems of overt or inapparent malnutrition. However, these deficits would be supplied if the diet were normal. In helping this family to understand its nutritional needs, the health worker will be most likely to encounter such problems as unawareness, lack of education, discouragement, lack of zest in life, bewilderment (particularly in the foreign-born), poverty, or food prejudices so deep-seated that they may not have been dispelled by the nutrition education offered through such activities as the child nutrition project in public schools,

the school lunch program,[1] and mass media programs for television.[2]

The family requiring therapeutic dietary modification. This is the family in which one or more members require modification of the diet. As part of the treatment for disease, the nutritionist and the nurse will also need to counsel the mother concerning the principles of the therapeutic diet prescribed and the meaning of these principles in terms of food to be served. The nurse will discuss, in terms of the total family situation, ways of fitting the patient's requirements into the family meals. As an example, the husband may have chronic heart disease for which the physician has prescribed restriction of sodium intake. The health worker may suggest that as the wife prepares the food for her family she remove the portion to be served to the husband before she adds salt to the remainder that is to be served to the family. The health worker and the wife may also discuss ways of seasoning the husband's food with herbs, spices, or condiments that do not contain sodium. Another example is a child with diabetes. The nutritionist who is called on to counsel the mother of such a child may need to take into consideration the family budget, the tastes and emotional needs of the patient's siblings, and perhaps a complex of additional factors to help the mother find a way to shift the diabetic child from a diet of sweets, for example, to other foods supplying the needed nutrients.

315

PROCEDURE FOR FAMILY DIET COUNSELING

Methods. In family diet counseling the nutritionist or the nurse must start by applying the initial principle of all counseling—begin where persons are. It is vital in counseling that a helping relationship first be established based on mutual trust before any active interchange to build desired behavior can occur.[3,4]

The next step is to learn the family's situation and values and to identify the nutritional needs. This can be accomplished by an interview in which a family nutrition history is taken. A standard form may be used for this purpose. Many forms have been used in such interviewing, of which the following are examples.

TWENTY-FOUR HOUR RECALL. Each member of the family is asked to recall every item of food taken during the preceding 24 hours.[5,6]

FOOD RECORDS. A record is kept for 24 hours or longer of all items eaten and drunk.[7]

STRUCTURED SCHEDULE FOR MEAL PATTERNS. A questionnaire or interview schedule is used, which lists each common meal item in the cultural pattern. For example, dinner may include the entrée, a starch accompaniment, a green or yellow vegetable, salad, bread, dessert, and beverage.

ACTIVITY-ASSOCIATED GENERAL DAY'S FOOD PATTERN. Perhaps one of the simplest and most helpful methods for both the interviewer and the family respondent (usually the mother) is the activity-associated general day's food pattern. Since for most people eating is related to activity or work throughout the day, making use of the association between the two gives the interviewer and the mother a structure—a beginning, a middle, and an end—and provides a series of mnemonics on which to flesh out the greater detail that will permit constructive counseling. A general form on which such an interview might be based is given on p. 317.

Diet history and analysis. By using such an interviewing schedule as the activity-associated general day's food pattern, three basic steps may be followed in performing a family nutrition analysis.

1. A general pattern of the day's activity and food intake should be obtained. The interview may begin with questions such as, "About what time do you usually get up in the morning? After you get up do you usually have something to eat? Can you give me examples of what you might have?" When this phase has been fully explored, the mother in the family or the patient in a hospital or clinic setting is led slowly through the usual routine for the day. Sometimes labels for informal meals are omitted so that the informant will remember to mention food that was eaten but not considered a meal. ("In the middle of the day do you usually have something to eat? Can you give me some examples?") Since family dinner is usually a more structured meal, it is reviewed carefully an item at a time, from the first dish served through the main dish, the dessert, and each of the various accompaniments. With respect to each item, the questions are asked in terms of general habit—food item, form, frequency, preparation, portion, seasoning—not in terms of a specific day's food intake. Sometimes pictures or models of portion sizes may be helpful in arriving at a clear picture of the family's general habits of food use.

2. The day's pattern should be checked by nutrient groups. A cross-check by nutrient groups helps to tally the day's use of given types of food. By referring to a crosslist of food items that have been categorized according to nutrient groups, the general use of the basic nutrients is tallied.

   a. *Protein foods*—milk, meat, fish, poultry, egg, cheese
   b. *Fruits and vegetables*—vitamin C and A sources, citrus and substitutes, deep green and yellow vegetables, raw and cooked fruits and vegetables, how cooked
   c. *Cereal grains and bread*—whole grain or enriched, forms used, frequency

Nutrition history

Activity-associated general day's food pattern

Name _____ Date _____

Height _____ Weight kg _____ Weight lb _____ Age _____

Ideal weight _____

Referral
Diagnosis
Diet order

Members of household

Occupation

Recreation, physical activity

Present food intake

	Place	*Hour*	*Frequency, form, and amount checklist*
Breakfast			Milk
			Cheese
			Meat
			Fish
Noon meal			Poultry
			Eggs
			Cream
			Butter, margarine
Evening meal			Other fats
			Vegetables, green
			Vegetables, other
			Fruits (citrus)
Extra meals			Legumes
			Potato
			Bread—kind
Summary			Sugar
			Desserts
			Beverages
			Alcohol
			Vitamins
			Candy

Nutritional analysis sheet		
Food intake **(family member, clinic patient)**	**Dietary guide** **(basic four food groups and** **main nutrient contributions of each)**	**Analysis of food intake**
Milk group		
Meat group		
Vegetable-fruit group		
Bread-cereal group		
Miscellaneous additions		

   d. *Desserts and beverages* — coffee, tea, soft drinks, alcohol

   e. *Miscellaneous snack items* — candy, chips, nuts, cookies

   f. *Nutrient supplements* — vitamins and minerals

As this cross-check is made, the questions asked will reflect back to the patient his original responses concerning the frequency of use of an item and the form in which it is consumed. ("Let's see now, tell me if this is about right. You mentioned drinking milk at dinner, but not at any other time. Would you say, then,

that you usually drink one glass of milk a day?") Weighted phrases such as "only one" or "plenty of," approving or disapproving tones or facial expressions, and the like should be avoided, as they tend to imply judgments and prevent straightforward responses.

Throughout such an interview, important clues to food attitudes and values are being communicated. The interviewer should carefully note these and remember them for later thought and possible exploration. If the interviewer's manner throughout has been interested and accepting, the information received should

Table 15-1. Daily dietary guide—the basic four food groups

Food group	Main nutrients	Daily amounts*
Milk		
Milk, cheese, ice cream, or other products made with whole or skimmed milk	Calcium Protein Riboflavin	Children under 9: 2-3 cups Children 9-12: 3 or more cups Teen-agers: 4 or more cups 4/5 Adults: 2 or more cups Pregnant women: 3 or more cups Nursing mothers: 4 or more cups (1 cup = 8 oz fluid milk or designated milk equivalent†)
Meats		

Beef, veal, lamb, pork, poultry, fish, eggs	Protein
	Iron
	Thiamin
		2 or more servings
		Count as 1 serving:
		    2-3 oz of lean, boneless, cooked meat, poultry, or fish
		    2 eggs

Alternates: dry beans, dry peas, nuts, peanut butter	Niacin Riboflavin	1 cup cooked dry beans or peas 4 tbsp peanut butter
Vegetables and fruits		4 or more servings Count as 1 serving: ½ cup of vegetable or fruit or a portion such as 1 medium apple, banana, orange, potato, or ½ a medium grapefuit, melon Include
	Vitamin A	A dark-green or deep-yellow vegetable or fruit rich in vitamin A at least every other day
	Vitamin C (ascorbic acid)	A citrus fruit or other fruit or vegetable rich in vitamin C daily
	Smaller amounts of other vitamins and minerals	Other vegetables and fruits including potatoes
Bread and cereals		4 or more servings of whole grain, enriched or restored Count as 1 serving:
	Thiamin Niacin Riboflavin Iron Protein	1 slice of bread 1 oz (1 cup) ready to eat cereal, flake or puff varieties ½-¾ cup cooked cereal ½-¾ cup cooked pastes (macaroni, spaghetti, noodles) Crackers: 5 saltines, 2 squares graham crackers, etc.

*Use additional amounts of these foods or added butter, margarine, oils, sugars, etc., as desired or needed.
†Milk equivalents: 1 oz cheddar cheese, 3 servings cottage cheese, 1 cup fluid skimmed milk, 1 cup buttermilk, ½ cup dry skimmed milk powder, 1 cup ice milk, 1⅔ cups ice cream, ½ cup evaporated milk.

be valid and straightforward. If the health worker is judgmental and authoritarian, the patient will probably only say what he thinks the health worker wants to hear, not what the true situation may be.

3. The general food pattern thus obtained should be analyzed by a dietary guide. Various dietary guides may be used as a measure of basic nutritional adequacy. Perhaps the most familiar guide is the list known as the basic four food groups (Table 15-1). Although this basic guide has limitations and often needs adapting, as in the evaluation and modification provided by King,[8] it may provide a useful, general tool for analyzing dietary adequacy. This guide groups food according to major nutrient components contributed to the daily diet and gives the general quantity needed for nutritional adequacy in terms of numbers of servings for different ages or circumstances, such as pregnancy and lactation.

Exploration of specific modifications. By recasting the general food pattern into categories, the patient may easily place the food intake and the basic four food groups guide side by side, so that the practitioner and the patient can analyze them together (p. 318). Together they may explore the possible additions or modifications needed and discuss a plan by which these nutrients may best be obtained. (See food plans at different cost levels, pp. 328-334.)

Inculcation of basic nutritional concepts. Using the patient's general nutritional analysis as a base, the health worker may clarify or reinforce an understanding of basic nutritional concepts (p. 301). A number of helpful tools, resource materials, and visual aids have been developed for use in teaching these concepts. Health workers may select from these materials or they may develop their own teaching materials on the basis of such guides, adapting them to each family's needs, abilities, and desires. Many helpful tools are available from community health resources.

Follow-through plans. After the nutritionist

and the patient have arrived at a definite plan for initial action that is expected to alter the food pattern, arrangements will be made with the patient for specific follow-up. This may take the form of return visits to the home, visits by the patient to the clinic or community health center, or consultation as needed with other members of the health team (physician, nutritionist, social worker, or other). The health worker may continue to help the patient and family with meal plans, marketing, economical buying, and suggestions for preparation of specific foods. Follow-up work requires patience, persistence, and a steady recollection of the goal. Imagination and good humor are invaluable. One step must be taken at a time. Throughout the whole process of guiding the patient and family in applied nutrition, the health worker will give support, help with adjustments of the plan, provide reinforcement of prior learning, and continue to add new learning opportunities as the family's needs develop.

FAMILY FOOD ECONOMICS— NEEDS AND COSTS

The basic responsibility for providing nourishing meals for the family usually rests with the mother or wife. To a great extent her self-esteem is bound up in her image of herself in the role of food provider, and she spends a large proportion of her time in activities related to this function. Often she is under the pressure of conflict between her desire to keep her family healthy by serving an adequate and balanced supply of foods and her limitation of financial resources for buying food.

The American family faces a vast array of tempting and colorful items in the supermarket and food costs that can be bewildering. If young parents have had little preparation for homemaking, they have even more difficulty managing to make ends meet. The average family in the United States spends about 20% of its income on food. About one third to one half of this money may be spent for such luxury items

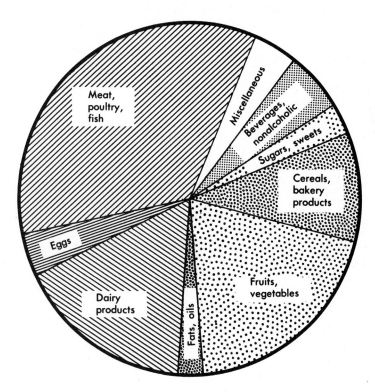

Fig. 15-1. The family food dollar, showing the approximate relative amount of money spent on common food items. (Data from Nationwide USDA Surveys, 1963-1966 and 1977-1978.)

Table 15-2. Bargains in the basic four food groups*

Food group	Usually less expensive, more food value for the money	Usually more expensive, less food value for the money
Milk products	Concentrated, fluid and dry nonfat milk, buttermilk, evaporated	Fluid whole milk, chocolate drink, condensed milk, sweet or sour cream
	Milk cheddar, Swiss, cottage cheese	Sharp cheddar, Roquefort or blue, grated or sliced cheese, cream cheese, yogurt
	Ice milk, imitation ice milk, imitation ice cream	Ice cream, sherbet
Meats		
Meat	Good and standard grades	Prime and choice grades
	Less tender cuts	Tender cuts
	Home-cooked meats	Canned meats, sliced luncheon meats
	Pork or beef liver, heart, kidney, tongue	Calf liver
Poultry	Stewing chickens, whole broiler-fryers, large turkeys	Poultry parts, specialty products, canned poultry, small turkeys
Fish	Rock cod, butterfish, other fresh fish in season, frozen fillets, steaks, and sticks	Salmon, crab, lobster, prawns, shrimp, oysters
Eggs	Grade A	Grade AA
Beans, peas, and lentils	Dried beans, peas, lentils	Canned baked beans, soups
Nuts	Peanut butter, walnuts, other nuts in shell	Pecans, cashews, shelled nuts, prepared nuts
Vegetables, fruits	Local vegetables and fruits in season	Out-of-season vegetables and fruits, unusual vegetables and fruits, those in short supply
Vitamin A rich	Carrots, collards, sweet potatoes, green leafy vegetables, spinach, pumpkin, winter squash, broccoli, and in season cantaloupe, apricots, persimmons	Tomatoes, brussels sprouts, asparagus, peaches, watermelon, papaya, banana, tangerine
Vitamin C rich	Oranges, grapefruit and their juice, cabbage, greens, green pepper, cantaloupe, strawberries, tomatoes, broccoli in season	Tangerines, apples, bananas, peaches, pears
Others	Medium-sized potatoes, nonbaking types	Baking potatoes, new potatoes, canned or frozen potatoes, potato chips
	Romaine, leaf lettuce	Iceberg lettuce, frozen specialty packs of vegetables
Bread, cereals	Whole wheat and enriched flour	Stone-ground, unenriched, and cake flour
	Whole grain and enriched breads	French, Vienna, other specialty breads, hard rolls
	Homemade rolls and coffee cake	Ready-made rolls and coffee cakes, frozen or partially baked products
	Whole grain or restored uncooked cereals	Ready-to-eat cereals, puffed, sugar-coated
	Graham crackers, whole grain wafers	Zwieback, specialty crackers and wafers
	Enriched uncooked macaroni, spaghetti, noodles	Unenriched, canned, or frozen macaroni, spaghetti, noodles
	Brown rice, converted rice	Quick-cooking, seasoned, or canned rice

*Cook, F., Groppe, C., and Ferree, M.: Balance food values and cents, Berkeley, Calif., 1970, University of California Agricultural Extension Service, Pub. HXT-42, pp. 6-7.

as expensive cuts of meats, out-of-season fresh fruits and vegetables, and other special foods. Nutritious, attractive meals can be had for less. It is the need to achieve this that faces the low-income family. Often the public health worker or the nutritionist is asked to counsel with such a family about ways to get the most nutrition from their limited food dollars. Sometimes the financial need is even more pronounced, and the health worker must help plan with a family in circumstances of extreme poverty.

U.S. family food use and costs. More specifically, just how much food does the average American family use and what money value does this amount of food represent? A previous U.S. Department of Agriculture nationwide survey indicated that the average family divides its food dollar as indicated in Fig. 15-1. This same general division continues today.

"Basic four" food bargains. The objective in wise food buying for the family is to obtain optimal nutritional value for money spent on food. The basic four food groups may serve as a guide for examples of ways in which food bargains, nutritionally speaking, may be obtained with careful planning. In Table 15-2 the food choices in the less expensive column are compared with those in the more expensive column.

Food buying guides

Today's American family spends more time shopping for food than cooking it. Food marketing is big business, and buying food for a family may seem to be a more intricate affair than the preparation of it at home. A large American supermarket may stock 8,000 or more different food items, and more are being added daily. A single food item may be marketed in a dozen different ways at as many different prices. Frequently in family diet counseling and in talking with patients about special modified diets, the health worker will observe that the family places greatest stress on their need for help in food buying.

Factors affecting family food costs. A number of factors influence the way in which a family divides its food dollar. The health care worker will explore these factors with the family in helping them outline their family food plan:

1. Family income
2. The number, sex, ages, and general activities of the family members
3. Whether any part of the family food is produced or preserved at home (gardening, canning, freezing)
4. The likes and dislikes of family members; special family dishes
5. Special dietary needs of any family member
6. The time, transportation, and energy available to the family for shopping and food preparation
7. The skill and experience the family has in family food management (planning, shopping, storing, preparing)
8. The storage and cooking facilities in the home
9. The amount and kind of entertaining, if any, the family does
10. The number of meals eaten away from home
11. The value the family places on food and eating

Economy buying suggestions. In each basic food group, suggestions for wise, economical buying may be explored with the family.

MEATS, FISH, POULTRY, EGGS. Since meat is commonly one of the more costly food items, considerable study should be given to how it is graded, cut, processed, and marketed. Excellent learning material is available through the local county home advisor, U.S. Department of Agriculture Extension Service.

1. The homemaker should buy cuts of meat that give the most lean meat for the money and should avoid paying for large amounts of gristle, bone, and fat.
2. The meat grade should be checked. The

lower grades provide good quality, less fat, and cost less. Meat on the U.S. market is usually graded according to quality and ratio of fat to lean. *USDA Prime* is of excellent quality and flavor. It is tender and moist and the fat well marbleized (distributed, striated) through the lean meat. It is not often seen in markets serving the general public, since it goes mostly to the hotel and restaurant trade. *USDA Choice* is of very good quality. It is popular because of the moderate amount of fat that is distributed through the lean portion. This is the grade usually found in most retail markets. *USDA Good* is of good quality and is relatively tender. It is preferred by consumers who desire a lower ratio of fat to lean. *USDA Standard* is acceptable quality. It comes from animals under 48 months of age and has a very thin covering of fat and high proportion of lean. It is a good buy. *USDA Commercial* is less tender but is of acceptable quality. It comes from older animals and has less fat than the higher grades. It is often a very good buy, but is seldom seen in retail markets. It goes mostly to meat products processing plants. *USDA Utility, Cutter,* and *Canner* are the three lowest grades, and they are used only in processed meat products.

3. The less costly meats have just as much food value as the higher cost cuts, and although they are less tender and juicy then the costlier cuts, they can be made equally tender and flavorful by cooking them slowly using methods that involve water or steam, such as pot-roasting or braising.

4. Grades of ground meat that sell at lower cost can be used, but the amount of fat should not be excessive. Some states (for example, California) have laws providing that all ground fresh beef may contain no more than 30% fat and that all meat used must be skeletal meat (edible meat of striated muscle originally attached to bones). In these states no organ meats, coloring, cereal, or preservatives may be added. Specific label names indicate the following:

   a. Ground beef or hamburger—only fresh beef containing no more than 30% fat may be sold under this label

   b. Ground chuck or round—must be only chuck roast or round with no more than 30% fat; usually contains less

   c. Pork sausage—ground pork with no more than 50% fat

5. Organ meats (liver, kidney, heart) are nutritious *bargains*. They should be used often. A good cookbook will have correct and appetizing ways of preparing them for family acceptance (for example, liver loaf [part liver, part ground beef] with Spanish sauce, stuffed and baked heart, and beef and kidney pie). Other variety meats include brains, tongue, sweetbreads (thymus gland from veal or very young beef; this gland disappears with maturity), and tripe (the plain or smooth lining, especially the pocket-shaped part from the end, of the cow's second stomach).

6. Poultry should be bought as the whole bird. Usually the larger, more mature birds cost less than young broilers and fryers and can be made equally tender by longer, moist cooking methods (braising, stewing, fricasseeing) or by pressure cooking.

7. Fish is usually a good buy since it is sold in cuts that contain little or no waste. Shellfish is more costly; fresh fish in season is less expensive.

8. Less expensive packed styles of canned fish should be used. For example, salmon species are usually priced according to color. Chinook, King, and Sockeye (Red) are deepest in color and cost more; Choho (Silver), Pink, and Chum (or Keta) are lighter colored, have less oil, and usually cost less. Tuna is packed according to size of pieces. Fancy or solid pack (large pieces) is most expensive; chunk style is made up of moderate-sized pieces and is moderate in price; flake or grated style consists of smaller pieces and is cheapest in price.

9. Eggs are sold according to grade and size, neither of which is related to food value. It is therefore advantageous to buy the least expen-

sive. Egg grades are AA, A, B, and C. Differentiation into these grades is based on such qualities as firmness of the egg white, appearance, and delicacy of flavor. The AA and A grades are better for poaching, frying, and cooking in the shell; lower grades are equally good for general cooking, scrambling, and omelets. The size classifications are based on weight per dozen: Jumbo (30 oz per dozen), Extra Large (27 oz per dozen), Large (24 oz per dozen), Medium (21 oz per dozen), Small (18 oz per dozen), and Peewee (pullet eggs, 15 oz per dozen). This classification has no relation to food value or quality. Shell color (white, brown, or speckled) varies with species and breeds of poultry and has no effect on egg quality.

MILK, CHEESE. Milk and milk products are bargains in nutrition. It is hard to get enough calcium and riboflavin without including dairy products in the diet.

1. Fluid skimmed milk, buttermilk, and canned evaporated milk cost less than fresh, whole, fluid milk. So-called low-fat milks are 2% butterfat (whole milk is 4% butterfat). To make them, part of the butterfat is removed from whole milk and dry milk solids are added. Low-fat milk contains 135 calories per 8-oz cup; whole milk contains 170 calories per cup; skim milk contains 80 calories per cup.

2. Nonfat dry milk is the best bargain of all forms. Reconstituted with water, it gives a fluid skimmed milk at less than half the cost of fresh fluid skimmed milk. Dry skimmed milk can be used in innumerable ways in cooking to add valuable nutrition.

3. Milk should be bought at the store. In most cities a family pays from 1 to 3 cents more per quart for delivery. However, some milk-delivery firms charge less than this per quart for large numbers of quarts delivered regularly.

4. If the family size warrants it, milk should be bought in large containers. Fluid milk sometimes costs less in the half-gallon on large bulk containers than in the quart container.

5. If cheese is used often, it should be bought in bulk. It costs less and keeps better. Cheese standards set by the Food and Drug Administration are based on percentage of fat and moisture. The most commonly used, cheddar cheese (American, Daisy, Longhorn), is 50% fat and 30% moisture. The spread cheeses and imported cheeses are more expensive.

6. Cottage cheese is an unripened, soft-curd (80% moisture) and hence is rapidly perishable. It should be bought only as used to avoid waste resulting from spoilage. The buyer should not be misled by the statement on the label that a cottage cheese is low in calories. Regular re-creamed cottage cheese contains not more than 4% milkfat; "low calorie" contains about 2% milkfat. The difference in calories is slight. One-half cup of regular recreamed cottage cheese provides 120 calories; the same amount of "low calorie" (partially recreamed) cottage cheese provides 100 calories.

VEGETABLES, FRUITS. Vegetables and fruits are the main sources of vitamins A and C, two nutrients found in community surveys to be most often lacking in the average American diet.

1. Fresh vegetables and fruits should be bought in season. Except for unpredictable crop shortages or surpluses, prices go through seasonal cycles according to supply. For example, citrus fruits usually cost less during the winter; fresh garden vegetables cost less during the summer, except for winter garden vegetables such as cabbage, winter squash, and sweet potatoes.

2. When one buys fresh produce, pieces that are firm, crisp, and heavy for their size should be selected. Fresh vegetables and fruits that are of medium size are usually better buys than large, of which more may need to be discarded.

3. The buyer should distinguish between types of defect. Small surface defects do not affect the eating quality or food value of fruits and vegetables, and pieces so blemished may cost less. Many or deep defects cause more

waste, as does decay that is even slightly evident.

4. If an item of fresh produce is sold by either weight or count, the resulting price per item should be computed by each method to find the one that costs less.

5. Fancy grades in canned vegetables and fruits should be avoided. Grading is based on shape, size, and perfection of pieces. Lower grades contain small, broken, or imperfect pieces, but are equal to higher grades in food value and are therefore good buys.

6. If family size warrants, fruits and vegetables should be bought in large cans. For example, the No. 3 cylinder can (46 fl. oz; 3 lb, 3 oz; or 5¾ cups) is the "economy family size" in fruit and vegetable juices, pork and beans, and so on. It yields from 10 to 12 servings. The size of can for fruits and vegetables that is stocked in largest quantities on market shelves is No. 303, which contains 2 cups, or 4 servings. Labels should be carefully checked for servings per unit. The largest (institutional) size can, No. 10, contains from 12 to 13 cups, or 25 servings.

7. Dehydrated foods vary in price. Dried beans, peas, and lentils are excellent food buys. Specialty dried foods, such as potatoes, are usually more expensive than the fresh product.

8. Frozen vegetables and fruits are usually more expensive than fresh or canned; however, specials and large family size packages should be compared weight for weight with canned or fresh produce in season.

9. Vegetables should be cooked with care. Excess cooking water and time destroy or eliminate vitamins and minerals and rob the vegetable of color and texture. Such unappetizing food often goes uneaten by the family, hence causes costly waste.

10. If the homemaker knows the produce person at the market, he or she can sometimes get good, usable produce that has been discarded on certain days as a fresh supply comes in. It will need careful checking and much cutting away of defective parts, but often it costs nothing except the time and effort in handling the crates and culling the material.

BREAD, CEREALS. Cereals are bargains in nutrition. Milled cereals are now commonly enriched. Grains have earned the title "staff of life," and people in many parts of the world today subsist almost entirely on them. They are found in American markets in many forms and are usually an economy food.

1. Grains should be brought in bulk for cheaper cost. However, adequate storage should be planned (room temperature or cool place, in tight container) to avoid waste resulting from spoilage by dust, moisture, or insects.

2. Whole grain or enriched cereal products should be purchased to ensure the content of B-complex vitamins and calcium and iron.

3. Unusual forms of grain should be tried. For example, bulgur is cooked and dried wheat with outer bran removed and the remaining kernels cooked to the desired size. Dry, cracked bulgur keeps well in a porous container in a cool place. It has a toastlike color, is rich in wheat flavor, is equal in food value to whole wheat, and makes an economical addition to the family menus for variety.

4. Regular, enriched white rice should be bought. Any processing or specialty preparation increases the cost.

5. To avoid costly waste of breads and cereals resulting from careless handling, dry cereals should be stored in a cool, dry place. The package should be closed tightly after each use. For long storage of bread, it should be frozen or placed in the refrigerator.

Menu planning to save money. As an example of the economy that can be effected by food choices for family meals, two menus are compared in Table 15-3. Both menus use essentially the same foods, but the cost difference resulted from selecting the best buys in each case.

Table 15-3. One menu at two cost levels for family of four (father and mother 33 years of age, boy 11, girl 8)*

Meal	Menu 1 (more costly)	Menu 2 (less costly)
Breakfast	Grapefruit juice (frozen)	Grapefruit juice (canned)
	Ready-to-eat cereal (oat)	Oatmeal
	Poached eggs (large)	Poached eggs (medium size)
	Enriched English muffins	Whole wheat toast
	Butter	Margarine
	Coffee (name brand)	Coffee (store brand)
	Milk for all (fluid, nonfat)	Milk for all (concentrated)
Lunch	Onion soup (canned)	Onion soup (dehydrated)
	Tuna salad sandwiches (chunk style tuna)	Tuna salad sandwiches (grated style tuna)
	Cabbage slaw (ready-made)	Cabbage slaw (homemade)
	Peaches (heavy syrup)	Peaches (light syrup)
	Milk for all (fluid whole for father and fluid nonfat for others)	Milk for all (concentrated)
Dinner	Cubed steaks	Individual meat loaves with potatoes and carrots
	Baked potatoes	
	Frozen carrots	
	Tossed green salad with French dressing (commercial)	Romaine salad with vinegar and oil dressing (homemade)
	Whole wheat brown-and-serve rolls	Hot whole wheat bread slices
	Butter	Margarine
	Frozen apple pie (commercial)	Baked apples
	Milk for all (whole, fluid)	Milk for all (concentrated)
	Coffee for adults (name brand)	Coffee for adults (store brand)

*Cook, F., Groppe, C., and Ferree, M.: Balance food values and cents, Berkeley, Calif., 1970, University of California Agricultural Extension Service, Pub. HXT-42, pp. 8-9.

Summary of good marketing and food handling practices

Planning ahead. The homemaker should use market guides, plan general menus, keep a kitchen supply check list, and make out a market list ahead according to location of items in a regularly visited market. Such planning helps to avert "impulse buying" and extra trips. Completely unplanned purchases account for over half of the items bought in supermarkets!

Buying wisely. The homemaker should know the market, market items, packaging, grades, brands, portion yields, measures, and food value in a market unit. The homemaker should watch for sales and buy in quantity if it effects a saving and if he or she can store and use the food. The homemaker should be cautious in selecting "convenience" foods. The added time saving may not be worth the added cost.

Storing food safely. The kitchen waste that

results from food spoilage and misuse should be controlled. Food should be conserved by storing items according to their nature and utilization. Dry storage, covered containers, and refrigeration should be used as needed. After a food package has been opened and part of its contents has been consumed, the opened package with the remaining food should be kept on the front of a shelf for early use. To avoid plate waste only the amount needed by the family should be cooked, and leftovers should be used intelligently.

Cooking food well. Maximum food value should be retained, but food should also be prepared with imagination and good sense. Zest and appeal can be given to dishes by using a variety of seasonings and combinations. However much the homemaker may have learned about nutrition, members of the family usually eat because they are hungry or because the food looks and tastes good—not because it is nutritious.

A most helpful food marketing guide has been prepared by Black and her associates for price-conscious families. The great variety of information presented can aid persons in becoming active, informed consumers.[10]

FOOD PLANS ACCORDING TO FAMILY INCOME

Except perhaps for the small group of very wealthy, most American families live under socioeconomic pressures, especially in a period of inflation. The problems of middle-income and low-income families differ only relatively. Health workers, if they are to provide realistic and useful assistance in health care to the individual family in these categories, will need to understand the background of economic pressures and the types of problems that result.

Middle-income groups

General socioeconomic pressures. A number of socioeconomic pressures create problems for middle-class families. Early marriage and young parenthood, incomplete education, continuing education (especially graduate and professional education), low job status, and low beginning salaries all exert financial pressures on young couples beginning to establish their homes. In their attempts to meet these pressures, most middle-income families assume increasing debt. For example, a previous study conducted in 1962 to 1963 by the U.S. Federal Reserve Board[11], and still representative despite current inflation, revealed that 8 out of 10 American households in which the head was under 35 years of age owed personal debt averaging $1,000, of which $700 was installment debt; meeting payments was a problem for some. Nine of every ten homes owned by American families in this young age group were mortgaged. This wide pattern of incurring and paying off debt is a normal part of the financial activities of the young; it becomes less important as they grow older.

Lack of preparation for family adjustments or unrealistic attitudes may also create problems for young couples. For example, the wife and mother may be a teenager accustomed to the standard of living that characterized her parents' home, which her young husband cannot, of course, maintain. In the past she may have had little motive or opportunity to learn skills in home and food management that would have enabled her to make optimum use of the money available. As a result, the couple's small income is misused, whereas intelligently planned spending would provide better food at less cost. In the course of professional work, particularly in the prenatal clinic, the nutritionist or the nurse frequently encounters a bewildered and anxious young wife who welcomes sympathetic understanding and counsel in these practical areas.

As family size increases and children grow older, the food bills increase as do the other financial commitments of the family. Job in-

Table 15-4. Moderate-cost family food plan

Sex-age group*	Milk, cheese, ice cream‡ (qt)	Meat, poultry, fish§		Eggs (no.)	Dry beans, peas, nuts		Flour, cereals, baked goods‖		Citrus fruit, tomatoes		Dark green and deep yellow vegetables		Potatoes		Other vegetables and fruits		Fats, oils		Sugars, sweets	
		lb	oz		lb	oz	lb	oz	lb	oz	lb	oz	lb	oz	lb	oz	lb	oz	lb	oz
Children																				
7 mo-1 yr	5	1	8	6	0	0	0	14	1	8	0	4	0	8	1	8	0	1	0	2
1-3 yr	5	2	4	6	0	1	1	4	1	8	0	4	0	12	2	12	0	4	0	4
3-6 yr	5	2	12	6	0	1	1	12	2	0	0	4	1	0	4	0	0	6	0	8
6-9 yr	5	3	4	7	0	2	2	8	2	4	0	8	1	12	4	12	0	10	0	14
Girls																				
9-12 yr	5½	4	4	7	0	4	2	8	2	8	0	12	2	0	5	8	0	8	0	12
12-15 yr	7	4	8	7	0	4	2	8	2	8	1	0	2	4	5	12	0	12	0	14
15-20 yr	7	4	8	7	0	4	2	4	2	8	1	4	2	0	5	8	0	8	0	12
Boys																				
9-12 yr	5½	4	4	7	0	4	2	12	2	4	0	12	2	4	5	8	0	10	0	14
12-15 yr	7	4	12	7	0	4	4	0	2	4	0	12	3	0	6	0	0	14	1	0
15-20 yr	7	5	4	7	0	6	4	8	2	8	0	12	4	0	6	8	1	2	1	2
Women																				
20-35 yr	3½	4	12	8	0	4	2	4	2	4	1	8	1	8	5	12	0	8	0	14
35-55 yr	3½	4	12	8	0	4	2	4	2	4	1	8	1	4	5	0	0	6	0	8
55-75 yr	3½	4	4	6	0	2	1	8	2	4	0	12	1	4	4	4	0	6	0	8
75 yr and over	3½	3	8	6	0	2	1	4	2	4	0	12	1	0	3	12	0	4	0	8
Pregnant¶	5½	5	8	8	0	4	2	12	3	4	2	0	1	8	5	12	0	6	0	8
Lactating¶	8	5	8	8	0	4	3	12	3	8	1	8	2	12	6	4	0	12	0	12
Men																				
20-35 yr	3½	5	0	7	0	4	4	0	2	4	0	12	3	0	6	8	1	0	1	4
35-55 yr	3½	4	12	7	0	4	3	8	2	4	0	12	2	8	5	12	0	14	1	0
55-75 yr	3½	4	8	7	0	2	2	8	2	4	0	12	2	4	5	8	0	12	0	14
75 yr and over	3½	4	8	7	0	2	2	4	2	4	0	12	2	0	5	4	0	8	0	12

*Age groups include the persons of the first age listed up to but not including those of the second age listed.
†Food as purchased or brought into the kitchen from garden or farm.
‡Fluid whole milk, or its calcium equivalent in cheese, evaporated milk, dry milk, or ice cream.
§Bacon and salt pork should not exceed ⅓ lb for each 5 lb of meat group.
‖Weight in terms of flour and cereal. Count 1½ lb bread as 1 lb flour.
¶Three additional quarts of milk are suggested for pregnant and lactating teenagers.

Table 15-5. Low-cost family food plan

Sex-age group*	Milk, cheese, ice cream‡ (qt)	Meat, poultry, fish§ lb	oz	Eggs (no.)	Dry beans, peas, nuts lb	oz	Flour, cereals, baked goods‖ lb	oz	Citrus fruit, tomatoes lb	oz	Dark green and deep yellow vegetables lb	oz	Potatoes lb	oz	Other vegetables and fruits lb	oz	Fats, oils lb	oz	Sugars, sweets lb	oz
Children																				
7 mo-1 yr	4	1	4	5	0	0	1	0	1	8	0	4	0	8	1	0	0	1	0	2
1-3 yr	4	1	12	5	0	1	1	8	1	8	0	4	0	12	2	4	0	4	0	4
3-6 yr	4	2	0	5	0	2	2	0	1	12	0	4	1	4	3	4	0	6	0	6
6-9 yr	4	2	4	6	0	4	2	12	2	0	0	8	2	4	4	4	0	8	0	10
Girls																				
9-12 yr	5½	2	8	7	0	6	2	8	2	4	0	12	2	4	5	0	0	8	0	10
12-15 yr	7	2	8	7	0	6	2	12	2	4	1	0	2	8	5	0	0	8	0	12
15-20 yr	7	2	12	7	0	6	2	8	2	4	1	4	2	4	4	12	0	6	0	10
Boys																				
9-12 yr	5½	2	8	6	0	6	3	0	2	0	0	12	2	8	5	0	0	8	0	12
12-15 yr	7	2	8	6	0	6	4	4	2	0	0	12	3	4	5	4	0	12	0	12
15-20 yr	7	3	8	6	0	6	4	12	2	0	0	12	4	4	5	8	0	14	0	14
Women																				
20-35 yr	3½	3	4	7	0	6	2	8	1	12	1	8	2	0	5	0	0	6	0	10
35-55 yr	3½	3	4	7	0	6	2	4	1	12	1	8	1	8	4	8	0	4	0	10
55-75 yr	3½	2	8	5	0	4	2	0	2	0	1	0	1	4	3	12	0	4	0	6
75 yr and over	3½	2	4	5	0	4	1	8	2	0	1	0	1	4	3	0	0	4	0	4
Pregnant¶	5½	3	12	7	0	6	2	12	3	4	2	0	1	8	5	8	0	6	0	6
Lactating¶	8	3	12	7	0	6	3	12	3	4	1	8	3	4	5	8	0	10	0	10
Men																				
20-35 yr	3½	3	8	6	0	6	4	4	1	12	0	12	3	4	5	8	0	12	1	0
35-55 yr	3½	3	4	6	0	6	3	12	1	12	0	12	3	0	5	0	0	10	0	12
55-75 yr	3½	3	0	6	0	4	2	12	1	12	0	12	2	4	4	8	0	10	0	10
75 yr and over	3½	2	12	6	0	4	2	8	1	8	0	12	2	0	4	4	0	8	0	8

*Age groups include the persons of the first age listed up to but not including those of the second age listed.
†Food as purchased or brought into the kitchen from garden or farm.
‡Fluid whole milk, or its calcium equivalent in cheese, evaporated milk, dry milk, or ice cream.
§Bacon and salt pork should not exceed ⅓ lb for each 5 lb of meat group.
‖Weight in terms of flour and cereal. Count 1½ lb bread as 1 lb flour.
¶Three additional quarts of milk are suggested for pregnant and lactating teenagers.

security and lessened income may be problems as age advances. Forced early retirement, limited pension funds, fixed incomes in the face of rising costs, and cost of chronic illness may add to the financial problems of older families.

Family food plans. To aid the health worker in counseling with families or in working with community groups, several *Family Food Plans* have been prepared by the U.S. Department of Agriculture, Consumer and Food Economics Research Division.[12] Five basic plans on different cost levels with additional variations are available: (1) liberal plan, (2) moderate plan, (3) low-cost plan and (4) thrifty plan.[13] The moderate and low-cost plans, often used to guide families of moderate income, are shown in Tables 15-4 and 15-5.

Low-income groups—the problem of poverty

Tremendous problems exist among the poor. At times they seem almost insurmountable. It is small wonder that a "culture of poverty" develops among the poor, which too often walls them off from the rest of society more completely than would physical barriers. These families are poor not only in income, but also in other aspects of their lives. They live in dilapidated, overcrowded buildings. Their education is usually inadequate in quality and quantity; and they have little or no access to educational opportunities. As a result, they are poorly prepared for jobs and often must make a day-to-day living at unskilled labor. They are poor in opportunity for contact with middle-class and upper-class groups. Often there is little beauty in their barren lives and even less hope.

Characteristics of the poor. As a result of the extreme pressures arising from their living conditions, poverty-stricken persons and families develop attitudes and characteristics that influence their use of community health services. Health workers must understand and appreciate these characteristics if they are to work

with these families and if they are to avoid impossible directives *on* them. Since imposing directives reinforces the character problems that obstruct health development, it is to be avoided as far as possible.

The traits that characterize the discouraged poor manifest themselves in many ways and in many individual forms; but experienced, sensitive health workers identify them essentially as feelings of *isolation, powerlessness,* and *insecurity.*[14]

ISOLATION. Strong feelings of alienation are common among the poor. In many communities, few, if any, channels of communication are open between the lowest income groups and the rest of society. Almost no opportunity exists for participation in community activities and organizations or for any meaningful dialogue and achievement of bridges of understanding. Many poor persons respond to such alienation by further withdrawal. Feeling isolated and alone, they conclude that no one is really concerned about their situation. The hazards to health that are inherent in poor housing and poor nutrition are compounded by alienation from the sources of help that would be available in the community if they were to attempt to make use of them.

POWERLESSNESS. It is ironic that often these persons most exposed to risks and emergencies have the least resources and power for coping with them. Extreme frustration is inevitable. Many a poor person becomes overwhelmed with a sense of helplessness. Why try, he concludes, if he has no control over the situation? Why plan if he has no future different from today? In such a day-to-day struggle to exist, the dispirited poor often see little value in long-range preventive health measures.

INSECURITY. Subjected to forces outside his control, the poor person has no security. A large proportion of the lowest economic class work by the day, if at all; and their unskilled labor is highly expendable. If such a person is sick and cannot work, he usually faces loss of employment rather than sick leave. In his effort to supply his family's needs, he is vulnerable to spurious schemes and enticing webs that can lead him into legal and still deeper financial problems. The impact of these pressures of insecurity and anxiety may incapacitate him. The appearance of detachment and lethargy that the health worker sees may only be a defense mechanism by which some poor persons attempt to cope with intolerable personal situations. Such an individual is so frozen with concern that he may appear to care about nothing. The coping mechanism of another poor person in the same situation may be totally different. He may respond with hostility. The openly hostile poor strike out at the helping source because they see it as part of the power structure they have come to view as towering and formidable. As part of this power structure, the source of help appears to them to be an enemy to be distrusted, rather than a friend to whom to look for help.

In such a setting, where hunger may be a constant companion, food—which has for the poor person the same deep psychologic and emotional connotations that it has for all—assumes even greater meaning than it has for persons who rarely know hunger. For people in a chronic state of insecurity, food can be a very serious matter involving the total person.

Role of the health worker. How may the health care practitioner work with individuals and families conditioned by years or generations of a culture of poverty? In the face of such overpowering feelings of isolation, helplessness, and insecurity, what attitudes must health workers have if they are to help them? What methods and approaches are most likely to reach them and supply their needs?

The basic principles of learning and health teaching discussed in the previous chapter can be helpful. Several seem particularly pertinent.

SELF-AWARENESS. Health care workers who have not explored their own feelings about these people and who have not come to a realistic awareness of their class values and attitudes are ill-equipped to work effectively in such a situation. If they are to be agents of *change,* a true "helping vehicle" (the beautiful phrase coined by Lucile Matthews[14] of the U.S. Children's Bureau), they must first have some understanding of the poor person and his broad social milieu, or themselves, and of their own cultural conditioning.

RAPPORT. Genuine warmth, interest, friendliness, and kindness grow from the inside out. They cannot be put on from the outside as one would put on a cloak. Rapport is that feeling of relationship between persons, which is born of mutual respect, regard, and trust. This sense of relationship gives both helper and helped a deep feeling of working *together.* Its most basic ingredient is concern for people and for persons—positive orientation toward the human race in general and a love and concern for individuals in particular.

ACCEPTANCE. Acceptance is another way of stating the principle that one must begin where the patient is. To begin to help, the health care worker must accept the person as he is in his situation as it exists. The worker must be concerned with the patient's concerns. It may be necessary to work with other team specialists through a veritable maze of factors before one individual is ready to accept or even to consider the health practice or the diet counsel that he needs or that is desired for him. The health practitioner may have to spend much time, for example, in coming to understand the meaning of food to this person before he or she can begin to explore practical dietary matters with him.

LISTENING. Here, more than elsewhere, the art of listening—positive, active, creative listening—is vital. The patient must tell his story in his own way. There must be no interruptions with distracting statements or questions, no deflecting of the conversation to someone else's problems. This listening must also be observant. Sequence of statements, subjects introduced, areas of intense feelings, and areas ignored give clues to needs. Throughout, the health worker

Table 15-6. Thrifty family food plan (designed for temporary use when funds are limited or when food stamps are available)

Sex-age group*	Milk, cheese, ice cream‡ (qt)	Meat, poultry, fish§		Eggs (no.)	Dry beans, peas, nuts		Flour, cereals, baked goods‖		Citrus fruit, tomatoes		Dark green and deep yellow vegetables		Potatoes		Other vegetables and fruits		Fats, oils		Sugars, sweets	
		lb	oz		lb	oz	lb	oz	lb	oz	lb	oz	lb	oz	lb	oz	lb	oz	lb	oz
Children																				
7 mo-1 yr	4	1	0	4	0	0	1	0	1	0	0	4	0	12	1	0	0	2	0	2
1-3 yr	4	1	4	4	0	1	1	12	1	0	0	4	1	0	2	0	0	4	0	4
3-6 yr	3½	1	8	4	0	4	2	4	1	4	0	4	1	8	2	8	0	6	0	6
6-9 yr	3½	1	12	5	0	6	3	0	1	8	0	8	2	8	3	0	0	10	0	10
Girls																				
9-12 yr	5	1	12	5	0	10	2	12	1	12	0	12	2	8	3	4	0	8	0	10
12-15 yr	6	2	0	6	0	10	3	0	1	12	1	0	3	0	3	8	0	10	0	10
15-20 yr	6	2	0	6	0	8	2	12	1	12	1	4	2	8	3	4	0	8	0	10
Boys																				
9-12 yr	5	2	0	5	0	8	3	4	1	8	0	12	2	12	3	4	0	10	0	10
12-15 yr	6	2	0	5	0	10	4	4	1	12	0	13	3	8	3	8	0	14	0	12
15-20 yr	6	2	8	5	0	10	5	0	1	12	0	12	4	12	3	8	1	0	0	14
Women																				
20-35 yr	3	1	12	6	0	10	2	12	1	8	1	8	2	12	3	0	0	8	0	12
35-55 yr	3	1	12	6	0	10	2	8	1	8	1	8	2	8	2	12	0	6	0	8
55-75 yr	3	1	8	4	0	6	2	0	1	12	1	0	2	8	2	12	0	6	0	6
75 yr and over	3	1	4	4	0	6	1	12	1	12	1	0	2	0	2	4	0	4	0	6
Pregnant¶	5½	2	0	7	0	10	3	0	3	0	2	0	2	8	4	8	0	6	0	6
Lactating¶	8	2	0	6	0	10	4	0	3	0	1	8	3	12	4	8	0	12	0	12
Men																				
20-35 yr	3	2	0	5	0	8	4	8	1	8	0	12	4	4	3	8	0	14	1	2
35-55 yr	3	1	12	5	0	8	4	4	1	8	0	13	3	8	3	4	0	12	0	14
55-75 yr	3	1	8	5	0	6	3	4	1	8	0	12	2	12	3	0	0	12	0	10
75 yr and over	3	1	8	5	0	6	3	0	1	8	0	12	2	8	2	12	0	10	0	6

*Age groups include the persons of the first age listed up to but not including those of the second age listed.
†Food as purchased or brought into the kitchen from garden or farm.
‡Fluid whole milk, or its calcium equivalent in cheese, evaporated milk, dry milk, or ice cream.
§Bacon and salt pork should not exceed ⅓ lb for each 5 lb of meat group.
‖Weight in terms of flour and cereal. Count 1½ lb bread as 1 lb flour.
¶Three additional quarts of milk are suggested for pregnant and lactating teenagers.

Table 15-7. Market basket for lower cost family food plan*

Food group	Food items included
Milk, cheese	Only nonfat dry milk, cheese
Meat, fish, poultry	Stewing beef, ground beef, salt pork, sausage, chicken, fish
Beans, peas, nuts	Dried beans, peanut butter
Flour, cereals, baked goods	Large proportion of flour and cornmeal; only cereals for cooking (no ready-to-eat cereals); rice and macaroni products; bread, crackers, and some sweet crackers
Citrus fruits, tomatoes	Canned orange juice, some fresh oranges, canned tomatoes
Potatoes	Only fresh potatoes (no processed)
Dark green and deep yellow vegetables	Sweet potatoes and carrots
Other vegetables and fruits	Cabbage, onions, bananas, apples; canned apples, corn, fruit juce, dried prunes
Fats, oils	Margarine, lard, and salad dressings
Sugars, sweets	Sugar, syrup, jelly
Accessories	A few seasonings; no soft drinks

*Peterkin, B. B.: Low-cost food plan—choices influence cost, Fam. Econ. Rev., March, 1967, pp. 7-9.

must sensitively guide and create a relaxed, nonthreatening atmosphere in a setting where the patient feels free to talk. *And the health worker must listen.* The reason that some frustrated people finally take their problems to the streets may well be that *no one listens to them unless they do.*

Methods. In light of the factors in the impact of the socioeconomic background, the conditioning that a culture of poverty builds in a person, and the rigid, removed, sterile, antiseptic setting in which most community health agencies operate, it is no wonder that so many of their well-intentioned efforts fail. New methods, approaches, and realistic and creative ideas are needed.

Many low-income families are being helped to better health through better food habits developed through community projects conducted in cooperation between the U.S. Federal Extension Service and the state extension service. One such project was conducted in the state of Alabama, in five Alabama counties. Its objectives were to develop and test methods for filling three basic needs: (1) reaching and teaching of young families, (2) provision of educational materials related to family financial management, nutrition, housing, and child development, and (3) training of nonprofessional aides to work with poor families under professional guidance and supervision. "Program aides" were employed.[15] These aides were mature, compassionate women without professional backgrounds, who were trained and supervised by nutritionists and home economists. They established contact with low-income, hard-to-reach families and taught them better ways of simple homemaking. In previous projects with similar goals, trained helpers such as home aides, health aides, or nurses' aides have been used. But they have usually gone into the home to perform a homemaking service while the mother is ill or unable to function. The program aides in the Alabama project were taught by the health professionals of the extension service not to do things *for* homemakers, but to help homemakers *help themselves*. The program aides did not decide what would be done, and did not do it for the family. They taught the homemakers how to perform a simple task, prepare a simple food, or make a simple garment—starting with problems that seem important *to the homemakers*. The focus of the program was on education and self-development, rather than on personal help. It provided an effort to break the chain of frustration and dependence. Each program aide kept a working log, which was in effect a diary of her relationships with those persons assigned to her. In some of these logs, the depth of quality in these personal, close-working relationships between aide and homemaker are poignantly revealed.

Reports of results are encouraging. Some of the families reached through the program lived in rural areas, some on the fringes of small towns, and some in urban, low-rent, public housing. Through intensive personal work in the family and in small discussion groups the aides substantially helped many young families. Of these young homemakers, 40% now use better buying practices than before, 44% have acquired skills in food preparation, and 42% have improved the eating habits of their families. In those families reported to show improvement, the meals are better balanced, better use is made of government-donated foods, or federal food stamps are spent more intelligently. In many instances food storage and kitchen equipment have been improved, the family's consumption of milk has increased, and gardens have been planted.[16]

Thrifty food plans. The lowest cost family food plan developed by the U.S. Department of Agriculture is the *Thrifty Family Food Plan* (Table 15-6), designed as a guide for counselors who help homemakers with very low income. Sample menus and market lists have been provided for families on food stamps and others who wish to use the thrifty food plan to economize on food.[17,18] However, current evaluations of this plan indicate that menus based on it cannot always assure nutritional adequacy.[19] Perhaps a revision of the plan based on a modified basic four food groups plan[8] would be helpful.

Low-cost food plans at still lower cost. In a further attempt to meet the requirements of very low income families, the USDA Low-Cost Food Plan (p. 330) has been tested by nutritionists to see if careful buying could reduce its costs still further. The resulting guide in Table 15-7 is given as an example of a very low-cost market basket.

CASE STUDY 5
The multiplying problems of poverty in a black ghetto family

Mary Johnson, aged 30, managed a small smile as she opened the door to welcome Mrs. Baker, the public health nutritionist. Mrs. Baker was her own age, had children of her own, and in the few times she had come to visit, Mary Johnson had finally begun to believe that someone really cared about her family and the struggle they were having to survive. Things had been so hard for so long and now seemed even more hopeless ever since Jim's accident.

James and Mary Johnson had spent their lives, it seemed, caught in the crushing grind of poverty. The hardships, indignities, and injustices of their childhood in the rural South, from generations of tenant farming, had etched themselves deeply in their minds and hearts. It had made them determined to try to seek a better life elsewhere for themselves and their children. Mary and James had managed to move to this large city in the north, but life here in the black ghetto was scarcely any better. James had found it difficult to find work, for he had had limited educational opportunity and had no marketable skills or trade. He went from place to place doing all sorts of odd jobs. Finally, however, he had gotten a job with a construction company. Now there seemed to be a glimmer of hope for learning a trade in night school and working up to something better. His foreman liked him and was going to help him.

As the number of children increased and there were more of them to feed, however, James became increasingly desperate. They always seemed to live a marginal existence on the brink of despair.

Then the accident happened. One day, preoccupied with worry over his family, James had not seen a large skull-cracker of the demolition crew swinging out of control. He did not jump clear in time as the men working next to him had, and the heavy metal ball struck him, breaking his back and leaving his legs paralyzed. Now, at 32, he was a paraplegic, embittered, blaming himself for his family's bleak existence. He had been in the hospital for many months and then received care at the rehabilitation center. His doctor had told him he thought he would be able to go home in the next few weeks if some plans could be made for his care there.

On today's visit Mrs. Baker had planned to talk with Mrs. Johnson about Mr. Johnson's rehabilitation care and more about the children's needs. She had made a number of observations on her previous visit and wanted to explore these observations with Mrs. Johnson. She knew that food was a basic problem in the family. As she looked at Mary Johnson today she seemed even thinner, and Mrs. Baker wondered how often she had gone without food herself to feed the children. Hunger was a constant companion.

After her visit last week, Mrs. Baker had jotted down these initial observations. There were six children. Gloria, aged 15, a pretty girl, was pregnant, expecting her baby in a short time. Despite a swollen look to her ankles, face, and hands, she seemed essentially underweight. Mrs. Baker wondered what, if any, prenatal care she had received. Was there indication of impending toxemia?

Bobby, aged 14, was small and thin. Mary had described him before as "our little fighter." Sensitive about his size, it seemed he was always in fights with the other children at school. The week before Mary said she had found some marijuana in his pockets, but when she had asked him about it, he had angrily stormed out of the house and was gone for two days. Now Mary was worried about what group he might be with.

Billy, aged 8, had obviously bowed legs, was quiet and withdrawn. Mary said he had very little appetite. Sally, aged 5, sat listlessly in a corner during all of Mrs. Baker's first visit, clutching a rag dog, sucking her thumb. She seemed to have no energy. Joseph, aged 18 months, clung to his mother and drank some milk from a bottle. Mary said he still used his bottle and scarcely ate any other food beside the milk.

The new baby, Arthur, was 6 months old. Mary had started nursing him, but after James' accident she had put him on bottle feeding because she had to go back to her old job to help feed the family. Gloria had been looking after the younger children, but now other arrangements would have to be made.

As the two women sat down together on the worn couch and began to talk, Mrs. Baker reached over and took Mary's hand. She was a warm, compassionate woman and had decided to become a nutritionist to help people in need. There was certainly need here.

"There are sources of help, Mrs. Johnson," she said. "We'll try to work things out together." Already she was thinking of other members of the health team at the health office who could assist them.

Questions to guide your inquiry

1. List the data you think significant for each member of the Johnson family. Include each of the children and the parents.
2. What additional data do you think are needed to identify their problems and help find solutions? What sources or methods would you use to obtain these data?
3. What nutritional problems do you think may be present in each family member? Give the scientific basis for each problem.
4. In relation to each problem, what goal do you think the nurse and Mrs. Johnson might set together? Why?
5. What would your plan of care for each family member include? What are the scientific reasons for your action?
6. Suppose the nutritionist, Mrs. Baker, carried out the actions you suggest for each member of the Johnson family. What results would you anticipate? Why?
7. What follow-up care for the family would you plan with Mrs. Johnson? Why?
8. Throughout your work with the Johnson family, what health workers would you involve? In what way? Why?
9. What community resources would you use? In what way?
10. In general, what types of families require nutritional counseling?
11. What are some ways of identifying the nutritional needs of a family?
12. What is "an activity-associated general day's food pattern" (p. 316)? How would you use this approach in taking a nutrition history? How would you make a nutritional analysis of your findings?
13. Consider the nutritional needs of the Johnson family and the basic amounts of food required to meet these needs. Consider this to apply after Mr. Johnson returns home. Using the lower cost food plan (Table 15-5), make out a list of the food needed by the family for a week and check its cost in a local food market. Indicate as a result what the total food cost for this family would be for one week.
14. What are some economy buying suggestions you could give Mrs. Johnson?
15. What federal food assistance programs exist in the United States to help poor families? Investigate the operation of these programs in your community. What deficiencies, inadequacies, or problems do you find in these programs? What solutions can you propose?
16. What characteristics and attitudes develop among poor persons as a result of the pressures they experience in a daily struggle to survive?
17. What attitudes must health workers have if they are to help poor families like the Johnsons? Why?
18. What new methods or approaches can you suggest for improving the health care, especially nutrional care, of low-income families? Are any of these methods or approaches being used in your community? If not, is there anything you may do to help initiate them?

REFERENCES
Specific

1. Maretzki, A. N.: A perspective on nutrition education and training, J. Nutr. Educ. **11**:176, Oct.-Dec., 1979.
2. Shannon, B., Thurman, G., and Schiff, W.: Food-ene: a pilot TV show on nutrition issues, J. Nutr. Educ. **11**:15, Jan.-March, 1979.
3. Danish, S. J.: Developing helping relationships in dietetic counseling, J. Am. Diet. Assoc. **67**:107, Aug., 1975.
4. Myers, M. L., Ling, L., Spragg, D., and Stein, P.: Guidelines for diet counseling, J. Am. Diet. Assoc. **66**:571, June, 1975.
5. Frank, G. C., Berenson, G. S., Schilling, P. E., et al.: Adapting the 24-hr. recall for epidemiologic studies of school children, J. Am. Diet. Assoc. **71**:26, July, 1977.
6. Report: The validity of 24-hour dietary recalls, Nutr. Rev. **34**:310, 1976.
7. Gersovitz, M., Madden, J. P., and Smiciklas-Write, H.: Validity of the 24-hr. dietary recall and seven-day record for group comparison, J. Am. Diet. Assoc. **73**:48, July, 1978.
8. King, J., et al.: Evaluation and modification of the basic four food guide, J. Nutr. Educ. **10**:27, 1978.
9. Williams, S. R.: Nutritional guidance in prenatal care. In Worthington, B., Vermeersch, J., and Williams, S. R.: Nutrition in pregnancy and lactation, ed. 2, St. Louis, 1981, The C. V. Mosby Co., p. 68.
10. Black, H.: The Berkeley co-op food book, Palo Alto, Calif., 1980, Bull Publishing Co.
11. Projector, D. S., and Weiss, G. S.: Survey of financial characteristics of consumers, Board of Governors of the Federal Reserve System, 1966; Schoenberg, J. K., et al.: Size and composition of consumer savings, Federal Reserve Bulletin, 1967.
12. Family food plans, Hyattsville, Md., 1975 rev., Agricultural Research Division, U.S. Dept. of Agriculture.
13. Peterkin, B., Chassy, J., and Kerr, R.: The thrifty food plan, Hyattsville, Md., 1975, U.S. Dept. of Agriculture, Agricultural Research Service.
14. Matthews, L. I.: Principles of interview and patient counseling, J. Am. Diet. Assoc. **50**:469, 1967.
15. Spindler, E. B.: "Program aides" for work with low-income families, J. Am. Diet. Assoc. **50**:478, June, 1967.
16. Oliver, M.: Pilot study in Alabama, J. Am. Diet. Assoc. **50**:483, 1967.
17. Cromwell, C., and McGreary, B.: Economical meals for the month, U.S. Dept. of Agriculture, Agricultural Research Service, Family Economics Review, Hyattsville, Md., Fall, 1975.
18. U.S. Dept. of Agriculture, Agricultural Research Service: Food for thrifty families, Washington, D.C., Sept., 1976.
19. Lane, S., and Vermeersch, J.: Evaluation of the thrifty food plan, J. Nutr. Educ. **11**:96, April-June, 1979.

General

Andrew, B. J.: Interviewing and counseling skills, J. Am. Diet. Assoc. **66**:576, June, 1975.

Block, I.: The health of the poor, New York, 1969, Public Affairs Pamphlet No. 435, USDHEW.

Cason, D., and Wagner, M. G.: The changing role of the service professional within the ghetto, J. Am. Diet. Assoc. **60**:21, 1970.

Coles, R.: Children of crisis, New York, 1967, 1970, 1971, 1972, Atlantic Press.

Coles, R., and Clayton, A.: Still hungry in America, New York, 1969, New American Library.

Danish, S. J.: Developing helping relationships in dietetic counseling, J. Am. Diet. Assoc. **67**:107, 1975.

Danish, S. J., and Hauer, A. L.: Helping skills: a basic training program, New York, 1973, Human Services Press.

Danish, S. J., Ginsberg, M. R., Terrell, A., Hammond, M. I., and Adams, S. O.: The anatomy of a dietetic counseling interview, J. Am. Diet. Assoc. **75**:626, Dec., 1979.

Eshleman, R. E., and McCloy, K. B.: The changing face of community nutrition, Fam. Commun. Health **1**:1, Feb., 1979.

Food and Nutrition Board, National Research Council: Recommended dietary allowances, ed. 9, National Academy of Sciences, Washington, D.C., 1980.

Garrett, A. M.: Interviewing—its principles and methods, ed. 25, New York, 1966, Family Service Association of America.

Glanz, K.: Dietitians' effectiveness and patient compliance with dietary regimens, J. Am. Diet. Assoc. **75**:631, Dec., 1979.

Hunt, I. F., Luke, L. S., Murphy, N. J., Gomez, J., and Smith, J. C., Jr.: Nutrient estimates from computerized questionnaires vs. 24-hr. recall interviews, J. Am. Diet. Assoc. **74**:656, June, 1979.

Kotz, N.: Let them eat promises; the politics of hunger in America, Englewood Cliffs, N.J., 1969, Prentice-Hall, Inc.

Ling, L., et al.: Guidelines for diet counseling, J. Am. Diet. Assoc. **66**:571, 1975.

Lowenberg, M., and Lucas, B.: Feeding families and children—1776 to 1976, J. Am. Diet. Assoc. **68**:207, 1976.

Lowenstein, F. W.: Preliminary clinical and anthropometric findings from the first health and nutrition examination survey, Am. J. Clin. Nutr. **29**:918, 1976.

Mahoney, M. J., and Caggiula, A. W.: Applying behavioral methods to nutrition counseling, J. Am. Diet. Assoc. **72**:372, April, 1978.

Mason, M., Wenberg, B. G., and Welsch, P. K.: The dynamics of clinical dietetics, New York, 1977, John Wiley & Sons, Inc.

Moore, M. C., Judlin, B. C., and Kennemur, P. M.: Using graduated food models in taking dietary histories, J. Am. Diet. Assoc. **51:**447, Nov., 1967.

Ohlson, M. A.: The philosophy of dietary counseling, J. Am. Diet. Assoc. **63:**13, July, 1975.

Perspectives in practice: dietary counseling in ambulatory care, J. Am. Diet. Assoc. **68:**246, 1976.

Report of the Citizens' Board of Inquiry into Hunger and Malnutrition in the United States, Hunger, U.S.A., Washington, D.C., 1968, New Community Press.

Schaefer, A. E., and Johnson, E. C.: Are we well fed? . . . The search for the answer, Nutr. Today **4:**2, 1969.

Witschi, J., Porter, D., Vogel, S., et al.: A computer-based dietary counseling system, J. Am. Diet. Assoc. **69:**385, Oct., 1976.

16

Nutritional deficiency diseases

Out of evident necessity, in its organized beginnings public health work was directed primarily toward the control of communicable disease in humans. One of the early manuals, provided a half century ago (1917) for its workers by the American Public Health Association, was oriented to the fulfillment of this need.[1] In the years since that time, communicable disease has come increasingly under control, at least in developed areas of the world. A pronounced shifting of emphasis in public health is now occurring. The primary world health problem today is *malnutrition*. The shift in emphasis to this problem was marked by the association's publication in 1960 of a companion manual, *Control of Malnutrition in Man*.[2]

Worldwide recognition of the public health significance of the nutritional diseases has continued to grow. Observation and experience, however, have also brought deepened awareness of two important interrelated facts: (1) food *alone* is not the answer and (2) a high standard of living does not necessarily solve the problem—even in the midst of plenty, malnutrition exists.

As the nutritional deficiency diseases are explored in this chapter, the following questions can be used as a guide. This brief discussion is intended to provide only an initial impetus; it is hoped that the material presented here will stimulate a continued concern and investigation.

First, the general, overall problem should be considered:

1. *The problem*. What is malnutrition? What is its extent and significance in world health today?
2. *Its ecology*. Why does malnutrition exist? What factors combine and interact to cause it?

Second, as each of the basic nutritional deficiency diseases is discussed, these related factors should be considered:

1. *Identification*. What is the nature of the disease? What are its clinical manifestations or associated laboratory findings?
2. *Etiology*. What specific nutritional deficiency is involved? On what type of diet does this disease occur?
3. *Occurrence*. In what inner and outer environment does this disease occur? In persons of what age? Of which sex? Living in what sort of community? In what parts of the world?
4. *Control*. What methods of control are effective in prevention and treatment of this disease?

It will be helpful to look back at the chapters in Part One in which each of the involved nutrients is discussed in detail for a review of the nutrient chemistry. In this chapter a knowledge of that chemistry will be applied to the clinical disease picture and its public health significance.

MALNUTRITION—WORLD HEALTH PROBLEM
Definitions

Malnutrition. Malnutrition at its fundamental biologic level is inadequate supply of nutrients to the cell. A lack of essential nutrients at the cellular level, however, is the result of a complex web of factors: psychologic, personal, social, cultural, economic, political, and educational.[3] Each of these factors is a more or less important cause of malnutrition at a given time and place, for a given individual. If these variables are only temporarily adverse, the malnutrition may be acute and may be alleviated rapidly, leaving no long-standing results or harm to life. But if these variables are continuously adverse and unrelieved, malnutrition becomes chronic. Irreparable harm to life follows, and eventually death ensues.

On a biologic level, nutritional deficiency diseases may be classified as primary or secondary, according to the availability of the nutrient.

Primary deficiency disease. A primary deficiency disease is a disease that results directly from dietary lack of a specific essential nutrient. For example, scurvy results if the diet is deficient in vitamin C; beriberi results if the diet is deficient in thiamin. The primary deficiency diseases are the subject of this chapter.

Secondary deficiency disease. A secondary deficiency disease is a disease that results from the inability of the body to use a specific nutrient properly. Such inability may result from either of two general types of failure: (1) failure to absorb the nutrient from the alimentary tract into the blood or (2) failure to metabolize the nutrient normally after it has been absorbed. For example, the malabsorption syndrome is characterized by failure of absorption of fats through the intestinal wall, so that fat is lost in the stool. Phenylketonuria is the inability of the body to metabolize the essential amino acid phenylalanine, so that phenylalanine is lost in the urine. Secondary deficiency disease will be discussed in later chapters.

Extent of malnutrition

Human misery and waste of human life from malnutrition, more stark in some regions than in others, occur in both world hemispheres. These effects are more profound and widespread in less developed areas of the world but are present in the more developed nations also.[4] The course that is already set by a mounting population must collide with the less rapidly growing (and in many areas, diminishing) food supplies. Because of the increasing complexity of society, many persons have only begun to glimpse the magnitude of future needs. The problem is further compounded by the fact that population growth rates often are highest in those countries that can least afford to maintain them. For example, the population of Latin America is the most rapidly growing in the world. It leads all other major regions of the world, with an annual 2.9% population increase. Within this area the fastest growing subregion is Mexico and the six Central American countries, in which the yearly growth rate is 3.4%. At this growth rate the population of these Middle American countries will increase 66% between 1970 and 1985.[5] Compare this growth rate with that of the world population— 2% a year—or of North America—1%.[6]

In many areas the dangerous race between population growth and the rate of increase in food supply is already being lost. In Latin America, for example, during the last two decades total food production has increased 69%. But the more rapid expansion in population is actually causing a decreasing per capita food supply.[7]

Infant and child mortality and morbidity provide an index to the extent of general malnutrition. In Latin America in the 1- to 4-year age group the death rate is 20 to 30 times as high as in the United States and Canada (Fig. 16-1). In some areas the rate is even 50% higher. If

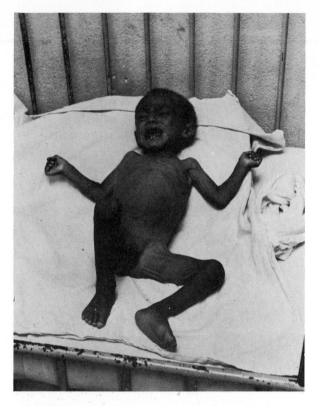

Fig. 16-1. A child in Guatemala suffering from acute malnutrition. Many young children in Latin America die each year from lack of food. (FAO photograph by Y. Nagata.)

the rates of infant and child mortality in Latin America were as low as those in the United States and Canada, 250,000 fewer children in this age group would die each year.[8]

Still more disturbing examples could be cited for other regions in the world, such as parts of Africa, India, the Orient, and the Middle East (Fig. 16-2). The problem is urgent. It is becoming more so.

Even in America, the wealthiest of nations, malnutrition exists. The National Nutrition Survey, conducted in 10 selected states by the U.S. Department of Health, Education, and Welfare, found nutrition deficiencies in hunger areas similar to those existing in underdeveloped countries. The report indicated growth re-

tardation from hunger in 15% of all the children surveyed; one third of the children under 6 had low hemoglobin levels; one third had unacceptable levels of vitamin A. Among children and adults, 35% to 55% had deficiencies of vitamin C; more than 16% had serious protein deficiencies. Tooth decay was widespread; 18% said that it hurt to chew or bite food. Even protein-calorie malnutrition diseases such as kwashiorkor and marasmus were found in the survey.[9,10] Also, from late 1969 to late 1970, for example, the University of Colorado Medical Center reported the admission of seven children with kwashiorkor and several dozen with marasmus. Many hospitals in urban centers can report similar incidences.

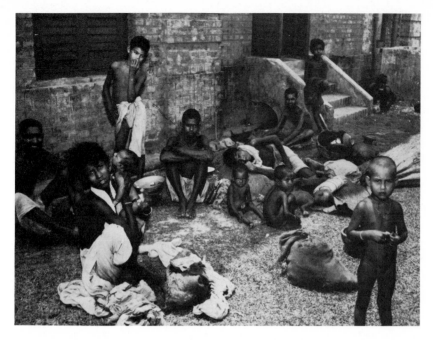

Fig. 16-2. Famine victims in East Pakistan. (FAO photograph by W. Williams.)

THE ECOLOGY OF MALNUTRITION

The word "ecology" comes from a Greek word *oikos,* meaning "house." Just as there are many factors and forces within a family's house that interact to influence its members, so there is an even more vast complex of interrelated forces housed in a biologic system that produces disease. Many factors work together to produce malnutrition. A disease caused by malnutrition may exist in many varieties, many degrees, and many combinations. It is often complicated by the presence of other diseases, such as tuberculosis, intestinal parasites, or skin sepsis. A synergism is, in fact, known to exist between malnutrition and infection. Each compounds the other, and together they cause more serious illness than either would bring alone. For example, a common infectious disease of childhood such as measles, which would otherwise be mild, in a severely malnourished child

may cause death. Infectious diarrhea is a common complication of kwashiorkor and may be the irreversible factor that causes death.

Some of the many related causes of malnutrition can be classed under the three factors that are classically cited by the epidemiologist as the triad of variables that influences disease: (1) *agent,* (2) *host,* and (3) *environment.*

Agent. The agent that is the fundamental cause of a malnutrition disease is *a lack of food.* Because of this lack, certain nutrients in food that are essential to the sustenance of cellular activity are missing. Various factors may cause or modify this lack of food:

1. *Food quantity.* The total quantity of food ingested may be below the level required to maintain the body tissues. The food deficiency may be partial or complete, seasonal or constant.

2. *Imbalance between community food sup-*

ply and need. The amount of food available per person may be reduced by natural disaster (drought, flood) or by man-made disaster (war, overpopulation, poor distribution, poverty).

3. *Food quality.* The food available may be of poor physical quality or biologic value.

4. *Food timing.* Food may not be present (as in infant and child feeding) when needed, in proper balance.

Host. The host is the person—infant, child, adult—who suffers from malnutrition. Various characteristics in the host may influence the disease:

1. *Presence of other disease.* Infections, allergies, metabolic diseases, gastrointestinal diseases, and so on compound the course of malnutrition.

2. *Increased dietary needs.* Any physiologic cause of stress such as growth, pregnancy, lactation, injury, illness, or physical labor increases the demand for nutrients.

3. *Congenital defects.* Premature birth or anatomic defects such as cleft palate influence food intake.

4. *Personal factors.* Ignorance of food needs or food values, carelessness, lack of education, emotional problems, indolence, poor habits, and anorexia influence the kind and amount of food consumed.

Environment. Many environmental factors influence malnutrition. Some are close at hand and may be controlled by the individual. Many more far-reaching ones are too enormous, too powerful, and too remote in their source to be influenced by a single person. Mass action and extensive study are needed to deal with these problems. The following are some of the environmental problems:

1. *Sanitation.* Food contamination causes food loss and produces disease, thus compounding malnutrition.

2. *Culture.* Traditional food habits and customs may hinder nutrition.

3. *Social factors.* Interrelated social problems, such as those created by poverty,

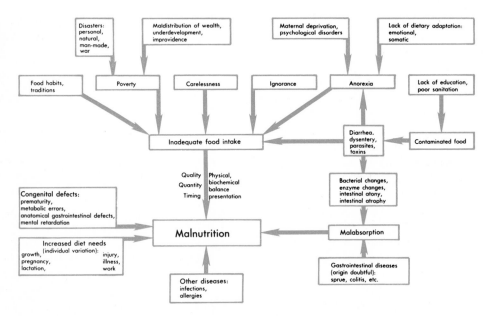

Fig. 16-3. The multiple etiology of malnutrition. (Adapted from Williams, C. D.: Malnutrition, Lancet **2**:342, 1962.)

racial discrimination, inadequate housing, and family disintegration, may contribute to lack of food and to malnutrition.

4. *Psychologic factors.* An example of the many psychologic problems that may contribute to malnutrition is maternal deprivation, which may lead to actual or felt rejection of a child and inadequate feeding.

5. *Economic and political structure.* The economic and political system of a region controls the power structure, governs administrative policy, and controls channels of food supply and form.

6. *Agriculture.* Geography, climate, food technology, and methods of agriculture influence food supply. What food can and will be produced is determined by the natural resources and their degree of development.

The interaction of some of these factors leading to malnutrition may be visualized in Fig. 16-3.

PROTEIN-CALORIE MALNUTRITION (PCM)

Millions of children throughout the world are exposed to various degrees of protein-calorie malnutrition. It is a health problem of major proportions, which causes a high rate of morbidity and death in children. Its long-range effects in those who survive are still incompletely understood. Ritchie Calder,[11] a widely known British writer on science and international affairs, voiced the question in the minds of many health workers, "Are the world's malnourished children of today already being maimed in frame and brain as citizens of 1984?" If the suspicions of many investigators are correct, such as those held by D. B. Jelliffe[12] as a result of his work in Uganda, East Africa, many undernourished populations will prove unable to achieve their full mental, social, and behavioral potential because of a possible long-term effect on brain growth. Should this effect be confirmed, it adds another compelling

reason for making an extended effort to combat this widespread public health problem.[13,14]

In protein-calorie malnutrition a broad clinical spectrum exists between *kwashiorkor* on the one hand and *marasmus* on the other, with many continuous overlapping conditions in between where features of both are found.[15] Although considerable variability is seen, distinctions usually are based on the nature of the dietary deficiency. In kwashiorkor, calories may be sufficient but protein is lacking; in marasmus, both calories and protein are deficient.

Kwashiorkor

Identification. The name *kwashiorkor* was first used by Cecily Williams, in describing her classic observations and work in the early 1930s with children in Ghana (then known as the Gold Coast).[16] The word comes from the Ghan language and may have several meanings, all usually associated with the mystique of jealousy between siblings and of physical sickness. It means "the sickness the older child gets when the next baby is born." Sometimes the name "kwashiorkor" is given to the younger child; when his older sibling becomes ill, his sickness is said to be caused by the birth of the second child. Originally a related meaning of "redness" (derived from the characteristic color of the skin in this disease, which results from depigmentation) was attached to the word, but it is now believed that this interpretation is less correct.

The name is appropriate, for kwashiorkor is the syndrome that develops in a child who, after being weaned from the breast at about the age of 1 year, on the birth of the next sibling is given a diet consisting largely of starchy gruels or sugar water. Such a sequence of events is typical of many cultures in the underdeveloped parts of the world. Before he was weaned the infant received, in the breast milk, protein and calories adequate for growth. The sharply curtailed diet, based on such starchy foods as tubers (manioc, cassava) or grains (maize), may

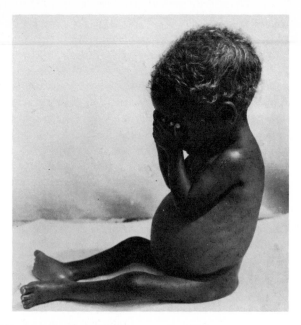

Fig. 16-4. A little African child suffering from kwashiorkor. Note uncurled, graying hair, edema, and skin lesions. (FAO photograph by M. Autret.)

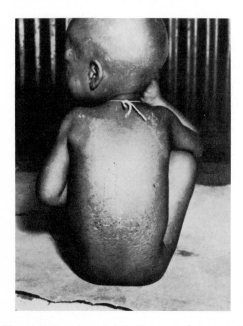

Fig. 16-5. The characteristic "flaky-paint" dermatosis of kwashiorkor.

supply adequate calories as carbohydrate, but its protein content is qualitatively and quantitatively inadequate. Various clinical pictures are determined by local food patterns, involving different degrees of calorie and vitamin deficiencies.

GENERAL SYMPTOMS. The classical syndrome of kwashiorkor comprises retardation of growth and development with peevish mental apathy (Fig. 16-4), edema, muscular wasting, depigmentation of hair and skin, characteristic scaly changes in skin texture (a "flaky paint" dermatosis, Fig. 16-5), hypoalbuminemia, reversible fatty infiltration of the liver, atrophy of the acini of the pancreas with reduction of the enzymatic activity of the duodenal juice, diarrhea, and moderate anemia (usually normochromic, but occasionally slightly macrocytic). Frequently associated are infections and severe vitamin A deficiency, resulting in permanent blindness. Serious deterioration of patients with kwashiorkor is caused by infections and diarrhea.

FLUID AND ELECTROLYTES. A consistent characteristic of kwashiorkor is the specific disturbance in water and electrolyte metabolism. Total body water increases, and there is marked reduction of total body potassium and retention of sodium. The sodium partially replaces the last of the intracellular potassium, a derangement that critically affects important cell enzyme systems that are normally dependent on potassium. Factors probably responsible for these fluid and electrolyte disturbances are hypoalbuminemia, endocrine dysfunction, and circulatory failure. A magnesium deficit, similar to that of potassium, has also been described and may also affect cell enzyme function.

FAT METABOLISM. An abnormality of blood lipid transport has also been found in kwashiorkor, which may account for the extremely low levels of vitamin A (the primary fat-soluble vitamin) that characterize the syndrome. There are also alterations in fat synthesis and catabolism. Some studies indicate probable deficiency of essential fatty acids.

PROTEIN METABOLISM. An extreme protein depletion reaches different degrees in different organs and tissues. Those tissues with faster protein turnover (such as the mucosa and secretory glands in the gastrointestinal system) are affected most. Protein concentrations important to metabolic function, as in enzymes and blood plasma, are greatly disturbed, and there is an extreme decrease in plasma free amino acids.

VITAMINS AND MINERALS. Blood levels of vitamins, especially vitamin A, are low. The overall decrease in metabolism, and therefore in the metabolic demand for vitamins, may be so profound that clinical signs of vitamin deficiency may not appear. A similar relationship appears to exist in most cases for iron and copper.

Etiology. Kwashiorkor results from protein malnutrition. Specifically it results from insufficient quantity or quality of protein (usually both) to meet the demands of growth and cell repair in the presence of more nearly adequate amounts of calories, usually from starchy foodstuffs. Hunger demands calories, not necessarily protein; and protein foods are more expensive and difficult to produce than starchy foods. Protein deficiency is therefore the lot of a major part of the underprivileged world. Protein *quality* refers to the capacity of a given protein, gram for gram, to promote growth and cell repair. This capacity is usually expressed in terms of biologic value (B.V.). The biologic value of a given protein is dependent on the total nitrogen content per 100 calories and the amino acid pattern per gram of nitrogen. Thus a high-quality protein food supplies essential amino acids in the relative amounts required (see amino acid proportionality pattern, p. 67) and supplies in addition sufficient nitrogen for synthesis of the nonessential amino acids that the body needs to build for its own use, and for synthesis of tissue protein and other nitrogen-containing compounds.

Occurrence. Kwashiorkor is usually seen in children in the postweaning years, ages 1 to 4. Particularly in certain areas such as South Africa and Trinidad, where urban mothers practice early weaning so that they may return to paid jobs, it may be seen in younger infants. Kwashiorkor occurs in tropical and subtropical areas, usually in regions where economic, social, and cultural factors combine to make sufficient protein unavailable to the child. It has been shown to be, and continues to be, a public health problem in 19 of the 21 countries of the Americas, in all of the countries and territories of Africa south of the Sahara, in India, and in most countries of the Middle and Far East.[17]

Control. Prevention depends on solution of the socioeconomic factors that underlie the disease. A twofold program adapted to meet individual community needs must include (1) education concerning improved available sources of dietary protein (skimmed milk powder, legumes, fish meal) and (2) motivation to provide adequate food and means for procuring it.

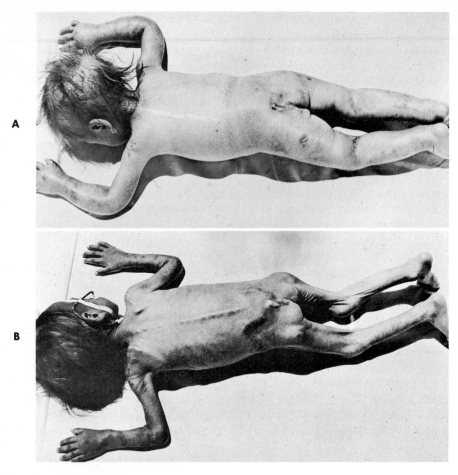

Fig. 16-6. A, Two-year-old child being treated for kwashiorkor. **B,** Two weeks after beginning treatment, edema has disappeared and skin lesions have improved. Note the muscular wasting that had been concealed by the edema. (Courtesy Pan American Sanitary Bureau, Regional Office of The World Health Organization.)

TREATMENT. During the first 24 hours of therapy, correction of water and potassium depletion should have priority, especially if diarrhea has been severe. Such correction may prevent sudden death from heart failure. A potassium-containing electrolyte solution such as Darrow's solution is given orally, unless vomiting necessitates intravenous administration. Transfusion of blood and plasma may also be required in severe cases. Beginning on the second day, skimmed milk (usually dry) is given, in a dilu-

tion yielding first 10 calories per 30 ml (1 oz), then 15. In cases of aggravated digestive disturbance, a formula of lactic acid in fresh skimmed milk (12.5 ml lactic acid to each 30 ml of milk) may be used. The size and spacing of feedings are calculated on the basis of individual need. The aim is to provide a protein intake of about 50 g per day (150 g of dried skimmed milk). Whole milk should be avoided during the first week because fat is poorly tolerated and may cause diarrhea. Apathetic children usually require hand feeding. Diuresis occurring after about seven days of treatment indicates a favorable response to initial therapy (Fig. 16-6). Thereafter the caloric content of the diet is increased by the addition of mixed foods suitable to the child's age, which also supply sufficient vitamins and minerals. To give vitamin concentrates during these first two weeks is unnecessary and may even be dangerous.

Marasmus

Identification. The word marasmus comes from the Greek word *marasmos,* which means "wasting." It is applied to the state of chronic total undernutrition in children, which represents a deficiency of both protein and calories in various degrees of severity and produces a gradual wasting away of body tissue with general emaciation.

GENERAL SYMPTOMS. Marasmus is characterized by gross underweight. Some children appear almost cadaverous—a living skeleton, skin and bones. There is atrophy of both muscle mass and subcutaneous fat, giving a shrunken, wizened, "old man" appearance to the face (Fig. 16-7), in contrast to the fat, rounded cheeks of children with kwashiorkor. There is little or no dermatosis or depigmentation. Edema is minimal or absent. Diarrhea is common. It may result from infection or from pathogenic microorganisms in the stools, or there may be preexisting nutritional diarrhea complicated by superimposed infection. Growth rate declines progressively; there are both physical stunting and mental and emotional impairment. The infant sleeps restlessly, is fretful, apathetic, and withdrawn. Body temperature may be subnormal because of the absence of the insulation that is normally provided by subcutaneous fat, and the child must be kept warm. Metabolic activity is minimal; the heart is weak and urine is scanty; prostration is common.

FLUID AND ELECTROLYTES. As in kwashiorkor, sodium depeletion may occur, especially if diarrhea persists. Little or no water retention is present, in contrast to the gross edema of kwashiorkor.

FAT METABOLISM. In marasmus, fat absorption, as demonstrated by normal vitamin A absorption, appears to be somewhat less impaired than in kwashiorkor. The enzyme systems for digestion, mechanism for transport of fat through intestinal wall, and sufficiency of lipid transport protein are conserved for a longer period in this disease.

PROTEIN METABOLISM. Although serum protein levels are diminished, they are higher than those in kwashiorkor. As general wasting occurs and metabolism approaches basal levels (because amino acids are not provided either endogenously from muscle catabolism or exogenously by the diet), the liver suffers acute and severe protein depletion and loss of its amino acid pool.

VITAMINS AND MINERALS. Body stores gradually decline. However, absorption of vitamin A remains normal for some time in contrast to the depressed absorption in kwashiorkor.

HORMONES. Glucocorticoid secretion remains high in marasmus and is low in kwashiorkor. This important distinction explains many of the differences between the syndromes. When glucocorticoid secretion fails, kwashiorkor develops rapidly, although the exact mechanism of this failure, which follows when caloric intake greatly exceeds that of protein, is unknown.

Etiology. Marasmus is caused by chronic dietary undernutrition, both of calories and of protein; gradual deterioration of body function and atrophy result. Usually deprivation is complete—food, general physical care, and emotional care are all lacking. Such profound deprivation may be found in three basic circumstances. The parents may be poor, and they are often ignorant of food values, so that they do not seek proper food. The parents may have severe mental or emotional problems. This is especially dangerous for the child when the mother is disturbed. She may reject the child and fail to give it care. There may be other

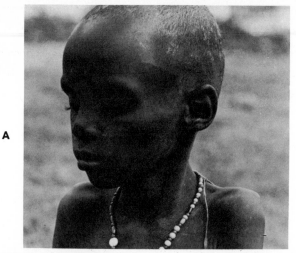

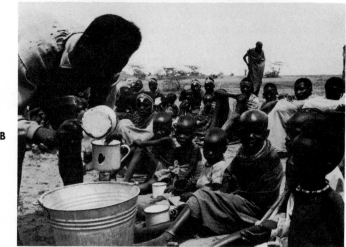

Fig. 16-7. A, African boy suffering from marasmus. His eyesight is poor, and his body is emaciated. **B,** The boy's village in Kenya. Victims of famine caused by drought. This soup, brought in twice a week by Red Cross volunteers, is the only nourishing food available. (FAO photographs by Pierre Pittet.)

disease, such as tuberculosis, chronic gastro-enteritis, dysentery, infectious diarrhea, or parasites, with concomitant lack of proper medical care. All these conditions thrive in poor socioeconomic settings, and the child is caught in these circumstances.

Occurrence. Marasmus is most common in infants 6 to 18 months of age. It occurs in slum conditions in any country where socioeconomic

deprivation breeds such diseases. In tropical and subtropical areas it occurs in much the same pattern in underdeveloped countries as does kwashiorkor.

Control. Prevention depends on eradicating the underlying causes of the disease, and thus on solution of the socioeconomic problems. Treatment follows much the same pattern as that given for kwashiorkor, with initial correc-

Table 16-1. General comparison of symptoms in kwashiorkor and marasmus

Symptom	Kwashiorkor	Marasmus
Growth retardation	X	X
Underweight	X (masked by edema)	X
Apathy, behavioral changes	X	X
Edema	X	—
Muscular wasting	X	X
Depigmentation	X	—
Dermatosis	X	—
Hypoalbuminemia	X	—
Fatty liver	X	—
Diarrhea	X	X
Moderate anemia	X	X
Infection (usual)	X	X
Potassium and electrolyte imbalance (hypokalemia)	X	X
Abnormal fat metabolism	X	—
Low vitamin A absorption	X	—
Protein depletion	X	X
Low body temperature	—	X
Glucocorticoids	—	X

tion of electrolyte imbalances and a gradual refeeding program. Since rejection and total deprivation are commonly a part of the etiologic picture, treatment also involves gradually holding the infant, as tenderness of his body allows, keeping the child warm, and the provision of much loving care.

Table 16-1 gives a comparison of the symptoms of kwashiorkor and marasmus.

VITAMIN DEFICIENCY DISEASES
Xerophthalmia

Identification. Xerophthalmia (Gr. *xēros,* dry; *ophthalmos,* eye) is a disease of the eye in which the cornea and conjunctiva become dry. It results from extreme deficiency of vitamin A. The dryness is a consequence of metaplasia of the conjunctiva, causing roughness. Metaplasia of the paraocular glands leads to a loss of their secretions. Infection usually follows. Early signs are drying, roughness, and wrinkling of the conjunctiva, swelling and redness of the lids, and pain and photophobia. Dry, lusterless patches may be seen on the conjunctiva, and triangular, whitish, foamy spots (Bitot's spots) occur at the limbus conjunctivae. The cornea loses sensitivity and becomes clouded, and ulcers may form. If the disease is untreated, the cornea softens (keratomalacia) and perforation may occur, resulting in total blindness.

Night blindness (inability to see in dim light) may also result from lack of vitamin A and is an early sign of deficiency. Its manifestations vary in degree. A dark-adaptation test is used to determine the rate at which a person's vision is recovered after the visual purple in the retina has been bleached by bright light (see p. 86).

Skin changes also appear in vitamin A deficiency (see Fig. 6-1). The skin becomes dry and rough. Papular eruptions occur at the sites of hair follicles, usually on the skin of the thighs and the upper arms, and spread to abdomen and back. The term *phrynoderma* or "toad's skin" has been given to these dermal changes.

Epithelial tissue changes may also occur in prolonged vitamin A deficiency. Degeneration or atrophy of mucous linings in the gastrointestinal and urinary systems becomes involved, and structural changes have been described in the enamel of teeth and in the nervous system. Histologic studies reveal atrophy of glandular tissue and hyperkeratosis.

Etiology. The clinical manifestations are the result of a deficiency of preformed vitamin A and its precursor, carotene. Vitamin A is found in animal foods such as liver, dairy fat, and eggs, and as carotene in plant foods such as green leafy vegetables, carrots, sweet potatoes, mango, artichokes, and papaya.

The deficiency of vitamin A may be caused by inadequate diet source (primary deficiency) or a disorder that leads to poor absorption or to poor conversion of carotene (conditional deficiency).

Occurrence. Vitamin A deficiency is one of the commonest nutritional deficiency states. Keratomalacia is typically observed in young children. It is still a major cause of blindness in certain underdeveloped countries. For example, in Indonesia many thousands of cases occur each year, and the World Health Organization (WHO) estimates that 5% of all the children in Indonesia have impaired vision or are blind because of vitamin A deficiency.[18] In fact the entire child population there has existed over the years on such a borderline vitamin A level that on one occasion when a large quantity of free skimmed milk was distributed, the increased protein intake caused xerophthalmia and keratomalacia by increasing the attendant requirement for vitamin A. The distribution of the skimmed milk had to be halted until vitamin A capsules could be obtained and given with it.[19] If whole milk had been given, this would not have happened, since natural vitamin A would have been consumed in the cream. Economic factors made the use of skimmed milk necessary.

Control. Prevention is based on education concerning food sources of vitamin A and the inclusion of more fruits and vegetables in the diet. Treatment is administration of vitamin A in doses determined by the severity of the clinical condition. Caution should be observed to avoid hypervitaminosis A from excessive intake. Acute hypervitaminosis A can occur only with a single massive dose (over 1 million IU) and is therefore seldom seen. Chronic states have been observed in children who received large amounts (about 100,000 IU per day) of vitamin A concentrate over some months. The symptoms of such intoxication are anorexia, growth failure, irritability, skeletal lesions with pain in extremities and periosteal bone thickening, skin itching, fissures at mouth and nose corners, coarsening of hair, and alopecia. The symptoms disappear promptly when the excessive intake is discontinued.

Beriberi

Identification. The clinical picture of beriberi varies according to the age of the patient and the body tissues primarily affected, but the neuromuscular system is usually involved. The two general types of beriberi are infantile beriberi and adult beriberi.

Infantile beriberi, occurring during the first year of life, is characterized by various symptoms in different cases: convulsive disorders, abrupt onset, respiratory difficulties, and gastrointestinal problems such as constipation and vomiting. Terminal symptoms in severe cases include cyanosis, dyspnea, and tachycardia; sudden death occurs a few hours after onset.[20]

Adult beriberi, usually seen in young adults who are experiencing additional physiologic stress such as pregnancy and lactation, may be either a dry or wet form, according to the absence or presence of edema. The symptoms usually result from involvement of the peripheral nerves and related muscle function. First, there may be tingling and numbness of extremities, leg muscle cramps, and later involvement of muscles of the forearms, thighs, and abdomi-

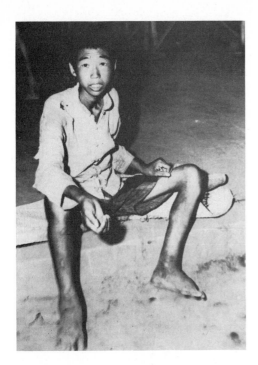

Fig. 16-8. Chinese refugee boy suffering from multiple nutritional deficiencies. Note the edema in feet and legs, characteristic of wet beriberi. (UNRRA photograph released by FAO.)

nal wall. Paralysis may result. As the heart muscle becomes involved, cardiorespiratory symptoms follow quickly—palpitation, tachycardia, dyspnea, cyanosis, and circulatory collapse. Vomiting and constipation are usually present. The edema in wet beriberi begins in the legs and progresses upward (Fig. 16-8).

LABORATORY FINDINGS. Since thiamin functions primarily as a coenzyme in glucose metabolism (especially in the conversion of pyruvic acid, see p. 103), laboratory findings in the deficiency disease are related to levels of pyruvic acid and thiamin. There is increased concentration of pyruvic acid in the blood, and decreased levels of body thiamin are noted in urine, circulating blood, and secretions such as breast milk of nursing mothers. Thiamin test loads are used to indicate general body stores.

Etiology. Beriberi is caused by a deficiency of thiamin. Diets based principally on refined cereal grains, such as the polished rice diet found in the Orient, are deficient in thiamin and contribute to development of the disease. A patient may have subsisted on minimal body thiamin stores until additional physiologic needs (pregnancy and lactation) increased the requirement for thiamin. When these increased requirements were not met, the disease ensued. Infection and gastrointestinal disturbances affecting absorption may also be precipitating factors.

Occurrence. In children, beriberi occurs mainly during the first year of life. It is seen more often in young adults than in the aged. Persons of both sexes are about equally likely to be affected, except that women are made somewhat more susceptible during the physiologic stress of pregnancy and lactation. The disease usually is found among low-income groups or those ignorant of the need for an adequate diet. Beriberi is endemic in many areas of the world such as Japan, Indonesia, China, Malaya, India, Burma, the Phillippines, and Brazil. For example, in Thailand, Burma, and Vietnam, it continues to be a major cause of death among infants two to five months of age.[21] Its incidence is actually increasing in some parts of Asia, such as Thailand, where gasoline-driven rice mills have replaced handpounding in small villages. The motor-driven rice mills remove more of the hull and the thiamin-containing germ of the grain; pregnant women therefore eat less thiamin in their food, and mothers secrete less in their milk.[22]

In the Western world, beriberi usually occurs in the milder form and may be associated with other disease. It may occur in poverty-stricken areas in conjunction with general states of malnutrition or among persons with alcoholism, in pregnant women with a history of poor diet, in the inmates of some prisons, or in hospitals for the chronically ill geriatric patient or for the mentally ill.

Control. Prevention of beriberi is based on improvement in economics and education. The aim of such measures is to supply diets adequate in thiamin. General measures of control include laws governing refinement of cereal grains and their enrichment, use of parboiled or converted rice where it is accepted, use of thiamin tablets, brewer's yeast, or extract of rice polishings (''tikitiki'') by members of stress groups in the population (expectant and nursing mothers), and education concerning wider food choices and cooking methods to minimize loss of thiamin.

TREATMENT. In acute infantile beriberi, parenterally administered thiamin is given immediately, 10 to 25 mg daily. After severe symptoms subside and orally administered thiamin is tolerated, it is continued in oral form at the rate of from 10 to 30 mg daily until the patient is free of symptoms. Lactating mothers with latent or manifest symptoms should be given 25 to 50 mg thiamin daily. Both mother and child should continue to receive supplementary thiamin and, in addition, other B-complex vitamins (niacin, pyridoxine, and riboflavin). The diet should be rich in thiamin-containing foods.

Ariboflavinosis

Identification. *Ariboflavinosis* is the term given to a general group of clinical manifestations that characterize the state of riboflavin deficiency. These characteristic findings include seborrheic dermatitis, cheilosis, and eye lesions. *Seborrheic dermatitis* is localized to skin folds, as in the groin area, behind the ears, the edges of the nose, and canthi (angles at either end of the slit between the eyelids). The skin becomes reddened and covered with small, greasy flakes. Hard sebaceous plugs may develop and project from pores on the nose, cheeks, or forehead. *Cheilosis* is a swelling and reddening of the lips, giving a chapped appearance, with fissures developing at the corners of the mouth. These fissured lesions extend onto the facial skin, rather than into the oral mucosa. Scars of previous lesions are sometimes seen also. *Eye lesions* are less frequently seen. They include photophobia and itching—a feeling of

irritation frequently described as ''sand in the eyes.'' The conjunctiva is engorged, there is constant water secretion (lacrimation: L., *lacrima,* tear), and capillary overgrowth occurs around the cornea.

Etiology. Diets deficient in riboflavin, one of the B-complex vitamins, induce these symptoms. Such diets are lacking in animal protein foods such as milk, meat, or fish; and in leafy vegetables and legumes—all sources of riboflavin. Riboflavin deficiency frequently develops in association with deficiencies of other B-complex vitamins such as niacin and thiamin, in situations of poverty, ignorance, chronic alcoholism, or illness such as prolonged diarrhea.

Occurrence. Riboflavin deficiency occurs in many underdeveloped areas, such as parts of Africa, Asia, India, Indonesia, the Caribbean, and Newfoundland. It is rarely seen in the United States, although it was formerly a public health problem in the southern states.

Control. A supply of foods containing adequate amounts of riboflavin is basic to prevention. Riboflavin is easily destroyed by exposure to light. Such good sources as milk must be protected from excessive exposure to light to ensure retention of their riboflavin content. Other sources that may be incorporated into the diet in any of various forms include cheese, meats, whole grain or enriched cereals, eggs, legumes, nuts, and most vegetables. Foods used as staples in a given country (wheat flour, cornmeal, rice, bread) may be the focus of an enrichment program. In the United States such basic foods are usually enriched with riboflavin.

Acute ariboflavinosis is treated by the oral administration of 10 to 20 mg of riboflavin daily, divided into several doses, replacement of attendant vitamin deficiencies by the administration of other vitamins, and a generally well-balanced diet containing from 3,000 to 3,500 calories.

Pellagra

Identification. Clinical manifestations of pellagra, a disease resulting from niacin deficiency, are of four types. *Gastrointestinal disturbances* include anorexia, general indigestion, weight loss, and diarrhea (which is often severe). *Stomatitis* is a swelling and reddening of the tongue, with hypertrophy, then atrophy, of the papillae. The entire buccal mucosa becomes involved with reddening, a burning sensation, and tissue erosion. *Dermatitis* is a highly characteristic sign of pellagra. The lesions resemble burned areas and become much more painful upon exposure to sunlight. The dermatitis occurs most often on exposed portions of the skin (hands, forearms, feet, lower legs, neck, and face), but may also be seen in skin folds, where the surface is subject to irritation, as around the scrotum, vulvae, and anus. Infection often occurs as the lesions rupture. Healing leaves darkly pigmented areas. *Neurologic change* includes mental apathy, depression, and anxiety of various degrees. In extreme cases, serious disorientation, confusion, and dementia may occur.

Etiology. Pellagra is caused by a deficiency of niacin (a B-complex vitamin) and the amino acid tryptophan, a precursor of niacin. Upon its conversion in the body, about 60 mg of tryptophan yields 1 mg of niacin; hence 60 mg of tryptophan is called a "niacin equivalent." The incidence of pellagra is especially high in populations whose staple food is corn, because corn is low in both tryptophan and niacin.[23] Pellagra may also be a conditioned response complicating other chronic disease involving diarrhea or poor food intake, or in chronic alcoholism with associated general malnutrition.

Occurrence. In the southern United States, especially in rural areas, pellagra was formerly widespread. Howver, since wheat flour, cornmeal, and other grains have been enriched, and since the general diet has been improved, pellagra is seen only occasionally in areas of poverty or in association with other disease affecting food intake or food utilization. Pellagra still occurs in parts of Egypt, Romania, and southern Yugoslavia, mostly in rural areas and villages where the diet tends to be little varied.

Control. Pellagra is prevented by a diet adequate in tryptophan and niacin. The dietary recommendation is stated in terms of niacin equivalents (17 to 21 mg equivalents daily) to include tryptophan sources as well as preformed niacin. Nutrition education should focus on available food sources, enrichment possibilities (especially for cornmeal, because it is often the staple food of patients with this disease), and dietary variety. Agricultural improvements to extend livestock production and crop diversification are fundamental to maintenance of adequate dietary resources.

Patients with acute pellagra require large amounts of niacin, usually as much as 300 to 500 mg or more of niacinamide daily. Usually a multivitamin preparation is given also, and a balanced diet furnishing about 3,000 calories, adequate amounts of good quality protein, and foods rich in niacin.

Pyridoxine (vitamin B_6) deficiency

Identification. A deficiency of pyridoxine has been reported to cause convulsions and hypochromic anemia in infants. Adults with multiple vitamin deficiency states characterized by muscle weakness and fatigue have responded to pyridoxine therapy. Additional proof of the effects of pyridoxine deficiency on the nervous system is the fact that an antagonist of pyridoxine, isonicotinic acid hydrazide (isoniazid), which is used in the treatment of pulmonary tuberculosis, causes peripheral neuritis and occasional convulsions. The hypochromic anemia occurring with these neurologic symptoms is thought to be caused by alteration of cellular metabolism of vitamin B_6.

When the diet is deficient in pyridoxine or when the metabolism of vitamin B_6 is obstructed by an antagonist such as isoniazid, products of abnormal metabolism of the amino acid tryptophan (such as xanthurenic acid) appear in the urine. A tryptophan-load test (giving 10 g of the amino acid in water or fruit juice, then measuring the urinary output of xanthurenic acid) may therefore be used to determine the presence of pyridoxine deficiency. Women in the latter half of pregnancy, as well as those using oral contraceptive agents, may evidence vitamin B_6 deficiencies in response to such tests, yet give no clinical evidence of deficiency.

Etiology. Since vitamin B_6 occurs in many natural foods, a deficiency is unlikely to occur in persons taking a well-balanced diet. The only instances of deficiency that have been reported occurred in infants fed a prepared formula in which the pyridoxine content had been destroyed by autoclaving. The convulsions that followed were quickly controlled by administration of vitamin B_6.

Control. The best prevention of pyridoxine deficiency is a mixed diet made up of a wide variety of foods. About 2 mg of the vitamin a day is adequate for body needs. Additional pyridoxine (5 to 10 mg) may be required during pregnancy to counteract the altered tryptophan metabolism, and 50 to 100 mg is needed for protection against the neuritis experienced during treatment with pyridoxine antagonists for other diseases.

Folic acid deficiency (megaloblastic anemia)

Identification. A deficiency of folic acid in human beings produces a macrocytic anemia associated with megaloblastic arrest in red blood cell production. Production of white blood cells and platelets is also hindered. Clinical manifestations include (1) the weakness and pallor usually associated with anemias and (2) degeneration of surface mucosal tissue, resulting in ulceration and secondary infections, sore tongue, and gastrointestinal disturbances such as diarrhea and poor fat absorption. A similar type of megaloblastic anemia occurs with the deficiency of vitamin B_{12} that is secondary to pernicious anemia. Folic acid deficiency anemia may be distinguished by trial therapy. If the anemia is the result of a deficiency of folic acid, a reticulocyte response will be evident within seven to ten days after administration

of folic acid, and blood values will return to normal.

Etiology. Folic acid deficiency may be caused by one of several factors: (1) a primary dietary lack, (2) poor intestinal absorption of the vitamin, or (3) increased metabolic demands, such as during late pregnancy and the rapid growth of early infancy, and in concurrent ascorbic acid deficiency.

The diets of persons evidencing nutritional folic acid deficiency are particularly lacking in animal protein foods and green vegetables. These should be supplied from adequate and varied food sources.

Occurrence. Folic acid deficiency occurs usually in conjunction with general malnutrition. The pregnant woman is especially susceptible. The infant also is at risk because of the increased physiological stress of growth, because of infections, or because of ascorbic acid deficiency resulting from a poor diet.

Although reports vary, some women using oral contraceptive agents have low serum folate levels but do not display clinical signs of folic acid deficiency anemia. However, of greater significance may be the fact that women frequently become pregnant upon discontinuing the pill, and it is well known that the pregnant woman tends to develop folic acid deficiency. Thus the reduced preconception tissue stores of folic acid may be a predisposing factor.

Control. Generally, diets that supply adequate amounts of the other B-complex vitamins will be adequate in folic acid also. Doses of 5 to 20 mg of folic acid may be given in cases of deficiency. The most intelligent approach to protection against the anemia of folic acid deficiency is the use of a well-balanced, varied diet providing optimal overall nutrition.

Vitamin B_{12} deficiency (pernicious anemia)

Identification. Clinical manifestations of pernicious anemia are anorexia, nausea, vomiting, diarrhea, abdominal pain, and weight loss. General signs of anemia are present—weakness, dyspnea, and palpitation. There may be a characteristic lemon yellow tinge to the skin, and the liver and spleen may enlarge. Some patients may experience spinal cord degeneration, which produces difficulty in walking, in sense of position, and in vibratory sense in the legs. Characteristic changes in the development of red blood cells result in a wide variety of abnormal sizes and shapes. The normal free gastric hydrochloric acid is absent.

Etiology. The vitamin B_{12} deficiency of pernicious anemia is secondary to an inherent lack of intrinsic factor in the gastric juice. The cause of this defect is not known; heredity is thought to be a factor.

Occurrence. Pernicious anemia occurs most often in middle-aged persons. Seldom is it seen in those under 30 years of age. The rates of occurrence in the two sexes do not differ. It seems to be more common in persons having type A blood than in those having type O blood, and to be more common in white-skinned than in dark-skinned persons.

Control. No means of preventing pernicious anemia is known; however, it may be treated effectively by injecting doses of vitamin B_{12} to bypass the absorption defect. The anemia may also be relieved by the administration of folic acid, but this form of therapy is contraindicated because it fails to control the degenerative changes in the central nervous system.

Iron medication or giving blood by transfusion is usually unnecessary. Rest and a high-protein diet supplemented with a multivitamin preparation are supportive measures.

Scurvy

Identification. Scurvy is a nutritional deficiency disease directly associated with a lack of vitamin C (ascorbic acid). The antiscorbutic activity of the vitamin has been well established.[24-26] Scurvy develops after the body tissue stores of ascorbic acid have been exhausted.

CLINICAL MANIFESTATIONS. Since ascorbic acid performs many vital physiologic functions, related especially to formation of connective tissue, collagen, and the integrity of capillary walls (see p. 124), the clinical manifestations of scurvy involve tissue deterioration and changes of hemorrhagic origin.

SKIN. The skin becomes dry, rough, and often has a dingy brown color. Scaly, raised areas, called perifollicular hyperkeratotic papules, develop around the hair follicles in the skin. The follicular hemorrhages develop around these papules (see Fig. 7-4). These skin changes usually occur in the arms and legs, the buttocks, and the back. Purpura (L., ''purple''), hemorrhaging into the skin that produces a reddish purple discoloration with the appearance of a bruise, appears first on the lower extremities and then spreads upward. Pinpoint hemorrhages produce small red spots called petechiae, which may coalesce into areas of purpura and finally, if large enough, into even larger areas called ecchymoses (Gr. *ek,* out; *chymos, juice*). Sometimes a whole extremity may be involved with extravasated blood.

MUSCLES. Deep hemorrhages in the muscle tissue may produce brawny areas of induration, resulting from hardening and thickening of the tissue. Phlebothrombosis (clotting in a vein) may follow.

JOINTS. Scurvy may also be manifested by hemorrhages into the cavities of joints, which cause local heat, painful swelling, and immobility. This condition is called *hemarthrosis*. The joint pain causes scorbutic infants to lie in a characteristic position, supine with the knees partially flexed and the thighs externally rotated —the only position of comfort. This is sometimes called the scorbutic pose.

GUMS. The gums are spongy, friable, grossly swollen, and bleed easily at the slightest touch. As tissue hemorrhaging continues, thromboses form in the blood vessels and infarcts occur, producing blue-red discoloration. The teeth become loosened and may fall out. Infection is frequent.

FAILURE OF WOUND HEALING. Any trauma, even small, produces ulcerated areas. New wounds fail to heal, or if they are apparently healed, they break open again under the slightest stress.

ANEMIA. Anemia usually accompanies scurvy. It is partially caused by hemorrhagic blood loss, but also by the faulty metabolic interrelationships of vitamin C with folic acid and with iron. Concurrent deficiency of other nutrients also contributes to the anemia.

AGE VARIANCE. Since the clinical picture of scurvy is modified by growth, the manifestations vary with the patient's age.

Adult scurvy is characterized by general weakness, lassitude, irritability, and vague, dull, aching pains in the muscles and joints of the lower extremities. There may be weight loss and dyspnea. The classic hemorrhagic changes occur in skin, muscles, and gums. The levels of vitamin C in the blood and urine are below normal.

Infantile scurvy differs from that found in adults because the reaction to vitamin C deficiency in the growing bones of children differs from that in the mature bones of adults. The growing ends of long bones in infants and children are particularly affected by insufficiency of vitamin C. Microscopic fractures, small defects or cracks, occur, associated with bleeding into the subperiosteal space. These defects progress to separation of the epiphyses and malformation of the bone, as calcified cartilage that has not been destroyed or withdrawn as in the normal process, piles up in the zone of provisional calcification. This gives the long bone the shape of a club. Characteristic changes occur also in the growing ribs. Because of the pull of the respiratory muscles, the costochondral junctions are deformed. The central part of the chest is sunken, and there is a sharp prominence of the bony ends of the ribs (costochondral beading).

Etiology. Scurvy results directly from a dietary lack of vitamin C. The most concentrated food sources of this vitamin are citrus fruits, tomatoes, and odd plants such as the acerola, a cherrylike fruit grown in tropical regions. Additional sources include other fruits and vegetables such as berries and potatoes. Human milk has an appreciable vitamin C content (4 to 8 mg/dl). Commercially prepared cows' milk, however, has almost none, since this vitamin is destroyed by pasteurization and other processing. Breast-fed infants therefore secure a sufficient supply of vitamin C, whereas bottle-fed infants require vitamin C supplementation.

Scurvy is most likely to occur in persons subsisting on limited, monotonous diets. Three groups are most at risk: (1) infants fed processed cows' milk and little else, with no vitamin supplementation, (2) persons living alone, preparing their own meals, subsisting on little more than cereals, bread, and milk, and (3) psychoneurotic individuals eating bizarre diets; for example, a case of advanced scurvy was reported in a 36-year-old woman who had been following a ritualistic Zen macrobiotic diet.[27]

Occurrence. Normally, infants are born with vitamin C adequate for several months, so that infantile scurvy rarely occurs before the age of 4 months. Peak incidence is at about 9 months of age, with some cases occurring at about 2 years of age. Under normal conditions, after age 2, children usually eat enough of the adult diet to prevent the clinical disease. However, certain groups of children are at greater risk, for example, institutionalized or defective children. Among adults, scurvy occurs more frequently in the aged because diets are more likely to be insufficient.

As the American public has become better informed about food values, ascorbic acid supplementation, and available food sources, the incidence of scurvy has greatly decreased in the United States. However, as recently as 1955 a rise in the incidence of scurvy in Canada led the American Academy of Pediatrics to conduct a survey in the United States, which revealed 713 pediatric cases of scurvy and a hospital admission rate of about one patient with scurvy in every 3,300 admissions.[28]

Control. Scurvy can be prevented by a well-balanced diet that includes some primary sources of vitamin C, such as citrus fruits, or a wide variety of secondary sources in fruits and vegetables (leafy greens, potatoes). Cases of frank scurvy respond quickly and dramatically to therapeutic doses of vitamin C of about 200 mg or more daily. For example, all bleeding ceases in 24 hours, gums heal in three or four days, and a leg that has been ecchymotic from hip to heel becomes normal in three weeks on such a regimen.

Rickets

Identification. Rickets, a disease directly related to impaired metabolism of calcium and phosphorus, is manifested in defective bone growth and changes in the body musculature. The impaired mineral metabolism in rickets may have many causes, but by far the commonest cause is a deficiency of vitamin D. The vitamin D may be preformed in food or formed in the body (the skin) through the action of short ultraviolet radiations such as those in sunlight. Vitamin D is necessary for the absorption of calcium and phosphorus and for their deposit in bone tissue.

CLINICAL MANIFESTATIONS. Characteristic clinical manifestations of rickets result from failure of calcification of the growing portions of bones. The resultant rarefaction of bone tissue may be observed by comparing X-rays of rachitic bones with x-rays of corresponding normal bones. The involved bones are deformed by the stress of weight bearing or even by the normal pull of attached muscles. Characteristic musculoskeletal and metabolic changes in rickets include the following.

HEAD. The head appears large because of the development of thickened areas in the temporal and parietal regions of the skull. The top of the skull appears flat and is often depressed toward the middle. These skull deformities result from a person's lying supine: the continued weight of the brain pressing on the back of the skull causes thinning of the bones and flattening of the back of the head. Such areas of softening in cranial bones are called areas of *craniotabes*.

LEGS AND ARMS. When the child begins to sit erect, the effect of gravity on the legs in the sitting position is to pull the epiphyses out of position. Bizarre deformities then develop in several different planes. The result is a combination of bowed thighs and knock-knees. In addition, a deformity called ''saber skin'' (anterior curving just above the ankle) may occur in the lower end of the tibia as it is tilted backward by the weight of the foot while the child is lying or sitting. Because of his muscular weakness, when the child is sitting, he attempts to support his trunk with his outstretched, pronated hands. This pressure causes a knobbing deformity at the wrists and a bowing of the arms. Later, when standing or walking is attempted, the weight of the child's body causes further bowing of the legs (see Fig. 6-2).

RIBS. The costochondral junctions become enlarged, and knobs form. These appear as rows resembling strings of beads, which run parallel to the sternum and curve outward toward the lower end of the thorax. This beaded effect is the characteristic ''rachitic rosary.'' With time, bending of the ribs and cartilage occurs, which interferes with normal expansion of the chest during respiration. A funnel-shaped depression develops in the lower end of the sternum, in addition to the overall ''pigeon-breasted'' effect produced by the rickets.

SPINE. Because his muscles are lax and hypotonic, the infant tends to slump when he tries to sit up. Gradual curving of the spine may follow, leading to kyphosis (Gr., ''humpback'').

ABDOMEN. The lax muscles of the abdomen and intestines may bring about protuberance of the abdomen (Fig. 16-9). Constipation often results from the intestinal atony.

TEETH. Infantile rickets does not affect the first temporary teeth, because these are fairly well-developed at birth; but the dentition of permanent teeth, which are forming during this

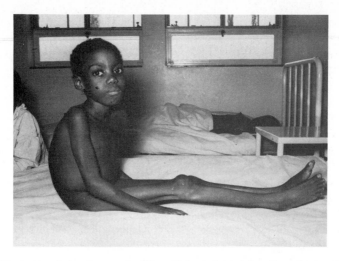

Fig. 16-9. African girl suffering from malnutrition. Note skeletal deformities of spine (kyphosis) and protuberant abdomen often seen in rickets. (FAO photograph by Pierre Pittet.)

period, may be affected with resultant alteration in the tooth structure.

TETANY. The impaired balance of calcium and phosphorus in the body fluids—lowering of the blood calcium, or decrease in the availability of calcium—may produce tetany in the rachitic patient. During the healing period, as calcium is withdrawn from the blood for bone mineralization, the blood calcium may be diminished and may remain low. This lowered level alone may not be sufficient to produce overt tetany, but the stress of a superimposed febrile illness may cause the latent tetany to become manifest in convulsions.

Etiology. In full-term infants, rickets is most commonly produced by a deficiency of vitamin D. In premature infants, deficiencies of calcium and phosphorus contribute to the development of the disease. Since a large amount of the fetal skeleton is mineralized during the last trimester of pregnancy, the body of a baby born four weeks prematurely contains only a little more than half the total calcium present in the normal full-term infant. In addition, the premature infant is smaller than the full-term infant and so has a more limited food capacity. Finally, hu-

man milk rarely can supply his demands for calcium. In these combined circumstances his rapid growth and slow rate of calcification may cause early, severe rickets. His milk should be fortified both with dried skimmed milk, to provide sufficient usable mineral to prevent rickets, and with supplementary vitamin D, necessary for utilization of these minerals.

Refractory forms of rickets have been observed, some of which are genetically acquired. A variety of signs appear in different members of the same family.[29] The clinical picture is similar; retarded growth and skeletal deformities occur. However, these unusual forms may be differentiated by their great resistance to vitamin D therapy. For example, a case has been reported in which the serum vitamin D levels were about 20 times greater than normal, and 1 million units of vitamin D daily were required for healing, with a necessary maintenance dose thereafter of 440,000 units daily.[30]

Occurrence. Vitamin D–deficiency rickets is observed most frequently in infants between the ages of 6 and 18 months. Rarely does it have its onset after the first two to three years of life. Other forms of rickets are usually first observed after their early period. In all forms, however, disturbance of calcium-phosphorus metabolism is the direct cause of the disease. In the north temperate zone, vitamin D–deficiency rickets has its onset most frequently in the spring. It is unusual in the tropics, where the body is exposed to more sunlight. It occurs more often in dark-skinned races, whose skin pigmentation inhibits the passage of ultraviolet rays. The customary diet of persons in the frigid zone is protective against rickets, since it contains fish oils and animal fat sources of vitamin D. In regions where breast feeding is practiced, the incidence is also reduced, chiefly because the ratio of calcium to phosphorus in human milk is lower than in cows' milk, not because there is a significant difference in the vitamin D content of the two milks.

Control. Supplementation of the diet with vitamin D effectively controls rickets. Exposure to sunlight is also effective, but in many areas this is seasonal and limited, thus uncertain as a source of the vitamin. Calcium and phosphorus adequate for human infants are supplied by either human milk or a diluted cows' milk formula. The milk enrichment program presently followed in the United States, in which each quart of milk is fortified with 400 IU of vitamin D, has greatly reduced the incidence of vitamin D–deficiency rickets; nevertheless, the disease is still seen despite these preventive measures.

Recovery from rickets follows the usual therapeutic dose of 2,000 to 4,000 units of vitamin D. Extreme skeletal deformities are occasionally corrected surgically, although certain deformities are not amenable to treatment. Many of these decrease with time, however.

Hemorrhagic disease of the newborn (vitamin K deficiency)

Identification. Since vitamin K is fairly widespread in nature, especially in green leaves of various kinds (spinach, cabbage, cauliflower), and is also synthesized by intestinal bacteria, a deficiency is relatively uncommon in adults. Exceptions may exist in patients who lack bile (necessary for the absorption of vitamin K) or in those with intestinal diseases (sprue or chronic diarrhea), which hinder its absorption. However, newborn infants lack stores of vitamin K at birth, have a sterile gastrointestinal tract and hence no bacterial synthesis, and do not obtain an adequate dietary supply in milk. Therefore there is a fall in prothrombin activity in the blood during the first few days of life, and life-endangering hemorrhages may result.

Etiology. Vitamin K is necessary to the synthesis of prothrombin by the liver (p. 97). If this first stage in the blood clotting mechanism does not proceed, hemorrhaging may result.

Occurrence. Some authorities have estimated that possibly one in every 1,000 newborn infants dies from hemorrhage preventable by treatment with vitamin K. Milder hemorrhage, preventable by treatment, is believed to have a much higher incidence.

Control. Hemorrhagic disease of the newborn can be prevented by giving parenterally small doses of water-soluble vitamin K analogues to newborn infants. Excess amounts of vitamin K may be toxic, even lethal. The Council on Drugs of the American Medical Association has recommended single doses of the water-soluble analogues equivalent to 1 mg of synthetic vitamin K for prophylaxis and treatment.[31]

MINERAL-DEFICIENCY DISEASES
Tetany

Identification. Tetany, first described by Armand Trousseau (1801-1865), is characterized by neuromuscular irritability, which manifests itself in various degrees of intermittent tonic muscle spasm, usually paroxysmal in nature and involving the extremities. Convulsive seizures may follow. The three major manifestations of tetany are the following:

1. *Carpopedal spasm* (Gr. *karpos,* L. *carpus,*

wrist; L. *pedalis,* foot). Tonic contracture of the hands and feet is the most characteristic sign of tetany. In carpal spasm the thumb is drawn into the cupped palm, the wrist is flexed, and the hands are abducted. The fingers are flexed at the metacarpophalangeal joints but are extended at the more distal joints. This posture of the hand may be produced in patients with latent tetany by maintaining a firm, constricting grip on the patient's upper arm for two or three minutes. The appearance of carpal spasm (Trousseau's sign) is evidence of latent tetany. In manifest tetany such spasms occur spontaneously; they may be transitory or may continue for days at a time. In the pedal spasm the sole of the foot is cupped and the toes are flexed inward. Both the arms and legs may be abducted and rigidly flexed.

2. *Laryngospasm.* The abductor muscles of the larynx spasmodically contract, producing *inspiratory stridor* (L. *stridor,* harsh sound), usually a high-pitched, crowing sound, heard as the patient breathes in. In extreme cases this spasmodic impedance of breathing may cause deep cyanosis; on rare occasions death has occurred during an attack.

3. *Convulsions.* Generalized convulsions may occur at long or short intervals. The patient (usually an infant) becomes unconscious. The body is in a rigidly tonic state with intermittent clonic jerkings. The hands are tightly clenched and held in the carpospasmodic position.

Etiology *(serum calcium to phosphorus ratio).* Any condition that lowers the blood calcium or decreases the availability of the calcium that is present in the blood or produces alkalosis may cause tetany. Ionized calcium, phosphate, carbon dioxide, and the acidity of the blood serum exist together in a relationship that may be expressed as follows:

$$\frac{Ca \times HPO_4 \times HCO_3}{pH} = K$$

K is constant. This indicates that if the carbon dioxide and the pH remain constant, the product of the calcium content (normally 10 to 11 mg/dl) and of the phosphate content (normally 3.0 to 3.5 mg/dl) of the serum must be constant between 30 and 40. In tetany, the calcium content drops to 6 mg/dl, and the phosphate rises to 5 or 6 mg/dl to maintain the constant product. (See calcium to phosphorus ratio, p. 135.)

Clinical forms of tetany must be classified according to these blood ratios.

Hypocalcemic tetany is produced by a decrease in the serum calcium. Tetany of the newborn may be the result of temporary hypofunction of the parathyroid glands; initial feedings of whole cows' milk, with its relatively high phosphate content, give too heavy a phosphate load for renal clearance. In response to the increased serum phosphate, serum calcium falls to maintain the constant calcium to phosphorus product. This state is sometimes called milk tetany of the newborn. A number of rare disorders, such as vitamin D–resistant rickets and renal tubular lesions, may produce hypocalcemia and therefore potential tetany.

Hyperventilation tetany is produced by overbreathing, which results in respiratory alkalosis (see p. 194). The pH of the blood and the relationships between blood carbon dioxide, calcium, and phosphorus are upset, thus disturbing the balance that is necessary to maintenance of the constant product.

Gastric tetany results from loss of chloride ions. Such loss may occur in excess vomiting, in repeated gastric lavage, in pyloric stenosis, or in high intestinal obstruction. As a result of the chloride loss the serum chloride is reduced and the bicarbonate elevated, increasing the blood pH and its carbon dioxide content (see metabolic alkalosis, pp. 194-195).

Bicarbonate tetany occasionally results from excess oral or intravenous intake of sodium bicarbonate, which elevates both the blood pH and the blood carbon dioxide content. Administering bicarbonate in the presence of vomiting or renal insufficiency is extremely dangerous.

Control. The control of tetany depends on control of the causative circumstance or condition. Primary attention is given to removing the cause or resolving the underlying disturbance. Calcium or ammonium chloride may be given orally if vomiting has subsided. The orally administered dose usually does not take adequate effect in less than 24 hours. For immediate control an injection of magnesium sulfate (10% solution, 1 mg/kg body weight) may be given intramuscularly. Any respiratory depressant effects may be counteracted by parenteral injection of a soluble calcium salt such as calcium lactate or calcium gluconate. The latter may also be given intramuscularly.

Osteomalacia and osteoporosis

Identification and etiology. Both osteomalacia and osteoporosis are diseases of impaired calcium and phosphorus metabolism with resulting changes in bone formation. They may be distinguished according to cause and result.

Osteomalacia is the adult form of rickets. It is caused by a deficiency of vitamin D, calcium, or phosphorus in the diet; or by a deficiency of the vitamin D that is produced by exposure to sunlight, especially during periods of increased physiologic need as in pregnancy and lactation; or by factors that hinder the proper metabolism of vitamin D, calcium, and phosphorus. Such a hindering factor may be a defect in renal tubular reabsorption, resulting in imbalances in serum calcium or phosphorus; a malabsorption syndrome such as sprue or steatorrhea, which makes calcium unavailable to the body, and allows it to be lost in the feces; or resistance to vitamin D. Secondary hyperparathyroidism also contributes to the developing disease state.[32] The most common primary contributing factors are (1) failure to absorb calcium, as in prolonged steatorrhea or uremia, with excess fecal excretion or calcium phosphate and (2) general malnutrition and dietary deficiency of calcium and vitamin D during the stress demands of pregnancy and lactation. The resulting osteomalacia is a softening of the bones caused by their demineralization, accompanied by general weakness and aching.

Osteoporosis is a metabolic disorder that usually occurs in persons older than 50 years, especially women after the menopause. The latter is called involutional or postmenopausal osteoporosis. It is believed to be caused by the age-related decline in secretions of anabolic hormones by the sex glands and pituitary glands. No doubt other factors also contribute, such as lack of stimulating exercise and malnutrition, especially protein malnutrition. The result is a decrease in bone-forming activity (ossification) with a consequent reduction in the amount of bone, although the composition of the bone remains normal. Hypercalcinuria may occur, especially when prolonged immobilization is a factor, and renal calculi frequently develop. Manifestations include weakness, anorexia, hip and back pain, muscle tenderness and cramping, stooped posture, decreased height because of shrinkage of the spine, and a tendency of the bones to fracture easily.

Occurrence. In addition to its frequency in postmenopausal women, osteomalacia occurs in adults during periods of extreme malnutrition and semistarvation, such as in war or famine. Pregnant women are a high-risk group because of their increased needs, especially those who have undergone several pregnancies while taking an inadequate diet. Osteomalacia of pregnancy and lactation is endemic in India and the Middle East because the practice of purdah confines women indoors, which gives them very little exposure to sunlight.

Control. Prevention of osteomalacia is based on adequate dietary provision of calcium, phosphorus, and vitamin D and treatment for any disease or other factor that prevents the proper utilization of these nutrients. The intake of these nutrients must be increased during pregnancy and lactation. Immediate treatment with therapeutic doses of vitamin D, as in rickets, is indicated. Establishment of overall dietary improvement should follow.

Osteoporosis is combated by the administration of combined male and female hormones. Dietary intake of vitamin D, calcium, and protein should be increased. Treatment has also included the use of fluoride.[33]

Iron-deficiency anemia

Identification. The general clinical manifestations of iron-deficiency anemia are similar to those of all types of anemia: weakness, pallor, fatigability (a sense of being ''dead-tired''), headache, and palpitation. If the anemia becomes more severe, there may be increased shortness of breath and some degree of cardiac enlargement. In time, some persons with chronic iron-deficiency anemia adapt their level of work to their hematologic status and live at this reduced level of activity.

CLINICAL MANIFESTATIONS. Distinctive signs of iron-deficiency anemia include the following.

NAILS. The fingernails of many patients become brittle and flat and develop longitudinal ridges. In some cases the changes are so marked that the nails are concave instead of normally convex, so that they appear spoon shaped—a condition called *koilonychia*, (Gr. *koilos,* hollow; *onyx, onych,* nail). The nail beds are pale.

TONGUE AND MOUTH. A papillary atrophy of the tongue is seen in about half the patients, and some have fissures at the corners of the mouth. The mouth is sore, and in severe cases there may occasionally be some difficulty in swallowing (the Plummer-Vinson syndrome).

GASTROINTESTINAL. Gastritis, achlorhydria, and gastric atrophy are common. Other complaints include anorexia, flatulence, epigastric distress, and constipation. The liver and spleen may be enlarged.

HANDS AND FEET. Some patients experience numbness and tingling of the hands and feet, but these symptoms are less pronounced than in pernicious anemia.

LABORATORY FINDINGS. In iron-deficiency anemia the red blood cells contain less than the normal amount of hemoglobin; they are small and pale (microcytic hypochromic anemia). The total hemoglobin level is always below normal and is more strikingly reduced than is the red blood cell count. The erythrocyte count may even be about normal (4.5 to 5.5 million per cubic millimeter) while the hemoglobin value is as low as 5 g/dl (normal range, 14 ± 2 g/dl for women; 16 ± 2 g/dl for men). The serum iron level is low, and the total iron-binding protein level is above normal.

Etiology. Since iron performs important physiologic functions in oxygen transport and cellular respiration, the body guards its small supply, using it over and over again. In conditions of physiologic stress such as growth, menstruation, pregnancy, or hemorrhage (often compounded by poor diet and impaired absorption), a negative iron balance may develop. Anemia is the result.

INFANTS AND CHILDREN. The body of a newborn infant contains about 500 mg of iron. When the normal person has reached maturity, this amount has increased by 2.5 to 4.5 g. This represents an average increase of 0.35 to 0.60 mg per day! The infant is vulnerable to iron deficiency because milk is a poor source of iron. The premature infant, especially if born to a malnourished mother, is in even greater jeopardy, since he lacks the normal quantity of iron stores present at birth in tissues, particularly in the liver and blood.

WOMEN IN THEIR REPRODUCTIVE YEARS. During normal menstruation a woman loses from 35 to 70 ml of blood per period, representing a total loss of iron in hemoglobin of 15 to 25 mg. Over the span of her reproductive years the normal woman has a continuous average iron loss of 0.5 to 1.0 mg per day. Without adequate replacement in her diet she is obviously in a precarious state of iron balance. Pregnancy deprives her of still further iron. The net iron demand of a full-term pregnancy has been conservatively estimated to be from 500 to 700 mg. It is evident that frequent, multiple pregnancies take their toll and must lead to iron deficiency if precautionary iron therapy is not given.

BLOOD LOSS. Acute hemorrhage is an evident emergency for which the patient usually receives immediate blood replacement. Chronic blood loss, especially gradual, occult gastrointestinal bleeding, may go unnoticed and drain the body reserves. Parasitic infections of the intestines may also cause a continuous blood loss.

POOR ABSORPTION. Diseases such as chronic diarrhea, infection, sprue, steatorrhea, or celiac disease hinder absorption of iron. These often compound such stress situations as growth and pregnancy and increase the iron need.

POOR DIET. A diet high in cereal content and low in animal protein and green vegetables is usually low in iron. Unfortunately this is the common dietary pattern of many people who lack the money, means, or knowledge necessary to improve their diets. During such periods the iron deficiency is compensated in some degree by increased efficiency of iron absorption (p. 150).

Occurrence. Iron deficiency anemia is a world health problem. It occurs in all countries, but is particularly prevalent (affecting in some areas as many as 20% of the population) in the Middle East, northern Africa, and Asia. The high-risk groups in any population are children, women in their reproductive years, and those suffering from chronic illness and infection.

Control. Where it can be achieved, correction of the factors that increase the requirement for iron (numerous pregnancies, parasitic infections, and so on) makes a significant contribution to the control of iron-deficiency anemia. The enrichment of cereals by iron should be considered, especially where cereals are the staple food. Optimal diet and supplementation of the diet with iron are important during periods of stress such as growth and pregnancy.

Treatment of iron-deficiency anemia consists of giving a simple ferrous salt, such as ferrous sulfate or ferrous gluconate. The gastrointestinal difficulties that attend the ingestion of an iron salt may be minimized by taking it after meals so that it is mixed with the food in the stomach. Causes of any abnormal blood loss should also be sought and corrected.

Goiter

Identification. Goiter (L. *guttur,* throat) is enlargement of the thyroid gland. The normal thyroid gland is about the size and shape of a lima bean. In states of iodine deficiency the gland undergoes compensatory enlargement and may reach many times its normal size, until it becomes plainly visible at a distance of several feet (Fig. 16-10).

SIMPLE GOITER. In simple goiter, compensatory mechanisms may suffice to produce adequate amounts of thyroxine (the thyroid hormone), so that hypothyroidism may not cause general symptoms and signs resulting from metabolic imbalance. The goiter is then manifest only in mechanical problems, such as the local disfigurement, compression of the trachea with consequent hoarseness of the voice, chronic nonproductive cough, possible difficulty or discomfort in swallowing, or congestion of the face.

CRETINISM. In areas where the soil is poor in iodine and goiter has affected a number of generations, severe iodine deficiency in mothers produces an endemic form of cretinism in the offspring, characterized by stunted growth, dwarfism, and various degrees of mental retardation. This profound result of continued iodine deficiency was recognized as long ago as 1871 by C. H. Flagge, an English physician. "Goiter is the earlier effect of the endemic influence; cretinism shows itself when the action of that influence is intensified by operating on more than one generation."[34]

Etiology. Simple goiter is the result of failure of the thyroid gland to receive sufficient iodine to maintain its normal structure and function

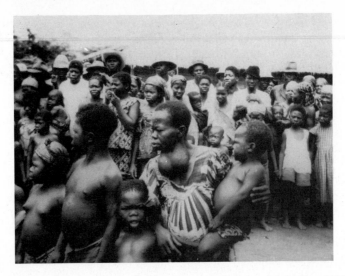

Fig. 16-10. Goiter and hyperthyroidism among children and adults in central Africa. (FAO photograph by Marcel Ganzin.)

(Fig. 8-4). Thyroxine is 65% iodine. When adequate iodine is not present, the gland's compensatory effort to produce the needed hormone results in its enlargement.

The dietary lack of iodine may be due to environmental factors—a deficiency of the mineral in soil and water. The deficiency may also be caused by factors that make the dietary iodine unavailable by interfering with its absorption or metabolism. Such goitrogenic substances are found in cabbage, brussels sprouts, soybeans, peanuts, turnips, and rutabagas. Further causes of deficiency are conditions such as chronic infection that increase the iodine requirement.

Occurrence. Goiter may occur in persons of any age. After puberty the incidence is somewhat greater in girls. In areas where examination of school children reveals a 5% to 10% incidence, goiter is a significant public health problem. In countries where the use of iodized salt has become an accepted public health practice, the incidence of goiter has been greatly reduced.

Control. Goiter may be prevented by a sufficient supply of iodine in the diet. The most practical means of ensuring adequate intake is the iodization of table salt. A content of 1 part iodine to 10,000 to 20,000 parts of salt is recommended in the western hemisphere; lower levels are used in Europe. Prevention is more effective than treatment; in longstanding goiter, treatment has little effect, because the chronic fibrosis is not reversible. Iodine may be administered to vulnerable groups (children, pregnant and lactating women), but is only a temporary measure.

METHODS OF COMBATING MALNUTRITION

Malnutrition is the world's primary health problem. How shall it be solved? It is evident that the problem is complex and that there are no simple answers. The discussion must end as it began with a restatement of the twofold premise: (1) supplying food alone is not the answer and (2) the problem is not confined to economically deprived populations.

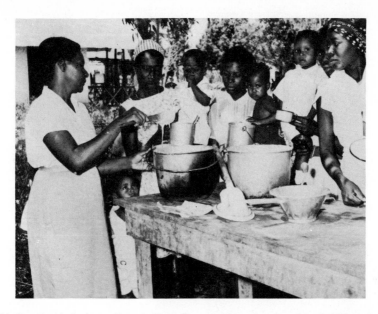

Fig. 16-11. Practical help for mothers in Haiti. Recuperation of malnourished children is aided not only by giving badly needed food, but also by teaching mothers the rudiments of nutrition and proper food preparation.

Requirements for solution of the problem of malnutrition

An approach to the problem of malnutrition must embrace three basic factors: medical care, health education, and responsibility of the persons involved.

Medical care. A direct attack involving case finding, clinical diagnosis, and treatment is a primary concern. All the resources of the medical team are needed for this aspect of the approach. But treating malnutrition and then sending the patient back into the environment that produced it is like putting a strip of adhesive bandage over a cancer.

Long-range control and prevention must focus on education and responsibility.

Health education. In addition to medical treatment, a balanced program must include nutritional rehabilitation and health education. The education must begin with the health personnel. At times it seems that a few members

of the health professions, whether working in the United States or in a foreign country, become encased in a crystallized rigidity, unable to learn from what meets the eye. Education must also reach the patients themselves, their parents and families, and the public. It must constantly develop to accommodate the constant changes in people, in the circumstances of their lives, in food products, and in scientific knowledge. It must be person centered and practical (Fig. 16-11). The principles discussed in the previous chapter apply here. Often the most significant care in such situations is personal teaching and supportive encouragement.

Responsibility. Ultimately the success of any efforts to combat malnutrition in a community must rest on a developed sense of responsibility in the people involved. The responsibility for providing sound, relevant health care rests with members of the health

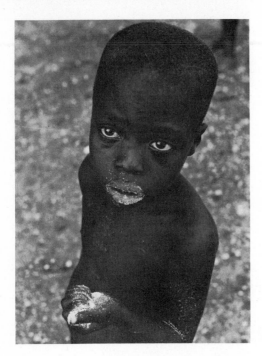

Fig. 16-12. A child eating a mouthful of maize flour at an FAO food distribution center in northern Dahomey. Recent drought in Dahomey and Togo brought famine to the area and necessitated aid from world health groups. (FAO photograph by C. Bavagnoli.)

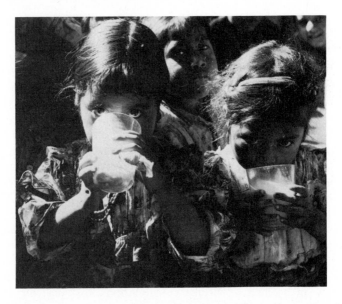

Fig. 16-13. Guatemalan children drinking Incaparina at school. After much experimentation, the Institute of Nutrition of Central America and Panama (INCAP) has succeeded in developing Incaparina, an inexpensive protein product of high nutritive value. It is now well liked and widely used in Central America. (WHO photograph by Todd Webb.)

professions. The responsibility for helping to provide a safe and adequate food supply, to explore food enrichment laws, agricultural methods, marketing practices, consolidation of control programs, supporting research, education, and technical development rests with the persons who form and administer the economic and political structure of the country. Responsibility for meeting health needs in daily life at the local level rests with community leaders. Responsibility for meeting personal and family health needs, for maintaining interest in good nutrition, for making certain that information is correct and clearly understood, and for carrying out the discipline that is required for the development of sound food habits rests with individuals and with the heads of families.

World health groups such as WHO, the Food and Agriculture Organization, UNICEF, and others are actively and earnestly engaged in the mammoth task of combating malnutrition (Fig. 16-12). Many other national and local groups in the United States and other countries are working toward the same goals. Food supplements such as the protein substance "Incaparina," which was developed by the Institute of Nutrition for Central America and Panama (INCAP) in Guatemala City are being studied and used to add needed nutrients to inadequate regional diets (Fig. 16-13). Research and education programs are helping to provide knowledge and tools.

Ultimately the welfare of a nation rests on the health of its people. George Herbert, an English poet who lived from 1593 to 1633 wrote, "Whatsoever was the father of a disease, an ill diet was the mother." He was far wiser than even he knew!

CASE STUDY 6
World health problem No. 1: malnutrition

In the West African village where her Peace Corps group was working in a small clinic, Laura Jensen had seen many health needs among the people. As a nutritionist on the team of medical workers assigned there, she had helped to care for persons with a number of diseases and conditions, for the underlying problem in most of them was malnutrition. The children seemed to be the most vulnerable. Many who managed to survive infancy did not live past the first few years of life.

There was little Mbugwa, for example, with whom Laura had spent many long anxious hours in the early critical time of his illness. When his mother first brought him to the clinic he was almost stuporous. He was about 18 to 20 months old, Laura learned from his mother, but he was small for his age. There seemed to be little or no muscle development, and his body was bloated and swollen. The usual tight mat of black curls on his head was gone, and instead his hair lay flat, straight, and graying. His skin was rough with cracking scales formed in many places. Large, ulcerous lesions had developed around many of the skin folds, especially in the area of his buttocks, where they were irritated by his severe diarrhea.

When Dr. Burrows, with Laura's help, examined him and did some blood tests, he found muscular wasting, gross edema, an enlarged liver, anemia, and hypoalbuminemia. The diarrhea had caused a severe hypokalemia. Dr. Burrows' first concern was correction of the water and electrolyte imbalance.

After Mbugwa responded to the fluid and electrolyte therapy during the first day, Laura began a careful refeeding plan. On the seventh day diuresis indicated that he was improving but revealed his sparse little bony frame beneath. Gradually, however, as Laura's feeding plan continued, Mbugwa's strength returned and he began to gain weight.

Laura's biggest concern now was devising some means of teaching Mbugwa's mother how to care for him and helping her learn to prepare and to feed him the foods he needed. This seemed to be a greater task than that of providing the initial medical care. The health team realized that the underlying causes of Mbugwa's illness were far deeper and more complex. Laura reminded them, when they discussed Mbugwa's needs, that the problem of nutrition is the result of a vast array of interrelated forces: cultural, social, political, economic, physiologic, psychologic, geographic, biologic, and others. Lest they be too discouraged at the results of their efforts, Laura also said that there were no simple solutions, but that they had a responsibility to do what they could where they were.

Questions to guide your inquiry

1. What name has been given to the disease syndrome from which Mbugwa suffered? What is the significance of this name?
2. What is the specific nutritional deficiency involved in the etiology of the disease?
3. Account for the related symptoms of enlarged fatty liver, hypoalbuminemia, edema and ascites, depigmentation, and typical skin changes or dermatosis.
4. When infectious diarrhea compounded Mbugwa's illness, why did he develop a critical fluid and electrolyte imbalance? Why is there potassium loss in prolonged diarrhea?
5. What changes occur in fat and protein metabolism as the disease progresses?
6. How would you identify and describe the three main stages of treatment?
7. Why would it be dangerous to give vitamin concentrates in the first two weeks of treatment?
8. What is marasmus? How does it differ from kwashiorkor?
9. What is protein-calorie malnutrition (PCM) such a worldwide health problem?
10. What did Laura mean when she said that there were no simple solutions? What are some of the interrelated factors that make the problem a complex one?
11. Outline a teaching plan that would be realistic for Laura to use in helping Mbugwa's mother learn how to care for him and feed him properly.
12. What are some of the world health organizations that provide resources for care and teaching in the area of nutritional problems in world health? Investigate some of the work these organizations are doing, such as by writing for materials describing their work.

REFERENCES
Specific

1. Emerson, H., editor: Control of communicable diseases in man, New York, 1917, The American Public Health Association.
2. Nordseik, F. W., editor: Control of malnutrition in man, New York, 1960, The American Public Health Association.
3. Gussow, J. D.: The feeding web: issues in nutritional ecology, Palo Alto, Calif., 1978, Bull Publishing Co.
4. Berg, A. D.: The nutrition factor: its role in national development, Washington, D.C., 1973, The Brookings Institution.
5. El-Badry, M. A.: Latin American population prospects in the next fifteen years, Popul. Studies **25**(2): 183, 1971.
6. Commission on Population Growth and the American Future: Population growth and America's future, Washington, D.C., 1971, U.S. Government Printing Office.
7. The state of food and agriculture, 1965. Review of second postwar decade, 1965, Food and Agriculture Organization.
8. Health Conditions in the Americas (1961-62), Pub. No. 104, 1964, prepared for the Meeting of the Directing Council, Pan American Health Organization/World Health Organization.
9. Shaefer, A. E., and Johnson, O. C.: Are we well fed? . . . The search for the answer, Nutr. Today **4**(1):2, 1969.
10. U.S. Department of Health, Education, and Welfare: Ten-state nutrition survey, 1968-1970, DHEW Pub. (HSM) 72-8134, Center for Disease Control, Atlanta, 1972.
11. Calder, R.: Proceedings of meeting on nutrition of the preschool child, Washington, D.C., 1965, National Academy of Sciences.
12. Jelliffe, D. B.: Effect of malnutrition on behavioral and social development, Proceedings, Western Hemisphere Nutrition Congress, Chicago, 1965, American Medical Association.
13. Scrimshaw, N. S., and Gordon, J. E., editors: Malnutrition, learning, and behavior, Cambridge, Mass., 1968, Massachusetts Institute of Technology Press.
14. Winick, M.: Malnutrition and brain development, J. Pediatr. **74**(5):667, 1969.
15. Rao, K. S.: Evolution of kwashiorkor and marasmus, Lancet **1**:709, 1974.
16. Williams, C. D.: Kwashiorkor: a nutritional disease of children associated with a maize diet, Lancet **2:** 1151, 1935.
17. Scrimshaw, N. S., and Béhar, M.: World-wide occurrence protein malnutrition, Fed. Proc. **18**(suppl. 3, pt. 2):82, 1959.
18. Joint FAO/WHO Expert Committee on Nutrition: Fourth report, WHO Tech. Rep. Ser. 97, 1955.
19. Oamen, H. A. P. C.: Clinical experience on hypovitaminosis A, nutritional disease. In Kinny, T. D., and Follis, R. H., Jr., editors: Proceedings of Conference on Beriberi, Endemic Goiter and Hypovitaminosis A, Fed. Proc. **17**(suppl. 2, pt. 2):162, 1958.
20. Burgess, R. C.: Beriberi, 6. Special problems concerning beriberi, B. Infantile beriberi, Fed. Proc. **17**(suppl. 2, pt. 2):39, 1958.
21. Schaefer, A. E.: Nutritional deficiencies in developing countries, J. Am. Diet. Assoc. **42**:295, 1963.
22. Scrimshaw, N. S.: Malnutrition and the health of children, J. Am. Diet. Assoc. **42**:203, 1963.
23. Roe, D. A.: Plague of corn, a social history of pellagra, Ithaca, N.Y., 1973, Cornell University Press.
24. Burns, J. J., editor: Vitamin C, Ann. N.Y. Acad. Sci. **92**:1, 1961.
25. Tolbert, B. M.: Report on the second year of research on ascorbic acid, biological function and chemistry, Contract No. DA-49-193-MD-2611, Office of the Surgeon General, U.S. Army, 1966.
26. Wagner, A. F., and Folkers, K.: Vitamins and coenzymes, New York, 1961, Interscience, p. 208.
27. Sherlock, P., and Rothschild, E. O.: Scurvy produced by a Zen macrobiotic diet, J.A.M.A. **199**:794, 1967.
28. Fraser, D.: Nutritional problems in North America, Proceedings, Western Hemisphere Nutrition Congress — 1965, Council on Foods and Nutrition, Chicago, 1966, American Medical Association.
29. Fraser, D.: Clinical manifestations of genetic aberrations of calcium and phosphorus metabolism, J.A.M.A. **176**:281, 1961.
30. Bakwin, H., et al.: Refractory rickets, Am. J. Dis. Child. **59**:560, 1940.
31. Council on Drugs: Doses of water-soluble vitamin A analogues in hemorrhagic disease of the newborn, J.A.M.A. **164**:1331, 1957.
32. Rizui, S. N. A., and Vaishnava, H.: Secondary hyperparathyroidism in nutritional osteomalacia, J. Indian Med. Assoc. **64**:199, 1975.
33. Jowsey, J., Riggs, B. L., and Kelly, P. J.: Longterm experience with fluoride and fluoride combination treatment of osteoporosis. In Kuhlencordt, F., and Kruse, H., editors: Calcium metabolism, bone and metabolic bone disease, New York, 1973, Springer-Verlag, New York, Inc.
34. Flagge, C. H.: On sporadic cretinism occurring in England, Medico-Chirurgical Transactions **54**:155, 1871.

General

Akbarian, M., Yankopoulos, N. A., and Abelmann, W. H.: Hemodynamic studies in beriberi heart disease, Am. J. Med. **41**:197, 1966.
Baum, J. L., and Rao, G.: Keratomalacia in the cachectic hospitalized patient, Am. J. Ophthalmol. **82**:435, 1976.

Black, I.: The health of the poor, New York Public Affairs Pamphlet No. 435, 1969.

Blackburn, G. L., and Bistrian, B. R.: Nutritional support resources in hospital practice. In Schneider, H. A., Anderson, C. E., and Coursin, D. B., editors: Nutritional support of medical practice, New York, 1977, Harper & Row, Publishers.

Butterworth, C. E., and Blackburn, G. L.: Hospital malnutrition and how to assess the nutritional status of a patient, Nutr. Today **10:**18, March-April, 1975.

Cerqueira, M. T., et al.: A comparison of mass media techniques and a direct method for nutrition education in rural Mexico, J. Nutr. Educ. **11:**133, July-Sept., 1979.

Coles, R., and Clayton, A.: Still hungry in America, New York, 1969, New American Library.

Dayton, D. H.: Early malnutrition and human development, Children **16**(6):211, 1969.

Goiter and iodine deficiency, Nutr. Rev. **22:**169, 1964.

Gordon, J. E.: Chairman, Subcommittee on Communicable Disease, Control of communicable disease in man, ed. 9, New York, 1960, American Public Health Association.

John, T. J., Blazovich, J., Lightner, E. S., et al.: Kwashiorkor not associated with poverty, J. Pediatr. **90:**730, May, 1977.

Kotz, N.: Let them eat promises: the politics of hunger in America, Englewood Cliffs, N.J., 1969, Prentice-Hall, Inc.

Larkin, F. A., Perri, K. P., Bursick, J. H., et al.: Etiology of growth failure in a clinic population, J. Am. Diet. Assoc. **69:**506, Nov., 1976.

Lozoff, B., and Fanaroff, A. A.: Kwashiorkor in Cleveland, Am. J. Dis. Child. **129:**710, 1975.

Report of the Citizens' Board of Inquiry into Hunger and Malnutrition in the United States, Hunger, U.S.A., Washington, D.C., 1968, New Community Press.

Review: Lymphocyte number and function in protein malnutrition, Nutr. Rev. **34:**208, 1976.

Scrimshaw, N. S.: Synergism of malnutrition and infection, J.A.M.A. **212:**1685, 1970.

Sydenstricker, V. P.: The history of pellagra, its recognition as a disorder of nutrition and its conquest, Am. J. Clin. Nutr. **6:**409, 1958.

Tobias, A. L., and Van Itallie, T. B.: Nutritional problems of hospitalized patients, J. Am. Diet. Assoc. **71:**253, Sept., 1977.

Walker, A. R. P.: Osteoporosis and calcium deficiency, Am. J. Clin. Nutr. **16:**327, 1965.

Williams, C. D.: Self-help and nutrition—real needs of underdeveloped countries, Lancet **1:**323, Feb. 13, 1954.

Williams, C. D.: Malnutrition, Lancet **2:**342, 1962.

Williams, C. D.: Maternal and child health services in developing countries, Lancet **1:**345, 1964.

Williams, C. D.: What is health education? Lancet **1:** 1205, 1966.

Williams, C. D.: Grassroots nutrition—or consumer participation, J. Am. Diet. Assoc. **63:**125, Aug., 1973.

Williams, R. R.: Can we eradicate the classical deficiency diseases? J. Am. Diet. Assoc. **36:**31, 1960.

NUTRITION IN
THE HEALTH CARE SPECIALTY

Not only in public health nutrition and nursing, but also in other health care specialties, the clinical specialist will seek to identify the nutritional needs of patients and to explore with them ways of meeting these needs. In Part Three, five of the specialty areas related to the life cycle will be considered, and in respect to each, ways will be discussed in which concern for significant nutritional needs can be integrated into total patient care.

The first three chapters of this part are concerned with the principles of nutrition as applied to the normal physiologic stress periods of gestation, lactation, and normal growth and development—to the well-being of mothers and children. In maternity care the first concern is antepartum care, the nutritional demands of pregnancy; then in postpartum care the practitioner is concerned with helping the new mother sustain lactation and initiate the first feedings of her newborn infant. In Chapter 17, "Nutrition during Pregnancy and Lactation," these needs are explored, the difficulties in setting nutritional standards are discussed, and some realistic guidelines for patient care are established.

In pediatric care the practitioner is concerned with providing for the needs of children during each stage of growth from infancy through adolescence. In Chapter 18, "Nutrition for Growth and Development: Infancy, Childhood, and Adolescence," these needs are traced through each stage of development. Throughout, food and feeding are viewed not only as being essential to physical growth but also as being an intimate part of the total human developmental process. Chapter 19, "Nutritional Therapy in Childhood Diseases," reviews general therapeutic nutritional needs in diseases such as those of the gastrointestinal system that affect digestion and absorption and genetic diseases that affect metabolism of key nutrients.

The remaining three chapters of this unit identify nutritional components of patient care in geriatrics, rehabilitation, and psychiatric care. In each instance the emphasis is on individual patients and families, their unique experience and needs, and the health worker's discovery together with the patient of how basic principles of nutrition, the meanings of food and feedings, may be applied in ways that will help move toward personal health and fulfillment.

17

Nutrition during pregnancy and lactation

Human reproduction involves complex processes of rapid, specialized growth. Both mother and child possess tremendous powers of adaptation that enable them to meet the demands of this growth. Gestation has well been called "the epitome of purposeful growth."

Because the maintenance of the health of body tissues is dependent on certain essential chemical nutrients in food, it is evident that the development of the infant is directly related to the diet of the mother. However, experience has shown that widely differing diets have sustained individual mothers through successful pregnancies, and the medical literature has reported conflicting and controversial observations concerning the nutritional requirements during pregnancy. Thus the thoughtful practitioner or student might well ask: What reasonable basis is there for establishing nutritional recommendations for my prenatal patient? What metabolic stress does the process of gestation place on the mother? How does this stress compare with that of lactation? What effects do complications of pregnancy have on the nutritional needs of the mother? As a guide in the practitioner's search for answers that may be applied realistically to patient care, it will be well to consider some of the background studies in the physiology of gestation and lactation as they relate to nutritional needs. The following questions should be used to guide further study:

1. What influence does maternal nutrition have on the outcome of pregnancy?

2. How does the physiology of gestation relate to antepartum nutritional needs? How may these needs be met through food choices?

3. How may general dietary problems associated with pregnancy best be met?

4. How should the diet be managed in complications of pregnancy?

5. What are the nutritional needs of the lactating mother?

6. What place does nutrition education have in maternity nursing?

THE RELATION OF NUTRITION AND PREGNANCY
Background

For centuries, in all cultures, a great body of folklore has surrounded pregnancy. Many traditional practices and diets have been followed, which have had little basis in fact, and much clinical advice was based only on supposition. Early in this century, for example, a German obstetrician named Ludwig Prochownick constructed the notion that semistarvation of the mother was really a blessing in disguise because it would produce a small baby of light weight who would be easier to deliver. Thus he proposed a diet low in calories, low in carbohydrate and protein, and restricted in water and salt.[1] Incredible as it seems in retrospect, despite the lack of any scientific evidence to support such ideas, this general view became implanted in obstetric textbooks and in obstetric practice, passed on from one generation of physicians to the next. Two erroneous assumptions grew and formed the basis of fallacious theories: (1) the "parasite theory"—whatever the fetus needs it will draw from the stores of the mother despite the maternal diet—and (2) the "maternal instinct theory"—whatever the fetus needs the mother will instinctively crave and consume.

Clinical observations and scientific studies in the following years, however, began to refute these false ideas. In 1929 Honora Acosta-Sison, a leading obstetrician in the Philippines, noted the vital relationship between the state of nutrition of the mother and the birth weight of the child.[2] A few years later a British scientist, Edward Mellanby, recognized the role of scientific nutrition in protecting the mother from complications of pregnancy.[3] Subsequent work of an American physician in the southern United States reinforced the relation of malnutrition among the pregnant poor women there to a higher incidence of fetal-maternal diseases and deaths.[4-7] This work in the South by Ross was reinforced by similar reports from another internist in Boston, Strauss, of his work demonstrating the effectiveness of a high-protein, high-vitamin, optimal diet in combating toxemia.[8] Strauss's observations were confirmed by other clinicians in similar situations.[9] It was about this same time in the mid-1930s that Toverud of Norway reduced the incidence of low-birth-weight babies in his carefully supervised group to 2.2% with emphasis on nutritional care. He expressed his working hypothesis that "a child is nutritionally nine months old at birth."[10]

During the 1940s, two studies further reinforced the basis of sound nutrition as a correlate with a successful outcome of pregnancy. In Toronto, Canada, Ebbs and co-workers[11] based their study on the diets of pregnant women, using records of food intake during one week. Half of the women were judged by their records to have "poor diets; below the recommended

standards." Within this group of women with "poor diets" a subgroup received, from the fourth month to term, a food supplement that raised their nutritional level to optimum standards. Without knowing to which group or subgroup each woman belonged, the clinic's obstetrician and pediatrician rated the pregnancies, labors, postpartum periods, and babies as good, fair, poor, or bad—depending on minor complaints or major complications. The results revealed that 36% of the women on "poor diet" had poor or bad prenatal ratings, whereas only 9% of the women who received the supplement that raised the nutritional intake had poor or bad ratings.

In Boston, Burke and co-workers at the Harvard School of Public Health and the Boston Lying-in Hospital,[12] conducted a similar study showing a high correlation of the prenatal diet with reproductive performance. Burke used a detailed dietary questionnaire to interview a number of pregnant women and rated their diets according to the recommended dietary allowances of the National Research Council (NRC), and then compared these ratings to the outcome of their pregnancies. She reported that most of the superior infants were born to mothers with good to excellent diets. All stillborn, all premature, all "functionally immature," all but one of the infants who died within a few days of birth, and a majority of those born with morbid congenital defects were delivered by women whose diets had been inadequate during gestation. These studies were substantiated by reports at this same time from Scotland.[13]

In the 1950s, Ferguson documented still further the severe and widespread malnutrition among the South's pregnant poor and its relationship to infant and maternal disease and death.[14] His work was done in Mississippi, a state that reports one of the highest infant and maternal mortality rates in the United States. Similar results were reported by Jeans and co-workers of a large group of low-income pregnant women living in a rural state.[15] A series of reports during this same period[16] led to disillusionment in some quarters because they seemed to present conflicting evidence. However, subsequent analysis indicated some misleading interpretations based on methodologic problems of failure to control for such variables as race or age or parity.[17]

In the 1960s and early 1970s, data published by Brewer based on his work with clinic populations in New Orleans, Miami, and California presented evidence that a vigorous program of sound nutrition with adequate protein of high biologic value, sufficient calories to spare protein for tissue synthesis, and enough salt and other essential regulatory agents of vitamins and minerals could dramatically reduce the incidence of maternal and infant disease and low birth weight.[18-22] Brewer's data indicate that such a nutritious diet producing a generous weight gain during pregnancy can in fact remarkably reduce the number of low birth weight babies. In 1,500 pregnancies among a lower economic group of women, the prematurity rate (birth weight below 2,500 g) was 2.2%, repeating the results of Toverud in 1938 and Ebbs in 1942. Even among 318 primipara from 14 to 21 years of age, always a higher risk group, Brewer reported a prematurity rate of only 2.8%. When these numbers are compared with the national U.S. average of 8.2% (1968) and 15% among lower income black women, the data become all the more significant. Commenting on the Brewer data, Lowe indicates that the United States may have failed to reduce its infant mortality rate and failed to stop the rising prematurity rate (factors of life in no other advanced nation) because of *iatrogenic* factors—a direct challenge to traditional European and American obstetric practice of demanding constraint on weight gain by calorie restriction (which always carries with it nutrient curtailment), a limitation on salt intake, and the use of saline diuretics. None of these restrictions was used in the Brewer series. Thus Lowe concludes that the change desired in the alarming national statistics may well lie in prenatal regimen and that real progress can be made *merely by feeding pregnant women*.[23]

This conclusion is substantiated by the work of Primrose and Higgins in Montreal, Canada.[24] In their study at the Montreal Diet Dispensary among a group of low-income women, a program of nutrition education and food supplementation was used to demonstrate the effectiveness of adequate nutrition in decreasing the incidence of toxemia during pregnancy and prematurity and morbidity among the newborn, and in reducing infant mortality. Nutrient requirements for protein and calories were determined on an individual basis and included an assessment for specific conditions of protein deficiency and underweight and for special conditions of stress in addition to those for normal needs. The average estimated daily requirement for calories, based on individual need and Canada's Food Guide, was 3,009 calories, 93% of which was actually reached by subjects in the study. The average estimated protein requirement was 107 g; 95% of this intake goal (100 g) was met by the subjects on the average. Even for the group of mothers aged 17 years or younger the incidence of prematurity was only 3.3%. Of the total cases in the study (1,362) the average weight gain during pregnancy was 11 kg (25 lb).

Considerations in determining needs

It is evident from this increasing amount of data and from the wide experience of many clinicians that maternal nutrition *is* critically important to both mother and fetus. Two factors seem responsible for this change in awareness and attitude of greater concern: (1) the rapidly expanding knowledge of the role of nutrition in the prevention and treatment of disease and (2) the realization that the numbers of stillbirths and infant deaths in the United States and Canada are much higher than one would expect. Low birth weight is now known to be associated with increased risk of neonatal death (i.e., within the first 28 days of life), and malnutrition is a factor contributing to the relatively large group of infants with perinatal handicaps and congenital injuries or who fail to grow and develop normally.

These concerns led to the formation of the Committee on Maternal Nutrition of the NRC, whose definitive report, *Maternal Nutrition and the Course of Human Pregnancy,* the result of three years' study, has been published.[25] This report clearly shows the need for change in traditional practices of care, the abandonment of unscientific, unfounded notions, for a new approach, a positive approach, to the dietary management of pregnancy. Based on these findings, subsequent guides for assessment of maternal nutrition, for use by physicians, nutritionists, dietitians, and nurses providing prenatal care, have been developed by the American College of Obstetrics and Gynecology and the American Dietetic Association.[26-28]

From the overwhelming evidence involved in the Maternal Nutrition Committee's deliberations and report, as well as statements in the resulting guidelines for practice, several important considerations emerge as determinants of nutritional requirements during pregnancy.

Age and parity of the mother. The teenage mother adds her own needs presented by her continuing growth to those introduced by her pregnancy. At the other end of the reproductive span, hazards increase with age. The number of pregnancies and the intervals between them influence the needs of the mother and the outcome of pregnancy.

Preconception nutrition. The mother brings to gestation all of her previous life experiences, including her diet. Her general health and fitness and her state of nutrition at the time of her infant's conception are products of her lifelong dietary habits and possibly of generations before her own conception. The woman is the product of the growth that has preceded.

Complex metabolic interactions of gestation. Although three distinct biologic entities are involved in pregnancy—the mother, the fetus, and the placenta—together they form a unique biologic *synergism* (p. 379). Constant metabolic interactions go on among them. Their functions, while being unique, are at the same time *interdependent.* Any number of variables therefore may combine in ways that make the determination of general needs difficult.

Individual needs and adaptations. Individual nutritional needs vary with time and circumstance; although homeostatic mechanisms appear to operate with special efficiency during pregnancy, special conditions of stress are placed on nutrient requirements in addition to those for normal needs.

Answer to the problem

Three basic concepts provide the framework for assessing maternal nutrition needs.

Perinatal concept. The prefix "peri" comes from the Greek root meaning "around, about, or surrounding." As knowledge and understanding increase, it is evident that the whole of the individual's life experiences surrounding the pregnancy must be considered. The nutritional status developed over previous years of living and the establishment of reserves for possible future pregnancies are both important.

Life continuum concept. The concept of the life continuum naturally follows the perinatal concept. Each child becomes a part of the ongoing continuum of life. Through the food she eats, each mother gives to her unborn child the nourishment required to initiate and sustain fetal growth; but she carries over the same nutritional principles in her feeding and teaching of the growing child—principles that he in turn internalizes and passes on to his child. Perhaps it should be said, that *she* in turn passes on to *her* child, for it is the nutritional development of the girl child that is of particular concern in this case; she is the potential mother of future generations.

Synergism concept. The word "synergism" comes from two Greek roots, "syn," meaning with or together, and "ergon," meaning work. Thus synergism is a term used to describe biologic systems in which the cooperative action of two or more factors produces a total effect greater than and *different from* the mere sum of their parts. In short, *a new whole* is created by the unified, joint effort of blending the parts, in which each part potentiates the action of the other. Of the many biologic and physiologic interactions providing examples of synergism, pregnancy is a prime case in point. Maternal organism, fetus, and placenta all combine to create a new whole, not existing before, and producing a total effect greater than and different from the sum of their parts, all for the purpose of sustaining and nurturing the pregnancy and its offspring. Physiologic parameters change therefore during this synergistic response to the pregnancy (e.g., blood volume increases, cardiac output increases, ventilation rate and tidal volume increase), and physiologic norms of the nonpregnant woman do not apply, nor can the normal physiologic adjustments of pregnancy be viewed as pathologic with application of treatment procedures for that same type of response to an abnormal state. For example, the physiologic generalized edema of pregnancy is a normal protective response, not to be confused with or treated as abnormal edema in other states (such as in congestive heart failure, for instance). The protective response of general edema is indicated by Hytten in his report of a study of 24,000 pregnancies in Aberdeen in which he found edema to be associated with enhanced reproductive performance. He concluded that edema in late pregnancy is a benign, healthy phenomenon in the absence of toxemia, that is, in the adequately nourished woman.[29]

NUTRITION IN PREGNANCY
Physiology of gestation
Fetal development

The development of the fetus undergoes three distinct morphologic phases: implantation, differentiation of major organs and tissues, and the intensive growth period.

Implantation (first two weeks). Prior to conception the endometrium, the membrane that lines the uterus, is prepared for the reception of the ovum by thickening and developing an increased blood supply. The fertilized ovum develops into a sphere called the *blastocyst,* which has an inner and an outer layer of cells. The outer layer of cells will later contribute to the formation of the placenta, which will carry nutrients from the mother to the fetus and waste products from the fetus into the maternal circulation for disposal. Because they are related to nourishment, these cells are called "trophoblasts" (Gr. *trophe,* nourishment; *blastos,* germ or cell). They develop within nine to ten days of fertilization of the ovum. The blastocyst imbeds itself in the endometrium, which invaginates to receive it. Here it is anchored by the trophoblasts. The trophoblasts also differentiate into two layers. One layer, in intimate relationship with the uterus, maintains important nutrient relationships with the mother. The ovum rapidly increases in size, largely as a result of the growth of the second layer, the *syncytium* (Gr. *syn,* with; *kytos,* cell), so named because it consists of cells whose protoplasm is continuous with that of the contiguous cells. The syncytium develops from the trophoblast; the syncytial trophoblast is that layer of the trophoblast which is in closest relation to the uterus. It is a highly structured, highly complex tissue, which becomes an important part of the placenta, where it helps to provide nourishment to the growing fetus. An idea of its complexity can be gained from the fact that this tissue is similar to the visceral epithelium in Bowman's capsule (surrounding the renal glomerulus) and in the convoluted tubules. This complex development represents an adaptation to the need for rapid transport of fluid and solute nutrients. By the completion of seven to ten days' development the cell mass (now the embryonic disc) is ready to differentiate into a thick plate of primitive ectoderm and an underlying layer of endoderm.

Differentiation of major organs and tissues (two to eight weeks). During the second phase of fetal development, rapid, dramatic changes take place in the developing embryo. The three basic layers of tissue (the "germ layers") are formed—ectoderm, mesoderm, and endoderm (Gr., *ektos,* outside; *mesos,* middle; *endon,* within; *derma,* skin). These three germ layers give rise to the various organs and tissues of the body in very specific ways. From the ectoderm come the entire nervous system and the epidermis. From the endoderm develop the lining of the gastrointestinal tract and such derivative organs as the liver, pancreas, and thyroid. From the mesoderm come the skeleton, connective tissues, the vascular and urogenital systems, the dermis, and most of the skeletal and smooth muscles. By the seventh week the body has begun to take form. Although the head remains large relative to the size of the body during the embryonic period, the body has begun to grow rapidly also. By now the neck can be recognized, the tail filament has disappeared, and by the end of the seventh or eighth week, the embryo can be identified as human. It is evident that with such rapid development of specialized cells, the nutritional status that the mother brings to conception and to these crucial early weeks is significant in the successful outcome of the pregnancy.

Intensive growth period (eight weeks to term). From the eighth week on the changes are less dramatic but equally vital to the entire future life of the developing human being. The specialized tissues continue to develop and grow during this period of most rapid fetal growth. There is also intensive *maternal* physiologic growth during this period; the mother's body undergoes nutritional reconditioning, and reserves are laid down to meet the demands of approaching labor, the period immediately following labor, and lactation.

Placenta

Definition and function. The placenta (L. "a flat cake") is an oval, spongy structure, which at term is 15 to 17.5 cm (6 to 7 in) in diameter and weighs about 450 g (1 lb). It is expelled following parturition and is then commonly called the afterbirth. The placenta is a complex, highly specialized organ. Its primary function is to transport and store oxygen and nutrients from the mother to the developing fetus and to return the end products of fetal metabolism to the maternal blood. In a highly selective manner the fetus draws its nutrients for growth and development from the placental stores supplied by the mother. From the time the fertilized egg is implanted in the uterus to full maturation and birth, the fetus depends for these functions entirely on this specialized placental structure. The placenta consists of physiologic divisions, specialized in function, and particularly adapted to serve each of these essential purposes.

Specialized functional parts. The specialized functional parts of the placenta are the fetal portion, the maternal portion, and the intervillous spaces.

FETAL PORTION (CHORION FRONDOSUM). The essential parenchyma (functional part of an organ as distinguished from its purely structural parts) of the placenta is its trophoblast. Soon after implantation of the fertilized ovum the highly invasive trophoblast penetrates the endometrium. It develops a functional outer shell or layer of cells called the syncytium. From the syncytium develop small villous protrusions; the surfaces of the villi are covered with even finer projections called microvilli. A similar structure in the small intestine provides maximum absorbing surface. This placental network of villi is adapted to serve the same purpose. The fetal portion of the placenta is called the *chorion,* and the projections are called the chorionic villi. Some villi extend to the endometrium as anchoring villi, but the majority end freely and continue to divide as the placenta develops, thus increasing the total absorbing surface.

MATERNAL PORTION (DECIDUA BASALIS). The name comes from the Latin word *decidua,* "falling off" (a tissue that will fall off after parturition), and the Latin and Greek root *basis,* the "base or lowest part." As the invasion of the endometrium continues, maternal blood vessels are tapped, and vacuoles in the cytoplasm coalesce to form larger *lacunae* (L. *lacuna,* a pit). The lacunae are hollow spaces that soon fill with blood from the endometrial arteries and veins. These spaces join and form a labyrinth of channels and columns lined with the highly selective, functional, trophoblast cells. These cells, the major agents for nutrition and homeostasis, are the survival links for the fetus.

INTERVILLOUS SPACES. As Ramsey's[30] beautiful, classic radiographic work clearly shows, like so many minute springs or fountains, vertical maternal arteries push blood, in funnel-shaped spurts, up from the floor of the decidua basalis. The blood flows around the chorionic villi that lie free in the intervillous spaces, bathing their surfaces and exchanging metabolic material. Then, as maternal blood pressure dissipates, the blood is dispersed laterally into endometrial veins. The intervillous spaces serve as the depot of transfer, and the chorionic villi serve as the agents of transfer. Through highly selective transport mechanisms similar to those operating in the small intestine and in the kidney, essential metabolic substances move across the trophoblast membrane by three basic mechanisms. Most of the small molecules (water, oxygen, electrolytes) move across membranes in this manner according to need and are guided by osmotic pressures (passive diffusion). Somewhat larger molecules (nutrients such as dextrose, amino acids, vitamins), primarily for nutrition, move across the membrane by specialized carrier systems of active

transport. Some of the larger molecules such as proteins are absorbed by means of an invaginating process called pinocytosis (see p. 215). In view of this highly selective transport activity provided by the placental membrane, perhaps the common term "placental barrier" is misleading. A better term may be "placental membrane."

Maternal nutrient needs

What nutrients must the mother take to supply the fetus and her own changing body optimally for this critical gestation period?

During the first trimester (the first three months), the fetus is small and undergoes differentiation, so that the mother's relative nutrient requirements are increased slowly from normal adult needs. These nutrients are, however, essential during this vital period; only the *quantitative* need for them is not yet greatly increased. The importance of a diet that contains balanced portions of essential nutrients according to individually assessed quantities continues into the second trimester.

The last three months of pregnancy is the period during which a greater *amount* of key nutrients is required by the fetus, as it lays down stores for growth. This need for increased amounts of certain nutrients is indicated by the recommended daily allowances outlined by the NRC (Table 17-1). It should be remembered that although the recommended allowances provide a margin of safety above minimal requirements to allow for variations of need, some individuals require more for optimal nutrition. For example, the reference woman in the table is aged 18 to 35 years, weighs 58 kg (128 lb), is 160 cm (64 in) tall, lives in a temperate climate, and is a normally active, healthy woman. Obviously, variations from this state would need to be considered. The increased quantitative need for nourishment by pregnant adolescents should be noted. The need for individual counseling and for correct use of these recommenda-

Table 17-1. Recommended daily dietary allowances of some selected nutrients for pregnancy and lactation (National Research Council, 1980 revision)

Nutrients	Nonpregnant girl 12-14 yr 47 kg (103 lb)	Nonpregnant girl 14-18 yr 55 kg (120 lb)	Nonpregnant woman 25 yr 58 kg (128 lb)	Pregnancy Added need	Pregnancy Girl 12-14 yr	Pregnancy Girl 14-18 yr	Pregnancy Woman 25 yr	Lactation (850 ml daily) Added need	Lactation Girl 12-14 yr	Lactation Girl 14-18 yr	Lactation Woman 25 yr
Calories	2,200	2,100	2,000	300	2,500	2,400	2,300	500	2,700	2,600	2,500
Protein (g)	46	46	44	30	76	76	74	20	66	68	64
Calcium (g)	1.2	1.2	0.8	0.4	1.6	1.6	1.2	0.4	1.6	1.6	1.2
Iron (mg)	18	18	18	‡	18+	18+	18+	‡	18+	18+	18+
Vitamin A (RE)*	800	800	800	200	1,000	1,000	1,000	400	1,200	1,200	1,200
Thiamin (mg)	1.1	1.1	1.0	0.4	1.5	1.5	1.4	0.5	1.6	1.6	1.5
Riboflavin (mg)	1.3	1.3	1.2	0.3	1.6	1.6	1.5	0.5	1.8	1.8	1.7
Niacin equivalent and tryptophan (mg)	15	14	13	2	17	16	15	5	20	19	18
Ascorbic acid (mg)	50	60	60	20	70	80	80	40	90	100	100
Vitamin D (μg)†	10	10	5	5	15	15	10	5	15	15	10

*Retinol equivalents.
†Cholecalciferol; 10 μg equals 400 IU vitamin D.
‡Required iron supplement 30-60 mg.

tions as guidelines is clearly stated by the NRC: "They are not called 'requirements' because they are not intended to represent merely literal (minimal) requirements of average individuals, but to cover substantially the individual variations in the requirements of normal people." In considering the needs of the normal pregnant woman, therefore, the nutrient elements should be reviewed in terms of the general amount of increased intake indicated, why this increase is recommended, and how it may be obtained in basic foods.

Protein. An additional daily allowance of 30 g of protein is recommended throughout pregnancy, raising the 44 g required by the normal nonpregnant woman to at least 74 g daily.

This represents an increase of about 66% or two thirds. For a large number of high-risk or active women, however, as cited studies have shown, more protein is needed—nearer 100 g or about double their previous intake.

Protein, with its essential constituent, nitrogen, is the nutritional element that is basic to growth. Nitrogen balance studies give some indication of the large amounts of nitrogen used by the mother and child during pregnancy. Study of fetal tissue composition reveals that during the last half of gestation the amount of nitrogen stored by the embryo rises from approximately 0.9 to 55.9 g. The mature placenta at term has stored about 17 g of nitrogen; the amniotic fluid contains 1 g. An estimated 17 g

Table 17-2. Daily food plan for pregnancy and lactation

Food	Nonpregnant woman	Pregnancy	Lactation
Milk, cheese, ice cream, skimmed or buttermilk (food made with milk can supply part of requirement)	2 cups	3-4 cups	4-5 cups
Meat (lean meat, fish, poultry, cheese, occasional dried beans or peas)	1 serving (3-4 oz)	2 servings (6-8 oz); include liver frequently	2½ servings (8 oz)
Eggs	1	1-2	1-2
Vegetable* (dark green or deep yellow)	1 serving	1 serving	1-2 servings
Vitamin C–rich food* Good source—citrus fruit, berries, cantaloupe Fair source—tomatoes, cabbage, greens, potatoes in skin	1 good source or 2 fair sources	1 good source and 1 fair source or 2 good sources	1 good source and 1 fair source or 2 good sources
Other vegetables and fruits	1 serving	2 servings	2 servings
Bread† and cereals (enriched or whole grain)	3 servings	4-5 servings	5 servings
Butter or fortified margarine	As desired or needed for calories	As desired or needed for calories	As desired or needed for calories

*Use some raw daily.
†One slice of bread equals 1 serving.

of nitrogen is incorporated in the developing maternal breast tissue, nearly 40 g in the increased uterine tissue. In addition a maternal reserve of 200 to 350 g is stored for the approaching losses during labor and parturition (from 300 to 500 ml or more of blood may be lost during delivery) and in preparation for the physiologic demand of lactation.

In summary, more protein is essential to meet the demands posed by the rapid growth of the fetus; by the enlargement of the uterus, mammary glands, and placenta; by the increase in maternal circulating blood volume and the subsequent demand for increased plasma protein to maintain colloidal osmotic pressure; and by the formation of amniotic fluid and storage reserves for labor, delivery, and lactation.

Milk, meat, egg, and cheese are complete protein foods of high biologic value. Protein-rich foods also contribute other nutrients such as calcium, iron, and B vitamins. The amounts of these foods that would supply the quantities of protein needed are indicated in the recommended daily food plan (Table 17-2). Additional protein may be obtained from legumes, whole grains, and nuts.

Calories. Calories should be sufficient to meet energy and nutrient demands and to spare protein for tissue building. Classic studies indicate that a minimum of 36 calories per kilogram of body weight is required for efficient use of protein during pregnancy.[31] Although only 300 calories additional to the amount ingested by the nonpregnant woman is recommended by the NRC, representing about a 10% to 15% increase over the usual previous intake, this amount is insufficient for many active or nutritionally deficient women, who may easily need as much as 2,500 to 3,000 calories. The emphasis should be a positive one on ample calories to ensure nutrient and energy needs, not a negative idea of restricting calories.

Minerals. The increased need for calcium and iron should be particularly emphasized throughout pregnancy.

CALCIUM. It is recommended that the woman during gestation increase her daily calcium intake by 0.4 g. Since the suggested intake for the nonpregnant woman is 0.8 g, the total daily intake during pregnancy should be 1.2 g. This is about a 50% increase.

The importance of calcium to the mother and fetus is suggested by the size of the increase that is recommended. Calcium is the essential element for the construction and maintenance of bones and teeth. It is also an important constituent of the blood clotting mechanism (p. 97) and is used in normal muscle action and other essential metabolic activities. Balance studies indicate that the calcium used by the maternal organism increases from about 4 g at the middle of pregnancy to about 30 g at term. Fetal tissue studies reveal an increase in the quantity of calcium stored, from about 1 g at the middle of gestation to about 23 g at term. For rapid mineralization of skeletal tissue during this final period of growth, more calcium is essential.

Dairy products are a primary source of calcium. Therefore some increase in milk or equivalent milk foods (cheese, ice cream, skimmed milk powder used in cooking) is recommended. Additional calcium is obtained in whole or enriched cereal grain and in green leafy vegetables. Because an occasional woman in the latter part of pregnancy may experience cramping of the muscles of the legs (induced, perhaps, by a transitory imbalance in the serum calcium or phosphorus ratio and the relatively high phosphorus content of milk), some health workers routinely advise pregnant women to drink no milk. If she eliminates milk altogether from her diet, the woman deletes an excellent source of other important nutrients, including protein, riboflavin, and vitamin A. To control the minor complaint of muscular cramping, would it not be more reasonable to simply indicate to her the amount of milk (3 to 4 cups) or *equivalent milk foods* that will supply her needs? Perhaps this patient likes milk or wants to use it in cooking. To take her calcium in this form would satisfy both the patient and her adviser.

IRON. A woman should maintain a daily intake of 18 mg of iron throughout her childbearing years. This amount would replenish menstrual losses and restore tissue and liver reserves after each pregnancy. To meet the iron needs of pregnancy, iron supplements to dietary sources are usually recommended. This need for iron may be appreciated by adding up the "iron cost" of a pregnancy:

Extra iron used in	
Products of conception	370 mg
Maternal blood increase	+290
TOTAL	660
Less iron "saved" by	
Cessation of menstruation	−120
TOTAL	540
	(more with multiple births)

Thus with increased demands for iron with insufficient maternal stores and inadequate provision through the usual diet, a daily supplement of 30 to 60 mg of iron has been recommended by the NRC Report on Maternity Nutrition.

The increase in maternal circulating blood volume during pregnancy has been estimated to be from 40% to 50%, or more with multiple births. Iron is essential to the formation of hemoglobin; an adequate supply of this mineral is therefore important to maintain the mother's hemoglobin level. If low preconception stores are suspected, if there is a history of anemia, or if there is doubt concerning adequate dietary iron sources, iron supplementation is needed. Iron is also needed for fetal development, especially for storage of reserve in the liver. About a three to four months' supply of iron is stored in the developing fetal liver to supply the infant's need after birth; this is necessary because his first food, milk, lacks iron. Adequate maternal iron stores also fortify the mother against the blood losses at delivery.

Liver contains far more iron than any other food. Women who dislike liver may be encouraged to use it more frequently by suggestions concerning appetizing ways of serving it. Other meat, dried beans, dried fruit, green vegetables, eggs, and enriched cereals are additional sources of iron.

Vitamins. Increased amounts of vitamins A, B, C, and D are recommended during pregnancy.

VITAMIN A. A daily increase of 200 μg retinol equivalents (RE) is recommended for pregnancy (about a 25% increase over the usual adult intake). Vitamin A is an essential factor in cell development, maintenance of the integrity of epithelial tissue, tooth formation (p. 88), normal bone growth, and vision. Liver, egg yolk, butter or fortified margarine, dark green and yellow vegetables, and fruits are good food sources.

B VITAMINS. There is an especially increased need for B vitamins during pregnancy. These are usually supplied by a well-balanced diet. When the physician doubts that the pregnant woman is taking an adequate diet, he or she may find it necessary to prescribe supplements. This B vitamins are important as coenzyme factors in a number of metabolic activities, energy production, function of muscle and nerve tissue, and therefore play key roles in increased metabolic activities of pregnancy.

There is an increased metabolic demand for folic acid during pregnancy. Folic acid deficiency usually occurs in conjunction with general malnutrition, making the pregnant woman in high-risk, low socioeconomic conditions especially susceptible. A specific megaloblastic anemia caused by maternal folate deficiency sometimes occurs and warrants attention to supplementation of the diet with folic acid, particularly where such needs are greater, as in chronic hemolytic anemia and multiple pregnancy. The NRC report recommends a daily supplement of 400 μg of folic acid to prevent such deficiencies.

VITAMIN C. Special emphasis must be laid on

the pregnant woman's need for ascorbic acid. A daily increase of 20 mg is recommended. Added to the adult recommendation of 60 mg, this makes a recommended daily total of 80 mg during pregnancy, or a 25% increase. Ascorbic acid is exceedingly important to the growing organism. It is essential to the formation of intercellular cement substance in developing connective tissue and vascular systems. It also increases the absorption of the iron that is needed for the increasing quantities of hemoglobin. The expectant mother should be encouraged to eat additional quantities of foods that are common sources of vitamin C, such as citrus fruit, berries, melon, and cabbage.

VITAMIN D. Adults who lead active lives entailing adequate exposure to sunlight probably need little additional source of vitamin D. However, during pregnancy the increased need for calcium and phosphorus presented by the developing fetal skeletal tissue necessitates additional vitamin D to promote the absorption and utilization of these minerals. Four hundred IU of vitamin D, or 15 μg of cholecalciferol, is recommended for pregnancy. Frequently supplementary vitamin D is ordered by the physician. Food sources include fortified milk, butter, liver, egg yolk, and fortified margarine.

Daily food pattern. A diet consisting of a variety of foods can supply needed nutrients and can make eating a pleasure. The increased quantities of essential nutrients needed during pregnancy may be met by intelligently planning around a daily food plan, using the key foods suggested. Such a daily food pattern is suggested in Table 17-2 and may be used as a helpful guide. Additional food may be added according to energy and nutrient needs.

GENERAL DIETARY PROBLEMS
Gastrointestinal problems

During pregnancy, several gastrointestinal difficulties may be encountered. These are highly individual in form and extent and will require individual counseling or control. Usu-

ally the complaints are relatively minor; but if they persist or become extreme, they will need attention from the physician. These problems include the following.

Nausea and vomiting. Nausea and vomiting are usually mild and transitory and limited to early pregnancy. It is commonly called "morning sickness," because it occurs more often upon rising than later in the day. A number of factors may contribute to this condition. Some are physiologic; they are traceable to the hormonal changes that occur in early pregnancy. These changes are probably accentuated in some patients by psychologic factors, various situational tensions, or anxieties concerning the pregnancy itself. Simple treatment usually suffices to improve food toleration. Small, frequent meals, fairly dry, and consisting chiefly of easily digested energy foods such as carbohydrates are most readily tolerated. Liquids are best taken between meals instead of with food. If the condition develops to *hyperemesis* (severe, prolonged, persistent vomiting), the physician will probably hospitalize the patient and feed her intravenously to avoid complications.

Constipation. Constipation is seldom more than minor. The pressure of the enlarging uterus on the lower portion of the intestine, in addition to the hormonal muscle relaxant effect on the gastrointestinal tract during pregnancy, may make elimination somewhat difficult. Increased fluid intake and use of naturally laxative foods such as whole grains with added bran, dried fruits (especially prunes and figs), other fruits, and juices usually induce regularity. Laxatives should be avoided; they should not be used except under the physician's supervision.

Weight gain in pregnancy

Optimal weight gain of the mother during pregnancy makes an important contribution to a successful course and outcome. The concept of caloric restrictions to avoid large total weight gains and to avoid toxemia is without foundation, having found its way into textbooks of obstetrics and widely followed by the medical profession despite lack of scientific basis. Not only has such a practice not proved helpful, it has imposed much harm. Evidence has mounted from many sources that women produce healthy babies within a wide range of total weight gain. In one large group of women who gained in excess of 14 kg (30 lb) during pregnancy, 91% had no difficulties at all.[1] Hytten indicates that the range of weight change in pregnancy may vary from very little or none to a gain of 27 kg (60 lb) or more, and that a normal outcome may be found in that range.[32]

The important consideration lies in the *quality* of the gain and the foods consumed to bring it about, rather than on a restriction on the quantity of weight gained. Also, there has been failure to distinguish between weight gained as a result of edema and that due to deposition of fat—maternal stores laid down for energy to sustain fetal growth during the latter part of pregnancy and energy for lactation to follow. About 2 to 4 kg (4 to 8 lb) of fat is commonly deposited for these stores, presumably as the result of stimulus by progesterone acting centrally to reset a "lipostat" in the hypothalamus. When the pregnancy is over, the lipostat reverts to its usual nonpregnant level, and the added fat is lost. The average weight of the products of a normal pregnancy are given below.

Products	Weight
Fetus	3,400 g (7.5 lb)
Placenta	450 g (1 lb)
Amniotic fluid	900 g (2 lb)
Uterus (weight increase)	1,100 g (2.5 lb)
Breast tissue (weight increase)	1,400 g (3 lb)
Blood volume (weight increase)	1,800 g (4 lb) (1,500 ml)
Maternal stores	1,800 to 3,600 g (4 to 8 lb)
TOTAL	11,000 to 13,000 g (11 to 13 kg; 24 to 28 lb)

Clearly, therefore, severe caloric restriction is unphysiologic and potentially harmful to the developing fetus and the mother. It is inevitably accompanied by restriction of vitally needed nutrients essential to the growth process going on. Weight reduction should never be undertaken during pregnancy. To the contrary, sufficient weight gain should be encouraged with the use of a nourishing, well-balanced diet as outlined.

Rate of weight gain. About 900 to 1,800 g (2 to 4 lb) is an average gain during the first trimester. Thereafter, about 450 g (1 lb) a week during the remainder of the pregnancy is usual. There is no scientific justification for routinely limiting weight gain to lesser amounts. It is only unusual patterns of gain, such as a sudden sharp increase in weight after the twentieth week of pregnancy, which may indicate excessive, not normal, water retention that should be watched.

Sodium restriction. Just as with restriction of calories, routine restriction of sodium is unphysiologic and unfounded. Physicians who prescribe diets low in calories and low in salt are placing pregnant women and their offspring at disadvantage and unnecessary risk. Robinson reported a clinical study in London in which a superior reproductive performance was observed in a group of pregnant women advised to use salt as compared with a group placed on a low-salt diet.[33] Greater use of protein usually accompanies use of salt—cheeses, meats, fish, and natural sodium in milk, for example. These observations are further supported by the work of Pike, indicating the need for sodium during pregnancy and the harm to maternal-fetal health by restricting salt.[34-37] Combined with the added injury of routine use of diuretics, such a program places the pregnant woman and the fetus in double jeopardy. Chesley indicates that diuretics have no value in the prevention and treatment of preeclampsia, because the problem is not with the sodium ion but with the role of plasma proteins in hypovolemia.[38] The NRC report labels such routine use of salt-free diets and diuretics as potentially dangerous.[25]

COMPLICATIONS OF PREGNANCY
Anemia

Anemia is common during pregnancy. Clinicians report that about 10% of the patients in large prenatal clinics in the United States have hemoglobin concentrations of less than 10 g/dl and a hematocrit reading below 32. Anemia is, of course, more prevalent among the poor, many of whom live on diets barely adequate for subsistence; but anemia is by no means restricted to the lower economic groups. Disregarding some of the hereditary anemias, some of the more common acquired types encountered in pregnancy are categorized here according to their cause.

Iron-deficiency anemia. A deficiency of iron is by far the most common cause of anemia in pregnancy. The cost of a single normal pregnancy in iron stores is large (from 500 to 800 mg). Of this amount, nearly 300 mg is used by the fetus; the remainder is utilized in the expansion of maternal red cell volume and hemoglobin mass. This total iron requirement exceeds the available reserves in the average woman. Studies have indicated that most women in the United States have low stores of iron.[39] The additional amount of iron needed during pregnancy may be made up in some women by increased dietary intake and increased efficiency of absorption; but in other women the iron level is borderline prior to pregnancy and insufficient to meet the augmented requirement. Anemia results. Usually the requirements of the fetus, which increase during the last trimester, will continue to be met by transfer of the iron across the placenta; it is the mother who will suffer the iron deficiency. Daily doses of 200 mg of an iron compound given orally are usually adequate for treatment. This oral therapy should be continued for three to six months after the anemia has been corrected in order to replenish the depleted stores. Meanwhile, ways of including more iron-rich foods in her diet should be explored with the patient.

Hemorrhagic anemia. Anemia caused by blood loss is more likely to occur during the puerperium than during gestation. Blood loss may occur earlier, however, as a result of abortion or ruptured tubal pregnancy. Most patients undergoing these physiologic disasters receive blood by transfusion, but iron therapy may be indicated in addition to support the formation of hemoglobin needed for adequate replacement.

Megaloblastic anemia. Megaloblastic anemia of pregnancy almost always results from folic acid deficiency. An analysis of the diet of these women usually reveals that they eat few if any vegetables (especially green leafy ones) and seldom take animal protein. Manifestations include intensification of nausea, vomiting, and anorexia. As the anemia progresses, the anorexia is more marked, thus further compounding the nutritional deficiency. The folic acid requirement of the adult woman, estimated by Herbert[40] and other investigators to be from 50 to 100 μg per day, is considerably increased by pregnancy,[41-44] as well as by the use of oral contraceptives during interconception periods, probably due to hormonal inhibition of folate absorption and metabolism.[45] During pregnancy, both trophoblast and the fetus are sensitive to folic acid inhibitors, and therefore probably have high metabolic requirements for folic acid and its derivatives. The placenta and the fetus appear to concentrate folic acid efficiently, since the fetus may have an adequate store while the mother is severely deficient in the compound. Pritchard[46] has reported one case in which the hemoglobin levels of the newborn infant were 18 g or more per deciliter, while the maternal levels were as low as 3.6 g/dl.

Toxemia

Where humans lack precise knowledge, they often must proceed on the basis of inference; but the human tendency to allow assumption to become dogma sometimes impedes the discovery of fact. In their development over the years, medicine, nursing, and nutrition have not been free from such errors. Certain assumptions about "the enigma of obstetrics"—toxemia—probably afford an example. Toxemia of pregnancy is still called by man "the disease of theories." Over the years the literature has abounded with conflicting views and open controversy concerning its etiology and treatment. Eastman and Hellman,[47] for example, reviewed 13 separate theories of the etiology of toxemia.

Brewer[18-22,48] and a number of other clinicians[49-51] have presented clinical and laboratory evidence that toxemia is a disease of malnutrition, and that the malnutrition affects the liver and its metabolic activities. Certainly, as Mengert and Tweedie,[52] Higgins,[53] and others[54] have stressed, toxemia is classically associated with poverty; it has been encountered most often in women subsisting on inadequate diets who have little or no medical care. The urgency of combating this disease is evident from a few statistics. Toxemia occurs in 6% to 7% of all pregnancies. It accounts for the majority of all maternal deaths (about 1,000 deaths annually in the United States), and for the majority of all deaths of newborn infants (some 30,000 stillbirths and neonatal deaths per year). Most of these deaths could be prevented by good prenatal care, which inherently includes attention to sound nutrition. Many studies such as those discussed in the beginning of this chapter indicate that a general state of good nutrition, which a woman *brings to her pregnancy and maintains throughout it,* provides her with optimal resources for adapting to the physiologic stress of gestation. Her fitness during pregnancy is a direct function of her past nutrition and her optimal nutrition during pregnancy.

Classification and clinical manifestations. Toxemia is generally classified and defined according to its manifestations. It is usually seen in the third trimester, toward term. Among its clinical manifestations are hypertension, edema, albuminuria, and, in severe cases, convulsions and coma.

The broad descriptive classification of toxemia outlined by the American Committee on Maternal Welfare (revised 1952) is widely used:

I. Acute toxemia of pregnancy (onset after the twenty-fourth week)
   A. Preeclampsia
      1. Mild
      2. Severe
   B. Eclampsia (convulsions or coma; usually both when associated with hypertension, proteinuria, edema)

II. Chronic hypertensive (vascular) disease with pregnancy
   A. Without superimposed acute toxemia or edema
      1. Hypertension known to exist before beginning of the pregnancy
      2. Hypertension discovered during the pregnancy (earlier than the twenty-fourth week and persisting into the postpartum period)
   B. With superimposed acute toxemia

Treatment. Specific treatment varies according to the patient's symptoms and needs. Optimal nutrition is a fundamental aspect of therapy. Emphasis is laid on protein foods of high biologic value and sources of vitamins and minerals for correction and maintenance of metabolic balance.

Preexisting chronic conditions

Preexisting conditions such as diabetes and heart disease are managed during pregnancy according to the general principles of care related to pregnancy and to the particular disease (pp. 606 and 710). A comprehensive review of the management of diabetes, heart disease, and other complications of pregnancy has been provided by Williams.[55] With the physiologic stress of pregnancy added to that of disease, closer medical and nutritional supervision is required. The pregnancy and the preexisting disease affect each other and enhance the difficulty of control. The therapeutic responsibility is frequently shared by internist, obstetrician, and nutritionist. With close observation of mother and child, cooperation by the patient, and good nutritional and nursing care, complications are minimized.

NUTRITION DURING LACTATION

The physiologic stress of lactation is even greater than that of pregnancy. The lactating mother consequently requires more dietary additions than does the pregnant woman. A comparison between the nutritional needs and daily food pattern of women in these two states may be made in Tables 17-1 and 17-2.

Nutritional needs

The basic nutritional requirements during pregnancy persist throughout lactation, with the following additions.

Protein. An increase of 20 g over the quantity recommended for the nonpregnant woman is recommended during lactation, making a total daily protein allowance of about 66 g.

Calories. The greatest recommended increase is in calories. Two hundred calories daily more than in the prenatal diet (500 calories more than the usual adult allowance) is needed for lactation, making a daily total of about 2,500 calories.

This additional recommendation of 500 calories for the overall total lactation process is based on three factors:

1. *Milk content.* An average daily milk production for lactating women is 850 ml (30 oz). Human milk has a caloric value of about 20 calories per ounce. Thus these 30 oz of milk have a value of 600 calories.
2. *Milk production.* The metabolic work involved in producing this amount of milk utilizes from 400 to 420 calories.
3. *Maternal adipose tissue storage.* The additional energy need for lactation is drawn from maternal adipose tissue stores laid down during pregnancy in normal preparation for lactation to follow in the maternal cycle. Depending on the adequacy of these stores, additional energy input (calories) may be needed in the lactating woman's daily diet.

Minerals. The quantities of calcium and iron required by the lactating mother are not greater than those needed during pregnancy. The increased amount of calcium that was required during gestation for mineralization of the fetal skeleton is now diverted into the mother's milk. Iron, since it is not a principal mineral component of milk, need not be increased for milk production per se.

Vitamins. An increased quantity of vitamin C above that recommended for the pregnant woman is recommended for the lactating mother. An increase of 40 mg over the nonpregnant woman's need is recommended, making her total ascorbic acid requirements 100 mg daily. Increases over the mother's prepartum intake are recommended also in vitamin A and the B-complex vitamins riboflavin and niacin (about a one-third increase over the quantities taken during pregnancy). These vitamins are important coenzyme factors in cell respiration, glucose oxidation, and energy metabolism; the quantities needed therefore invariably increase as calorie intake increases.

Fluids. A practice sometimes neglected, because fluids may not be considered a nutrient, but which is highly significant to adequate milk production, is the increased intake of fluids. Water and beverages such as juices, tea, coffee, and milk all add to the fluid necessary to produce milk, a fluid tissue.

Rest and relaxation. In addition to the augmented diet, the mother who would breast-feed her baby requires rest, moderate exercise, and relaxation. Often the nurse may help the mother by counseling with her about her new family situation; together they may develop plans to accommodate these needs.

Summary concept. Throughout the experience of pregnancy and lactation, intelligent care is based on general nutritional fitness and attention to individual needs. And these are but a continuation of a woman's lifetime nutritional experience.

CASE STUDY 7
"You're going to have a baby, Mrs. Barton"

Jane Barton, aged 19, clutched the laboratory requisition sheets and information booklet the clinic nurse had given her a moment ago. The elevator ride to the first floor seemed forever. Tears smarted in her eyes, and feelings of panic and anger welled up within. Her husband, Bill, aged 21, was equally quiet. "I guess it was a surprise to him, too," Jane thought. "I know he blames me, and I do myself, for forgetting my pills." She could still hear the doctor's words after he finished examining her. "You're going to have a baby, Mrs. Barton."

All the old stories her mother had told her while she was growing up about the difficulties she had had with Jane filled her mind. Jane was an only child, and her mother had communicated much of her own maternal insecurity and fear to Jane.

The elevator reached the ground floor and they walked out into the lobby. By now Jane could not control herself and the sobs came. She crumpled the papers in her hand and threw the torn pieces in a corner wastebasket as she ran from the building. "No! No! No! Not now!"

Bill and Jane Barton were sophomores at the university in town. They had decided to get married during their freshman year. Their parents had wanted them to finish school first but finally agreed to help with their school costs. They would have to meet their living expenses on their own. They both got part-time jobs, rented a small apartment in a student housing village, and were barely making it on a tight budget. However, Bill and Jane were serious students. Both wanted to be doctors, and they knew that this meant more years of study. A family would have to wait quite a while, they had agreed. But now Jane's fears were real. They certainly hadn't planned for this baby now. What would they do? How would they manage?

The next day Dr. Berlyn called the clinical nutritionist and the prenatal clinic nurse to arrange a team conference about helping the Bartons. The receptionist in the clinic lobby had seen Jane's upset state as she left the building, retrieved the crumpled and torn lab slips from the wastebasket, and taken them to Dr. Berlyn. The health care team arranged a special appointment for Jane and Bill to discuss their needs, provide support, and plan care. Here they talked a long time about the experience of having a baby, about Jane's needs for care, and especially her need for Bill's support. After they had talked, Jane felt a little less frightened by the whole prospect. She and Bill were pleased about the educational program that was part of the prenatal care in the clinic, group discussions where young couples could talk with each other and the staff about their problems and adjustments to parenthood. In these sessions the parents learned a great deal about pregnancy, labor and delivery, care of the baby, and themselves. Jane and Bill agreed to come the next night. The subject was to be Nutritional Needs of Pregnancy, led by the nutritionist.

"I can see I certainly need that," answered Jane. "With our tight schedule, meals have been pretty haphazard snacks. I really know nothing about what's good for you. I never had any responsibilities at home when I was growing up. I don't know anything about food buying or cooking, and I've always been too busy with my schoolwork to try to learn. But I have someone else to consider now, and with our budget it will take some real planning."

As the months of planning and preparation went by, Jane and Bill become regular participants in the maternity care program at the clinic. Their interest and involvement grew. It was a family-centered program in which both were involved. Toward the latter part of Jane's pregnancy one of the discussion groups led by the nutritionist was on Infant Feeding. By this time Jane had decided that she wanted to breast-feed her baby and wait until the child was older to begin her classes again at the university.

Continued.

CASE STUDY 7

"You're going to have a baby, Mrs. Barton"—cont'd

When the time for her labor and delivery came, it turned out to be a profound experience for Jane and for Bill. He was with her all the way, coaching her breathing during labor, holding her hand tightly during delivery. Dr. Berlyn and the nurses were a great support, too. Their son arrived strong and well, vigorous, and with a lusty cry. Jane and Bill looked at him and at each other. They knew they had grown a great deal in the past months and that this was only the beginning. They would all continue to grow together.

Questions to guide your inquiry (Refer also to Chapter 14.)

1. What do you think some of Jane's needs were in the beginning of her pregnancy?
2. If you were the nutritionist or the nurse helping to plan Jane's maternity care, what processes would you use to handle and clarify her needs?
3. What health professionals do you think should participate in the team planning for a maternity care educational program, such as the one in which Jane and Bill were involved? What role or specific activities do you see each health team member carrying out in such a program?
4. What aspects of the human personality are involved in learning? How do these apply in Jane and Bill's situation?
5. What basic principles of learning and health teaching would you use in planning and conducting this maternity care educational program? Illustrate these principles by describing what understandings and actions you would use to help the Bartons.
6. What does the word awareness mean to you? Why is this a key characteristic for a successful teacher? In what ways do you think the health team here demonstrated this basic characteristic?
7. In the initial interview with Jane in planning her maternity care, including her nutritional needs, what things do you think the nutritionist and Jane would explore together? Why would optimum nutrients, especially protein, key vitamins, minerals, and sufficient calories, be more important considerations than weight control?
8. Outline what you think Jane's daily food pattern probably was, and analyze it in terms of her nutritional needs for pregnancy.
9. List the changes in Jane's food habits that you think would be needed, and outline a basic diet plan for her.
10. What practical problems do you think Jane would have in following her diet plan? What suggested solutions could you offer her?
11. Outline a teaching plan for group instruction for the session on Nutritional Needs for Pregnancy that Jane and Bill were attending. Include the following:
    a. Objectives
    b. Main discussion points
    c. Methods of teaching, learning experiences for the group, means of achieving group involvement
    d. Materials or resources
    e. Carry-over or follow-up plans
    f. Evaluation
12. Make a similar plan for the later class they attended on Infant Feeding.
13. What particular suggestions concerning breast-feeding do you think would be helpful to Jane?

REFERENCES
Specific

1. Shank, R. E.: A chink in our armor, Nutr. Today **5**(2): 2, 1970.
2. Acosta-Sison, H.: Relation between state of nutrition of the mother and the birth weight of the fetus, J. Philippine I. Med. Assoc. **9**:174, 1929.
3. Mellanby, E.: Nutrition and child-bearing, Lancet **2**:1131, 1933.
4. Ross, R. A.: Relation of vitamin deficiency to the toxemias of pregnancy, Southern Med. J. **28**:120, 1935.
5. Ross, R. A.: Factors of probable significance in causation of toxemias of pregnancy, Southern Med. Surg. **102**:613, 1940.
6. Ross, R. A.: Late toxemias of pregnancy: the number one obstetrical problem of the South, Am. J. Obstet. Gynecol. **54**:723, 1947.
7. Ross, R. A.: Toxemia of pregnancy: socioeconomic background, Med. Ann. DC **28**:493, 1959.
8. Strauss, M. B.: Observations on the etiology of toxemias of pregnancy. The relationship of nutritional deficiency, hypoproteinemia and elevated venous pressure to water retention during pregnancy, Am. J. Med. Sci. **190**:811, 1935.
9. Dodge, E. F., and Frost, T. T.: Plasma proteins and toxemia, J.A.M.A. **111**:1898, 1938.
10. Toverud, G.: The influence of nutrition on the course of pregnancy, Milbank Mem. Fund Quart. **28**:7, 1950. Reviewed with pertinent comments by N. Eastman, Obstet. Gynecol. Sur. **5**:482, 1950.
11. Ebbs, J. H., Tisdall, E. F., and Scott, W. A.: The influence of prenatal diet on the mother and the child, J. Nutr. **22**:515, 1941.
12. Burke, B. S., Beal, V. A., Kirkwood, S. B., and Stuart, H. C.: Nutrition studies during pregnancy, Am. J. Obstet. Gynecol. **46**:38, July, 1943.
13. Cameron, C. S., and Graham, S.: Antenatal diet and its influence on still-births and prematurity, Glasgow Med. J. **24**:1, 1944.
14. Ferguson, J. H., and Keaton, A.: Studies of the diets of pregnant women in Mississippi. I. The ingestion of clay and laundry starch, New Orleans Med. Surg. J. **102**:460, 1950. II. Diet patterns, New Orleans Med. Surg. J. **103**:81, 1950.
15. Jeans, P. C., Smith, M. B., and Stearns, G.: Incidence of prematurity in relation to maternal nutrition, J. Am. Diet. Assoc. **31**:576, 1955.
16. McGanity, W. J., et al.: Vanderbilt cooperative study of maternal and infant nutrition. XII. Effect of reproductive cycle on nutritional status and requirements, J.A.M.A. **168**:2138, 1958.
17. Terris, M.: The epidemiology of prematurity: studies of specific etiologic factors. In Chipman, S. S., editor: Research methodology and needs in perinatal studies, Springfield, Ill., 1966, Charles C Thomas, Publisher.
18. Brewer, T. H.: Limitations of diuretic therapy in the management of severe toxemia: the significance of hypoalbuminea, Am. J. Obstet. Gynecol. **83**:1352, 1962.
19. Brewer, T. H.: Metabolic toxemia of late pregnancy: a disease of malnutrition, Springfield, Ill., 1966, Charles C Thomas, Publisher.
20. Brewer, T. H.: Metabolic toxemia of late pregnancy: a disease entity, Gynaecologia (Basel) **167**:1, 1969.
21. Brewer, T. H.: Human pregnancy nutrition: an examination of traditional assumptions, Aust. N. Z. J. Obstet. Gynaecol. **10**:87, 1970.
22. Brewer, T. H.: Disease and social class. In Brown, M., editor: The social responsibility of the scientist, New York, 1971, Macmillan Publishing Co., Inc.
23. Lowe, C. U.: Research in infant nutrition: the untapped well, Am. J. Clin. Nutr. **25**:245, 1972.
24. Primrose, T., and Higgins, A.: A study in human antepartum nutrition, J. Reprod. Med. **7**:257, 1972.
24a. Higgins, A.: Montreal diet dispensary study. In Proceedings of Workshop on Nutritional Supplementation and Outcome of Pregnancy, Washington, D.C., 1973, National Academy of Sciences.
25. Food and Nutrition Board, Committee on Maternal Nutrition, National Research Council: Maternal nutrition and the course of human pregnancy, Washington, D.C., 1970, National Academy of Sciences.
26. American College of Obstetrics and Gynecology, Committee on Nutrition: Nutrition in maternal health care, Chicago, 1974.
27. American College of Obstetrics and Gynecology, Task Force on Nutrition: Assessment of maternal nutrition, Chicago, 1978.
28. Brennan, R. E., Caldwell, M., and Rickard, K. A.: Assessment of maternal nutrition, J. Am. Diet. Assoc. **75**:152, Aug., 1979.
29. Hytten, F. E.: Oedema in pregnancy. In Rippmann, E. T., editor: Die Spätgestose, Basel, 1970, Schwabe and Co.
30. Ramsey, E., Corner, G. W., and Donner, M. W.: Serial and cineradiographic visualization of maternal circulation in the primate (hemochorial) placenta, Am. J. Obstet. Gynecol. **86**:213, 1963.
31. Oldham, H., and Sheft, B. B.: Effect of calorie intake on nitrogen utilization during pregnancy, J. Am. Diet. Assoc. **27**:847, 1951.
32. Hytten, F. E., and Leitch, I.: The physiology of human pregnancy, Oxford, 1964, Blackwell Scientific Publications.
33. Robinson, M.: Salt in pregnancy, Lancet **1**:178, 1958.
34. Pike, R.: Sodium intake during pregnancy, J. Am. Diet. Assoc. **44**:176, 1964.

35. Pike, R.: Further evidence of deleterious effects produced by sodium restriction during pregnancy, Am. J. Clin. Nutr. **23:**883, 1970.

36. Pike, R., and Yao, C.: Increased sodium chloride appetite during pregnancy in the rat, J. Nutr. **101:** 169, 1971.

37. Pike, R., and Smiciklas, H.: A reappraisal of sodium restriction during pregnancy, Int. J. Gynaecol. Obstet. **10:**1, 1972.

38. Chesley, L. C.: Plasma and red cell volume, Am. J. Obstet. Gynecol. **112:**449, 1972.

39. Pritchard, J. A., and Mason, R. A.: Iron stores of normal adults and replenishment with oral iron therapy, J.A.M.A. **190:**897, 1964.

40. Herbert, V.: Minimal daily adult folate requirement, Arch. Intern. Med. **110:**649, 1962.

41. Kitay, D. Z.: Folic acid deficiency in pregnancy, Am. J. Obstet. Gynecol. **104:**1067, 1969.

42. Kitay, D. Z., and Harbort, R. A.: Iron and folic acid deficiency in pregnancy, Clin. Perinatol. **2:**255, 1975.

43. Rothman, D.: Folic acid in pregnancy, Am. J. Obstet. Gynecol. **108:**149, 1970.

44. Zuspan, F. P., et al.: Anemia in pregnancy, J. Reprod. Med. **6:**13, 1971.

45. Shojania, A. M., Hornady, G. J., and Barnes, P. H.: The effect of oral contraceptives on folate metabolism, Am. J. Obstet. Gynecol. **111:**782, 1971.

46. Pritchard, J. A.: Megaloblastic anemia during pregnancy and the puerperium, Am. J. Obstet. Gynecol. **83:**1004, 1962.

47. Eastman, N. J., and Hellman, L. M.: Williams' obstetrics, ed. 13, New York, 1966, Appleton-Century-Crofts.

48. Brewer, T. H.: Role of malnutrition in preeclampsia and eclampsia, Am. J. Obstet. Gynecol. **125:**281, 1976.

49. Sheehan, H. L., and Lynch, J. B.: Pathology of toxemia in pregnancy, Baltimore, 1973, The Williams & Wilkins Co.

50. Call, M., and Lorentzen, D.: Rupture of the liver associated with toxemia, Obstet. Gynecol. **25:**466, 1965.

51. Maqueo, M., Ayala, L., and Cervantes, L.: Nutritional status and liver function in toxemia of pregnancy, Obstet. Gynecol. **23:**222, 1964.

52. Mengert, W. F., and Tweedie, J. A.: Acute vasospastic toxemia: therapeutic nihilism, Obstet. Gynecol. **24:**662, 1964.

53. Higgins, A. C.: Nutritional status and the outcome of pregnancy, J. Can. Diet. Assoc. **37:**17, 1976.

54. National Research Council, Committee on Maternal Nutrition: Maternal nutrition and the outcome of pregnancy, Washington, D.C., 1970, National Academy of Sciences, chap. 2.

55. Williams, S. R.: Nutritional therapy in special conditions of pregnancy. In Worthington, B., Vermeersch, J., and Williams, S. R.: Nutrition in pregnancy and lactation, ed. 2, St. Louis, 1981, The C. V. Mosby Co.

General

NUTRITION AND PREGNANCY

Adams, S. O., Barr, G. D., and Huenemann, R. L.: Effect of nutritional supplementation in pregnancy. I. Effect on outcome of pregnancy, J. Am. Diet. Assoc. **72:**144, 1978.

Adams, S. O., Huenemann, R. L., Bruvold, W. H., and Barr, G. D.: Effect of nutritional supplementation in pregnancy. II. Effect on diet, J. Am. Diet. Assoc. **73:** 630, Dec., 1978.

American College of Obstetrics and Gynecology, Committee on Nutrition: Nutrition in maternal health care, Chicago, 1974.

American College of Obstetrics and Gynecology: Task force report. Nutrition assessment of maternal nutrition, Chicago, 1978.

Appel, J. A., and King, J. C.: Energy needs during pregnancy and lactation. In Williams, S. R., and Dickman, S. R., editors: Nutrition and health promotion, Fam. Commun. Health **1:**7, Feb., 1979.

Babson, S. G., Pernoll, M. L., Benda, G. I., and Simpson, K.: Diagnosis and management of the fetus and neonate at risk, ed. 4, St. Louis, 1979, The C. V. Mosby Co.

Benjamin, F., Bassen, F. A., and Meyer, L. M.: Serum levels of folic acid, B_{12}, and Fe in anemia of pregnancy, Am. J. Obstet. Gynecol. **96:**310, 1966.

Blackman, M. L., and Calloway, D. H.: Energy expenditure of pregnant adolescents, J. Am. Diet. Assoc. **65:** 24, 1974.

Blumenthal, I.: Diet and diuretics in pregnancy and subsequent growth of offspring, Br. Med. J. **2:**733, 1976.

Bowering, J., et al.: Role of EFNEP aides in improving diets of pregnant women, J. Nutr. Educ. **8:**111, 1976.

Brennan, R. E., Caldwell, M., and Rickard, K. A.: Assessment of maternal nutrition, J. Am. Diet. Assoc. **75:** 152, Aug., 1979.

Clarren, S. K., and Smith, D. W.: The fetal alcohol syndrome, N. Engl. J. Med. **298:**1063, 1978.

Fielding, J. E., and Yankauer, A.: The pregnant drinker, Am. J. Public Health, **68:**836, Sept., 1978.

Food, pregnancy, and family health: American College of Obstetrics and Gynecology, Pub. No. R-37, Chicago, 1976.

Hanson, J. W., Streissguth, A. P., and Smith, D. W.: The effects of moderate alcohol consumption during pregnancy on fetal growth and morphogenesis, J. Pediatr. **92:**457, 1978.

Higgins, A.: Montreal diet dispensary study. In Proceedings of Workshop on Nutritional Supplementation and Outcome of Pregnancy, Washington, D.C., 1973, National Academy of Sciences.

Hunt, I. F., Jacob, M., Ostegard, N. J., et al.: Effect of nutrition education on the nutritional status of low income pregnant women of Mexican descent, Am. J. Clin. Nutr. **29:**675, 1976.

Hytten, F. E., and Leitch, I.: The physiology of human pregnancy, ed. 2, Oxford, 1971, Blackwell Scientific Publications.

Jacobson, H. N.: Diet in pregnancy: new perspectives, N. Engl. J. Med. **297:**1051, 1977.

Johnson, E. M., and Schwartz, N. E.: Physicians' opinions and counseling practices in maternal and infant nutrition, J.A.D.A. **73:**246, Sept., 1978.

Kaminetsky, H. A., Langer, A., Baker, H., et al.: The effect of nutrition in teenage gravidas on pregnancy and the status of the neonate. I. A nutritional profile, Am. J. Obstet. Gynecol. **115:**639, 1973.

Laboratory indices of nutritional status in pregnancy, National Academy of Sciences, Pub. No. F-427, Washington, D.C., 1977.

Light, H. K., and Festner, G.: Maternal concerns during pregnancy, Am. J. Obstet. Gynecol. **118:**46, 1974.

Lindheimer, M. D., editor: Hypertension in pregnancy: an invitational symposium, J. Reprod. Med. **8**(3):97, 1972.

Orr, R. D., and Simmons, J. J.: Nutritional care in pregnancy, J. Am. Diet. Assoc. **75:**126, Aug., 1979.

Snowman, M. K., and Dibble, M. V.: Nutrition component in a comprehensive child development program, J. Am. Diet. Assoc. **74:**119, Feb., 1979.

Weigley, E. S.: The pregnant adolescent: a review of nutritional resources and programs, J. Am. Diet. Assoc. **66:**588, 1975.

DIABETES IN PREGNANCY

Beard, R. W., and Oakley, N. W.: The fetus of the diabetic. In Beard, R. W., and Nathanielsz, P. W., editors: Fetal physiology and medicine, New York, 1976, W. B. Saunders Co.

Green, J. W.: Diabetes mellitus in pregnancy, Obstet. Gynecol. **46:**6, 1975.

Gugliucci, C. L., O'Sullivan, M. J., Opperman, W., et al.: Intensive care of the pregnant diabetic, Am. J. Obstet. Gynecol. **125:**435, 1976.

Jouganatos, D. M., and Gabbe, S. G.: Diabetes in pregnancy: metabolic changes and current management, J. Am. Diet. Assoc. **73:**168, Aug., 1978.

Karlsson, K., and Kjellmer, I.: The outcome of diabetic pregnancies in relation to mother's blood sugar level, Am. J. Obstet. Gynecol. **112:**213, 1972.

Spearing, G. J.: Diabetes in pregnancy, J. Hum. Nutr. **31:**329, Oct., 1977.

Tsai, A., Rueler, J., and Rubenstein, A.: Diabetes and pregnancy, J. Reprod. Med. **11:**23, 1973.

Tyson, J. E., and Hock, R. A.: Gestational and pregestational diabetes: an approach to therapy, Am. J. Obstet. Gynecol. **125:**1009, 1976.

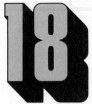

Nutrition for growth and development: infancy, childhood, and adolescence

Growth may essentially be defined as an increase in size. Biologic growth of an organism takes place through cell multiplication. Development is the associated process in which growing tissues and organs take on increased complexity of function. Thus since both processes are part of one whole, the combined terms *growth and development* form a unitary concept that indicates the magnitude and quality of maturational changes.

At birth the newborn infant displays evidence in form and function of the tremendous growth and development that has already taken place during his fetal life. He brings to the beginning of the life cycle the heritage of generations before him and the physical resources provided by the maternal organism. It is upon this heritage and these resources that his total life experience will make an indelible imprint. Therefore the molding of growth and development factors in these early impressionistic years is of vital import.

Physiologic growth is dependent on special chemical nutrients in the food a person eats and the biochemical processes of metabolism that supply the right elements in the right place, at the right time, for the formation and maintenance of body tissues. However, human growth and development involves far more than the physical process alone. It encompasses social and psychologic influences and relationships, the whole of the environment and culture that nurtures the individual growth potential. Food

and feeding during these highly significant years do not, indeed cannot, exist apart from this broader, overall concept of growth and development. The *whole* process produces the *whole* person. This study therefore will use this conceptual approach. Within this framework food and feeding will be considered as a part of the whole development of the child. Age group nutritional needs and the food that supplies them will be adapted to the general psychosocial as well as physical maturation normally achieved at that age. These related questions may be helpful guides for study:

1. What is the normal physical growth pattern for children?
2. In what ways may growth of children be determined? What general nutritional problems do U.S. surveys reveal?
3. What psychosocial problems face the growing child? What related developmental tasks does he learn in each age period? How are these related to food and feeding?
4. What are the basic nutritional needs for normal growth and development of children?
5. How may these combined physical and psychosocial needs in each age group be met in food choices and feeding practices?

Throughout the study it should be remembered that although the discussion is in terms of general needs at a given age level, wide individual variations exist within normal ranges. Thus in the care of children the practitioner should never lose sight of the individual child and his own unique needs and growth potentials.

GROWTH AND DEVELOPMENT

Normal life cycle growth pattern. The normal human life cycle follows four general phases of overall growth.

INFANCY. During the first year the infant grows rapidly, the rate tapering off somewhat in the latter half of the year. At age 6 months he will probably have doubled his birth weight and at 1 year may have tripled it. Thus a baby weighing 3 kg (7 lb) at birth will weigh approximately 6 kg (14 lb) at 6 months and about 9.5 kg (21 lb) at 1 year of age.

LATENT PERIOD OF CHILDHOOD. During the years between infancy and adolescence, the rate of growth slows and becomes erratic. At some periods there are plateaus; at others, small spurts of growth. The overall rate, being erratic, affects appetite accordingly; at times a child will have little or no appetite, and at others he will eat voraciously.

ADOLESCENCE. The second rapid growth spurt occurs during adolescence in association with the manifold physical changes of puberty. Because of the hormonal influences, multiple body changes occur including development of long bones, sex characteristics, and fat and muscle mass.

ADULT. In the final phase of the normal life cycle, growth levels off in the adult plateau and gradually declines during senescence.

Physical growth. There is a wide variance in the physical growth of children. In clinical practice a child's pattern of growth is compared with percentile growth curves derived from measurement of numbers of children throughout the growth years. Formerly used growth charts have not been satisfactory for current use as they were based on data from only two small biased groups of children in Boston (Stuart) and Iowa (Meredith).[1,2] Recently, however, new contemporary growth charts have been developed by the National Center for Health Statistics (NCHS) reflecting growth patterns in children today.[3] These improved charts are based on more valid data from large numbers of a nationally representative sample of children. Two age intervals are used: birth to 36 months and 2 to 18 years, with separate curves for boys and for girls.

By using these NCHS growth charts and other clinical standards as reference, several basic measures of physical growth may be assessed.

WEIGHT AND HEIGHT. Weight and height are the common general measures of physical growth. They form, however, a crude index without giving finer details of individual variations. Generally, as the child's growth is supervised, his weight and height are compared with the percentile measures of weight and height for his age on the growth chart.

BODY MEASUREMENTS. In addition to general weight and height, several body measurements are helpful indicators of growth. These include the recumbent length of the infant and small child as compared with the standing height as he grows older. Also, head circumference is a valuable measure in infants but is seldom taken routinely after 3 years of age. Other circumference measures are those of the chest, the abdomen, and the leg at its maximal girth of the calf. An additional measure is that of pelvic breadth, which is taken with a broad sliding caliper. Other measurements made with calipers may include skin fold thicknesses. Longitudinal growth studies in research centers employ many measures of development (Fig. 18-1).

CLINICAL SIGNS. Various clinical signs of optimal growth may be observed as measures. These include general vitality; a sense of well-being; posture; the condition of gums and teeth, skin, hair, and eyes; development of muscles; and nervous control. A number of these clinical

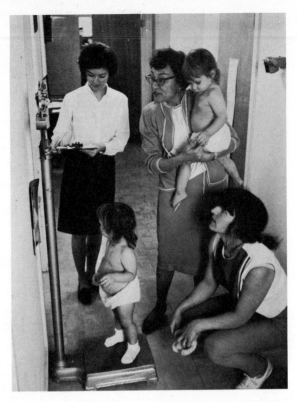

Fig. 18-1. Growth and development study being conducted at the University of California in Berkeley. Here weight of twins in the study is being recorded. Many other measures are taken, some by use of calipers.

signs and observations of nutritional status are summarized in Table 18-1.

LABORATORY DATA. In addition, finer measures are obtained by various laboratory tests. These include studies of blood and urine to determine levels of vitamins, hemoglobin, and so on. X-rays of the bones in the hand and wrists may also be taken to indicate degree of ossification.

NUTRITIONAL ANALYSIS. A measure of the growth of a child may be based on a nutritional analysis of his general eating habits. A diet history form and an analysis chart such as those suggested for use in family diet counseling (pp. 317-318) may be used.

Mental growth. Measures of mental growth

usually involve abilities in communication and the development in ability to handle abstract and symbolic material in thinking. The child originally thinks very literally. As he develops in mental capacity, he increasingly can handle more than single ideas and develop constructive concepts.

Emotional growth. Emotional growth is measured in the capacity for love and affection, the ability to handle frustration and its anxieties, to control aggressive impulses, and to channel hostility from destructive to constructive activities.

Social and cultural growth. Social development of a child is measured in terms of his ability to relate to others and to participate in

Table 18-1. Clinical signs of nutritional status

	Good	Poor
General appearance	Alert, responsive	Listless, apathetic, cachexic
Hair	Shiny, lustrous; healthy scalp	Stringy, dull, brittle, dry, depigmented
Neck (glands)	No enlargement	Thyroid enlarged
Skin (face and neck)	Smooth, slightly moist, good color, reddish pink mucous membranes	Greasy, discolored, scaly
Eyes	Bright, clear; no fatigue circles beneath	Dryness, signs of infection, increased vascularity, glassiness, thickened conjunctiva
Lips	Good color, moist	Dry, scaly, swollen; angular lesions (stomatitis)
Tongue	Good pink color, surface papillae present, no lesions	Papillary atrophy, smooth appearance; swollen, red, beefy (glossitis)
Gums	Good pink color; no swelling or bleeding, firm	Marginal redness or swelling, receding, spongy
Teeth	Straight, no crowding, well-shaped jaw, clean, no discoloration	Unfilled caries, absent teeth, worn surfaces, mottled, malposition
Skin (general)	Smooth, slightly moist, good color	Rough, dry, scaly, pale, pigmented, irritated, petechia, bruises
Abdomen	Flat	Swollen
Legs, feet	No tenderness, weakness, or swelling; good color	Edema, tender calf, tingling, weakness
Skeleton	No malformations	Bowlegs, knock-knees, chest deformity at diaphragm, beaded ribs, prominent scapulae
Weight	Normal for height, age, body build	Overweight or underweight
Posture	Erect, arms and legs straight, abdomen in, chest out	Sagging shoulders, sunken chest, humped back
Muscles	Well developed, firm	Flaccid, poor tone; undeveloped, tender
Nervous control	Good attention span for age; does not cry easily, not irritable or restless	Inattentive, irritable
Gastrointestinal function	Good appetite and digestion; normal, regular elimination	Anorexia, indigestion, constipation or diarrhea
General vitality	Endurance, energetic, sleeps well at night; vigorous	Easily fatigued, no energy, falls asleep in school, looks tired, apathetic

group living in his culture. These social and cultural behaviors he learns first through his relationships with his parents, then with his family. As his horizon broadens, he develops relationships with those outside the family, with friends, and with those in the community. For this reason a child's play in his early years is a highly purposeful activity.

NUTRITIONAL REQUIREMENTS

Calories—total energy needs. During childhood the demand for calories is relatively great. However, there is much variation in need with age and condition. For example, approximately 50% of the 5-year-old's calories are needed for basal metabolic requirements. Another 5% is involved in the specific dynamic action of food, which includes the various metabolic processes involved in the digestion, absorption, and metabolism of food substances. Therefore 55% of his calories are involved in the metabolic activities of basal metabolism and food digestion. Physical activity requires 25% of his calories, growth needs 12%, and 8% is represented in fecal loss. In recent revisions of the National Research Council (NRC) for nutrient recommendations, the caloric allowances were reduced for children. The reduced general activity of children in an industrialized society requires fewer calories. Of these calories, carbohydrate is the main energy source. It is important also as a protein sparer to ensure that protein vital for growth will not be diverted for energy needs. Fat calories are important, although caution should be exercised against an excess. Certain fatty acids are essential, especially linoleic acid. A characteristic eczema has been observed in infants whose diets were deficient in linoleic acid.

Protein. Protein is the *growth element* of the body. It supplies the essential amino acids that are necessary for formation and maintenance of muscle and nerve tissue and bone matrix. Protein also serves as an integral part of most body fluids and secretions such as enzymes, hormones, lymph, and plasma. As stated in the chapter on protein, these essential amino acids have to be supplied in proper amounts, proportion, and timing for tissue protein to be synthesized (p. 60).

The final determinant for the protein requirement of a child is his overall growth pattern. His requirements per unit of body weight gradually decrease. For example, during the first six months of life he requires 2.2 g of protein per kilogram of body weight. This amount relative to body weight gradually decreases until adulthood, when his protein need is 0.8 g/kg of body weight. By and large the healthy, active, growing child will consume his needed amount of calories and proteins in the variety of food provided him.

Water—body content and consumption. Water is second only to oxygen as a prerequisite for life. The human need for water is well estab-

Table 18-2. Approximate daily requirements of children for calories, protein, and water*

Age in years	Calories†		Protein (g/kg‡)	Water †	
	per kg	per lb		ml/kg	oz/lb
Infancy§	110	50	2.0-3.5	150	2¼
1-3	100	45	2.0-2.5	125	2.0–
4-6	90	41	3.0	100	1½
7-9	80	36	2.8	75	1.0+
10-12	70	32	2.0	75	1.0+
13-15	60	27	1.7	50	¾
16-19	50	23	1.5+	50	¾
Adult	40	18	1.0	50	¾

*Nelson, W. E., editor: Textbook of pediatrics, Philadelphia, 1969, W. B. Saunders Co., p. 109.
†At least 10% variation.
‡To convert g/kg to g/lb, divide by 2 and subtract 10% of the quotient. Thus 4 g/kg is equivalent to 1.8 g/lb.
§Needs during the first weeks are lower; during the first six months they are relatively higher than during the last six months.

lished. The infant need, however, is even greater than that of the adult. The infant's body content of water, for example, is from 70% to 75% of his body weight, whereas in the adult, water comprises only from 60% to 65% of the total body weight. Also in the infant a relatively large amount of the total water is outside the cell and thus is more easily lost.

The infant's requirement for water is related to the caloric intake and the specific gravity of the urine. Generally an infant consumes daily an amount of water equivalent to 10% to 15% of his body weight. The adult consumes daily an amount of water equivalent to 2% to 4% of his body weight. The approximate daily requirements of children for water, calories, and protein are outlined in Table 18-2.

Minerals. A number of minerals relate to special body function and are essential in body metabolism. Two minerals particularly vital to the growing child are calcium and iron.

CALCIUM. Calcium is necessary for the rapid bone mineralization that takes place during growth. In the newborn infant only the central sections of large bones are mineralized. An X-ray taken at this time would give the appearance of a collection of disconnected, separate bones. Calcium is also needed for the developing teeth, for muscle contraction, nerve irritability, blood coagulation, and the action of the heart muscle.

IRON. Iron is necessary for the formation of hemoglobin. Iron is also used as a component of several oxidative enzymes. Since the infant's fetal store is diminished in three to four months and his basic food, milk, lacks iron, the infant soon needs solid food additions to supply iron. Such foods as meat, enriched cereal, and egg yolk accomplish this.

Vitamins. In the chapters on vitamins it was learned that a large number are essential for growth and maintenance. In fact the word vitamin refers to their essential character. They were so named because they are necessary to life and play many key roles in body metab-

olism. There are several vitamins for which growth requirements have been set.

VITAMIN A. Vitamin A is a necessary constituent of the substance in the eye, visual purple, that regulates adaptations to light and dark. It is also used in bone and tooth development and in the formation and maturation of epithelial tissues such as the skin, the eye, and in the digestive, respiratory, urinary, and reproductive tracts.

B-COMPLEX VITAMINS. The main B-complex vitamins include thiamin, niacin, and riboflavin.

THIAMIN. Thiamin is directly related to carbohydrate metabolism, hence to caloric intake. As caloric needs increase, thiamin needs increase. It is evident then that thiamin needs accompany the caloric demands for energy. Thiamin function as an important coenzyme factor, especially in the oxidation of pyruvic acid, and therefore is important to energy production for use in body activity and metabolic work. In growth there is increased anabolic activity and increased physical activity, both of which increase energy demands.

NIACIN. Niacin is also an important coenzyme factor in metabolic activities. It is required for cellular oxidation.

RIBOFLAVIN. Riboflavin also acts as a coenzyme factor in metabolism, in reactions involving amino acids and fatty acids as well as carbohydrates. Table 18-3 shows that beginning with the preadolescent period there is a difference in requirements of riboflavin for boys as compared with those for girls. Usually the requirements for boys are greater because of their increasing size and change in muscle mass and body weight.

OTHER B VITAMINS. Several B vitamins are associated with the proper formation of red blood cells and therefore are important during growth. These include cobalamin, pyridoxine, and folic acid.

COBALAMIN (VITAMIN B_{12}). A deficiency of vitamin B_{12} is associated with juvenile pernicious

Table 18-3. Recommended daily dietary allowances for growth (National Research

	Age (yr)	Weight		Height		Energy (kcal)	Protein (g)	Fat-soluble vitamins			
								Vit. A		Vit. D	Vit. E
		kg	lb	cm	in			μg RE	IU	(μg*)	(mgαTE)
Infants	Birth-0.5	6	13	60	24	kg × 115	kg × 2.2	420	1,400	10	3
	0.5-1	9	20	71	28	kg × 105	kg × 2.0	400	2,000	10	4
Children	1-3	13	29	90	35	1,300	23	400	2,000	10	5
	4-6	20	44	112	44	1,700	30	500	2,500	10	6
	7-10	28	62	132	52	2,400	34	700	3,300	10	7
Males	11-14	45	99	157	62	2,700	45	1,000	5,000	10	8
	15-18	66	145	176	69	2,800	56	1,000	5,000	10	10
Females	11-14	46	101	157	62	2,200	46	800	4,000	10	8
	15-18	55	120	163	64	2,100	46	800	4,000	10	8

*As cholecalciferol; 10 μg cholecalciferol = 400 IU vitamin D.

anemia resulting from a defect in the absorption of the vitamin because of an absence of the necessary intrinsic factor in the gastric juice.

PYRIDOXINE (VITAMIN B₆). A deficiency of pyridoxine is associated with nerve and muscle irritability and hypochromic anemia.

FOLIC ACID (FOLACIN). A deficiency of folic acid is associated with megaloblastic anemia, especially in infancy.

VITAMIN C. Vitamin C plays an important role in the growth period in several ways:

1. It participates in the formation of intercellular cement substance in all tissues. In this role vitamin C is especially needed in the rapidly growing tissue of a child.
2. It facilitates the absorption of essential iron.
3. It participates actively in a number of other general metabolic activities including mineralization and enzyme systems. For example, ascorbic acid is probably a coenzyme in the metabolism of phenylalanine and tyrosine, both of which are important amino acids for growth.

VITAMIN D. Vitamin D (cholecalciferol) is essential during growth for the absorption and utilization of calcium and phosphorus needed for bone development. It regulates the absorption of these minerals, probably by affecting the permeability of intestinal membranes. It also aids in the anchoring of the minerals in the bone by regulating the level of serum alkaline phosphatase.

VITAMIN K. Vitamin K is essential in the formation of prothrombin by the liver (p. 97), an initial element in the blood-clotting mechanism. A lack of vitamin K is not usually a dietary problem, because it is synthesized by intestinal microorganisms. However, since the newborn lacks these microorganisms at birth, he is usually given vitamin K to avoid any hemorrhagic tendencies.

VITAMIN E. Although no definitive mechanisms are as yet determined, current research indicates possible growth-associated functions of vitamin E, perhaps in relation to muscle metabolism and to erythrocyte fragility (p. 94).

Council 1980 revision)

	Water-soluble vitamins						Minerals					
Vit. C (mg)	Fola-cin (μg)	Nia-cin (mg)	Ribo-flavin (mg)	Thia-min (mg)	Vit. B_6 (mg)	Vit. B_{12} (μg)	Cal-cium (mg)	Phos-phorus (mg)	Iodine (μg)	Iron (mg)	Mag-nesium (mg)	Zinc (mg)
35	30	6	0.4	0.3	0.3	0.5	360	240	40	10	50	3
35	45	8	0.6	0.5	0.6	1.5	540	360	50	15	70	5
45	100	9	0.8	0.7	0.9	2.0	800	800	70	15	150	10
45	200	11	1.0	0.9	1.3	2.5	800	800	90	10	200	10
45	300	16	1.4	1.2	1.6	3.0	800	800	120	10	250	10
50	400	18	1.6	1.4	1.8	3.0	1,200	1,200	150	18	350	15
60	400	18	1.7	1.4	2.0	3.0	1,200	1,200	150	18	400	15
50	400	15	1.3	1.1	1.8	3.0	1,200	1,200	150	18	300	15
60	400	14	1.3	1.1	2.0	3.0	1,200	1,200	150	18	300	15

Hypervitaminoses A and D. Hypervitaminoses A and D (pp. 90 and 93) are possibilities when excess amounts of the vitamins are given for prolonged periods because of a misunderstanding, ignorance, or carelessness. Parents should be counseled to use only the amount directed and no more. Symptoms of toxicity from excess vitamin A include anorexia, slow growth, drying and cracking of the skin, enlargement of the liver and the spleen, swelling and pain of long bones, and bone fragility. Symptoms of toxicity from excess vitamin D include nausea, diarrhea, weight loss, polyuria, nocturia, and eventually calcification of soft tissues, including those of renal tubules, blood vessels, bronchi, stomach, and heart.

Summary of nutritional needs. A summary of the nutritional needs for growth is presented in Table 18-3, as recommended by the NRC in their 1980 revisions. Since the original publication of these recommendations in 1943, the NRC has made seven revisions as new knowledge has been gained from research. In Table 18-3 a summary of the 1980 dietary allowances is given for study. In the allowances of protein the recommendations are based on basal calorie requirements, the generally good quality of protein in an average American diet, with appropriate increments for growth on the basis that gain in body weight is 18% protein. Some allowance is then added to cover individual variability within a large population.

These overall allowances include safety margins to cover individual variations in healthy, normal children. As such they are *guidelines* for needed amounts of nutrients that can be attained with a variety of common foods.

AGE GROUP NEEDS

Throughout the human life cycle, food and feeding not only serve to meet nutritional requirements for growth and physical maintenance, but they also relate intimately to personal psychosocial development. The nutritional age group needs of children cannot be understood apart from the child's overall maturation as a person. Erik Erikson[4-6] has contributed much insight to an understanding of this pattern of human growth and its critical periods of development. Erikson has identified eight stages in man's growth, and a basic psychosocial problem or crisis with which one struggles at each stage. The developmental problem at each stage has a positive ego value and a conflicting negative counterpart:

Infancy—trust versus distrust

Toddler—autonomy versus shame and doubt

Preschooler—initiative versus guilt

School-aged child—industry versus inferiority

Adolescent—identity versus role confusion

Young adult—intimacy versus isolation

Adult—generativity versus stagnation

Old age—ego integrity versus despair

Given favorable circumstances a growing child develops the positive aspect of his developmental problem at each life stage and therefore builds increasing strength to meet the next crisis. However, the struggle at any age is not forever won at that point. A residue of the negative remains, and in periods of stress, such as during illness, regression in some degree usually occurs. But as the child gains mastery at each stage of development, assisted by significant relationships of a positive nature surrounding him, integration of self-controls takes place. Various related developmental tasks surround each of these stages and its core problem. These are learnings that when accomplished contribute to successful resolution of the core problem. Therefore these developmental tasks are integrated and associated with the normal physical maturation at that point. In each of these stages of childhood, food choices and feeding practices are related to the general age group characteristics.

Infancy (birth to 1 year)
The premature infant

Physical characteristics. Although premature infants vary in weight and development, a child is usually considered premature if he is born at fewer than 270 days of gestation or if he weighs less than 2,500 g (5.5 lb). The premature infant lacks the nutritional and developmental resources provided in the final weeks of normal gestation. Thus he faces survival hazards. He is a fragile, unfinished product. He has much more water and less protein and minerals per kilogram of body weight than the full-term baby. There is little subcutaneous fat, and his bones are poorly calcified. The neuromuscular system is incompletely developed, making normal sucking reflexes weak or absent. The digestive ability and renal function may be limited. The immature liver lacks adequate iron stores and developed metabolic enzyme systems.

Food and feeding. Despite these handicaps, however, relatively simple feeding routines are usually effective, and good growth may be expected if the child is also kept warm and free from infection.

TYPE OF MILK. Breast milk alone is seldom adequate because it lacks sufficient protein for the rapid growth of the premature infant. Fat is poorly tolerated because of the immature digestive apparatus. Therefore the usual milk of choice is skimmed or partially skimmed diluted cow's milk with added carbohydrate as needed. This may be supplemented by breast milk should the mother desire. Until the infant is strong enough to nurse at the mother's breast, the milk may be expressed manually or with a common hand breast pump. Feedings are usually delayed 24 to 36 hours following birth. The comparative inactivity and low heat production of the infant plus his relatively large body water content reduce his immediate need for calories. Also his weakness and the danger of aspiration make some feeding delay advisable. The first feedings are usually sterile 5% to 10% solutions of glucose in water. A few milliliters are given at frequent intervals, gradually building up the amount and adding small amounts of milk formula.

Generally one needs to proceed more slowly with smaller infants and never to hurry with any. Usually by the time an infant is a week old, he should be receiving about 25 to 30 calories per kilogram—approximately 30 ml of formula per kilogram per day (50 to 60 calories per pound—approximately 2½ oz of formula per pound per day). There is increased need for supplement of vitamins C and D; approximately 35 to 50 mg of ascorbic acid and 500 to 1,000 IU of vitamin D are usually given during the second and third weeks respectively, depending on individual need. Ascorbic acid is needed for the intermediate metabolism of phenylalanine, an amino acid essential to growth. Vitamin D is needed for the rapid mineralization of bones.

Methods of feeding will vary with the infant's strength and the nurse's experience. The feedings may be given by medicine dropper, by bottle with a soft nipple having larger than usual holes, or by gavage. Care must be taken in all methods to avoid aspiration. This is especially true with the gavage method. A small soft plastic tube with a rounded tip is used in gavage feeding to avoid tissue trauma, and there are two holes on either side of the tip. The tube is passed through the nose until 2.5 cm (1 in) of the lower end is in the stomach. Proper depth placement in the stomach is guided by markings on the tube made according to the measure of the individual infant. Correct anatomic placement is tested by placing the free end in water. If bubbles appear in the water, the tube is in the trachea. It should be withdrawn immediately and reinserted. Careful control of amount of feeding and rate of flow is necessary.

An excellent review of the nutritional needs of premature and low-birth-weight infants has been provided by the Committee on Nutrition of the American Academy of Pediatrics.[7]

The full-term infant

Physical characteristics. The growth rate during infancy is rapid. Consequently energy requirements are high. The full-term infant has the ability to digest and absorb proteins, a moderate amount of fat, and simple carbohydrates. He has some difficulty with starch since amylase, the starch-splitting enzyme, is not being produced. However, as starch is intro-duced, this enzyme functions. His renal system functions well, but he needs more water relative to his size than an adult does to manage renal excretion. Teeth do not erupt until about the fourth month, so his initial food is liquid or semiliquid. He has limited nutritional stores from gestation, especially in iron; therefore he needs supplements of vitamins and minerals, first in concentrate and later in solid food additions to his milk. The *newborn's rooting reflex* and his somewhat recessed lower jaw are natural adaptations for feeding at the breast.

Psychosocial development. The core psychosocial problem in infancy is the development of *trust versus distrust*. Feeding is his main means of establishing human relationships. The close mother-infant relationship in the feeding process fills his basic need to build trust. The need for sucking and the development of oral organs, lips and mouth, as sensory organs represent adaptations to ensure an adequate early food intake. As a result food becomes the infant's general means of exploring his environment. As muscular coordination involving the tongue and the swallowing reflex develops, he will gradually learn to eat a variety of semisolid foods when they are started at about 6 months of age. As he grows he will begin to evidence a desire to help feed himself. If his needs for food and love are fulfilled in this early relationship with the mother and in broadening relationships with other family members, trust is developed. He evidences this trust by an increasing capacity to wait for his feedings while they are being prepared.

Breast feeding. The ideal food for the young infant, certainly for the first six months of life, is human milk. It has specific characteristics that match the infant's nutritional requirements during the first year of life.[8-10] The process of breast feeding today, as in times past, is successfully initiated and maintained by 99% of women who try.[11]

The female breasts, or mammary glands, are highly specialized secretory organs. They are composed of glandular tissue, fat, and connective tissue. The glandular tissue is composed of 15 to 20 lobes, each containing many smaller units called *lobules*. In the lobules, secretory cells called *alveoli* or *acini* form milk from the materials supplied to them by a rich capillary system in the connective tissue. During pregnancy the breast is prepared for lactation. The alveoli enlarge and multiply and toward the end of the prenatal period secrete a thin yellowish fluid called *colostrum*. After delivery the breast secretion is colostrum for two to four days (10 to 40 ml a day) until milk production begins about the third day. This colostrum provides some initial nutrition for the infant. It contains more protein and minerals than breast milk but less carbohydrate and fat. It is also thought to impart helpful antibodies to the newborn.

The first milk is a transition form from colostrum; it gradually assumes the composition and form of mature breast milk by the third or fourth week. Milk is produced under the stimulation of a hormone, *prolactin,* produced by the anterior pituitary gland. After the milk is formed in the mammary lobules by the clusters of secretory cells (the acini or alveoli), it is carried through converging branches of the lactiferous ducts to reservoir spaces under the *areola,* the pigmented area of the skin surrounding the nipple. These reservoir spaces for the milk are called *ampullae*. From 15 to 20 excretory lactiferous ducts carry the milk from the ampullae out the surface of the nipple. Other pituitary hormones, principally *oxytocin* and to a lesser extent *vasopressin,* stimulate the ejections of the milk from the aveloli to the ducts, releasing it so the baby can obtain it. This is commonly called the let down reflex. It causes a tingling sensation in the breast and the flow of milk. The initial sucking of the baby stimulates this reflex.

FEEDING TECHNIQUES. The rooting reflex of the newborn, his oral needs for sucking, and his basic hunger drive usually make breast feeding simple for the healthy relaxed mother who is nutritionally sustained by an adequate diet for milk production. Several suggestions to the

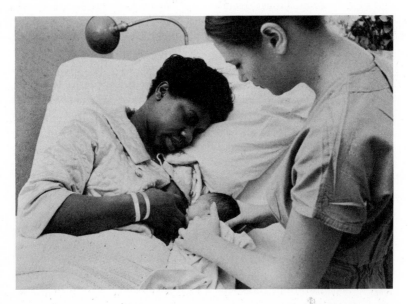

Fig. 18-2. Breast feeding the newborn infant. Note that the nurse, in assisting the mother, avoids touching the infant's outer cheek so as not to counteract his natural rooting reflex at the touch of the breast.

mother who chooses to nurse her baby may be helpful.

1. She should assume the position that is most relaxing. It may be reclining in bed initially (Fig. 18-2). Later a rocker or other comfortable chair with arm support and a low foot stool usually provide support.

2. The baby should be cradled in her arms in a semireclining position against the breast. The warm touch of the breast on his cheek will stimulate the natural rooting reflex, causing him to turn his head *toward* the direction of the touch and to begin sucking motions with his mouth. Therefore his outer cheek should not be touched with the hand in an effort to turn his head toward the breast. This only confuses him; the reflex causes him to turn his head away from the breast toward the hand.

3. The baby should grasp most of the areola in his mouth, not merely the outer tip of the nipple. This wider grasp compresses the ampullae underneath the areola and expresses the milk. If he grasps only the tip of the nipple, his mouth will clamp off the milk flow instead and may cause nipple irritation.

4. In the beginning both breasts may be used at one feeding. After lactation is established, probably alternate breasts will be used for each feeding.

5. Usually a hungry infant will get his fill of milk in about the first five minutes of nursing, but he may continue for some 20 minutes. He has had a sufficient amount and is obviously satisfied when he stops nursing and is disinterested in more.

6. Feedings may be given according to the hunger needs of the baby. Usually these will be at closer intervals for the newborn, perhaps every two to three hours. About three- to four-hour intervals will suffice as he develops.

7. After each feeding the baby should be held erect on the mother's shoulder to allow him to expel swallowed air. Sometimes this is necessary during the feeding also or after he has been back in his crib.

8. After lactation is established, an occasional bottle feeding may replace the breast feeding if the mother desires or has need to be away.

9. No particular food per se in the mother's diet influences milk production or disturbs the infant. The mother's basic needs are for specific nutrients and fluids as outlined in the lactation diet on pp. 383 and 390.

CARE OF THE BREASTS. A properly fitting brassiere should be worn day and night to provide adequate support. It should be changed daily to a clean one. A folded clean white cloth or disposable pad placed inside the brassiere will absorb any milk that may leak between feedings. Plastic brassiere liners should be avoided because they curtail air circulation and prevent adequate drying of the nipple area.

Plain water is best for cleansing. Soap and alcohol are too drying; boric acid should not be used. The nipples should be dried well.

If difficulty with nipples should occur (cracking or infection), the milk may be expressed with a hand breast pump and fed to the baby in bottles for a few days until the nipples heal. A nipple shield is sometimes satisfactorily used while healing occurs.

The advantages of breast feeding and guidance for lactating mothers have been outlined in depth by Taylor and Worthington.[12] An understanding of these advantages should serve to develop an increasing support for breast feeding among professionals and mothers alike.

Bottle feeding. Artificial feeding of cow's milk formula by bottle may be preferred by some mothers. A comparison of the composition of human milk and cow's milk gives the basis for the formula ingredients, since the objective is to modify the cow's milk to make its nutrient proportions similar to those in human milk. The basic differences in protein, carbohydrate, and minerals are shown in Table 18-4.

Cow's milk contains about twice as much protein and about six times as much mineral matter as does human milk. This is not surpris-

Table 18-4. Comparison of human milk and cow's milk*

	Human milk	Whole cow's milk
Water (%)	87-88	83-88
Protein (%)	1.0-1.5	3.2-4.1
Lactalbumin	0.7-0.8	0.5
Casein	0.4-0.5	3.0
Sugar (lactose) (%)	6.5-7.5	4.5-5.0
Fat (%)	3.5-4.0	3.5-5.2
	(more oleic acid and fewer of the volatile fatty acids)	
Minerals (%)	0.15-0.25	0.7-0.75
Calcium	0.034-0.045	0.179-0.222
Phosphorus	0.015-0.04	0.09-0.196
Magnesium	0.005-0.006	0.013-0.019
Sodium	0.011-0.019	0.05-0.06
Potassium	0.048-0.065	0.138-0.172
Iron	0.0001	0.00004
Vitamins (per deciliter)		
A (IU)	60-500	80-220[†]
D (IU)	0.4-10.0	0.3-4.4[†] (+400/L [1 qt])
C (IU)	1.2-10.8	0.9-1.4[†]
Thiamin (mg)	0.002-0.036	0.03-0.04[†]
Riboflavin (mg)	0.015-0.080	0.10-0.26[†]
Niacin (mg)	0.10-0.20	0.10
Digestion		Occurs less rapidly
Emptying of stomach		Occurs less rapidly
Curd	Soft, flacculent	Hard, large
Calories per 30 ml (1 oz)	20	29

*Adapted from Nelson, W. E., editor: Textbook of pediatrics, Philadelphia, 1969, W. B. Saunders Co., p. 135. (Data assembled from a number of sources.)
†Pasteurized.

ing because the growth rate of the calf, for whom cow's milk was intended, is much greater than that of the infant. The calf is running about shortly after birth and reaches maturity in a matter of months, whereas it takes a year to get a human offspring on his feet and years more for him to reach full physical growth. Human milk, on the other hand, has more carbohydrate than cow's milk. Therefore for use in infant feeding the cow's milk is modified in two ways. It is diluted with water to re- duce the protein and mineral salts, and it is mixed with a simple sugar to increase the carbohydrate content. The sugar may be in the form of corn syrup, granulated sugar, or a special sugar for infants such as Dextrimaltose. A basic 24-hour formula pattern is given in Table 18-5.

FORMULA PREPARATION AND STERILIZATION. Keeping the area of preparation, the utensils, and the hands clean is simple initial sanitation. The clean utensils and the ingredients should

Table 18-5. Basic 24-hour formula

Age	Milliliters of whole milk per kilogram body weight per day	Ounces of whole milk per pound body weight per day	Sugar*	Water
First 2 weeks	22	1½ (¾ oz evap.)	14 g (½ oz; 1 tbsp)†	Add amount neces-
2 weeks to 2 months	22-30	1½ to 2 (1 oz evap.)	21-28 g (¾-1 oz; 2 tbsp)†	sary to bring total solution to
After 2 months	30	2 (1 oz evap.)	28 g (1 oz; 2 tbsp)†	amount required

*May be granulated, corn syrup, or malt-dextrin preparation.
†2 tbsp granulated sugar or corn syrup = 28 g (1 oz); 4 tbsp Dextrimaltose = 28 g (1 oz).

Table 18-6. Suggested schedule on an approximate four-hour basis

Age	Milliliters per feeding	Ounces per feeding	Number of feedings	Time of feedings
1 week	60-90	2 to 3	6	6, 10, 2, 6, 10, 2
2-4 weeks	90-150	3 to 5	6	6, 10, 2, 6, 10, 2
2-3 months	120-180	4 to 6	5	6, 10, 2, 6, 10
4-5 months	150-210	5 to 7	5	6, 10, 2, 6, 10
6-7 months	210-240	7 to 8	4	6, 10, 2, 6
8-12 months	240*	8	3	7, 12, 6

*120 ml (4 oz) milk may be given midafternoon.

be assembled. Canned evaporated milk is commonly used with a simple sugar such as corn syrup for making a home formula. Tap water in the indicated amount is added to the correct amount of sugar and milk. After the formula has been measured and mixed, it is poured into clean bottles in the amount needed for each feeding. The bottles are capped and sterilized according to direction. The terminal method of sterilization is usually preferred because it is simpler than the aseptic technique and is less likely to permit contamination in handling. In the so-called aseptic technique the equipment is sterilized first. The formula is made in a sterile container with boiled water, then poured into sterile bottles. It is highly doubtful that in the average kitchen this technique would actually be aseptic.

More often today a commercial formula may be used rather than a home-prepared one when the bottle-feeding method is chosen by the mother. A number of such products are marketed, so care should be taken in selection and use.

FEEDING TECHNIQUES. The child should be cradled in the arm as in breast feeding. The close human touch and warmth are important. The bottle should be inclined to keep the nipple

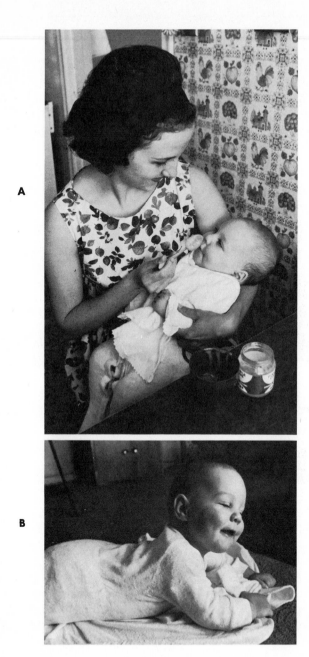

Fig. 18-3. A, This 6-month-old boy is beginning to take a variety of solid food additions and is developing wide tastes. Here feeding has become a bond of relationship between mother and child and is serving not only as a source of physical growth but also of psychosocial development. **B,** Optimum physical development and security are evident, the result of sound nutrition and loving care.

filled with milk to minimize the swallowing of air.

When the infant is obviously satisfied, he should not be forced to accept more milk, regardless of the amount remaining in the bottle. Often the roots of childhood obesity may lie in such forced feeding practices. A healthy infant will take what he needs; he should be the guide. A suggested schedule of feedings is given in Table 18-6.

After the infant has been fed, he should be held erect against the mother's shoulder to expel any swallowed air.

Solid food additions. Today nutritional and medical authorities are generally agreed that for the first six months of life the optimal single food for the infant is human milk, with solid foods being added as supplementary nutrition after 6 months of age. Until that time the infant does not need any additional foods nor is he

Table 18-7. Guideline for addition of solid foods to infant's diet during the first year*

When to start	Foods added	Feeding
First month	Vitamins A, D, and C in multivitamin preparation (according to prescription)	Once daily at a feeding time
Fifth to sixth month	Cereal and strained cooked fruit	10 AM and 6 PM
	Egg yolk (at first, hard boiled and sieved, soft boiled or poached later)	
	Strained cooked vegetable and strained meat	2 PM
	Zweiback or hard toast	At any feeding
Seventh to ninth month	Meat: beef, lamb, or liver (broiled or baked and finely chopped)	10 AM or 6 PM
	Potato: baked or boiled and mashed or sieved	
Suggested meal plan for age 8 months to 1 year or older		
7 AM	Milk	240 ml (8 oz)
	Cereal	2-3 tbsp
	Strained fruit	2-3 tbsp
	Zweiback or dry toast	
12 NOON	Milk	240 ml (8 oz)
	Vegetables	2-3 tbsp
	Chopped meat or one whole egg	
	Puddings or cooked fruit	2-3 tbsp
3 PM	Milk	120 ml (4 oz)
	Toast, zweiback, or crackers	
6 PM	Milk	240 ml (8 oz)
	Whole egg or chopped meat	
	Potato, baked or mashed	2 tbsp
	Pudding or cooked fruit	2-3 tbsp
	Zweiback or toast	

*Semisolid foods should be given immediately before milk feeeding. One or two teaspoons should be given at first. If food is accepted and tolerated well, the amount should be increased to 1 to 2 tbsp per feeding.
Note: Banana or cottage cheese may be used as substitution for any meal.

fully able to handle them. On the contrary, such early excess feeding contributes frequently to childhood obesity.

When solid foods are added to the infant's diet, beginning at about 6 months of age, there is no one specific sequence of food additions that must be followed. Individual responses and needs may be a basis for choices, with food becoming a source of enjoyment and bonding of warm family relationships (Fig. 18-3). Although a variety of commercial baby foods are available, some mothers choose to prepare their own. This can easily be done by cooking and straining vegetables and fruits, freezing a batch at a time in ice cube trays, then storing the cubes in plastic bags in the freezer. A single cube can then be reheated conveniently for use at a feeding. Cereals are usually added first with a little milk, then fruits and vegetables, egg, potato, and meat. Small amounts are given initially and are usually offered before the milk feeding. Over time the child will be introduced to a wide variety of foods and develop an enjoyment of a large number of them.

In general, then, two factors seem to be guiding principles. *Necessary nutrients* are the needs, not any one food per se. The general direction of a physician to a mother that she give her child "table foods" without exploration of what "table food" at home is may be giving an unwise prescription, depending on the level of the household hygiene or the family food pattern. Some more specific individual assessment and guidance may be indicated. *Food is a basis of learning.* Theoretically, if additional nutrients in concentrated form were given to the child, he could get along well only on milk during his infancy. However, food serves not only for physical sustenance but also supplies other personal and cultural needs. The addition of foods characteristic of a culture is a basis of teaching a cultural pattern of eating. On this foundation the child will continue to base his food habits. Good food habits begin early in life and may be continued as the child grows older.

A guideline for the addition of solid foods to the infant's diet is given in Table 18-7. Individual practices will vary widely around this sequence. By the time a child is approximately 8 or 9 months old, he should have attained a fairly good ability to eat so-called family foods, chopped, cooked foods, simply seasoned, without recourse to a large number of special infant foods.

Childhood
Toddler (1 to 3 years)

Physical characteristics and growth. Following the first year the child's growth rate slows. Although his rate of gain is less, the pattern of growth produces significant changes in his body form. His legs become longer. He begins losing his baby fat. There is less body water and more water in the cells. He begins to look and feel less like a baby and more like a child. There are fewer energy demands because of the slackened growth. However, important muscle development takes place. Muscle mass development accounts for about one half of the total gain during this period. As the child begins to walk and stand erect, more muscle is needed to strengthen the body. There is special need, for example, for big muscles of the back, the buttocks, and the thighs. The overall rate of skeletal growth slows, but there is more deposit of mineral rather than great lengthening of bones. The increased mineralization strengthens the bones to support the increasing weight. The child has six to eight teeth at the beginning of the toddler period. Most of his deciduous teeth have erupted by the time he is 3 years of age.

Psychosocial development. The toddler's psychosocial development is pronounced. The core problem with which he struggles is the conflict between *autonomy and shame.* He has an increasing sense of self—of "I"—of being a person, distinct and individual, apart from his mother, not just an extension of her. As his physical mobility increases, he has an increasing sense of independence. His growing curiosity leads to much exploration of his environment. Increasingly his mouth is his means of exploring. Touch is important to him. It is his means of learning what objects are like. Often his constant use of ''no'' is not perverse negativism as much as it is his struggle with his ego needs in conflict with his mother's efforts to control him. He wants to do more and more for himself, and his attention span is fairly short because of his increasing diversion of interest to other things around him.

Food and feeding. Calorie needs are not high during the toddler age. They increase very slowly; an increase of only 300 to 500 calories is required over the two-year span. At about 1 year of age he needs approximately 1,000 calories, and only 1,300 to 1,500 calories by the time he is 3 years old. From age 1 to 2 some children do not eat as many calories as they did in the second half of infancy. Knowledge of the child's decreased need for calories and of his struggle for autonomy, which often involves refusal of food, will help a mother avoid conflict with a toddler about eating.

Protein needs are relatively large in comparison to caloric needs. The child requires about 450 mg of protein per kilogram of body weight (1 g/lb). There is rapid growth of muscle and other body tissues. At least half of this protein should be of animal origin, since animal protein has high biologic value. Calcium and phosphorus are also needed for bone mineralization. The bones are strengthening to keep pace with the muscle development and increasing activity. Two to three cups of milk are sufficient for the child's needs. Sometimes excess milk intake, a habit carried over from infancy, may exclude some solid foods from the diet. As a result the child may be lacking iron and develop a ''milk anemia.'' On the other hand, a child may dislike milk, and milk solids may be used in soups, custards, or puddings, and dry milk can be used in cereals, mashed potatoes, meat loaf, and so on. A variety of food should be offered the child, avoiding an emphasis on refined sweets.

These should be reserved for special occasions, not for habitual use or bribe mechanisms to get a child to eat.

In summary two factors are important for the mother to know, understand, and practice during this period: (1) The child needs fewer calories but more protein and mineral matter for growth. Hence a variety of foods should be offered in smaller amounts to provide key nutrients. (2) The child is struggling for autonomy. This struggle often takes the form of refusal of food and a desire to do things for himself before he is fully able to do them completely. If the mother offers a variety of foods in small amounts and supports and encourages some degree of food choice and self-feeding in the child's own ceremonial manner, eating can be a pleasant, positive means of development. It can help satisfy his growing need for independence and his desire for ritual. The mother needs to maintain a calm, relaxed attitude of sympathetic interest, to understand his struggle and give help where needed, but to avoid both overprotection and excessive rigidity.

Preschool child (3 to 6 years)

Physical characteristics and growth. Physical growth continues in spurts. On occasion the child bounds with energy; his play is hard play—running, jumping, testing new physical resources. At other times he will sit for increasing periods of time engrossed in passive types of activities. His mental capacities are developing. He is doing more thinking and is exploring his environment. Specific nutrients need emphasis.

Protein requirements continue to be relatively high. The preschool child needs about 30 g of good quality protein daily, such as is found in milk, meat, egg, and cheese. He continues to need calcium and iron for storage. Since U.S. surveys indicate that vitamins A and C are likely to be lacking in the diets of preschool and growing children, a variety of fruits and vegetables should be provided.

Psychosocial development. Each age period builds on the previous one. The toddler who has been given the physical and psychosocial resources by understanding and able parents has a foundation on which the preschool period builds. The child is continuing to form life patterns in attitudes and basic eating habits as a result of his social and emotional experiences. The twofold guiding principle for parents remains the same—to provide the right food to meet physical needs and the right climate to promote and support social and emotional growth.

The core problem with which the preschool child struggles during these ages is essentially that of *initiative versus guilt*. He is beginning to develop the superego (the conscience). As his powers of locomotion increase, he has increasing imagination and curiosity. This very capacity often leads him into troubled feelings about this changing attitudes, especially toward his parents. This is a period of increasing imitation and of sex identification. The little boy will imitate the father. The little girl will imitate the mother. In their play, much of this becomes evident in the use of grown-up clothes and role playing in domestic stituations. Eating therefore assumes greater social aspects. The family meal time is an important means of this socialization and sex identification The children imitate their parents and others at the table. Depending upon the example of the parents and other family members, this may be negative rather than positive training.

Food and feeding. Of all the food groups, vegetables usually are less well liked by most children, yet they contain vitamins and minerals needed for growth. Consideration given to the way they are prepared and served is valuable. Children like crisp raw vegetables better than cooked ones. They have a keen sense of taste. Flavor and texture are important. They usually dislike strong vegetables such as cabbage and onions. Tough strings cause problems. Tough parts are hard to manage and should be removed. For example, it is easy to break a crisp piece of celery and remove the strings before giving it to the child. Children also react to consistency of vegetables. Because they prefer their foods lukewarm, some foods may remain on their plates and become dry and gummy and hence are refused. Children usually prefer single foods to combination dishes such as casseroles or stews. In such combinations the foods lose their identity, and flavors are intermingled. The child prefers a single food that he can identify and that has retained its characteristic texture, color, and form. He likes food he can eat with his fingers. Frequently when appetites lag, fruit may be substituted for vegetables. Often a variety of raw fruit and raw vegetables cut in finger-size pieces and offered to a child for his own selection provides a resource of needed nutrition. Fruit in a gelatin base is usually liked, and if a child has a choice in selecting the color of the gelatin, often it is accepted more readily.

Because of his developing social and emotional needs, the preschool child frequently follows food jags that may last for several days. However, this is usually short lived and of no major concern.

It is helpful when the child can set his own goals in quantity of foods. His portions need to be relatively small. Often if he can pour his own milk from a small pitcher into a small glass, he consumes a greater amount. The quantity of milk needed usually declines during these years. The child will consume 2 to 3, rarely 4, cups of milk during the day. Smaller children like their milk more lukewarm, not icy cold. Also, they prefer it in small glasses that hold about ½ to ¾ of a cup, rather than in large adult-size glasses. Meat should be tender, easy to chew or cut; hence ground meat is popular.

The preschool period is one of increasing growth for the child. Lifetime food habits are forming. Food continues to play an important part in developing his personality. Group eating becomes significant as a means of socialization. The child learns to control strong dislikes at the family table or in group situations away from home. He may be involved in nursery or play-school situations in which he eats with other children. Here he learns a widening variety of food habits and forms new social relationships.

School-age child (6 to 12 years)

Physical characteristics and growth. The school-age period has been called the latent period of growth. The rate of growth slows, and body changes occur gradually. Resources, however, are being laid down for the growth needs to come in the adolescent period; sometimes it has been called the lull before the storm. By now the body type is established. Growth rates will vary widely within this period. Girls usually outdistance boys by the latter part of the period.

Psychosocial development. The core problem with which the child struggles during these years is the tension between *industry and inferiority*. There is increasing mental development and ability to work out problems. With widening horizons, new school experiences, and challenging learning opportunities the child is involved in activities that develop his sense of adequacy and accomplishment. He develops his ability to cooperate in group activities. He begins moving from a dependence on parental standards toward standards of his peers in preparation for his own coming maturity. Pressures are generated for self-control of his changing body. These pressures produce changes in previously learned habits, and the negative attitudes that are sometimes asserted are but evidence of these struggles for growing independence. There is a temporary disorganization of previous learning and developed personality, a sort of loosening up of the personality pattern for the inevitable changes ahead in adolescence. A number of years ago an insightful observer[13] called the latter part of this period the "soaking the beans before you cook them." It is a diffuse period of gangs, of cliques, of hero worship, of pensive day dreaming, of emotional stresses, of learning to get along with other children.

Food and feeding. The slowed rate of growth during this latent period results in a gradual decline in the food requirement per unit of body weight. This decline continues up to the latter part of the period, when there is a gradual increase in need because reserves are being laid down for the demands of the approaching adolescent period. Likes and dislikes are a product of earlier years and continue in patterns set previously. Family attitudes are imitated. There is an increasing interest and participation in other activities, which compete with mealtimes. The breakfast meal may be inadequate for the young child whose growth and developmental maturation lead a working mother to give the child more responsibility, often leaving him alone to prepare food for himself. In such situations, meals are makeshift or nonexistent. The school lunch program provides a nourishing noon meal for many children who would not otherwise have one. Midafternoon snacking is common. The snack may be sweets of empty calories, or it may be an opportunity for additional needed nourishment.

Food behavior reflects the child's developmental changes. Manners and punctuality at meals sometimes are a family problem. The source of conflict usually comes from unrealistic parental expectations, expecting adult manners from a child. Too often parents may seek to train children by constant correction at the table, rather than setting the example in their own behavior. In these years of imitation, children learn more from a good example lived before them daily than from constant negative fault finding or correction. Such a negative approach is hurtful in the child's struggle against inferiority feelings, especially when it occurs before people who are significant to the child—his teacher or his peers. Often, however, the school-age child has increasing exposure to positive learning opportunities in the classroom, where nutrition is integrated in other activities. Also he can observe many food attitudes and taste new foods in a group school lunch program that he may not accept otherwise.

Adolescence (12 to 18 years)

Physical characteristics and growth. During the adolescent period, with the onset of puberty, the final growth spurt of childhood occurs. Maturation during this period varies so widely that chronologic age as a reference point for discussing growth ceases to be useful, if indeed it ever was. *Physiologic age* becomes more important in dealing with individual boys and girls. It accounts for wide fluctuations in metabolic rates, in food requirements, in scholastic capacity, and even in illness. These capacities can be more realistically viewed only in physiologic growth terms.

The body changes in the adolescent period result from hormonal influences regulating the development of the sex characteristics. The rate at which these changes occur varies widely and is particularly distinct in growth patterns that emerge between the sexes. A 13-year-old girl, for example, who is past puberty is about two years ahead of a boy the same age in development—sometimes she feels as if it were five.

Other physical growth differences emerge

Table 18-8. Tool for summarizing growth and development needs of children

Age group	Core psychosocial problem	Growth and development characteristics	Food and feeding
Infant (Birth to 1 yr)	Trust vs. distrust		
Toddler (1-3 yr)	Autonomy vs. shame and doubt		
Preschool child (3-6 yr)	Initiative vs. guilt		
School-age child (6-12 yr)	Industry vs. inferiority		
Adolescent (12-18 yr)	Identity vs. diffusion		

Table 18-9. Food intake for good nutrition according to food groups and the average size of servings at different age levels*

Food group	Servings per day	Average size of servings at each age level					
		1 year	2-3 years	4-5 years	6-9 years	10-12 years	13-15 years
Milk and cheese (1.5 oz cheese = 1 cup milk)	4	½ cup	½-¾ cups	¾ cup	¾-1 cup	1 cup	1 cup
Meat group (protein foods)	At least 3						
Egg		1 egg	1 egg	1 egg	1 egg	1 egg	1 egg
Lean meat, fish, poultry (liver once a week)		2 tbsp	2 tbsp	4 tbsp	2-3 oz (4-6 tbsp)	3-4 oz	4 oz or more
Peanut butter		1 tbsp	1 tbsp	2 tbsp	2-3 tbsp	3 tbsp	3 tbsp
Fruits and vegetables	At least 4, including:						
Vitamin C source (citrus fruit, berries, tomato, cabbage, cantaloupe)	1 or more (twice as much tomato as citrus)	⅓ cup citrus	½ cup	½ cup	1 med. orange	1 med. orange	1 med. orange
Vitamin A source (green or yellow fruits and vegetables)	1 or more	2 tbsp	3 tbsp	4 tbsp (¼ cup)	¼ cup	⅓ cup	¾ cup
Other vegetables (potato, legumes) or	2 or more	2 tbsp	3 tbsp	4 tbsp	⅓ cup	½ cup	¾ cup
Other fruits (apple, banana)		¼ cup	⅓ cup	½ cup	1 medium	1 medium	1 medium
Cereals (whole grain or enriched)	At least 4						
Bread		½ slice	1 slice	1½ slices	1-2 slices	2 slices	2 slices
Ready-to-eat cereals		½ oz	¾ oz	1 oz	1 oz	1 oz	1 oz
Cooked cereal (including pastes, rice, etc.)		¼ cup	⅓ cup	½ cup	½ cup	¾ cup	1 cup or more
Fats and carbohydrates	To meet caloric needs						
Butter, margarine, mayonnaise, oils: 1 tbsp = 100 calories		1 tbsp	1 tbsp	1 tbsp	2 tbsp	2 tbsp	2-4 tbsp
Desserts and sweets 100 calorie portions: ⅓ cup pudding or ice cream, Two 3-inch cookies. 1 oz cake, 1⅓ oz pie, 2 tbsp jelly, jam, honey, sugar		1 portion	1½ portions	1½ portions	3 portions	3 portions	3 to 6 portions

*Bennett, M., and Hansen, A.: Nutritional requirements. In Nelson, W., editor: Textbook of pediatrics, Philadelphia, 1969, W. B. Saunders Co., p. 123.

between the sexes. In the girl there is an increasing amount of subcutaneous fat deposit, particularly in the abdominal area. The hip breadth increases, and the bony pelvis widens in preparation for reproduction. A pelvic girdle of subcutaneous fat results. This is often a source of anxiety to many figure-conscious young girls. In the boy, physical growth is manifest more in an increased muscle mass and in long-bone growth. His growth spurt is slower than that of the girl, but he soon passes her in weight and height, and at age 18 weighs about 63 kg (140 lb).

Reaction to disease. During this transitional period of rapid growth the physical resistance of the adolescent to infectious disease seems lessened. Usually the incidence of disease and the individual reaction to it is related to the physical nutritional resources the adolescent has to meet metabolic demands of the pubertal growth period. Also, increased activity of sweat glands and lack of good skin care make acne of face and back a common and vexing problem.

Psychosocial development. Adolescence is an ambivalent period full of stresses and strains. On the one hand the child looks back to the securities of earlier childhood. On the other hand, he reaches for the maturity of adulthood. The core problem with which the adolescent struggles is that of *identity versus diffusion*. The search for self begun in early childhood reaches a climax in the identity crisis of the teen years. The profound body changes associated with sexual development cause changes in body image and resulting tensions in maturing boys and girls. Individual variance is great in response to these tensions, depending upon the resources that have been provided for them in their earlier developmental years. In American society adolescent children continue to have problems in a rigid school system that groups them only by an arbitrary chronologic age rather than by a plan that considers their physiologic

and mental ages. Frustrations are often generated during this period in many adolescents and no doubt have an effect on their adult lives.

The identity crisis of the teen years, largely revolving around sexual development and preparation for an adult role in a complex society, produces many psychologic, emotional, and social tensions. The period of rapid physical growth is relatively short, only two to three years. However, the attendant psychosocial development continues over a longer period. The pressure for peer group acceptance is strong, and fads in dress and food habits are common. Also, in a technically developed society such as in the United States, where high values are placed on education and achievement, prolonged preparation for careers often delays marriage and establishment of the new family far beyond the initiation of the reproductive years. Social tensions and family conflicts are created. These conflicts may have nutritional consequences as the teenager eats away from home more often and develops a snacking pattern of his own food choices.

Food and feeding. *Caloric* needs increase with the metabolic demands of growth and energy expenditure. Although individual needs vary, girls consume fewer calories than boys (from 1,800 to 2,500 a day; boys need 2,500 to 3,500 a day). Sometimes the large appetite characteristic of this growth period leads an adolescent to satisfy his hunger with snack foods high in sugar and fat and to slight essential protein foods.

Protein needs for adolescent growth are great, especially during the pubertal changes in both sexes and for the developing muscle mass in boys. From 50 to 60 g of protein sustains daily needs and maintains nitrogen reserves.

Minerals particularly needed are calcium and iron. Bone growth demands calcium. Menstrual iron losses in the adolescent girl predispose her to simple iron-deficiency anemia. In some areas where iodized salt use does not ensure sufficient iodine for the increased thyroid activity associated with growth, a deficiency state may result.

Vitamins are necessary regulators of metabolic activity. The B vitamins are needed in increased amounts, especially by boys, to meet the extra demands of energy metabolism and muscle tissue development. Intakes of needed vitamin C and vitamin A may be low because of erratic food intake.

Eating habits. Physical and psychosocial pressures influence eating habits. By and large the adolescent boy fares better than the girl. His large appetite and the sheer volume of food it leads him to consume usually assure his intake of adequate nutrients. The adolescent girl, however, is less fortunate. Most U.S. surveys show her to be most vulnerable to nutritional deficiencies in comparison to other age-sex groups in the general population. Two factors combine to help produce this result: (1) Because of her physiologic sex differences associated with fat deposits during this period and her comparative lack of physical activity, she may gain excess weight easily. (2) Social pressures and personal tensions concerning figure control will sometimes cause her to follow unwise self-imposed crash diets for weight loss. As a result she may be malnourished at the very time in her life when her body is laying down reserves for coming reproduction. The hazards of such eating habits to her future course during potential pregnancies is clearly indicated in the studies relating preconception nutritional status to the outcome of gestation (pp. 375-377).

SUMMARY OF NEEDS FOR GROWTH

Throughout human growth, therefore, it is apparent that nutritional resources to meet physical growth are conditioned by the food habits and feeding practices that are psychosocially and culturally derived. Large numbers of growing children have these resources and arrive at adulthood vigorous and happy. Unfortunately, many others do not.

Helpful tools to use in reviewing these developmental needs for growth are given in Tables 18-8 and 18-9. In Table 18-8 a brief summary of each age group may be filled in, relating the core psychosocial problem and its related developmental characteristics and physical maturation to food and feeding needs for each state of growth. As a result of this study, practitioners and students should have a more realistic, sound *working knowledge* of normal growth and development needs, which will enable them to help young children who are struggling to grow up and parents who are trying to guide them.

CASE STUDY 8

A community nutrition program for teenagers

Susan Cummings, a graduate dietetic intern in clinical nutrition, was about to undertake a new learning experience. Along with several other members of her class she had been asked by her clinical professor to assist in planning and conducting some of the group sections in a special conference—Food for Teen Fitness—being held for all the city's high schools on the campus of a state college. Students from a number of the health professions—nutrition, medicine, dentistry, nursing, and social work—had been asked to participate.

One of the first things each of the participating students groups had been asked to do was to write a brief article to be printed in an advance bulletin for distribution in the high schools. The bulletin was to publicize the conference and stimulate interest in attending. Susan's group met several times to get ideas for their article and to develop them. Finally after much discussion and revision they completed their piece and entitled it "Teenage Nutrition: A Seeming Paradox." In it they tried to answer the basic question, "Why is it that officials always seem so concerned about the food habits of teenagers when we seem on the whole to be a pretty healthy group? What's the real story?"

The next task Susan and her committee faced was planning their group sessions for the conference. They met with participating students from the other health professions, as well as members of the student steering committee from the high schools. It was an exciting brain-storming session, with a sections meeting afterward in smaller groups to organize the individual sessions. The large group decided on three main topics:

1. Physical Fitness—
   Result of Good Nutrition
2. Food Problems of Teenagers
3. Snacks for Good Nutrition

Then the group responsible for each topic met separately to plan their section meeting. Susan's committee was divided, with representatives on each of the three planning groups.

When the big day finally arrived, Susan and a friend had the usual "preperformance jitters" about speaking in their respective sessions meetings. But they also felt confident, because they knew they had planned well. And it had been great fun working with students from all the other schools.

The conference was indeed a success. A large crowd attended, and the discussions were lively, realistic, intelligent, and probing. Susan learned a great deal; she was glad she had had such an opportunity.

Questions to guide your inquiry

1. Consider the title of the article Susan's group wrote for the conference bulletin. What answers would you have included in such an article, and what background evidence would you use?
2. What main points would you have included in the group discussion of the topic, Physical Fitness— Result of Good Nutrition? What questions would you ask about each point? What methods or materials would you have planned to involve the group?
3. What main points would you have included in the group discussion of the second topic, Food Problems of Teenagers? What questions would you ask about each point? What methods or materials would you have planned to involve the group?
4. What main points would you have included in the group discussion of the third topic, Snacks for Good Nutrition? What questions would you ask about each point? What methods or materials would you have planned to involve the group?
5. What physical characteristics and growths occur in the adolescent period?
6. What core psychosocial problem does the adolescent struggle with? What are some of the causes of this problem, and in what ways does it manifest itself?
7. What effect does this physical and psychosocial development have on the nutritional needs and food habits of teenagers?
8. List some of your own personal observations of food habits of teenagers. How would you rate these habits nutritionally?
9. List some snacks for teenagers that would be interesting and tasteful and contribute to nutrition.

REFERENCES
Specific

1. Stuart, H. C., and Meredith, H. V.: Use of body measurements in the school health program, Am. J. Public Health **36:**1365, 1948.
2. Reed, R. B., and Stuart, H. C.: Patterns of growth in height and weight from birth to eighteen years of age, Pediatrics **24:**904, 1957.
3. National Center for Health Statistics, HCHS growth charts, 1976. Monthly vital statistics, report, vol. 25, no. 3, suppl. (HRA) 76-1120, Health Resources Administration, Rockville, Md., June, 1976.
4. Erikson, E.: Youth and the life cycle, Children **7:**43, 1960.
5. Erickson, E.: Childhood and society, ed. 2, New York, 1963, W. W. Norton & Co., Inc., pp. 247-274.
6. Duvall, E. V.: Family development, ed. 2, Philadelphia, 1962, J. B. Lippincott Co.
7. American Academy of Pediatrics, Committee on Nutrition: Nutritional needs of low-birth-weight infants, Pediatrics **60:**519, Oct., 1977.
8. Hall, B.: Changing composition of human milk and early development of appetite control, Lancet **1:**779, 1975.
9. Foman, S. J.: Infant nutrition, ed. 2, Philadelphia, 1974, W. B. Saunders Co.
10. American Academy of Pediatrics, Committee on Nutrition: Commentary on breast feeding and infant formulas, including proposed standards for formulas, Pediatrics **57:**278, 1976.
11. Worthington, B. S.: Lactation, human milk, and nutritional considerations. In Worthington, B. S., Vermeersch, J., and Williams, S. R.: Nutrition in pregnancy and lactation, ed. 2, St. Louis, 1981, The C. V. Mosby Co.
12. Taylor, L. E., and Worthington, B. S.: Guidance for lactating mothers. In Worthington, B. S., Vermeersch, J., and Williams, S. R., Nutrition in pregnancy and lactation, ed. 2, St. Louis, 1981, The C. V. Mosby Co.
13. Redl, F.: Preadolescents: what makes them tick? Child Study **21:**44, 1933-1934.

General
GENERAL NUTRITION

Birch, H. G., and Gussow, J. D.: Disadvantaged children: health, nutrition, and school failure, New York, 1970, Harcourt Brace Jovanovich, Inc.

Center for Disease Control, Ten-state nutrition survey, 1968-1970, Washington, D.C., U.S. Dept. of Health, Education, and Welfare, Pub. No. (HSM) 72-8130-34, 1972.

Food and Nutrition Board: Recommended dietary allowances, ed. 9, Pub. No. 1980, National Academy of Sciences, National Research Council, Washington, D.C., 1980.

Kallen, D. J.: Nutrition, development and social behavior, DHEW Pub. No. (NIH) 73-242, Washington, D.C., 1973.

Martin, E.: Robert's nutrition work with children, Chicago, 1954, University of Chicago Press.

Nelson, W. E., editor: Textbook of pediatrics, ed. 8, Philadelphia, 1964, W. B. Saunders Co.

Preliminary findings of the first health and nutrition examination survey (HANES), 1971-1972: dietary intake and biochemical findings, DHEW Pub. No. (HRA) 74-1219-1, 1974.

Read, M. S.: Malnutrition, hunger, and behavior. I. Malnutrition and learning. II. Hunger, school feeding programs, and behavior, J. Am. Diet. Assoc. **63:**379, 1973.

Stefferud, A., editor: Food, the yearbook of agriculture, 1959, Washington, D.C., 1959, U.S. Dept. of Agriculture; also 1979.

Stone, L. J., and Church, J.: Childhood and adolescence, ed. 3, New York, 1973, Random House, Inc.

Williams, S. R., and Dickman, S. R., editors: Nutrition and health promotion, Fam. Commun. Health, vol. 1, no. 4, Feb., 1979.

INFANCY

American Academy of Pediatrics, Committee on Nutrition: Iron supplementation for infants, Pediatrics **58:**765, 1976.

Anderson, T. A.: Commercial infant foods: content and composition, Pediatr. Clin. North Am. **24:**37, 1977.

Brachemyre, P., and Schreiner, R. L.: Late metabolic acidosis of the premature infant, J. Am. Diet. Assoc. **72:**298, March, 1978.

Deeming, S. B., and Weber, C. W.: Trace minerals in commercially prepared baby foods, J. Am. Diet. Assoc. **75:**149, Aug., 1979.

Foman, S. J.: Infant nutrition, ed. 2, Philadelphia, 1974, W. B. Saunders Co.

Foman, S. J.: What are infants fed in the United States? Pediatrics **56:**350, 1975.

Hall, B.: Changing composition of human milk and early development of an appetite control, Lancet **1:**779, 1975.

Jelliffe, D. B., and Jelliffe, E. F. P.: Nutrition and human milk, Postgrad. Med. **60:**153, 1976.

Johnson, E. M., and Schwartz, N. E.: Physicians' opinions and counseling practices in maternal and infant nutrition, J.A.D.A. **73**(3):246, 1978.

Lackey, C. J.: International symposium on infant and child feeding, Nutr. Today **13:**11, Nov.-Dec., 1978.

Lakdawala, D. R., and Wildowson, E. M.: Vitamin D in human milk, Lancet **1:**167, 1977.

Lamm, E., Delaney, J., and Dwyer, J. T.: Economy in the feeding of infants, Pediatr. Clin. North Am. **24:**71, 1977.

McMillan, J. A., and Landaw, S. A., and Oski, F. A.: Iron sufficiency in breast-fed infants and the availability of iron from human milk, Pediatrics **58:**686, 1976.

Milton, S. E., and Fox, H. M.: Nebraska physicians' attitudes and practices in the field of infant feeding and nutrition, J. Am. Diet. Assoc. **73:**416, Oct., 1978.

Morse, W., Sims, L. S., and Guthrie, H. A.: Mothers' compliance with physicians' recommendations on infant feeding, J. Am. Diet. Assoc. **75:**140, Aug., 1979.

Ounsted, M., and Sleigh, G.: The infant's self-regulation of food intake and weight gain, Lancet **1:**1393, 1975.

Overfeeding in the first year of life, Nutr. Rev. **31:**116, 1973.

Owen, G. M., Kram, K. M., Garry, P. J., et al.: A study of nutritional status of pre-school children in the United States, 1968-1970, Pediatrics **53**(suppl.):597, 1974.

Picciano, M. F., and Guthrie, H. A.: Copper, iron and zinc contents of mature human milk, Am. J. Clin. Nutr. **29:**242, 1976.

Pipes, P.: When should semisolid foods be fed to infants? J. Nutr. Educ. **9:**57, 1977.

Potter, J. M., and Nestel, P. J.: The effects of dietary fatty acids and cholesterol on the milk lipids of lactating women and the plasma cholesterol of breast-fed infants, Am. J. Clin. Nutr. **29:**54, 1976.

White paper on infant feeding practices, Washington, D.C., 1974, Center for Science in the Public Interest.

Worthington, B. S., Vermeersch, J. A., and Williams, S. R.: Nutrition in pregnancy and lactation, ed. 2, St. Louis, 1981, The C. V. Mosby Co.

CHILDHOOD

Brown, G., Wyse, B. W., and Hansen, R. G.: A nutrient density-nutrition education program for elementary schools, J. Nutr. Educ. **11:**31, Jan.-March, 1979.

Burt, J. V., and Hertzler, A. A.: Parental influence on the child's food preference, J. Nutr. Educ. **10:**127, July-Sept., 1978.

Caliendo, M. A., Sanjur, D., Wright, J., et al.: Nutritional status of preschool children: an ecologic analysis, J. Am. Diet. Assoc. **71:**20, July, 1977.

Chang, A., Kayman, S., McCoy, E., and Parziale, L.: Nutrition services in child day care centers, J. Am. Diet. Assoc. **74:**356, March, 1979.

Dwyer, J. T., Palumbo, R., Valadian, I., and Reed, R. B.: Preschoolers on alternate life-style diets: associations between size and dietary indexes with diets limited in types of animal foods, J. Am. Diet. Assoc. **72:**264, March, 1978.

Fisk, D.: A successful program for changing children's eating habits, Nutr. Today **14:**6, May-June, 1979.

Fryer, B. A., Lamkin, G. H., Vivian, V. V. M., et al.: Growth of preschool children in the north central region, J. Am. Diet. Assoc. **60:**30, Jan., 1972.

Larkin, F. A., Perri, K. P., Bursick, J. H., et al.: Etiology of growth failure in a clinic population, J. Am. Diet. Assoc. **69:**506, Nov., 1976.

Martin, J.: School nutrition programs in perspective, J. Am. Diet. Assoc. **73:**389, Oct., 1978.

Sims, L. S., and Morris, P. M.: Nutritional status of preschoolers, J. Am. Diet. Assoc. **64:**592, 1974.

Snowman, M. K., and Dibble, M. V.: Nutrition component in a comprehensive child development program, J. Am. Diet. Assoc. **74:**119, Feb., 1979.

Yperman, A. M., and Vermeersch, J. A.: Factors associated with children's food habits, J. Nutr. Educ. **11:**72, April-June, 1979.

ADOLESCENCE

Gains, E., and Daniel, W., Jr.: Dietary iron intakes of adolescents, J. Am. Diet. Assoc. **65:**275, 1974.

Huenemann, R., Shapiro, L., Hampton, M., et al.: A longitudinal study of gross body composition and body conformation and their association with food and activity in a teen-age population: view of teen-age subjects on body conformation, food, and activity, Am. J. Clin. Nutr. **18:**325, 1966.

Huenemann, R., Shapiro, L., Hampton, M., et al.: Teenagers' activities and attitudes toward activity, J. Am. Diet. Assoc. **51:**433, Nov., 1967.

Huenemann, R., Hampton, M., Behnke, A., Shapiro, L., and Mitchell, B.: Teenage nutrition and physique, Springfield, Ill., 1974, Charles C Thomas, Publisher.

Law, H. M., Lewis, H. F., Grant, V. C., et al.: Sophomore high school students' attitudes toward school lunch, J. Am. Diet. Assoc. **60:**38, Jan., 1972.

McKigney, J. I., and Munro, H. N.: Nutrient requirements in adolescence, Bethesda, Md., National Institutes of Health, NICHD Office of Research Reporting, DHEW Pub. No. (NIH) 76-771, 1976.

Schorr, B. C., Sanjur, D., and Erickson, E. C.: Teen-age food habits, J. Am. Diet. Assoc. **61:**415, Oct., 1972.

ATHLETICS

Hanley, D. F., Jr.: Athletic training—and how diet affects it, Nutr. Today **14:**5, Nov.-Dec., 1979.

Hanley, D. F., Jr.: Basic diet guidance for athletes, Nutr. Today **14:**22, Nov.-Dec., 1979.

Hursh, L. M.: Practical hints about feeding athletes, Nutr. Today **14:**5, Nov.-Dec., 1979.

Lewis, S., and Gutin, B.: Nutrition and endurance, Am. J. Clin. Nutr. **26:**1011, 1973.

Slovic, P.: What helps the long-distance runner run? Nutr. Today **10:**18, 1975.

Smith, N. J.: Food for sport, Palo Alto, Calif., 1976, Bull Publishing Co.

Smith, N. J.: Gaining and losing weight in athletics, J.A.M.A. **236:**149, 1976.

Vitousek, S. H.: Is more better? (athletic performance), Nutr. Today **14:**10, Nov.-Dec., 1979.

19 Nutritional therapy in childhood diseases

The child's reaction to illness is conditioned by his past experiences and the common growth and development patterns of childhood. Sick or well, all children struggle to accomplish indispensable tasks of physical and psychosocial development. As Erikson[1] points out, however, during illness some degree of regression occurs. Therefore in exploring patient needs and planning relevant care, not only must the particular age group needs of the child be considered, but also individual responses to the experience of illness according to unique personal resources.

Nutritional therapy will play an important role in the care of a child. Basic normal nutritional needs of the particular growth period, as outlined in the previous chapter, will take on added significance as a foundational resource for meeting the physiologic stress of disease. These food factors need to be assured in the diet. In some instances, dietary modifications will need to be made to accommodate a particular disease condition. The alert, observant, and sensitive practitioner will find many opportunities to provide learning experiences for children and their parents in the principles of health care. A fundamental part of this health care is good nutrition.

Therefore the general needs of the hospitalized child will be looked at first, and in the light of these basic needs the factors involved in planning personal nutritional care will be considered. With this background a few of the diseases involving nutritional consideration will be used as examples of adjusting normal nutritional needs for therapeutic care.

This study will revolve around the following questions:

1. What role does nutritional therapy play in meeting the needs of ill children?
2. What nutritional therapy is used in the management of gastrointestinal problems of infants and children?
3. What are genetic diseases? How are they related to nutrients?
4. What is the basic genetic defect in phenylketonuria and galactosemia? How are the results of these defects managed in the child's diet? What are the public health implications?
5. What are the principles of care in juvenile diabetes?
6. What is the wise approach in childhood to nutritional care of common public health problems such as obesity and dental caries?

THE HOSPITALIZED CHILD

Good patient care essentially centers on two factors: (1) determining the needs of the patient and (2) planning wise action to meet these needs. Many health care practices considered helpful of themselves are not necessarily helpful to a particular patient in a particular situation. This is especially true in the care of children. But here health care workers have an added responsibility. They must be able to communicate with children. This ability comes from knowing children and caring about their concerns. It is based on an indefinable quality of feeling for them that enables the worker to establish contact with a child who is often inarticulate, emotionally disoriented, and physically ill. A consideration of the basic needs of the ill, hospitalized child is an essential first step. Then plans for nutritional care will be an integral part of total care.

Basic needs of ill children

Physical care. Quality medical care and supervision are primary considerations. The child is hospitalized at the direction of his physician, who carries the medical responsibility for the child's health. He or she relies heavily, however, on other members of the health team in the total care of the child, particularly on the nutritionist or dietitian and the nurse for supportive care. Often it is the high quality of this care by sensitive, skilled, attuned practitioners that makes the difference in the child's illness and helps him to recovery of health again. A major aspect of nutritional care will be close observation of the child's food attitudes and intake and fluid intake and careful recording of these observations for analysis by the health care team (Fig. 19-1; see also Table 18-2).

Emotional support. The hospitalized child

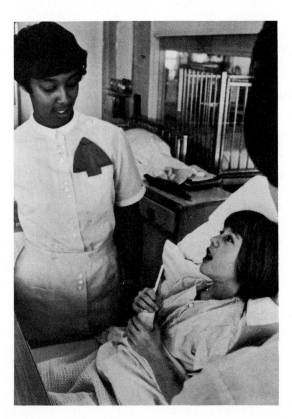

Fig. 19-1. Adequate fluid intake is essential for children, especially during illness. Here student nurses encourage a child to drink some orange juice.

usually has anxieties and fears. These anxieties may stem from separation from his family, especially his mother, and from his fears concerning his illness and its treatment. A number of factors influence a child's adjustment to hospitalization. These include his age, how ill he is, the kind of care he receives, and the inner personal resources he may have developed thus far from all his past experiences that enable him to cope with his present situation. His particular life experiences may have given him few resources to meet this added crisis. He may be malnourished or lack emotional strength and control. To meet such situations, practitioners must have an understanding of the child's emotional needs and provide wise ways of meeting them.

Optimal nutrition. Food is an essential principle in physical and emotional recovery from illness. It is a fundamental means of metabolic return to health, even in this age of miracle drugs. Sometimes this simple fact is forgotten. The biochemical base of health functions at the cellular level through the media of innumerable chemicals and their metabolic interactions. These chemicals or their precursors must be obtained in food. The problem in nutritional care of children therefore is twofold. The necessary food must be provided, and the food must be eaten by the child. Usually in a qualified hospital there is adequate administration and trained personnel equipped to accomplish the first aim. The crux of the problem is more often the second need—the acceptance of the food by the child. This aspect of the problem becomes the responsibility mainly of the clinical nutritionist or dietitian and the nurse.

Plans for nutritional care

In planning for the nutritional care of the child, personal needs must be considered—general age group needs, any necessary diet modifications, and the individual child and family.

Age group needs. What age is the child and in what stage of growth? What related developmental age group needs is he struggling with just now? How are these in any way related to feeding, to food, and to fluid intake?

Diet modifications. What is the illness? Is it long or short term? Does it hinder eating ability in any way? Does it require any dietary modifications? If so, what changes and why? Have these needs been discussed by the dietitian or nutritionist with the health care team?

The child's acceptance of food. Up to this point in the exploration of the child's needs it may be evident that the food is well planned and prepared. But if the child does not eat it, it does him no good. On the child's acceptance of the food hinges the success of his nutritional care. Granted that hospital food is usually not exactly like mother's home cooking, it still can be made appetizing and interesting to stimulate lagging appetites. Exploration of the child's reason or reasons for not eating and ingenuity in ways of presenting the food will pay great dividends.

Reasons for food rejection. A number of things may contribute to the child's poor appetite and refusal of food.

ILLNESS. The child may be too ill or weak to eat. He may have some physical intolerance for the food. He may require liquid or soft food, food substitutions, or gentle help in feeding.

ANXIETY. The child may be tense and frightened because of separation from his family, especially his mother. The strange and unfamiliar surroundings may frighten him. He may be concerned about his illness and its outcome. Involving his parents in plans for his care or helping to make arrangements for his mother to be with him usually provides needed security and support. Also, helping him to talk about his fears, understanding and accepting him and his fears, and providing simple, brief explanations of his care and his treatment as needed all help to reduce his anxiety, to gain his confidence, and to give him added resources with which to cope.

PRESENTATION OF FOOD. Often the child rejects food because of the way in which it is presented to him. For example, an ill 2-year-old is confronted with a tray full of wan food and man-sized utensils unceremoniously planted before him by a large, forbidding, strange adult with the command, "Now eat!" and is overwhelmed. Worse yet, force-feeding a child who has inner conflicts only adds more trauma. Some children already wear battle scars of home combat with an adult over food!

Ways of achieving food acceptance. Nutritionists, dietitians, nurses, and physicians experienced in caring for children have devised numerous ways of presenting food. Basically these ways of helping a child to eat revolve around two related factors—self-selection and a warm mealtime atmosphere.

SELF-SELECTION. Allowing a child to have some degree of choice in his food is helpful. Following the early classic experience of Davis[2] with children's self-selection of foods, the staff of the same Chicago hospital in which those experiments took place brought food in sufficient variety to the pediatric ward in a heated conveyor. The children were allowed to select their food from the items displayed.[3] Another hospital in Colorado capitalized on its western heritage and converted their pediatric food cart into a "chuck wagon" outfitted with all the covered wagon trimmings. Periodically the "chuck wagon" travels to the pediatric ward

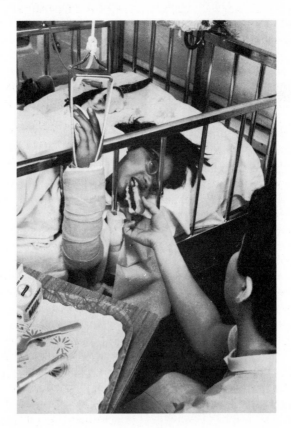

Fig. 19-2. Child with fractured arm is assisted in eating by student nurse.

and the adolescent areas of the hospital for evening "chow time." A "cowboy," assisted by nurses and a dietitian, dispenses food selected by the young patients.[4] Several other children's hospitals have planned cafeteria service and group eating for all their ambulatory patients. Although such activities may not be possible in all hospitals, a selective menu from which the child, with guidance, may help select his own food is a step in that direction. Some consideration of a child's likes and dislikes, with encouragement in convalescence to try new tastes in foods, also helps achieve food acceptance.

WARM MEALTIME ATMOSPHERE. The manner in which the food is served and a warm atmosphere at mealtime are major influences on the child's reaction. The following factors may help to build this atmosphere:

1. *Personnel.* The warm, supportive manner of the personnel serving the food is of inestimable value. They must know the children and have a feeling for them. Food is served attractively in proper-sized, small portions and in correct, child-sized utensils. Bed patients are made as comfortable as possible and assisted as needed (Fig. 19-2).

2. *Group eating.* Often ambulatory patients may eat at small tables in family style. Interest is heightened if the children are involved in the preparation; for example, setting the table, serving as host and hostess, passing the food, and refilling serving dishes as needed. Nurses, dietitians, or physicians may eat with the children occasionally and find in sharing food not only a means of observing and learning more about their patients, but also an important vehicle of establishing feeling relationships with them.

3. *Festive days.* Observance of holidays and birthdays with special food or favors or decorations will help to interest children and give support.

4. *Familiar food.* Consideration should be given to ethnic food habits. Sometimes a familiar food or dish from home that is not contraindicated by the child's illness will stimulate his appetite and interest in eating and secure for him needed nourishment. Preparing food and ethnic dishes to which the child is accustomed or flavoring food according to his familiar tastes are helpful to a child, especially one confined to bed for an extended period.

Family involvement. Exploration of the child's home eating habits with his mother and of the ways she prepares and serves his food will give helpful background for planning the child's nutritional care while he is in the hospital. Also, such discussions provide an opportunity for parents to express their own anxieties about the child and lead to mutual learning concerning normal growth and developmental needs of children. If the child requires any special diet modifications, these needs may also be discussed with the parents, helping them to explore ways the child's needs may be fitted in with family eating habits.

GASTROINTESTINAL PROBLEMS OF INFANTS AND CHILDREN
General disturbances

Infantile colic. Infantile colic is the name given to paroxysmal intermittent periods of loud, continuous crying. It is not uncommon in newborns and lasts no longer than the third month. It is usually seen only in firstborn infants and seldom in their subsequent siblings. Because it occurs rather routinely in the evening hours between five or six o'clock and midnight, medical and nursing care is usually better directed toward the ragged nerves of the new inexperienced parents than to the infant himself. It is a self-limiting difficulty, ending spontaneously during the first three months. However, to young, tense parents this brief interval of time may seem an eternity.

Treatment usually involves careful history taking, discovering attitudes and feeding practices. The child may be underfed and simply screaming because he is hungry, or he may be overfed by a zealous young mother and have abdominal discomfort. In other cases his formula may be rapidly changed from day to day by an experimenting mother. (One young mother changed her baby's formula seven times in as many days). Also the common pacifier is much more in vogue, with the blessing of most pediatricians. At least the pacifier has the value of closing the opening from which the cacophony emanates. Mostly, however, treatment involves explanation and moral support to the parents, with reassurance that their child is growing normally. They may take courage from the knowledge that such an active, energetic child with high neuromotor function often develops faster than his more passive peers. He may hold up his head, walk, sit, and talk sooner. He has excellent energy potential for becoming a vigorous and vocal adult. One tongue-in-cheek reviewer has called such a baby "one having the pent-up energy of a born protester and a larynx of unquestioned competence."[5]

Simple functional vomiting. Regurgitation, or "spitting up," is common in most young infants. Its cause is usually gastric distention from overfeeding or from air-swallowing during feeding or crying. Related factors may be ineffective burping and leaving the baby in a supine position rather than a prone position after feeding. Also, overactivity and semiacrobatics at the hands of doting fathers and grandparents soon after he has been fed may stimulate regurgitation. Temperature of the feeding may be a factor, as feedings that are too hot may induce vomiting. Milk at room temperature is better tolerated, and even cold feedings have evoked no difficulty in a number of infants.[6] Again, simple attention to possible causative factors and reassurance to the young mother will provide adequate care.

Constipation. The old adage, "It is not what he eats, but what eats him!" is correctly applied

to constipation. Dietary manipulation is often not a fundamental cure but simply a helpful adjunct. *Psychogenic* constipation may occur during the ages 1 to 2 while the child is being toilet trained. Sometimes a compulsive anal-fixated mother, who believes in an arbitrary timetable of elimination ("a daily bowel movement is absolutely essential to health") imposes stringent toilet disciplines on the child, scolding him for failure and rewarding him for perfect performance. The child soon learns that he can suppress the natural impulse to defecate, and he uses this power as a weapon in his conflict with his mother. In time the habit weakens normal peristalsis. Stools become dry and difficult to pass. Correction of the problem involves adjustment of the parent-child relationship and a resulting easing of the conflict and tensions. The mother needs to learn two simple physiologic facts: (1) toxins are not absorbed from fecal material, and therefore (2) a *daily* stool is not essential to the child's health.

Occasional simple physiologic constipation is usually transient. It is aided by moderately reducing the milk intake, increasing the carbohydrate intake, increasing fruits and vegetables, and increasing the water intake.

Diarrhea

Fluid and electrolytes. Diarrhea in infants may be a more serious problem, especially if it is prolonged and associated with infection. Because of his relatively high water content and his large area of intestinal mucosa in proportion to body surface area, the infant's fluid and electrolyte reserves may be rapidly depleted. The sequence of steps leading to dehydration should be reviewed in Chapter 9, Water and Electrolytes. Common mild diarrhea usually responds to simple treatment. This consists of reducing the food intake, especially of carbohydrate and fat in the formula, and increasing the water intake, sometimes including in it oral electrolyte replacements. More serious forms involving infection and producing marked dehydration and acidosis are medical emergencies calling for immediate parenteral fluid and electrolyte therapy. The loss of potassium can be dangerous, since hypokalemia affects action of the heart muscle.

Oral feedings. After initial essential replacement of fluid and electrolytes and when the infant is able to take oral feedings more readily, they are resumed. Water, glucose, and balanced salt solutions may be used, followed by milk mixtures, breast milk, or substitutes such as Probana (a high-protein formula with banana powder) or Nutramigen (a casein hydrolysate free of galactose) as stool volume decreases. Calories are increased to normal requirements as soon as possible. Such agents as pectin and kaolin may thicken the stools, but most authorities agree they have little or no therapeutic usefulness in severe infant diarrhea. Although views differ, pediatricians generally discount the previous practice of completely starving patients with acute diarrhea, a practice that was based on the erroneous belief that avoidance of oral intake put the bowels at rest.[7] Also, tea should not be given to the child. The xanthines in tea stimulate and excite children and in some cases cause diuresis, which in turn only aggravates the fluid imbalance.

Celiac (malabsorption) syndrome

Identification. In 1889 a London physician named Gee observed a number of malnourished patients having a diarrheal disease and distended abdomens. He gave the name *celiac* to the general clinical syndrome, from the Greek word *kolia,* meaning "belly" or "abdomen." For several decades thereafter, confusion existed among a number of conditions with the same four basic symptoms, all of which were clinical manifestations of intestinal malabsorption: (1) general malnutrition, (2) multiple, foul, bulky, foamy, greasy stools, (3) distended abdomen, due to an accumulation of improperly

digested food material and inadequately absorbed food material and due to abnormal gas accumulations, and (4) secondary vitamin deficiencies.

Etiologic classification. Beginning in the 1930s, with advances in knowledge, it became clear that the term *celiac* covered not one but a group of entities, each distinguished by its etiology, but having the same general clinical manifestations of intestinal malabsorption and hence steatorrhea. Three basic contributions of knowledge have helped to clarify these disease entities. In the late 1930s Anderson and others[8,9] distinguished *cystic fibrosis of the pancreas* as a separate disease entity by the absence of pancreatic enzymes in the duodenal juice. A group of Dutch workers[10] in the early 1950s identified a separate *gluten-induced enteropathy* as a leading cause of the syndrome in children. In the mid-1950s Shiner[11,12] developed a peroral biopsy technique. Using a flexible tube with a suction-guillotine tip, small tissue samples of the intestinal mucosa could be obtained for microscopic study. Electron micrographs of these tissues have consistently shown an eroded mucosal surface without the number or form of villi normally seen and with sparse microvilli. This erosion effectively reduces the absorbing surface areas as much as 95%. As a result of these and other studies the various diseases of the malabsorption syndrome have been grouped according to etiology. The general causes of steatorrhea are given in the following outline*:

A. Impaired digestion of fat
   1. Inadequate lipolysis due to absence of pancreatic lipase
      a. Cystic fibrosis of pancreas
      b. Congenital hypoplasia of exocrine pancreas
      c. Dietary protein deficiency

---

*Nelson, W. E., editor: Textbook of pediatrics, ed. 8, Philadelphia, 1964, W. B. Saunders Co., p. 723.

2. Inadequate emulsification of fat due to exclusion of bile from intestine
   a. Atresia of bile ducts
   b. Obstructive jaundice (e.g., viral hepatitis)
B. Impaired absorption of fat
  1. Inadequate length of small bowel or increased transport time
   a. Extensive surgical resection
   b. Intestinal fistulas
   c. Increased intestinal motility due to diarrhea
  2. Obstruction of intestinal lymphatics
   a. Exudative enteropathy due to lymphatic anomalies
   b. Tuberculosis
   c. Hodgkin's disease
   d. Lymphosarcoma
  3. Inflammatory disease or involvement of intestinal mucosa in systemic diseases
   a. Intestinal infections and infestations
   b. Regional enteritis
   c. Ulcerative colitis
   d. Gaucher's disease
   e. Niemann-Pick disease
   f. Scleroderma
  4. Biochemical dysfunction of mucosal cells
   a. Gluten-induced enteropathy
   b. Parenteral diarrhea (in infancy)
   c. Severe starvation
C. Basic mechanism obscure*
  1. Incomplete obstruction of intestinal tract (malrotation, stenosis, blind-loop syndrome, etc.)
  2. Idiopathic steatorrhea
  3. Gastrointestinal allergy
  4. Acanthocytosis
  5. Hypoparathyroidism
  6. Sugar-splitting enzyme deficiencies

The principal causes of the celiac syndromes are cystic fibrosis of the pancreas, gluten-induced celiac disease, idiopathic celiac disease or steatorrhea, and exudative enteropathy. These conditions are characterized by excessive intestinal loss of serum protein, often with ab-

---

*Familial dysautonomia (Riley-Day syndrome) and ganglioneuroma may be responsible for diarrhea, but it has not been established whether steatorrhea occurs.

normalities of the intestinal lymphatics. A still useful summary of these disease entities has been outlined by Di Sant' Agnese and Jones.[13] The two entities most commonly encountered in children are (1) gluten-induced enteropathy, and (2) cystic fibrosis of the pancreas.

Gluten-induced enteropathy (celiac disease)

Etiology. The celiac syndrome seen in children is apparently caused by an enzymatic defect or metabolic error in the intestinal mucosal cells brought out by wheat or rye gluten. It is thought to be a genetic defect, although the mechanism is unknown. In adults the condition is known as nontropical sprue. In the process of the disease the villi of the intestinal mucosa atrophy, greatly reducing the absorptive and secretory surface. Tissue changes occur in the mucosal cells, which brings on pathologic lesions of varying sorts. Whether these mucosal changes are reversible or not is controversial. Efforts of some investigators to return patients to regular diets after initial improvement on a low-gluten regimen have been successful in a few cases with children, but the majority (mostly adults) have not responded. Most of the children seem to recover from the overt disease by school age. Apparently, however, the disease process is in remission, since it may appear again in adult years. Most adults with sprue give a history of having had celiac disease in childhood.

The protein *gluten* is found mainly in wheat and rye. It is composed of two fractions, *glutenin* and *gliadin*. The gliadin fraction is mainly responsible for the malabsorption in gluten-induced enteropathy. About 47% of the weight of the wheat gliadin has been identified as the amino acid *glutamine*. Studies of this amino acid seem to implicate it in the biochemical defect. It is now apparent that the steatorrhea is a secondary manifestation caused by the primary biochemical reaction to gliadin in sensitive patients.

Clinical symptoms. In children who develop gluten-induced celiac disease the onset usually occurs between the ages of 6 and 18 months, with symptoms appearing later in those who were breast-fed babies. It usually begins with a chronic course, which may suddenly be worsened by a celiac crisis, usually triggered by an infection. This is a severe episode of dehydration and acidosis in whcih there are large, watery stools and copious vomiting. It is an acute medical emergency. There is chronic diarrhea with passage of characteristic foul, foamy, bulky, greasy stools. About 80% of the ingested fat appears in the stools, usually in the form of soaps and fatty acids. There is progressive malnutrition with signs of deficiency states secondary to the malabsorption—anemia, rickets, and an increased bleeding tendency. The abdomen is grossly distended. There is loss of subcutaneous fat tissue, leaving the buttocks flattened and wrinkled with folds of skin. The child takes on the emaciated, apathetic, and fretful appearance of malnutrition.

Idiopathic steatorrhea is the term given to the disease clinically identical to gluten-induced enteropathy. It is sometimes called idiopathic celiac disease, a source of frequent confusion. The only distinction is in etiology. Idiopathic steatorrhea is *not* induced by gluten and hence does not respond to a clinical trial with a low-gluten regimen.

Dietary management of gluten-induced enteropathy would be better defined as *low-gluten* rather than *gluten-free,* because it is impossible to remove all the gluten completely, and there is evidence that a small amount of gluten is tolerated by most patients.[14] Wheat and rye are the main sources of gluten, and gluten is also present in oats and barley. Therefore these four grains (wheat, rye, oats, and barley) are eliminated from the diet. Corn and rice are the substitute grains used. The offending grains are obvious in cereal form, but they are also used as ingredients (thickeners or fillers) in many commercial products. Therefore specific instructions must be outlined to the child's parents, giving the principal omissions in each main food group, a basic meal pattern, and recipes for food preparation.[15] Commercial products involving gluten and careful label-reading habits should be discussed.

Good dietary management varies according to the age of the child, his clinical status, and pathologic conditions. Generally, however, the course of treatment will follow the stages outlined on p. 432 during the acute and follow-up phases with infants and young children. For continuing use, a dietary program such as the guideline above may be followed. A still useful and excellent summary of the practical details of dietary management of patients with the celiac syndrome has been outlined by Mike.[18]

Cystic fibrosis of the pancreas

Identification and clinical manifestations. Cystic fibrosis is a generalized hereditary disease of children that involves the exocrine glands and affects many tissues and organs. In past years its prognosis was poor. Few children with early disease survived past 10 years of age. However, with better knowledge of the disease and improved diagnostic tests, clinical treatment, and antibiotic therapy, prognosis has improved. Cystic fibrosis usually produces characteristic clinical manifestations:

1. Pancreatic deficiency with greatly diminished digestion of food caused by the absence of pancreatic enzymes: amylase, which is responsible for hydrolysis of starch; trypsin, chymotrypsin, and carboxypeptidase, which digest proteins; and lipase, the primary fat hydrolyzing enzyme. It is the lack of pancreatic lipase that creates the greatest problem with malabsorption and subsequent steatorrhea. This problem leads in turn to the loss of fat-soluble vitamins, as well as other essential nutrients such as iron. There is also an increased loss of bile

General clinical dietary management during acute and follow-up phases of celiac disease in infants and young children

Stage I

Celiac crisis—1 to 3 days

Intravenous replacement therapy of fluid and electrolytes

Stage II

Initial oral feedings—1 to 6 months (depending on patient's initial condition and individual response)

High-protein, low-fat, starch-free feedings (until diagnosis of gluten-induced enteropathy is clearly established, all types of starch are omitted)

Formulas

1. Protein milk with glucose and banana powder
2. Skimmed milk (Probana or Hi Pro)

According to age of child, add simple carbohydrate foods for additional caloric requirements—fruit juice, *ripe* banana, cooked or canned fruit in syrup (pureed), such as applesauce; protein—strained meat, beginning with beef and liver

Stage III

Gradual liberalization of diet—indefinite period depending on individual clinical course; form of food will remain soft or pureed

Meats—lean (no fat); add seafood with caution

Eggs

Vegetables, pureed

Fruits, pureed—fruit ices, fruit whips

Cereal—corn and rice (small amounts)

Miscellaneous—gelatin desserts, honey, sugar

General meal pattern

Breakfast

Fruit juice (citrus or apple)

Fruit (ripe banana or other pureed or soft fruit)

Egg (no added fat)

Low-fat cottage cheese or meat (strained or finely ground), if desired

Formula

Lunch

Lean meat (strained or finely ground)

Vegetable—cooked (strained, or chopped, depending on age)

Fruit—cooked, stewed, or soft

(Starch: 1 small serving—corn or rice cereal)

Formula

Dinner

Meat, strained (may substitute cottage cheese or egg)

Vegetable (strained or chopped, depending on age)

Dessert—gelatin desserts or fruit

Formula

Evening

Formula

Between meal feedings—depending on appetite

Table 19-1. Principles of dietary management for patients with cystic fibrosis

Principle	Reason
High calorie	Energy demands of growth and compensation for fecal losses; large appetite usually ensures acceptance of increased amounts of food
High protein	Usually tolerated in large amounts; excess above normal growth needs required to compensate for losses
Moderate carbohydrate	Starch less well tolerated, simple sugars easily assimilated
Low to moderate fat, as tolerated	Fat poorly absorbed, but tolerance varies widely
Generous salt	Food generously salted to replace sweat losses; salt supplements in hot weather
Vitamins	Double doses of multivitamins in water-soluble form (vitamin E supplements sometimes used as low blood levels of the vitamin have been observed); vitamin K supplements with prolonged antibiotic therapy
Pancreatic enzymes	Large amounts given by mouth with each meal (may be mixed with cereal or applesauce for infants) to compensate for pancreatic deficiency—powdered pancreas extract containing steapsin, trypsin, and amylopsin (Pancreatin, or other pancreatic extracts such as Cotazyme or Viokase).

acids, with fecal bile acid secretion being as much as twice the normal amount.[19]

2. Malfunction of mucus-producing glands with accumulation of thick viscid secretions and subsequent respiratory difficulty and chronic pulmonary disease.

3. Abnormally high electrolyte levels in secretions of the sweat glands.

4. Possible cirrhosis of the liver arising from biliary obstruction and increased by malnutrition or infection.

Treatment therefore is based on three factors: (1) control of respiratory infection, (2) relief from the effects of extremely viscid bronchial secretions, and (3) maintenance of nutrition. The digestive deficiency and malabsorption character of cystic fibrosis are evident in the nature of the child's stools. They are similar to those in celiac disease (typically bulky, mushy, greasy, foul, foamy), but they also contain more undigested food. Only about half (50% to 60%) of the child's food is absorbed. Thus the child with cystic fibrosis has a much more voracious appetite.

Dietary management. The basic objective of nutritional therapy is to compensate for the large loss of nutrient material resulting from the insufficiency of pancreatic enzymes. Apparently protein hydrolysates, split fats (emulsified, simple fats), and simple sugars are assimilated readily. There is a wide variation, however, in tolerance for fat, and the amount of fat intake is usually prescribed according to the character of the stools. A more readily absorbed fat preparation, a vegetable oil made of short- and medium-chain triglycerides (MCT) may be used for food preparation. Large increases of protein seem to be well tolerated and are needed for replacement of losses and for growth.

Dietary programs for cystic fibrosis are similar to those outlined for celiac disease, the food used varying in form according to the age of the child. The diet differs, however, in that gluten sources need not be restricted, and, of course, there is greater emphasis on quantity of food. The important principles of dietary management for patients with cystic fibrosis are summarized in Table 19-1.

Low-gluten diet for patients with celiac disease

Diet principles

1. Calories—High, usually about 20% above normal requirement, to compensate for fecal loss
2. Protein—high, usually 6 to 8 g/kg body weight
3. Fat—low, but not fat-free, because of impaired absorption
4. Carbohydrate—simple, easily digested sugars (fruits, vegetables) should provide about one half of the calories
5. Feedings—small, frequent feedings during ill periods; afternoon snack for older children
6. Texture—smooth, soft, avoiding irritating roughage initially, using strained foods longer than usual for age, adding whole foods as tolerated and according to age of child
7. Vitamins—supplements of B vitamins, vitamins A and B in water-miscible forms, and vitamin C
8. Minerals—iron supplements if anemia present

Food groups	Foods to use	Foods to avoid
Milk	Milk (plain or flavored with chocolate or cocoa) Buttermilk	Malted milk; preparations such as Coco-malt, Hemo, Postum, Nestle's chocolate
Meat or substitute	Lean meat, trimmed well of fat Eggs, cheese Poultry, fish Creamy peanut butter (if tolerated)	Fat meats (sausage, pork) Luncheon meats, corned beef, frankfurters, all common prepared meat products with any possible wheat filler Duck, goose Smoked salmon Meat prepared with bread, crackers, or flour
Fruits and juices	All cooked and canned fruits and juices Frozen or fresh fruits as tolerated, avoiding skins and seeds	Prunes, plums (unless tolerated)
Vegetables	All cooked, frozen, canned as tolerated (prepared *without* wheat, rye, oat, or barley products); raw as tolerated	Any causing individual discomfort All prepared with wheat, rye, oat, or barley products
Cereals	Corn or rice	Wheat, rye, oat, barley; any product containing these cereals
Breads, flours, cereal products	Breads, pancakes, or waffles made with suggested flours (cornmeal, cornstarch; rice, soybean, lima, potato, buckwheat)	All bread or cracker products made with gluten, wheat, rye, oat, barley, macaroni, noodles, spaghetti, any sauces, soups, or gravies, prepared with gluten flour, wheat, rye, oat, or barley
Soups	Broth, bouillon (no fat, cream; no thickening with wheat, rye, oat, or barley products); soups and sauces may be thickened with cornstarch	All soups containing wheat, rye, oat, or barley products

Low-gluten diet for patients with celiac disease—cont'd		
Food groups	**Foods to use**	**Foods to avoid**
Desserts	Cornstarch, rice, or tapioca puddings; custard, fruit ice, plain ice milk, sherbet, gelatin desserts, fruit whips; special cakes or cookies made with allowed flours only	Pies, cookies, cakes, doughnuts, ice cream, prepared mixes
Fats and oils	Cottonseed, corn, soybean, or olive oil Olives French dressing; true mayonnaise or other dressing made with cornstarch Limited amounts of butter, margarine	Meat fat, bacon, lard Salad dressings or mayonnaise thickened with flour (check label) Coconut or oil Excessive chocolate Nuts
Sugars and sweets	All sugars, syrups, honey, molasses, jellies Marshmallows or sauce	Candies containing wheat, rye, oat, or barley products Avoid excessive use of high-fat candy (most candy bars)
Seasonings	As desired, soy sauce	Fat seasonings or gluten products not allowed
Vitamins	Aqueous multivitamins; B complex	

Cleft palate

Feeding difficulties in infants and young children may result from abnormalities in the structure of the mouth. When the parts of the upper jaw and of the palate separating the mouth and nasal cavity do not fuse properly during fetal development, the anatomic abnormality creates difficult feeding problems. The premaxillary and maxillary processes normally fuse early in gestation (between the fifth and eighth week of intrauterine life), and fusion of the palate is completed about one month later. If this fusion fails to occur, cleft lip (harelip) or cleft palate results. Since the infant is unable to suck adequately, early feedings are tiring and lengthy. A softened nipple with enlarged opening, through which the infant can obtain milk by a chewing motion, is helpful. In some instances a medicine dropper or gavage feedings may be used initially. The infant should be held in an upright position and fed slowly, in small amounts, to avoid aspiration. There should be brief rest periods and frequent burping to expel the large amount of air swallowed. If acid foods such as orange juice are irritating, ascorbic acid supplement is usually prescribed. As solid foods are added, they may be mixed with milk in the bottle and given in gruel or thickened form through a large nipple opening.

Surgical repair of a cleft palate is usually carried out over the growth years, depending on the extent of the deformity and the growth of the child. During this period the child may be cared for by a group of specialists to handle his overall development. This group may be found in larger medical centers and is called the cleft palate team. Preparation for surgery demands good nutritional status. Following surgery, special nutritional and nursing care is essential. The infant or child is usually fed a fluid or semifluid diet by use of a medicine dropper or a spoon. Great care must be exercised to protect the suture line and avoid any strain.

GENETIC DISEASES
Genetic inheritance concept

The concept of "inborn errors of metabolism" was first postulated by Sir Archibald Garrod in 1908. Although he probably had no clear conception of enzyme action, he pointed the way to a large number of conditions known today as genetic diseases that result from an inherited autosomal recessive mutant gene.

Definitions. The following is a review of the meanings of some key terms involved in the basic concept of genetic disease:

1. A *chromosome* is a rod-shaped body developed in the cell nucleus. Each human cell contains 46 chromosomes arranged in 23 pairs. One pair forms the sex chromosomes carrying the sex trait, and the remaining 22 pairs control the other various characteristics of the cell and of the individual.

2. *Autosomes* are any of the chromosomes other than the sex characteristics.

3. *Genes* (Gr. *gennan,* to produce) are self-reproducing particles in the cells, located at definite individual points (loci) on chromosomes. Each gene is a long, double-stranded molecule (helix) of DNA *(deoxyribonucleic acid),* with a special arrangement of its components—its so-called genetic code (see p. 60).

A *mutant gene* (L. *mutare,* to change) is an altered form of a gene that can be transmitted to the offspring. Why genes mutate is not known. Probably temperature, irradiation, or infection is involved. A mutant gene is an abnormal gene that keeps on reproducing itself in successive generations.

4. The genes on the respective pairs of chromosomes are almost identical with each other, so they too form pairs, or so-called links

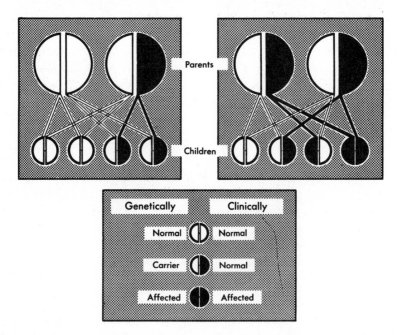

Fig. 19-3. Pattern of genetic disease. Transmission of recessive traits follows Mendel's law. If two carriers marry, one child will be normal, one child will manifest the trait, and two children will be carriers.

of genes. A gene trait is *recessive* (does not manifest itself) if it does not match its partner. The recessive gene must be carried by both parents to cause a defect.

5. *Heterozygote* is an individual in whom the members of one or more gene pairs are unlike. Such a person is called a "carrier" of that trait, but he does not manifest its symptoms. Transmission of recessive traits to successive generations follows the pattern established by Mendel (Fig. 19-3). If two carriers marry, the risk for each birth is 25% manifest trait, 50% carriers, 25% normal (neither carrier nor manifesting the trait).

Genetic control of heredity and cell function

Control of heredity. When the human ovum (female sex cell) is fertilized by the sperm (male sex cell), the fertilized ovum from which the new individual develops contains 46 chromosomes, 23 contributed by the sperm cell from the father and 23 contributed by the ovum from the mother. These 46 chromosomes align themselves in 23 pairs in the fertilized ovum, and with each successive cell division (mitosis) by which growth occurs in the new life, these same pairs of chromosomes are duplicated in the nucleus and become a part of the new cell. Thus the gene pattern of the original chromosomes received at conception from the parents remains to determine the offspring's inherited traits of sex, physical appearance, eye color, and so on.

Control of cell function. The genes not only control common hereditary characteristics in this manner but also control the metabolic function of the cell by their control of the synthesis of specific metabolic enzymes. There are 1,000 or more protein enzymes that control essentially all the chemical reactions that take place in cells. Each one of these enzymes is a *specific* protein synthesized by a *specific* DNA pattern in a *specific* gene (see p. 75). Therefore when a specific gene is abnormal (mutant), the en-

zyme whose synthesis it controls cannot be made. And in turn the metabolic reaction controlled by that enzyme cannot take place. The result is a genetic disease manifesting symptoms relative to those reaction products. Two such diseases are *phenylketonuria* and *galactosemia*.

Phenylketonuria (PKU)

Metabolic defect. Phenylketonuria was first observed in 1934 by a Norwegian biochemist and physician, Asbjorn Fölling. It is a genetic disease resulting from a mutant autosomal recessive gene. The normal gene controls the synthesis of the liver enzyme *phenylalanine hydroxylase,* which oxidizes *phenylalanine,* an essential amino acid, to *tyrosine,* another amino acid. Since the gene is defective, the enzyme cannot be produced, and the reaction does not proceed normally (Fig. 19-4). Phenylalanine accumulates in the blood, and its alternate metabolites, the phenyl acids, are excreted in the urine. One of these acids, *phenylpyruvic acid,* is a phenylketone; hence the name phenylketonuria. This acid gives the characteristic green color reaction with ferric chloride (the basis for the "diaper test" of the infant's urine to detect the presence of phenylketonuria).

Clinical symptoms. The most profound effect that may occur in untreated phenylketonuria is mental retardation. The IQ is usually below 50, and most frequently under 20. The damage to the central nervous system probably occurs within the first two years. The child may learn to walk, but few learn to talk. There is increased motor irritability, hyperactivity, convulsive seizures, and bizarre behavior—disorientation, failure to respond to strong stimuli, catatoniclike positions, fright reactions, and screaming episodes.

Because tyrosine is used in the production of the pigment material *melanin,* phenylketonuria children usually have blond or light brown hair and blue eyes. The skin is fair and susceptible to eczema. Tyrosine also is involved in the pro-

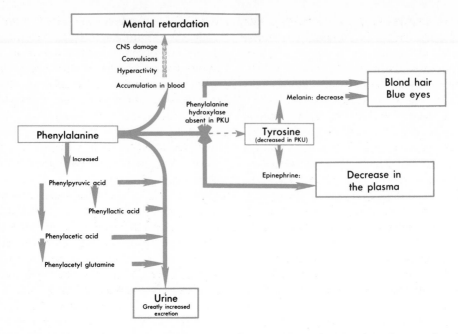

Fig. 19-4. The metabolic error in phenylketonuria. Because of the absence of the enzyme phenyl-alanine hydroxylase, the essential amino acid phenylalanine cannot be converted to tyrosine.

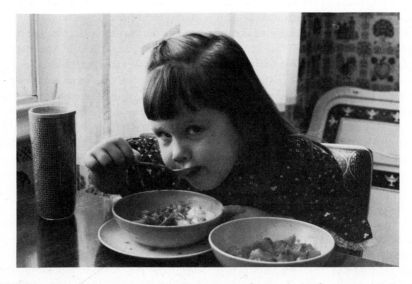

Fig. 19-5. PKU. This child is a delightful, perfectly developed 2-year-old. Screened and diagnosed at birth, she has eaten a carefully controlled low-phenylalanine diet and is growing normally.

duction of epinephrine by the adrenal gland, accounting for the low blood level of epinephrine in the child.

The urine frequently has a strong musty odor from the presence of large amounts of phenylacetic acid (Fig. 19-4). Sometimes this is the first thing the mother notices, leading her to seek a physician's care. This was the case in the initial discovery of the disease when a mother of two mentally retarded children complained of this unusual odor in the children's urine and called it to Fölling's attention, thus stimulating his active interest and study of the disease.

Dietary management. Treatment of phenylketonuria is dietary. A low-phenylalanine diet is used to reduce the serum phenylalanine and prevent the high levels that cause the clinical symptoms, especially the central nervous system damage. Since phenylalanine is an essential amino acid necessary for growth, it cannot be totally removed from the diet. Blood levels of phenylalanine are constantly monitored by the nutritionist or the physician, and the nutritionist calculates the diet to allow the limited amount of phenylalanine, usually between 10 and 20 mg/kg body weight (the diet of a normal child contains 100 to 200 mg of phenylalanine per kilogram body weight). This amount will maintain the blood levels within acceptable ranges (2 to 6 mg/dl) to prevent symptoms. Normal phenylalanine blood levels range from 1 to 3 mg/dl blood. In the untreated phenylketonuric child they may run as high as 60 times this.

MILK SUBSTITUTE FORMULA. Milk has a relatively high phenylalanine content, so the first need for the infant is a milk substitute. The formula is usually made from Lofenalac, a special casein hydrolysate balanced with fats, carbohydrates, vitamins, and minerals. One measure of Lofenalac powder in 60 ml (2 oz) of water makes a formula of 20 calories per 30 ml (1 oz) and is well accepted by the infant. A small designated measure of milk may be added to the Lofenalac formula to adjust the phenylalanine content.

LOW-PHENYLALANINE DIET. As the child grows (Fig. 19-5), solid foods are added to the diet as calculated according to their phenylalanine content. These food additions are selected from a list of phenylalanine food exchange groups or equivalents. The diet is prescribed by the nutritionist or physician according to the child's blood phenylalanine test.[20] The food plan is then calculated and outlined by the nutritionist in terms of numbers of food choices allowed daily from each food group. Then a meal pattern of feedings is made out for the mother to follow. The phenylalanine food exchange groups forming the basis of the low-phenylalanine diet are outlined in Table 19-2. It is not known yet how long such a diet must be continued. One clinician has suggested it may be possible to relax the dietary controls as early as age 4,[21] and subsequent tests in the use of a moderately relaxed diet with children ages 4 to 16 have shown all of them doing well.[22] For social reasons some clinics advise parents to discontinue the diets for boys when they enter school, but to continue it for girls since dietary management will be even more important in these patients during childbearing.[23,24] However, at present it is probably wise to continue the diet at least until the child is 6 to 8 years old.

Family counseling. Since dietary management of phenylketonuria (PKU) is the only known effective method of treatment, it is essential that initial education of the parents be as comprehensive and supportive as possible. A number of teaching guides and materials are available.[20] The parents charged with the care of a phenylketonuric child face physical, emotional, and financial tension. Depending on their personal resources and strength in all three areas, the course may be stormy or relatively stable. They must understand and accept the absolute necessity of following the diet carefully, so patient and understanding teaching must be done. Frequent home visits by the nutritionist or nurse may be a source of guidance and support as the child grows older (Fig. 19-6). Other family members and any subsequent siblings should be tested for phenylketonuria also.

Table 19-2. Food lists for use with low-phenylalanine diet*

Food	Amount	Phenylala-nine (mg)	Protein (g)	Cal-ories
Vegetables				
(Each serving listed contains approximately 15 mg phenylalanine)				
Baby and junior				
Beets	7 tbsp	15	1.1	35
Carrots	7 tbsp	15	0.7	28
Creamed spinach	1 tbsp	16	0.4	6
Green beans	2 tbsp	15	0.3	7
Squash	4 tbsp	14	0.4	14
Sweet potato	4 tbsp	15	0.7	42
Table vegetables				
Asparagus, cooked	1 stalk	12	0.6	4
Beans, green, cooked	4 tbsp (¼ cup)	14	0.6	9
Beans, yellow, wax, cooked	4 tbsp (¼ cup)	15	0.6	9
Bean sprouts, mung, cooked	2 tbsp	18	0.6	5
Beets, cooked	8 tbsp (½ cup)	14	0.8	34
Beet greens, cooked	1 tbsp	14	0.2	3
Broccoli, cooked	1 tbsp	11	0.3	3
Brussels sprouts, cooked	1 medium	16	0.6	5
Cabbage, raw, shredded	8 tbsp (½ cup)	15	0.7	12
Cabbage, cooked	5 tbsp (⅓ cup)	16	0.8	12
Carrots, raw	⅙ large (¼ cup)	16	0.5	16
Carrots, cooked	8 tbsp (½ cup)	17	0.5	23
Cauliflower, cooked	3 tbsp	18	0.6	6
Celery, cooked, diced†	4 tbsp (¼ cup)	15	0.4	6
Celery, raw†	1 stalk, 8-inch	16	0.5	7
Chard leaves, cooked	2 tbsp	19	0.6	6
Collards, cooked	1 tbsp	16	0.5	5
Cucumber slices, raw	8 slices, ⅛ inch thick	16	0.7	12
Eggplant, diced, raw	3 tbsp	18	0.4	9
Kale, cooked	2 tbsp	20	0.5	5
Lettuce†	3 small leaves	13	0.4	5
Mushrooms, cooked†	2 tbsp	14	0.4	35
Mushrooms, fresh†	2 small	16	0.5	3
Mustard greens, cooked	2 tbsp	18	0.6	6
Okra, cooked†	2 pods, 3-inch	13	0.4	7
Onion, raw, chopped	5 tbsp (⅓ cup)	14	0.5	20
Onion, cooked	4 tbsp (¼ cup)	14	0.5	19
Onion, young scallion	5, 5-inch long	14	0.5	23
Parsley, raw, chopped†	3 tbsp	13	0.4	5

*Bureau of Public Health Nutrition of the California State Department of Public Health: PKU, a diet guide for parents of children with phenylketonuria, 1969 revision, Berkeley, Calif., pp. 7-11.
†Phenylalanine calculated as 3.3% of total protein.
‡Phenylalanine calculated as 2.6% of total protein.
§Low phenylalanine recipes in Phenylalanine-restricted diet recipe book, Berkeley, Calif., 1972, State of California Dept. of Public Health.

Table 19-2. Food lists for use with low-phenylalanine diet—cont'd

Food	Amount	Phenylala-nine (mg)	Protein (g)	Cal-ories
Vegetables—cont'd				
Parsnips, cooked, diced†	3 tbsp	13	0.3	18
Peas	1 tbsp	15	0.4	5
Peppers, raw, chopped†	4 tbsp	13	0.4	12
Pickles, dill	8 slices, ⅛ inch thick	16	0.7	12
Pumpkin, cooked	4 tbsp (¼ cup)	14	0.5	16
Radishes, red, small†	4	13	0.4	8
Rutabagas, cooked	2 tbsp	16	0.3	10
Spinach, cooked	1 tbsp	15	0.4	3
Squash, summer, cooked	8 tbsp (½ cup)	16	0.6	16
Squash, winter, cooked	3 tbsp	16	0.6	14
Tomato, raw	½ small	14	0.5	10
Tomato, cooked	4 tbsp (¼ cup)	15	0.6	10
Tomato juice	4 tbsp (¼ cup)	17	0.6	12
Tomato catsup	2 tbsp	17	0.6	34
Turnip greens, cooked	1 tbsp	18	0.4	4
Turnips, diced, cooked	5 tbsp (⅓ cup)	16	0.4	12
Soups (condensed)				
Asparagus	1½ tbsp	16	0.5	14
Beef broth	1 tbsp	14	0.5	3
Celery	2 tbsp	18	0.4	19
Minestrone	1 tbsp	17	1.5	25
Mushroom	1 tbsp	11	0.2	17
Onion	1 tbsp	14	0.6	8
Tomato	1 tbsp	11	0.2	11
Vegetarian vegetable	1½ tbsp	17	0.4	14
Fruits				
(Each serving listed contains approximately 15 mg phenylalanine)				
Baby and junior				
Applesauce	11 tbsp	15	0.3	137
Applesauce and apricots	10 tbsp	15	0.4	128
Applesauce and pineapple	10 tbsp	15	0.3	110
Apricots with tapioca	12½ tbsp	15	0.5	146
Bananas	8 tbsp (½ cup)	14	0.6	97
Bananas and pineapple	10 tbsp	14	0.4	117
Peaches	9½ tbsp	16	0.7	117
Pears	14 tbsp	15	0.6	136
Pears and pineapple	14 tbsp	15	0.8	146
Plums with tapioca	11 tbsp	15	0.5	149
Prunes with tapioca	9½ tbsp	14	0.4	119
Fruit juices				
Apricot nectar	6 oz (¾ cup)	14	0.6	102
Cranberry juice	12 oz (1½ cups)	15	0.6	39
Grape juice	4 oz (½ cup)	14	0.5	80

Continued.

Table 19-2. Food lists for use with low-phenylalanine diet—cont'd

Food	Amount	Phenylala-nine (mg)	Protein (g)	Cal-ories
Fruits—cont'd				
Grapefruit juice	8 oz (1 cup)	16	1.2	104
Orange juice	6 oz (¾ cup)	16	1.2	84
Peach nectar	5 oz (⅔ cup)	15	0.5	75
Pineapple juice	6 oz (¾ cup)	16	0.6	90
Prune juice	4 oz (½ cup)	16	0.5	84
Table fruits				
Apple, raw	2 med. 2½-inch diam.	16	0.6	160
Applesauce	16 tbsp (1 cup)	16	0.6	273
Apricots, raw	1 medium	12	0.5	25
Apricots, canned	2 med. 2 tbsp syrup	14	0.6	80
Avocado, cubed or mashed‡	5 tbsp (⅓ cup)	16	0.6	80
Banana, raw, sliced	5 tbsp (¼ cup)	15	0.5	66
Blackberries, raw‡	5 tbsp (⅓ cup)	14	0.6	25
Blackberries, canned in syrup‡	5 tbsp (⅓ cup)	13	0.5	55
Blueberries, raw or frozen‡	12 tbsp (¾ cup)	16	0.6	60
Blueberries, canned in syrup‡	10 tbsp	16	0.6	140
Boysenberries, frozen, sweet‡	8 tbsp (½ cup)	16	0.6	72
Cantaloupe, diced	⅙ medium	13	0.4	19
Cherries, sweet, canned in syrup‡	8 tbsp (½ cup)	16	0.6	104
Dates, pitted, chopped	3 tbsp	18	0.7	96
Figs, raw‡	1 large	18	0.7	40
Figs, canned in syrup‡	2 figs in 4 tsp syrup	16	0.6	90
Figs, dried‡	1 small	16	0.6	40
Fruit cocktail‡	12 tbsp (¾ cup)	16	0.6	120
Grapefruit, raw	½ medium	11	0.5	41
Grapes, American type	8 grapes	14	0.5	24
Grapes, American slipskin	5 tbsp (⅓ cup)	16	0.6	25
Grapes, Thompson seedless	8 tbsp (½ cup)	13	0.8	64
Guava, raw‡	½ medium	13	0.5	35
Honeydew melon‡	¼ small 5-inch melon	13	0.5	32
Mango, raw‡	1 small	18	0.7	66
Nectarines, raw	1-2 inches high, 2 inches diam.	15	0.4	45
Oranges, raw	1 medium 3 inches diam. or ⅔ cup sections	15	1.5	73
Papayas, raw‡	¼ med. or ½ cup	14	0.6	36
Peaches, raw	1 medium	15	0.5	46
Peaches, canned in syrup	2 medium halves	18	0.6	88
Pears, raw	1, 3 × 2½ inches	14	1.3	100
Pears, canned in syrup	2 med. halves, 2 tbsp syrup	14	1.3	78
Pineapple, raw‡	16 tbsp (1 cup)	16	0.6	80
Pineapple, canned in syrup‡	2 small slices	13	0.5	93
Plums, raw	½ 2-inch plum	12	0.3	15

Table 19-2. Food lists for use with low-phenylalanine diet—cont'd

Food	Amount	Phenylala-nine (mg)	Protein (g)	Cal-ories
Fruits—cont'd				
Plums, canned in syrup	3-2 tbsp syrup	16	0.5	91
Prunes, dried	2 large	14	0.4	54
Raisins, dried seedless	2 tbsp	14	0.5	54
Raspberries, raw‡	5 tbsp (⅓ cup)	13	0.5	25
Raspberries, canned in syrup‡	6 tbsp	14	0.5	78
Strawberries, raw‡	10 large	16	0.6	32
Strawberries, frozen‡	6 tbsp	14	0.5	108
Tangerines	1½ large	15	1.2	66
Watermelon‡	½ cup cubes	13	0.5	28
Breads and cereals				
(Each serving listed contains approximately 30 mg phenylalanine)				
Baby and junior				
Cereals, ready to serve				
Barley	3 tbsp	32	0.8	24
Oatmeal	2 tbsp	35	1.2	28
Rice	5 tbsp (⅓ cup)	30	0.6	40
Wheat	2 tbsp	30	0.6	17
Creamed corn	3 tbsp	30	0.5	27
Sweet potatoes (Gerber's)	3 tbsp	32	0.5	31
Table foods				
Cereals, cooked				
Cornmeal	4 tbsp (¼ cup)	29	0.6	29
Cream of rice	4 tbsp (¼ cup)	35	0.7	34
Cream of Wheat	2 tbsp	27	0.6	16
Farina	2 tbsp	25	0.5	18
Malt-o-Meal	2 tbsp	27	0.5	17
Oatmeal	2 tbsp	32	0.7	18
Pettijohns	2 tbsp	24	0.5	19
Ralston	2 tbsp	34	0.7	18
Rice, brown or white	4 tbsp (¼ cup)	35	0.7	34
Wheatena	2 tbsp	27	0.5	19
Cereals, ready to serve				
Alpha Bits	4 tbsp (¼ cup)	32	0.6	28
Cheerios	3 tbsp	32	0.6	20
Corn Chex	7 tbsp	31	0.7	39
Cornfetti	5 tbsp (⅓ cup)	31	0.6	46
Cornflakes	5 tbsp (⅓ cup)	29	0.6	30
Crispy Critters	4 tbsp (¼ cup)	30	0.6	28
Kix	5 tbsp (⅓ cup)	28	0.6	31
Krumbles	3 tbsp	32	0.7	26
Rice Chex	6 tbsp	32	0.7	49
Rice flakes	5 tbsp (⅓ cup)	33	0.6	32
Rice Krispies	6 tbsp	30	0.6	40

Continued.

Table 19-2. Food lists for use with low-phenylalanine diet—cont'd

Food	Amount	Phenylala-nine (mg)	Protein (g)	Cal-ories
Breads and cereals—cont'd				
Rice, puffed	12 tbsp (³/₄ cup)	30	0.6	38
Sugar Crisp, puffed wheat	4 tbsp (¹/₄ cup)	30	0.6	46
Sugar Frosted Flakes	5 tbsp (¹/₃ cup)	29	0.6	55
Wheat Chex	10 biscuits	30	0.6	22
Wheaties	3 tbsp	26	0.5	20
Wheat, puffed	6 tbsp	30	0.6	16
Crackers				
Arrowroot cookies	1¹/₂	33	0.7	31
Barnum Animal	5	30	0.6	45
Graham (65/lb)	1	26	0.5	30
Ritz (no cheese)	2	24	0.5	34
Saltines (140/lb)	2	29	0.6	28
Tortilla, corn	¹/₂ (6-inch diam.)	32	0.8	32
Wheat Thins (248/lb)	5	30	0.6	45
Zweiback	²/₃ biscuit	30	0.6	21
Corn, cooked	2 tbsp	32	0.7	17
Hominy	2 tbsp	32	0.7	17
Macaroni, cooked	1¹/₂ tbsp	34	0.6	19
Noodles, cooked	1¹/₂ tbsp	30	0.6	19
Popcorn, popped	5 tbsp (¹/₃ cup)	31	0.6	17
Potato chips	6 chips, 2-inch diam.	29	0.7	68
Potato, Irish, cooked	3 tbsp	33	0.8	31
Spaghetti, cooked	2 tbsp	33	0.6	21
Sweet potato, cooked	2 tbsp	25	0.4	31
Fats				
(Each serving listed contains approximately 5 mg phenylalanine)				
Butter	1 tbsp	5	0.1	100
French dressing, commercial	1 tbsp	5	0.1	59
Margarine	1 tbsp	5	0.1	100
Mayonnaise, commercial	¹/₂ tbsp	5	0.1	30
Olives, green or ripe	1 medium	5	0.1	12
Desserts				
(Each serving listed contains approximately 30 mg phenylalanine)				
Cake§	¹/₁₂ of cake			
Cookies Rice flour§	2			
Corn starch§	2			
Cookies, Arrowroot	1¹/₂			
Ice cream				
Chocolate§	²/₃ cup			
Pineapple§	²/₃ cup			
Strawberry§	²/₃ cup			

Table 19-2. Food lists for use with low-phenylalanine diet—cont'd

Food	Amount	Phenylala-nine (mg)	Protein (g)	Cal-ories
Desserts—cont'd				
Jell-O	⅓ cup			
Puddings§	½ cup			
Sauce, Hershey	2 tbsp			
Wafers, sugar, Nabisco	5			
Free foods				
Apple juice				
Beverages, carbonated				
Gingerbread§				
Guava butter				
Candy				
Butterscotch				
Cream mints				
Fondant				
Gumdrops				
Hard				
Jelly beans				
Lollipops				
Cherries, maraschino				
Fruit ices (if no more than ½ cup used daily)				
Jell-Quik				
Jellies				
Kool-Aid				
Lemonade				
Molasses				
Oil				
Pepper, black, ground				
Popsicles, with artificial fruit flavor				
Rich's Topping				
Salt				
Shortening, vegetable				
Soy sauce				
Sugar, brown, white, or confectioner's				
Syrups, corn or maple				
Tang				

The physician and the nutritionist carry primary responsibility on the clinical care team, with supportive care by the nurse as well as the biochemist providing laboratory services. Together with wise parents, this team provides initial and continuing care so that the phenylketonuric child will grow and develop normally. Such a child, diagnosed at birth by widespread screening programs, has a healthy and happy adulthood ahead, instead of the profound disease consequences he would probably have experienced so few years ago.

Public health implications. Phenylketonuria screening surveys have shown that the con-

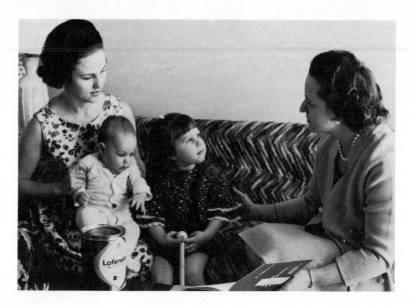

Fig. 19-6. Home visits by the nutritionist support this young mother's fine care of her 2-year-old daughter, a phenylketonuric child screened at birth. Careful, understanding diet control has enabled this child to develop normally in all respects. Here she sits between her mother and the nutritionist, interested and alert. The infant, a boy, is normal.

dition occurs more frequently than originally estimated. These surveys indicate an incidence of about one in every 10,000 births. The possibilities of severe mental retardation from undiagnosed and untreated phenylketonuria make public health implications obvious. A number of tests have been developed to detect the disease. They are listed on p. 447.

The more recent, sensitive tests of blood samples have been the basis of laws in several states making mandatory the screening of all newborns for phenylketonuria. The inhibition assay test, developed by Guthrie,[25-27] is a highly specific blood test, sensitive as early as the third day of life. A simple heel puncture is made and the blood is absorbed on specially treated absorbing paper. Another definitive blood test is the fluorimetric procedure developed by McCaman and Robins.[28] For some time, in California both of these tests have been approved for use under the regulations that are now part of the State Administrative Code, Ti-

tle 17. These amendments, which make phenylketonuria screening mandatory throughout the state for all newborns, were signed into law in 1965 and became effective January 1, 1966.

Tyrosinosis

A similar genetic disease, tyrosinosis, having high gene frequency among people of French Canadian descent,[29] is characterized by elevated plasma and urinary tyrosine and by an increase in urinary phenolic acids. It is caused by the missing enzyme *para-hydroxyphenylpyruvic acid oxidase,* which converts para-hydroxyphenylpyruvic acid (pHPPA), a metabolic product in the normal pathway of tyrosine oxidation, into homogentisic acid in the liver. The resulting increases in tyrosine and its metabolites in body fluids and tissues account for the clinical manifestations. These clinical problems include cirrhosis of the liver, hypophosphatemia, rickets, renal tubular damage, and mental retardation.[30]

TO PROBE FURTHER
Tests used in phenylketonuria

Test	Method	Use
Urine tests		
Diaper test	10% ferric chloride dropped on freshly wet diaper. Green spot is positive, indicates probable PKU.	Cheap. Useful in screening large groups of infants, but not of value until the infant is at least 6 weeks of age.
Phenistix* test	Prepared test stick pressed against wet diaper or dipped in urine. Green color reaction indicates probable PKU.	Simple; more accurate than diaper test. Useful in screening large groups of infants, but not of value until after infant is 6 weeks old.
Dinitrophenyl-hydrazine (DNPH) test†	0.5 to 1.0 ml of urine placed in test tube and equal amount of DNPH solution added. Immediate pale yellow-orange color reaction is negative. A gradual change to opaque bright yellow is positive and indicates probable PKU.	Cheap, accurate, but more complicated than diaper test or Phenistix; most useful in clinical setting to confirm these tests.
Blood serum phenylalanine tests		
Guthrie inhibition assay method‡	Drops of blood placed on filter paper. Lab uses a bacterial growth inhibition test. Level above 8 mg phenylalanine per deciliter blood diagnostic of PKU.	Effective in newborn period. Used also to monitor PKU diet. Blood easily obtained by heel or finger puncture. Inexpensive; used for wide-scale screening.
LaDu-Michael method§	5 ml of blood; serum separated and tested for phenylalanine. Level above 8 mg/dl. blood indicates PKU. In PKU patients, level above 8 to 12 mg phenylalanine per deciliter blood indicates loss of dietary control.	Useful diagnostic tool, and to monitor PKU diet. Requires blood drawn from patient, and the lab method is difficult (test not available in many labs).
McCaman and Robins fluorometric method‖	5 ml of blood; serum separated and tested for phenylalanine. Level above 8 mg indicates PKU or loss of dietary control.	Diagnostic and diet monitoring tool. Lab procedure more simple than LaDu-Michael method. Test not available in many labs.

*Manufactured by Ames Co., Elkhart, Ind.
†Centerwall, W., and Centerwall, S.: Phenylketonuria, U.S. Children's Bureau, Pub. No. 338, Washington, D.C., 1961, Government Printing Office.
‡Guthrie, R.: Blood screening for phenylketonuria, J.A.M.A. **178**:863, 1961.
§LaDu, B., and Michael, P.: An enzymatic spectrophotometric method for the determination of phenylalanine in blood, J. Lab. Clin. Med. **55**:491, 1960.
‖McCaman, M., and Robins, E.: Fluorometric method for the determination of phenylalanine in the serum, J. Lab. Clin. Med. **59**:885, 1962.

Treatment centers on dietary management designed to remove tyrosine and its precursor, phenylalanine, from the diet. Principles such as those used in treatment of PKU are followed: (1) use of a milk substitute, a commercial product made from a casein hydrolysate from which most of the phenylalanine and tyrosine has been removed, and (2) addition of selected foods from carefully calculated food lists according to content of both amino acids—phenylalanine and tyrosine.[31] Clinical experience with several patients showing elevated serum methionine levels as well has led some practitioners to restrict this amino acid also. Food lists reflecting restriction of these three amino acids—phenylalanine, tyrosine, and methionine—are provided.[32]

Galactosemia

Metabolic defect. Galactosemia is also a genetic disease caused by a missing enzyme. The metabolic defect, transmitted by a single autosomal recessive gene, is illustrated in Fig. 19-7. The incidence of galactosemia is lower than that of phenylketonuria. It occurs about once in 25,000 to 50,000 births.

The missing enzyme, *galactose-1-phosphate uridyl transferase,* is one of three enzymes that control steps in the conversion of galactose to glucose. Milk, the infant's first food, contains a large amount of the disaccharide lactose (milk sugar), which is acted on by the intestinal digestive enzyme *lactase* (see p. 20) to produce th monosaccharides glucose and galactose. After galactose is initially combined with phosphate to begin the metabolic conversion to glucose, it cannot proceed further in the galactosemic infant. Galactose-l-phosphate and galactose rapidly accumulate in the blood and in various body tissues.

Clinical symptoms. The excess tissue accumulations of galactose cause rapid damage to the untreated infant. The child fails to thrive, and clinical evidences are apparent soon after birth. Liver damage brings jaundice, hepatomegaly with cirrhosis, enlargement of the spleen, and ascites. Death usually results from hepatic failure. If the infant survives, the continuing tissue damage and accompanying hypoglycemia in the optic lens and the brain cause cataracts and mental retardation.

Dietary management. The main indirect source of dietary galactose is milk. Therefore *all* forms of milk and lactose must be removed from the diet. In this instance a galactose-*free* diet can be used. Although galactose is part of certain body structures, the needed amounts can be synthesized by the body. The milk substitute

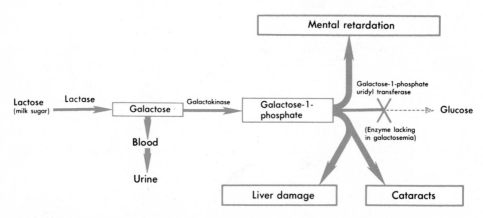

Fig. 19-7. Metabolic error in galactosemia. Because of the absence of the enzyme galactose-1-phosphate uridyl transferase, galactose cannot be converted to glucose.

usually used for infant feeding is Nutramigen, a complete protein hydrolysate that is free of galactose. Careful attention must be given to avoid lactose from other food sources as solid foods are added to the infant's diet. An outline of foods to use and to avoid is given on p. 451. Parents must be carefully instructed to check labels on all commercial products. Table 19-3 gives products that normally contain lactose. Even drugs contain lactose occasionally as an ingredient.

Public health implications. Although original estimates place the incidence of galactosemia at one in every 25,000 to 50,000 births, there is evidence that it may not be so rare. Asymptomatic carriers have been detected in families of galactosemic children and in other individuals. Also, continuing reports give increasing incidence. The severe and rapid effects of the disease and the profound effects on body organs and tissues, especially on the brain, make attention to early diagnosis at birth and subsequent careful treatment with a galactose-free diet mandatory. Tests have been developed for such immediate screening. Cord blood may be used immediately after birth to establish a diagnosis, using a simple test for galactose-1-phosphate activity in erythrocytes. Children detected may be carefully observed with continuing blood tests every two to three months to monitor the diet.[33] Since a carrier can also be identified by a lowered enzyme level in the red cells, it may be advisable to eliminate lactose from the prenatal diet of a mother detected as a carrier.

Maple syrup urine disease (MSUD)

Another rare genetic disease among the aminoacidurias is maple syrup urine disease, so called because of the sensory and physical

---

Table 19-3. Typical uses of lactose*

Ascorbic acid and citric acid mixtures	Monosodium glutamate extender
Buttermilk	Party dips
Cakes and sweet rolls	Penicillin and other antibiotics
Canned and frozen fruits and vegetables	Pharmaceutical bulking agents, fillers, and excipients
Caramels, fudge, and tableted candies	
Cheese foods and spreads	Pie crusts and fillings
Cookies and cookie sandwich fillings	Powdered coffee cream
Cordials and liqueurs	Powdered soft drinks
Cottage cheese and cottage cheese dressings	Puddings
Dietetic and diabetic preparations	Salad dressings
Dried soups	Sherbets, frozen desserts, and ices
Easter egg dyes and dye carrier	Simulated mother's milk; infant food formulas
Fireworks, flares, and pyrotechnics	Sour cream
French fries and corn curls	Spice blends
Frozen cultures	Starter cultures
Health and geriatric foods	Sweetened condensed milk
High-solids ice cream	Sweetness reducers in icings, candies, preserves, and fruit pie fillings
Instant coffee	
Instant potatoes	Tablets (food and pharmaceutical)
Meat products	Tinctures
Modified skimmed milk	Vitamin and mineral mixtures

*Koch, R., et al.: Nutrition in the treatment of galactosemia, J. Am. Diet. Assoc. **43:**221, 1963.

characteristics of the urine. It is an autosomal recessive inborn error of metabolism involving a deficiency of the oxidative decarboxylation of the keto acids derived from the three essential branched-chain amino acids—leucine, isoleucine, and valine. The only treatment is dietary restriction of these three amino acids. Helpful food guides for this difficult diet have been prepared by Acosta and Elsas[34] and expanded by Bell and others[35] to provide more variety in food choices. Tabulated food lists are available from these excellent sources.

Lactose intolerance

A deficiency of any one of the disaccharidases in the intestine—lactase, sucrase, maltase, or isomaltase—may produce a wide range of gastrointestinal problems and abdominal pain because the specific sugar involved cannot be digested. Of these clinical problems, lactose intolerance is perhaps the most common.[36] It is frequently seen in adults and may also occur in children. A diet similar to that used for galactosemia is required. Milk and all products containing lactose are carefully avoided. For children a milk substitute is used—Nutramigen, soy milk, or a meat base formula.

Juvenile diabetes
Dietary management

Diabetes and its current management is discussed in Chapter 25. Several principles, however, of the care of diabetes occurring in children are important to emphasize here.

The child with diabetes must not be viewed as a "little adult." In fact the two forms of diabetes as seen in children and in adults are so different as to warrant the use of two different names. The cause of juvenile diabetes is different, treatment is different and more complicated, and the prognosis is far more critical.[37-39]

Pediatricians usually hold one of three opinions concerning a philosophy of diet management for diabetic children. These are rigid diet control, the "free" diet, and the moderate approach.

Rigid diet control. This approach perhaps arises from experience in previous years, before development of more sensitive and varied types of insulin to meet individual needs, and from the more severe nature of the disease in children. A rigid, calculated, and weighed diet (weighed on gram scale) is prescribed and followed in some clinics.[40] Pediatricians who still follow this approach apparently feel that the more brittle, labile form of diabetes in children, as compared with its more stable form in adults, requires this rigid supervision. In such programs, urine sugars are carefully checked frequently, with a sugar-free urine the criterion as a measure for control.

"Free" diet. Quotation marks are needed around the word "free," because most pediatricians who use this term do not mean *absolutely* free. However, they do seem to feel that a somewhat unlimited approach to diet (food as the child desires or has appetite for) should be followed. Insulin is usually adjusted to cover the food intake, and some sugar spillage in the urine is allowed. The rationale given for such an approach is the psychologic benefit it has for the child.

Moderate approach. The more moderate approach, avoiding the tension of extreme rigidity on the one hand, and the inconsistencies of a purely "free" regimen on the other, is followed by the majority of pediatricians and nutritionists. This approach is based on two realistic principles: (1) the normal physical and psychosocial growth and development needs of the child and (2) the nature of diabetes in children and the needs it imposes for balance and consistent habits.

NORMAL NUTRITIONAL NEEDS FOR GROWTH AND DEVELOPMENT. During the formative growth years an optimum nutritional base is essential to health. These physiologic needs for growth and the psychosocial developmental paths that accompany each stage of normal development

Foods that may be included or should be excluded in a galactose-free diet*

Food categories	Foods included	Foods excluded†
Milk and milk products	None; Nutramigen and soybean milks used as milk substitutes	All milk of any species and all products containing milk, as skim, dried, evaporated, condensed; yogurt; cheese; ice cream; sherbet; malted milk
Legumes	All may be included if facilities are available for monitoring erythrocyte galactose-1-phosphate	
Meat, fish, and fowl	Plain beef, chicken, fish, turkey, lamb, veal, pork, and ham	Creamed or breaded meat, fish or fowl; sausage products, such as weiners, liver sausage cold cuts containing milk; organ meats, such as liver, pancreas, and brain
Eggs	All	None
Vegetables	Artichokes, asparagus, beets, broccoli, cabbage, carrots, cauliflower, celery, chard, corn, cucumber, eggplant, green beans, kale, lettuce, mustard, okra, onions, parsley, parsnips, pumpkin, rutabagas, spinach, squash, tomatoes	Sugar beets, peas, lima beans; creamed, breaded or buttered vegetables; canned or frozen vegetables; corn curls (if lactose is added during processing)
Potatoes and substitutes	White and sweet potatoes, yams, macaroni, noodles, spaghetti, rice	Any creamed, breaded, or buttered; French fried or instant potatoes if lactose is added during processing
Breads and cereals	Any that do not contain milk or milk products‡	Prepared mixes, such as muffins, biscuits, waffles, pancakes; some dry cereals; Instant Cream of Wheat. *Read labels carefully.*
Fats	Margarines and dressings that do not contain milk or milk products; oils, shortenings; bacon	Margarines and dressings containing milk or milk products; butter; cream; cream cheese
Soups	Clear soups; vegetable soups that do not contain peas or lima beans; consommés	Cream soups, chowders, commercially prepared soups containing lactose
Desserts	Water and fruit ices; gelatin; angel food cake; homemade cakes, pies, cookies made from acceptable ingredients	Commercial cakes, cookies, and mixes; custard, puddings, ice cream made with milk; any containing chocolate
Fruits	All fresh; canned or frozen that are not processed with lactose	Any canned or frozen processed with lactose
Miscellaneous	Nuts and nut butters, unbuttered popcorn, olives, pure sugar candy, jelly or marmalade, sugar, corn syrup, plain chocolate, dry cocoa	Gravy, white sauce; milk chocolate, toffee, peppermints, butterscotch, caramels, molasses; instant coffee, powdered soft drinks, monosodium glutamate, some spice blends, chewing gum

*Koch, R., et al.: Nutrition in the treatment of galactosemia, J. Am. Diet. Assoc. **43:**220, 1963.

†In all instances, labels should be read carefully, and any product that contains milk, lactose, casein, whey, dry milk solids, or curds should be omitted.

‡In each area, bakeries should be contacted and a list of acceptable products made available.

Table 19-4. Teaching plan and record for diabetic child and parents*

Patient's name _____

	Discussion	Return explanation	Demonstration	Return demonstration	Date	P = Parents C = Child **Remarks**
Conference with physician						
Provide educational materials on diabetes						
Nature of diabetes						
Acidosis						
Insulin shock						
Collecting and testing urine						
Method used at home						
Giving insulin injections						
Type of insulin						
Site of injection						
Rotation of injection sites						
Procedure						
Mixing insulin						
Equipment for insulin (same as home)						
List of equipment to buy						
Cost and where purchased (review comparison costs of all equipment)						
Diet						
Diet history, assessment, and food plan: nutritionist						
School						

*I am indebted to my colleague and friend Marian Yeaw, R.N., pediatric nursing instructor, for this comprehensive and useful tool to guide the education program of a diabetic child and his family.

Table 19-4. Teaching plan and record for diabetic child and parents—cont'd

Patient's name	Discussion	Return explanation	Demonstration	Return demonstration	Date	P = Parents C = Child **Remarks**
Home						
Exercise						
Gym and sports						
Hygiene						
Feet						
Skin						
Time schedule arranged with family						
Home routine						
Weekends						
Diabetic camp (purpose, costs, application, procedure)						
"Forecast"						
Medic Alert (purpose, application, procedure)						
School						
Conference with school nurse						
Testing urine						
Giving insulin						
Reference materials						

have been outlined in the previous chapter. The normal nutritional needs of the child are fundamental.

ACCOMMODATIONS TO DIABETES. The insulin-sensitive type of diabetes in children appears different from diabetes that occurs in adults in their middle or older years of life. The child developing diabetes is likely to be undernourished when the disease is first discovered. It usually runs a more labile course and requires closer consideration and consistent, sound, self-care by the patient and family. Also the erratic pattern of physical activity in children and the emotional struggles of obtaining maturity impose additional needs for sympathetic guidance, balance, and control.

NUTRIENT RATIO. A balanced diet for children includes adequate quantities of protein, carbohydrate, and fat to meet growth and energy demands.

PROTEIN. Optimal levels for growth are about 1.8 g/kg body weight for children under 3 years of age, and 1 g/kg body weight for older children. Protein should contribute about 20% of the total calories.

CALORIES. Calories should be sufficient for activity and growth. Carbohydrates should contribute about 50% of the total calories to supply the major source of energy, with the majority of this amount coming from complex carbohydrates—starch, with its fiber content intact. Fat should be sufficient but not excessive, *moderation* being the key. As the child grows older, weight control will be an important part of general care, and dietary habits of moderation in the use of fat will be helpful to that end. Also, because carbohydrate and fat metabolisms are so intimately associated and interrelated (see p. 30), both factors are well considered together in the management of diabetes.

VITAMINS AND MINERALS. Optimal intake of vitamins and minerals should be assured for the metabolic requirements of growth. A well-planned and consistently followed balanced diet should supply these needs. Occasionally, however, where adequate diet may be questionable or a greater margin of safety is desirable, the physician may prescribe supplements.

DISTRIBUTION OF MEALS. The distribution of food through the day should be based on the absorption rate and activity of the insulin used and on the general family meal pattern. Usually these needs are met with three fairly equal meals at breakfast, lunch, and dinner, with an added afternoon and evening snack. A midmorning snack may also be required by a younger child.

REGULARITY AND PORTION SIZES. The establishment of regular habits and a routine schedule are important factors in early and continuing stabilization of the diabetes. Day-to-day needs and activities will influence the schedule, but these may be accommodated in the day's balanced plan. The three balance factors are always food, insulin, and exercise, with additional considerations during periods of infection.

EXCHANGE SYSTEM OF DIETARY CONTROL. For some three decades a system of dietary control based on food equivalents has been in common use throughout the United States for planning diabetic diets.[41] This plan is based on the concept that if foods are of fairly equal composition, it does not matter which of them is used. Thus foods commonly used are grouped according to like composition, and these groups are called "exchange groups." The diet plan outlines for the mother and the child a meal pattern based on the number of choices from each of the food groups for each meal. With such a plan, flexibility and freedom of choice within the food groups are possible, all the while maintaining the consistency of habit necessary for control. A listing of these exchange food groups is given on pp. 546-550. A new revision of the food exchange groups, mainly incorporating low saturated fat modifications, has been issued.[42]

Teaching program for juvenile diabetes

The keystone of treatment and the basis of continuing care should be an early, thorough, and understanding teaching program for the child and his family. There should be no discounting of the fact that the child has diabetes, but at the same time it should not be used as a crutch or excuse to deprive the child of developing normal responsibility and maturity along with his peers. That he is essentially a "normal" healthy person, given the wise control of his diabetes, is an important concept to grasp. He is not primarily a diabetic child—he is a normally growing and developing child who has diabetes. There is a great difference in the two perspectives.

Time of instruction. Many later problems in control may be avoided by careful and thorough instruction at the initial development of the diabetes. Time spent in the beginning often saves time and tears later. Parents and child need time and opportunity to accept their new situation and make adequate psychologic adjustment to it. By and large, mature adjustment to any problem is aided by sound knowledge of its nature. This is especially true in the care of juvenile diabetes; the essential aim is to build in the patient as he grows an independence from the physician for ordinary day-to-day care of the diabetes and to develop in him a mature sense of responsibility and self-direction. In the last analysis the welfare of the person with diabetes—as with almost all persons—is in his own hands.

Content of instruction. The instructions should include basic needs for routine care: (1) an understanding of diabetes, (2) a realistic diet plan to meet normal needs, provide a basis for balance of the diabetes, and fit in with family food patterns, (3) techniques of insulin administration and minor adjustment, (4) urine testing for sugar, (5) the keeping of reasonable daily records according to need, (6) personal cleanliness and skin care, (7) recognition of early signs of insulin shock and how to treat it, and (8) recognition of early signs of acidosis and the need for immediate medical care.

A check list for planning such a teaching program as is followed in many clinics is given in Table 19-4. Active involvement of the patient and his family in practice sessions and feedback discussion is essential.

FOOD ALLERGIES IN INFANTS AND CHILDREN

The care of the allergic child is often frustrating and formidable for both the child and his parents. A wide variety of environmental, emotional, and physical factors influence the child's reaction, and a suitable regimen is sometimes difficult to find. Since sensitivity to protein substances is a common basis of the allergy, the early foods of infants and children are frequent offenders. Children tend to become less allergic to food sources as they grow older and respond more to inhalent allergens.

Milk. Cows' milk has long been and continues to be the most common cause of allergic disease in young infants. Park's classic 1920 case of an infant with violent vomiting reactions to minute amounts of milk is well known. The child's severe response was only overcome by a long, gradual desensitizing program, beginning at 6 weeks of age with a single drop of diluted cows' milk and bringing the child to a tolerance for 0.5 L (1 pt) of milk a day by the time he was 3 years old. Other such reports of violent reactions are found in the literature. Current observation, continuing former clinical experience,[43] indicates that milk allergy occurs in 1% to 2% of all infants and accounts for some 30% of the cases among allergic infants.

The allergy to milk usually causes gastrointestinal difficulties such as vomiting, diarrhea, and colic. The problem is generally identified by clinical symptoms, family history, and a trial on a milk-free diet, using a substitute formula such as a soybean preparation (for example, Sobee) or a meat formula. However, pediatricians agree generally that there may be a tendency among some clinicians to overdiagnose milk allergy in infants and children with diarrhea, colic, irritability, and skin rash. Thus a remission of symptoms on a milk-free diet should always be followed by a trial on milk again to determine if it does indeed cause the symptoms to reappear. Only then should the child be labeled as allergic to milk.[44] Sometimes lactose intolerance may be confused with milk allergy.[45]

Other frequent responses among infants allergic to milk are skin problems, such as rashes or eczema, and respiratory difficulties, such as wheezing or runny nose. Often these symptoms appear and disappear spontaneously, regardless of dietary changes. But they tend to be more often caused by food if gastrointestinal problems are also present with them.

Eggs, wheat, and other foods. The albumin in egg white is a potential allergen, and hence is usually added to the infant's diet following earlier use of egg yolk. Wheat is also a fairly common food allergen among allergic children. The specific biochemical sensitivity to gluten (a protein found in wheat) in the child with gluten-induced celiac disease (p. 430) may be considered an example, although the biochemical defects in the mucosal cell in celiac disease probably represent a different sensitivity mechanism.

Dietary management. In an allergic child's diet, foods are usually added slowly, common offenders being excluded in early feedings. In some cases a series of diagnostic diets, such as the Rowe Elimination Diets (p. 457), may be used to identify the offending food. Each of the four basic diets is used for a trial period. If no change occurs in the allergic condition, the patient is given the next diet. If, however, on a given diet the patient's symptoms improve, it is assumed that the offending food is not in that diet list. Then foods are added one at a time to test the patient's response. If a given food causes return of the allergy, the food is then identified as an offending allergen and is eliminated from use. Guidance in the substitution of special food products and in the use of special recipes should be provided for the child's mother by the nutritionist and the nurse.

The following is a general hypoallergy diet list of foods that should be avoided:

Eggs	Bacon
Fish	Citrus fruits
Wheat	Nuts
Strawberries	Peanut butter
Tomatoes	Chocolate
Pork	Pineapple
Milk* or milk products	

*Use soybean milk substitute.

Family education. The education of the parents and family of an allergic child should include a knowledge and understanding of the allergic state and the many factors that influence it. If specific foods have been definitely identified as offenders, careful guidance to the mother to eliminate these from the child's diet will follow. Discussion of the food's common use in daily meal patterns and its occurrence in a number of commercial products and other hidden sources will make label reading and attention to recipes of prime consideration.[46] As the child grows older, the allergic reaction to the given food may wane, and it may be gradually readded to the diet.

Food additives. As food processing expands and the use of a wide variety of food additives increases, a greater number of allergic reactions to these chemicals is being encountered by clinicians. The full scope and magnitude of the problem for the allergist is indeed great, since the Food Protection Committee of the National Research Council lists 13 classes of additives, which include over 2,700 individual items. Feingold outlines diagnosis and treatment procedures for reactions to a number of food colors, sweeteners, and flavors and suggests a relationship of this type of sensitivity in some children to hyperactivity.[47,48] The Feingold hypothesis is being tested clinically with inconclusive results at this point. A review of these studies and the difficulties inherent in such a research problem have been carefully outlined by Abrams.[49]

OBESITY IN CHILDREN

Great variations in weight and height occur among normal, healthy children. Therefore it is somewhat difficult to establish criteria for a definition of obesity in children. Moreover, the important contribution of Bruch[50] states that in some cases the state of obesity may be an important resolution in the child's personality of deep-seated psychiatric problems. Nonetheless, reports indicate that approximately 10% of the

Rowe Elimination Diets*—straight lines enclose foods in the cereal-free elimination diets 1, 2, and 3, a commonly used combination

Diet 1	Diet 2	Diet 3	Diet 4
Rice	Corn	Tapioca	Milk†
Tapioca	Rye	White potato	Tapioca
Rice biscuit	Corn pone	Breads made of any	Cane sugar
Rice bread	Corn-rye muffin	combination of soy,	
	Rye bread	lima and potato	
	Ry-Krisp	starch and tapioca	
		flours	
Lettuce	Beets	Tomato	
Chard	Squash	Carrot	
Spinach	Artichoke	Lima beans	
Carrot	Asparagus	String beans	
Sweet potato or yam			
		Peas	
Lamb	Chicken (no hens)	Beef	
	Bacon	Bacon	
Lemon	Pineapple	Lemon	
Grapefruit	Peach	Grapefruit	
Pears	Apricot	Peach	
	Prune	Apricot	
Cane sugar	Cane or beet sugar	Cane sugar	
Sesame oil	Mazola oil	Sesame oil	
Olive oil‡	Sesame oil	Soybean oil	
Salt	Salt	Salt	
Gelatin, plain or flavored with lime or lemon	Gelatin, plain or flavored with pineapple	Gelatin, plain or flavored with lime or lemon	
Maple syrup or syrup made with cane sugar flavored with maple	Karo corn syrup White vinegar	Maple syrup or syrup made with cane sugar flavored with maple	
Royal baking powder	Royal baking powder	Royal baking powder	
Baking soda	Baking soda	Baking soda	
Cream of tartar	Cream of tartar	Cream of tartar	
Vanilla extract	Vanilla extract	Vanilla extract	
Lemon extract		Lemon extract	

*Rowe, A. H.: Elimination diets and the patient's allergies, ed. 2, Philadelphia, 1944, Lea & Febiger.
†Milk should be taken up to 2 to 3 L (2 to 3 qt) per day. Plain cottage cheese and cream may be used. Tapioca cooked with milk and milk sugar may be taken.
‡Allergy to it may occur with or without allergy to olive pollen. Mazola oil may be used if corn allergy is not present.

children in the United States are obese.[51] Later reports confirm these findings. Also, from a preventive medicine point of view the development of obesity in childhood is a significant factor in avoiding problems in adulthood associated with the overweight state. The problem of obesity in children is complex. An increased understanding may be gained by clarification of words used in discussing obesity, by considering some of the causes for its development, and by comparing the basic types of obesity.

Associated definitions. In view of the controversy and divergent opinion concerning exact terminology, the Committee on Nutrition of the American Academy of Pediatrics gave the following definitions for terms used:

Hunger—a biologic phenomenon predominantly learned and unconditioned

Appetite—a learned response usually in intimate association with the memory of past food experiences

Anorexia—absence of desire for food in circumstances where one might ordinarily anticipate such a desire

Satiety—the lack of desire to eat that ensues after eating, predominantly determined by postingestion factors

Palatability—related to preingestion factors such as taste, aroma, texture, appearance, color, and temperature and association with past experiences

Causes of obesity

Cultural factors. Many cultural factors condition food intake (p. 267). There is much seasonal emphasis, such as the Christmas and Thanksgiving feasts, and emphasis on eating certain foods at certain times, all of which habits are culturally derived. Also, meal patterns are different in different cultures. The three-meals-a-day pattern is a cultural one, not a biologic necessity. Some indication exists that less food more often may be better to control weight than larger meals less frequently. However, there needs to be some consideration of the type and frequency of the snacks. Too often among growing children these foods tend to be rich in carbohydrate and relatively low in content of other nutrients and only serve to give excess calorie intake.

Body needs and food habits. Sometimes the classic experiments of Davis[2,3] are called on to support the contention that children will eat what they need. However, some difficulty exists in interpretation of these studies. Apparently the children in her group were only offered "good" foods, and they had no opportunity to select an imbalanced diet. Also these children seem to have spent some time in tasting the food before settling down to more restricted use of their preferred foods, which suggests that *learning* rather than *instinct* guided their choice. Observation and research indicate that new habits do form in accordance with body needs but that old established habits persist as regulators of food selection, even after the need for those habits is no longer present.

Excessive parental concern with appetite. The normal growth pattern follows a rapid period of growth during the first year with a comparative decrease in food intake during the latent childhood years as a result of the normal slowed and erratic growth pattern. Frequently during these periods mothers express dissatisfaction with the amount of food their children eat. As a result they tend to overfeed them, pushing food at periods of time when such an intake is not needed for growth.[51,52]

Decreased physical activity. There is also evidence from research and observation that in the age of automation there is a decreasing amount of physical activity among growing children. The California study of Huenemann's group[53,54] emphasizes this aspect of developing obesity in children. Her results showed that American teenagers today are less active than adolescents of former years and frequently evidence little interest in becoming more active.

Types of obesity

The pattern of the growth years and the study of developing obesity during these years point to two types of obesity.

Developmental obesity. Studies indicate that at birth, fat accounts for about 12% of the infant's body weight.[55] During the middle of the first year there is usually more fat in males than in females. By the time the infant is 1 year old, fat accounts for about 24% of the body weight. As the child continues to grow through the childhood years, this general percent of fat remains essentially constant, relative to the desired weight for height and age. Heald and Hollander[56] indicate that the peak for onset of juvenile obesity occurs during the first four years of the child's life and that it is established by the time the child is 11 years old. About the twelfth year the percent of body fat increases in girls, and the development of lean body mass begins to rise sharply in boys.

The developmental form of obesity begins early in life. The cells become supersaturated with fat, and additional cells are recruited from connective tissue for fat deposit. With the increasing weight, additional bone and muscle cells must also increase to help carry the load. As a result these children are usually taller, have an advanced bone age, and have been obese since infancy. Their percentage of lean body mass is high and so also is the fat deposit.

Reactive obesity. The reactive type of obesity usually results from intense and oft-repeated episodes of emotional stress. As a result of the stress period the child overeats and his weight often assumes an up-and-down type of pattern. His body composition is high in fat but not in the lean body mass observed in the developmental type of obesity.

Implications for food practices during growth years

Several implications of these studies and observations appear reasonable in considering feeding patterns of the early growth years.

Fat content of infant formulas and quantity fed. With the knowledge regarding the rapid growth of the first year and the normal laying down of fat during that period, questions can be raised concerning the fat content of infant diets and formulas. The attitude of mothers who insist on the emptying of the bottle with every feeding of formula beyond the infant's obvious desire for food can also be questioned. Breast feeding is recommended for infants at least during the first six months of life, with additions of solid foods beginning at 6 months of age.

Sex differences in early years. If the sex differences at the early age of 2 or 3 years in calorie expenditure are considered, it should be realized that all toddlers are not going to eat the same amount of food. The basal metabolic rate is higher in the male than in the female during the second and third years of life. Therefore parents should be prepared for very early differences among young boys and young girls.

Overfeeding in preschool years. Overfeeding during the years of slow growth can make a large contribution to the development of continuing obesity. The peak onset of developmental types of obesity is during these early years. Mothers of young children would be well advised to offer them the enjoyment of a wide variety of food in realistic portion sizes.

Decreased activity of elementary school years. Prior to the beginning of the school years the child engages in much strenuous physical play, testing his developing strength and motor capacity. Usually this is more independent spontaneous activity and there is not yet a set schedule for the day. With the continuing experiences of school the child becomes more sedentary in his recreational pattern as well as his school activities. This great change in energy expenditure during ages 7 to 11 calls for guidance from mothers concerning food intake habits.

Adolescent sex differences in body composition. The increasing tendency for fat deposit in the teenage girl, in comparison to greater increase in lean body mass in the teenage boy, makes weight control a greater problem for the girl. Guidance from parents in a supportive, accepting manner, especially for young girls, is needed.

DENTAL CARIES

Incidence. Dental decay is a prevalent disease among young children. Almost no one escapes it. According to surveys, over 99% of the children in the United States at one time or another are affected by it, and there seems to be little pattern to its incidence. It is found in well-fed and in undernourished children. Perhaps because it is so common and seldom causes grave problems, it is often dismissed with indifference or ignored. Yet it remains and continues to disfigure, cause pain, and cost money.

Etiology. Three factors combine to produce tooth decay—the susceptible host, oral bacteria, and diet.

THE SUSCEPTIBLE HOST. Inherent differences in caries susceptibility vary widely among individual children. Some of these are hereditary differences in the anatomic characteristics of the tooth, but the ultimate form is influenced by interrelationships between these inherited characteristics and the environment that sustains its development during its formative period. Since teeth once formed are stable structures, it is evident that this positive nutritional influence can have effect only during growth and development of the enamel-forming organ and the tooth bud. Certain vitamins and minerals, especially vitamins A and D, calcium, and phosphorus, play a part during this period (see p. 88). Studies indicate that fluoride ingestion during this period may have a direct influence on tooth formation.[57]

ORAL BACTERIA. In humans, streptococci comprise the highest number of bacteria in the dental plaque, the gelatinous coating of the teeth. They seem to have a particular affinity for carbohydrates and act upon them rapidly. It has been shown in controlled tests that only 13 minutes after carbohydrate was present as a substrate, streptococci alone lowered the pH of the dental plaque from 6.0 to 5.0.[58] However, the oral flora is complex, and bacterial effects can vary because of symbiosis between two or more microorganisms. It is their substrate that is mandatory for the metabolism of caries-producing organisms. This substrate is carbohydrate.

DIET. As *carbohydrate* food accumulates in the mouth, it provides the necessary media for the normal growth of acidogenic microorganisms that cause tooth decay. In sites of greatest food particle retention around the teeth and on food textures that adhere and remain more readily (sticky, gummy), the bacterial activity is greatest. Persistent and continuous eating of adhesive carbohydrates, therefore, is a prime factor in tooth decay. The most convincing proof of this fact comes from an earlier five-year study in Sweden[59,60] in which a steady, controlled diet situation at a constant caloric level was maintained with a group of institutionalized patients. Over the years different variables were added at different times. Supplementation of vitamins and minerals produced no difference. But the addition of carbohydrates brought about marked changes. One group eating bread containing 50 g of sugar once a day had no caries increase. However, when this same amount was distributed through the day at four different times, definite increase in caries did occur. Also a large amount of carbohydrate (300 g) taken in liquid form with meals produced no change, but when this same amount was given as milk chocolate four times a day between meals, the incidence of caries was greater and increased even more when caramels were used. During every period when the candy was withdrawn, the caries attack rate decreased.

The other dietary element that has a large influence on dental caries is *fluoride*. Repeated studies consistently confirm about 60% reduction in the incidence of dental caries in children, both in prenatal and postnatal exposure to fluoridated water. A significant extensive project on the dental caries activity in children from 11 areas in five western states (Oregon, Idaho, Montana, Utah, and Washington) found the one most significant factor was the fluorides in the water supplies. Dental caries rates in the children consuming the fluoridated water were less than half those in the children whose water was fluoride-free.[61,62]

Dietary implication. While the problem of dental caries is by no means solved, recent advances in the knowledge of nutrition and its relationship to caries provide helpful steps in that direction.[63,64] Two nutritional factors seem apparent. *Adhesive carbohydrates* (sweets, candy bars, caramels) consumed at frequent intervals *do* increase dental caries. Also, carbohydrates in liquid form are less cariogenic than those in solid form. *Fluoridated public water supplies do* decrease dental caries rates, although this practice still remains a source of controversy in many communities.

CASE STUDY 9
Teena's family adapts to phenylketonuria

Carla Anderson, aged 20, and her husband Bob, aged 22, had happily anticipated the birth of their first child. Bob had even made a cradle in his workshop in the garage. Carla's pregnancy had gone well, and her delivery was without difficulty. They had a lovely little girl, they were told, and they named her Christine.

After the baby was born, when Carla was back in her room on the postpartum ward resting, she and Bob were talking about their plans, wondering why they hadn't seen the baby yet. When Dr. Simmons came in from the hospital nursery they had a feeling, from the look on his face, that something must be wrong. Carla couldn't seem to find her voice, and Bob asked about the baby. Dr. Simmons said there had been a test done that was routine for all newborns there and that rarely showed a positive result. But Teena's test had been that rare positive one. She had phenylketonuria, he said.

For a moment there was silence in the room. The word—that strange word—seemed to hang heavy between them. Then Bob finally asked, "What does that mean?"

Dr. Simmons explained that Teena had inherited a rare gene that meant she couldn't handle a certain substance in her food. As a result her diet would have to be carefully controlled to keep that substance at a low level. Then he turned to Carla. "One of the main food sources of this substance is milk, Mrs. Anderson, so I'm afraid you won't be able to breast-feed your baby as you had planned. I'll have to prescribe a special preparation for you to use in making her formula. The nutritionist will be helping you with some instructions about it."

They talked further for a few moments, but Carla seemed to hear very little else that was said. Finally Dr. Simmons had to leave. Bob and Carla were quiet for a long while. When Bob spoke he said slowly, "Something she inherited? Well, whatever care Teena needs, I'll see that she gets it." Carla nodded. The days and months that lay ahead were to test their maturity.

Before Carla left the hospital the nutritionist showed her the material she was to get for Teena's formula and gave her instructions for obtaining it. Bob purchased several cans of the powder to have ready at home.

The first few weeks went fairly well. The nutritionist and the pediatrician had frequent blood samples taken to keep a close watch on Teena's responses to her feedings, and the nutritionist carefully calculated Teena's special formula needs. The laboratory technician would prick Teena's tiny little heel and absorb a small bit of blood on some specially treated absorbent paper.

Later, when Teena began to need some solid food in addition to her formula, the nutritionist outlined for Carla a careful plan to restrict Teena's diet to a specifically calculated amount of phenylalanine and no more. By now Carla knew quite a bit about the disease and what phenylalanine was, because she and Bob had read all they could find about it. The nutritionist also gave Carla a booklet to keep for reference that explained the diet plan in further detail. On one of Carla's visits to the clinic with Teena the nutritionist went over a number of recipes and food-preparation suggestions to add interest and variety.

Teena was a beautiful child. Her nature was sunny and outgoing. She seemed to thrive on the diet Carla planned with the nutritionist and followed carefully every day. Especially did Teena thrive on the mature love and understanding that Carla and Bob gave her. When she was 2 years old she was perfectly developed for her age, accustomed to the foods Carla prepared for her, and aware that she must not eat anything else. About this time, and after much genetic counseling with Dr. Simmons, Carla and Bob decided to have one more child. The second child was a boy whose PKU screening

---

CASE STUDY 9
Teena's family adapts to phenylketonuria—cont'd

---

test at birth was negative. This was their family now, Carla decided—these two beautiful, healthy children. Both were healthy because Teena's needs had been learned immediately at birth, and her mature young parents had provided for her the wise care and love she needed to grow normally— physically and emotionally. She was indeed a fortunate child.

Questions to guide your inquiry

1. What is meant by the term "inborn errors of metabolism" on the concept of genetic disease?
2. What is phenylketonuria? What is an inherited autosomal recessive gene?
3. What is the metabolic defect in phenylketonuria?
4. What are the symptoms? Relate these to the metabolic defect.
5. What specific treatment is indicated? How is the diet managed?
6. What special milk substitute formula was given to Carla for Teena's feedings? Obtain some printed descriptive material from the manufacturer and if possible obtain some of the powder and taste a solution of it.
7. How is the diet managed when solid foods begin to be used?
8. What counseling help do you think a family with a PKU child would need?
9. Plan a day's menu suitable for Teena when she was 2 years old. (See Appendix L and Table 19-2.)
10. What is the public health significance of phenylketonuria?
11. What blood test was the health care team probably using on Teena? What are some other urine and blood tests used in screening or monitoring PKU?
12. Compare and contrast the genetic disease galactosemia with PKU.

CASE STUDY 10
Mark learns about food and his asthma

Five-year-old Mark Campbell was a thin child, small for his age. He lay quietly in bed holding a yellow stuffed Pooh Bear with a red jacket. He was audibly wheezing when Miss Bancroft, his nurse, came in with his lunch tray. Mark had been brought to the children's ward at the hospital the week before with a respiratory infection that had brought on an asthma attack.

Mark was an only child. He lived in a small apartment in the city with his mother. His parents had been divorced during the past year, for which Mrs. Campbell blamed his father's alcoholism. During their six years of marriage they had moved constantly, since Mr. Campbell had found it difficult to keep one job very long. Mark had started school this fall, attending kindergarten for a half-day morning session and staying at the day-care center next to the school grounds during the afternoon. He received his lunch at the day-care center. His mother worked as a secretary in the city and would pick him up from the day-care center on her way home from work each day.

Continued.

CASE STUDY 10

Mark learns about food and his asthma—cont'd

During Mark's hospitalization he had had no visitors except his mother. She usually came by for a brief visit after work each day. She explained that they did not know many people, since they had just moved to the city when the new school year began so that she and Mark could try to start a new life for themselves.

Since Mark had been in the hospital, Dr. Ashland had called in an allergy consultant. As soon as Mark's infection was cleared up they wanted to arrange a complete workup in the allergy clinic to diagnose the cause of his asthma and outline his treatment. They suspected food allergies as the primary cause.

Mrs. Campbell said Mark had had no real difficulty until now, and she could contribute very little medical history, except for a brief period when he was an infant when the doctor told her he seemed to be allergic to certain foods. But she had never followed it up because they had moved again.

While Mark was in the hospital, Dr. Ashland had placed him on a general hypoallergy diet until his allergy could be studied further after he was over the infection. However, Mark's appetite was poor, and he had eaten very little. The clinical dietitian, Mrs. Stewart, came often to see Mark and directed his nutritional therapy, working closely with his pediatrician. Miss Bancroft also stayed with him a great deal and encouraged him to eat as best he could.

During the last few days in the hospital before Mark was ready to go home the health care team talked several times with Mark's mother, exploring ways of arranging his care. Mrs. Campbell was able to take some leave time from her work to be with him while they went through the tests in the allergy clinic.

Before Mark was discharged from the hospital, Mrs. Stewart, the clinical dietitian, reviewed his diet needs with Mrs. Campbell. Because of the severity of Mark's asthma attack the clinical nutrition specialist and allergy specialist who were to continue his care thought it best that Mark follow a careful diet when he went home, until they could diagnose his specific allergens. It was the cereal-free Rowe Elimination Diets 1, 2, and 3. Miss Bancroft set up Mark's follow-up appointments in the allergy clinic and the nutrition clinic.

Questions to guide your inquiry

1. In planning Mark's nutritional care during his hospitalization, what significant factors should be considered?
2. What effect do you think environmental, emotional, and physical factors may have had on Mark's illness?
3. Identify Mark's nutritional needs: (a) the basic nutritional needs of a 5-year-old boy and (b) Mark's particular food problems.
4. What solutions would you propose to the problems you identified above? What specific nutritional care actions could Mrs. Stewart, the clinical dietitian, plan? How could she involve other persons, such as Mark's mother and other health team members?
5. Plan a day's diet for Mark while he was in the hospital on the hypoallergy diet. What milk substitute would you use?
6. Outline the teaching plan you would use to help Mark and his mother plan his diet after his return home. How would you suggest his noon meal and snacks be controlled after he returns to school and the day-care center?

CASE STUDY 10

Mark learns about food and his asthma—cont'd

7. What type of tests might be used in the allergy clinic to help diagnose the specific allergens in Mark's case?

8. When the clinical nutrition specialist and the allergy specialist spoke with Mark's mother in the hospital before his discharge, they told her that in the clinic they would be using three basic tools to help determine what foods Mark might be allergic to: a detailed food history, food records, and the Rowe Elimination Diets. Describe how you think each of these tools would be used and what purpose they would serve.

9. Once the specific food allergens have been diagnosed, what sort of a family education plan would you conduct for Mark and his mother? Outline the basic knowledge and understandings you think they should have and the practical means of controlling food products selection, preparation, and feeding.

CASE STUDY 11

Carl's adaptive survival with cystic fibrosis

Carl Harrington, aged 16, entered the hospital two weeks ago with pneumonia, but his was not an ordinary pneumonia. He had not only survived early childhood with a serious generalized hereditary disease but had developed a realistic and mature attitude toward himself and his life situation that few healthy teenagers achieve.

Carl was born prematurely, weighing 2,300 g (5 lb). He showed poor weight gain and had frequent respiratory infections. Soon his breathing developed a sort of snorting, gurgling pattern. His stools increased in frequency and were large, foul, and contained undigested food material. When he was 9 months old, the diagnosis was certain. He had cystic fibrosis.

Then followed years of frequent hospitalizations—numerous bouts with pneumonia, pneumonitis, bronchitis, fever, cough, difficulty in breathing from the heavy bronchial secretions. Despite all this, however, Carl, a bright student, had kept up his school work, so that all the time he missed had put him only two years behind his normal grade level.

Carl is the seventh of nine children in a large Irish-Catholic family. His father is a businessman in a suburban community, and the family lives in a modest but comfortable home. Carl has received much support from his family. The oldest child died at 3 months of age with cystic fibrosis, and Carl's attitude is that he is just glad he had the disease now, when it can be treated, rather than when his oldest brother was born.

Carl has made many adaptive responses. For example, he is thin—weighs only 48 kg (106 lb) when the normal weight for his age and height is about 63 kg (140 lb)—has little muscle development, and tires easily, so he can't participate in sports as a player, as other boys can. Instead, he has transferred this desire to taking a position as manager of the ball team rather than playing. His mother's attitude toward him is not overprotective nor permissive. He has many friends, a number of whom have come to visit him during this hospitalization.

Continued.

CASE STUDY 11
Carl's adaptive survival with cystic fibrosis—cont'd

Miss Spencer, Carl's nurse, carried his lunch tray into his room, checking to see if the extra salt packets ordered were there. Carl was coughing when she entered, and as the spell subsided he lay back, fatigued from the effort it expended. He usually had a good appetite, but it was still an effort sometimes to get in the large amount of food and fluids that he needed. She knew, she thought to herself, that she would have to devise ways to increase his intake of both. As she put his tray down she took the Cotazym (pancrelipase) capsules and a glass of water and handed them to Carl. He was always good about taking his medications because he realized how important they were to his survival. Sometimes when she was a little late bringing them in—for example, with his Theragram tablets and his vitamin E—he asked about them. She still remembered how difficult it was to give him injections because of his wasted muscles. Even now there was a reddened area on his hip that she needed to massage frequently to help stimulate circulation.

Miss Spencer was also reviewing in her mind some of the things she wanted to talk about with the clinical dietitian who was taking care of Carl's nutritional therapy and visiting with him each day, and with Carl's mother when she came to visit him this afternoon.

Questions to guide your inquiry

1. What is cystic fibrosis? What clinical effects produced by the disease process was Carl having?
2. What are the basic goals of treatment in cystic fibrosis?
3. Why is vigorous nutritional therapy such an important part of Carl's care?
4. What would be an appropriate diet order for Carl? Give the rationale for each factor.
5. Identify Carl's nutritional needs: basic nutritional requirements for a 16-year-old boy, adolescent psychosocial needs in relation to food and feeding, and Carl's specific needs and feeding problems.
6. What would be a realistic plan of care to help Carl obtain the large amount of calories and protein he needs? Consider actions related to food forms, health teaching, and supportive encouragement.
7. Outline a day's food plan for Carl. Check the amount of protein and calories to ensure the extra that he needs. How much extra does he require? Why?
8. What vitamin supplement may Carl require because of his prolonged antibiotic therapy? Why?
9. Why would Carl require therapeutic dosages of multivitamins, including the B complex? Why would he need to have these in water-soluble form?
10. Why does Carl receive 100 IU of vitamin E each day?
11. Why does Carl require extra salt tablets in hot weather?

REFERENCES
Specific

1. Erikson, E.: Childhood and society, ed. 2, New York, 1963, W. W. Norton & Co., Inc., pp. 247-274.
2. Davis, C. M.: Self-selection of diet by newly weaned infants, Am. J. Dis. Child. **36:**651, 1928.
3. Davis, C. M.: A practical application of some lessons of the self-selection of diet study to the feeding of children in hospitals, Am. J. Dis. Child. **46:**743, 1933.
4. Chuck wagon for the pediatric floor, J. Am. Diet. Assoc. **51:**432, 1967.
5. Current aspects of infant nutrition in daily practice, Evansville, Ind., 1962, Mead Johnson & Co., p. 1.
6. Holt, L. E., Jr., Davies, E. A., Hasselmeyer, E. G., and Adams, A. O.: A study of premature infants fed cold formulas, J. Pediat. **61:**556, 1962.
7. Keitel, H. G.: Pitfalls in clinical practice. I, Pediat. Clin. North Am. **12**(1):1965.
8. Andersen, D. H.: Cystic fibrosis of the pancreas and its relation to celiac disease, Am. J. Dis. Child. **56:** 344, 1938.
9. Anderson, D. H.: Cystic fibrosis of the pancreas and

its relation to celiac disease, Am. J. Dis. Child. **56:** 344, 1938.

10. Dicke, W. K., Weijer, H. A., and Van de Kamer, J. H.: Caeliac disease. 2. The presence in wheat of a factor having a deleterious effect in cases of caeliac disease, Acta Paediat. **42:**34, 1953.
11. Shiner, M.: Duodenal biopsy, Lancet **1:**17, 1956.
12. Rubin, C. E., Brandborg, L. L., Phelps, P. C., and Taylor, H. C., Jr.: Studies of celiac disease. I. The apparent identical and specific nature of the duodenal and proximal jejunial lesion is celiac disease and idiopathic sprue, Gastroenterology **38:**28, 1960.
13. Di Sant' Agnese, P. A., and Jones, W. O.: The celiac syndrome in pediatrics, J.A.M.A. **180:**308, 1962.
14. Weijers, H. A., Van de Kamer, J. H., and Dicke, W. K.: Celiac disease. In Advances in pediatrics, vol. 9, Chicago, 1957, Year Book Publishers.
15. Hjortland, M., et al.: Low gluten diet with tested recipes, Clinical Research Unit, University of Michigan, Ann Arbor, Mich., 1973.
16. Nishita, K. D.: A yeast-leavened, rice-flour bread, J. Am. Diet. Assoc. **70:**397, April, 1977.
17. Smith, E. B.: Development of recipes for low-protein, gluten-free bread, J. Am. Diet. Assoc. **65:**50, 1974.
18. Mike, E. M.: Practical dietary management of patients with the celiac syndrome, Am. J. Clin. Nutr. **7:**463, 1959.
19. Barry, M. M.: Cystic fibrosis, J. Am. Diet. Assoc. **75:**446, Oct., 1979.
20. Acosta, P. B., Wenz, E., and Williamson, M.: Methods of dietary inception in infants with PKU, J. Am. Diet. Assoc. **72:**164, Feb., 1978.
21. Horner, F. A., Streamer, C. W., Alejandrino, L. L., Reed, L. H., and Ibbott, F.: Termination of dietary treatment of phenylketonuria, N. Engl. J. Med. **226:** 79, 1962.
22. Beckner, A. S., Centerwall, W. R., and Holt, L.: Effects of rapid increase of phenylalanine intake in older PKU children, J. Am. Diet. Assoc. **69:**148, Aug., 1976.
23. Kang, E. S., Sollee, N. D., and Gerald, P. S.: Results of treatment and termination of the diet in phenylketonuria, Pediatrics **46:**881, 1970.
24. Yu, J. S., and O'Halloran, M. T.: Children of mothers with phenylketonuria, Lancet **1:**210, 1970.
25. Guthrie, R.: Letters to the journal—blood screening for phenylketonuria, J.A.M.A. **178:**863, 1961.
26. Guthrie, R., and Susi, A.: A simple phenylalanine method for detecting phenylketonuria in large populations of newborn infants, Pediatrics **32:**338, 1963.
27. Guthrie, R., and Whitney, S.: Phenylketonuria: detection in the newborn infant as a routine hospital procedure, Children's Bureau, U.S. Dept. Health, Education, and Welfare, Washington, D.C., 1965, Government Printing Office.
28. McCaman, M. W., and Robins, E.: Fluorimetric method for the determination of phenylalanine in serum, J. Lab. Clin. Med. **59:**885, 1962.
29. Scriver, C. R., LaRochelle, J., and Silverberg, M.: Hereditary tyrosinemia and tyrosyluria in a French Canadian geographic isolate, Am. J. Dis. Chil. **113:** 41, 1967.
30. Kogut, M. D., Shaw, K. N., and Donnell, G. N.: Tyrosinosis, Am. J. Dis. Child. **113:**47, 1967.
31. Hill, A., Nordin, P. M., and Zaleski, W. A.: Dietary treatment of tyrosinosis, J. Am. Diet. Assoc. **56**(4): 308, 1970.
32. Michols, K., Matalon, R., and Wong, P. W.: Dietary treatment of tyrosinemia type I, J. Am. Diet. Assoc. **73:**507, Nov., 1978.
33. Kirkman, H. N., and Maxwell, E. S.: Enzymatic estimation of erythrocytic galactose-1-phosphate, J. Lab. Clin. Med. **56:**161, 1960.
34. Acosta, P. B., and Elsas, L. J.: Dietary treatment of branched chain ketoaciduria (MSUD). In Dietary management of inherited metabolic disease: phenylketonuria, glactosemia, tyrosinemia, homocystinuria, maple syrup urine disease, Atlanta, 1976, ACELMU Publishers.
35. Bell, L., Chao, E., and Milne, J.: Dietary management of maple-sirup-urine disease; extension of equivalency systems, J. Am. Diet. Assoc. **74:**357, March, 1979.
36. Kretchmer, N.: Lactose and lactase, Sci. Am. **227**(4): 70, 1972.
37. Jackson, R. L.: The child with diabetes, Nutr. Today **6**(2):2, 1971.
38. Jackson, R. L.: Insulin-dependent diabetes in children and young adults, Nutr. Today **14:**26, Nov.-Dec., 1979.
39. Lum, B. O. L.: Preventing ketoacidosis in the child with juvenile-onset diabetes, J. Am. Diet. Assoc. **69:**157, 1967.
40. Traisman, H. S.: Management of juvenile diabetes mellitus, ed. 3, St. Louis, 1980, The C. V. Mosby Co.
41. Caso, E. K., and Stare, F. J.: Simplified method for calculating diabetic diets, J.A.M.A. **113:**169, 1947.
42. American Diabetes Association: Exchange lists for meal planning, New York, 1976.
43. Bachmann, K., and Dees, S. C.: Milk allergy. II. Observations on incidence and symptoms of allergy and milk in allergic children, Pediatrics **20:**400, 1957.
44. Keitel, H. G.: Pitfalls in clinical practice. I, Pediat. Clin. North Am. **12**(1):27, 1965.
45. Garza, C., and Scrimshaw, N. S.: Relationship of lactose intolerance to milk intolerance in young children, Am. J. Clin. Nutr. **29:**192, 1976.
46. Conrad, M.: Allergy cooking, New York, 1971, Pyramid Books.

47. Feingold, B. F.: Recognition of food additives as a cause of symptoms of allergy, Ann. Aller. **26**:309, 1968.

48. Feingold, B. F.: Why your child is hyperactive, New York, 1975, Random House, Inc.

49. Abrams, B. F., et al.: Perspectives in clinical research: a review of research controversies surrounding the Feingold diet, Fam. Commun. Health **1**:93-113, Feb., 1979.

50. Bruch, H.: The importance of overweight, New York, 1957, W. W. Norton & Co., Inc.

51. Winick, M.: Childhood obesity, Nutr. Today **9**(3): 6, 1974.

52. Himes, J. H.: Infant feeding practices and obesity, J. Am. Diet. Assoc. **75**:122, Aug., 1979.

53. Huenemann, R., Shapiro, L., Hampton, M., et al.: Teen-ager's activities and attitudes toward activity, J. Am. Diet. Assoc. **51**:433, Nov., 1967.

54. Huenemann, R., et al.: Teenage nutrition and physique, Springfield, Ill., 1974, Charles C Thomas, Publisher.

55. Wallace, W. M.: Why and how are children fat? Pediatrics **34**:303, 1964.

56. Heald, F. P., and Hollander, R. J.: The relationship between obesity and adolescence and early growth, J. Pediat. **67**:35, 1965.

57. Brudevold, F.: Chemical composition of the teeth in relation to caries. In Sognnaes, R. F., editor: Chemistry and prevention of dental caries, Springfield, Ill., 1962, Charles C Thomas, Publisher, pp. 32-88.

58. Gibbons, R. J., Socransky, S. S., DeAraujo, W. C., et al.: Studies of the predominant cultivable microbiota of dental plaque, Arch. Oral Biol. **9**:365, 1964.

59. Stralfors, A.: Investigations into the bacterial chemistry of dental plaques, Odont. T. **58**:151, 1950.

60. Gustafsson, B. E.: Vipeholm dental caries study; effects of different levels of carbohydrate intake on caries activity of 436 individuals observed for 5 years, Acta Odont. Scand. **11**:232, 1954.

61. Tank, G., and Starvick, C. A.: Dental caries experience of school children in Corvallis, Oregon, after 7 years of fluoridation of water, J. Pediat. **58**:528, 1961.

62. Tank, G., and Starvick, C. A.: Caries experience of children one to six years old in two Oregon communities (Corvallis and Albany). I. Effect of fluoride on caries experience and eruption of teeth, J.A.D.A. **69**: 749, 1964.

63. Nizel, A. E.: Nutrition in preventive dentistry: science and practice, Philadelphia, 1972, W. B. Saunders Co.

64. DePaola, D. P., and Alfano, M. C.: Diet and oral health, Nutr. Today **12**:6, May-June, 1977.

General
THE HOSPITALIZED CHILD

Nelson, W. E., editor: Textbook of pediatrics, ed. 8, Philadelphia, 1964, W. B. Saunders Co.

Nutrition, growth and illness in children, Nutr. Rev. **20**: 101, 1962.

Palmer, S., and Thompson, R. J., Jr.: Nutrition: an integral component in the health care of children. The interdisciplinary team in action, J. Am. Diet. Assoc. **69**:138, Aug., 1976.

Rose, M. H.: Communicating with children, Nurs. Outlook **9**:428, 1961.

ALLERGY

Garza, C., and Scrimshaw, N. S.: Relationship of lactose intolerance to milk intolerance in young children, Am. J. Clin. Nutr. **29**:192, 1976.

Harper, P. H., Goyette, C. H., and Conners, C. K.: Nutrient intakes of children on the hyperkinesis diet, **73**: 515, Nov., 1978.

Kolata, C. B.: Childhood hyper-activity: A new look at treatment and causes, Science **199**:515, 1978.

Sobotka, T. J.: Hyperkinesis and food additives: a review of experimental work, FDA By-lines **8**:165, 1978.

Speer, F.: Food allergy, Littleton, Mass., 1978, PSG Publishing Co.

GENERAL GASTROINTESTINAL PROBLEMS AND CELIAC DISEASE, CYSTIC FIBROSIS, AND CLEFT LIP AND PALATE

Anderson, D. H., and Mike, E. M.: Diet therapy in the celiac syndrome, J. Am. Diet. Assoc. **31**:340, 1955.

Arvanitakis, C.: Diet therapy in gastrointestinal disease: a commentary, **75**:449, Oct., 1979.

Barry, M. M.: Cystic fibrosis, J. Am. Diet. Assoc. **75**: 446, Oct., 1979.

Berry, S. D., et al.: Dietary supplement and nutrition in children with cystic fibrosis, Am. J. Dis. Child. **129**:165, 1975.

Gayton, W. F., Friedman, S. B., Tavormina, J. F., et al.: Children with cystic fibrosis, Pediatrics **59**:888, 1977.

MacCollum, D. W., and Richardson, S. O.: Care of the child with cleft lip and cleft palate, Am. J. Nurs. **58**:211, 1958.

Nishita, K. D.: A yeast-leavened, rice-flour bread, J. Am. Diet. Assoc. **70**:397, April, 1977.

Schwachman, H.: Gastrointestinal manifestations of cystic fibrosis, Pediatr. Clin. North Am. **22**:787, 1975.

Smith, E. B.: Development of recipes for low-protein, gluten-free bread, J. Am. Diet. Assoc. **65**:50, 1974.

Strober, W., Falchuk, Z. M., Rogentine, G. N., et al.: The pathogenesis of gluten-sensitive enteropathy, Ann. Intern. Med. **83**:242, 1975.

Weijers, H. A., and Van de Kamer, J. H.: Some considerations of celiac disease, Am. J. Clin. Nutr. **17**:51, 1965.

Zickefoose, M.: Feeding the child with a cleft palate, J. Am. Diet. Assoc. **36**:129, 1960.

PHENYLKETONURIA, GALACTOSEMIA, AND OTHER GENETIC DISEASES

Acosta, P. B., and Centerwall, W. R.: Phenylketonuria: dietary management, J. Am. Diet. Assoc. **36**:206, 1960.

Acosta, P. B., et al.: PKU—a guide to management, Berkeley, Calif., 1972, California State Dept. of Public Health.

Acosta, P. B., and Elsas, L. J.: Dietary management of inherited metabolic disease: phenylketonuria, galactosemia, tyrosinemia, homocystinuria, maple syrup urine disease, Atlanta, 1976, ACELMU Publishers.

Acosta, P. B., Wenz, E., and Williamson, M.: Methods of dietary inception in infants with PKU, J. Am. Diet. Assoc. **72**:164, Feb., 1978.

Beckner, A. S., Centerwall, W. R., and Halt, L.: Effects of rapid increase of phenylalanine intake in older PKU children, J. Am. Diet. Assoc. **69**:148, Aug., 1976.

Bell, L., Chao, E., and Milne, J.: Dietary management of maple-sirup-urine disease: extension of equivalency systems, J. Am. Diet. Assoc. **74**:357, March, 1979.

Berry, H. K., Hunt, M. M., and Sutherland, B. K.: Amino acid balance in the treatment of phenylketonuria, J. Am. Diet. Assoc. **58**(3):210, 1971.

Bureau of Public Health Nutrition of the California State Dept. of Public Health: The phenylalanine-restricted diet; a diet guide for parents of children with phenylalanine (booklets), Berkeley, Calif., 1966.

Centerwall, W. R.: Phenylketonuria, J. Am. Diet. Assoc. **36**:201, 1960.

Dahlqvist, A.: Disaccharide intolerance, J.A.M.A. **195**:225, 1966.

Fincke, M. L.: Inborn errors of metabolism, J. Am. Diet. Assoc. **46**:280, 1965.

Guest, G. M.: Hereditary galactose disease, J.A.M.A. **168**:2015, 1958.

Koch, R., Dobson, J., and Williamson, M.: Research design for the collaborative study of children treated for phenylketonuria, Los Angeles Children's Hospital, Los Angeles, 1970.

Koch, R., et al.: Galactosemia. In Kelley, V. C., editor: Metabolic, endocrine, and genetic disorders of children, Hagerstown, Md., 1974, Harper & Row, Publishers.

Koch, R., Acosta, P., Ragsdale, N., et al.: Nutrition in the treatment of galactosemia, J. Am. Diet. Assoc. **43**:216, 1963.

Koch, R., Acosta, P., Ragsdale, N., et al.: Nutrition in the treatment of phenylketonuria, J. Am. Diet. Assoc. **43**:212, 1963.

Lindquist, B., and Meeuwisse, G.: Diets in disaccharidase deficiency and defective monosaccharide absorption, J. Am. Diet. Assoc. **48**:307, 1966.

Marino, M. A.: Developing and testing a programmed instruction unit on PKU, J. Am. Diet. Assoc. **76**:29, Jan., 1980.

Michals, K., Matalon, R., and Wong, P. W.: Dietary treatment of tyrosinemia type I: importance of methionine restriction, J. Am. Diet. Assoc. **73**:507, Nov., 1978.

Pueschel, S. M., Yeatman, S., and Hum, C.: Discontinuing the phenylalanine-restricted diet in young children with PKU. Psychological aspects, J. Am. Diet. Assoc. **70**:506, May, 1977.

Scriver, C. R., and Rasenberg, L. E.: Amino acid metabolism and its disorders, Philadelphia, 1973, W. B. Saunders Co.

Shroyer, K.: Our encounter with PKU, Calif. Med. **113**:94, 1970.

Stacey, H.: Coordination of long-term care of PKU children, J. Am. Diet. Assoc. **42**:311, 1963.

Umbarger, B.: Phenylketonuria: dietary treatment, Am. J. Nurs. **64**:96, 1964.

Wright, S. W.: Phenylketonuria, J.A.M.A. **165**:2079, 1957.

JUVENILE DIABETES

Hooker, A. D.: Camping and the diabetic child, J. Am. Diet. Assoc. **37**:143, 1960.

Jackson, R. L.: The child with diabetes, Nutr. Today **6**(2):2, 1971.

Jackson, R. L.: Insulin-dependent diabetes in children and young adults, Nutr. Today **14**:26, Nov.-Dec., 1979.

Koukal, S. M., and Parham, E. S.: A family learning experience to serve the juvenile patient with diabetes, J. Am. Diet. Assoc. **72**:411, April, 1978.

Lum, B. O. L.: Nutrition education for the child with diabetes, Diabetes Educator **1**:6, June, 1975.

Lum, B. O. L.: Preventing ketoacidosis in the child with juvenile-onset diabetes mellitus, J. Am. Diet. Assoc. **69**:157, Aug., 1976.

Prater, B., Denton, N., and Fisher, K.: Food and you: nutrition in diabetes, Intermountain Regional Medical Program, University of Utah, Salt Lake City, 1970.

Travis, L. B.: An instructional aid on juvenile diabetes mellitus, ed. 5, Galveston, Tex., 1978, Department of Pediatrics, University of Texas Medical Branch.

OBESITY

Crawford, P. B., Hankin, J. H., and Huenemann, R. L.: Environmental factors associated with preschool obesity.

III. Dietary intakes, eating patterns, and anthropometric measurements, J. Am. Diet. Assoc. **72:**589, June, 1978.

D'Augelli, A. R., and Smiciklas-Wright, H.: The case for primary prevention of overweight through the family, J. Nutr. Educ. **10:**76, April-June, 1978.

Gross, I., Wheeler, M., and Hess, K.: The treatment of obesity in adolescents using behavioral self-control, Clin. Pediatr. **15:**920, 1976.

Heald, F. P., and Khan, M. A.: Teenage obesity, Pediatr. Clin. North Am. **20:**807, 1973.

Himes, J. H.: Infant feeding practices and obesity, J. Am. Diet. Assoc. **75:**122, Aug., 1979.

Huenemann, R. L.: Environmental factors associated with preschool obesity, J. Am. Diet. Assoc. **64:**580, 1974.

Kaufmann, N. A., Posnauski, P., and Guggenheim, K.: Eating habits and opinions of teenagers on nutrition and obesity, J. Am. Diet. Assoc. **66:**264, 1975.

Salans, L. B., Cushman, S. W., and Weismann, R. E.: Studies of human adipose tissue: adipose cell size and number in non-obese and obese patients, J. Clin. Invest. **52:**929, 1973.

Smiciklas-Wright, H., and D'Augelli, A. R.: Primary prevention for overweight: Preschool Eating Pattern (PEP) Program, J. Am. Diet. Assoc. **72:**626, June, 1978.

Weil, W. B.: Current controversies in childhood obesity, J. Pediatr. **91:**175, 1977.

Winick, M.: Childhood obesity, Nutr. Today **9:**6, 1974.

DENTAL HEALTH

Alfano, M. C., and DePaola, D. P., editors: Nutrition, Dent. Clin. North Am. vol. 20, no. 3, 1976.

Bibby, B. G.: Cariogenicity of foods, J.A.M.A. **177:**316, Aug. 5, 1961.

DePaola, D. P., and Alfano, M. C.: Triphasic nutritional analysis and dietary counseling, Dent. Clin. North Am. **20:**613, 1976.

DePaola, D. P., and Alfano, M. C.: Diet and oral health, Nutr. Today **12:**6, May-June, 1977.

DePaola, D. P., Modraw, C. L., and Wittemann, J. K.: An integrated nutrition education program for dental students, J. Nutr. Educ. **10:**160, Oct.-Dec., 1978.

DiOrio, L. P., and Madsen, K. O.: A personalized program educating the patient in the prevention of dental disease, Chicago, 1972, March Publishing Co.

Fluoridation is here to stay, J. Am. Diet. Assoc. **65:**578, 1962.

Lackey, H. B.: Developing a "nutrition nook" in a dental office, J. Nutr. Educ. **8:**34, Jan.-March, 1976.

McBean, L. D., and Speckmann, E. W.: A review: the importance of nutrition in oral health, J. Am. Dent. Assoc. **89:**109, 1974.

Miller, J. A.: Protecting those pearly whites, Science News, **116:**394, Dec. 8, 1979.

Nizel, A. E., and Shulman, J. S.: Interaction of dietetics and nutrition with dentistry, J. Am. Diet. Assoc. **55:**470, Nov., 1969.

Nizel, A. E.: Nutrition in preventive dentistry: science and practice, Philadelphia, 1972, W. B. Saunders Co.

Odom, J. G., DePaola, D. P., and Robbins, A. E.: Clinical nutrition education for dental students: a conjoint approach, J. Am. Diet. Assoc. **72:**56, Jan., 1978.

Robinson, L. G., et al.: Nutrition counseling and children's dental health, J. Nutr. Educ. **8:**33, Jan.-March, 1976.

Rowe, N. H., Garn, S. M., Coark, D. C., and Guire, K. E.: The effect of age, sex, race and economic status on dental caries experience of the permanent dentition, Pediatrics **57:**457, 1976.

Tank, G.: Recent advances in nutrition and dental caries, J. Am. Diet. Assoc. **46:**293, 1965.

20 Nutrition for the aging and the aged

The previous three chapters have formed a unit on maternal-child health. In these chapters the human life cycle has been reviewed from the point of conception through the prenatal period to birth, and continuing through the growth and development years of childhood to maturity. In the care of individuals in each of these stages of growth these basic human developmental needs have been related to optimal nutritional care. This chapter views the middle and later years of the life span in the same way—as part of the whole growth pattern. Each phase of development along the way has meaning only in relation to the whole.

Following the tumultuous adolescent years from age 13 to 18, when youth in American society are struggling with the core problem of identity versus identity diffusion, of learning who they are and where they are going, three more basic stages in a human's life span, as identified by Erikson (see p. 404), complete human development.

Young adulthood (ages 18 to 40). In the years of young adulthood the individual, now launched on his own, must resolve the core problem of *intimacy versus isolation*. If he achieves his goal, he is able to build an intimate relationship leading to marriage or self-fulfillment in other personal relationships. But if he fails to do so, he becomes increasingly isolated from others. These are the years of career beginnings, of establishing one's own home, of parenthood, of starting young children on

their way through the same life stages, and of early struggles to make one's way in the world.

Middle adulthood (ages 40 to 60). In the years of adulthood, the core problem the individual faces is *generativity versus self-absorption*. The children have now grown and gone to make their own lives in turn. These are the years of the "empty nest," the coming-to-terms with what life has offered, and of finding expression for stored learning in passing on life's teachings. It is a regeneration of one life in the lives of young persons following the same way. To the degree that these inner struggles are not won, there is increasing self-absorption, a turning-in on one's self, and a withering rather than a regenerating.

Older adulthood (ages 60 to 80-plus). In the last stage of life (old age, senescence) the final core problem is resolved between *integrity versus despair*. Depending on one's resources at this point, there is either a predominant sense of wholeness and completeness, or a sense of distaste, of bitterness, of revulsion, and of wondering what life was all about. If the outcome of life's basic experiences and problems has been positive, the individual arrives at old age a rich person—rich in wisdom of the years. Building on each previous level, his psychosocial growth has reached its positive human resolution.

Not all elderly patients will be able to say with Browning at this point that this is the "best of life for which the first was made." Some of them will not have resolved the core psychosocial conflicts and struggles with which they wrestled in previous stages. They arrive at middle and later years poorly equipped to deal with the adjustments and health problems that may face them. Many others, however, will have been enriched by life's experiences in their maturing process. They will bring enrichment to the health professional in turn, and the resulting relationship will be mutually rewarding.

As the developmental needs of individuals in these middle and later years are studied and integration of nutrition into patient care and total health care is sought, the following questions should be considered:

1. What social and economic problems does the aging person face in American society?
2. What is the biologic nature of the aging process? Is it the same in all aging persons?
3. What is the role of nutrition in the aging process? Are needs for specific nutrients changed in any way?
4. What clinical problems may aging individuals encounter? How is nutrition related to these problems?
5. What practical daily living problems might the aged patient have related to eating?
6. Are there community resources available to help meet the aged person's needs?

Two important concepts should develop, therefore, as a result of this study: (1) aging is an *individual* process and (2) aging is a part of a *total life* process. These two basic concepts will govern all other aspects of need during these years—biologic, nutritional, socioeconomic, psychosocial, and spiritual.

GERONTOLOGY AND GERIATRICS— APPROACH TO THE STUDY OF AGING

Several terms are used in discussing the middle and later years of life. A clarification in meaning will be helpful.

Gerontology and geriatrics. The word *gerontology* comes from two Greek words, *geron* meaning "old man," and *logos* meaning "study of." It is the study of the process of aging and its phenomena. The word *geriatrics* comes also from the Greek word *geron,* and from *iatrike,* meaning "medical treatment." It is the study and treatment of diseases of old age. Geriatrics therefore is a fairly narrow medical term. For purposes of this study the idea behind the much broader term "gerontology" will be used.

Aging and the aged. The two terms aging and aged have comparative yet distinct meanings. *Aging* is a life process. The age of a person or an object is from the point of its beginning existence to the present time. Thus human aging is the total life process. It begins at conception and ends at death. It may be somewhat startling to think that even now every person is aging, and has been since the moment of conception. But it is a biologic truth. *Aged* refers to one who is old. He has arrived near the end of the aging process and bears visible physical signs of the gradual process of decline. Sometimes people are spoken of as young-old (those in the ages 60 to 75) and of old-old (those over 75) because marked distinctions may exist among persons in these two age brackets.

Senescence and senile. Senescence comes from a Latin verb *senescere,* which means "to grow old." It refers to the process of growing old or, more specifically, to the later period of life, old age. It is similar to the Latin root for adolescence, for example, which means "to grow up," or the later period of attaining physical maturity. The word *senile* is from the Latin word *senilis,* which simply means "old." However, common usage has given it a negative clinical connotation, a meaning that should not be attached to *normal* old age.

The pattern emerges of a life continuum. Aging is a positive concept. It encompasses the whole of life, and each period has its own unique potentials and fulfillments. The period of middle and later years is no exception. Its own particular capacities can be lived to the fullest. These are attitudes the health care workers may have opportunity to help support in their patients.

SOCIOECONOMIC AND PSYCHOLOGIC FACTORS

The increasing industrialization and urbanization of American society, the complexity of the culture it is building, and the changes in age distribution in the population have all brought about changes in the life of the aging person in the United States today.

Population changes. Not only has the general population been increasing rapidly, but significant shifts have also occurred in the age distribution. Increasing longevity has produced a larger number of persons in the older age group. More people are living longer. By 1975, 12%, or over 22 million, of the American population were 65 years of age or over, with proportionate increases expected in succeeding years. However, biostatisticians such as Yerushalmy[1] point out that there is need for more knowledge of *qualitative* longevity, how the interdependence of biologic and environmental factors affects the quality of the lengthened life. Quantitative statistics alone do not reveal the many subtle individual differences. He raises significant questions such as: Do stressful experiences at one period of life have a measurable effect on subsequent survival? Do repeated exposures to physical and mental stresses in early life leave their mark on the individual?

In general this increased longevity is influenced by two factors, medical care and improved living standards.

MEDICAL CARE. The great progress in care of infants and children has reduced infant mortality, controlled communicable diseases, and improved child care. The increased availability and quality of medical care during adult years is also a factor in health during the maturing years. But there has been relatively limited progress in control of chronic disease in old age.

IMPROVED LIVING STANDARDS. With an increasing national economy and affluence, the general U.S. living standards are high. For many, this factor has led to increased education, better housing, and improved nutrition during the growth and early adult years. In older age, however, problems in socioeconomic status increase for many. The factors that have contributed to the increased number of older persons in the population have medical, social, and economic implications.

Social and economic factors. America's increasing industrialization and subsequent changing social attitudes have affected the position of the older person in American society. Economic insecurity creates pressures. An increasing policy of early retirement in industry and employment difficulties with advancing age create financial pressures. Changing social attitudes toward the elderly person and his capacities have increased institutional care and segregation in living situations. The older person is often removed from the stimulus of involvement in the activities of society.

Psychologic factors. Financial pressures and a decreasing sense of acceptance and accomplishment have developed in many old persons anxieties and a loss of personal values. Many feel inadequate. They do not have a sense of belonging, of self-esteem, or of achievement. They are often lonely, restless, unhappy, and uncertain. The experiences of visiting nurses working with elderly persons in the community have led them to identify basic common personal needs. Austin[2] has previously summarized these well; they continue to hold true today:

1. An income and economic security through socially useful and personally satisfying means
2. A sense of *maximum* personal effectiveness
3. A suitable place in which to live
4. The spending of leisure time constructively
5. A sense of positive and well-integrated

social relationships within the family and the community

6. A sense of achieving and maintaining spiritual values and goals

BIOLOGIC NATURE OF THE AGING PROCESS

Biologic changes. From a biologic standpoint there is limited knowledge of the process of aging. The general biologic process extends over the entire life span and is conditioned by experiences that have gone on before. In the later ages, however, there is a cell loss and reduced cell metabolism. Studies[3,4] have shown that during the ages 30 to 90 there is gradual reduction in the performance capacity of most organ systems. For example, the speed of conducting a nerve impulse diminishes by 15%, the rate of blood flow through the kidney is reduced 65%, and the resting cardiac output is reduced by 30%. The pulmonary function (the maximum voluntary ventilatory capacity) is reduced 60%, and there is a reduced recovery rate following a displacing stimulus. For example, in a glucose tolerance test the blood sugar level takes longer to return to normal, and the pulse rate and respiration after exercise take longer to return to normal.

There seems to be an overall, gradual reduction in the body's reserve capacities, an important cause of which is the gradual reduction of cellular units (for example, nephrons are lost from the kidney as functioning units; there is a loss of pulmonary functional tissue). Some resulting physiologic factors may affect food patterns. For example, there may be a diminished secretion of digestive juices, a decreased motility of the gastrointestinal tract, and decreased absorption and utilization of nutrients.

Individuality of the process. The biologic changes are general. Persons in the advancing years of life will display a wide variety of individual reaction. Each person bears the imprint of his individual trauma and accumulation of

disease experience. This has a direct effect on his individual aging process. Therefore specific needs of individuals must always be remembered and considered when discussing general aging and general nutritional needs. It seems, therefore, that the greatest influence of nutrition on the aging process takes place in earlier years. Nutrition's most effective role is in the growth and middle years, which prepare the individual to meet the gradually declining metabolic processes of old age.

NUTRITIONAL REQUIREMENTS
Calories

Standard allowances. The reduced basal energy requirement, caused by losses in functioning protoplasm, and the reduced physical activity combine to create less demand for calories in advancing age. The statement of the Food and Agriculture Organization indicates a reduction in calories of approximately 7.5% for each decade past age 25. The standard allowances of the National Research Council (NRC) are based on estimates of a decrease in metabolic activity of about 5%. The average estimate is an approximate caloric requirement of 1,800 calories. Men may require more—about 2,200 calories.

These standards seem to be borne out by various studies of the food intake patterns of older people. For example, in the earlier San Mateo County study in California there was a reported caloric intake for men aged 50 to 70 of 2,165 to 2,618 calories, and an intake for women the same ages of 1,586 to 1,780 calories.[5] Other reports indicate the caloric intake of aged women living at home to be approximately 1,500 calories.

However, there are major gaps in our knowledge of nutrient allowances for the elderly. Munro reviews current nutritional status of older people, especially of those already old, and indicates an urgent need in determining nutritional requirements for the elderly is to assess the allowances for each nutrient as age advances.[4] Also, because the range and living situations are wide among older adults, there is need for much more information on the daily life activities of older people and the degree of energy that they may be capable of expending. The calorie requirements are highly individual, according to activity. Primary consideration must also be given to the living status of the individual and the degree of his or her activity in various phases of life. Perhaps the simplest criterion for judging adequacy of caloric intake is the maintenance of *normal* weight.

Carbohydrates. Generally about 50% to 60% of the total calories should be provided in the form of carbohydrate and about 20% to 30% as fat, mainly plant fats. Otherwise, part of the protein will be diverted for use as energy rather than tissue maintenance. The label "nonprotective" or "empty" that is frequently put on carbohydrate and fat foods is not entirely correct. They perform important functions in providing energy and protecting protein for tissue metabolic activities. The optimum amount of carbohydrate intake is unknown, but it is usually recommended that about 50% of the calories come from carbohydrate foods. Easily absorbable sugars are not contraindicated, and there is usually no disturbance in carbohydrate metabolism. The fasting blood sugar level has been found to be essentially normal in the aged.[6] There should be a fairly free choice of carbohydrate foods according to individual digestion or metabolism situations.

Fats. Fats usually contribute about 20% of the total calories. They provide a source of energy, important fat-soluble vitamins, and essential fatty acids. A reasonable objective is the avoidance of large quantities of fat with more emphasis on the quality of fat consumed. The digestion and absorption of fats may be delayed in the elderly person, but they are not greatly disturbed with age. There is no need to be unduly restrictive. Enough fat for meal palatability aids appetite. Fat loads, however, should be avoided because of the delayed absorption capacity in elderly persons.

Protein

Standard allowances. The NRC recommends a continuation of the daily protein intake for the aging individual at the same adult allowance given for age 25—0.8 g/kg body weight. Even this amount provides an allowance for a wide variation in individual needs. Also, although there may be increased need for protein during illness or convalescence or after a wasting disease, the overall mass of actively metabolizing tissue decreases with age. There usually is no increased requirement for protein per se under normal circumstances. The difficulty in establishing precise protein requirements is evidenced by the conflicting reports of studies. Some of the data obtained from population groups in institutions may have some questionable applications to relatively healthy persons living a fairly active life at home, engaged in business, professional, and social interests. Most investigators agree, however, that age itself does not alter adult protein needs.

Protein value. Needs are influenced by (1) the biologic value of the protein (the quantity and ratio of its amino acids) and (2) adequate caloric value of the diet. It is estimated that one fourth to one half of the protein intake should come from animal sources with the remainder from plant protein sources. If animal and plant protein foods are consumed at the same meal, there is better utilization of the incomplete plant protein for tissue synthesis, because the lacking amino acids may be supplied by the animal protein foods. It is estimated that protein should supply from 15% to 20% of the day's total calories. For healthy adults there is usually no need for supplemental amino acid preparations as some food faddists may claim. They are expensive, unpalatable, irritating, impractical, and an inefficient source of available nitrogen.

Vitamins

The sale of so-called geriatric vitamin preparations, especially of the B complex, implies that the requirement for them increases with age. There may be gradually decreasing tissue stores with normal aging, but long-term studies show no difference in requirement from that for normal adults. The problem in some individual cases may stem from inadequate normal intake rather than from an increased need. A well-selected, mixed diet should supply all the essential vitamins in normally needed quantities. Increased therapeutic needs in illness should be evaluated on an individual basis.

Minerals

There is also no need for increased minerals in normal aging. The same adult allowances are sufficient on a continuing basis and are supplied by a well-balanced diet. Two essential minerals that may be lacking in poor diets, however, are iron and calcium. Encouragement may need to be given to some individuals to ensure adequate dietary sources among their daily food choices.

Water

The need for water varies with environment. A liberal intake should be assured, with thirst as the general guide.

CLINICAL NEEDS

Chronic illness such as heart disease (see Chapter 28) often creates additional problems for aging persons. Also, although physiologic needs for nutrients do not increase with age, other environmental factors may contribute to illness and produce clinical needs.

Malnutrition

By and large, poor dietary habits in young adulthood, as with any other personal habits, tend to be set and accentuated in older age. Although surveys show on the average adequate total calorie intakes, there is frequent evidence of inadequate distribution of these calories in food choices. For example, there may be fewer animal proteins (meat, egg,

cheese, milk), more use of grain and other starch in breads and cereals, fewer vegetables and fruits, and more sweets and desserts (even to the extent of about 20% of the day's calories). Also, older persons are frequently prey to claims of food faddists concerning restorative food products, tonics, regulators, and so on.

Causes of malnutrition. Numerous factors may contribute to developing malnutrition in an elderly person.

ORAL PROBLEMS. Poor teeth or poorly fitting dentures may make chewing difficult. However, it must be remembered that a denture can only be as successful as the health of the tissue on which it rests. Also, an analysis of the three stages of eating food—biting, chewing, and swallowing—will provide a basis for helping the new denture wearer adjust to his prosthesis.[7] Poor appetite and limited financial means for adequate dental care may discourage efforts to seek improvement of the situation. Also, buccal mucosa changes in the mouth and decrease or change of quality in salivary secretions may cause difficulty in eating.

GASTROINTESTINAL PROBLEMS. Numerous gastrointestinal complaints, from vague indigestion to specific disease (peptic ulcer, diverticulitis), sometimes effectively reduce food intake and curtail the needed nutrients. A variety of other acute or chronic illnesses may limit food intake or utilization.

PERSONAL FACTORS. Financial resources may be limited with little money available to purchase needed food. There may be a lack of knowledge of the food needed for a well-balanced diet. Boredom, loneliness, anxiety, insecurity, and apathy compound the problem. Especially if an older person lives alone, the social value of eating is gone. Also, he may lack adequate cooking, refrigeration, or storage facilities and have no means for transportation to obtain food and bring it back to his home. Often a vicious cycle ensues—his funds are low, he hesitates to spend, goes without, builds increasing weakness and lethargy, which leads to still less interest and incentive. Finally, he is ill.

Implications for patient care. The malnourished older patient needs much understanding care and support to build improved eating habits. Helpful attitudes and actions by practitioners are based on an understanding and realistic approach.

FOOD HABITS SHOULD BE ANALYZED CAREFULLY. The practitioner must listen well to learn the patient's attitudes and precise situation and its limiting factors. Nutritional needs can be met with a variety of foods, and suggestions can be adapted to fit his particular needs and personal situation, as well as his desires. Suggestions should be administered in a practical and realistic manner.

THE PRACTITIONER SHOULD NOT MORALIZE. ''Eat this because it is good for you'' should be struck from every nurse's, nutritionist's, and physician's vocabulary. It has little possible value for any patient, much less one who is struggling to maintain his personal integrity and self-esteem.

INTEREST SHOULD BE ENCOURAGED IN FOOD VARIETY AND SEASONING. A bland and unattractive diet is presumed by many to be necessary for all elderly persons. It is not. A variety of food and adventure with new foods, tastes, and seasonings often prove to be the needed stimuli for poor appetite and lack of interest in eating. Sometimes smaller amounts of these foods and more frequent meals are helpful.

Obesity

In a different sense, obesity may be considered a form of malnutrition. It is a potential health hazard, indicated in a number of degenerative diseases. In fact, Mayer[8] indicates that the prevention of obesity in earlier growth years may be the major nutritional measure one may take in preparation for old age.

Causes of obesity. Many of the same living situations and emotional factors may cause obesity by contributing to compensatory overeating or poor food choices. Also, there is usually decreased physical activity, and the maintenance calorie requirement is lessened.

Individual approach. Discouraging reports come from clinicians attempting weight reduction programs with older persons. It is difficult to change long-standing habits or long-standing obesity. Certainly in most cases a reasonable approach should be followed with no drastic measures or diet, planning only for a slow, gradual loss. Because individual calorie requirements vary widely and individual personalities and problems are unique, personal and realistic planning with the individual patient, followed by supportive guidance and encouragement, usually pays the greatest dividends.

COMMUNITY RESOURCES
Professional organizations

The American Geriatrics Society. The American Geriatrics Society was organized in 1942. Physicians engaged in the medical care of elderly patients promote research to advance scientific knowledge of the aging process and the treatment of its diseases. A number of nurses and other health professionals are associate members. The society publishes the *American Journal of Geriatrics*.

The Gerontological Society, Incorporated. The Gerontological Society was organized in 1944. This society has a broader base of interest in all aspects of aging and a wider membership of interested health professionals. The Committee on Aging of this group has stimulated increased interest among other related organizations and community and government agencies in the problems of the aging person in our society. The organization publishes the *Journal of Gerontology*.

The local community groups representing other health professions such as the Medical Society, the nursing organizations, and the Dietetic Association sponsor a variety of programs to help meet the needs of the aged people in their respective communities. For example, the Dial-a-Dietitian program of the Dietetic Association provides sound information concerning nutritional needs.

Government agencies

Federal legislation. The impact in the United States of the initial federal legislation covering aid to elderly persons for medical care under the Social Security Act can hardly be minimized. Over the past few years this medicare bill (Title XIX) has increased the demand for high-quality medical care and its availability to elderly persons. The pressure on community nursing homes, hospitals, and related medical care resources has long been felt. Revisions and clarifications are needed concerning the type of care being provided, the professional person providing the service, and the place it is being provided. Additional medical assistance programs in a number of states augment the community resources on the state and local level.

Department of Health, Education, and Welfare. In August of 1950 the first national conference on aging was held in Washington, D.C. As a result of this beginning activity and stimulus of interest, in 1956 the President appointed a federal council on aging to coordinate and broaden federal activities under the Department of Health, Education, and Welfare. This council publishes the newsletter *Aging* and provides many other resource materials for community workers.

Thirty-five hundred delegates met in Washington, D.C., November 28 to December 2, for the second (1971) White House Conference on Aging.[9] A number of recommendations emerged from efforts to construct a national policy on aging. Recommendations on aging also developed from the 1968 White House Conference on Food, Nutrition, and Health.[10] The third national (U.S.) conference on aging will be held in 1981.

Department of Agriculture. The Department of Agriculture through its Agriculture Extension Services in state universities and county home advisors on the local level provides much practical aid for elderly persons and community workers.

Public health departments. Skilled health professionals work in the community through local and state public health departments. Much health guidance for elderly persons is available through their resources. Many chronic disease programs or related programs are in operation.

Nutritionists in private practice. An increasing number of practicing nutritionists with advanced skills, education, and clinical experience are available in communities. They provide individual primary care and serve as consultants to a variety of community agencies.

Volunteer organizations

Many activities of volunteer health organizations such as the Heart Association and the Diabetes Association relate to the needs of older persons. Also, two particular national organizations sponsor local community groups: (1) Senior Citizens of America, organized in 1954, and (2) American Society for the Aged, Incorporated, organized in 1955. Additional resources are provided in some larger urban centers, such as the Meals-on-Wheels program, which prepares and delivers hot meals to persons in need of such services, who are referred to the group by their physicians.

Industry

A number of industry-related groups such as the Dairy Council and pharmaceutical firms provide educational materials and sponsor research and workshops.

CASE STUDY 12
The patient with congestive heart failure

Mr. and Mrs. Poulos, aged 75 and 73 respectively, have lived for some years in a small, third-floor walk-up apartment in a large city. They have a small income, barely enough to meet expenses if they plan carefully, based entirely on their Social Security checks. They have no hospitalization insurance and know very little about medicare enrollment. They have no relatives nearby. Their two married sons live in a distant city and have had little contact with their parents in recent years.

For some time Mr. Poulos has been almost incapacitated with arthritis. He has had increasing difficulty walking and caring for himself. Mrs. Poulos had been in fairly good health, although she has had a little hypertension in previous years. She has remarked to the neighbors in their apartment building that she is grateful for her own good health so that she is able to take care of Mr. Poulos as he grows older. They are members of a Greek Orthodox church within walking distance of their apartment, to which Mrs. Poulos goes frequently to services. For some time, however, Mr. Poulos has not been able to go with her. A small grocery store had been located in the neighborhood, but in the past year the owner had not been able to continue his business and it had closed. The nearest large supermarket was quite a distance from their apartment. However, Mrs. Poulos has been managing on the city bus, buying very few things at a time so that she could carry them back to the apartment.

Lately, however, she noticed some shortness of breath when she climbed the stairs back to the apartment or walked the few blocks to their neighborhood church. She attributed this to her moderately increased weight (she was a short woman—152 cm (5 ft, 1 in)—and weighed 63 kg (140 lb). She commented to her neighbor that she knew she would need to lose weight.

Mrs. Poulos had made a small effort in the past to reduce her weight but had found it difficult since she was fond of the Greek foods to which she had been accustomed all her life. Especially did they have frequently the salty cheeses—feta, caceri, and cephalotyri. One of their favorite dishes, for example, was mousaka, with its layers of potato and vegetables with cheese and spices, covered with a flaky thin pastry. Lately she had cooked this more frequently for Mr. Poulos because he had asked for it on numerous occasions. She still made loaves of the delicious bread that they both enjoyed and that was such a large part of every meal. They were also particularly fond of tyropetta and spanacopetta, in which she used generous amounts of the cheese of which they were both so fond.

On special occasions, such as holidays, Mrs. Poulos made the very delicious pastry, baklavas, brushed with butter and sprinkled with nuts, sugar, spices and served covered with syrup. In fact, much of the Pouloses' life centered around their cultural food dishes these days, because Mrs. Poulos felt there was very little else she could do. She had always received a great deal of enjoyment from cooking. Often they would call their neighbor in the next apartment, a younger single woman, to share their food with them.

Today, walking back the two blocks from their church, Mrs. Poulos noticed increased difficulty breathing. As she started to climb the steps to their apartment she could scarcely lift one foot above the other. She sat down on one of the steps and rested for a while and then tried to walk some more. Finally she reached the apartment, after resting several times along the stairway. Inside the apartment she had increasing difficulty getting her breath. Mr. Poulos, not knowing what else to do, went next door to call their neighbor. When the neighbor returned with him, she recognized the distress Mrs. Poulos was experiencing because her mother had had similar difficulty. She called the county hospital, since Mr. and Mrs. Poulos had no routine medical care or regular physician, and arranged to have Mrs. Poulos taken to the hospital for treatment.

Continued.

CASE STUDY 12
The patient with congestive heart failure—cont'd

At the hospital, Mrs. Poulos was taken into the emergency room for care. Mr. Poulos waited in the hallway, anxiously wringing his hands and saying to the neighbor who had come with them, "She's always seemed so well and has been our mainstay, taking care of both of us. What will happen to us now? What if I lose her? What will I do?"

After the doctor's initial examination of Mrs. Poulos, he instituted therapy to relieve her breathing. His initial diagnosis was listed as congestive heart failure and arteriosclerotic heart disease with hypertrophy. He instituted diuretic therapy, Mercuhydrin injection, and an oral chlorothiazide. He also ordered some potassium chloride and sedatives. She was taken to a bed on the medical ward, where the doctor began to administer digoxin. He asked that the head of her bed be elevated, and discussed with the clinical dietitian a diet plan limiting sodium to 500 mg.

After Mrs. Poulos appeared to be resting and responding somewhat to initial therapy, the doctor talked with Mr. Poulos and assured him that she was in good hands and would be cared for. He suggested that Mr. Poulos get some rest at home and return in the morning if he wished. The neighbor said someone would be close by to be with him, and she assured him that she and the other neighbors in the building would take care of him.

Mrs. Poulos spent a fairly restful night, although she was having some difficulty. Her breathing as well as her color were improved. As she continued to improve, the dietitian maintained her nutritional therapy of 1,200 calories, 500 mg sodium. Later, Mr. Poulos returned to the hospital, having been brought again by the neighbor to visit his wife. He was still greatly concerned and apprehensive and insisted on sitting in the ward by the bed although his extreme tension seemed to upset Mrs. Poulos considerably. She was worried about how he would be taken care of now that she was ill.

Mrs. Poulos ate poorly the first meals that were brought to her that day, as she had little appetite and felt nauseated. As the days went by, however, she responded increasingly to her overall medical treatment and her nutritional therapy through the personal care of the clinical dietitian so that by the end of the first week her dietary sodium intake was increased to 1,000 mg. After the second week the doctor felt that she had improved sufficiently to leave the hospital.

But the question now centered on her means of home care or continued care in some extended-care facility. It would be imperative that she continue carefully on the medications and the 1,200-calorie, 1,000-mg sodium diet. Several conferences were held to discuss what means of care could be provided for her. The health team explored several possibilities and helped to arrange with Mr. Poulos for her continuing care. The health team also discussed Mr. Poulos's needs in making arrangements for both of them.

Questions to guide your inquiry
(Refer also to Chapters 13 and 28.)

1. What is congestive heart failure?
2. What physiologic factors—imbalances in normal homeostatic mechanisms for fluid and electrolyte balance—cause the major problem of edema?
3. Describe the sequence of events involving the metabolism of sodium, potassium, and water that produces and compounds the problem of cardiac edema.
4. What was the general goal of the plan of therapy for Mrs. Poulos? By what means was this achieved?
5. How does chlorothiazide achieve its diuretic action? Why did the doctor order potassium chloride?
6. What foods could Mrs. Poulos use as good sources of potassium to ensure adequate replacement?

CASE STUDY 12
The patient with congestive heart failure—cont'd

7. Digoxin is a glycoside derivative of digitalis. What is a glycoside?
8. In planning care for Mrs. Poulos, what problems do you think the health team might identify? What is the scientific basis for these problems?
9. What solutions would you propose? Why?
10. What are Mrs. Poulos's nutritional needs? What are her basic age group needs? What are her specific needs, as a result of her illness?
11. What additional personal factors would need to be considered in planning to meet Mrs. Poulos's nutritional needs? What are some of the characteristics of Greek food habits?
12. How would the health team involve other persons in initial plans for Mrs. Poulos's care? Husband? Neighbor? Community resources?
13. What is the common amount of sodium in an average adult diet? What are the major sources of dietary sodium?
14. What levels of sodium restriction are outlined in the American Heart Association diets in common use in the United States? What are the characteristics of each of these four levels of sodium restriction?
15. Do you think Mrs. Poulos would find difficulty in accepting her low-sodium diet? Why?
16. How do you think the clinical dietitian might help make her hospital diet more palatable?
17. Outline a day's menu for Mrs. Poulos on her 1,200-calorie, 1,000-mg sodium diet.
18. What problems are there in Mrs. Poulos's continuing care after she leaves the hospital?
19. What solutions do you think the health team members may use? Why?
20. What community resources might they use?
21. What teaching materials or approaches do you think would be useful in helping Mrs. Poulos continue her diet at home?
22. What practical problems would face Mrs. Poulos in buying her food and getting it into the home when she is at home? What is the Meals-on-Wheels program in many large American cities (p. 478)? How might this be used to help Mrs. Poulos? Investigate any possible programs for the elderly in your own community that would be helpful to patients in Mrs. Poulos's situation.

REFERENCES
Specific

1. Yerushalmy, J.: Factors in human longevity, Am. J. Public Health **53:**148, 1963.
2. Austin, C. L.: The basic six needs of the aging, Nurs. Outlook **7:**138, 1959.
3. Shock, N. W.: Physiological aspects of aging, J. Am. Diet. Assoc. **56:**491, June, 1970.
4. Munro, H. N.: Major gaps in nutrient allowances: the status of the elderly, J. Am. Diet. Assoc. **76:**137, Feb., 1980.
5. Morgan, A. F.: The San Mateo study of the nutritional status of the aging, Calif. Health **13:**65, 1955.
6. Horwitt, M. K.: Dietary requirements of the aged, J. Am. Diet. Assoc. **29:**433, 1953.
7. Nizel, A. E.: Food and nutrition for the new denture wearer, particularly the geriatric patient. In Nizel, A.

E., editor: The science of nutrition and its application in clinical dentistry, Philadelphia, 1966, W. B. Saunders Co.
8. Mayer, J.: Nutrition in the aged, Postgrad. Med. **32:** 394, 1962.
9. Donnelly, M. M.: The White House Conference on Aging, J. Am. Diet. Assoc. **60**(2):103, 1972.
10. Report of Panel II-4: Aging. In White House Conference on Food, Nutrition, and Health, Final Report, Washington, D.C., 1970, Government Printing Office.

General

Anderson, E. L.: Eating patterns before and after dentures, J. Am. Diet. Assoc. **58**(5):421, 1971.
Brown, P. T., Bergan, J. G., Parsons, E. P., et al.: Dietary status of elderly people: rural, independent-living men

and women vs. nursing home residents, Am. J. Diet. Assoc. **71**:41, July, 1977.

Campbell, V. A., and Dodds, M. L.: Collecting dietary information from groups of older people, J. Am. Diet. Assoc. **51**:29, 1967.

Chope, H. G.: Relation of nutrition to health in aging persons—a four-year follow-up of a study in San Mateo County, Calif. Med. **81**:335, 1954.

Elwood, T. W.: Nutritional concerns of the elderly, J. Nutr. Educ. **7**:50, 1975.

Farmer, F. A., editor: Nutrition of the aged, Calgary, Alberta, 1977, University of Calgary Press.

Fitzgibbons, J. J., and Garcia, P. A.: TV, PSAs, nutrition and the elderly, J. Nutr. Educ. **9**:114, July-Sept., 1977.

Food and Agriculture Organization of the United Nations, Calorie Requirements, FAO Nutritional Studies No. 5.

Gerontological Society: Working with older people. II. Biological, psychological, and sociological aspects of aging, Washington, D.C., 1970, Government Printing Office.

Granick, S., and Patterson, R., editors: Human aging. II. An eleven year follow-up biomedical and behavioral study, Pub. No. (HSM) 71-9037, Washington, D.C., 1972, Government Printing Office.

Grotkowski, M. L., and Sims, L. S.: Nutritional knowledge, attitudes, and dietary practices of elderly, J. Am. Diet. Assoc. **72**:499, May, 1978.

Holmes, D.: Nutrition and health-screening services for the elderly, J. Am. Diet. Assoc. **60**(4):301, 1972.

Howell, S. C., and Loeb, M. B.: Nutrition and aging: a monograph for practitioners, St. Louis, 1969, Gerontological Society.

Kohrs, M. B.: The nutrition program for older Americans: evaluation and recommendations, J. Am. Diet. Assoc. **75**:543, Nov., 1979.

Kohrs, M. B., O'Hanlon, P., Krause, G., and Nordstrom, J.: Title VII—nutrition program for the elderly. II. Relation of socioeconomic factors to one day's nutrient intake, J. Am. Diet. Assoc. **75**:537, Nov., 1979.

Lasswell, A. B., and Curry, K. R.: Curriculum development for instructing the elderly in nutrition, J. Nutr. Educ. **11**:14, Jan.-March, 1979.

Lau, D.: Elderly nutrition research: a major project underway at the University of Toronto, J. Can. Diet. Assoc. **39**:198, 1978.

Munro, H. N.: Major gaps in nutrient allowances. The status of the elderly, J. Am. Diet. Assoc. **76**:137, Feb., 1980.

Munro, H. N., and Young, V. R.: Protein metabolism in the elderly, Postgrad. Med. **63**:143, 1978.

Neugarten, B. L.: Middle age and aging: a reader in social psychology, Chicago, 1968, University of Chicago Press.

Nutrition and Human Needs, Part 14: Nutrition and the Aged, Hearings before the Select Committee on Nutrition and Human Needs of the United States Senate, Ninetieth Congress, Second Session, and Ninety-First Congress, First Session, September 9, 10 and 11, 1969, Washington, D.C., 1969.

O'Hanlon, P., and Kohrs, M. B.: Dietary studies of older Americans, Am. J. Clin. Nutr. **31**:1257, 1978.

Pelcovits, J.: Nutrition to meet the human needs of older Americans, J. Am. Diet. Assoc. **60**(4):293, 1972.

Phillips, E.: Meal a la car, Nurs. Outlook **8**:76, 1960.

Rae, J., and Burke, A. L.: Counseling the elderly on nutrition in a community health care system, J. Am. Geriat. Soc. **26**:130, 1978.

Report: Committee on Guidelines for Home Delivered Meals, National Council on the Aging, Inc., Am. J. Pub. Health (suppl.), 1965.

Riley, M. W., et al.: Aging and society. I. An inventory of research findings, 1968; II. Aging and the practicing professions, New York, 1969, Russell Sage Foundation.

Shannon, B., and Smiciklas-Wright, H.: Nutrition education in relation to needs of the elderly, J. Nutr. Educ. **11**:85, April-June, 1979.

Shock, N. W.: Physiologic aspects of aging, J. Am. Diet. Assoc. **56**(6):491, 1970.

Steinkamp, R. C.: Resurvey of an aging population—fourteen year follow-up, J. Am. Diet. Assoc. **46**:103, 1965.

Stiedemann, M., Jansen, C., and Harrill, I.: Nutritional status of elderly men and women, J. Am. Diet. Assoc. **73**:132, 1978.

Tappel, A. L.: Where old age begins, Nutr. Today **2**(4): 2, 1967.

Townsend, C.: Old age: the last segregation, New York, 1970, Grossman Publishers.

Troll, L. E.: Eating and aging, J. Am. Diet. Assoc. **59**(5): 456, 1971.

Vaughn, M. E.: An agency nutritionist looks at home health care under Medicare, J. Am. Diet Assoc. **51**: 146, 1967.

Watkin, D. M.: Nutrition for the aging and the aged. In Goodhurt, R. S., and Shils, M. E., editors: Modern nutrition in health and disease, ed. 6, Philadelphia, 1980, Lea & Febiger, p. 781.

Weinberg, J.: Psychological implications of the nutritional needs of the elderly, J. Am. Diet. Assoc. **60**(4):293, 1972.

Wells, C. E.: Nutrition programs under the Older Americans Act. Am. J. Clin. Nutr. **26**:1127, 1973.

Zanni, E., Calloway, D. H., and Zezulka, A. Y.: Protein requirements of elderly men, J. Nutr. **109**:513, 1979.

21 Nutrition in rehabilitation

At any one of the stages of the normal growth and development span of human life, in addition to common human developmental struggles, an individual may face the added stress of a disabling physical condition or mental illness and need special care. It is usually a situation of more or less profound trauma and calls for tremendous recourses on the patient's part to cope with the condition. These patients are essentially the same persons with the same basic age group needs as the practitioner or student has encountered in previous study and will care for on other clinical services. Here, however, they face added physical and psychologic problems. Such a situation requires of the physician, the nutritionist, the nurse, and the physical therapist special knowledge and skills, sympathetic insights, and personal strengths.

Nursing and physical care of patients undergoing such severe difficulties involves certain nutritional components. In this chapter nutritional principles in rehabilitation care will be identified and practical means offered to apply them in the necessary daily activity of eating.

The following are questions to which realistic answers will be sought:

1. What positive concept underlies all of rehabilitation nursing? How does this concept affect nutrition and feeding?
2. What social, economic, and psychologic problems does the patient face?
3. How does the physical problem affect nu-

tritional needs? What solutions are there for practical eating problems?
4. What special clinical problems may require particular dietary management?

GOALS AND METHODS

Rehabilitation is both a concept and a process. It involves a positive philosophy based on optimum potential and a cooperative approach built on a learning objective.

A positive concept. Basic to an understanding of rehabilitation needs is the concept of the patient's optimum potential. Rehabilitation specialists see the patient not primarily from the usual view of the public of what his disability prevents him for doing; rather they consider what maximum function his disability will allow him to achieve. There is an important difference in perspective and philosophy. One breeds increasing dependence and is negative. The other is a reaching for independence and is positive.

Specialists in rehabilitative medicine speak of this positive role as being both *preventive* and *restorative*.[1] Many of the techniques of care that have been developed are designed to prevent further disability and also to restore maximum potential use. Both of these key principles of prevention and restoration apply also to nutritional care.

A team approach. How is the twin goal embodied in this concept to be realized? In some cases, obstacles seem almost insurmountable. Often the patient's initial reaction is one of defeat. Certainly he cannot accomplish the goal alone. Such a complex and complicated endeavor requires a *team* approach. Several skilled health specialists lend their particular training, insights, and resources to identify specific needs and seek solutions. This *multidisciplinary* team of specialists, under the direction of the physiatrist—a specialist in physical medicine—includes psychiatrists, clinical and social psychologists, nurses, social workers, physical therapists, occupational therapists, speech therapists, nutritionists, special school teachers for handicapped children, and others according to special needs such as orthopedists, plastic surgeons, dentists, and orthodontists. Additional health workers such as licensed vocational nurses, hospital aides, volunteers, and vocational counselors provide essential services.

The most important member of the health team, however, is the patient himself, and with him, his family. The patient is the focus of the team effort. Goal setting is always done *with,* not for, the patient and his family. These three therefore—the health specialists, the patient, and the patient's family—together form a greater health team. It is a shared undertaking.

SOCIOECONOMIC AND PSYCHOLOGIC FACTORS

Social attitudes. The all-too-common attitude of society toward a disabled person is one of overprotection or avoidance. Some people are repelled by gross deformities. Others completely ignore them. The first attitude builds dependence and sometimes smothers the all-important *will* of the patient to fight against the odds that surround him and develop self-acceptance. The second attitude creates problems in everyday living. Like the left-handed child who finds himself in a world built for right-handed people, the disabled person faces doorways not built for wheelchairs, stairs, curb-

ings, and a multitude of articles encountered in everyday living all designed for simple neuromotor controls that he lacks. One of these simple, everyday activities that sometimes becomes a monumental task for the disabled person is *eating*—and food he must have.

Increasingly, however, through the work of many realistic, accepting, and knowledgeable people the public is being educated to the fact that disabled persons are human beings and that they do have potential with which they can find useful and productive roles in society. Perhaps in the process some doorways will be widened and some ramps built, as well as some minds opened and some attitudes lifted.

Economic problems. Rehabilitation care is a long and costly process. A major area of exploration for the health team is one of financial resources and assistance needed. Also, continuing long-term economic problems will revolve around employment capabilities or earning capacities or the means for providing care.

Living situations. The disabled person faces many practical problems of everyday living. Whether the individual needs institutional care or can maintain independent living, perhaps with an attendant, depends on a number of physical and situational factors. If with help he is able to maintain his own home, the necessary special equipment for maximum self-care and his additional care by the attendant must be provided.

Psychologic barriers. Tremendous psychologic adjustment is required of the disabled person to resolve the problems he faces. The trauma to self-image as well as to the physical body and the regressive tendency that he must struggle against constantly may leave him withdrawn, defeated, and exhausted. Often personality changes occur during the rehabilitation process. The patient's inner strength and resources, as well as his physical stamina, are tested and tried, and, depending on the nature of his coping resources and defenses, he will be able to function or not. Much of the health team's keen insight and concern are directed toward supporting the patient in *his* efforts to meet his own needs. That many disabled persons do achieve this goal is evident by the repeated monumental achievements these persons attain despite—or perhaps because of—their difficulties.

BASIC PRINCIPLES OF NUTRITIONAL CARE

Two basic principles of nutritional care evolve from the goals of rehabilitation—prevention and restoration.

Prevention of malnutrition

Calories. The rehabilitation process of physical therapy often involves hard work. The patient may tire easily, and his energy must be sufficient to meet the demands. Excess calories, however, must be avoided to prevent obesity. Also sufficient energy for metabolic tissue demands is important.

Protein. Tissue and organ integrity is a bulwark against skin breakdown, decubitus ulcers, infections, and negative nitrogen balance. Protein in optimum quantity and quality must be assured in the diet. Essential amino acids are required for tissue synthesis. Negative nitrogen balance is often seen in disabled persons, especially in the early stages following the initial injury. The negative balance occurs because the rate of breakdown of tissue proteins (catabolism) exceeds that of building them up (anabolism) (see p. 59). It almost always occurs after spinal cord injury. The metabolic process usually follows three stages:

1. *Early catabolic period*—peaks about two weeks after the injury and may remain for several more weeks; nitrogen replacement needs are high, and usually plasma transfusions are required

2. *Late catabolic period*—nitrogen excretions lessen; this period may remain for some weeks or months, especially if it is complicated by infections or decubiti

3. *Positive nitrogen balance period*—finally reached after protein therapy by dietary means and clearing of any infection or ulcers; sometimes as much as 150 to 300 g of protein is required daily, and protein supplements will need to be used

Carbohydrates. The proper metabolism of carbohydrate may also be impaired in the early stages following a severe injury. The oxidation of glucose by the cell is dependent on the presence of the specific enzyme glucokinase. This enzyme controls the initial phosphorylation reaction that attaches phosphate to glucose (p. 25). Without being phosphorylated, glucose cannot be oxidized for energy. The activity of glucokinase and other similar enzymes is in turn controlled by hormone regulators from the pituitary and the adrenal cortex and from the pancreatic islet cells (insulin). The increased activity of the pituitary and in turn the adrenal gland, following the stress of injury (p. 189), inhibits the proper functioning of the cellular enzyme systems and prevents adequate phosphorylation and oxidation of glucose. More breakdown of tissue protein and fat occurs to provide needed energy, thus effectively adding further to the negative nitrogen balance. Sufficient carbohydrate foods are therefore important in the diet to help provide needed energy.

Fats. Essential fatty acids (linoleic acid) are needed by the body for its metabolism and have also been associated with skin integrity, especially in children. The National Research Council recommends for adults that about 20% to 30% of the total day's calories be supplied by fats and that 1% of the total calories be essential fatty acids. Enough fat for food palatability aids appetite, which tends to be poor in the course of long, confining illness.

Vitamins and minerals. Optimum intake for metabolic activity and nutritional maintenance is essential. The normal age group allowances are adequate unless therapeutic needs such as anemia indicate individual increases. In some rehabilitation centers, however, multivitamin preparations are given routinely as insurance against deficiencies. How necessary this is may be questionable; however, all steps warranted to maintain optimum nutrition should be taken as the physician and the nutritionist deem wise.

Restoration of eating ability

Maximum use is made of individual available motor resources. These resources are aided by self-feeding devices as needed.

ACTIVITIES OF DAILY LIVING— EATING

The achievement of nutritional goals rests upon adequate food intake. The achievement of rehabilitation goals rests upon development of maximum individual potential. Eating, therefore, is an important part of learning. Persons with disabilities affecting use of the upper body and extremities will have need for retraining as much as is possible to manage the daily task of eating. Four considerations are involved in planning such a teaching program. These are the basic principles of specific individual need and related equipment, the use of self-help devices, the learning process, and a satisfactory place to eat.

Principles

Determining specific individual needs. How much can the patient do? What use does he have of his hands, and what reaching capacity does he have? Also, what ability does he have to get to the place in which he wants to eat? What muscles are involved? What muscle development or aid does he need?

Providing equipment to meet needs. What specific self-help devices does his particular disability require? How may these be procured or constructed? What tables or trays or other items are needed? For home use, what storage facilities might the necessary equipment require?

Self-help devices

Food textures. You may have heard at one time or another this little rhyme:

> Don't puree the food if ground will do;
> Don't grind the food if chopped will do;
> Don't chop the food if whole will do;
> Do all you can to make them chew.*

It is important to keep the patient as independent as possible for as long as possible, particularly in the personal activity of eating.

The food should be kept as nearly "regular" food as the individual patient can handle. Besides the physical benefit of needed bulk and some degree of chewing (even "gumming"), the patient gets an added psychologic boost from not having to eat baby food. Many toothless patients can manage most stews, soft fish and poultry, or moist meatloaf without difficulty. If foods do have to be pureed, patients would prefer having the regular food put through a sieve or blender, rather than eating commercial baby food.

Grasping and holding devices. With the proper approach and attitudes and with the help of a few simple, well-planned devices, many patients can bridge the gap between discouraging dependency and independent self-help. These devices may well make the difference between utter frustration and a renewed interest in eating. Some of these self-help devices for eating include the following.

HANDCUFF WITH PALM POCKET TO HOLD EATING UTENSIL. The handcuff is made of wide elastic to fit over the back of the hand. The palm piece has a pocket or slot formed by sewing together two pieces of leather, leaving an opening into which the fork or spoon handle fits.

---

*I am indebted to my friend and colleague, Delores Nyhus, late Nutrition Consultant, California Department of Public Health, for this pointed reminder that pureed foods have little valid use in adult diets and in this case are self-defeating in result.

THICKENED HANDLE. When painful fingers or weakened muscles make it difficult to grasp objects, often simply thickening the handle of the utensils will enable the patient to manage holding his fork, spoon, or knife. The following are suggested ways of thickening the handle:

1. Foam rubber strips wrapped around handles
2. Handle inserted into center space of large-sized foam rubber or plastic hair curlers after removal of the clip part
3. Use of bicycle handlebar grip after wrapping to make a still larger handle
4. Use of file handle attached for length as well as thickness

All these gadgets can be removed for washing of the utensil.

LENGTHENED HANDLE. If range of motion is limited, handles may be lengthened, or the direction of the tines of the fork or the bowl of the spoon can be altered. Some of these long-handled utensils are also collapsible for carrying.

CURVED KNIFE. A knife with a curved blade to cut meat and other food is useful for a patient with weak hands or a patient who has only one hand. These knives are sometimes called rocker knives.

Plate modifications. Plate guards that attach to the side of the plate or scoop-type dishes and spoons are available to enable to patient to corner his food rather than have it go round and round as he tries to get it up. Often simple rounded bowls or ones with straight edges, such as Pyrex baking dishes, can help him just as well. Also the dish should be stationed firmly. It can be anchored with ordinary suction cups or adhesive tape, or a tray insert can be made by cutting out holes or building up rims to fit dishes.

Devices to aid drinking. Liquids often present difficulty, not only in swallowing, but also in grasping and lifting the container. Thus the container should be as lightweight as possible.

DRINKING STRAWS AND STRAW HOLDERS. When a patient cannot use his hands or has difficulty in using a glass, the problem of grasping and lifting can be eliminated by the wise use and placement of drinking straws. Usually plastic tubing can be purchased in about 150 cm (5 ft) lengths and cut to any desired size, then bent to the most satisfactory angle for approach to the mouth. Two simple devices will help to stabilize the straw in the glass: (1) a "bulldog clip" can be clamped to the glass and the straw fitted through or (2) a common pencil clip can be used the same way on the edge of the glass with the straw fitted through the space ordinarily provided for the pencil.

COASTERS OR JACKETS FOR GLASSES. If a patient can achieve some degree of grasp and lift of the glass, simple coasters or jackets fitted over the glass will often help him to hold on to it better. These can be crocheted or straw matted or stocking type. The rougher surface, free of moisture, will give him a more secure grip. And where color is used, it adds a bright note to the tray or to the table.

TILT AND SWALLOW. The swallowing reflex is frequently diminished or absent in disabled persons. The reflex may be enhanced, however, by the use of an ice collar or by brushing the neck with a small brush (such as a small paint brush) just before eating. The liquid should be placed behind the front teeth, and the patient should slowly tilt his head back and swallow. He can learn this routine as the nurse goes over it several times with him, saying "Tilt and swallow . . . tilt and swallow . . . tilt and swallow. . . ."

Cups. Cups should have large enough handles for the entire hand to be placed in it so that the cup can be grasped more securely. They should be made of lightweight material that does not conduct heat.

Paper cups are difficult to manage and should not be attempted. Some patients, however, want to practice despite extensive hand involvement from high cervical traumatic lesions. All materials used should be unbreakable to reduce the patient's fear and anxiety.

The learning process

Learning to eat is often a frustrating and tedious process for the disabled person. However, it is worth the effort. A more independent patient, doing as much as possible to help himself, is a happier patient.

Evaluation of patient's abilities. The patient's ability to move effectively, to use his hands, and to reach for things must be evaluated. He should be helped into the most comfortable position or helped to get to the place where he wants to eat. The nurse should acquaint the patient with the various utensils and tableware, their nature, the materials from which they are made, their shapes, possible adjustments, and uses they serve. Additional special equipment and devices may be necessary to facilitate the use of the hands.

Usually it is easier to start with the spoon and work up to the use of forks and knives.

Arm support. The nurse should see that the patient has good forearm support, perhaps with his elbows on the table. Some patients may need more elaborate support such as a rocker splint.

Use of real food. Applesauce is a good food to start with, because it is easily managed and the temperature does not matter. It is good either warm or cold. As the learning process proceeds, there should be a happy medium in the consistency of food as patients try to feed themselves. Foods should not be too soft (liquid or gruel consistency) or too dry. For example, mashed potatoes, fairly firm puddings, and other such foods adhere more easily to the utensils. But such foods as rice or green peas may prove difficult to manage. If it sticks together and sticks to the utensil, it is easier to eat.

Continued use of devices. Later on, the devices may be discarded, or their use may be necessary on a permanent basis. In this case the patient may use a small plastic bag to carry them, and he may want to include a large napkin as protection against spills.

A place to eat

The table. From the beginning the table is the best place to use for eating, if it is at all possible. It helps to develop skills and has psychologic value. The nurse should help the patient assume the best posture possible for reaching.

The bed. If the patient is eating in bed, he must have adequate support. An overbed table should be provided for the tray. Trays should be used that are stable and do not tip.

A wheelchair. When the patient is eating in a wheelchair, an overbed table or the regular wheelchair tray may be used. Frequently wheelchair patients enjoy eating out-of-doors when weather permits, to have the social value in eating together. A regular table with legs spaced apart to give room for the wheelchair may be used also. The height of the table should be sufficient to allow the arms of the wheelchair underneath it, so that the patient may get close enough to the table for comfort.

CLINICAL PROBLEMS

Injuries producing prolonged immobility or enervation or muscles controlling normal elimination create additional problems for some disabled persons. With adequate medical and nursing care, much difficulty can be avoided.

Elimination

Constipation. Constipation and fecal impaction occur frequently following disabling illnesses and injuries. Careful attention to simple measures is imperative.

FLUID INTAKE. Adequate fluid intake is an important nutritional principle at all times, both in health and in disease. It becomes of prime significance in disabling injuries. Assuming a normal renal function, 2 to 3 L of total fluid intake daily should be assured. Water should be placed in convenient reach of the patient. If he cannot use his upper extremities in cases of severe disability, a plastic water bottle may be arranged with a drinking tube fixed in place, and positioned at the bedside so that the patient may take frequent sips. In some rehabilitation centers a 2.5 cm (1 in) layer of water in the bottom of the bottle is first frozen; then the bottle is filled with water and attached at the bedside. This practice helps to keep the water cool and makes it more tasteful to the patient.

Careful records of fluid intake should be kept and continuing supportive encouragement given to the patient to assure an adequate amount of fluid intake.

ELIMINATION AIDS. According to the physician's direction, additional aids to elimination may be used, such as wetting agents to maintain a soft stool or occasional bulk-producing agents when natural bulk in foods is limited or impossible. Intravenous or tube feeding may be necessary in early stages after injury, but a return to a regular diet should follow as soon as possible to aid normal peristalsis. Glycerine suppositories or a suppository of bisacodyl (Dulcolax) may be ordered by the physician in constipation problems involving impaction. These should only be used under medical supervision.

Bowel and bladder training. Fluid intake is an important aspect of a bowel and bladder training program. Such training should be encouraged when possible to give the patient a greater degree of independence, particularly if he has employment potential. A bowel training program to establish regular evacuation, similar to that used in many rehabilitation centers, follows:

BOWEL REHABILITATION ROUTINE

1. Daily intake of adequate fluids should be maintained (2 to 3 L); a record should be kept to ensure knowledge of optimum amount.
2. A diet high in natural residue foods should be given.
3. A regular time should be scheduled for defecation. In rehabilitation centers this may be in the evening. For a home patient the more practical time may be in the morning.
4. According to the individual schedule, 120 ml (4 oz) prune juice (a little lemon juice improves the flavor and is also an elimination aid) should be given about 12 hours before the scheduled defecation time. For the evening evacuation plan the prune juice would be taken before or with breakfast. For the morning evacuation plan it would be taken the night before.
5. Twenty to thirty minutes before the scheduled evacuation time, glycerine suppositories (one or two according to individual need) should be inserted. These should be placed well above the internal sphincter, at least 6.5 cm (2½ in) into the rectum, against the rectal mucosa.
6. The patient should be placed in a relaxed sitting position on the toilet or bedside commode. Care should be taken to see that he has adequate support as needed.
7. The schedule and recording of results should be maintained with no interruption by enemas.

Renal calculi

Prolonged enforced immobilization and certain paralytic disorders usually cause calcium withdrawal from the bones.[1] Apparently, bone integrity and homeostasis, a balance between calcium accretions and calcium withdrawal, are maintained by a combination of weight bearing and muscle tension. The needed muscle tension comes from the natural pull on origin and insertions of muscles produced by normal motion and activity. When the operation of these factors is prevented by paralyzing or immobilizing injuries or by treatment such as extensive body casting, bone calcium withdrawal increases. This imbalance produces excessive urinary excretions of calcium and consequent danger of stone formation.

Early use of tube feeding or subsequent regular dietary management should give attention to the calcium content of the diet. In prolonged inactivity it may need to be reduced and a low-calcium regimen (about 400 to 500 mg of calcium) followed. In less severe cases the average normal adult intake of calcium (about 800 mg) is sufficient. In any case, *excess* calcium should be avoided, and individual therapeutic needs should be treated accordingly. A review of the metabolism of calcium in Chapter 8, and of diet therapy for renal calculi in Chapter 29, will help clarify these nutritional principles.

Obesity

Perhaps the one most common nutritional problem in rehabilitation is obesity. Even a small amount of excess weight in patients with severe disabilities may hinder their progress. If caloric intake is not adapted to energy expenditure level, a gradual gain in weight will follow. Individual need is important. The amount of possible exercise and activity varies. Thus weight control by a balanced diet, adjusting its caloric value to the need of the patient, is essential.

Overweight patients should have sufficient calorie reduction to effect a gradual weight loss. Stringent weight reduction programs are usually unwise and should be used with caution. A 1,200 calorie diet may be effective to bring about the desired results. In some cases, however (such as elderly paralyzed patients), a diet as low as 800 calories may be required to reduce weight. In these cases strict attention must be given to dietary nutrient intake with supplementary vitamins and minerals given as needed.

Indiscriminate fasting programs are unwise. Important protein tissue (muscle mass) needed in the rehabilitation program may be lost, especially by the more inactive patients. Also a large part of the loss in such a program is only temporary water loss. However, some clinicians feel that there may be some possible advantage in a fasting program in cases of extreme obesity, built on noncaloric fluids, vitamins, and physical activity.[2]

The nutritional principles of weight control and various dietary reduction programs are given in greater detail in Chapter 24.

CASE STUDY 13
The patient with a cerebrovascular accident

It was as Dr. Grant had feared. One morning not long after the health center case conference, Mr. Harris had arisen and begun to prepare to go to work. Mrs. Harris was in the kitchen preparing breakfast for the family. She heard a noise in the bathroom like someone falling. She ran to see what was the matter and found Mr. Harris unconscious on the bathroom floor. There was no evidence of vomiting or incontinence.

Immediately she called Dr. Grant at the health center, and an ambulance was sent to bring Mr. Harris to the hospital. At the hospital Dr. Grant examined him. He was still unconscious. His tongue deviated to the right. There was a flaccid paralysis on the right side, but the left side appeared normal. There was a pinprick response on the left side, but a questionable response on the right side. The Babinski and Chaddock reflexes were absent on both sides. During the examination Mr. Harris regained consciousness. He seemed confused, disorientated, and apprehensive. His blood pressure was 190/100, and his pulse was rapid. Dr. Grant wrote in the chart: impression—cerebral hemorrhage, left-middle cerebral artery prefrontal area with massive extension; paralysis, right side; aphasia.

Dr. Grant ordered further tests, including BUN, FBS, and serum cholesterol. He also ordered an intravenous infusion started, composed of 500 ml 2.5% dextrose in 0.45% saline, every eight hours, with the flow regulated so that each 500 ml would take eight hours to run in. He also ordered that Mr. Harris was to have clear fluids by mouth as tolerated.

After he had concluded the examination and Mr. Harris was transferred to a room on the medical ward, Dr. Grant went out to the hallway where Mrs. Harris was waiting anxiously. He gave her a brief summary of his findings and encouraged her. He made arrangements for her to remain with Mr. Harris according to his need.

Later on in the day Mr. Harris was able to take a few sips of water, although he had a little difficulty swallowing it. His nurse, Miss Jensen, assisted him carefully. She noticed that there was drooling from his mouth, which caused him a great deal of concern. He tried to make motions with his hand and appeared anxious about his condition. Miss Jensen brought him a pencil and pad, but Mrs. Harris said that he was right-handed. Miss Jensen encouraged him to try printing with his left hand. The nurse noted a little later that the initial laboratory report had been returned and was in the chart. She read BUN—16 mg/dl; FBS—140 mg/dl; cholesterol—290. She also noticed that additional laboratory work had been ordered and the results returned. They were hemoglobin—14; hematocrit—40; CO_2-combining power—60 volumes per deciliter serum; sodium—135; potassium—4.2; chloride—98.

The following day Mr. Harris was able to take a full liquid diet, which Miss Jensen fed to him carefully. Dr. Grant discontinued the intravenous infusion, since Mr. Harris was able to take some liquids by mouth. Miss Jensen noted that Mr. Harris had had no bowel movement, and she wondered what provision might be made to help his elimination problem.

On the fourth day Mr. Harris was able to take some solid food, and Miss Jensen helped him with his soft diet. She arranged the foods attractively on his tray and fed him carefully to avoid causing choking. By the end of two weeks Mr. Harris was able to take a full diet. The clinical dietitian, Miss Bennett, developed aids by which Mr. Harris could help to feed himself.

After four weeks Dr. Grant decided it would be helpful to Mr. Harris if he were transferred to the rehabilitation center where he could have full advantage of the therapy facilities available there. Miss Jensen helped prepare him for the trip, and he was moved by ambulance.

Continued.

CASE STUDY 13

The patient with a cerebrovascular accident—cont'd

At the rehabilitation center the health team conferred concerning Mr. Harris's therapy needs. A vigorous program of physical therapy and speech therapy was initiated. The nutritionist and the nurse worked with Mr. Harris to help him learn to feed himself with the use of self-help feeding devices. They also gave attention to the types of food that he could handle more easily. Mr. Harris was considerably overweight still, so the nutritionist continued him on a reduction-level diet of 1,500 calories and indicated that a good amount of protein was to be included.

Gradually Mr. Harris responded to the supportive and vigorous program of care in which he participated at the rehabilitation center. In six months' time he was walking with a cane. He had also regained in large measure his ability to speak. When he was ready to go home, arrangements were made with Mrs. Harris for his care at home. Occasional visits by the public health nurse, nutritionist, social worker, and physical therapist helped to support Mrs. Harris. Dr. Grant also made arrangements for a work evaluation for Mr. Harris and helped him in determining his capacities for a limited job situation.

Mr. Harris continued to lose weight gradually, although he was still at this point over his optimum weight. However, he had been able to stop smoking, as the doctor had long urged him to do.

Questions to guide your inquiry

1. What is a cerebrovascular accident? Account for the symptoms Mr. Harris displayed.
2. What were Mr. Harris's initial nutritional needs? How were these met?
3. When Mr. Harris was able to take liquid and later solid foods by mouth, what feeding problems did he present? What solutions would you propose to meet these problems? Why?
4. What dietary means can you propose for helping to alleviate Mr. Harris' bowel problem?
5. After Mr. Harris was moved to the rehabilitation center, what major problems would the health team identify concerning his care?
6. What solutions to these problems would you propose? Why?
7. What are the goals and methods of rehabilitation?
8. Why is the patient considered to be the most important member of the health team in a rehabilitation program? What role should the patient's family play in his rehabilitation? Why?
9. What social attitudes may create problems for the disabled person?
10. What economic problems might the Harris family face as a result of Mr. Harris's illness? What possible solutions might be found to meet this problem?
11. What are some of the psychologic problems that the disabled person faces? What psychologic problems do you think Mr. Harris might be facing? What help do you think the nurse and other members of the health team can be in meeting these needs?
12. What are the basic principles of nutritional care for a disabled person in rehabilitation?
13. Why should an overweight person such as Mr. Harris be turned frequently in the early stages?
14. Why is protein such an important part of the diet for a person in rehabilitation therapy?
15. What principles would govern the health team at the rehabilitation center in determining Mr. Harris's self-help needs for eating?
16. Describe some of the self-help devices that Mr. Harris might find useful to help him in eating and drinking.
17. What factors would the nutritionist and the nurse consider in helping Mr. Harris learn how to care for himself, especially to feed himself?
18. When Mr. Harris went home from the rehabilitation center, what problems might there have been in his home care?
19. What solutions do you propose for meeting these problems? How would you involve the members of the health team, such as the public health nurse, the social worker, the physical therapist, and the nutritionist? How would you involve the family?

REFERENCES
Specific

1. Aegerter, E. E., and Kirkpatrick, J. A.: Orthopedic diseases, ed. 4, Philadelphia, 1975, W. B. Saunders Co., p. 32.
2. Hirschberg, G. G., Lewis, L., and Thomas, D.: Rehabilitation: a manual for the care of the disabled and elderly, Philadelphia, 1964, J. B. Lippincott Co., p. 6.

General

Arthritis—the basic facts, New York, 1976, The Arthritis Foundation.

Bienenstock, H., and Fernando, K. R.: Arthritis in the elderly: an overview, Med. Clin. North Am. **60:**1173, 1976.

Boroch, R. M.: Elements of rehabilitation in nursing: an introduction, St. Louis, 1976, The C. V. Mosby Co.

Hirschberg, G. G., Lewis, L., and Thomas, D.: Rehabilitation, a manual for the care of the disabled and elderly, Philadelphia, 1964, J. B. Lippincott Co.

Hyman, L. R., Boner, G., Thomas, J. C., et al.: Immobilization hypercalcemia, Am. J. Dis. Child. **124:**723, 1972.

Katz, W. A.: Rheumatic diseases: diagnosis and management, Philadelphia, 1977, J. B. Lippincott Co.

Kaye, R. L., and Pemberton, R. E.: Treatment of rheumatoid arthritis, Arch. Intern. Med. **136:**1023, 1976.

Klinger, J. L., Frieden, F. H., and Sullivan, R. A.: Mealtime manual for the aged and handicapped, New York, 1970, Simon & Schuster, Inc.

Larson, C. B., and Gould, M.: Orthopedic nursing, ed. 9, St. Louis, 1978, The C. V. Mosby Co.

Lawton, E. B.: Activities of daily living for physical rehabilitation, New York, 1963, McGraw-Hill Book Co.

Lowman, E. W., and Klinger, J. L.: Aids to independent living—self-help for the handicapped, New York, 1969, McGraw-Hill Book Co.

May, E. E., Wagonner, N. R., and Boettke, E. M.: Homemaking for the handicapped, New York, 1966, Dodd, Mead, & Co.

Rusk, H. A.: Nutrition in the fourth phase of medical care, Nutr. Today **5**(3):24, 1970.

Rusk, H. A.: Rehabilitation medicine, ed. 4, St. Louis, 1977, The C. V. Mosby Co.

Self-help devices for rehabilitation (booklet), Institute of Physical Medicine and Rehabilitation, New York University, Bellvue Medical Center, New York, 1975 (rev.).

Symposium on arthritis in older persons, J. Am. Geriatr. Soc. **25:**49, 1977.

Wheeler, V. H.: Planning kitchens for handicapped homemakers, Rehabilitation Monograph 27, New York, 1965, Institute of Rehabilitation Medicine, New York University Medical Center.

Wolf, A. W., Chuinard, R. G., Riggins, R. S., et al.: Immobilization hypercalcemia. A case report and review of the literature, Clin. Orthop. **118:**124, 1976.

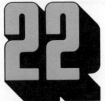 **Nutrition in psychiatric care**

Psychiatric principles are not confined merely to the care of patients with manifest mental illness. They are an integral part of all health care. In education for all the health professions these fundamental mental health principles are introduced in the beginning of the student's general clinical experience, although they may not always be identified as such at that time. They continue to be woven throughout the professional education process and form a large base for all clinical practice. Perhaps the only difference in the application of these principles in the care of patients with mental illness is that the basic human psychologic need is much more acute at this point and has led to pathologic symptoms, thus making the principles of care that much more evident.

The human being gains certain masteries and controls and coping mechanisms at each stage of his individual development. These strengths vary with individuals according to their unique life experiences and relationships. However, everyone deals with the same essential human problems of self—the problems of meaning, relationship, and communication. Over the years numerous psychiatrists and psychologists have added insights concerning these basic human needs. For example, Jurgen Ruesch[1,2] has developed a theory and approach to mental illness basically around success or failure in communication. Carl Rogers[3] has focused attention on the patient and his own essential capacities for psychologic growth.

Increasingly, medicine, nutrition, and nursing have based their approaches to general patient care on psychiatric principles. Nutrition, as an essential part of all total patient care, is applied, therefore, in the light of these basic human needs. Many of these relationships between food and feeding and individual psychosocial needs have been developed in the previous chapters. They will focus here on the patient with mental illness, the goals and methods of psychiatric care, the problems the psychiatric patient faces in the community, and the many opportunities the practitioner finds to apply principles of nutrition to day-to-day care.

The same principles stated at the beginning of Chapter 21, Nutrition in Rehabilitation, apply to psychiatric care. Realistic answers should be sought to the following questions:

1. How do rehabilitation principles apply to psychiatric care?
2. What social attitudes, economic problems, and psychologic barriers does the patient with mental illness face?
3. What are the basic principles of nutritional care of psychiatric patients? What practical approaches may help overcome feeding problems?
4. What special clinical problems may involve particular dietary management?

GOALS AND METHODS

A positive concept. As in rehabilitation, psychiatric care is based on a positive concept of the healing potential within the patient himself. To this end the psychiatric hospital community seeks to establish a therapeutic environment to support the patient in his effort to regain health.

A team approach. The skills of many health professionals are used in a group effort to work *with* the patient and guide his way back to health. He is the focus of the team. They work with him in individual and group relationships and many of their techniques are based on the therapeutic value of this human relationship of finding meaning in human experience through relating to another person. The psychiatric health team is guided by the psychiatrist who coordinates the overall plan for individual patient care. Other specialists who work with him in this effort include clinical psychologists, clinical nutritionists, nurses, social workers, technicians, vocational nurses, aides, occupational and recreational therapists, and others. The food service dietitian in the psychiatric hospital is also a special resource person to the psychiatric team and is in a key position to help make experiences with food have meaningful therapeutic value for the individual patients.

SOCIOECONOMIC AND PSYCHOLOGIC FACTORS

Many interrelated socioeconomic and psychologic factors surround the psychiatric patient and account for his responses. Human behavior has causes, both rational and irrational, and can be understood if its background is known.

Social attitudes. Although social attitudes toward mental illness are increasingly more enlightened, they still convey a negative stigma of guilt, shame, or fear. Many feel that mental illness is something to be hidden as if one were less a person because of his illness. Moreover, many attitudes prevail in American society today such as prejudice, discrimination, segregation, injustice, and lack of communication, all of which devalue and alienate the individual.

These unaccepting and somewhat moralistic views create problems for the patient and for those who would help him in his effort to function in society again.

Economic problems. Because of negative social attitudes the patient faces economic problems in future employment and in finding a productive role in his group. Also, anxieties concerning the cost of psychiatric care may prevent the patient having need for such care from seeking it. In addition, such burdens may create anxieties that further complicate his treatment and cause him to respond to his environment in a negative way.

Care facilities. Some of the related social problems involve facilities for care of the person with mental illness. Public education concerning mental health is helping to bridge the gap, and many community counseling activities are being provided for those in need. Supportive nutritional programs in day treatment centers are helping to provide knowledge and social skills in food selection, handling, and preparation.[4] There are clinics for treatment of alcoholism, family case work, pastoral counseling, marital counseling, work through the courts with juvenile offenders, and public health programs. For the most part, however, the initial clinical care of patients with mental illness will concern those hospitalized in psychiatric institutions. Through many activities of daily living in this group situation the practitioners will relate to patients and aid in their recoveries. One of these basic activities is nutritional—eating.

BASIC PRINCIPLES OF NUTRITIONAL CARE

The same two basic principles of nutritional care that governed activities in rehabilitation also operate in the care of psychiatric patients.

Prevention of malnutrition

Many surveys and general observations have indicated that patients in hospitals for the mentally ill, especially in large, overcrowded state hospitals, frequency suffer from varying degrees of malnutrition. Because the number of personnel is often inadequate and the patients' needs are so great, a far from ideal environment sometimes prevails. Persons with severe illness and consequent eating problems may not receive the close attention and care they require to help them eat. The resulting chronic malnutrition adds to their generally poor state of health and in turn to their mental illness. Sometimes these groups of patients are called "the forgotten back ward," a label that indicates their great need for care. That even these seemingly hopeless situations are amenable to improvement, however, is evident through the experience of one large state hospital. A few concerned staff members with help from interested volunteers from the community found that a custodial ward could be changed to a treatment ward and self-respect restored for patients and aides.[5]

Although general mental illness per se does not require an increase in nutrients, some research has been done on the therapeutic value of megadoses of certain vitamins and minerals for individuals apparently requiring more than the recommended allowances perhaps due to variances in rate of oxidation in the metabolic pathways producing energy.[6] However, a task force established by the American Psychiatric Association to investigate the curative megadose claims, especially for niacin, found no evidence to support the theory and practice of orthomolecular psychiatrists.[7] Whatever the individual need, the value of sound nutrition lies in the contribution it makes to general physical health and the increasing sense of strength and well-being such a state gives an individual to aid his efforts to recovery.

Restoration of eating abilities and satisfactions

The positive goal of nutritional care is achieved through restoration of the disturbed patient's ability to eat and to receive both physical and emotional satisfaction from his food. Often with increased interest in eating comes increased interest in other aspects of his environment, and positive steps are taken toward health.

APPLICATION OF NUTRITIONAL PRINCIPLES IN PATIENT CARE
Food as a therapeutic tool

In the discussion of influences on eating habits in Chapter 13 it was found that a great many cultural, social, and psychologic factors influence response to food. Certain foods and food patterns have meaning largely as a result of past experiences in human relationships. From earliest infancy, food is a vehicle of relationship, first between the infant and his mother, then between the growing child and his family, and finally between the adult and his wider social relationships in the enlarging community. Food is one of the earliest means of building trust. Early feeding experiences can either build warmth, satisfaction, comfort, and a sense of being cared for, or they can build anxiety, frustration, and a sense of rejection and neglect. These are the sorts of underlying psychic patterns that become perpetuated with age and adult relationships. In the mentally ill person they become even more exaggerated by the kind of interpersonal relations the person is now maintaining. If early feeding experiences were negative, they may express themselves in negative attitudes toward food and toward the person offering it.

Thus because food does carry meaning— often great symbolic meaning—for the patient, the nature of it and the way it is offered can have great therapeutic significance. Often it is simply the persistent sympathetic manner in which a nurse helps a person to eat that says to him "I care," and helps him to overcome his projected feelings.

Feeding problems

A number of feeding problems may exist among psychiatric patients. Solutions for these problems must be found individually by understanding the factors behind such food behavior.

Refusal to eat. Severely disturbed patients may reject food completely, not because they are unwilling to eat but because their illness makes eating on their own initiative impossible.

The extreme form of inability to eat, *anorexia nervosa,* is a somewhat uncommon psychophysiologic reaction seen mostly in adolescent girls or young adult single women. As described by Sir William Gull in his original classic papers (1858, 1874),[8] these patients are usually of high intelligence, introverted, perfectionistic, compulsive, and overly sensitive. Their response to food is one of revulsion and disgust with vomiting usually following any forced feeding. Sometimes there is a preceding history of the opposite reaction to food, overeating and obesity, followed with shame at being fat. Usually there is hostility in parental relations at home, especially with the mother, or in sibling rivalry and jealousy. Occasionally a pregnancy fantasy may have triggered the desire to ''diet,'' with complete refusal of food developing as a result. Bruch has termed this distorted body image and its accompanying eating disorder ''the golden cage'' virtually imprisoning the patient.[9] She warns against the use of punitive behavior modification methods of treatment, as patients may feel tricked into letting go control over their bodies and their lives, with a resulting pervasive sense of personal ineffectiveness, a root problem in the development of the anorexia nervosa in the first place.[10] During hospitalization and treatment with psychotherapy the nurse may give support to the patient by offering intimate personal attention at meals. Often this is done in many small ways. The nurse may at first be able to feed the patient in an unhurried and accepting manner, gradually encouraging self-feeding. Small doses of insulin before meals may sometimes be a part of the treatment to stimulate need and desire for food. Some patients, however, will require tube feeding.

Refusal to eat in other patients may have a number of conscious and unconscious psychologic roots. It may stem from a suicidal death wish. It may result from feelings of guilt or personal unworthiness with the denial of food as the means of self-punishment. The patient's delusional beliefs that the food is poisoned, that he has no stomach to hold or digest it, or that he is eating various body parts may cause him to reject the food. Hallucinations such as hearing voices commanding no food intake or preoccupation, depression, withdrawal, and catatonic states may influence the patient's reaction to food and make it impossible for him to eat.

APPROACH. The patient's physical survival, however, depends on food. On his own he would starve. He must have nourishment. Treatment is aimed at seeking to determine the reasons for his rejection of food and to support all individual efforts in retraining to eat. If tube feeding must be used as a last lifesaving resort, the procedure should be done in a therapeutic manner—*never* in a punitive manner. Since the nursing aim is to help the patient assume responsibility for his own eating, there should be a consistent approach involving patience and understanding. The patient should be involved in the care plan, given the reasons for it, and helped to see that he is accepted and cared for as a person. His refusal to eat must be recognized as his inability to do otherwise, not as a perverse unwillingness to do so. As a relationship of confidence and trust builds, the patient may be led to become more actively involved in self-feeding and eventually in group eating.

Reluctant or anxious eating behavior. The anxious patient finds decision making difficult. As a result, food intake may be inadequate because in his confusion he hesitates and questions whether he should eat or not, what items he should eat, and how much he should eat. He takes a long time over his food, eats very slowly, if at all, and resists being hurried or pushed. Sometimes he may hide food, give it away, or try to bargain with the nurse to avoid pressures concerning eating.

In caring for such patients the wise nurse and nutritionist will recognize that through such seemingly reluctant food behavior the patient is trying to communicate other unmet personal needs. By accepting the behavior as such a reflection, therefore, the nurse may help him to express his real needs and explore with him actions or activities that will help to meet these needs. The nurse may need to help feed him at first, giving support and assurance as the patient assumes more and more of the responsibility for food choices, and helping him toward the social value of group eating as soon as he is able.

Bizarre food behavior. Other bizarre food behavior may take the form of general destructiveness or personal untidiness. The patient may throw food or dishes; he may grab at other patient's food. He may mix all his food up on his plate, play with it, drop it on the floor. He may eat his food in an unconventional manner— spitting it up, stuffing it in his mouth, gulping it down.

Again the nurse will approach such a patient with an effort to understand the personal needs expressed by such behavior. Punitive reactions or disgust only reinforce his behavior and worsen his condition. In periods of destructiveness, brief use of paper food containers may be helpful. The essential aim of nursing care, however, is to help the patient get personal and social satisfactions from the experience of eating and to assume an increasing responsibility for achieving this goal.

Food and food service. Administrative and medical personnel in psychiatric hospitals are increasingly recognizing the therapeutic value of good food served in pleasant, comfortable, and attractive surroundings. Cafeterias that offer a variety of food choices are being used to help develop the patient's confidence in his ability to make decisions. In many hospitals the food is appetizing, attractive, and tasteful. Old drab dining rooms with long bare tables and benches are being replaced by colorful rooms with draperies, wall pictures, and modern small tables and comfortable chairs. In these situations, eating becomes a major support of therapy and a way of sharing with the patient a meaningful activity, one that is vital to his welfare. Around the dining table in small group situations the patient finds in sharing food a way of relating to others. Such experiences strengthen his efforts to reach out for personal relationships and give him a foundation for future satisfying relations with others.

NUTRITIONAL THERAPY IN CLINICAL PROBLEMS
Alcoholism

Alcoholism is a disease, often expressing symptoms of underlying emotional difficulties. Experienced psychiatric personnel point out that it often represents problems of hostility, rejection, or excessive dependency. The problem of alcoholism is particularly associated with large cities and continues to be a grave health problem in the United States.

Often malnutrition compounds the basic psychosocial problem of the alcoholic, and physical health deteriorates. The medical program of treatment will include optimum nutritional therapy and help in building better food habits. Usually the diet is poor. The person frequently skips meals, using alcohol instead, or goes without food for longer periods of time during drinking bouts. As a result, the body is depleted of needed nutrients especially proteins and vitamins. Increased amounts of protein, carbohydrates, and vitamins should be given, unless advanced liver disease calls for a reduced protein intake (see Chapter 27).

General care. In providing care and in discussions with the patient concerning nutritional needs, the nutritionist and the nurse will remember the principles of learning (Chapter 14). An individual must learn for himself and accept the responsibility of his own personal choices in the light of facts presented. The patient's basic need is to develop self-respect and responsibility. The practitioners will therefore avoid moralistic judgments but will provide sound, straightforward information. They will give emotional support with acceptance and understanding. To the question once asked a psychiatric social worker, ''Do you hold your patient's hand?'' her wisdom borne of much experience in helping alcoholics gave the reply, ''Yes, and we let go finger by finger.''[11]

Korsakoff's psychosis. Acutely ill hospitalized patients, suffering from the effect of prolonged alcoholism, may display symptoms of Korsakoff's psychosis. This syndrome is named for the Russian physician Sergei Korsakoff, who first described its clinical nature in 1887. Because of the nutritional deficiency imposed by excess alcohol intake, especially of the vitamins thiamin and niacin, degenerative changes occur in the long peripheral nerves and the nerve cells of the cerebral cortex. A neuritis develops with pain and tingling in the feet and legs. The calves of the legs are tender to pressure, and foot drop occurs. The leg muscles may even atrophy and produce painful contractures. The patient is treated initially with intravenous glucose solutions containing large amounts of thiamin chloride and nicotinic acid. Electrolytes and fluids are also given to combat dehydration and to increase the alkaline reserves. Insulin may be used to accelerate the metabolism of the alcohol of the body. As the patient is able to take oral feeding, he is given large amounts of fluid (3,000 to 4,000 ml daily), much of it as orange juice and milk. If symptoms of impending hepatic coma occur, he is changed to a low-protein or protein-free diet with large amounts of carbohydrate. These symptoms are not confined, however, to alcoholism and may occur in other vitamin B deficiency states from other causes.

Insulin coma therapy in schizophrenia

Insulin shock therapy may sometimes be used as a treatment for schizophrenia in supportive preparation for psychotherapy. It was initially developed and used in the early 1930s, and although not in as common use today, it has been considered by some clinicians as an effective therapy in this type of mental disorder. Patients are carefully selected according to their physical condition and age, and most of them are over 40 years old. The patient is given injections of insulin beginning with about 40 units daily and continuing until the desired coma stage is reached. He is held in this stage for 30 to 60 minutes. If the coma deepens during this period, it is terminated immediately. Over a period of weeks the course of treatment may involve 30 to 40 comas, depending on individual need and response. The amount of regular crystalline insulin necessary to produce the coma generally varies from 80 to 600 units. The coma is terminated by an injection (0.25 to 0.50 mg) of glucagon (p. 25). During the period of treatment the staff team maintains close contact with the patient, and opportunity for closer therapeutic communication is experienced.

Nursing care is essential to help prepare the patient for the treatment, explaining its general nature and effectiveness. The nurse should be well versed in the symptoms of insulin shock and the levels of coma and be alert to the progress of the desired coma stage. A quiet therapeutic environment should be maintained during the awakening periods. The first meal following a treatment may be high in carbohydrate to replenish glycogen stores and blood glucose levels.

Mental retardation

Nutritional care of mentally retarded children is based on meeting the physical growth and development needs of the individual child according to his age-group needs. These growth needs have been outlined in Chapter 18. Sometimes in the presence of profound disabilities, concern for the child's disability may overshadow his basic physical needs, and care for these primary needs may be neglected. Approaches to feeding will be adapted to each child's need, with emotional support or physical aid as he may require.

Particular disabilities may require additional nutritional care. In *cerebral palsy,* for example, the uncontrollable body motions of *athetoids* necessitate a diet high in calories for simple physical maintenance. (Athetoid motions are repeated involuntary muscular distortions of the limbs—legs, arms, hands, fingers—and sometimes involve the entire body. They are caused by the brain lesion.) Also the child with cerebral palsy may have great difficulty chewing and swallowing. Anorexia or obesity may be additional complications requiring individual nutritional planning.

General clinical situation involving the central nervous system

Chorea. Chorea is an infectious disease of the central nervous system and affects both the brain cortex and the basal ganglia. Chorea is believed to be caused by the same organism that causes rheumatic fever. Danger lies in involvement of valvular heart disease. The child displays muscular incoordination in jerky, involuntary movements. A quiet environment of physical and mental rest is essential. The diet should be of high nutritional quality and may require extra calories because of the hyperactivity.

Delirium from general systemic infection. Delirium from systemic infection is seen more often in general hospitals, but it may be observed on psychiatric wards. The patient requires a high fluid intake (3,000 to 5,000 ml daily). Cool beverages and fruit juices are desirable. The calories should be high, and the food texture should be liquid to soft. Caution must be exercised in feeding to prevent choking.

Traumatic coma. Following injury to the brain a patient may remain in coma for a number of days. Usually tube feedings (Chapter 30) are required to sustain his nutritional requirements.

Cerebral arteriosclerosis. In older patients damage to brain function may occur from arteriosclerosis. The diet may be modified in fat or sodium according to individual situations. In any case it should be of optimum general nutrition. The brain damage may involve paralysis—a cerebrovascular accident (''stroke'')—and the patient will need to be fed. An unhurried, patient, kind approach to the feeding of these patients is a highly significant part of their nursing care.

Epilepsy. The general term epilepsy (Gr. *epilepsia,* a seizing) refers to several types of recurrent seizures of varying intensities produced by excessive neuronal discharges in different parts of the brain. It may be caused by a number of cerebral and general physical disorders. Usually drug therapy controls the convulsive seizures, and there is no dietary modification required. However, for those children who do not tolerate the drugs or whose seizures cannot be controlled with these medications, treatment may sometimes involve a *ketogenic* diet, one high in fat content and relatively low in carbohydrate sufficient to produce a pronounced state of ketosis.[12,13] Because of the large amount of fat the diet is unpleasant, even to the point of nausea. It is therefore difficult to maintain and hence is not frequently used.

CASE STUDY 14
The patient with psychiatric problems

The clinical nutritionist, Dr. Susan Walker, glanced at her watch to note that it was time for Mrs. Adams's appointment in the nutrition clinic at the medical center. The medical record lay open before her on the desk where she had been reviewing all the pertinent medical data. It was evident that Mrs. Adams had a chronic heart condition, atherosclerotic cardiovascular disease with hypertension. More specifically, however, Dr. Walker was concerned about Mrs. Adams's psychiatric problems.

A few days before, Dr. Stone, one of the clinical psychologists in the psychiatry department, had come to confer with Dr. Walker about Mrs. Adams. He discussed his concerns for her nutritional status and his desire to include this approach as part of her support therapy. Dr. Stone had been seeing Mrs. Adams in outpatient therapy for a number of months since her discharge from the psychiatric ward of the county hospital where she had been hospitalized following a suicide attempt. She was suffering from depression and paranoia but was beginning to respond to Dr. Stone's very supportive and skilled care. He was now seeing her weekly in the clinic, since she had been able to return to her small apartment where she lived alone. He wanted to refer her to Dr. Walker for nutritional support therapy, since she had lost weight and was eating poorly, and also to extend her personal contacts to provide emotional support. The two therapists agreed that Dr. Walker would make a special appointment for Mrs. Adams and that they would continue to see her on alternating weekly follow-up visits.

Dr. Walker looked forward to working with Dr. Stone, as she had many times before, since the counseling aspect of her work as a clinical nutrition specialist was especially important to her. All through her graduate work in nutritional science and her clinical dietetic internship she had made it a point to take extra work in counseling. Now it was proving to be particularly helpful in her clinical practice.

When Dr. Walker called Mrs. Adams personally to make the special appointment, she thought Mrs. Adams sounded pleased and interested in coming in to the clinic for a nutrition conference. She was careful to give Mrs. Adams very detailed instructions about the location of the clinic and the purpose of her visit.

When the receptionist called to say that Mrs. Adams had arrived, Dr. Walker called her from the waiting room and helped to make her comfortable in her office. At first Mrs. Adams seemed hesitant, but gradually began to respond to Dr. Walker's warm manner, although she retained her quiet pattern of speaking. As the interview continued, Dr. Walker learned that Mrs. Adams was 69 years old, a widow for the past three years, with two married sons living in distant cities whom she seldom saw. She had no close friends, lived alone in a small studio apartment, and had no personal transportation. She had begun to feel more secure on the city bus and was now trying to take the bus to the nearest market and carry her few groceries home. She said she had very little energy for or interest in food preparation. She only left the apartment to come to the clinic and to make her occasional trips to the market. She was 163 cm (5 ft, 5 in) tall with a normal weight of 57 kg (125 lb). Since her husband died, however, and her present illness began to worsen, she had lost weight to her present level of 43 kg (95 lb). Since Christmas was only five days away, Dr. Walker asked if she had any plans for a Christmas dinner with friends or neighbors. She quietly answered, "No, there is no one. It will be just another day, I guess."

Even the history Mrs. Adams gave of her food habits was sparse: breakfast—coffee and a piece of toast; lunch—a peanut butter sandwich; dinner—a frozen TV dinner that she heated in a small oven. When asked what she usually did after dinner, Mrs. Adams answered, "I just go to bed."

Continued.

CASE STUDY 14
The patient with psychiatric problems—cont'd

Dr. Walker explored some simple beginning steps Mrs. Adams might take to broaden her food choices and preparation and made arrangements for the first of her follow-up visits the following week. As Mrs. Adams left, Dr. Walker made a note to see if she could involve her in a community Christmas dinner in the neighborhood senior center near where she lived.

The following week on the day of Mrs. Adams's follow-up appointment, Dr. Walker's office phone rang. It was Mrs. Adams, calling from her room in the adjoining hospital building to tell Dr. Walker that she would be unable to keep her appointment, since she had been admitted to the hospital Christmas Eve following her collapse at home, suffering from dehydration. Surprisingly her voice sounded almost cheerful as she said she was feeling much better and expected to be going home in a few days. Dr. Walker said she would be right over to the ward to see her.

With a puzzled expression Dr. Walker slowly replaced the telephone. "Maybe this was the way she has been able to avoid being alone at Christmas," she thought as a smile came over her face and she hurried out the door to go over to the ward.

Questions to guide your inquiry (Refer also to Chapters 13 to 15, 20, and 23.)

1. What nutritional problems can you identify? How are they related to Mrs. Adams's current medical and psychiatric situation? How are they related to her social living situation?
2. What solutions to these needs can you propose? What data do you need to collect and assess? How would you obtain this data?
3. In developing a plan of care for Mrs. Adams, what do you think may be more immediate goals? Long-term goals? How do you think you might plan with Mrs. Adams to work toward these goals?
4. How would you involve other resource persons in this plan of care?
5. How may food be used as a therapeutic tool in mental illness?
6. What are some practical ways you might help Mrs. Adams to become more involved with food as a nutritional support as well as an emotional support to broaden her social contacts?
7. What community nutrition programs are available for older persons living alone in Mrs. Adams's situation? Investigate any such program operating in your community, make a visit to see its operation, and interview the dietitian in charge.

REFERENCES
Specific

1. Ruesch, J., and Bateson, G.: Communication, the social matrix of psychiatry, New York, 1951, W. W. Norton & Co., Inc.
2. Ruesch, J., and Kees, W.: Nonverbal communication, Los Angeles, 1959, University of California Press.
3. Rogers, C.: Client-centered therapy, Boston, 1957, Houghton Mifflin Co.
4. Johnson, C. A., Haney, C. E., Flowers, B., et al.: Dietitians help mental patients "make it on the outside," J. Am. Diet. Assoc. **70:**513, May, 1977.
5. Ruhlman, R. G., and Ishiyama, T.: Remedy for the forgotten back ward, Am. J. Nurs. **64:**109, 1964.
6. Watson, G.: Nutrition and your mind, New York, 1971, Harper & Row, Publishers.
7. American Psychiatry Association: Task Force report 7. Megavitamin and orthomolecular therapy in psychiatry, Washington, D.C., 1973.
8. Gull, W. W.: Anorexia nervosa, Trans. Clin. Soc. (London) **7:**22, 1874.
9. Bruch, H.: The golden cage: the enigma of anorexia nervosa, Cambridge, Mass., 1978, Harvard University Press.
10. Bruch, H.: Perils of behavior modification in treatment of anorexia nervosa, J.A.M.A. **230:**1419, 1974.
11. Peltenburg, C. M.: Casework with the alcoholic patient, Social Casework **37:**81, 1956.

12. Lasser, J. L., and Brush, M. K.: An improved ketogenic diet for treatment of epilepsy, J. Am. Diet. Assoc. **63**:281, March, 1973.
13. Signore, J. M.: Ketogenic diet containing medium-chain triglycerides, J. Am. Diet. Assoc. **62**:285, March, 1973.

General

Axelrod, J.: Neurotransmitters, Sci. Am. **230**:58, June, 1974.

Bruch, H.: Eating disorders, obesity, anorexia nervosa, and the person within, New York, 1973, Basic Books, Inc., Publishers.

Calvert, S. D., Vivian, V. M., and Calvert, G. P.: Dietary adequacy, feeding practices, and eating behavior of children with Down's syndrome, J. Am. Diet. Assoc. **69**:152, Aug., 1976.

Cravioto, J., Hambraeus, L., and Vahlquist, B., editors: Early malnutrition and mental development, Swedish Nutrition Foundation XII, Uppsala, Sweden, 1974, Almqvist & Wiksell.

Davis, K. L., Berger, P. A., and Hollister, L. E.: Choline for tardive dyskinesia, N. Engl. J. Med. **293**:152, 1975.

Dempsey, G. M., et al.: Treatment of excessive weight gain in patients taking lithium, Am. J. Psychiatry **133**:1082, 1976.

Dobbing, J.: Nutrition and brain development. In Hegsted, D. M., et al.: Present knowledge of nutrition, ed. 4, New York, 1976, The Nutrition Foundation, p. 453.

Dodson, W. E., et al.: Management of seizure disorders: selected aspects, II, J. Pediatr. **89**:695, 1976.

Donnelly, M.: White House Conference on Aging, J. Am. Diet. Assoc. **60**:103, 1972.

Fernstrom, J. D.: How food affects your brain, Nutr. Action **6**:5, Dec., 1979.

Fernstrom, J. D., and Wurtman, R. J.: Nutrition and the brain, Sci. Am. **230**:84, 1974.

Freedman, A. M., Kaplan, H. I., and Sadock, B. J., editors: Comprehensive textbook of psychiatry, ed. 2, Baltimore, 1975, The Williams & Wilkins Co.

Garrett, A.: Interviewing: its principles and methods, New York, 1942, Family Service Association of America.

Halmi, K. A., Powers, P., and Cunningham, S.: Treatment of anorexia nervosa with behavior modification, Arch. Gen. Psychiatry **32**:93, 1975.

Howard, R. B., and Herbold, N. H.: Nutrition in clinical care, New York, 1978, McGraw-Hill Book Co.

Iber, F. L.: In alcoholism, the liver sets the pace, Nutr. Today **6**:2, Jan.-Feb., 1971.

Iverson, L. L.: The chemistry of the brain, Sci. Am. **241**:134, Sept., 1979.

Iverson, S. D., and Iverson, L. L.: Behavioral pharmacology, Oxford, England, 1979, Oxford University Press.

Kolata, G. B.: Brain biochemistry: effects of diet, Science **192**:41, 1976.

Lipton, M. A., and Kane, F. J., Jr.: Psychiatry. In Schneider, H. A., Anderson, C. E., and Coursin, D. B., editors: Nutritional support of medical practice, New York, 1977, Harper & Row, Publishers, p. 463.

Lucas, A. R., Duncan, J. W., and Pieus, V.: The treatment of anorexia nervosa, Am. J. Psychiatry **133**:1034, 1976.

Mereness, D., and Taylor, C. M.: Essentials of psychiatric nursing, ed. 10, St. Louis, 1978, The C. V. Mosby Co.

Norman, E. C.: Mental health consultation in nutrition, J. Am. Diet. Assoc. **63**:30, 1973.

Shaw, S., and Lieber, C. S.: Nutrition and alcoholism. In Goodhart, R. S., and Shils, M. E.: Modern nutrition in health and disease, ed. 6, Philadelphia, 1980, Lea & Febiger, p. 1220.

Singer, I., and Rotenberg, D.: Mechanisms of lithium action, N. Engl. J. Med. **289**:254, 1973.

Varda, V. A., Bartok, B. R., and Slowie, L. A.: Nutritional therapy of patients receiving lithium carbonate, J. Am. Diet. Assoc. **74**:149, Feb., 1979.

Weinberg, J.: Psychological aspects of aging, J. Am. Diet. Assoc. **60**:293, 1972.

Wurtman, R. J., and Fernstrom, J. D.: Effects of the diet on brain transmitters, Nutr. Rev. **32**:193, 1974.

part four

NUTRITION AND CLINICAL CARE

23 Principles of nutritional assessment and therapy in patient care

ROLE OF NUTRITION IN CLINICAL CARE

Persons face acute illness or chronic disease and its treatment in a variety of settings—the acute care hospital, the long-term rehabilitation center, the extended care facility, the clinic, the private care office, the home. Indeed the continuum of care may encompass all these places at different points in an individual's experience with a health problem. In all instances, however, nutritional care is fundamental, both as support for any medical treatment being given and as a primary therapy in itself. Clearly defined comprehensive nutritional assessment and appropriate nutritional therapy based on identified needs and sound clinical judgment and expertise of the nutritionist will provide an essential component for success of medical treatment, recovery from illness or injury, continuing health promotion and maintenance, and control of health care costs.

The discussion here focuses on the comprehensive care of the patient's nutritional needs in the hospital, the clinic, the office, or the home. Wherever the place of care, the principles of clinical nutrition outlined will provide the basis for planning nutritional care in any setting. Whatever the need, the practitioners, the patient, and the family work together to support the healing process and promote health through responsible, informed self-care by the patient. In this team effort the nutritionist or clinical dietitian, as the clinical nutrition specialist, carries the primary responsibility with the patient and the physician for nutritional care. The nurse and other practitioners participate in team support as needed.

THE HOSPITALIZED OR AMBULATORY PATIENT—FACTORS IN CARE

The basis of care given all patients is the need each individual presents in the course of illness and its medical treatment. In her excellent book *Newer Dimensions of Patient Care*[1] Brown has stressed the positive concepts that the environment of the general hospital or medical center *can* be therapeutic, that staff motivation and competence *can* be improved, and—most important of all—that *patients are people,* by which she does not mean the idea of "collective people" but rather the very human dimension of *individual persons.* Sometimes in the idealistic and diffuse "service to humanity" notions, health team members may forget that *individual persons* are cared for, one at a time, and that each one is unique. Thus to give good patient care they need to understand factors at work in the patient and in the hospital setting that influence reactions. On this basis they may be able to identify personal health needs and plan individual care to meet these needs.

The patient

From a personal perspective the uninitiated patient in the hospital milieu often faces a formidable environment. Illness and anxieties create psychologic tensions, and various coping mechanisms result. Also the patient brings to the experience personal socioeconomic and cultural molding and, in whatever nature and degree they may have been developed, spiritual resources. Each is a *whole* person. Physical, physiologic and biochemical, psychologic, social and economic, and cultural factors are part of the whole and need to be considered in the total care of the patient.

Physical factors

One of the physician's first acts is to examine the patient physically and conduct a medical workup. This is an imperative initial step in planning medical care. Likewise the clinical nutritionist/dietitian must collect and assess all data pertinent to nutritional status and needs and use them as a basis for making nutritional diagnoses and planning valid nutritional therapy. Careful clinical observations of physical details such as age, sex, general physical condition, and presence and degree of signs and symptoms of illness will aid the skilled nutritionist making sound nutritional care decisions with the patient and the family.

The clinical nutritionist/dietitian especially must *know* the patient as a person if relevant and valid nutritional care is to be planned. Evidence of an appalling amount of hospital-iatrogenic malnutrition in general hospital and in long-term care facilities has been brought out in several surveys.[2-7] As newly nutrition-conscious physicians, nurses, and other health team members are aware, this all-too-prevalent health problem has serious professional and legal implications.

Awareness of this problem of present and potential malnutrition with its costs and threat to health has led to current professional concern reflected in regulations for hospital accreditation. The consistent practice of nutrition assessment for hospital as well as clinic patients is needed, with follow-up nutritional care and documentation in every case. These are vital responsibilities of the clinical nutritionist.

Psychologic factors

The stress an individual faces causes him to use the various mental mechanisms developed during the growing years in an attempt to relieve tension. These mechanisms are often the only means of making a painful situation psychologically tolerable.

Depression. Responses may vary from a quiet downheartedness, feelings of general pessimism, inadequacy, and discouragement, to hopeless despair. The patient is quiet, restrained, and inhibited.

Repression. The patient may completely repress painful aspects of the environment, pushing them out of conscious awareness. They remain within, however, and may manifest their influence in various personality traits.

Suppression. Undesired strivings not possible in the present situation may be suppressed by the patient on a more conscious level, only to have them come out later, perhaps in a different form of behavior.

Identification. The patient may find support through identifying with persons or associations in the environment. He may *transfer* a past role image to the nurse, for example, his mother; or he may be able to project his feelings as warmth and empathy for another patient; or he may *introject* (direct to himself) aspects of another person's personality.

Reaction-formation. Sometimes inappropriate perfectionistic or rigid responses may be observed. These may be reactions formed as opposites of the natural desire in the circumstance.

Compensation. Inadequacies or inabilities in one area may lead to compensating developments in another. This is often observed in patients with physical disabilities, for example, who have developed other capacities in remarkable ways. In some cases the loss of prestige and self-esteem that often accompanies the indignities of the patient role will lead a patient to compensate with boastings or constant commands for attention.

Rationalization. Perhaps more operative in everyone is the mental mechanism of rationalizing to prevent guilt feelings or loss of self-respect. It is the well-known "sour grapes" response. After first responding to something without clear motives, a person then offers "reasons" for his act, presentable and reasonable motives to excuse his behavior. These usually have a portion of truth in them and are hence admissible to his conscience. Such rationalization often serves a useful protective function to the psyche and gives comfort.

Substitution. To combat frustration, if one desired goal is not obtainable, the patient may substitute an alternative gratification. Sometimes it does not necessitate a changed goal but a different means of achieving it.

Displacement. Sometimes a deeper anxiety is handled by transferring the emotional feeling from its real object to a substitute object. This may take the form of phobias, such as that associated with extreme cleanliness in constant hand washing, or of symbolization. Food sometimes serves as such a symbol, and the patient may use it as his language of communication.

Projection. A common defense mechanism is a person's attributing to others traits in himself that he dislikes. A person's severe criticism of another's weak points may indicate the presence of these very weaknesses in himself.

Withdrawal. If the situation remains unresolved and too stressful, the patient may withdraw. Mild withdrawal protects one's resources but can develop to undesirable extremes and prevent the healthy involvement of the patient in his own recovery.

Social and economic factors

Family. Persons live in families, be they near or far or no longer present. These family relationships, derived or present, directly influence the patient's development and his present living situation.

Group memberships. Memberships in various community group situations outside the family also influence a patient's responses or provide supportive group resources for him. These groups may be businesses or professional, volunteer service groups, social, civic, or religious groups.

Occupation. Occupational roles in society develop related behavior patterns. One's occupation also determines a person's social class status and income level (pp. 273-274).

Financial resources. Direct pressures may result from anxieties concerning the high cost of medical care and limited personal financial resources to pay the bills. Often help may be worked out for some source of financial assistance through consultation with the social workers on the hospital staff.

Housing. The patient's living situation may have been a factor in his illness. It may still offer problems in planning his continuing care.

Cultural factors

A person is a direct product of his culture, ethnic and religious, and bears the imprint of its values, attitudes, and behaviors. Within the broad culture there are also significant influential subculture groups (p. 273).

The hospital or clinic setting

The hospital or clinic setting itself imposes other limiting factors on the patient. Often he is no longer a person; he is a case. If he is hospitalized, no matter what his illness, he is immediately bedbound, and stripped of clothing and other personal identification, and all rights of decision or independent action are removed. Even such a homely and necessary task as going to the toilet is listed on his chart as a "privilege." He is punctured, plumbed, and palpated with innumerable, fearsome-looking gadgets and machines, with little or no explanation of what is happening. Or he is repeatedly given lectures as if he has no knowledge at all.

The often complicated structure of the modern community hospital and extended outpatient clinics, especially in larger cities, bewilders and confuses many patients. It is both a medical complex devoting its energies and resources to healing and at the same time a large social community with many overt and subtle networks of relationships.

Complex medical center. Many departments contribute specialized medical and allied services. Numerous medical specialty groups work with laboratory, X-ray, nursing service, dietary, social service, pharmacy, publications, medical records, library, and other groups. Also, necessary departments to carry on the day-to-day business of the medical center include accounting, reception, maintenance, central supply, purchasing, housekeeping, and many others. During hospitalization a representative procession of these persons file in and out of the patient's room with a confusing and often conflicting array of requests and a denial of privacy. Through a labyrinth of corridors, doorways, and elevators he may be wheeled or escorted by or to these various hospital staff members for vague and undefined purposes.

The hospital or clinic hierarchy. Among the many groups of persons comprising the medical center's staff and personnel there are numerous intrarelationships and interrelationships. Sometimes the patient may find himself caught in the middle of conflicts between these groups, and his interests suffer. A distinct hospital hierarchy assigns status rights and privileges, eating areas, use of facilities, with an infinite number of admission symbols ranging from the dangling stethoscope to the enveloping gown or lab coat. In his popular book *Games People Play* psychiatrist Eric Berne describes many of the common human patterns in social relationships, maneuvers, and manipulations. Stein[8] sees the easily recognizable flow of communication between physicians and nurses as the "doctor-nurse game." This is perhaps a necessary relationship played by both to preserve the physician's psychic strength for the responsibility he carries for the patient's life.

That such forces do operate in many complex medical center communities is evident by what Brown calls "competing chain of command" between medical and hospital administrations.[1] Increasingly, however, positive changes are being made. Cooperative group efforts are helping to meet personal needs of the staff for recognition and a sense of accomplishment and at the same time provide for the patient the high quality of care he must have.

The health team. One such positive change is the increasing use of the health team in the various aspects of the patient's care. This approach, described in previous chapters, recognizes the unique contribution of special skills and knowledge and the value to the patient and to the health workers of a team effort. In the care of the patient, key persons related to his day-to-day welfare include the physician, the nurse, the dietitian, the social worker, and in many places the hospital chaplain, who is specially trained in pastoral counseling. Provision in many medical centers for such a significant new health team member indicates the close relationship of human spiritual needs to mental health and to physical health. Public health workshops for representatives from both groups —mental health and religion—are being held in many centers to discuss common areas of patients' needs to which both may contribute insights and resources.

Many other administrative level conferences and other small group sessions are being organized in many hospitals to facilitate communication between these groups and improve patient care (Fig. 23-1).

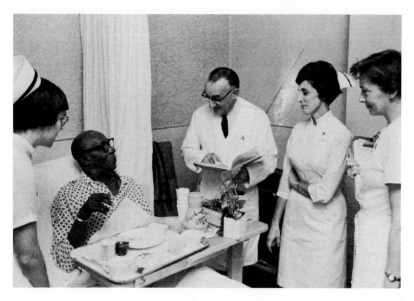

Fig. 23-1. The health team on ward rounds. Here the physician, nurse, dietitian, and student nurse confer with a patient recovering from a coronary occlusion.

NUTRITIONAL ASSESSMENT
Patient's health needs—nutritional assessment and diagnosis

In the setting provided by the individual medical center, with its strengths and despite its shortcomings, the nutritionist or clinical dietitian must care for the patient's nutritional needs in relation to medical and nursing care. The diagnosis of the patient's nutritional care needs will be the nutritionist's initial responsibility. A broad base of related information about the patient's nutritional status, food habits, and life situation provides the data necessary for making valid initial assessments. Useful background knowledge may come from a variety of sources such as the patient, the patient's chart, the family or other relatives or friends, oral or written communication with other hospital personnel or surrounding staff, and related research. Thus the basic dictum in nutritional practice, too often overlooked in routine procedures, is evident: to be valid, nutritional care must be person centered, based on initial and continuing identified needs, and updated constantly with the patient.

Continuity of care spectrum

The concept of continuity of care therefore becomes fundamental to providing successful therapy and avoiding the fragmentation of services that too often results in large complex medical centers. A helpful approach is to view the patient in terms of past experiences, present situation, and probable future course or plans. The following outline may be used in this approach as a guide:

I. Influence of past experience on present needs (Interviewing is an important communicative skill in patient care [Fig. 23-2]. Here the skill is history-taking to obtain needed information relevant to the patient's care.)
   A. Social history: general socioeconomic and cultural background (family, living situation, occupations, and any other important individual information)
   B. Medical history: previous illnesses, surgery,

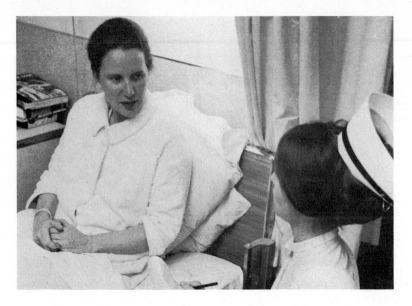

Fig. 23-2. Interviewing of patient to plan personal care.

reactions (including drug sensitivities), hospitalization, treatments
C. Nutrition history and analysis: general diet habits, marketing and cooking methods, food behavior, likes, dislikes, food meanings; typical day's food intake, and analysis of nutritional status (Review the discussion in Chapter 15 to provide background materials for nutrition history and analysis.)
II. Present needs
A. General needs of hospitalized patients
  1. Physical safety and comfort needs
  2. Basic physiologic needs
     a. Nutrition (including water and electrolytes)
     b. Hygiene: cleanliness, elimination
     c. Rest, sleep
     d. Exercise, body mechanics
  3. Basic psychosocial needs
     a. Minimum stress: nonthreatening environment
     b. Effective communication, meaning
     c. Integrity, fulfillment
B. Patient care needs of present illness (classic picture and individual patient response)
  1. Nature of the illness and its effect on the body, clinical signs and symptoms
  2. Tests, treatments, and medications; patient responses
  3. Diet therapy: specific order, rationale for each principle, and foods affected; meals planned (selected menu), mode of food service and any needs for eating aids; patient response
III. Future needs for continuing patient care
A. The plan of continuing medical care
B. Care facilities: home, relative, nursing home
C. If indicated, a person responsible for care, to discuss the patient's care plans: family member, visiting nurse, home aide

An additional summary guide for assessment and care of nutritional needs to assure comprehensive continuity of patient care is provided in Tool A.

Methods of nutrition assessment

The basic methods used in clinical nutrition assessment may be categorized in four groups: anthropometric measures, biochemical tests, clinical observations, and dietary evaluations including diet-drug interactions. The basic methods have been called by some practitioners

TOOL A

Guide for assessment and care of nutrition needs*

I. Assess nutrition needs
  A. The person
    1. Who he is: age, sex, family occupational role, culture, socioeconomic status, personal characteristics, limitations, strengths
    2. Where he is: physical setting—place of care, its possibilities and limitations; personal setting—mental, psychologic, emotional, and physical, in relation to health or disease, adaptation
    3. His nutritional status: food habits and general nutritional analysis (pp. 316-318), clinical observations and signs (Table 23-3)
  B. The disease or normal physiologic stress (such as pregnancy and growth)
    1. The general disease or physiologic process: anatomy and physiology, signs and symptoms, general treatment or management, pathology, course, prognosis
    2. Patient's unique experience with the disease or physiologic stress: duration, intensity, medical management, prior diet therapy, adaptation, problems and solutions, knowledge of disease and its care—source, form, attitude, behavior response
II. Identify and define problems and develop plan of care
  A. Explore present needs
    1. Day-to-day nutritional support: maintenance, optimum intake, basic nutritional requirements
    2. Nutritional therapy: treatment by modified diet
    3. Teaching: basic nutrition knowledge or principles of special diet modifications
  B. Explore future needs
    1. Continuity of care: home, responsible significant others, extended-care facility
    2. Plan for medical management: health team conferences, nursing team conferences
    3. Plan for nutritional care: diet modifications, practical food management (family situation, living alone, degree of disability, etc.), follow-up diet counseling and nutrition education, community resources
III. Carry out plan of care
  A. Physical, psychosocial responses: diet and its meaning
  B. Teaching plan: materials needed, content, sequence, methods, approaches, plan for evaluation
  C. Records of action for study
IV. Check results
  A. Follow-up care: planned with patient, family, and health team
  B. Reinforcement to strengthen learning
  C. Revision: as needed

*Williams, S. R.: Essentials of nutrition and diet therapy, ed. 2, St. Louis, 1978, The C. V. Mosby Co.

the "ABCD's of nutrition assessment" to indicate their fundamental role in determining nutritional needs and planning patient/client care. Although a broad number of tests may be used for research purposes in a large facility with access to highly sophisticated equipment, the procedures outlined below provide a good base in general clinical practice for assessing and monitoring a patient's nutritional status and planning nutritional therapy, maintenance, and rehabilitation.

Anthropometric measures. Skill gained through careful practice is necessary to minimize the margin of error in making body measurements. A recent survey conducted by the Center for Disease Control of the U.S. Department of Health, Education, and Welfare indicated that errors result from inaccurate instruments, poor technique, or inaccurate readings and recording of data.[9] Thus selection and maintenance of proper equipment and attention to careful technique are essential to securing valid data.

The basic anthropometric measures used in general clinical practice are weight, height, mid-upper-arm circumference, triceps skinfold thickness, and the derived value for mid-upper-arm muscle circumference. The subscapula skinfold thickness is sometimes measured also. These data provide an assessment of skeletal muscle mass, a major protein compartment of the body:

1. *Weight.* It is necessary to use regular clinic beam scales with nondetachable weights. An additional weight attachment is available for weighing very obese persons. Metric scales with readings to the nearest 20 g provide more specific data. All scales should be checked frequently and calibrated at three- to four-month intervals for continued accuracy. Hospitalized patients should be weighed at consistent times, for example, before breakfast after the bladder has been emptied. Clinic patients should be weighed without shoes in light indoor clothing or examining gown.

After careful reading and recording of the patient's weight, obtain information about the usual body weight and check standards for ideal body weight. Interpret present weight in terms of percent of usual and ideal body weight. Check for any significant weight loss: 1% to 2% in past week, 5% over past month, 7.5% during previous three months, or 10% in past six months. These amounts of weight loss are significant; more than this rate of loss can be severe. Values charted in the patient's record should indicate percent of weight change.

2. *Height.* If possible use a fixed measuring stick or tape on a true vertical flat wall or a rigid, free-standing instrument with a movable block squared at a true right angle against the vertical flat surface that can be moved down to the exact crown of the patient's head. If this device is not available, the movable measuring rod on the platform clinic scales may be used with reasonable accuracy. The patient should stand as straight as possible, without shoes or cap, heels together, looking straight ahead. The heels, buttocks, shoulders, and head should be touching the wall or vertical surface of the measuring rod. Read the measure carefully and compare with previous recordings to detect possible errors or to note growth of children. Metric measures of height in centimeters provide more accurate data.

3. *Mid-upper-arm circumference.* Use a centimeter tape made of nonstretchable material such as metal, plastic, or fiberglass, not cloth or paper. On the nondominant arm, locate the midpoint of the upper arm: (1) have patient bend arm at the elbow, 90-degree angle with palm up, (2) place tape vertically on posterior side of arm, (3) mark arm midpoint between the acromial process of the scapula (bony protrusion on posterior of upper shoulder) and the olecranon process of the elbow (bony part of the elbow). Measure upper-arm circumference at this midpoint, securing tape snugly but not so tightly as to make indentation. Read and record measure accurately to the nearest tenth

Table 23-1. Ideal weight and urinary creatinine values for height (adults)*

Height (cm)	Females		Males	
	Weight (kg)	Creatinine (mg)	Weight (kg)	Creatinine (mg)
140	44.9			
141	45.4			
142	45.9			
143	46.4			
144	47.0			
145	47.5		51.9	
146	48.0		52.4	
147	48.6	828	52.9	
148	49.2		53.5	
149	49.8		54.0	
150	50.4	852	54.5	
151	51.0		55.0	
152	51.5		55.6	
153	52.0	878	56.1	
154	52.5		56.6	
155	53.1	901	57.2	
156	53.7		57.9	
157	54.3	922	58.6	1,284
158	54.9		59.3	
159	55.5		59.9	
160	56.2	949	60.5	1,325
161	56.9		61.1	
162	57.6		61.7	
163	58.3	979	62.3	1,362
164	58.9		62.9	
165	59.5	1,005	63.5	1,387
166	60.1		64.0	
167	60.7	1,040	64.6	1,421
168	61.4		65.2	
169	62.1		65.9	
170		1,075	66.6	1,465
171			67.3	
172			68.0	
173		1,111	68.7	1,516
174			69.4	
175		1,139	70.1	1,552
176			70.8	
177		1,169	71.6	1,589
178			72.4	
179			73.3	
180		1,204	74.2	1,639
181			75.0	
182			75.8	
183		1,241	76.5	1,692
184			77.3	
185			78.1	1,735
186			78.9	
187				1,776
188				
189				
190				1,826

*1959 Metropolitan Life Insurance Company Standards corrected for nude weight without shoe heels. Data from Jelliffe, D. B.: The assessment of the nutritional status of the community, Geneva, 1966, World Health Organization.

of a centimeter, comparing with previous measurements to note possible changes.

4. *Triceps skinfold thickness*. This measure provides an estimate of subcutaneous fat reserves and together with the midarm circumference at the same spot enables the practitioner to make a good estimate of the midarm muscle circumference as an indicator of the status of the skeletal muscle mass protein compartment. Use a standard millimeter skinfold caliper such as the Lange, Harpenden, or Holtain. If possible have patient stand with nondominant arm previously measured hanging loosely. Use thumb and forefinger to grasp a vertical pinch of the patient's skin and subcutaneous fat about 1 to 2 cm above the previously marked mid-upper-arm point. Pull the skinfold gently away from the underlying muscle. Place the caliper jaws over the lifted skinfold at the midpoint mark while maintaining the skinfold grasp. Read the measure of the compressed skinfold to the nearest full or fraction of a millimeter within 2 to 3 seconds after releasing the caliper extender. Avoid excessive pressure or delayed reading. For increased accuracy take three measures and use the mean for calculations. Record results and compare mean value with previous measures to note changes.

5. *Subscapula skinfold thickness*. If the subscapula skinfold is also measured, use the left side of the body. Locate the subscapula site just below the angle of the scapula and gently grasp a skinfold as before. Place the caliper jaws on a downward and lateral axis. Read and record the measure in the same manner described for the triceps measure.

6. *Mid-upper-arm muscle circumference*. This derived value gives an indirect measure of the body's skeletal muscle mass. First convert the triceps skinfold (TSF) mean value (millimeters) to centimeters (divide millimeter value by 10), then calculate the midarm muscle circumference (MAMC) by the following formula:

$$MAMC\,(cm) = MAC\,(cm) - 3.14 \times TSF\,(cm)$$

(If desired, the TSF can be left in millimeters as measured and the value of the π factor in the formula changed to 0.314.)

Interpretation of these anthropometric measures for monitoring of the patient's nutritional status is made by comparison of results as percent of standards provided in reference tables, such as those based on the classic international nutrition work of Jelliffe[10] or more recently developed American standards such as those by Frisancho.[11] Some examples of these standards are given in Tables 23-1 and 23-2.

Biochemical tests. A number of biochemical tests are available for studying nutritional status. Of these the most commonly used tests for assessing and monitoring nutritional status and planning nutritional therapy in clinical practice are the ones listed below. Results of laboratory data should always be interpreted by the standards for normal values established by the individual laboratory and its methods used. General ranges for normal values are given in standard texts. (Examples are given in Appendixes J and K.)

1. *Measures of plasma protein compartment*
   a. Basic: serum albumin, hemoglobin, hematocrit
   b. Additional: serum transferrin (or total

Table 23-2. Standards for anthropometric measures*

	Male	Female
Arm circumference (cm)	29.3	28.5
Triceps skinfold (mm)	12.5	16.5
Arm muscle circumference (cm)	25.3	23.2

*Data from Jelliffe, D. B.: The assessment of the nutritional status of the community, Geneva, 1966, World Health Organization.

iron-binding capacity [TIBC]); following is formula for deriving either value:

$$\text{Transferrin} = (0.8 \times \text{TIBC}) - 43$$

2. *Measures of immune system integrity, anergy*
   a. Basic: lymphocytes
   b. Additional: skin testing, delayed sensitivity to common recall antigens such as mumps, *Candida*, PPD, SK/SD. Skin tests are read at 24 and 48 hours, with greater than 5 mm considered positive and the presence of one positive test indicating intact immunity
3. *Measures of protein metabolism: 24-hour urine tests*

Table 23-3. Clinical signs of nutritional status*

Body area	Signs of good nutrition	Signs of poor nutrition
General appearance	Alert, responsive	Listless, apathetic, cachexic
Weight	Normal for height, age, body build	Overweight or underweight (special concern for underweight)
Posture	Erect, arms and legs straight	Sagging shoulders, sunken chest, humped back
Muscles	Well developed, firm, good tone, some fat under skin	Flaccid, poor tone, undeveloped, tender, "wasted" appearance, cannot walk properly
Nervous control	Good attention span, not irritable or restless, normal reflexes, psychological stability	Inattentive, irritable, confused, burning and tingling of hands and feet (paresthesia), loss of position and vibratory sense, weakness and tenderness of muscles (may result in inability to walk), decrease or loss of ankle and knee reflexes
Gastrointestinal function	Good appetite and digestion, normal regular elimination, no palpable organs or masses	Anorexia, indigestion, constipation or diarrhea, liver or spleen enlargement
Cardiovascular function	Normal heart rate and rhythm, no murmurs, normal blood pressure for age	Rapid heart rate (above 100 beats per minute tachycardia), enlarged heart, abnormal rhythm, elevated blood pressure
General vitality	Endurance, energetic, sleeps well, vigorous	Easily fatigued, no energy, falls asleep easily, looks tired, apathetic
Hair	Shiny, lustrous, firm, not easily plucked, healthy scalp	Stringy, dull, brittle, dry, thin and sparse, depigmented, can be easily plucked
Skin (general)	Smooth, slightly moist, good color	Rough, dry, scaly, pale, pigmented, irritated, bruises, petechiae
Face and neck	Skin color uniform, smooth, pink, healthy appearance, not swollen	Greasy, discolored, scaly, swollen, skin dark over cheeks and under eyes, lumpiness or flakiness of skin around nose and mouth
Lips	Smooth, good color, moist, not chapped or swollen	Dry, scaly, swollen, redness and swelling (cheilosis), or angular lesions at corners of the mouth or fissures or scars (stomatitis)

*Williams, S. R.: Nutritional guidance in prenatal care. In Worthington-Roberts, B., Vermeesch, J., and Williams, S. R.: Nutrition in pregnancy and lactation, St. Louis, 1981, The C. V. Mosby Co.

Continued.

Table 23-3. Clinical signs of nutritional status—cont'd

Body area	Signs of good nutrition	Signs of poor nutrition
Mouth, oral membranes	Reddish pink mucous membranes in oral cavity	Swollen, boggy oral mucous membranes
Gums	Good pink color, healthy, red, no swelling or bleeding	Spongy, bleed easily, marginal redness, inflamed, gums receding
Tongue	Good pink color or deep reddish in appearance, not swollen or smooth, surface papillae present, no lesion	Swelling, scarlet and raw, magenta color, beefy (glossitis), hyperemic and hypertrophic papillae, atrophic papillae
Teeth	No cavities, no pain, bright, straight, no crowding, well-shaped jaw, clean, no discoloration	Unfilled caries, absent teeth, worn surfaces, mottled (fluorosis), malpositioned
Eyes	Bright, clear, shiny, no sores at corner of eyelids, membranes moist and healthy pink color, no no prominent blood vessels or mount of tissue or sclera, no fatigue circles beneath	Eye membranes pale (pale conjunctivas), redness of membrane (conjunctival injection), dryness, signs of infection. Bitot's spots, redness and fissuring of eyelid corners (angular palpebritis), dryness of eye membrane (conjunctival xerosis), dull appearance of cornea (corneal xerosis), soft cornea (keratomalacia)
Neck (glands)	No enlargement	Thyroid enlarged
Nails	Firm, pink	Spoon shape (koilonychia), brittle, ridged
Legs, feet	No tenderness, weakness, or swelling; good color	Edema, tender calf, tingling, weakness
Skeleton	No malformations	Bowlegs, knock-knees, chest deformity at diaphragm, beaded ribs, prominent scapulas

a. Urinary creatinine: total 24-hour excretion interpreted in terms of ideal creatinine excretion for height, the creatinine-height index (CHI). Standard values are given in Table 23-1.

b. Urinary urea nitrogen: total 24-hour nitrogen excretion is used with calculated dietary nitrogen intake over same 24-hour period to determine the patient's nitrogen balance:

$$\text{Nitrogen balance} = \frac{\text{Protein intake}}{6.25} - (\text{Urinary urea nitrogen} + 4)$$

(The formula factor of 4 represents additional nitrogen loss through feces and skin.)

Clinical observations. Careful attention to physical signs of possible malnutrition provide an added dimension to the overall assessment of general nutritional status. A description of such signs is given in Table 23-3. Make a careful descriptive record of any such observations in the patient's medical record. Other physical data may include pulse rate, respiration, temperature, blood pressure. A study of the common procedures of a normal physical examination will provide useful background orientation.

Diet evaluation. A careful nutrition history is a fundamental component of nutrition assessment. In the nutrition assessment procedures outlined here the patient's diet evaluation will take two basic forms:

1. *Specific 24-hour food record.* During the

Nutrition history: activity-associated general day's food pattern*

Name _____ Date _____

Height _____ Weight (lb) _____ (kg) _____ Age _____

Ideal weight _____

Referral
Diagnosis
Diet order
Members of household
Occupation
Recreation, physical activity
Present food intake

	Place	Hour	Frequency, form, and amount checklist
Breakfast			Milk
			Cheese
			Meat
			Fish
Noon meal			Poultry
			Eggs
			Cream
			Butter, margarine
			Other fats
Evening meal			Vegetables, green
			Vegetables, other
			Fruits (citrus)
			Legumes
Extra meals			Potato
			Bread—kind
			Sugar
			Desserts
Summary			Beverages
			Alcohol
			Vitamins
			Candy

*Williams, S. R.: Essentials of nutrition and diet therapy, ed. 2, St. Louis, 1978, The C. V. Mosby Co.

TOOL B
Stages of nutrition interview*

I. The patient as a person
  A. Introduction
    1. Developing a relationship   Establishing rapport; putting the patient at ease; gaining the patient's confidence and trust; mutual trust
    2. Defining roles   Selling health worker's role as helper, health counselor, teacher; determining patient's role as learner and active participant in taking increasing responsibility for own learning and care according to individual capacity
    3. Determining the patient's health need or problem and related personal goals   Discovering whether the patient's goals are different than expected; deciding whether underlying objectives exist other than those concerning the immediate dietary problem
    4. Redefining objectives in light of patient's goals   Seeing counseling goals in terms of those of patient
  B. Patient profile   Who and what kind of person is the patient?
    1. Gathering physical data
      a. Age   How do these affect the health problem? How long has the problem existed? Has the patient known anyone with a similar problem?
      b. Height
      c. Weight—present and past history
      d. Experience with disease or weight problem
    2. Understanding the patient's setting   The patient's environment: social and economic factors involved
      a. Family   Identity of family (ethnic); number in family; who cooks, markets, etc.
      b. Work   Hours; extent of activity; effect on eating habits; education
      c. Social activity   Recreation: physical exercise
    3. Interpreting the patient's attitudes toward his disease or weight problem   How has the patient's experience with the problem influenced his belief about it? Have family members or friends influenced him? Fears, misconceptions, understanding

II. The patient's food habits
  A. Nutrition history
    1. Determining present food intake   What does the patient usually eat? Flavorings, seasonings, condiments, beverages, other relevant additions
    2. Learning place and time   Where and when does the patient eat? How do these affect what he eats? Can any times or places be changed or eliminated?

*Williams, S. R.: Essentials of nutrition and diet therapy, ed. 2, St. Louis, 1978, The C. V. Mosby Co.

TOOL B
Stages of nutrition interview—cont'd

3. Referring to checklist of various food groups and some individual foods	Keeping some form of reminder for the counselor to make sure that relevant foods have been covered
4. Determining who prepares the food and how	Possible consultation with the wife or mother
B. Physical exercise and recreation: activities associated with the patient's food habits	Work, school, social gatherings, travel
C. Food reactions: patient's likes, dislikes, intolerances, allergies	Could food be accepted in a different form or using another method of preparation? Possible substitutes?
III. Diet counseling	
A. Choosing the diet	What is the diet indicated by the health problem and outlined by the nutritionist? What form will be best understood by the patient?
B. Explaining the reasons for the diet	Why the increases in certain foods or restrictions on others; the effect of the disease on food; the effect of food on the disease
C. Planning a daily food pattern with the patient	Considering the patient's likes and dislikes, usual habits, and the restrictions because of the health problem; developing a dietary plan that fits into daily activities
D. Reviewing the diet and answering questions	Answering inquiries throughout interview but asking specifically for questions or feedback toward the end Does the patient understand?
IV. Termination of the interview	
A. Planning for follow-up	When will the patient be seen again? Encouraging him to record questions or problems that may develop to discuss next time
B. Recording the interview	Completing any needed charting of the interview Keeping any needed notes in records

24-hour period of urine collection for the creatinine and urea nitrogen excretion tests a specific and detailed record of all food intake by the patient is essential for determining total protein and energy values of the diet. The protein value is used in calculation of the nitrogen balance by the formula given above. The caloric value will give an indication of how well goals for energy input are being met. These goals are based on the energy expenditure demands of the patient's illness or health maintenance requirements.

2. Diet history. Knowledge of the patient's basic eating habits is necessary to determine possible nutritional deficiencies. In conjunction with the patient's living situation and related food attitudes and values, medical status, and treatment the diet history provides an essential base for personal nutrition counseling and planning care. The activity-associated day's food intake pattern given on p. 316 may guide the practitioner in obtaining a valid picture of food habits and eating behaviors. Tool B provides an outline to guide and analyze the nutrition interview.

In addition to food and nutrition information the practitioner must obtain drug therapy data from the medical record and the patient to determine any possible drug-nutrient interactions involved or teaching needed by the patient. A good updated pharmacology reference is a necessary tool for the clinical nutritionist or dietitian, as for all clinical practitioners.[12-14]

The patient's health care—a personal care plan

Communication skills. On the basis of data gathered and analyzed through the nutrition assessment procedures and knowledge of specific care relative to present illness and general needs, the nutritionist will determine an individually adapted personal care plan for the patient. It will need to be flexible. Results must be checked from day to day, even hour to hour during critical care, and the plan reevaluated according to need. Involvement of the patient in the plan is essential. Communication skills in interviewing and alert observation are vital parts of good patient care.

Points to consider. Generally therefore the valid patient-centered care plan will consider these points:

1. Identified needs
2. Goals related to specific needs
3. Relevant background knowledge
4. Related valid patient-centered care activity
5. Results

Nutritional needs will be a fundamental part of the total plan of care. They will be found as identified needs through careful comprehensive nutrition assessment. Priority of goals in relation to identified needs will be established with the patient. Related background knowledge will be based on the nutritionist's comprehensive command of nutritional sciences and clinical dietetics. The related patient care activities will involve nutrition assessment as needed using

methods described, planning comprehensive patient care and education, and following through with the patient and family to determine future care needs. In clinical conferences with the teaching dietitian or the clinical nutrition specialist and the physician these activities will be clarified and enlarged.

The patient's health care record— problem-oriented medical record by the health care team

Philosophy. The problem-oriented medical record (POMR), pioneered by Lawrence Weed[15] in his clinical practice and teaching at Cleveland Metropolitan General Hospital, incorporates a fundamental humanistic philosophy of personal patient care. As in any area of human behavior or practices, basic belief systems and attitudes determine actions. It is small wonder, therefore, that in the history of such personal activities as medical, nursing, and nutrition therapies in health care, widely varying and often incomplete or invalid practices have appeared. In many instances, impersonal and less-than-ideal care has resulted, frustrating many patients and practitioners alike. However, the POMR approach helps health care providers, especially in primary care, to recognize and apply two basic and profound philosophic positions concerning (1) the role of the patient and (2) the roles of the health care providers as a team.

ROLE OF THE PATIENT. By focusing on identified needs and problems of the patient in an organized fashion, health care workers are forced to acknowledge two facts: (1) it is the patient's health and welfare that is central, not that of any practitioner providing care, and (2) the ultimate decisions about his health and options for its care will be made by the patient himself or his family, not by the health care providers. Therefore client- or patient-centered care becomes paramount. It is the only valid care and so must include the patient's attitudes, perceptions, health practices, life style, socioeconomic-cultural-family background, education, and occupation.

ROLES OF THE HEALTH CARE PROVIDERS AS A TEAM. With the use of the problem-oriented record and its focus on clearly identified, specific, individual, patient care needs, the responsibilities of the primary care team—physician, nurse, nutritionist/dietitian—emerge. There is participation on the team of other specialists, such as social worker, pharmacist, or health educator as needed.

In essence the problem-oriented record represents a rather profound change in philosophy of health care, more so than was realized at its advent. It helps to deliver the individual patient's records, and hence his care, from the mystical realm of ''a private sanctum for the physician with a rigid caste system imposed upon others who might make entries''[16] to a far more valid and dynamic vehicle that helps to ensure quality care for all patients by recognizing all the patient's problems all the time and by coordinating the activities of all the health team members in personalized care.[17]

Procedures. At the initiation of either hospital or clinic care, procedures for establishing a problem-oriented medical record include the collection of a data base, the construction of a complete problem list with the initial plans for each problem, and the use of a continuing care structure for progress notes.

DATA BASE. A comprehensive data base is collected from the existing record to date by chart review (if the POMR system is being established for the first time) and by introductory information from the following sources: admission or registration data such as name, age, sex, race, referral source, patient's perception of purpose of visit or admission (chief complaint), place patient will receive primary care; and a brief patient profile from various histories taken at the time of visit or admission initiating current care. These important data include that obtained from histories such as family-marital-social, occupation-education, living situation,

financial status or health insurance coverages or assistance programs, and future plans. These data come from medical history, physical examination, laboratory tests, and nutrition history.

INITIAL COMPLETE PROBLEM LIST AND PLANS FOR EACH PROBLEM. On the basis of the data base collected a complete problem list is constructed with initial plans for each identified problem.

PROBLEM LIST. Individual problems may be identified according to several general categories:

1. *Established problems*—any identified problem (medical, nutritional, nursing, psychosocial, behavioral, economic, environmental) that concerns the patient or his health care providers and for which an initial plan will be written.

2. *Temporary problems*—any acute, short-term problems that have predictable resolutions without a major change in the ongoing therapy program (for example, an upper respiratory infection).

3. *Status-post problems*—any problems resolved prior to creation of the established problems list but that have left some anatomic, metabolic, or environmental change of concern to the patient or practitioner (for example, a postgastrectomy state).

3. *Allergy, sensitivity, intolerance problems*—problems involving various allergies, intolerances, or agent interactions (for example, lactose intolerance, specific food allergies, drug allergies, nutrient and drug interactions). It is obviously imperative that all health care providers on the team have easy access to drug, immunization, nutrition, and diet histories.

5. *Drug and diet problems*—any problems related to prior and current drug and diet therapy, including record of date on and off drug or diet and the specific purpose of each therapy with related patient responses.

PLANS FOR EACH PROBLEM. The initial plans for each problem will be constructed according to three specific areas of patient need:

1. *Diagnosis*—name of the problem with specific definition.
2. *Therapy*—specific treatment plans, including various aspects, such as medical, nursing, nutritional care, outlined by each respective specialist.
3. *Patient education*—careful inclusion of discussion, explanation, and educational activities concerning diagnosis and treatment plan to be conducted with patient or family.

CONTINUING CARE STRUCTURE. Following the establishment of a comprehensive data base as indicated, with construction of a related initial, complete, problem list with initial plans for each problem, the continuing care record will include two important ongoing activities: (1) keeping the problem list current and (2) charting progress notes according to a problem-related format (SOAP):

1. *Current problem list.* It is particularly vital that the problem list be contemporary. As the patient's care progresses, the problem list is maintained in an accurate, complete, and up-to-date manner by adding new problems as they develop (a new number is used for each new problem in order of adding) and deleting (by marking through) problems as they are resolved giving date and manner of resolution. (A previously assigned number is not used again for a new problem). This current, complete, problem

---

TOOL C
Problem-oriented records

   I. Data base: Information gained from initial histories, observations, tests, examinations, chart review
     A. Patient profile
     B. Past and present medical history
     C. Family and social history, life situation
     D. Nutrition history
  II. Problem list: Problems identified from data base and initial care plans for each problem
     A. Problems
        1. Established problems
        2. Temporary problems
        3. Status-post problems
        4. Allergies
        5. Medications
        6. Diet, nutrition
     B. Plans for care
        1. Diagnosis—including nutritional diagnosis
        2. Therapy—nutritional, drug, etc.
        3. Patient education—nutrition education, self-care needs
 III. Progress notes: Record of continuing care according to identified problems
     A. **S**ubjective—patient's perceived needs
     B. **O**bjective—specific data from tests, history, etc.
     C. **A**ssessment—interpretation of data and identified need
     D. **P**lan—new or continuing care plans related to data and assessment

list is always kept at the front of the chart and serves as a "table of contents" with cross-reference numbering. A copy of this list can also be kept by each practitioner on the primary care team in a personal office notebook as a constant reminder.

2. *Progress notes.* Rather than having a rambling, disorganized, or biased narrative that leaves health care practitioners on the team helplessly leafing chart pages, the POMR system of continuing care progress notes uses a structured format that succinctly organizes needed information, each element of which forms the easily remembered acronym SOAP:

S*ubjective:* Any new information gained from talking with the patient, that is, his perceived pain, tolerances, feelings about his health status or care; thus charted in "report language" as patient's statements, descriptions, reports.

O*bjective:* Any specific new data obtained from laboratory or X-ray tests, performance measures, nutrition analyses, physical findings, observations of behavior, and so on.

A*ssessment:* Interpretation or significance of these new data toward understanding of the problem as defined.

P*lan:* Any continuing or new diagnostic, therapeutic, or patient education activities to be carried out in relation to data and assessment above.

With use of the problem-oriented record system, each practitioner on the health care team is accountable for quality care and the charting of specific aspects of that care pertinent to each one's specific area of expertise and professional responsibility. Health care legislation concerning quality care audit is increasingly mandating such care as accurately recorded in an organized

---

TOOL D
Worksheet for planning patient care using the POMR method

Data base	Problem list	Initial plans	Continuing care
Given data Additional data needed	Goals Priorities	Diagnosis (precise) Therapy Patient education	Current problem list Progress record (SOAP)

manner. A system such as the POMR system will help health care workers provide patient care that is comprehensive and complete rather than fragmented and episodic, responsive and responsible rather than insensitive and impersonal. Furthermore, and perhaps this is a most important ingredient in our increasingly complex and changing world, it communicates human compassion to the patient in the simple message, "I care!"

For the concerned clinical practitioner and student a number of references on problem-oriented records are given at the end of the chapter under a special heading. These may be helpful for further study and adaptation to particular practice needs and settings. A summary of the POMR approach is given in Tool C, and a worksheet for planning patient care using the POMR method is given in Tool D.

NUTRITIONAL THERAPY
Basic concepts

Normal nutrition base. The primary concept of nutritional therapy should be reviewed again as stated in the introduction to Part Four. In nutrition counseling this is an important initial fact to grasp and to impart to patients and clients. For example, it is a great source of encouragement to the mother of a newly diagnosed diabetic child that the food plan will be based on individual growth and development needs and will use regular foods. Again a therapeutic diet is but a modification of normal nutrition, modified only insofar as the specific disease in the specific individual necessitates.

The disease application. The principles of a specific therapeutic diet will be based on modifications of the nutritional components of the normal diet. These changes may include the following:

1. Nutrients—modifications in one or more of the basic nutrients (protein, carbohydrate, fat, minerals, vitamins)
2. Energy—modification in energy value (calories)

3. Texture—modification in texture or seasoning (liquid, bland, low residue, and so on)

The individual patient adaptation. A diet may be theoretically correct and contain well-balanced food plans, but if these plans are unacceptable to the patient, they will not be followed. Careful planning *with* the patient, based on an initial interview to obtain a nutrition history and knowledge of general food habits, living conditions, and related factors is necessary. Thus the diet principles may be understood and motivation secured to follow through. It will be a workable plan adapted to individual needs and desires. Individual tailoring of the diet to individual needs is imperative to successful therapy.

Routine "house" diets. A schedule of routine "house" diets is followed in hospitals for those patients not requiring a so-called special diet modification. According to general patient need and tolerance the diet ordered may be liquid (clear liquid or full liquid, milk being used on the full liquid diet), soft (no raw foods, generally bland in seasoning), and regular (a full, normal for age diet). Occasionally an interval step between soft and regular will be used—the light diet. Table 23-4 indicates the usual progression and food choices in each stage.

Role of the nurse. The nurse works closely with the nutritionist/dietitian in supporting the nutritional care of patients. Skills in consultation and referral therefore are essential. At varying times, depending on need, the nurse may serve as coordinator, interpreter, or teacher.

COORDINATOR. Nurses are best able to coordinate any special services and treatments required because of their close relationship to patients and their more constant attendance. The nurse may be the one to help schedule activities to prevent conflicts or secure needed consultation for the patient with the social worker, the dietitian, or other member of the health team.

Table 23-4. Routine hospital diets

Food groups	Clear liquid	Full liquid	Soft	Light	General
Soup	Broth, bouillon	Same, plus strained soups	Same	All	All
Cereal			Refined cooked cereals, cornflakes, rice, noodles, macaroni, spaghetti	Same	All
Bread			White bread, crackers, Melba, Zwieback	Same, plus graham and rye bread	All
Protein foods		Milk, cream, milk drinks	Same, plus eggs (not fried), mild cheese, fowl, fish, sweetbreads, tender beef, veal, lamb, liver, bacon, gravy	Same	All
Vegetables			Potatoes—baked, mashed, creamed, steamed, escalloped; tender cooked whole bland vegetables (may be strained or pureed)	Same, cooked whole bland	All
Fruit and fruit juices	Bland juices	All fruit juices	Same, plus bland cooked fruit; peaches, pears, applesauce, peeled apricots, white cherries, bananas, orange and grapefruit sections without membrane	All	All
Desserts, gelatin	Plain gelatin, fruit ices	Same, plus sherbet, ice cream, puddings, custard	Same, plus plain sponge cakes, plain cookies, plain cake, simple puddings	Same	All
Miscellaneous	Ginger ale, carbonated water, coffee tea	Same	Same, plus butter or margarine, salt, pepper	Same	All

INTERPRETER. Because of a close relationship with the patient the nurse can help reduce his tension by careful, brief, easily understood explanations to him concerning his various treatments and plan of care. This will include basic interpretation of the therapeutic diet order from the nutritionist or the physician and resulting food selections on the tray.

TEACHER. The nurse's most significant role in nutritional care is that of teacher. There will be innumerable informal opportunities during daily nursing care for planned conversation about sound nutrition principles reinforcing the nutrition counseling of the nutritionist. In addition, according to patient situations the nurse may work with the dietitian during periods of instruction concerning the principles of therpeutic diet integrated with general health teaching about disease (Fig. 23-3). The nurse will work in close cooperation with the clinical nutritionist or dietitian and the physician to coordinate efforts with the medical and nutritional management of the patient's illness. At all times the nurse will work closely with the hospital's therapeutic dietitians to support and sup-

plement primary nutrition education from them. The dietitian will also be an excellent resource for teaching materials and needed nutrition information.

It is evident that learning about the patient's needs should be a continuing activity beginning with hospital admission. It should follow through and include plans for continuing application in the home environment. Follow-up care may be provided by the outpatient dietitian, by consulting nutritionists in community private practice, by public health nutritionists or nurses, or by referrals to various community resource groups.

That this optimum learning situation does not prevail in all hospitals is a concern of many clinical dietitians, nutritionists, nurses, and physicians. There are many reasons, and they vary in different situations. Several reasons, however, are pertinent here—the lack of nutrition in medical education, the negative attitude of many nurses about their own study and practice of nutrition, and the negative patient responses to their nutrition education efforts. A two-year study in California hospitals,[18]

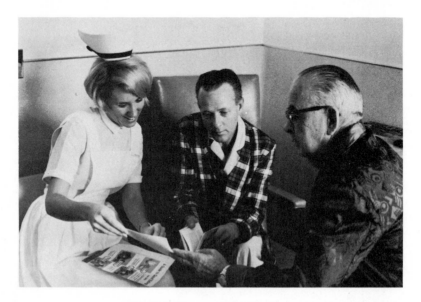

Fig. 23-3. The nurse as a teacher.

sociologic and anthropologic in orientation, not only indicated this fact of negative attitudes and responses but also that physician information was preferred even though it is often least informed in applied nutrition, that printed diet lists were the main means of conveying information to patients, and that the nurses closest to the patient placed the least priority value on nutrition in patient care.

SUMMARY

Perhaps through the different concepts and perspectives presented here, the clinical nutritionist or dietitian, the nurse, and the physician will be able to venture into new approaches as a team. The patient is their concern, and his care is their responsibility. Providing more patient-centered care through team effort with the dietitian/nutritionist and the physician will bring not only better care to the patient but also more satisfaction to the nurse. The newer dimensions of the comprehensive health care for the future demand such a collaborative approach.[19-22]

CASE STUDY 15

The patient with gastric cancer: nutritional assessment and therapy

Erlene Smith, aged 43, is a patient on the surgery ward, now eight days postoperative following her gastrectomy for treatment of gastric cancer. Prior to her surgery and the onset of her illness, Erlene had maintained a normal weight of 59 kg (130 lb), ideal for her medium frame height of 160 cm (5 ft, 4 in). Since her illness, however, she had been losing weight over the past four months. Nothing seemed to have any taste, and her appetite had lessened as her concern and anxiety about her condition had grown. Now her weight was down to 47 kg (104 lb), and there seemed to be no means of stopping the continued weight loss. Presently she was being given a postgastrectomy diet and was able to take 60 to 120 ml (2 to 4 oz) of milk every few hours with an added soft egg one or two times a day. She was counting up the amount of food she could tolerate, because she knew she must try to eat. Today, day 8 after her surgery, she had managed to get in 720 ml (24 oz) of milk and two eggs.

Erlene was interested in the measurements that the clinical nutritionist had come in to do a few hours before. She had written them down for Erlene so she could compare them with follow-up measures later to see what progress she was able to make. Erlene picked up the written note again to review it: nutrition assessment data—weight (without clothing save for the skimpy hospital gown) 47.3 kg (104 lb), height 162.6 cm (63¾ in), triceps skinfold 10 mm (1 cm), midarm circumference 17 cm. Afterward the nutritionist had calculated her midarm muscle circumference as she had explained to Erlene, as well as the protein and energy values in the food she had been able to eat.

When the nutritionist went out to the charting desk to enter her findings in Erlene's medical record, she reviewed the current laboratory test results and made a note of them: serum albumin 3.0 g/dl; TIBC 230 μg/dl; lymphocytes 1,200/mm^3 (23%); hematocrit 35%; hemoglobin 10.5 g/dl; and 24-hour urine: urea nitrogen 16 g, creatinine 1.75 g. Skin tests pending.

Quickly the nutritionist completed her calculations for the remaining assessment data—nitrogen balance for the day, transferrin, creatinine-height index—and entered them in the record. In preparation for her recommendation at the nutrition support team meeting for Erlene's nutritional management the nutritionist calculated Erlene's basal energy expenditure requirement as well as her added requirement for overcoming her catabolic condition. Together with her calculations for needed calories and protein, she also began to estimate Erlene's additional needs for vitamins and minerals, as well as to consider the best means of feeding her to meet these nutritional therapy requirements.

Later at the nutrition team conference the decision was made to begin parenteral nutrition. After the TPN began to provide the needed support, Erlene improved as evidenced by her follow-up nutritional assessment data. Soon she was discharged to continue the TPN at home along with a small amount of oral intake as time went by. In the weeks that followed, however, when she began her chemotherapy with the oncologist, she experienced much increased discomfort with sore mouth, nausea, and food intolerances. During this period she returned to the nutritionist's office for nutritional therapy and counseling and also attended the cancer team's patient group sessions along with her husband.

Questions to guide your inquiry (Refer also to Chapter 31.)

1. Using the format for a nutrition assessment data summary sheet from your hospital record forms, or a form of your own design, list all the data available concerning Erlene's nutritional status. What additional data would you consider useful? How would it be obtained?
2. What specific nutritional needs can you identify?

CASE STUDY 15

The patient with gastric cancer: nutritional assessment and therapy—cont'd

3. Consider the needs you have listed. What nutritional objective would you state as the priority at this time?
4. Check your list of all the assessment data. Explain each test in terms of its contribution to knowledge of Erlene's nutritional status, what each test is measuring, and the significance of the information it provides.
5. Calculate Erlene's nitrogen balance for day 8. What is its significance? Why is this an important key test in nutrition assessment?
6. What is transferrin? Calculate this value for Erlene.
7. What is creatinine? How does the creatinine-height index reflect nutritional status? What is Erlene's index?
8. Interpret Erlene's anthropometric data, including her midarm muscle circumference you have calculated.
9. What skin tests were probably ordered for Erlene? Why? How would these results contribute to assessment of her nutritional status and therapy needs?
10. State the reasons, as you see them from the data gathered, that the nutrition team made the decision to use TPN as a feeding modality.
11. What later nutritional problems do you see facing Erlene and her care team? What solutions can you propose? What persons would you involve?

REFERENCES
Specific

1. Brown, E. L.: Newer dimensions of patient care, New York, 1964, Russell Sage Foundation.
2. Butterworth, C. E.: The skeleton in the hospital closet, Nutr. Today **9:**4, March-April, 1974.
3. Blackburn, G. L., and Bistrian, B.: A report from Boston, Nutr. Today **9:**30, May-June, 1974.
4. Butterworth, C. E., and Blackburn, G. L.: Hospital malnutrition, Nutr. Today **10:**8, March-April, 1975.
5. Bistrian, B. R., Blackburn, G. L., Hallowell, E., et al.: Protein status of general surgical patients, J.A.M.A. **230:**858, 1974.
6. Bistrian, B. R., Blackburn, G. L., Vitale, J., et al.: Prevalence of malnutrition in general medical patients, J.A.M.A. **235:**1567, 1976.
7. Blackburn, G. L., et al.: Nutritional and metabolic assessment of the hospitalized patient, J. Parent. Enteral Nutr. **1:**11, 1977.
8. Stein, L. I.: The doctor-nurse game, Arch. Psychiatry **16:**699, 1967.
9. Sources of error in weighing and measuring children. In Center for Disease Control: Nutrition surveillance, U.S. Dept. of Health, Education, and Welfare Pub. No. (CDC) 76-8295, Atlanta, 1975, p. 6.
10. Jelliffe, D. B.: The assessment of the nutritional status of the community, Geneva, 1966, World Health Organization.
11. Frisancho, A. R.: Triceps skin fold and upper arm muscle size norms for assessment of nutrition status, Am. J. Clin. Nutr. **27**(10):1052, 1974.
12. Wang, R. I. H.: Practical drug therapy, Philadelphia, 1979, J. B. Lippincott Co.
13. Miller, R. R., and Greenblatt, D. J.: Handbook of drug therapy, New York, 1979, Elsevier North Holland, Inc.
14. American Hospital Formulary Service, American Society of Hospital Pharmacists: Publication and membership services, Washington, D.C., annual update.
15. Weed, L. L.: Medical records, medical education and patient care, Chicago, 1969, Year Book Medical Publishers, Inc.
16. Voytovich, A. E.: The dietitian/nutritionist and the problem-oriented medical record: a physician's viewpoint, J. Am. Diet. Assoc. **63:**639, Dec., 1973.
17. American Hospital Association: Recording nutritional information in medical records, Chicago, 1976.
18. Newton, M. E., Beal, M. E., and Strauss, A. L.: Nutritional aspects of nursing care, Nurs. Res. **16:** 46, 1967.

19. Graning, H. M.: The dietitian's role in "heads up" patient care, J. Am. Diet. Assoc. **56:**299, April, 1970.
20. Duval, M. K.: The challenge ahead, J. Am. Diet. Assoc. **60:**13, Jan., 1972.
21. Kocher, R. E.: New dimensions for dietetics in today's health care, J. Am. Diet. Assoc. **60:**17, Jan., 1972.
22. Kocher, R. E.: Monitoring nutritional care of the long-term patient, J. Am. Diet. Assoc. **67:**45, July, 1975.

General

American Dietetic Association: Patient nutritional care in long-term care facilities, Chicago, 1977.

Center for Disease Control: Nutrition surveillance, DHEW Pub. No. (CDC) 78-8295, March, 1977 (issued March, 1978).

Christakis, G., editor: Nutritional assessment in health programs, Washington, D.C., 1973, American Public Health Association.

Davidson, J. K., Delcher, H. K., and Englund, A.: Spin-off cost/benefits of expanded nutritional care, J. Am. Diet. Assoc. **75:**250, Sept., 1979.

Diet Therapy Section Committee: Guidelines for diet counseling, J. Am. Diet. Assoc. **66:**571, 1975.

Evans, S. N., Hsu, N., and Gormican, A.: Use of computers for dietary histories, J. Am. Diet. Assoc. **63:** 397, Oct., 1973.

Flynn, M., Keithly, D., and Colwill, J. M.: Nutrition in the education of the family physician, J. Am. Diet. Assoc. **65:**269, Sept., 1974.

Foman, S. J.: Nutritional disorders of children. Prevention, screening, and follow-up, DHEW Pub. No. (HSA) 76-5612, 1976.

Food and Nutrition Board, National Academy of Science, National Research Council: Recommended dietary allowances, rev. 1980.

Galbraith, A. L.: Hospital dietetics in transition, J. Am. Diet. Assoc. **67:**439, Nov., 1975.

Goodhart, R. S., and Shils, M. E., editors: Modern nutrition in health and disease, ed. 6, Philadelphia, 1980, Lea & Febiger.

Grant, A.: Nutritional assessment guidelines, Seattle, 1979, Anne Grant, Box 25057, Northgate Station, Seattle, Wash. 98125.

Guide for developing nutrition services in community health programs, DHEW Pub. No. (HSA) 78-5103, 1978.

Hallstrom, B. J., and Lauber, D. E.: Multidisciplinary manpower in the nutrition component of comprehensive health care delivery, J. Am. Diet. Assoc. **63:**23, July, 1973.

Halpern, S. L., editor: Quick reference to clinical nutrition, Philadelphia, 1979, J. B. Lippincott Co.

Hegsted, D. M.: Nutritional requirements in disease, J. Am. Diet. Assoc. **56:**303, April, 1970.

Hegsted, D. M.: Priorities in nutrition in the United States, J. Am. Diet. Assoc. **71:**9, July, 1977.

Howard, R. B., and Herbold, N. H.: Nutrition in clinical care, New York, 1978, McGraw-Hill Book Co.

Johnson, C. A.: The needs for better nutritional care: Who's responsible? J. Am. Diet. Assoc. **67:**219, Sept., 1975.

Karkect, J. M.: Viewpoint of the hospital dietitian, J. Am. Diet. Assoc. **68:**249, March, 1976.

Leverton, R. M.: The RDAs are not for amateurs, J. Am. Diet. Assoc. **66:**9, Jan., 1975.

Mahoney, M. J., and Caggiula, A. W.: Applying behavioral methods to nutrition counseling, J. Am. Diet. Assoc. **72:**372, April, 1978.

Mayer, J.: Time for reappraisal, J. Nutr. Educ. **7:**8, 1975.

Mead, M.: Comments on the division of labor in occupations concerned with food, J. Am. Diet. Assoc. **68:** 321, April, 1976.

Meiling, R. L.: The institutional system, Nutr. Today **9:**34, July-Aug., 1974.

Ohlson, M. A.: Philosophy of dietary counseling, J. Am. Diet. Assoc. **73:**13, July, 1973.

Ometer, J. L.: Documentation of nutritional care, J. Am. Diet. Assoc. **76:**35, Jan., 1980.

Pennington, J. A.: Dietary nutrient guide, Westport, Conn., 1976, AVI Pub. Co.

Preliminary findings of the first health and nutrition examination survey (HANES), United States, 1971-1972: Dietary intake and biochemical findings, DHEW Pub. No. (HRA) 74-1219-1, 1974.

Prevost, E. A., and Butterworth, C. E.: Nutritional care of hospitalized patients, Am. J. Clin. Nutr. **27:**432, 1974.

Schiller, M. R., and Vivian, V. M.: Role of the clinical dietitian, J. Am. Diet. Assoc. **65:**284, Sept., 1974.

Scialabba, M. A.: Functions of dietetic personnel in ambulatory care, J. Am. Diet. Assoc. **67:**545, Dec., 1975.

Shapiro, L. R.: Streamlining and implementing nutritional assessment: the dietary approach, J. Am. Diet. Assoc. **75:**230, Sept., 1979.

Spodnick, J. P.: Nutrition in the health maintenance organization, J. Am. Diet. Assoc. **61:**163, Aug., 1972.

Springer, N. S., and Segal, R. M.: Dietitians' attitudes toward advocacy, J. Am. Diet. Assoc. **67:**445, Nov., 1975.

Ten-State nutrition survey 1968-1970: Highlights, DHEW Pub. No. (HSM) 72-8134, 1972.

Tobias, A. L., and Van Itallie, T. B.: Nutritional problems of hospitalized patients, J. Am. Diet. Assoc. **71:**253, Sept., 1977.

Treacy, L. H.: The nutritionist in a comprehensive health care plan, J. Am. Diet. Assoc. **68:**253, March, 1976.

Wade, J. E.: Role of a clinical dietitian specialist on a nutrition support service, J. Am. Diet. Assoc. **70:**185, 1977.

Walters, F. M., and Crumley, S. J., editors: Patient care audit—a quality assurance procedure manual for dietitians, Chicago, 1978, American Dietetic Association.

PROBLEM-ORIENTED MEDICAL RECORDS

American Hospital Association: Recording nutritional information in medical records, Chicago, 1976.

Bjorn, J. C., and Cross, H. D.: Problem-oriented practice, Chicago, 1970, Modern Hospital Press.

The dietitian/nutritionist and the problem-oriented medical record, Parts I to III, J. Am. Diet. Assoc. **63:**639, Dec., 1973.

Fletcher, R. H.: Auditing problem-oriented records and traditional records, N. Engl. J. Med. **290:**829, 1974.

Froom, J. F.: Conversion to problem-oriented records in an established practice, Ann. Intern. Med. **78:**254, 1973.

Hurst, J. W.: Ten reasons why Lawrence Weed is right, N. Engl. J. Med. **284:**51, 1971.

Hurst, J. W., and Walker, H. K., editors: Quality control in health care—applications of a problem-oriented system, New York, 1974, Medcom, Inc.

Raker, R. E.: The problem-oriented medical record, Am. Family Phys. **10:**3, 100-111, 1974.

Swisher, S., and Enelow, A. J.: Interviewing and patient care, New York, 1972, Oxford University Press.

Walker, H. K., and Hurst, J. W.: Applying the problem-oriented system, New York, 1973, Medcom, Inc.

Weed, L. L.: Medical records, medical education, and patient care, Chicago, 1969, Year Book Medical Publishers, Inc.

Weed, L. L.: Quality control and the medical record, Arch. Intern. Med. **127:**101, 1971.

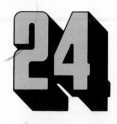

The problem of obesity and weight control

BASIS OF THE PROBLEM OF OBESITY

Obesity is a problem of affluent societies. Abundant statistical evidence indicts it as a health hazard. It increases the risk of a number of diseases such as diabetes mellitus, gout, gallbladder disease, coronary atherosclerosis, and hypertension. It complicates respiratory difficulties such as emphysema, chronic bronchitis, and asthma. It increases surgical risk, complicates pregnancy, and disturbs the growing adolescent. It reduces life expectancy.

Rare forms of obesity caused by disorders exist, but it is the so-called simple obesity constantly seen in everyday clinical practice that concerns both patient and practitioner. In the face of overwhelming and obvious evidence of its effect on health, the obesity problem continues to plague victims and health authorities alike, and efforts to combat it are largely frustrating to both. It soon becomes evident, therefore, that so-called simple obesity is not so simple after all. The enigma of the problem stems generally from two factors—its unsure definition and its multiple etiology.

Definitions

Ideal weight. The clinical term obesity is given to the presence of excess body weight (15% or more above the ideal weight). The problem, however, lies in defining the word "ideal." It is generally defined in reference to average weight according to height and frame, but in reality there is no such thing as an average person. Each person is individual, and normal values in healthy persons vary over a wide range. And how does one precisely measure *frame?* Research studies at the University of California's School of Public Health employing anthropometric methods to determine body build and composition use from 33 to 38 separate measures.[1] Also, tables of "ideal" weight usually use figures based on "average" activity. This factor too may be an unrealistic one. Individuals vary widely in the amount of their physical exercise, and the majority of them are becoming increasingly sedentary, as indicated by many studies and by general observation. An old general rule of thumb, however, for measuring ideal weight is for women, beginning with a height of 150 cm (5 ft) use 45 kg (100 lb), and add 2 kg (5 lb) for every 2.5 cm (1 in) over 150 cm; for men, beginning at 150 cm use 50 kg (110 lb), and add 2 kg for every 2.5 cm over 150 cm.

Types of obesity. Recognition of different types of obesity adds to the problem of definition. It is not merely a matter of total weight. The ratio of lean body mass (muscle) to body fat is involved. For example, a *developmental* type of obesity, beginning early in life and steadily continuing into adult years produces a higher ratio of lean body mass, whereas the *reactive* type associated with emotional stress of growth years produces an excess ratio of fat (p. 459). Therefore body composition must be considered in making more precise definitions. Tests being used today by researchers to measure this variation in body composition include

1. Anthropometric measures—measures size of body frame and body contours; skinfold thicknesses—measures subcutaneous or surface fat, adipose tissue
2. Water displacement—measures total fat content of the body
3. Radioactive potassium count—measures amount of lean body tissue
4. X-ray diffraction (shadows)—measures fat surrounding organs, minimal fat deposits

Etiology

The complexity of "simple" obesity is further increased by its multiple etiology. Among these factors are the following.

Physical factors. The basic physical laws of energy exchange (Chapter 8) account for obesity—an intake of more energy potential (calories) in food than output (calories) in total energy metabolism, including basal needs and physical activity. Table 24-1 indicates a general scheme for measuring basal energy needs and additions for activities. The statement concerning the balance of energy exchange, however, simple as it seems, is more complex. The maintenance level of calories varies widely with individuals in like circumstances. It is also influenced by their activity level. Numerous investigators report that obese subjects generally consume fewer calories than nonobese ones, but their activity level is usually lower also.[2] Obese sedentary persons, therefore, simply cannot afford to eat as much as their leaner counterparts.

Physiologic factors. The normal physiology of growth years contributes to accumulation of fat tissue deposits. Numerous studies and surveys[2-4] indicate there are critical periods for the development of obesity. For children the critical periods are early infancy and early stages of puberty.[5,6] For women a critical period is after age 21 because of less activity with no adjustment of caloric intake. Other times are during the first pregnancy and after menopause, due to the hormonal factors that are operating. For men a critical period is between the ages of 25 and 40, generally caused by decreasing activity with no consequent change in the large food habits formed during adolescence. Both men and women tend to gain weight after the age of 50 because of the lowered basal metabolic rate and decreased exercise, with failure to adjust calories accordingly.

Practical factors that influence physical obesity are the overfeeding of infants and children and lack of dietary adjustment by adults during periods of increased susceptibility to weight gain.

Table 24-1. General approximations for daily adult basal and activity energy needs

Basal energy needs (avg. 1 cal./kg/h)		Man (70 kg) calories 70 × 24 = 1,680	Woman (58 kg) calories 58 × 24 = 1,392
Activity energy needs			
Very sedentary	+20% basal	1,680 + 336 = 2,016	1,392 + 278 = 1,670
Sedentary	+30% basal	1,680 + 504 = 2,184	1,392 + 418 = 1,810
Moderately active	+40% basal	1,680 + 672 = 2,352	1,392 + 557 = 1,949
Very active	+50% basal	1,680 + 840 = 2,520	1,392 + 696 = 2,088

Inheritance factors. Some experimental studies with mice[7] seem to indicate a genetic factor in obesity, but the significance of these results for human obesity is unknown. It is true that obese children are more likely than non-obese children to have obese parents. Surveys indicate that where one parent is obese, approximately 40% of the offspring are obese; where both parents are obese, 80% of the offspring are obese. It is probable, however, that the familial influence is a situational one that molds food habits. Excessive food preparation and consumption is the normal family habit pattern, one that tends to be perpetuated in adulthood and passed on to successive generations.

Social factors. The class values placed on the obese state by different social groups will also influence the incidence of obesity. A study by Goldblatt's group at the University of Pennsylvania[8] surveyed 1,660 representative adults in an urban residential area. These subjects were grouped according to socioeconomic status, and their rates of obesity were compared. A greater number of obese persons were found in the lower socioeconomic status group than in the higher one. Also it was found that with increasing upward mobility the incidence of obesity declined; there was a more noticeable difference being seen in women than in men. With increasing social status the women moved from the "obese" to the "thin" category; the men moved from the "obese" to the "normal" category. These investigators concluded that movement *among* social classes as well as membership *in* a social class influences obesity. In the lower socioeconomic status groups, obesity was common and therefore considered normal, whereas greater social value was placed on the nonobese state in higher groups. The length of exposure to these values and their pressure on individuals determine their reaction to them.

Psychologic factors. The relation of emo-tional factors to obesity is well established. The obese state may well be the individual's protective resolution of deeper emotional problems. In such cases to remove it without providing an alternative and satisfying resolution may well create still further problems. Bruch[9] (p. 456) indicates from her many studies of children that such obesity problems may develop through the growth years when normal psychosocial struggles of children are not positively supported by the child's environment. Classic studies with college students at Cornell University revealed that success or failure in a weight reduction program could be predetermined by measures of the individual's degree of emotional stability.[10,11]

DIET THERAPY

By and large three general approaches to the control of obesity are found in clinic practice, depending on the orientation of the clinician and the type of patient and obesity with which he or she is dealing. These three approaches include (1) a metabolic basis, (2) general clinical care with reduction diet, and (3) adjunct behavioral therapies. For the type of obesity that has been labeled "intractable" or "biochemically resistant," the approach of some researchers is based theoretically on a postulated metabolic etiology.

Metabolic approach

Principles and rationale. The metabolic approach was illustrated by the research of Gordon's group some years ago at the University of Wisconsin Medical School.[12] Based on their studies and resulting theories, this group developed a dietary program around several metabolic principles:

1. Lipogenesis
   a. The close relation of glucose and fat metabolism, the conversion of glucose to fatty acid, and the subsequent formation of triglycerides

b. The influence of meal distribution (glucose load) on the conversion of glucose to fat

c. The influence of brief fasting on the breaking of this lipogenesis chain

2. Lipolysis—the influence of unsaturated fatty acids on the oxidation of saturated fat or body fat

3. Water metabolism—sodium and water retention (100 g of fat when oxidized yields 112 g of water)

DIET PLAN. The resulting diet therapy principles and rationale of the Gordon program are summarized in Table 24-2. The suggested dietary regimen such as may be used with medically selected and supervised patients in a clinical setting is given on p. 539.

Some clinics continue to use this approach, and a number of popular ''diet books'' perpetuate it in various forms periodically. However, it is not generally supported nor recommended for regular practice by current nutritional and medical authorities.

General clinical approach
Principles and rationale

In common practice the general approach to the control of simple obesity (excluding that form in subjects with more pronounced psychologic or metabolic problems) is based on the underlying energy exchange etiology and the patient's situational needs. It has three main principles:

1. Individual decision and support
2. Individual diet with calorie and situational adaptions
3. A planned follow-up program

Motivation and support. The degree of patient motivation is a prime factor. The initial interviews seek to determine individual needs, attitudes toward food, and the meaning food has for the patient. Recognition is given to the emo-

Table 24-2. Principles and rationale for the Gordon diet for treatment of obesity*

Diet principles			Rationale theory
1. Initial 48-hour total fast			Breaks the metabolic pattern of augmented lipogenesis (based on rat experiments)
2. Diet:	**g**	**Calories**	
High protein	100	400	High satiety value and specific dynamic action
Moderate fat	80	720	Satiety value; 15%-20% as UFA supplement
Low carbohydrate	50	200	Close relation of glucose to fat formation
TOTAL CALORIES		1,320	
3. Six-meal pattern (equal)			Reduce lipogenesis from smaller glucose loads
4. Low salt (2-3 g)			Water produced by fat oxidation; Slow disposal of sodium loads
5. Supplement of polyunsaturated fatty acids (vegetable oil); 15%-20% of fat calories			Accelerates oxidation of body fat

*Adapted from Gordon, E. S., et al.: A new concept in the treatment of obesity, J.A.M.A. **186:**50, 1963.

Table 24-3. Calorie adjustment required for weight loss

To lose 454 g (1 lb) a week—500 fewer calories daily

Basis of estimation
1 lb body fat	=	454 g
1 g pure fat	=	9 calories
1 g body fat	=	7.7 calories (some water in fat cells)
454 g × 9 calories per gram	=	4,086 calories per 454 g fat (pure fat)
454 g × 7.7 calories per gram	=	3,496 calories per 454 g body fat (or 3,500 calories)
500 calories × 7 days	=	3,500 calories = 454 g body fat.

Table 24-4. Weight reduction diets using the exchange system of dietary control

Food exchange group*	Approx. measure	800 calories	1,000 calories	1,200 calories	1,500 calories
Total number of exchanges per day					
Milk (nonfat)	1 cup	2	2	2	2
Vegetable A	As desired	Free	Free	Free	Free
Vegetable B	½ cup	1	1	1	1
Fruit	Varies	3	3	3	4
Bread	1 slice	1	3	4	4
Meat	28 g (1 oz)	6	6	7	9
Fat	1 tsp	1	1	2	4
Distribution of food exchanges					
Breakfast					
Fruit		1	1	1	1
Meat		1	1	1	1
Bread		1	1	1	1
Fat		1	1	1	1
Lunch and dinner					
Meat		2-3	2-3	3	4
Vegetable A		Any	Any	Any	Any
Vegetable A (either meal)		1	1	1	1
Bread		0	1	1-2	1-2
Fat		0	0	0-1	1-2
Fruit		1	1	1	1-2
Milk		1	1	1	1

*See Food Exchange Groups, pp. 546-550.

The Gordon diet for treatment of obesity*

Foods to include daily
1. One egg
2. Lean meat, 308 g (11 oz, cooked weight)
3. Margarine or oil or equivalent, 7 tsp
4. Skim milk, 2 cups
5. Fruit, 2 servings
6. Vegetables from list A†, 2-4 cups
7. Bread, ½ slice

Menu plan (minimum of six meals a day)

Breakfast	*Lunch*	*Dinner*
½ cup vitamin C fruit or juice	84 g (3 oz) meat	84 g (3 oz) meat
1 egg	vegetable A	vegetable A
28 g (1 oz) meat	1 tsp margarine	1 tsp margarine
1 tsp margarine	2 tsp corn oil	2 tsp corn oil
½ slice bread	coffee or tea	1 serving fruit
coffee or tea		coffee or tea
Midmorning	*Midafternoon*	*Evening*
1 cup skim milk	½ cup skim milk	½ cup skim milk
28 g (1 oz) meat	56 g (2 oz) meat	28 g (1 oz) meat

"Free" foods
1. Clear fat-free broth (homemade)
2. Unsweetened plain gelatin
3. Artificially sweetened gelatin products
4. Lemon
5. Vinegar
6. Spices and herbs
7. Carbonated beverages prepared with noncaloric sweeteners

Foods to avoid
1. Sugar, syrups, molasses, honey, candy, cake, cookies, ice cream, potato chips, crackers, gelatin products sweetened with sugar, puddings, pies, gravy, alcoholic beverages
2. Highly salted foods (use salt *lightly* in cooking; no added salt)
3. Any foods not included in the diet list above

*Adapted from Gordon, E. S., et al.: A new concept in the treatment of obesity, J.A.M.A. **186:**50, 1963.
†See Food Exchange Groups, pp. 546-550.

tional factors involved in a reduction program, and support is provided by the team of physician, nutritionist, and nurse to meet the patient's particular needs. Shame or scare tactics generally have no place in such a program.

Diet control. Control is based on two factors—an initial interview and an individual diet plan.

INITIAL INTERVIEW. On the basis of careful interviewing, the patient's food habits and situational factors are determined. A balanced diet is made out for the patient based on normal nutritional needs, and the calorie level is adjusted to meet his individual weight reduction requirement. One thousand fewer calories daily is the necessary adjustment to lose about 900 g (2 lb) a week; 500 fewer calories to lose 450 g (1 lb) a week. The basis of this calculation is

---

TO PROBE FURTHER
The exchange system of dietary control

The exchange system of dietary control, developed by professional organizations such as the American Dietetic Association, is based on a simple grouping of common foods according to generally equivalent nutritional values. This system may be used for any situation requiring caloric and food value control.

The foods are divided into six basic groups (some with subgroups), called the "exchange groups" (pp. 546-550). Each food item within a group or subgroup contains approximately the same food value as any other food item in that group, allowing for exchange within groups, thus providing for variety in food choices as well as food value control. Hence the term "food exchanges" is used to refer to food choices or servings. The total number of exchanges per day depends on individual nutritional needs, based on normal nutritional standards. Although there is some variation in the composition of foods within the exchange groups, for simplicity the following values for carbohydrate, protein, fat, and calories are used.

Food	Approximate Measure	Carbohydrate (g)	Protein (g)	Fat (g)	Calories
Milk exchanges	1 cup				
A (nonfat)		12	8	—	80
B (low fat)		12	8	5	125
C (full fat)		12	8	10	170
Vegetable exchanges					
A (low)	As desired	—	—	—	Negligible
B (medium)	½ cup	7	2	—	35
Fruit exchanges	Varies	10	—	—	40
Bread exchanges	1 slice	15	2	—	70
Meat exchanges	28 g (1 oz)				
A (lean)		—	7	3	55
B (medium fat)		—	7	6	78
C (high fat)		—	7	8	100
Fat exchanges	1 tsp				
A (unsaturated)		—	—	5	45
B (monounsaturated)		—	—	5	45
C (saturated)		—	—	5	45

given in Table 24-3. Usually the energy value of the adjusted diet will range between 800 and 1,500 calories.

INDIVIDUAL DIET PLAN USING EXCHANGE SYSTEM. Using the basic exchange system of dietary control given in Table 24-4, a meal pattern is made out with the patient that will meet his individual living situation, individual desires, and cultural patterns. Food choices for meals are taken from the Food Exchange Groups listed on pp. 546-550.

Follow-up program. A follow-up schedule of appointments is outlined, and its values are discussed with the patient. On subsequent clinical visits progress records are kept, problems discussed, and solutions to them mutually decided. Continuing support is given. A number of practical suggestions to dieters have evolved from much experience (p. 545). These may help the patient to anticipate needs, avoid pitfalls, and sustain his motivation.

Essential characteristics of sound diet for weight control

Experience in many clinics has shown that there are no real short cuts. In the face of many periods of discouragement the patient may be harried and vexed, tempted to grab for a plethora of pills, formulas, and fads. However, a sound dietary approach to weight control that holds hope of achieving a degree of *lasting* success must be based on five characteristics:

1. *Realistic goals.* Goals must be realistic in terms of overall loss and rate of loss.
2. *Calories lowered according to need.* The diet must be low enough in calories in relation to individual expenditure levels of energy to effect a gradual weight loss. Usually a rate of 450 to 900 g (1 to 2 lb) a week is recommended.
3. *Nutritional adequacy.* The diet must be nutritionally adequate. Lower caloric levels may need supplementation. The nutrient ratio should supply no less than 12% to 15% of the calories as protein; no

more than 35% of the calories as fat, with reduced intake of saturated fats; and the rest of the calories as carbohydrate, using little sucrose and including a variety of food sources.

4. *Culturally desirable.* The food plan must be enough like the cultural eating pattern of the individual to form the basis for *permanent* reeducation of his eating habits. In other words, he must be able to live with it.
5. *Calorie readjustment to maintain weight.* When the desired weight level is reached, the calories are adjusted accordingly, but the reeducation achieved in basic habits is the continuing means of weight control.

BEHAVIORAL APPROACHES

Increasingly practitioners in health care settings are recognizing the need to give attention to supportive therapies for weight control that focus on the behavioral aspects of the problem. Food behavior is rooted in many human experiences and associations and in varying life situations, often producing an addictive form of eating response or conditioning. In essence, behavior-oriented adjunct therapies help the obese person change such food and eating patterns through increased insight and understanding, motivation, and reconditioning. By changing associations with the undesirable habit patterns, a means of constructive action is often provided. Two such behavioral approaches to the problem of obesity and weight control are behavior modification and clinical hypnosis.

Behavior modification

Principles. Behavioral change and control through the techniques of behavior modification are based on the work of Skinner[13] in the field of behavioral psychology and his basic principle of operant conditioning. According to this principle, behavior *operates* on the environment to generate consequences. These consequences then are fed back through the sense organs and serve to reinforce the behavior even when no organic needs are involved. Other workers in the field, such as Bandura,[14] have developed these principles further and made numerous applications of them in clinical and educational settings. Thus an underlying philosophy of behavior modification comes from learning theory, with the assumption that if a behavior can be learned, it can be retrained, or if it is unlearned, it can be shaped and directed. Hence in the treatment of obesity behavior modification, activities are directed toward both control of ingestive behavior (the when, why, where, how, and how much of eating) and promotion of physical activity and energy expenditure, providing overall for a better total energy balance. Numerous references are provided at the end of this chapter to guide a needed increased focus on physical activity.

Techniques. As applied to the treatment of eating disorders and obesity, techniques of behavior modification are reviewed by a number of clinicians.[15,16] Also resource books such as those by Stuart and Davis,[17] Ferguson,[18] and Nash and Long[19] provide many helpful guides for use of these methods in individual and group settings. These techniques by and large seek to control eating behavior in its three aspects:

1. *Antecedents of the behavior.* What happens before and "cues" the behavior?
2. *Response behavior.* What happens during the eating behavior following the "cue"?
3. *Consequences of the behavior.* What happens after the eating behavior response that may serve to reinforce it?

A program of behavior modification in the treatment of obesity, therefore follows three basic progressive actions:

1. Define *specifically* the problem behavior and the desired behavior. This process clearly establishes operational objectives.
2. Record baseline behavior and analyze it carefully. What types of habit patterns emerge? What is the frequency and rate of their occurrence? What conditions

seem to "trigger" or signal the behavioral cues? What consequent events seem to maintain the habits (time and pace, place, persons, social responses, hunger before and after, emotional mood, etc.)?

3. Manage or "consequate" the situational forces surrounding the behavior. Set up controls of the external environmental contingencies, and proceed with a planned and monitored program involving choices and reinforcers for desired behavior. This management of the environment will involve control of situational forces related to antecedents, responses, and consequences of the behavior.

a. Antecedent behavior
(1) *Eliminate* as many cues for the problem behavior as possible. For example, control situational stimuli; put temptation out of reach; avoid contact with problem foods; make the problem behavior as difficult as possible, thus interrupting the chain of actions that achieve it.
(2) *Suppress* those cues for the problem behavior that cannot be entirely eliminated. For example, control social interactions that produce and maintain the problem behavior; provide positive reinforcement for the desired behavior; have a trusted person monitor eating patterns; minimize contact with excessive food; make small portions appear larger; control deprivation states.
(3) *Strengthen* those cues for the desired behavior that have positive functional value. For example, provide information concerning a wide array of appropriate food choices and amounts; provide food behavior aids for feedback and progress, such as records, diary, or log; spread appropriate foods in desirable meal and snack

pattern; make desirable foods as attractive as possible.

b. Response behavior
   (1) Slow the pace of eating. For example, suggest that the patient take only one bit at a time, placing utensil on plate until next bite or during intermittent one- to three-minute periods of conversation; suggest that the patient delay starting the meal when first seated.
   (2) Savor the food. Advise that the person chew slowly, allowing sensory feelings of taste and texture awareness to develop.

c. Consequence behavior
   (1) *Decelerate* the problem behavior. For example, respond neutrally to all negative deviations from the desired behavior, thus giving social reinforcement for adherence; focus on ultimate aversive consequences of the problem eating behavior in health problems.
   (2) *Accelerate* the desired behavior. For example, update the progress records daily; respond positively to all desired behavior; provide some sort of material reinforcement for positive behavior; provice social reinforcement for all constructive efforts to modify behavior.

d. Evaluate overall program continuously and terminally when specific objectives are reached.

Clinical hypnosis

Principles. Hypnotherapy in clinical practice has roots in early medicine. The word "hypnosis" was first coined by the Scottish physician James Braid from the Greek word *hypnos,* meaning sleep. This was an unfortunate choice of words, as he later recognized, since hypnosis was not sleep, but to the contrary was a state of altered consciousness, alertness, and concentration. Prior to the advent of anesthesia it was a major therapy used to control pain. It finds similar applications today in modern medicine and dentistry. It is especially used as adjunct behavioral therapy in internal medicine, obstetrics and pediatrics, psychiatry, and clinical psychology.

Principles underlying hypnosis are based on the adaptive response of the brain and central nervous system to specific ideas, images, and feelings presented in the context of specific patient needs. In the hypnoidal state there is a degree of dissociation that is characterized by selective inattention to surrounding stimuli with an inhibiting of cortical or critical thinking and a greater state of physical and mental relaxation. Since critical thinking is reduced in a motivated and supportive environment, with the aid of an operator or through learned techniques of autohypnosis, enhanced suggestibility for the desired behavior or pain control results. Thus the hypnotic state is self-achieved by the patient from personal desires, expectations, and needs through a state of selective attention and concentration to the problem. The capacity for such relaxation and concentration is within the patient. The clinician merely helps to bring it to the surface, acts as a trusted guide, and helps the patient learn techniques for autohypnosis, directed toward the patient's particular health need or difficulty.

Techniques. A number of techniques have been developed by workers in the field of clinical hypnosis. Generally they utilize the body's capacity for directed mental and physiologic functioning:

1. *Relaxation methods.* Greater states of relaxation may be achieved by progressive attention to various parts of the body, especially to respiration.[20] Jencks[21] gives many suggestions for breathing exercises to enhance sensory awareness and reduce stress.
2. *Meditation exercises.* Various forms of meditation have been used since ancient times to achieve mental and physical re-

laxation and concentration. Payne[22] provides a number of such approaches to increased sensory awareness and expanded consciousness.

3. *Imagery*. Visualization of mental images directed toward the patient's needs is an effective means of concentration and relaxation, with attention to related body functioning, health problem or behavior problem, or desired state of appearance or confidence or function. Applications of such mental exercises to weight control have been provided by Stern and Hoch.[23]

4. *Ideomotor movements*. Activities involving motor movements of hands or arms, for example, may be used as means of concentration or to help induce a more relaxed state.

5. *Autohypnosis*. Autogenic training can be given patients for concentrated practice in learning how to relax or deal more effectively with problems, physical or behavioral. Patients often develop their own suggestions and relaxation practice and sometimes find audiotapes they have made a continuing help. Jencks[24] provides a useful manual based on the work of Schultz.

Many more techniques may be found in standard references such as those by Kroger and Fezler.[25,26] Kroger gives a discussion, for example, of his own work with obese patients. Stanton[27] also provides a discussion of weight loss through hypnosis from his own clinical practice. Additional references for the concerned student or practitioner may be found at the end of this chapter under a special heading.

PREVENTIVE APPROACH

In the last analysis, in the approach to the problem of obesity and its control, it would seem that the most constructive work would be aimed at *prevention*.[28] Early nutrition education, positive food behavior and habit formation, and support to young mothers and children before the obese condition becomes a reality will help prevent many problems later in adulthood.

A comprehensive annotated list of references and resources on weight control and obesity has been prepared by the Society for Nutrition Education.[29] It can be obtained by writing to the Society in Berkeley, California.

TO PROBE FURTHER
Practical suggestions to dieters

Goals	Be realistic. Don't set your goals too high. Adapt your rate of loss to 450 to 900 g (1 to 2 lb) per week. If visible tools are helpful motivation techniques, use them.
Calories	Don't be an obsessive calorie counter. Simply become familiar with the food exchanges in your diet list and learn the general calorie values of some of your favorite home dishes so that you might occasionally make substitutions.
Plateaus	Anticipate plateaus. They happen to everyone. They are related to water accumulation as fat is lost. During these periods, increase your exercise to help you get started again.
Binges	Don't be discouraged when you break over and have a dietary binge. This too happens to most people. Simply keep them infrequent, and when possible, plan ahead for special occasions. Adjust the following day's diet or remaining part of the same day accordingly.
Special diet foods	There is no need to purchase special low-calorie foods. Learn to read labels carefully. Most special diet foods are expensive, and many are not much lower in calories than regular foods.
Home meals	Try to avoid a separate menu for yourself. Adapt your needs to the family meal, adjusting seasoning or method of preparing family dishes to lower caloric values of added fats and starches.
Eating away from home	Watch portions. When a guest, limit extras such as sauces and dressings, trim meat well. In restaurants select singly prepared items rather than combination dishes. Avoid items with heavy sauces or fat seasoning. Select fruit or sherbet as desserts rather than pastries.
Appetite control	Avoid dependence on appetite depressant medications. Usually they are only crutches. Beginning efforts to control appetite may be aided by nibbling on food from the free list or by saving over meal items for use between meals such as the fruit.
Meal pattern	Eat three or more meals a day. If you are used to three meals, then leave it at that. If you are helped by snacks between meals, then plan part of your day's allowance to account for them. The main thing is that you do not take all of your calories at one sitting. Avoid the all-too-common pattern of no breakfast, little or no lunch, and a huge dinner!

Food exchange groups

List 1: Milk exchanges (Cream portion of whole milk equals two fat exchanges. Hence 1 cup whole milk equals 1 cup skim milk plus two fat exchanges.)

Group A (nonfat)

Skim or nonfat milk	1 cup
Buttermilk	1 cup
Canned, evaporated skim milk	½ cup
Powdered, nonfat dry milk (before adding liquid)	⅓ cup
Yogurt made from skim milk (plain, unflavored)	1 cup

Group B (low fat)

Low-fat milk (2% butterfat)	1 cup
Yogurt made from low-fat milk (plain, unflavored)	1 cup

Group C (full fat)

Whole milk	1 cup
Canned, evaporated whole milk	½ cup
Powdered, whole dry milk (before adding liquid)	⅓ cup
Yogurt made from whole milk (plain, unflavored)	1 cup

List 2: Vegetable exchanges (As served plain, without fat, seasoning, or dressing. Any fat used is taken from the fat exchange allowance.)

Group A (In amounts commonly eaten, use as desired.)

Asparagus	Green pepper, chili pepper	Parsley
Bok choy, gai choy	Greens	Pimientos
Bamboo shoots	Beet	Radishes
Bean sprouts	Chard	Rhubarb
Broccoli	Collards	Sauerkraut
Brussels sprouts	Dandelion	String beans: green, yellow, wax
Cabbage	Escarole	Summer squash
Cauliflower	Kale	Tomato juice
Celery	Mustard	Tomatoes
Chicory	Spinach	Turnips
Chinese cabbage	Turnip	Vegetable juice, mixed
Cucumber	Lettuce: all varieties	Watercress
Eggplant	Mushrooms	Zucchini
Endive	Onions	

Group B (One serving equals ½ cup unless otherwise stated.)

Artichoke (1 medium)	Carrots (1 medium)	Okra (8-9 pods)
Beets	Green peas (⅓ cup)	Rutabagas

List 3: Fruit exchanges (Unsweetened: fresh, frozen, canned, cooked. One exchange is the portion indicated by the fruit.)

Berries		Other fruits	
Blackberries	½ cup	Apple	1 small
Blueberries	½ cup	Apple cider	⅓ cup
Raspberries	½ cup	Apple juice	⅓ cup
Strawberries	¾ cup	Applesauce	½ cup
Citrus fruits		Apricots	2 medium
Grapefruit	½ small	Banana	½ small
Grapefruit juice	½ cup	Cherries	10 large, 17 small
Orange	1 small	Fig	1 large
Orange juice	½ cup	Fruit cocktail	½ cup
Tangerine	1 medium	Grape juice	¼ cup
Melons		Grapes	10 medium
Cantaloupe	¼ medium	Kiwi fruit	1 medium
Honeydew	⅛ medium	Mango	½ small
Watermelon	1 cup diced (approx. ½ center slice)	Nectarine	1 small
		Papaya	⅓ medium, ½ small
Dried fruits		Peach	1 medium
Apricots	4 halves	Pear	1 medium
Dates	2 medium	Persimmon	1 medium
Figs	1 medium	Pineapple	½ cup; 1 round center slice
Peaches	2 halves		
Pears	2 halves	Pineapple juice	⅓ cup
Prunes	2 medium	Plums	2 medium
Raisins	2 tbsp	Prune juice	¼ cup
		Prunes, fresh	2 medium

List 4: Bread exchanges (Equivalent portions indicated by each item.)

Bread		Cereal	
Bagel	½	Bulgur, cooked	½ cup
Bread (loaf, average size slice)	1 slice	Cereal, cooked	½ cup
French		Cereal, dry (ready-to-eat, un-sweetened)	
Italian			
Pumpernickel		Bran flakes	½ cup
Raisin		Grape-nuts	¼ cup
Rye		Other (flake, puff)	¾ cup
White		Cornmeal, dry	2 tbsp
Whole wheat		Flour	2½ tbsp
Bread crumbs, dried	3 tbsp	Grits, cooked	½ cup
English muffin	½	Pasta, cooked (spaghetti, noodles, macaroni)	½ cup
Hamburger bun	½		
Roll, frankfurter	1	Popcorn (popped, no fat)	1½ cup
Roll, plain	1 small	Rice, cooked	½ cup
Tortilla (6 inches diameter)	1	Wheat germ, plain	3 tbsp

Continued.

Food exchange groups—cont'd

List 4: Bread exchanges—cont'd

Crackers

Arrowroot	3
Graham, 2½-inch square	2
Matzoth, 4 × 6 inches	1
Oyster crackers	20
Pretzels, 3⅛ × ⅛ inch	25
Round butter type crackers	6
Rye wafers, 2 × 3½ inches	3
Saltines	5
Soda crackers, 2½-inch square	3

Dried beans, peas, lentils

Beans, peas, lentils (dried and cooked)	⅓ cup
Baked beans, no pork	¼ cup

Starchy vegetables

Corn	⅓ cup
Corn on cob (6-inch ear)	½ ear
Lima beans	½ cup
Parsnips	½ cup
Potato, white	1 small
Potato, white mashed	½ cup
Pumpkin	1 cup
Sweet potato	½ small; ⅓ cup
Winter squash (acorn, butternut, banana)	½ cup

Yam	½ small; ⅓ cup

Prepared foods

Angel food cake (1½-inch cube or small slice)	1 slice
Biscuit, 2 inches diameter (omit 1 fat exchange)	1
Chips, potato or corn (omit 2 fat exchanges)	15
Corn muffin, 2-inch diameter (omit 1 fat exchange)	1
Cornbread, 2 × 2 × 1¼ inches (omit 1 fat exchange)	1 square
Crepe, 6 inches diameter (omit 1 fat exchange)	1
Ice milk, ½ cup scoop (omit 1 fat exchange)	1 scoop
Muffin, plain, 2 inches diameter (omit 1 fat exchange)	1
Pancakes, 4 inches diameter (omit 1 fat exchange)	1
Potatoes, french fried (length 2-3 inches (omit 1 fat exchange)	8 pieces
Sherbet, fruit ice, ½-cup scoop	1 scoop
Waffle, 4 inches diameter or (omit 1 fat exchange)	1

List 5: Meat exchanges

Group A (lean)

I. Lean meats, less tissue fat

Fish (any fresh or frozen)	28 g (1 oz)
Canned salmon, tuna, mackerel	¼ cup
Sardines, drained	3
Shellfish	
Clams, oysters, scallops	5
Crab, lobster	¼ cup
Poultry (no skin)	
Chicken, turkey, cornish hen, guinea hen, pheasant	28 g
Veal (any lean trimmed cut)	28 g

II. Lean meats, more tissue fat

Beef	28 g
Very lean young beef; chipped beef; lean cuts of chuck, flank steak, tender loin, plate ribs and skirt steak, round (top, bottom), rump, spare ribs, tripe	
Lamb	28 g
Lean cuts: leg, rib, sirloin, loin (roast, chops), shank, shoulder	

Food exchange groups—cont'd

List 5: Meat exchanges—cont'd

Pork	28 g (1 oz)	Parmesan	3 tbsp
Lean cuts of leg (rump, center shank), ham (smoked center cut)		Cottage cheese, recreamed	¼ cup
		Cholesterol foods	
III. Cheese	28 g	Egg	1
Cottage cheese	¼ cup	Organ meats	28 g
Dry curd		Liver, kidney, sweet-	
Low fat, partially re-creamed		breads, heart	
		Shrimp	5 large
Other cheeses	28 g	Other	
Less than 5% butterfat; partially skim milk		Peanut butter (omit 2 fat exchanges)	2 tbsp
Group B (medium fat)		Tofu	98 g (3½ oz)
Beef	28 g	*Group C (high fat)*	
Ground (15% fat), corned beef (canned)		Beef	28 g
Pork		Brisket (fresh or corned), ground (20% or more fat)	
Loin (roast, chops), shoulder arm (picnic), shoulder blade, Boston butt, Canadian bacon, boiled ham		Lamb breast	28 g
		Pork	28 g
		Spare ribs, back ribs, ground pork, sausage, country style ham, deviled ham	
Cheese		Cheese, cheddar types	28 g
Mozzarella, ricotta, Swiss, Jack, farmer's cheese, Neufchâtel		Cold cuts	1 slice
		Frankfurter	1 small
		Poultry	28 g
		Capon duck, goose	

List 6: Fat exchanges

Group A (polyunsaturated plant fats)		*Group B (monounsaturated plant fats)*	
Margarine,* soft (stick or tub)	1 tsp	Avocado	⅛
Mocha mix (cream substitute)	2 tbsp	Nuts	
Salad dressings*		Almonds	10 whole
French	1 tbsp	Peanuts	20 whole
Italian	1 tbsp	Pecans	2 whole
Mayonnaise	1 tsp	Olives	5 small
Seeds (sunflower, sesame, pumpkin)	1 tbsp	Vegetable oils (olive, peanut)	1 tsp
		Group C (saturated animal fats)	
Vegetable oils (safflower, corn, soy, cottonseed, sesame)	1 tsp	Butter	1 tsp
		Cheese spreads	1 tbsp
		Cream	
Walnuts	4-5 halves	Half & half (10% cream)	2 tbsp

*Made with safflower, corn, soy, cottonseed oil.

Continued.

Food exchange groups—cont'd

List 6: Fat exchanges—cont'd

Light (20% cream)	2 tbsp	Pork fat	
Heavy (40% cream)	1 tbsp	Bacon crisp	1 strip
Sour (light)	2 tbsp	Bacon fat	1 tsp
Cream cheese	1 tbsp	Lard	1 tsp
		Salt pork	¾-inch cube

Miscellaneous foods allowed as desired (negligible carbohydrate, protein, fat)

Artificial sweeteners, as permitted

Bouillon, broth, clear fat free

Catsup, mustard, horseradish, meat sauce

Coffee, tea

Cranberries, cranberry juice (unsweetened)

Garlic

Gelatin, plain or D-Zerta

Herbs and spices

Lemon, lime

Pickles, dill and sour

Salt and pepper

Vinegar

CASE STUDY 15
The obese patient with gallbladder disease

Roselle Romano, aged 45, had a reputation among her friends as being the best cook in her Italian neighborhood. She used only the finest imported olive oil from the old country in her frying and baking, and no insalata was complete without a good portion of it mixed with wine vinegar. Her pasta was always perfect, white mounds covered with bubbly tomato sauce and cheese or made with meat fillings.

"The only trouble is this weight of mine," Roselle thought, as she looked again at herself in the full mirror as she was dressing. Since her marriage and the six children in succession, she had been too busy with her increasing family to pay much attention to herself. She had weighed nearly 90 kg (200 lbs) ever since her last pregnancy. With her short height of 155 cm (5 ft, 2 in), her weight made her increasingly uncomfortable. She had begun to worry too about the pain that kept bothering her—a sharp pain in her abdomen, especially after she at a large meal. There was a fullness and a pressure that lingered. Several times the pain and distention had brought on vomiting.

One evening after dinner the pain was especially severe. Her husband insisted that she see the doctor the following day for a checkup, and she finally agreed. She knew she had just been putting it off.

The next day Roselle's oldest daughter took her to Dr. Barrett's office. After the doctor had examined Roselle, he gave her instructions for an X-ray test he wanted her to have done. When she returned several days later after the test, Dr. Barrett confirmed the diagnosis. She had an inflamed

---

CASE STUDY 15

The obese patient with gallbladder disease—cont'd

---

gallbladder from a chronic infection, and there were stones formed. Dr. Barrett said that she needed to have surgery. However, he wanted her to lose weight first, since her present weight would only add risks to the surgery. He asked her to see the clinic nutritionist about the weight control program and to follow her dietary instructions carefully.

Over the next few months Roselle attended the weight control group sessions faithfully. The nutritionist who conducted the group sessions provided much support and practical sound guidance. It was not easy to change some of her deep-rooted eating habits, excessive as they were. But she was motivated by her need for surgery and her desire to be healthy. The nutritionist had helped her plan a diet that would fit in with her family meal preparation with some calorie modification for herself.

Gradually Roselle's faithful efforts began to pay off. She slowly lost weight at the rate of about 1 kg (2 lb) per week. By the time the first six months' period was over she had almost reached the point that Dr. Barrett felt would allow him to proceed with the surgery.

Roselle was an inspiration and great encouragement to the other members of her group as they watched the progress she made. She also contributed many suggestions to the others of things she had learned in her own effort to adapt her eating habits around those of her family. She found, for example, that many foods could be cooked without the fat seasoning, with her good Italian herbs used just the same. Then after her portion was removed she would add the fat seasoning for the rest of the family. When a food was to be fried for the family, she would adapt the method of cooking of her portion, using oven methods of cooking. She found after a while that her foods could taste just as good with the use of her herbs and not so much of the olive oil.

Desserts had been a large factor in the Romano family dinner pattern, and Roselle still prepared these for the family. But she usually substituted some fruit for herself, and before long the desire for the sweets had diminished. She took great pride in her increasingly slender figure and the new clothes she was able to wear in smaller sizes. Her family was a great support to her also. Her husband particularly complimented her frequently and insisted that the food did not need as much fat seasoning anyway for the rest of them. She would never forget the day when her youngest son, Bill, aged 6, excitedly exclaimed when he gave her a hug, "Mama, now I can reach all the way around when I hug you!"

Finally the day came when Dr. Barrett felt it was wise to go ahead with surgery, and a date was scheduled for it. He gave Roselle instructions about admission to the hospital in preparation for the cholecystectomy. The day of her surgery, Roselle looked like a different person. She withstood the procedure in excellent fashion and was soon back in her room from the recovery room.

Gradually she was able to begin to take liquids and then a bit of food again. The doctor had ordered a low-fat diet for her, and her nurse explained why it was important that she still watch the fat in her diet, even though the gallbladder had now been removed. But this was no large problem for Roselle, because she had made adjustments in her eating habits in the preceding months of her weight reduction program. Now she did not desire to go back to her old excessive habits. She was pleased with her new self, and her friends commented on how changed a person she was. She began to get out more, to become involved in community organizations and activities in general. Her life became full and interesting. Her family agreed that living with her had been good before, but now it was even better.

Questions to guide your inquiry (Refer also to Chapter 27.)

1. What is the function of the gallbladder?

Continued.

CASE STUDY 15

The obese patient with gallbladder disease—cont'd

2. What are the components of liver bile? What is the difference between liver bile and gallbladder bile?
3. How much bile does the liver secrete daily? What is the capacity of the gallbladder? What is the concentrating power of the gallbladder?
4. What is the mechanism controlling the release of bile from the gallbladder into the small intestine? Describe the operation of this mechanism? What is the function of bile salts?
5. What was the X-ray test of gallbladder function Dr. Barrett ordered for Roselle? How is it done?
6. What is cholecystitis? Cholelithiasis?
7. What causes the formation of gallstones?
8. Account for the symptoms that Roselle experienced, especially after eating a full meal.
9. What role does obesity play in the development of gallbladder disease? Why?
10. What problems faced Roselle when the doctor indicated her need for weight reduction? What motivated her to follow through with the weight reduction program?
11. Suppose you were the nutritionist working with Roselle's group in the weight reduction program. Outline the topics to be discussed and the methods you would use to involve the group for several of the group sessions.
12. What sort of an approach do you think would be most useful in working with such a group of overweight persons?
13. What practical suggestions can you list for adapting dietary habits to conserve calories and bring about a weight loss?
14. What factors would the nutritionist have to keep in mind in planning a reduction program for Roselle? Why?
15. Occasionally Roselle's family went to a restaurant for a meal. What suggestions could you give her for eating away from home?
16. Roselle indicated that one of her difficulties was snacking between meals. What suggestions could you give her to meet this problem?
17. One of Roselle's friends told her that when she was attempting to lose weight she had to buy her food in a health food store. If Roselle asked you about the use of such "special diet" foods, how would you answer her?
18. Why do you think Roselle was able to succeed in her weight reduction efforts?
19. Why did Roselle need to continue a low-fat intake even after the gallbladder had been removed?
20. Why would the nurse observe Roselle's incision carefully and frequently after her surgery to be sure there was no excessive bleeding?

REFERENCES
Specific

1. Hampton, M. C., Huenemann, R. L., Shapiro, L. R., Mitchell, B. W., and Behnke, A. R.: A longitudinal study of gross body composition and body conformation and their association with food and activity in a teen-age population. II. Anthropometric evaluation of body build, Am. J. Clin. Nutr. **19:**422, 1966.

2. Huenemann, R. L., Shapiro, L. R., Hampton, M. C., and Mitchell, B. W.: Teen-agers' activities and attitudes toward activity, J. Am. Diet. Assoc. **51:**433, 1967.
3. Forbes, G. B.: Overnutrition for the children: blessing or curse? Nutr. Rev. **15:**193, 1957.
4. Heald, F. P., and Hollander, R. J.: The relationship

between obesity in adolescence and early growth, J. Pediatr. **67:**35, 1965.

5. Winick, M.: Childhood obesity, Nutr. Today **9:**6, May-June, 1974.

6. Hines, J. H.: Infant feeding practices and obesity, J. Am. Diet. Assoc. **75:**122, Aug., 1979.

7. Mayer, J.: An experimentalist's approach to the problem of obesity, J. Am. Diet. Assoc. **31:**230, 1955.

8. Goldblatt, P. B., Moore, M. E., and Stunkard, A. J.: Social factors in obesity, J.A.M.A. **192:**1039, 1965.

9. Bruch, H.: The importance of overweight, New York, 1957, W. W. Norton & Co., Inc.

10. Darling, C. D., and Summerskill, J.: Emotional factors in obesity and weight reduction, J. Am. Diet. Assoc. **29:**1204, 1953.

11. Young, C. M., et al.: Psychologic factors in weight control, Am. J. Clin. Nutr. **5:**186, 1957.

12. Gordon, E. S., Goldberg, M., and Chosey, G. J.: A new concept in the treatment of obesity, J.A.M.A. **186:**50, 1963.

13. Skinner, B. F.: The behavior of organisms, New York, 1961, Appleton-Century-Crofts.

14. Bandura, A.: Principles of behavior modification, New York, 1969, Holt, Rinehart and Winston.

15. Levitz, L. S.: Behavior therapy in treating obesity, J. Am. Diet. Assoc. **62:**22, Jan., 1973.

16. Stunkard, A. J.: New therapies for the eating disorders: behavior modification of obesity and anorexia nervosa, Arch. Gen. Psychiatry **76:**391, 1972.

17. Stuart, R. B., and Davis, B.: Slim chance in a fat world: behavioral control of obesity, Champaign, Ill., 1972, Research Press Co.

18. Ferguson, J. M.: Habits, not diets, Palo Alto, Calif., 1976, Bull Publishing Co.

19. Nash, J. D., and Long, L. O.: Taking charge of your weight and well-being, Palo Alto, Calif., 1978, Bull Publishing Co.

20. Benson, H.: The relaxation response, New York, 1976, Avon Books.

21. Jencks, B.: Respiration for relaxation, invigoration, and special accomplishment, Salt Lake City, 1974, Beata Jencks Pub.

22. Payne, B.: Getting there without drugs: techniques and theories for the expansion of consciousness, New York, 1973, The Viking Press.

23. Stern, F. M., and Hoch, R. S.: Mind trips to help you lose weight, New York, 1977, Playboy Press.

24. Jencks, B.: Exercise manual for J. H. Schultz's standare autogenic training and special formulas, Salt Lake City, 1973, Beata Jencks Pub.

25. Kroger, W. S.: Clinical and experimental hypnosis, ed. 2, Philadelphia, 1977, J. B. Lippincott Co.

26. Kroger, W. S., and Fezler, W. D.: Hypnosis and behavior modification: imagery conditioning, Philadelphia, 1976, J. B. Lippincott Co.

27. Stanton, H. E.: Weight loss through hypnosis, Am. J. Clin. Hypnosis **18:**2, Oct., 1975.

28. Smiciklas-Wright, H., and D'Augelli, A. R.: Primary prevention for overweight: preschool eating pattern (PEP) program, J. Am. Diet. Assoc. **72:**626, June, 1978.

29. Weight control and obesity, Nutrition Education Resources Series, No. 7, Society for Nutrition Education, 2140 Shattuck Avenue, Berkeley, Calif., 1975.

General

American Dietetic Association: Exchange lists for meal planning, rev. ed., Chicago, 1976.

Asher, W. L., editor: Treating the obese, New York, 1974, Medcom, Inc.

Bray, G. A., and Bethume, J. E., editors: Treatment and management of obesity, New York, 1974, Harper & Row, Publishers, Inc.

Bruch, H.: The importance of overweight, New York, 1957, W. W. Norton & Co., Inc.

Bruch, H.: Eating disorders: obesity, anorexia nervosa, and the person within, New York, 1973, Basic Books, Inc.

Dudleston, A. K., and Bennion, M.: Effect of diet and/or exercise on obese college women, J. Am. Diet. Assoc. **56**(2):119, 1970.

Dwyer, J. T., and Mayer, J.: Potential dieters: who are they? J. Am. Diet. Assoc. **56**(6):510, 1970.

Hampton, M. C., Huenemann, R. L., Shapiro, L. R., and Mitchell, B. W.: Caloric and nutrient intakes of teenagers, J. Am. Diet. Assoc. **50:**385, 1967.

Hegsted, D. M.: Energy needs and energy utilization, Nutr. Rev. **32:**33, 1974.

Leveille, G. A., and Romsas, D. R.: Meal eating and obesity, Nutr. Today **9:**4, 1974.

Lewis, K. J., and Doyle, M. D.: Nutrient intake and weight response of women on weight control diets, J. Am. Diet. Assoc. **56**(2):119, 1970.

Mann, G. V.: Obesity, the nutritional spook, Am. J. Public Health **61**(8):1491, 1971.

Mann, G. V.: The influence of obesity on health, N. Engl. J. Med. **291:**178, 226, 1974.

Mayer, J.: Overweight, Englewood Cliffs, N.J., 1968, Prentice-Hall, Inc.

Moxley, R. T., III, Pozefsky, T., and Lockwood, D. Y.: Protein nutrition and liver disease after jejunoileal bypass for morbid obesity, N. Engl. J. Med. **290:**921, 1974.

Mulcare, D. B., Dennin, H. F., and Drenick, E. J.: Effect of diet on malabsorption after small bowel by-pass, J. Am. Diet. Assoc. **57**(4):331, 1970.

Nash, J. D., and Long, L. O.: Taking charge of your weight and well-being, Palo Alto, Calif., 1978, Bull Publishing Co.

Pi-Sunyer, F. X.: Jejunoileal bypass surgery for obesity, Am. J. Clin. Nutr. **29:**409, 1976.

Rilin, R. S.: Treatment of obesity with hormones, N. Engl. J. Med. **292:**26, 1975.

Ruffer, W. A.: Two simple indexes for identifying obesity compared, J. Am. Diet. Assoc. **57**(4):326, 1970.

Salans, L. B., Cushman, S. W., and Weismann, R. E.: Studies of human adipose tissue: adipose cell size and number in non-obese and obese patients, J. Clin. Invest. **52:**929, 1973.

Schacter, A., and Rodin, J.: Obese humans and rats, Hillsdale, N.J., 1974, Lawrence Erlbaum Associates, Inc.

Silverstone, T., editor: Obesity: its pathogenesis and management, Acton, Mass., 1975, Publishing Sciences Group, Inc.

Spargo, J. A., Heald, F., and Peckos, P. S.: Adolescent obesity, Nutr. Today **1**(4):2, 1966.

Stein, M. R., Julis, R. E., Peck, C. C., et al.: Ineffectiveness of human chorionic gonadotropin in weight reduction: a double blind study, Am. J. Clin. Nutr. **29:**940, 1976.

Stunkard, A. J.: The pain of obesity, Palo Alto, Calif., 1976, Bull Publishing Co.

Sundaravalli, O. E., Shurpalekar, K. S., and Rao, M. N.: Inclusion of cellulose in calorie-restricted diets, J. Am. Diet. Assoc. **62:**41, Jan., 1973.

Symposium on jejunoileostomy for obesity, Am. J. Clin. Nutr. **30**(1), 1977.

Tullis, I. F., and Tullis, K. F.: Obesity. In Schneider, H. A., Anderson, C. E., and Coursin, D. B., editors: Nutritional support of medical practice, New York, 1977, Harper & Row, Publishers, Inc.

Van Itallie, T. B., and Campbell, R. G.: Multidisciplinary approach to the problem of obesity, J. Am. Diet. Assoc. **61:**384, Oct., 1972.

Young, C. M., Frankel, D. L., Scanlan, S. S., et al.: Frequency of feeding, weight reduction, and nutrient utilization, J. Am. Diet. Assoc. **59:**473, Nov., 1971.

Young, C. M., Scanlan, S. S., Topping, C. M., et al.: Frequency of feeding, weight reduction, and body composition, J. Am. Diet. Assoc. **59:**466, Nov., 1971.

BEHAVIOR MODIFICATION

Arnheim, R., et al.: Psychology today: an introduction, ed. 2, Del Mar, Calif., 1972, CRM Books.

Bandura, A.: Principles of behavior modification, New York, 1969, Holt, Rinehart & Winston.

Ferguson, J. M.: Habits, not diets, Palo Alto, Calif., 1976, Bull Publishing Co.

Ferguson, J.: Learning to eat: behavior modification for weight control, Palo Alto, Calif., 1975, Bull Publishing Co. (leader's manual and student's manual).

Grinker, J.: Behavioral and metabolic consequences of weight reduction, J. Am. Diet. Assoc. **62:**30, Jan., 1973.

Hamilton, C. L.: Physiologic control of food intake, J. Am. Diet. Assoc. **62:**34, Jan., 1973.

Ikeda, J.: For teenagers only: change your habits to change your shape, Palo Alto, Calif., 1978, Bull Publishing Co.

Jordan, H. A.: In defense of body weight, J. Am. Diet. Assoc. **62:**17, Jan., 1973.

Jordan, H. A., and Levitz, L. S.: Behavior modification in a self-help group, J. Am. Diet. Assoc. **62:**27, Jan., 1973.

Leitenberg, H., editor: Handbook of behavior modification and behavior therapy, Englewood Cliffs, N.J., 1976, Prentice-Hall, Inc.

Levitz, L. S.: Behavior therapy in treating obesity, J. Am. Diet. Assoc. **62:**22, Jan., 1973.

Mahoney, M. J., and Mahoney, K.: Permanent weight control: a total solution to the dieter's dilemma, New York, 1976, W. W. Norton & Co., Inc.

Skinner, B. F.: Walden two, New York, 1948, The Macmillan Co.

Skinner, B. F.: Beyond freedom and dignity, New York, 1971, Alfred A. Knopf, Inc.

Stuart, R. B., and Davis, B.: Slim chance in a fat world: behavioral control of obesity, Champaign, Ill., 1972, Research Press.

Weisenberg, M., and Fray, E.: What's missing in the treatment of obesity by behavior modification? J. Am. Diet. Assoc. **65:**410, Oct., 1974.

CLINICAL HYPNOSIS

American Journal of Clinical Hypnosis, American Society of Clinical Hypnosis, 2400 East Devon Ave., Suite 218, Des Plaines, Ill., 60018.

American Society of Clinical Hypnosis, Education and Research Foundation: A syllabus on hypnosis and handbook of therapeutic suggestions, Des Plaines, Ill., 1973.

Barber, T. X.: Hypnosis: a scientific approach, New York, 1969, Van Nostrand Reinhold Company.

Jencks, B.: Exercise manual for J. H. Schultz's standard autogenic training and special formulas, Salt Lake City, 1973, Beata Jencks Pub.

Jencks, B.: Respiration for relaxation, invigoration, and special accomplishment, Salt Lake City, 1974, Beata Jencks Pub.

Kroger, W. S.: Clinical and experimental hypnosis, Philadelphia, 1963, J. B. Lippincott Co.

Payne, B.: Getting there without drugs: techniques and theories for the expansion of consciousness, New York, 1973, The Viking Press.

Reyher, J.: Hypnosis, Des Plaines, Ill., 1970, American Society of Clinical Hypnosis.

Schultz, J. H., and Luthe, W.: Autogenic training, New York, 1959, Grune & Stratton, Inc.

Selye, H.: The stress of life, New York, 1956, McGraw-Hill Book Co.

Stanton, H. E.: Weight loss through hypnosis, Am. J. Clin. Hypnosis **18:**2, Oct., 1975.

Tart, C. T.: Altered states of consciousness, New York, 1969, John Wiley & Sons, Inc.

EXERCISE, PHYSICAL ACTIVITY

Bailey, C.: Fit or fat, Pleasant Hill, Calif., 1977, Covert Bailey Pub.

Batten, J.: The complete jogger, New York, 1977, Harcourt Brace Jovanovich, Inc.

Cooper, K.: The new aerobics, New York, 1970, Bantam Books, Inc.

Cooper, M., and Cooper, K.: Aerobics for women, New York, 1970, Bantam Books, Inc.

Fixx, J. E.: The complete book of running, New York, 1977, Random House, Inc.

Jeffrey, D. B., and Katz, R. C.: Take it off and keep it off, Englewood Cliffs, N.J., 1977, Prentice-Hall, Inc. (Spectrum Books).

Lewis, S., Haskell, W. L., Wood, P. D., et al.: Effects of physical activity on weight reduction in obese middle-aged women, Am. J. Clin. Nutr. **29:**151, Feb., 1976.

Mitchell, C.: The perfect exercise: the hop, skip and jump way to health, New York, 1976, Simon & Schuster, Inc.

Sharkey, B. J.: Physiological fitness and weight control, Missoula, Mont., 1974, Mountain Press Publishing Co.

Ullyot, J.: Women running, Mountain View, Calif., 1977, World Publications.

Unger, L.: Walking: the perfect exercise, San Luis Obispo, Calif., 1977, Impact Publishers, Inc.

Vodak, P.: Exercise: the why and the how, Palo Alto, Calif., 1980, Bull Publishing Co.

25 Diabetes mellitus

HISTORY

Diabetes is an ancient disease. Its symptoms have been found described on an Egyptian papyrus—the Ebers Papyrus—dating about 1500 BC. In the first century the Greek physician Aretaeus wrote of a malady in which the body "ate its own flesh" and gave off large quantities of urine. He gave it the name *diabetes,* from the Greek word meaning "siphon" or "to pass through." Much later, in the seventeenth century, the word *mellitus,* from the Latin word for honey, was added because of the sweet nature of the urine. This addition distinguished it from *diabetes insipidus* (p. 190), another disorder in which the passage of copious amounts of urine was observed.

Over the years many scientists and physicians continued to puzzle over the mystery of diabetes, but the cause remained obscure. For physicians and their patients these years could be called the "Diabetic Dark Ages." Patients had short lives and were maintained on a variety of semistarvation regimens.

A beginning clue pointing to the involvement of the pancreas in the disease was provided by a young German medical student, Paul Langerhans. He found special clusters of cells scattered about the pancreas, so-called cellular islands or islets. These cells were different from the rest of the tissue. Although their function was still then unknown, these islet cells were named for their young discoverer—the islets of Langerhans. Soon after, in 1922, two Canadian scientists following this lead, F. G. Banting and his assistant, C. H. Best, isolated and identified the special substance secreted by these islet cells. It proved to be a hormone that regulates the oxidation of blood sugar and helps convert it to heat and energy. They called the new hormone *insulin,* from the Latin word *insula* meaning "island." For his discovery, Banting received a Nobel Prize and was knighted by his government.

Upon the fundamental base of sound diet therapy, insulin now continues to be the tool of control for diabetes, but the underlying metabolic problem even yet is unsolved. Insulin assay tests developed to measure the level of insulin activity in the blood have found insulin-like activity (ILA) levels in early diabetes to be two or three times the normal insulin levels. Investigators have postulated that the insulin is present but bound with a protein, hence making it unavailable.[1] Diabetes therefore results from the lack of insulin; whether the lack is in production by the pancreatic islet cells or at the level of availability in the blood is not entirely clear.

DESCRIPTION
Clinical manifestations

Diabetes has been found to be a hereditary disease. It is defined in terms of the clinical symptoms produced as a result of the lack of insulin. These symptoms appear as the diabetes develops.

1. Initial complaints
   a. Increased thirst (polydipsia)
   b. Increased urination (polyuria)
   c. Increased hunger (polyphagia)
   d. Weight loss (maturity onset frequently is opposite—the patient may be obese)
2. Clinical laboratory test data
   a. Glycosuria (sugar in the urine)
   b. Hyperglycemia (elevated blood sugar level)
   c. Abnormal glucose tolerance tests (With a glucose load the blood sugar rises to a higher level and takes a longer period to return to normal.)
3. Other possible overt symptoms
   a. Blurred vision
   b. Skin irritation or infections
4. If the diabetes continues uncontrolled
   a. Fluid and electrolyte imbalance
   b. Acidosis (ketosis)
   c. Loss of strength (weakness)
   d. Coma

Because the apparent symptoms, glycosuria and hyperglycemia, are related to excess glucose, diabetes has been called a disease of carbohydrate metabolism. However, as more has been learned about the intimate interrelationships of carbohydrate metabolism with fat and protein metabolism, it is increasingly viewed as a general metabolic disorder resulting from an insulin lack (absolute, partial, or due to its unavailability) affecting more or less each of the basic nutrients, especially the interrelated metabolism of the two fuels, carbohydrate and fat, in the body's energy system.

Classification

Juvenile onset. In its juvenile form, diabetes develops fairly rapidly and is more severe and unstable; the child is usually underweight. Acidosis is fairly common, and insulin therapy is required (see p. 450).

Maturity onset. In its maturity onset form, diabetes develops more slowly, is usually milder and more stable, and the patient may

be overweight. Acidosis is infrequent, and the majority of patients are maintained on oral hypoglycemics and diet therapy or by diet therapy alone.

Metabolic pattern

Normal blood sugar controls. A knowledge of the controls for maintaining a normal blood sugar level (70 to 120 mg/dl) is essential to an understanding of the impairment of these controls in diabetes. The basic metabolism of carbohydrates in Chapter 2 should be reviewed carefully. In Fig. 25-1, these normal control routes may be visualized. Entry of blood glucose from dietary carbohydrates, protein, and fat and from liver glycogen (glycogenolysis) maintains a steady supply of blood glucose. To prevent a continued rise above 120 mg/dl, several routes of glucose use are active:

1. Conversion to glycogen for storage in the liver (glycogenesis)
2. Conversion to fat (lipogenesis) and storage in adipose tissue
3. Conversion to muscle glycogen
4. Cell oxidation for energy

Insulin. Although its precise role is not entirely clear, insulin has an effect on these control mechanisms. It is believed to function in several ways (p. 24):

1. It facilitates the transport of glucose through the cell membrane.
2. It enhances the conversion of glucose to glycogen and its storage in the liver (glycogenesis).
3. It stimulates the conversion of glucose to fat (lipogenesis).
4. It influences glucose oxidation through the main glycolytic pathway by aiding the necessary initial phosphorylation reaction catalyzed by the enzyme glucokinase.

Glucagon. Subsequently, another pancreatic hormone was discovered, secreted by the alpha cells in the islets of Langerhans. Insulin is produced by adjacent beta cells. The new hormone was given the name *glucagon* because

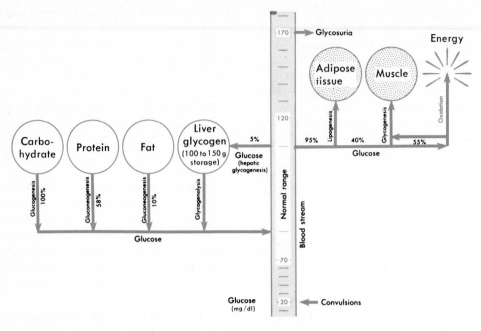

Fig. 25-1. Sources of blood glucose (food and stored glycogen) and normal routes of control.

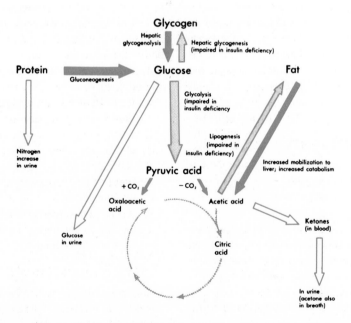

Fig. 25-2. Abnormal metabolism in uncontrolled diabetes. (From Harper, H. A.: Review of physiological chemistry, ed. 10, Los Altos, Calif., 1963, Lange Medical Publications.)

of its stimulating effect on *glycogenolysis,* the conversion of glycogen to glucose. It has an opposite action to insulin and is sometimes used to control more brittle or unstable diabetes. It acts as a counterbalance to excess insulin, that is, as treatment for insulin shock or hypoglycemic reactions.

Somatostatin. Recently a third hormone has been discovered that interacts with insulin and glucagon to control blood glucose levels. This is somatostatin, a hypothalamic hormone that suppresses the pancreatic hormones insulin and glucagon as needed to normalize blood glucose.[2,3]

Metabolic changes in diabetes. In uncontrolled diabetes, insulin is lacking to facilitate the operation of normal controls of the blood sugar level. Glucose cannot be oxidized properly through the main glycolytic pathway in the cell to furnish energy, and it therefore builds up in the blood (hyperglycemia). Fat formation (lipogenesis) is curtailed, and fat breakdown (lipolysis) increases, leading to excess ketone formation and accumulation (ketosis). The appearance of one of these ketones—*acetone*—in the urine indicates the development of ketosis. Tissue protein is also broken down in an effort to secure energy, causing weight loss and nitrogen excretion in the urine. These changes from normal metabolic pathways that operate in uncontrolled diabetes are illustrated in Fig. 25-2.

MEDICAL TREATMENT

Objectives of medical care. The physician and the clinical nutritionist have three basic objectives in the medical care of the diabetic patient.

The first objective is to maintain optimum nutrition. The patient's basic requirement is adequate nutrition for growth and development and the maintenance of an *ideal* weight. The leaner side of the average weight for height is wise, and any degree of overweight is to be avoided.

The second objective is to keep the patient relatively free of symptoms such as glycosuria and hyperglycemia.

The third is to prevent complications in tissues such as the eye (retinopathy), in nerve tissue (neuropathy), and in renal tissue (nephropathy). Coronary artery disease occurs in diabetics about four times as often as in the general population, and peripheral vascular disease occurs about 40 times as often. These chronic manifestations may be reduced by good care and control.

A fourth objective is increasingly being recognized and implemented by practitioners. This is the vital objective of sound, informed self-care by the person with diabetes, for ultimately the patient treats himself. More emphasis therefore is being placed on comprehensive diabetes education programs that build self-responsibility for good daily control.

Philosophies of control. Physicians vary as to their approaches to control measures. Some follow a philosophy of strict *chemical control,* seeking to constantly maintain a sugar-free urine. Others follow a more moderate *clinical control* approach, seeking to maintain the patient *relatively* free of clinical symptoms. Still others follow a *free control* approach, placing little or no control on the patient's diet and administering insulin if necessary accordingly. Whatever philosophy of diabetic management a particular physician may use, the basic *consistency* of habit prevails. Someone has expressed this important characterization as the three R's: *regulation, regularity,* and *routine.*

Whatever the individual practitioner's approach, the basic control of diabetes rests upon a balance of three important interrelated factors: (1) diet, (2) insulin, and (3) exercise.

DIET THERAPY
Nutritional needs: the diet prescription

The fundamental principles of the diet for an individual diabetic patient may be stated simply. *It is always based on the normal nutritional needs of that individual.* The personal diet is expressed in terms of total requirement of calories and a ratio of these calories in grams of carbohydrate, protein, and fat.

Calories. Calorie specifications are based on *ideal weight,* with allowances for physical activity or added stress, such as growth. If the patient is obese, as many adult diabetics are, then the diet prescription would indicate a sufficient reduction in calories to effect a gradual weight loss (about 1,200 to 1,500 calories per day). On the other hand, if the patient is a fast-growing, lean, adolescent boy, the calories may need to be as high as 4,000.

Carbohydrate. Current recommendations for carbohydrate are more liberal than in the past, both for energy needs and for smoother blood sugar control, with 50% to 55% of the total calories assigned here. However, the greater amount of the carbohydrate (about 40% of the total calories) should be used as complex carbohydrates (starches) that break down more slowly and release their available glucose over time. The remaining carbohydrate can be used as the simple sugars found in fruits, vegetables, and milk, which have a more immediate effect on the blood sugar level. The presence of fiber as in whole grains, fruits, and vegetables influences the transit time of the food mass and hence the rate of absorption of the available glucose (see p. 18). Refined sucrose or ''free' sugars should be avoided in habitual use. Sugar substitute sweeteners may be used with discretion.

Protein. Normal age group requirements for protein govern the amount indicated for the individual patient, with perhaps the optimum or upper range being the guidelines. About 20% of the total calories allotted to protein is a good general rule to follow.

Fat. Fat should always be used in moderation, with greater attention given to the control of saturated fats. This current recommendation is based on the general indication of a relationship between saturated fats and coronary artery disease and the greater risk factor of such

disease in diabetes. This relationship is the basis for the revised food exchange groups[6] used in planning diabetic diets (see p. 546). No more than 25% to 30% of the total calories should be given to fat, with about 15% of that total fat given to unsaturated fat and 15% to saturated fat.

In summary, the diabetic diet prescription is established as follows:

A. Calories—determination of energy needs based on sufficient calories to achieve and maintain ideal body weight and balance with exercise pattern.

B. Nutrient ratio
   1. *Carbohydrate* —50% of total calories. Convert to grams by dividing by its fuel factor of 4 (see p. 73). Use about 40% of the total calories as complex carbohydrate.
   2. *Protein* —20% of the total calories. Convert to grams by dividing by its fuel factor of 4.
   3. *Fat* —30% of the total calories, with about half each for saturated and unsaturated fat. Convert to grams by dividing by its fuel factor of 9.

Meal distribution

An important consideration is the distribution of the total diet through the day. This will be influenced by the type of control used—insulin, oral hypoglycemic agent, or diet alone.

Insulin. The schedule of the day's food intake pattern should be balanced with the type of insulin used and its pattern of absorption and activity peaks.

Short-acting insulin —regular crystalline, semilente. Short-acting insulins cover about a four-hour period of time and thus only the one meal following their use. These insulins are usually used in situations where short-term periods of control are indicated, such as in surgery, during labor and delivery, or in periods of illness. Also, for control of the more labile juvenile-onset diabetes, regular short-acting insulin may be mixed with the longer-acting insulin for smoother immediate control.

Medium-acting insulin—NPH (neutral protamine Hagedorn), lente, globin. NPH is the most widely used insulin preparation. Medium-acting insulins usually are given in the morning a half hour before breakfast, reach their peak of activity in eight to ten hours (about midafternoon), and last from 20 to 24 hours. The meal distribution may be considered a $1/5$, $2/5$, $2/5$ pattern, with allocations for a midafternoon and evening snack or with the snacks coming from lunch and dinner as three fairly equal meals. For some patients, particularly adult patients, the afternoon snack may not be as important, depending on the interval of time between lunch and dinner.

Long-acting insulin—PZI (protamine zinc insulin). PZI is rarely used now. Long-acting insulins require a more substantial evening meal and bedtime snack to cover the more prolonged period of activity through the sleep hours. The meal distribution is a $1/7$, $2/7$, $2/7$, $2/7$ pattern for each of the three meals and the bedtime snack.

MIXTURES OF INSULIN. Occasionally two types of insulin may be mixed in one syringe and given in one injection. For example, regular insulin may be mixed with NPH if more immediate morning coverage is required. In such cases a more substantial breakfast may be given and a midmorning snack as well as midafternoon and bedtime snacks. The morning snack is usually necessary only for the younger child.

Oral hypoglycemic drugs. Although there is some increased concern about their continued use, oral hypoglycemic agents may be used for some patients. General indications for the use of these medications include (1) maturity onset type of diabetes, (2) no history of ketosis or coma, and (3) presence of the diabetes for less than 10 years. Examples of these drugs are tolbutamide (Orinase), chlorpropamide (Diabinese), and acetohexamide (Dymelor). An additional oral hypoglycemic agent

phenformin (DBI), has been removed from the market because of some risks in its use indicated in recent research and clinical use. With oral medications a fairly even distribution of the diet is also important. These medications are thought to operate on the basis of stimulation they provide for the limited function of insulin-producing cells in the pancreas. There is insulin activity going on as a result of their use, and distribution of food to balance with this activity would naturally follow.

Diet alone. Even if the diabetes requires only diet control, there is still need to consider distribution through the day in a fairly consistent balance of meals. Since by definition in diabetes there is a limited tolerance for handling glucose, a load of glucose at any one point is to be avoided. There is better overall control with a balance of meals through the course of the day.

Diet management with exchange system

Recognizing the need for a more flexible and realistic approach to the dietary management of diabetes, a joint national committee with representatives from the American Diabetes Association and the American Dietetic Association formulated a system of dietary control based on the concept of food equivalents. This system of control was introduced in 1950. In this system, foods commonly used were grouped according to like nutrient composition and designated Food Exchange Groups. Six food groups were listed: milk, vegetables A and B, fruit, bread, meat, and fat. Within any one group, food items can be freely exchanged, since all foods in that group, in the portion indicated, are of approximately the same food value.

Since its introduction, the food exchange system has been widely accepted and used in health centers of all kinds for care and teaching of the diabetic patient. It has provided a simple and sound means of dietary regulation that is easily understood and flexible enough to meet a wide variety of living situations. The revised food lists incorporate the low saturated fat modification in subgroups and a few minor changes in vegetable groupings. Essentially, however, they are the same basic food groups in the food exchange system.[6]

The food exchange groups. The six food groups of the exchange system (see the food exchange groups listed on pp. 546-550 form the basic tools with which clinical nutritionists

may calculate diet needs and patients may learn to make wise food selections and substitutions. The composition and characteristics of these food groups are given in Table 25-1.

CALCULATION. Using the food exchange groupings, the nutritionist may easily calculate the individual diabetic patient's diet by a short method illustrated in Table 25-2.

Steps in calculation
1. Use the food groups and their designated nutrient values listed in Table 25-1 for

Table 25-1. Food exchange groups

| Food group | Unit of exchange | Composition | | | | Characteristic items |
		Carbo-hydrate (g)	Protein (g)	Fat (g)	Calories	
Milk	1 cup					Equivalents to 1 cup whole milk listed; 1 cup skim + 2 fat exchanges = whole milk
Skim		12	8	—	80	
Low fat		12	8	5	120	
Whole		12	8	10	170	
Vegetables						
A	As desired	—	—	—	—	Free use: 3% carbohydrate and below (tomatoes, green beans, leafy vegetables)
B*	½ cup	7	2	—	35	Medium carbohydrate: pod and root varieties (green peas, carrots)
Fruit	Varies	10	—	—	40	Fresh or canned without sugar Portion size varies with carbo-hydrate value of item; all portions equated at 10% carbohydrate
Bread	Varies; 1 slice bread	15	2	—	70	Variety of starch items, breads, cereals, vegetables; portions equal in carbohydrate value to 1 slice bread
Meat	28 g (1 oz)	—				Protein foods; exchange units equal to protein value of 28 g lean meat (cheese, egg, seafood)
Lean		—	7	2.5	50.5	
Medium fat		—	7	5	75	
Higher fat		—	7	7.5	95.5	
Fat	1 tsp					Fat food items equal to 1 tsp margarine (oil, mayonnaise, olives, avocados)
Polyunsaturated		—	—	5	45	
Monounsaturated		—	—	5	45	
Saturated		—	—	5	45	

*Eliminated in 1976 revised edition. However, in my own clinical practice I have retained this division for psychologic as well as physiologic reasons.

reference. Arrange the nutrient tabulation columns and the list of food exchange groups in the specific order given in Table 25-2.

2. Place the diet prescription (calories and grams of carbohydrate, protein, and fat derived as outlined on p. 560) in spaces indicated at tops of nutrient tabulation columns.

3. Make estimates of general use of the first three food items—milk, vegetable B (group A may be considered "free" and not calculated), and fruit. Base estimated allowances on general calorie level of diet, nature of food item, and its use by patient revealed in initial nutrition history.

4. Fill in nutrient values of the milk, vegetable B, and fruit items from values for single items given in Table 25-1.

5. Calculate the number of bread exchanges required to use the remaining carbohydrate in the diet prescription.
   a. Add the carbohydrate in the first three items (milk, vegetable, fruit), and subtract this amount from the day's total allowance of carbohydrate. The re-

maining carbohydrate will be used in bread exchanges.
   b. Divide the carbohydrate value of one bread exchange (15 g) into the remaining carbohydrate to be used. This will give the total number of bread exchanges. Fill in this number of exchanges and its nutrient values, both carbohydrate and protein, found by multiplying the single bread exchange values in Table 25-1.
   c. Total carbohydrate column. (Totals in each nutrient column within 3 to 4 g of indicated prescription are satisfactory.)

6. To calculate number of meat exchanges
   a. Add protein in items used thus far (milk, vegetable, bread). Subtract this amount from the day's total allowance of protein. The remaining protein will be used in meat exchanges.
   b. Divide the protein value of one meat exchange (7 g) into the remaining protein to be used. This will give the total number of meat exchanges. Fill in this number of exchanges and its nutrient

Table 25-2. Calculation of diabetic diet—short method using exchange system (2,200 calories)

Food group	Total day's exchanges	Carbo-hydrate (275 g)	Protein (82.5 g)	Fat (85.5 g)	Breakfast	Lunch	Dinner	Snacks PM	Snacks HS
Milk (low fat)	2	24	16	10	1				1
Vegetable A	As desired	—	—	—		As desired	As desired	As desired	
Vegetable B	1	7	2				1		
Fruit	5	50 / 81			1	1	1	1	1
Bread	13	195 / 276	26 / 44		3	3	3	2	2
Meat	6		42 / 86	30 / 40	1	2	3		
Fat, polyun-saturated	9			45 / 85	2	2	3	1	1

values, both protein and fat, found by multiplying the single meat exchange values in Table 25-1.

    c. Total protein column

7. To calculate the number of fat exchanges

    a. Add fat in items used thus far (milk, meat) and subtract from the day's total fat allowance.

    b. Divide value of one fat exchange (5 g) into the remaining fat to be used. This will give the total fat exchanges. Fill in this amount and its nutrient value.

    c. Total fat column

Meal pattern. The total number of exchanges calculated for each food group is distributed into the day's meal pattern to provide general overall distribution balance, cover any specific exercise periods, and balance with any oral medication or insulin used. (The example given above is the general pattern for use with medium-acting insulin.) If insulin is not used, as with many adult diabetics, meals should be divided fairly evenly, and a consistent pattern should be maintained.

Using the meal-snack pattern as a guide, the patient may make individual daily menus, choosing a variety of foods from the food exchange groups (pp. 546-550) in the amounts indicated in the food group lists and the basic meal pattern.

INDIVIDUAL ADAPTATION. Each patient's diet must be tailored to fit individual needs, living situation, and general eating habits. Therefore a careful diet history is an important first step in adapting the needed dietary pattern to the individual patient's life situation. If the diet is to be a useful therapeutic tool in the care of diabetes, it must be realistic and workable for each person on an individual basis.

Using the patient's diet history as a guide, the nutritionist outlines and discusses personal diabetic diet needs with the patient, determining what limited modifications of his present habits are wise. After the diet plan is in use,

follow-up counseling will determine any further adjustments or changes that are needed.

AMERICAN DIABETES ASSOCIATION DIETS. In the past, for the convenience of physicians, a series of nine diet plans had been outlined by the American Diabetes Association. These diets, ranging in caloric values from 1,200 to 3,000, are no longer issued or used, since they do not meet correct diet therapy recommendations as outlined here for nutrient ratios. Instead, personalized valid care can better be provided for patients with the service of a professional clinical nutritionist or dietitian by using the diet prescription and calculation method described above and the food exchange lists (p. 546) or the new revised listings adapted for individual need. The booklet "Exchange Lists for Meal Planning" is available from the American Diabetic Association or the local Diabetes Association affiliate or from the American Dietetic Association.

PATIENT EDUCATION

The key to satisfactory management of diabetes lies in sound, realistic patient education, initiated early and followed up as needed for reevaluation and reinforcement and support. A general admonition to stay away from starches and sweets is wholly inadequate and may well lead to bizarre food choices. Wise teaching based on a well-planned diet program is sound nutrition education. Frequently the nutrition of the whole family improves when the home meals are planned around the well-balanced outline given the diabetic member. Also, because the patient has a flexible plan that allows a variety of food choices, he is more likely to follow it and build the consistent food habits that give better long-range diabetic control.

What the diabetic patient must know

Education of the diabetic patient should include a thorough knowledge of all those factors that must be understood in order to assume responsible self-care. These factors are

1. The disease—general facts of diabetes, its nature, symptoms, and care
2. The diet—basic knowledge of food values, individual diet plan, and ways of using substitutes; practical guides in marketing and food preparation
3. Insulin or oral hypoglycemics—details of insulin administration and care of equipment or use of oral drugs; relation to food intake and exercise
4. Urine testing—methods of testing urine for sugar and acetone and recording of results
5. Exercise—its value in diabetic control and general health; its relation to balance with insulin and food
6. Skin care and hygiene—control of infection and maintenance of good circulation
7. Insulin shock—recognition of symptoms and knowledge of action to counteract those symptoms
8. Diabetic acidosis—recognition of symptoms and the need for immediate medical care
9. Personal identification—the necessity for a card or tag identifying diabetic needs, especially if on insulin
10. Educational resources—reading materials and community organizations providing services

Diet instructions
Methods

Individual counseling. The skilled personal diet counseling given a patient with newly diagnosed diabetes is the most valuable means of initiating a stable course. Regulation of the diabetes depends on securing the necessary cooperation of the patient and family. Sound knowledge is the basis of wise action and consistent habits. Therefore the initial dietary interview and the planning of the diet *with* the patient to meet individual needs are of primary importance.

Follow-up program. Follow-up interviews continue the learning process. Adjustments may be made, new material introduced, and former knowledge corrected or reinforced. Emotional support is provided for acceptance of the disease and the working-out of personal adjustments to its care. Involving other family members in the discussions strengthens the instructions and clarifies home needs.

Group instruction. Group instruction and discussion is a helpful adjunct to personal counseling. Classes are regularly held in many clinics. Physicians, clinical nutritionists and dietitians, and nurses share in the teaching responsibilities. The group discussions often reinforce personal decisions, and the exchange of ideas and experiences provides resources for learning.

Teaching materials

Visual aids and equipment. A number of audiovisual materials are available or can easily be constructed that enhance and clarify instruction. Wax, plastic, or cardboard food models help to picture portion sizes. Food models may also be prepared by dipping a measured portion of the real food (held in a strainer) into hot paraffin, then placing the mound of food on a cardboard circle to set and harden.[7] Later the hardened food portion may be encased in a thin film of plastic for cleanliness and protection. Different sizes of cups, glasses, and spoons will also help the patient to determine standard portion sizes.

Charts, diagrams, and pamphlets help to clarify factual material. Exhibits prepared around a basic facet of care provide additional background information. Films, filmstrips, and slides are useful for group discussion. Also, demonstration equipment for practice in insulin administration and urine testing is needed.

Programmed instruction. Teaching machines are used in some clinics to augment the patient education program. Usually this teaching method is well-accepted by patients and is effective. Although it cannot replace the necessary personal instruction—nor is it so intended—it is a helpful reinforcement, freeing the dietitian and the nurse from repetitive routine teaching so that they may do more creative work with patients. Some clinics are also expanding their education program to include the use of closed-circuit television in teaching.

Reading and reference material. A number of standard reference books have been provided for diabetic patients. Some of these are listed in the patient-education references at the end of this chapter.

Community resources. Other helpful pamphlets and booklets are provided by pharmaceutical firms, professional groups, and health organizations. Materials available from the American Diabetes Association are listed in the chapter references. Local chapters of the American Diabetes Association are active in many communities with annual detection drives, conferences, group meetings, and classes cooperatively sponsored by adult evening schools.

Medic Alert. An identification program for alerting medical personnel to the needs of persons with hidden health problems has been provided through the creative efforts of a California physician, Dr. Marion Collins. When his own daughter, a student nurse, suffered a near-fatal reaction to horse serum given in a routine postinjury tetanus injection, he designed for her an identifying metal disc to protect her from similar danger again in the course of routine care. Afterward he began to prepare identifying discs for his patients who had drug allergies or other hidden medical problems. In 1956 his plan was officially endorsed by the American College of Surgeons and is now a nonprofit service foundation with more than 150,000 American members and affiliated groups in a number of foreign countries.

The small stainless steel medallion, worn on a bracelet or necklace, carries the individual's assigned identification serial number, a brief warning of the medical problem, and a telephone number. The telephone number may be called collect, day or night, to reach the Central Answering Service in the foundation's Turlock, California, headquarters, where all members' records are on file and are available to medical personnel.

The small membership fee is paid only once. It includes the stainless steel medallion with emblem and a supplemental wallet card. Additional information may be obtained by writing Medic Alert Foundation International, Turlock, California 95380.

CASE STUDY 16

Kim and his family learn to live with diabetes

Kim Wong, aged 8, lived with his parents and two older brothers, ages 12 and 14, in San Francisco where Mr. Wong worked as a waiter in one of the fine Chinese restaurants. Kim was usually an active child, playing with his older brothers. The family was a very close one, and both sets of grandparents lived nearby. There were frequent large family gatherings.

Recently, however, Kim had begun to lose some of his usual energy. Mrs. Wong also noticed that his weight was steadily dropping, despite the fact that he seemed hungry all the time and was eating a great deal. He also was drinking more water than usual and urinating more frequently. One morning, when Kim said that he didn't feel well at all and couldn't go to school, his mother decided to take him to the doctor. At the office Dr. Barber examined Kim carefully, talked with Mrs. Wong, and did some simple urine and blood tests. As she had suspected, she found sugar in the urine and an elevated level in the blood.

When Dr. Barber told Mrs. Wong about the findings, she asked if there had been a family history of diabetes. Mrs. Wong answered that she was really not surprised. She had suspected this all along.

"Kim's father's diabetes was discovered just before we were married, when he went to have his examination and blood test." She smiled faintly. "In fact, we spent the time we had planned to be away on our honeymoon at the hospital and the doctor's office getting his diabetes regulated." She hesitated a moment and then went on, "I guess we just didn't want to face the fact that Kim had diabetes because we knew we had given it to him."

Dr. Barber made arrangements for Kim to be admitted to the hospital so that more definitive tests could be made and his diabetes could be regulated. She also wanted Kim and his family to have a careful plan of teaching during his hospital stay. After Kim was admitted to the hospital, the further tests on glucose tolerance did show an abnormal curve, and the fractional urine tests that were done through the days indicated an elevated and erratic pattern. There was also some positive testing for acetone in the urine.

Kim's reaction to his hospitalization was on the whole a positive one. Although he seemed a little bewildered by all the activities going on around him at first, he soon became accustomed to the hospital routine. His family visited often, his brothers brought him many of his things from home, and even his grandparents were there. He also received much support from the hospital staff. He responded well to treatment. His biggest concern, however, was with his food. He said he just never got enough, and besides, it wasn't like "our food" that mother made at home.

The clinical nutritionist, Mrs. Walker, assessed Kim's nutritional needs and started Kim's diet therapy at 1,600 calories because he was not as active just now. The diet would need to be built up gradually as his diabetes became more regulated and he needed more food. She indicated that the calories would be gradually increased to a maintenance level of about 2,000 for the present. Kim was to have three meals each day, with snacks between meals and in the evening. He was receiving 15 units of NPH insulin, plus 5 units of regular insulin. Gradually his urine tests, although still somewhat erratic, showed improvement.

The health care team taking care of Kim was aware that the educational aspect of his care was the key to his learning to live with his diabetes. This initial experience, the knowledge and skills gained from it, and even more the underlying attitudes developed during it would play a large part in determining how well Kim would be able to adapt to the disease and in general what the future course of the disease might be. In planning for the teaching that needed to be done, the clinical nutritionist talked with Mrs. Wong in detail about the family's food habits and with other members of the health team who had occasion to observe Kim and his reaction to his food in the hospital.

Continued.

During the next two weeks the health team worked with Kim and the Wongs in helping them learn the things they needed to know to control Kim's diabetes. A warm relationship developed. It was a good experience of a team effort on everyone's part. Mrs. Walker, the nutritionist, arranged several follow-up visits at the health center with Kim and Mrs. Wong to adjust Kim's diet as needed when he resumed his normal activities. She also contacted the school nurse at Kim's school and reviewed Kim's situation with her. Together they arranged for Kim to have the care he needed in any emergency that might arise. Kim's teacher at school was also involved in these conferences.

Questions to guide your inquiry
(Refer also to Chapter 19.)

1. What were the reasons for the initial symptoms Kim experienced at home?
2. What implications for counseling might exist because of the hereditary nature of the disease?
3. If Kim's mother had not been alert and taken him to the doctor when she did, what progression of Kim's symptoms might have occurred? Account for these progressive symptoms by the chain of metabolic imbalances occurring in uncontrolled diabetes.
4. In the initial therapy at the hospital, along with insulin, glucose, and diet, Dr. Barber also ordered daily tests on serum sodium and potassium levels. Why would close observance of these electrolyte levels be important and replacement therapy indicated?
5. In planning the overall educational program for Kim and his parents, Mrs. Walker listed all the items important for a person with diabetes to know. What would she have included in her list. Why?
6. Identify Kim's nutritional needs: (a) basic nutrition requirements for an 8-year-old boy and (b) Kim's specific needs or problems.
7. Outline the steps you would follow in teaching Kim and his parents about his diet. What is the role of the nutritionist in this plan? What are the nurse's responsibilities? What are the physician's responsibilities?
8. What cultural, social, or pyschologic factors would you need to consider in planning Kim's diet with his mother?
9. Outline a day's diet pattern and sample food plan (menu) for Kim to use at home after he returns to school on a 2,000 calorie diet. He is to continue three meals and three snacks.
10. What are some of the basic needs of ill children?
11. How may these basic needs of ill children, especially hospitalized children, be considered in planning for their nutritional care? What are some ways of achieving food acceptance?
12. What are the differences in juvenile diabetes, such as Kim's, and maturity-onset diabetes?
13. What are some of the basic opinions held by pediatricians concerning a philosophy of dietary management for diabetic children?
14. What are the basic principles of a moderate approach to dietary management of juvenile diabetes?
15. What is the general nature of the disease process in diabetes? How is the metabolism affected in the handling of carbohydrates? Protein? Fats?
16. Why must insulin be given by hypodermic injection rather than taken as an oral medication?
17. What is the relationship of the distribution of food through the day to the taking of insulin in the beginning of the day? Use Kim's insulin dosage, a mixture of NPH and regular insulin in one syringe, as an example of the balance he would need in his food pattern through the day. How would you explain this balance to Kim's mother?
18. What teaching materials or community resources would you involve in your educational plan for Kim and his family?

CASE STUDY 17
Control of diabetes in the midst of family problems

Rose Turrino, aged 45, learned two years ago that she had diabetes. In a routine checkup following a series of infections she had developed, her physician found sugar in a urine test. Her glucose tolerance test was positive, and fractional urine tests the following few weeks continued to show 1+ to 2+ sugar. The doctor had started her on oral hypoglycemic medication, chlorpropamide, morning and evening. Rose weighed 93 kg (205 lb) and was 163 cm (5 ft, 5 in) tall. However, she had not returned to the clinic as the doctor had instructed or followed up on his caution that she must lose weight. She did purchase the medications and promised to take them.

Mrs. Turrino was a warm, outgoing Italian woman whose life centered in her family. Her husband worked a rotating shift at an assembly plant nearby and so had to be away from the home a great deal of the time. Food played a large part in their family life, and Rose was known for her excellent Italian cooking. But money was scarce—Rose said there was barely enough for living expenses—although she managed somehow by careful planning.

Rose's three children had all been large babies, weighing between 4,000 and 4,500 g (9 and 10 lb) at birth. Now they were all teenagers. Robert was 19, and the girls, Linda and Laura, were 17 and 15. Rose was concerned about her children's problems of growing up in two cultures and in a changed world, a world that sometimes seemed strange to her.

Now Rose was in the hospital, recovering from diabetic acidosis. She explained that she had been too involved in her children's problems to care for herself. She had been inconsistent in taking her medication and had not followed her diet. In fact, she had even gained a few more pounds. When Robert had started using drugs—"pep pills," "speed," mescaline—and dropped out of school, it had been a great blow to her. But she realized now that she could not help her family by becoming ill herself.

She had responded well to treatment, however, and was now regulated on 40 units of NPH insulin and a diet of 1,200 calories. The clinical nutritionist again emphasized how important it was that she begin to lose weight and keep her appointments in the clinic for follow-up care and diabetes education, so that she could learn how to take care of herself.

Questions to guide your inquiry
(Also refer to Chapter 24.)

1. What factors do you think contributed to Rose's experience with acidosis? Why? What relation do these factors have to diabetes control?
2. What data given here about Rose as a person and about her disease do you think are significant in assessing her nutritional needs? Why?
3. What additional information would be important for you to have? Why? How would you obtain it?
4. On the basis of the information you have, what nutritional problems do you identify? What is the scientific basis for each problem?
5. What goals in relation to the problems identified do you think are important and realistic for the health team and Rose to establish?
6. Outline a plan of action to reach these goals. Consider present needs and future needs. Give scientific reasons for your actions.
7. What sort of response do you think Rose will make to her care plan? Why?
8. Why is a comprehensive educational program, including follow-up care, a vital component in the care of persons with diabetes?
9. What do you think such an educational program should include?
10. Outline a day's menu plan for Rose to use after she goes home. Include the basic food pattern (for 1,200 calories) from which you planned the menu.

Continued.

CASE STUDY 17
Control of diabetes in the midst of family problems—cont'd

11. What are the basic principles of diet management in control of diabetes? Give the reasons for each.
12. What practical problems will Rose have at home relating her own dietary needs to family needs? What solutions can you suggest?
13. Since Rose is on insulin, what distribution of her food through the day will be important for balance with the insulin activity?
14. What is the "exchange system" for dietary control? What are the food groups in this system?
15. Why is exercise important for Rose? What forms would you suggest?
16. What practical teaching-learning aids do you think would be helpful to Rose?
17. What community resources might she use?
18. Why is it so imperative that Rose lose weight?
19. Considering the background information you have about Rose, what factors do you think have contributed to her weight problem?
20. The nutritionist has indicated to Rose that she would like her to lose about 900 g (2 lb) a week. How many fewer calories daily will be necessary for Rose to eliminate from her usual intake to achieve this rate of loss?
21. What do you think would be a realistic weight goal for Rose?
22. Why is a program of follow-up appointments with the nutritionist important for a person in Rose's situation? What sort of activities may be involved in such follow-up conferences? What purpose would they serve?
23. Summarize the essential characteristics of a sound plan for weight control.

REFERENCES
Specific

1. Antoniades, H. N., Bougas, J. A., and Pyle, H. M.: Studies on the state of insulin in blood, N. Engl. J. Med. **267:**218, Aug. 2, 1962.
2. Gerich, J. E., Lorenzi, M., Bier, D. M., et al.: Prevention of human diabetic ketoacidosis by somatostatin. Evidence for an essential role of glucagon, N. Engl. J. Med. **292:**985, May 8, 1975.
3. Maugh, T. H.: Diabetes (III): new hormones promise more effective therapy, Science **188:**920, 1975.
4. West, K. M.: Prevention and therapy of diabetes mellitus, Nutr. Revi. **33:**193, 1975.
5. Wood, F. C., and Bierman, E. L.: New concepts in diabetic dietetics, Nutr. Today **7:**4, May-June, 1972.
6. American Diabetes Association: Exchange lists for meal planning, rev. ed., New York, 1976.
7. Moore, M. C., et al.: Using graduated food models in taking dietary histories, J. Am. Diet. Assoc. **51:**447, 1967.

General
DIABETES

Albrink, M. J.: Dietary and drug treatment of hyperlipidemia in diabetes, Diabetes **23:**913, 1974.
Cole, H. S., and Camerini-Davalos, R. A.: New concepts of the diet therapy of diabetes mellitus. In Halpern, S. L., editor: Quick reference to clinical nutrition, Philadelphia, 1979, J. B. Lippincott Co.
Eaton, R. P.: Evolving role of glucagon in human diabetes mellitus, Diabetes **24:**523, 1975.
Friedman, G. J.: Diet in treatment of diabetes mellitus. In Goodhart, R. S., and Shils, M. E., editors: Modern nutrition in health and disease, ed. 6, Philadelphia, 1980, Lea & Febiger.
Jackson, R. L.: The child with diabetes, Nutr. Today **6**(2):2, 1971.
Lum, B. O.: The learning environment, J. Am. Diet. Assoc. **69:**161, 1976.
Meissner, C., et al.: Antidiabetic action of somatostatin assessed by artificial pancreas, Diabetes **24:**988, 1975.

Miranda, P. M., and Horowitz, D. L.: High-fiber diets in the treatment of diabetes mellitus, Ann. Intern. Med. **88:**482, April, 1978.

Nuttall, F. Q., and Brunzell, J. D.: Commentary: principles of nutrition and dietary recommendations for individuals with diabetes mellitus, 1979, J. Am. Diet. Assoc. **75:**527, Nov., 1979.

Power, L.: New approaches to the old problem of diabetes education, J. Nutr. Educ. **5:**230, 1973.

Sharkey, T. P.: Diabetes mellitus—present problems and new research. I. Prevalence in the U.S. II. Obesity. III. Glucose tolerance and aging, J. Am. Diet. Assoc. **58**(3):201, 1971.

Sharkey, T. P.: Diabetes mellitus—present problems and new research. IV. The heart and vascular disease. V. Biochemical abnormalities in atherosclerosis, J. Am. Diet. Assoc. **58**(4):336, 1971.

Sharkey, T. P.: Diabetes mellitus—present problems and new research. VI. Nephropathy and neuropathy, J. Am. Diet. Assoc. **58**(5):442, 1971.

Sharkey, T. P.: Diabetes mellitus—present problems and new research. VII. Retinopathy. VIII. References, J. Am. Diet. Assoc. **58**(6):528, 1971.

Unger, R. H.: Glucagon and blood sugar, N. Engl. J. Med. **294:**1239, 1976.

Weinsier, R. L., Seeman, A., Herrera, M. G., et al.: Diet therapy of diabetes. Description of a successful methodologic approach to gaining diet adherence, Diabetes **23:**699, Aug., 1974.

West, K. M.: Diet therapy of diabetes: an analysis of failure, Ann. Intern. Med. **79:**425, 1973.

West, K. M.: Prevention and therapy of diabetes mellitus. In Hegsted, M., et al.: Nutrition reviews, present knowledge in nutrition, ed. 4, Washington, D.C., 1976, The Nutrition Foundation, Inc.

West, K. M.: Diabetes mellitus. In Schneider, H. A., Anderson, C. E., and Coursin, D. B., editors: Nutritional support of medical practice, New York, 1977, Harper & Row, Publishers.

Williams, S. R.: Pregnancy and diabetes. In Worthington-Roberts, B., Vermeersch, J., and Williams, S.: Nutrition in pregnancy and lactation, ed. 2, St. Louis, 1981, The C. V. Mosby Co.

Wyse, B. W.: Nutrient analysis of exchange lists for meal planning. I. Variation in nutrient levels. J. Am. Diet. Assoc. **75:**238, Sept., 1979.

PATIENT EDUCATION

ADA Forecast, magazine published bimonthly by the American Diabetes Assoc., Inc., 18 E. 48th St., New York, N.Y. 10017.

ADA Meal Planning Booklet, Exchange lists for meal planning, rev. ed., 1976, The American Diabetes Association. Also: Diabetic Diet Card for Physicians.

Cooper, K. H.: The new aerobics, New York, 1970, Bantam Books, Inc.

Danowski, T. S.: Diabetes as a way of life, ed. 2, New York, 1964, Howard-McCann, Inc.

Dolger, H., and Seeman, B.: How to live with diabetes, New York, 1965, W. W. Norton & Co., Inc. (Paperback edition, New York, 1973, Pyramid Books).

Duncan, G. G.: A modern pilgrim's progress—with further revelations—for diabetics, ed. 2, Philadelphia, 1967, W. B. Saunders Co.

Duncan, T. G., Lodewich, P. A., and Schatanoff, J.: The good life with diabetes, Philadelphia, 1973, The Garfield Duncan Research Foundation, Inc.

Ferguson, M. P.: An introduction to diabetes for the young child, Springfield, Ill., 1972, Charles C Thomas, Publisher.

Gormican, A.: Controlling diabetes with diet, Springfield, Ill., 1971, Charles C Thomas, Publisher.

Jones, J.: The calculating cook, San Francisco, 1972, 101 Productions, Inc.

Marble, A., White, P., Bradley, R. F., and Krall, L. P., editors: Joslin's diabetes mellitus, ed. 11, Philadelphia, 1971, Lea & Febiger.

Middleton, K., and Hess, M. A.: The art of cooking for the diabetic, Chicago, 1978, Contemporary Books, Inc.

Revell, D. T.: Gourmet recipes for diabetics, Springfield, Ill., 1971, Charles C Thomas, Publisher.

Rosenthal, H., and Rosenthal, J.: Diabetic care in pictures, Philadelphia, 1960, J. B. Lippincott Co.

Standford, E. D.: Feet first, Division of Nursing, Public Health Service, Washington, D.C., 1970, Government Printing Office.

Sussman, K., and Metz, R., editors: Diabetes mellitus, New York, 1975, American Diabetes Association.

Tani, G. W., and Hankin, J. H.: A self-learning unit for patients with diabetes, J. Am. Diet. Assoc. **58:**331, 1971.

Travis, L. B.: Juvenile diabetes mellitus: an instructional aid, ed. 5, Galveston, Tex., 1978, University of Texas.

26

Gastrointestinal diseases

GENERAL DIETARY CONSIDERATIONS

Personal needs. The gastrointestinal tract is a sensitive mirror of the individual human condition. Its physiologic functioning reflects both physical and psychologic conditioning. In adapting diet therapy for patients with gastrointestinal disorders, the practitioner is dealing not so much with a specific food item per se, as with the state of the body that receives it. There is far more truth than mere humor to the statement, "Surrounding every stomach there is a person."

Physiologic functions. The digestion and absorption of the food a person eats is accomplished in the gastrointestinal tract through a series of intimately related secretory and neuromuscular mechanisms. In Chapter 10 this normal network of functions was summarized and forms the basis for understanding general dietary modifications used in diseases that hinder the normal operation of these mechanisms.

Factors involved in diet therapy. Diet therapy for various gastrointestinal disorders, therefore, will be determined by a consideration of four basic factors involved. Three of these factors are physiologic:

1. The secretory functions that provide the necessary environment and agents for chemical digestion
2. The neuromuscular functions that provide the necessary motility for mechanical digestion and move the food mass along

3. The absorptive functions that enable the end products of digestion (the nutrients) to enter the body's circulation and nourish the cells

The fourth factor affects each of the others. It is the *psychologic influence*. The individual's particular emotional makeup and his manner of coping with life's day-to-day problems and challenges will often be reflected in the functions of his digestive tract. Here again, it is not what he eats, it's what is eating him that is important.

The principles of nutritional care in each of the gastrointestinal disorders discussed here will concern in some way (1) chemical secretions, (2) degree of motility, (3) absorbing mucosa, and (4) the person himself.

PEPTIC ULCER
Etiology

Peptic ulcer is the general term given to an eroded mucosal lesion in the stomach or the duodenum. Gastric ulcers are less common; most occur in the duodenal bulb where gastric contents emptying into the duodenum through the pyloric valve are most concentrated.

The fundamental cause of peptic ulcer is not clear. However, two factors seem to be involved: (1) the amount of gastric acid and pepsin secreted and (2) the degree of tissue resistance to withstand the digestive action of these secretions. In the development of gastric ulcers, although the presence of acid is essential, the degree of tissue sensitivity seems to be the paramount factor. In the patient with duodenal ulcer, excess production of acid and pepsin is the primary factor. In either case, hydrochloric acid in the gastric juice is generally acknowledged to be the essential factor in the development, perpetuation, and recurrence of peptic ulcer.

The psychogenic factor in peptic ulcer is variable. The so-called ulcer personality has been described in many texts. Although overdrawn perhaps in some sources, the ulcer-prone individual does tend to be anxious or tense, aggressive, and competitive. Peptic ulcer usually occurs in men between the ages of 20 and 50 years, a time of life when career and personal strivings may be at a peak.

Clinical manifestations

Increased gastric tone and painful hunger contractions when the stomach is empty are cardinal symptoms of peptic ulcer. The amount and concentration of hydrochloric acid is increased in duodenal ulcer, but may be normal in gastric ulcer. Nutritional deficiencies may be manifest in low plasma protein levels, anemia, and loss of weight. Hemorrhage may be the first sign of the ulcer in some patients. Confirmation of the diagnosis comes from clinical findings, X-ray tests, or visualization by gastroscopy.

General medical management

Three factors form the basis of medical care: (1) *drug therapy* and antacids, to counteract hypermotility and hypersecretions, (2) *rest,* both physical and mental, aided as needed by sedative therapy, and (3) *diet therapy,* to provide maximum restorative powers and prevent further tissue damage.

Diet therapy

The general term "bland" has been used to describe the various ulcer regimens found in common practice. The word comes from the

Latin word *blandus* meaning "a smooth tongue" or "soothing" and has taken on the connotation of something insipid, dull, uninteresting, and unattractive. Such meanings are all too often conveyed by the ulcer routines in many hospital diets that are nutritionally inadequate, esthetically repelling, scientifically unsound, and emotionally disturbing. That such a state need not be is increasingly made evident by research that indicates that the usual rigid and restrictive approach is based more on tradition and assumption than on scientific fact. Perhaps a better perspective may be gained by seeing the background development of diet therapy for peptic ulcer, the rationale given for the traditional conservative management, and the current challenge by the liberal individual approach.

History of dietary treatment for peptic ulcer. The roots of diet manipulation in the treatment of patients with peptic ulcer extend far back in medical history. As early as the first century, Celsus ordered smooth diets free of "acrid" food, and practitioners of the seventh century wrote of their belief in "special healing properties" of milk for patients with digestive disturbances. In the first half of the nineteenth century, peptic ulcer became established as a pathologic and clinical entity, and physicians generally advocated a liberal dietary regimen with frequent feedings.

However, in the later part of the nineteenth century a radical change developed in medical opinion concerning peptic ulcer treatment. The belief spread that food was harmful to the ulcer, and only complete rest—meaning an empty stomach—would allow the stomach to heal itself. Semistarvation regimens became the accepted practice among European physicians and were soon introduced in the United States.

In 1915 an American physician, Bertram Sippy,[1] broke the common practice of initial starvation treatment and established the beginning principles of continuous control of gastric acidity through diet and alkaline medication. However, his rigidly outlined program of milk and cream feedings with slow additions of single soft food items over a prolonged period of time allowed little variation for individual need to nutritional adequacy. Some increase in diet was made in 1935 by a Danish physician, Meulengracht,[2] who introduced a more liberal approach in feeding peptic ulcer patients, especially as treatment for hemorrhage. In the main, however, Sippy's regimen, although clearly establishing the important acid neutralizing principle of frequent feedings, continued to place rigid restrictions on the traditional dietary programs followed in common practice.

Traditional conservative dietary management. Although many changes in details of management have occurred since Sippy's day, his general restrictive pattern has been the mold for much of the traditional conservative management still used in some clinical settings today. This traditional diet therapy is based on several principles. The food must be both acid neutralizing and nonirritating.

ACID NEUTRALIZING. Therapy begins with milk and cream feedings every hour or so to neutralize free acid with milk protein, suppress gastric secretion with cream, and generally soothe the ulcer by coating it. These assumptions have not been supported by research.

There are gradual additions of soft bland foods over a period of time, keeping some food in the stomach at all times to mix with the acid to prevent its corrosive action on the ulcer. These bland foods are usually limited to choices of white toast or crackers, refined cereals, egg, mild cheeses, a few cooked pureed fruits and vegetables, and later, ground meat.

NONIRRITATING. The diet therapy is designed to eliminate chemical, mechanical, and thermal irritation.

CHEMICAL IRRITATION. Any food believed to stimulate gastric secretions is prohibited. These include highly seasoned foods, meat extractives, coffee, tea, alcohol, citrus fruit juices, fried foods, spices, and flavorings.

MECHANICAL IRRITATION. Any food believed to be abrasive in its effect on the ulcer is prohibited. These include all raw foods, plant fibers (strained fruits and vegetables are used), coarse or rough foods, whole grains, and "gas-forming" or strongly flavored foods.

THERMAL IRRITATION. Any very hot or cold food believed to irritate the lesion by its effect on surface blood vessels is prohibited. These include hot beverages and soups, frozen desserts or iced beverages.

After initial hourly milk and cream only, the diet is gradually increased as the ulcer heals. The routine usually follows a progressive four-stage pattern similar to that shown on pp. 576-578.

Liberal individual approach. Accumulating experience and research, however, has begun to challenge the validity of some of these beliefs. In the 1940s the classic experiments of Wolf and Wolff[3] with their fistulous subject demonstrated the influence of various environmental stimuli. The irritating effect of emotional tension was verified by their observations of engorged blood vessels of the stomach fistula mucosa, increased acid production, and active motility when the man was provoked and anxious. Wolf[4] later fed a variety of highly seasoned foods to a fistulous subject whose stomach and duodenum were normal and to a second patient with a gastric fistula who also had an active duodenal ulcer. No evidence of irritation to the gastric mucosa appeared in either subject. Wolf even applied several chemicals, including strong condiments, directly through the fistulas to the gastric mucosa of the two subjects. At the same time he also applied the same materials to the skin of their forearms. There was no remarkable effect on the gastric mucosa; the greater reaction was on the skin.

Several other English physicians followed up Wolf's studies with experiments of their own. Gill[5] reported a series of studies with chronic ulcer patients whose ulcers healed in four to eight weeks with placebo treatment of a daily injection of 1 ml of distilled water and no diet or exercise restrictions or medications. He concluded that ulcers healed not by manipulation of the various common therapies used but because "the man with the ulcer comes under the care of a physician who is able to transmit some of his own confidence to the patient." Larger groups of patients with gastric and duodenal ulcers were studied by Lawrence,[6] Todd,[7] and Doll's group.[8] In each instance the results were the same. They each concluded that the current concept of rigid dietary treatment was not verified as superior or sound therapy. Bland foods did not increase the rate of healing, nor was there any particular benefit from avoidance of all foods thought to be commonly irritating.

Studies by American physicians supported these results of English workers. Kramer[9] treated a group of clinic patients with duodenal ulcers with a routine schedule consisting of milk, antacid, and the regular ingestion of foods as desired. There was no dietary restriction. Each patient ate as he chose. Relief and healing in these patients was the same as with those on a strict bland diet. Miller and Berkowitz[10] demonstrated the same results in a large series of patients. Satisfactory healing in peptic ulcer disease was obtained on a much more liberal dietary regimen than is conventionally prescribed.

The question of food influence on gastric acidity and irritation has been investigated by several workers. Schneider's group[11] tested a number of spices and herbs on patients with active and healing ulcers and checked the responses by gastroscopy and personal patient reactions. There was no irritating effect from a number of common spices and herbs (allspice, caraway seeds, cinnamon, mace, paprika, thyme, sage) when they were used with foods. Only slight effects were noted by some patients from chili powder, nutmeg, mustard seeds, cloves, and black pepper. The effect of foods on the gastric acidity was studied by Saint-Hilaire's group.[12] The sight, smell, and taste of most food normally initiated gastric secretion. But no significant change in gastric pH was noted with any items, except in the case of alcohol, caffeine, meat extractives, and black pepper. Also no food is sufficiently acid of itself to effect a significant pH change or cause direct irritation of an ulcer.

Protein foods are effective buffering agents because of their amphoteric nature (p. 53). Milk has some buffering effect, but other protein foods seem to be as effective or more so. All proteins influence acid secretion, however, more than do carbohydrates and fats. Any form of fat tends to suppress gastric secretion and motility through the enterogastrone mechanism (p. 208). Volume of any food sufficient to exert antrum pressure stimulates gastric secretion through the gastrin mechanism (p. 208).

The routine omission of any fiber in the diet also seems to have no basis in fact. Individual modes of eating, improper mastication, and rapid consumption of meals are more involved as sources of irritation. Many clinicians, such as Shull,[13] contend from their experiences with individual patients that so-called coarse or rough foods, such as lettuce, raw fruits, celery, cabbage, and nuts, do not necessarily traumatize a peptic ulcer when they are properly chewed and mixed with saliva. Grinding or straining of food is needed only when teeth are poor or absent.

Foods labeled "gas formers" also are questionable routine omissions for all patients with peptic ulcers. Koch and Donaldson[14] found little consistency in the replies of 655 hospitalized patients concerning individual tolerances for standard foods such as onions, fried foods, cabbage, coffee, baked beans, orange juice, milk, nuts, and spices foods. Symptoms and responses varied widely among the patients, with no greater frequency of intolerance in those with gastrointestinal disease than in those with no disorder of the gastrointestinal tract. It was entirely a matter of individual response.

Graduated bland diet for peptic ulcer

General description

1. Avoid overeating at any one meal. It is better to eat smaller amounts more often.
2. Eat slowly and chew thoroughly. Sip liquids slowly, especially hot or cold ones.
3. Avoid worry, tension, argument, hurry, and fatigue, particularly at mealtime.
4. Avoid monotony in diet by varying the foods used as much as the diet allows.
5. Use no spices or seasonings except salt. Avoid concentrated sweets. Small amounts of sugar may be used.
6. Do not drink over a glass of liquid with each meal, but drink as much as desired between meals.
7. Take medications regularly as directed.
8. Follow all directions carefully and include only that part of the following diet list which is prescribed. Make the additions to the diet only as the physician advises it.
9. Maintain regular hours for eating, and take meals regularly.

Stage I

Food	Allowed	Not allowed
Milk	Regular or homogenized buttermilk	
Cream	Plain or mixed with milk	
Fats	Fresh butter or fortified margarine	Any others
Eggs	Boiled, poached, coddled; plain omelet or scrambled in double boiler; eggnog with vanilla only	Fried eggs
Cereals	Cooked refined or strained; oatmeal, cream of wheat, Farina, Wheatena, precooked infant cereals; also plain buttered noodles, macaroni, spaghetti, or white rice Dry cereals such as cornflakes, puffed rice, Rice Krispies, without bran	Whole grain cereals; cereals containing bran or shredded wheat
Desserts	Plain custard, Jell-O, rennet, plain cornstarch, tapioca or rice puddings; plain vanilla ice cream (if allowed to melt in mouth)	Any other
Bread	Enriched white; fine rye or fine whole wheat bread at least one day old (may be plain or toasted); soda crackers, zweibach, melba toast, hard rolls	Whole wheat and other whole grain bread; graham or coarse crackers; hot or fresh bread
Cheese	Cream, cottage cheese, mild processed American and Swiss	All other
Sweets	Jelly (clear, plain), honey, sugar (in moderation), strained cranberry sauce	Any other
Potato	White, baked, boiled, creamed; boiled or baked sweet potatoes or yams in moderate amounts	Any other

Graduated bland diet for peptic ulcer—cont'd

Stage I—cont'd

Food	Allowed	Not allowed
Cream soups	Homemade cream soups from the following pureed vegetables: asparagus spinach pea potato green bean tomato	Canned cream soups; soups from any other vegetables; dehydrated soups, chicken soups, broths, meat stock, bouillon

Stage II

Food	Allowed	Not allowed
Fruit juices	Strained orange juice, beginning with ¼ cup, diluted with water and taken at the end of the meal Later can be undiluted; prune juice if necessary for bowel regulation; grapefruit juice may be added later if tolerated	Any other
Plain cake	Angel food, sponge, pound, butter cake (without frosting)	Any cakes made with nuts, dates, spices, frostings
Vegetables (Group 1)	Winter squash, banana squash, or acorn squash; tomato juice if tolerated The following cooked and strained, or prepared infant strained vegetables; asparagus, peas, carrots, green beans, beets, spinach	Any other, also raw or coarse vegetables
Fruits (Group 1)	The following stewed, cooked fruits that have been strained (or prepared strained infant fruits): pear, peach, prune, apricot, applesauce	All other

Stage III

Food	Allowed	Not allowed
Fowl	Tender white or dark meat boiled, broiled, roasted, or baked; of turkey, chicken, squab, or pheasant	Fried, braised, or in any other form; skin, gristle, or fat
Fish	Fresh or frozen; boiled, broiled, or baked; scalded canned tuna or salmon; oysters, fresh or canned	Other canned fish or prepared in any other manner; smoked, pickled, preserved fish, crab, lobster, sardines
Meats	At first, only finely ground, plain beef; later, tender cuts of beef, veal, lamb; also liver, sweetbreads, brains (boiled, broiled, creamed, roasted)	Fried, smoked, pickled, cured; skin, gristle, fat, meats with tough fiber; delicatessen pork, ham, bacon, salami, weiners

Stage IV

Food	Allowed	Not allowed
Desserts	Prune or apricot whip; plain vanilla, chocolate, or sugar cookies or wafers; plain sherbet, water ices, ice cream, if eaten slowly; fine graham crackers	Rich pastries or pies, nuts, raisins, coconut; gingerbread, spice cake, candy

Continued.

Graduated bland diet for peptic ulcer—cont'd

Stage IV—cont'd

Food	Allowed	Not allowed
Vegetables (Group 2)	Tender whole cooked vegetables: asparagus, squash, carrots, spinach, peas, string beans, beets, mushrooms, tomatoes, peeled	Onions, celery, sauerkraut, cucumbers, peppers, turnips, radishes, cabbage, cauliflower, broccoli, brussels sprouts; any coarse vegetables; hull or fiber of green vegetables; salads or coleslaw
Fruits (Group 2)	Canned or cooked without skins or seeds: pear, apricot, peach, persimmon; Nectar from pear, peach, or apricot; juices of apple, grapefruit, or orange	
Beverages	Weak tea, weak cocoa, Sanka, Postum; plain milkshakes	Coffee, strong tea or coffee, iced drinks, soft drinks, alcoholic beverages of any kind
Miscellaneous	Homemade mayonnaise without spices; duck; crisp bacon; vegetable oils or shortening; less tender cuts of meat (properly prepared) such as beef round, cutlet; sour cream, yogurt; brown sugar, powdered sugar; mint jelly	Spices or condiments, pepper, horseradish, meat sauces, catsup, mustard, vinegar, pickles, relishes, olives; spicy foods of any kind; fried foods of any kind; gravies; hot cakes and other hot breads; chewing gum

BASIC PRINCIPLES OF LIBERAL DIETARY MANAGEMENT. In the light of studies such as the preceding and the accumulative experiences of many physicians in daily practice, what reasonable principles of diet therapy for peptic ulcer disease may be concluded? Certainly more extensive and controlled research will continue to give needed knowledge on which to base treatment and will aid in distinguishing between assumption and fact and between traditional belief and scientific finding. That sound dietary management does play an important part in total therapy is clear. But it seems equally clear that the individual must be the focus of treatment. It is not *an* ulcer; it is *his* ulcer. It is conditioned by his unique makeup and life situation, and the presence of the ulcer in turn affects the patient's life.

Therefore two basic principles guide the more liberal approach:

1. *The individual must be treated as such.* A careful initial history will give information about daily living situations, attitudes, food reactions, and tolerances. On the basis of such a history a reasonable and adequate dietary program *that he can follow* may be worked out.

2. *The activity of the patient's ulcer will influence dietary management.* During acute periods of active ulceration more vigorous treatment is necessary to control acidity and initiate healing. However, when pain disappears, feedings should be liberalized according to individual tolerance and desire, using a variety of foods. Optimum nutrition and emotional outlook—hence recovery—are more likely to be supported by such a program. During quiescent

periods and for long-term prophylaxis when the patient is asymptomatic, he fares best from judicious choice of a wide range of foods and the establishment of regular, unhurried eating habits.

Current clinical practice now seems to rest firmly upon the scientific principles undergirding the liberalized individual approach rather than the dogma of the past.[15,16] The American Dietetic Association has reinforced this approach in its position paper outlining a more rational basis for nutritional therapy in clinical practice and patient education.

Summary of general diet therapy. The following is a summary of the diet therapy principles for peptic ulcer:

1. There must be *optimum total nutrition* to support recovery and maintenance of health, based on individual needs and food tolerances.
2. *Protein* must be adequate for tissue healing needs and for buffering capacity.
3. *Fat* should be used in moderate amounts for suppression of gastric secretion and motility. Where cardiovascular disease is a concern, reduction of saturated fat may be desired and substitutions made of polyunsaturated fat.[18,19]
4. *Meal intervals and size* should be adequate to maintain individual control of gastric secretions. There should be frequent, small feedings during more active stress periods. Regular meals, moderate in size and sufficient in number for individual need, should be an established habit.
5. *Positive individual needs on a flexible program* rather than negative blanket restrictions on a rigid regimen should be the guide. In any event, picayune dictums and uncompromising prohibitions have no place. Objective research that eliminates prejudiced ideas and individual counseling that meets personal needs together form the keystone of wise peptic ulcer therapy.

A general dietary guide incorporating these nutritional therapy principles for a more liberal approach to control of peptic ulcer disease is given on p. 580.

INTESTINAL DISEASES
General functional disorders

General functional disorders of the intestine, such as "irritable colon," constipation, or diarrhea, are treated by attention to underlying cause and symptomatic care. Adjunct therapy with diet may involve fluid intake, modification of the diet's fiber content, and adjustment of specific foods according to individual tolerances.

Organic diseases

Organic diseases of the intestine may be classified in three general groups: (1) anatomic changes, as in diverticulosis, (2) malabsorption difficulties, as in sprue or celiac syndrome, and (3) inflammatory and infectious mucosal changes, as in ulcerative colitis or in Crohn's disease.

Diverticulosis and diverticulitis

Etiology. Diverticula (L. *diverticulare,* to turn aside) are small tubular sacs branching off from a main canal or cavity in the body. The formation of these small protrusions from the intestinal lumen, usually the colon, produces the condition diverticulosis. More often diverticulosis occurs in older people and develops at points of weakened musculature in the bowel wall.

Clinical manifestations. The condition is asymptomatic unless the diverticula become inflamed, a state called *diverticulitis.* Fecal residue causes increased irritation. There is pain and tenderness usually localized in the lower left side of the abdomen, nausea, vomiting, distention, and intestinal spasm accompanied by fever. If the process continues, intestinal obstruction or perforation may necessitate surgery.

Liberal food guide for peptic ulcer

General directions

1. Respect individual responses or tolerances to specific foods experienced at any given time, remembering that the same food may evoke different responses at different times depending on the stress factor.
2. Eat smaller meals more often, eat slowly, savor your food in a calm environment as much as possible.
3. Try to avoid caffeine beverages such as coffee, cola, and tea; also avoid alcohol.
4. Cut down on or quit smoking cigarettes—not only to help the ulcer but also to help food taste better.
5. Avoid excessive pepper on food or concentrated meat broths and extractives.
6. Avoid frequent use of aspirin or other drugs that may damage the stomach lining.

Foods	Recommended foods	Controlled foods
Bread, cereals (at least 4 servings daily)	Any whole grain or enriched bread, cereals, crackers, pasta	None
Vegetables (at least 2 servings daily)	Any vegetable, raw or cooked; vegetable juices	None
Potatoes, other starches	White potatoes, sweet potatoes, or yams, enriched rice, brown rice, corn, barley, millet, bulgur, pasta	Fried forms
Fruits (at least 2 servings daily)	Any fruit, raw or cooked; fruit juices	None
Milk, milk products (2 servings daily as desired)	Any form of milk or milk drink; yogurt; cheeses	None
Meats or substitutes (2 servings daily)	Poultry, fish and shellfish, lean meats; eggs, cheeses; legumes—dried beans and peas, lentils, soybeans; smooth peanut butter	Fried forms or too highly seasoned or fatty
Soups, stews	Mildly seasoned, less concentrated meat stock base; any cream soups	More highly seasoned or concentrated base
Desserts	Any desserts tolerated	Items containing nuts or coconut; fried pastries
Beverages	Decaffeinated coffee, cocoa, fruit drinks, mineral waters, noncola soft drinks; less strong tea with milk	Regular coffee, strong tea; colas, alcohol
Fats (use in moderation)	Margarine; butter, cream; vegetable oils; mild salad dressings, mayonnaise, oil and vinegar with herbs	Highly seasoned dressings
Sauces, gravies	Mildly flavored, less strong meat bases	Strongly seasoned, especially with pepper, hot peppers, and sauces
Miscellaneous	Salt in moderation (iodized); flavorings; herbs, spices; mustard, catsup, vinegar in moderation, as tolerated	Strongly flavored condiments; popcorn; nuts, coconut as tolerated

Treatment. During acute periods, oral feedings may be limited to liquids with gradual progression in texture. Follow-up diet therapy traditionally has been based on a low-residue regimen. Since during brief initial care such limited texture may be preferred a simple diet plan is available on p. 583. However, current studies and clinical practice have demonstrated better management of diverticular disease with a high-residue diet using more bran fiber.[20,21] For an extended discussion of dietary fiber and its relation to health and disease and applications to clinical needs, see pp. 16-18 in Chapter 2.

Malabsorption syndrome (sprue)

Etiology. The general classification of malabsorption conditions manifesting the common characteristics of steatorrhea is given on p. 429. Adult nontropical sprue is similar in nature to childhood celiac disease. In fact, most adults with sprue give a history of having had episodes of celiac disease as a child. A review of the discussion of celiac disease in Chapter 19 will be helpful here.

Clinical manifestations. The characteristic diarrhea in sprue consists of multiple foamy, malodorous, bulky, and greasy stools. Poor absorption of fat is evident in the large amounts appearing in the stools as soaps (saponification of fatty acids with calcium salts) and fatty acids. Poor absorption of iron produces a microcytic hypochromic anemia. In other persons a lack of folic acid will produce a macrocytic anemia. Poor absorption of vitamin K may lead to hemorrhagic tendencies. Poor calcium absorption may produce a disturbed serum calcium to phosphorus ratio with resulting tetany (p. 135). The condition varies widely among individuals with consequent differences in severity of symptoms and nature of treatment.

Treatment—diet therapy. Since the discovery that gluten is an important factor in the etiology of nontropical sprue (p. 429), the gluten-free or low-gluten diet has been widely used with marked remission of symptoms. Gluten is a protein found mainly in wheat, with additional amounts in rye and oat. The gliadin fraction of the gluten protein seems to be the offending agent in sensitive individuals (p. 430). A regimen similar to that used by many clinics is the wheat-, rye-, and oat-free diet given on p. 584. Compare this with the low-gluten diet therapy outlined for children in Chapter 19.

Ulcerative colitis

Etiology. The cause of ulcerative colitis, or the similar condition of Crohn's disease, is unknown, and no specific cure has been devised. However, treatment today is far more helpful than in years past, as it is based on a better understanding of the clinical types of the diseases and how the pathology involved develops. New drug therapy with more potent antibiotics and endocrine agents has improved the condition in many patients.

Ulcerative colitis usually occurs in young adulthood. In Hightower's classic study of 220 patients[22] the average age at onset for the men was 31 and for the women was 29. Some observers describe a psychogenic overlay in the development of the disease, with patients manifesting various degrees of anxiety and insecurity. However, this is by no means true in all cases.

Clinical manifestations. The common clinical manifestation is a chronic bloody diarrhea that occurs at night as well as during the day. Ulceration of the mucous membrane of the intestine leads to various associated nutritional problems such as anorexia, nutritional edema, anemia, avitaminosis, protein losses, negative nitrogen balance, dehydration, and electrolyte disturbances. There is weight loss, often general malnutrition, fever, skin lesions, and arthritic joint involvement.

Treatment. The management of patients with active but uncomplicated chronic ulcerative colitis involves the three important factors of rest, nutritional therapy, and sulfonamides. Steroid therapy has been helpful in controlling Crohn's disease. There must be vigorous nutritional therapy. Indeed, many physicians have identified nutrition as the key to successful medical treatment.

Diet therapy. Nutritional therapy for ulcerative colitis and Crohn's disease is based on restoration of nutrient deficits, prevention of local trauma to the inflamed area, and controlling less easily absorbed materials such as fats.[23] Medium-chain triglycerides, as in the commercial preparations Portagen or MCT oil, may be used instead of regular fats.

HIGH PROTEIN. The raw surface of the inflamed colon may be regarded as equivalent to an extensive wound or burn of the skin. There are massive losses of protein from the colon tissue by exudation and bleeding. Also, there are losses associated with impaired intestinal absorption. Only if adequate protein is provided for tissue synthesis can healing take place. The diet should supply from 120 to 150 g of protein per day. Protein supplements, such as between meal feedings using skim milk powder or one of the various commercial products available, are helpful to achieve the necessary intake. Tasteful ways of including protein foods of high biologic value (eggs, meat, cheese) must be devised. Milk causes some difficulty with many patients, so it is usually omitted at first, then gradually added in cooked form, such as cream soups or puddings.

HIGH CALORIE. At least 3,000 calories a day are needed to restore nutritional deficits from daily losses in the stools and the consequent weight loss. Also, only if sufficient calories are present to support and protect protein's main anabolic function will the negative nitrogen balance be overcome.

INCREASED MINERALS AND VITAMINS. When anemia is present, iron supplements may be ordered. However, in many patients oral iron preparations are poorly tolerated and blood transfusions are used instead. Extra vitamins associated with the healing process and with the metabolism of the increased calories and protein are especially needed. These are ascorbic acid and the B vitamins thiamin, riboflavin, and niacin. Usually additional supplements of these vitamins are ordered. Potassium therapy may also be indicated due to losses from diarrhea and tissue destruction.

LOW RESIDUE. To avoid irritation to the colon, the diet is fairly low in residue. In acute stages it may be almost residue free (based mainly on lean meat, rice, white bread, Italian pasta, strained cereal, cooked eggs, sugar, butter, and cream). The graduated low-residue diet (p. 585) may be used initially, with additional protein and calorie additions in interval feedings. As soon as tolerated, a full bland diet with high-protein feedings should be attained. Only heavy roughage need be avoided, as the primary concern is the positive supply of necessary nutrition in as appetizing a manner as possible.

Perhaps no other condition better illustrates the need for a close working relationship between physician, nurse, dietitian, and patient than does chronic ulcerative colitis. The appetite is poor, but adequate nutritional intake is imperative. In many creative ways, individually explored and implemented, the fundamental therapeutic needs must be met—through attractive, nourishing food, given with supportive warmth and encouragement.

Low-residue diet

Foods	Allowed	Not allowed
Beverages	Only 2 glasses of milk, if allowed, boiled or evaporated; fruit juices, coffee, tea, carbonated beverages	Alcohol
Eggs	Prepared in any manner, except fried	Fried eggs
Cheese	Cottage, cream, milk American, Tillamook (use in small amounts)	Highly flavored cheeses
Meat or poultry	Roasted, baked, or broiled tender beef, bacon, ham, lamb, liver, veal, fish, chicken, or turkey	Tough meats, pork; no fried or highly spiced meats
Soup	Bouillon, broth, strained cream soups from the foods allowed	Any others
Fats	Butter, margarine, oils, 30 ml (1 oz) cream daily	None
Vegetables	Canned or cooked strained vegetables, such as asparagus, beets, carrots, peas, pumpkin, squash, spinach, young string beans, tomato juice	Raw or whole cooked vegetables
Fruits	Strained fruit juices, cooked or canned apples, apricots, Royal Anne cherries, peaches, pears; dried fruit puree; ripe banana and avocado; all without skins or seeds	All other raw fruits, other cooked fruits
Bread and crackers	Refined bread, toast, rolls, crackers	Pancakes, waffles, whole grain bread or rolls
Cereals	Cooked cereal as Cream of Wheat, Maltomeal, strained oatmeal, cornmeal, cornflakes, puffed rice, Rice Krispies, puffed wheat	Whole grain cereals; other prepared cereals
Potatoes and substitute	Potatoes, white rice, macaroni, noodles, spaghetti	Fried potato, potato chips, brown rice
Desserts	Gelatin desserts, tapioca, angel food or sponge cake, plain custards, water ice or ice cream without fruit or nuts, rennet or simple puddings	Rich pastries, pies, anything with nuts or dried fruits
Sweets	Sugar, jelly, honey, syrups, gumdrops, hard candy, plain creams, milk chocolate	Other candy; jam, marmalade
Miscellaneous	Cream sauce, plain gravy, salt	Nuts, olives, popcorn, rich gravies, pepper, spices, vinegar

Gluten-free diet for nontropical sprue

Characteristics

1. All forms of wheat, rye, oat, buckwheat, and barley are omitted except gluten-free wheat starch (Cellu Products Co.).
2. All other foods are permitted freely, unless specified otherwise by the doctor.
3. The diet should be high in protein, calories, vitamins, and minerals.

Foods	Allowed	Not allowed
Milk (2 glasses or more)	As desired	
Cheese	Any, as desired	
Eggs (1 or 2 daily)	As desired	
Meat, fish, fowl (1 or 2 servings)	Any plain meat	Breaded, creamed, or with thickened gravy; no bread dressings
Soups	All clear and vegetable soups; cream soups thickened with cream, corn-starch, or potato flour only	No wheat flour thickened soup; no canned soup except clear broth
Vegetables (2 servings of green or yellow daily, at least)	As desired, except creamed	No cream sauce or breading
Fruits (at least 2 or 3 daily, including 1 citrus	As desired	
Bread	Only that made from rice, corn, or soybean flour, or gluten-free wheat starch	All bread, rolls, crackers, cake, and cookies made from wheat and rye, Ry-Krisp, muffins, biscuits, waffles, pancake flour, and other pre-pared mixes, rusks, Zwiebach, pretzels; any product containing oatmeal, barley, or buckwheat; no breaded food or food crumbs
Cereals	Cornflakes, cornmeal, hominy, rice, Rice Krispies, Puffed Rice, pre-cooked rice cereals	No wheat or rye cereals, wheat germ, barley, buckwheat, kasha
Pastes		No macaroni, spaghetti, noodles, dumplings
Desserts	Jell-O, fruit Jell-O, ice or sherbet, homemade ice cream, custard, junket, rice pudding, cornstarch pudding (homemade)	Cakes, cookies, pastry; commercial ice cream and ice cream cones; prepared mixes, puddings; home-made puddings thickened with wheat flour

CAUTION: Read labels on all packaged and prepared foods.

Gluten-free diet for nontropical sprue—cont'd

Foods	Allowed	Not allowed
Beverages	Milk, fruit juices, gingerale, cocoa (read label to see that no wheat flour has been added to cocoa or cocoa syrup); coffee (read labels on instant coffees to see that no wheat flour has been added), tea, carbonated beverages	Postum, malted milk, Ovaltine
Condiments and sweets	Salt; sugar, white or brown; molasses; jellies and jams; honey, corn syrup	Commercial candies containing cereal products (read labels)
Fats	Butter, margarine, oils	Commercial salad dressings, except pure mayonnaise (read labels)

Graduated low-residue diet for ulcerative colitis

General directions
1. Monotony in diet should be avoided by varying the foods as much as the diet prescription allows.
2. There is an individual variation in the tolerance to certain foods. If any of the foods in this diet disagrees with the patient, some change in the diet schedule may be required.

Foods	Allowed	Not allowed
Beverages	Carbonated drinks (not iced) in small amounts; coffee or substitutes, tea, special mixtures as prescribed	Milk in any form; fruit juices
Bread	Enriched white or fine rye bread, plain or toasted; plain or salted crackers, Zweibach, melba toast, plain muffins	Whole wheat, dark rye, pumpernickel, or any hot breads
Cereals	Cooked refined or strained—oatmeal, cream of wheat, cream of rice, Farina, Wheatena; precooked cereals; Pablum, Pabena, Cerevim Dry cereals without bran or shredded wheat; noodles, spaghetti, macaroni, plain rice	Cereals containing bran or shredded wheat; unrefined rice, hominy
Meat	Ground or tender beef, lamb, pork, veal; sweetbreads, brains, liver; may be baked, boiled, broiled or roasted; crisp bacon	Fried, smoked, pickled, or cured meats, meat with long fibers, gristle, skin, delicatessen rare meats

Continued.

Graduated low-residue diet for ulcerative colitis—cont'd

Foods	Allowed	Not allowed
Fish	Fresh fish, boiled, broiled, or baked; canned, scalded tuna or salmon; crab meat, oysters	Fried fish, lobster, other canned, smoked, pickled, preserved, or gefilte fish
Fowl	Any boiled, broiled, baked, or roasted	Gristle, skin, or fat; fried fowl
Eggs	Soft- or hard-boiled, poached, coddled, plain omelet, scrambled, creamed	Fried
Cheese	Cream, cottage, mild cheddar, or American	All other cheeses
Milk	None	
Fats	Butter, or margarine in limited amounts, cream for beverage or cereal; crisp bacon; plain gravies in small amounts	Any other
Soup	Bouillon, broth, meat or poultry; may add strained vegetable juices	Cream soup, vegetable soup
Vegetables	Potatoes without skins	All others
Fruits	None	All
Desserts	Plain angel food, butter, sponge or pound cakes, plain cookies, plain sherbet or water ice, plain ice cream, plain smooth puddings (rice, tapioca, bread, starch, custard), plain Jell-O in small quantities; gelatin flavored with coffee, strained fruit juices	Nuts, coconut, raisins
Sweets	Plain jelly, sugar, honey, syrup, plain hard canies, in *limited* amounts	Large amounts of any sweets, jam, or marmalade, candy with nuts or fruit, concentrated sweets, rich pastry or candy
Miscellaneous	Spices and seasonings in moderation	Nuts, olives, pickles, popcorn, horseradish, relishes

Additions

The following foods may be added, in order, only when prescribed. Add each food in small amounts at first until tolerance is assured.
1. Banana, ripe
2. Orange juice—strained and diluted at first—begin with ¼ glass at end of a main meal and gradually increase to full glass
3. Vegetable juice, including tomato—canned, or vegetable juices prepared in a blender and strained
4. Other fruit juices—as with orange juice
5. Vegetables—cooked and strained, or prepared strained baby vegetables
6. Fruits—cooked or stewed, and strained; or prepared strained baby fruits; canned pears; strained applesauce; baked apple without skin or seeds; no dates, figs, or other raw fruits
7. Milk—boiled for three minutes. May be served hot or cold. Begin with ½ glass once daily. May be used in creamed soups, creamed sauce, milk toast, or plain pancakes. Increase slow-

Graduated low-residue diet for ulcerative colitis—cont'd

Additions—cont'd

    ly to ½ glass three times daily and finally to one glass at a time as prescribed. May be used with flavoring nutrient powders or cream.

8. Vegetables—tender, whole cooked or canned, not strained. Gradually introduce asparagus tips, carrots, beets, spinach, squash, string beans, peas, and pumpkin. Avoid skin and seeds. No cabbage, cauliflower, onions, radishes, and turnips.
9. Raw, crisp lettuce (finely shredded); raw tomato; no other raw vegetables
10. Unboiled milk

CASE STUDY 18
Ralph Gregory's ulcer

Ralph Gregory, aged 40, owns and operates an interior decorating company that he has built into a successful chain of offices and display stores in several states. He has much creative, driving energy and works long hours planning innovative approaches and keeping in close touch with all his branch offices. Often this necessitates travel on extended buying trips and "trouble-shooting" visits to branch offices to settle problems that constantly arise. Lately his smoking has increased, along with his tensions, and his numerous business contacts and long hours have involved increased use of alcohol and coffee.

Ralph is married and has two teenaged sons. Some discord has developed at home because of his frequent absences and what his wife interprets as lack of concern for her and their sons. She feels the boys need their father especially now, and Ralph is rarely able to spend any time with them.

Recently Ralph began to develop a dull, gnawing pain in his upper abdomen that seemed to be relieved somewhat when he ate something. He tried to discount it as "just nerves" and used an increased amount of aspirin on his trips to relieve the accompanying headaches. Shortly after he returned home from one of his business trips the pain was unusually severe. He vomited bright red blood. His wife called their physician and, with the help of their sons, took him immediately to the hospital.

After initial treatment in the hospital with blood transfusions and intravenous fluids and electrolytes, including vitamin C, Mr. Gregory began to respond. Although he still felt weak and nauseous, he did not vomit again. However, he did pass several large "tarry" stools. Gradually he began to take sips of water, then a small amount of milk every hour with Gelusil between. The doctor added orange juice and full liquids as soon as Ralph could tolerate them. The patient continued to improve, and his diet was increased to a full soft diet according to toleration. By the end of the second week the doctor told Ralph he would be able to go home. But he cautioned him that he would have to watch his diet, eat regularly, eliminate regular coffee, and use between-meal food with added multivitamins. He would also have to eliminate his smoking and all alcoholic beverages and rest before returning to his work. Even then he would have to greatly curtail much of his former extensive activity. He was to return to see Dr. Blythe the next week.

Continued.

CASE STUDY 18
Ralph Gregory's ulcer—cont'd

As Ralph left the hospital with his wife, he indicated he was glad to be up so that he could look after things with his business, because a number of problems had arisen during his illness. "When are you going to learn, Ralph," his wife asked, "to let some of the other people handle a lot of that detail, and you take care of your health? You need to relax and enjoy life more."

Questions to guide your inquiry

1. The X-ray diagnosis of Ralph's illness was a gastric ulcer in the lesser curvature. What does this mean? Where are the majority of peptic ulcers located? Why?
2. What do you think are some of the factors involved in the development of Ralph's ulcer? What effect did these factors have?
3. Identify Ralph's basic nutritional needs.
4. Outline a teaching plan you would use to help Ralph with his diet. Would you include his wife? Why?
5. What practical problems might he face when he returns to his work? What solutions do you propose?
6. Ralph received medications including vitamin C and other multivitamins and iron. What is the role of this vitamin and mineral therapy in ulcer treatment?
7. Why would there be dietary emphasis on increased calories and protein with between-meal feedings?
8. Why would Ralph need to eliminate alcohol and coffee from his diet?
9. Which dietary approach do you consider most valid, the traditional conservative treatment or the liberal individual approach? Describe each of these methods of care, and give evidence to support your own selection.
10. Summarize the general diet therapy principles in peptic ulcer disease, and give the rationale for each principle.

CASE STUDY 19
Margaret has ulcerative colitis

Margaret Robbins, aged 34, lay back on her hospital bed, spent and exhausted. It seemed so difficult to regain her strength this time. It was the same cycle over and over again—the hated bloody diarrhea, continued weight loss, no appetite, a fever, swelling of her hands, face, and ankles. Even her joints ached. Then came the siege in the hospital where Dr. Towers's kind support and rigorous therapy had helped to stem the tide and build her up again. Sometimes she wondered, through all this, if she would ever be well again.

Although Margaret's condition had seemed worse lately, it had really started some years ago, a year or so after her marriage. Her mother had really been upset then, Margaret thought. But then she couldn't remember when her mother hadn't been upset with her. She could never seem to please her.

CASE STUDY 19

Margaret has ulcerative colitis—cont'd

"Maybe that was why Father just left when I was 4 years old," Margaret mused, "and never returned." Margaret barely remembered her father. He was a shadowy figure from her early childhood, of whom she cherished pleasant memories as a kind man. After he left, there was only Margaret and her mother, who never remarried. Men could never be trusted, Margaret's mother vowed after that.

Margaret grew up in a series of boarding houses as her mother moved from place to place working as a sales representative for a silverware company. In fact, it was in one such boarding house, the summer she was 18 and just out of high school, that she met Ray, a medical student rooming there. By summer's end they had eloped. Although Ray's family had been kind to her through the years, she never really felt they accepted her.

After Ray began his medical practice in his home town, it was even worse. All his family and friends were educated professional people, and she had only finished high school and had no family background. At first she was absorbed with their two children, a boy and a girl. But after the children were older and in high school, she determined she'd go to college, although she had to commute the 100-mile round trip each day to attend classes. She was determined to show Ray she could make the dean's list also, and she did.

Margaret would have graduated in only a few months if the wreck hadn't occurred. One day as she was driving home from the university, the car had skidded on a curve and turned over down an embankment. Luckily she was only bruised and shaken, but the car was a total loss. That was when this present siege of her colitis began again. Dr. Towers told her this time she would just have to rest for a long while and not try to push so hard to finish school.

Margaret opened her eyes again, and her thoughts were brought back to the present as her nurse came into her room to bring medications. So many pills, Margaret thought with a grimace. But the new, more potent drugs and also the vitamins that Dr. Towers was using were helping. Ray had tried to tell her what they were when he came by to see her last night after rounds with his own patients, but she was too tired to listen.

After she had swallowed all the pills, Margaret looked at the menu the clinical nutritionist, Mrs. Scott, had brought to her. Together they marked a few of the items that Mrs. Scott encouraged her to try. She had eaten more since Mrs. Scott had been helping her with her diet. She had begun to realize even more now, as a result, how important a part of her treatment the diet was. She had asked Mrs. Scott to talk with her further about how she might work out the needs of her diet when she was well enough to go home. Margaret's weight was coming up a little, and she was beginning to feel better.

Questions to guide your inquiry

1. What is ulcerative colitis? What causes it? How does it affect the colon?
2. What symptoms result? How do you account for these symptoms?
3. What factors in Margaret's life may have played a part in the development of her disease?
4. What additional information do you think would be useful to you in determining Margaret's needs? Why? What sources and means would you use to obtain it?
5. What nutritional problems do you think Margaret presents? What is the scientific basis for each?
6. What specific and realistic goals do you think the health team and Margaret may set in relation to her problems? Why?
7. Outline a plan of action you would use in seeking to meet Margaret's needs. Give the scientific basis for your actions.

Continued.

CASE STUDY 19
Margaret has ulcerative colitis—cont'd

8. From the information given here, what results would you anticipate from your actions? Why? What follow-up care would you plan as a result?

9. What other persons on the health team would you involve in Margaret's care? In What ways?

10. How would you involve her family?

11. In helping Margaret prepare to leave the hospital after she is better, what plans would you help her make for home care? What resources could you explore?

12. What are the general principles of treatment for ulcerative colitis and the reasons for each?

13. Why is vigorous nutritional therapy so essential? What is its basic goal?

14. What are the principles of the diet used to treat ulcerative colitis? Give the scientific basis for each principle.

15. Outline a day's diet for Margaret to meet her therapeutic needs. Calculate the calories and protein to ensure that she gets the necessary amounts.

16. What are some ways of getting extra amounts of protein into Margaret's diet?

17. What are some ways Mrs. Scott may help Margaret accept her diet and support her efforts to eat?

REFERENCES
Specific

1. Sippy, B. W.: Gastric and duodenal ulcers: medical cure by an efficient removal of gastric juice erosion, J.A.M.A. **64:**1625, 1915.

2. Meulengracht, E.: Treatment of haematemesis and melena with food: mortality, Lancet **2:**1220, 1935.

3. Wolf, S., and Wolff, H. G.: Human gastric function: experimental study of man and his stomach, ed. 2, London, 1947, Oxford University Press, pp. 187-191.

4. Wolf, S.: A clinical appraisal of the dietary management of peptic ulcer and ulcerative colitis, Am. J. Clin. Nutr. **2:**1, 1954.

5. Gill, A. M.: Pain and healing of peptic ulcer, Lancet **1:**291, 1947.

6. Lawrence, J. S.: Dietetic and other methods in treatment of peptic ulcer, Lancet **1:**481, 1952.

7. Todd, J. W.: Treatment of peptic ulcer, Lancet **1:** 291, 1952.

8. Doll, R., Friedlander, P., and Pygott, F.: Dietetic treatment of peptic ulcer, Lancet **1:**5, 1956.

9. Kramer, P.: Symposium on specific methods of treatment: medical treatment of peptic ulcer, Med. Clin. North Am. **39:**1381, 1955.

10. Miller, T. G., and Berkowitz, D.: Analysis of results of conservative peptic ulcer therapy, Gastroenterology **20:**353, 1955.

11. Schneider, M. A., DeLuca, V., Jr., and Gray, S. J.: The effect of spice ingestion upon the stomach, Am. J. Gastroenterol. **26:**722, 1956.

12. Saint-Hilaire, S., Lavers, M. K., Kennedy, J., and Code, C. F.: Gastric acid secretory value of different foods, Gastroenterology **39:**1, 1960.

13. Shull, H. J.: Diet in the management of peptic ulcer, J.A.M.A. **170:**1068, 1959.

14. Koch, J. F., and Donaldson, R. M.: A survey of food intolerances of hospitalized patients, N. Engl. J. Med. **271:**657, 1964.

15. Mendeloff, A. I.: What has been happening to the duodenal ulcer? Gastroenterology **67:**1020, 1974.

16. Grossman, M. I., Guth, P. H., Isenberg, J. I., et al.: A new look at peptic ulcer, Ann. Intern. Med. **84:** 57, Jan., 1976.

17. American Dietetic Association: Position paper on bland diet in the treatment of chronic duodenal ulcer disease, J. Am. Diet. Assoc. **59:**244, 1971.

18. Kinsell, L. W., et al.: Dietary considerations with regard to type of fat, Am. J. Clin. Nutr. **15:**198, 1964.

19. Hartroft, W. S.: The incidence of coronary artery disease in patients with Sippy diet, Am. J. Clin. Nutr. **15:**205, 1964.

20. Plumley, P. F., and Francis, B.: Dietary management of diverticular disease, J. Am. Diet. Assoc. **63:**527, Nov., 1973.

21. Idea exchange: Fiber in the diet, J. Am. Diet. Assoc. **66:**50, Jan., 1975.

22. Hightower, N. C., Jr., et al.: Chronic ulcerative colitis. I. Diagnostic considerations, Am. J. Dig. Dis. **3**(n.s.): 722, 1958.

23. Ament, M. E.: Inflammatory disease of the colon:

ulcerative colitis and Crohn's colitis, J. Pediatr. **86:** 322, 1975.

General

American Dietetic Association Position Paper on Bland Diet in the Treatment of Chronic Duodenal Ulcer Disease, J. Am. Diet. Assoc. **59**(3):244, 1971.

Benson, J. A.: Simple chronic constipation, Postgrad. Med. vol. 57, Jan., 1975.

Bockus, H. L.: Gastroenterology, ed. 3, Philadelphia, 1974, W. B. Saunders Co.

Broitman, S. A., and Zamcheck, N.: Nutrition in diseases of the GI tract: B. Nutrition in diseases of the intestines. In Goodhart, R. S., and Shills, M. E., editors: Modern nutrition in health and disease, Philadelphia, 1980, Lea & Febiger.

Burkitt, D. P.: Some diseases characteristic of modern western civilization, Br. Med. J. **1**:274, 1973.

Burkitt, D. P., Walker, A. R. P., and Painter, N. S.: Effect of dietary fiber on stools and transit-times, and its role in causation of disease, Lancet **2**:1408, 1972.

Caron, H. S., and Roth, H. P.: Popular beliefs about the peptic ulcer diet, J. Am. Diet. Assoc. **60**(4):306, 1972.

Castell, D. O.: Diet and the lower esophageal sphincter, Am. J. Clin. Nutr. **28**:1296, 1975.

Cohen, S., and Booth, G. H.: Gastric acid secretion and lower esophageal sphincter pressure in response to coffee and caffeine, N. Engl. J. Med. **293**:897, 1975.

Cooperman, A. M., editor: Peptic ulcer disease, Surg. Clin. North Am. **56**(6), 1976.

De Risi, L. L.: Starving in the midst of plenty: adult celiac disease, Am. J. Nurs. **70**(5):1048, 1970.

Farmer, R. G.: The protean manifestations of Crohn's disease, Postgrad. Med. **57**:129, 1975.

Feeley, R. M., Criner, P. E., and Slover, H. T.: Major fatty acids and proximate compositions of dairy products, J. Am. Diet. Assoc. **66**:140, 1975.

Fein, H. D.: Nutrition in diseases of the gastrointestinal tract: A. Diseases of the stomach including related areas in the esophagus and duodenum. In Goodhart, R. S., and Shills, M. E., editors: Modern nutrition in health and disease, Philadelphia, 1980, Lea & Febiger.

Ferry, G. D.: Nutrition and disorders of the colon. In Halpern, S. L., editor: Quick reference to clinical nutrition, Philadelphia, 1979, J. B. Lippincott Co.

Friedman, G. D., Siegelant, A. B., and Seltzer, C. C.: Cigarettes, alcohol, coffee, and peptic ulcer, N. Engl. J. Med. **290**:469, 1974.

Gallagher, C. R., Molleson, A. L., and Caldwell, J. H.: Lactose intolerance and fermented dairy products, J. Am. Diet. Assoc. **65**:418, 1974.

Goldstein, F.: Diet and colonic disease, J. Am. Diet. Assoc. **60**:499, 1972.

Greenberger, N. J., and Isselbacher, K. J.: Disorders of absorption. In Thorn, G. W., et al., editors: Harrison's principles of internal medicine, ed. 8, New York, 1977, McGraw-Hill Book Co.

Hanson, M.: Diet management for ulcerative colitis, Springfield., Ill., 1971, Charles C Thomas, Publisher.

Hightower, N. C.: Applied anatomy and physiology of the esophagus. In Bochus, H. L.: Gastroenterology, vol. 1, ed. 3, Philadelphia, 1974, W. B. Saunders Co.

Hjortland, M., et al.: Low gluten diet with tested recipes, Ann Arbor, Mich., 1973, The University of Michigan.

Ingelfinger, F. J.: Intestinal absorption, Nutr. Today **2**(1): 2, 1967.

Ingelfinger, F. J.: Gastric function, Nutr. Today **6**(5):2, 1971.

Ingelfinger, F. J.: The esophagus: how to swallow and belch and cope with heartburn, Nutr. Today **8**(1):4, 1973.

Ippoliti, A. F., Maxwell, V., and Isenberg, J. I.: The effect of various forms of milk on gastric acid secretion, Ann. Intern. Med. **84**:286, 1976.

Katz, A. J., and Falchuk, Z. M.: Current concepts in gluten sensitive enteropathy (celiac sprue), Pediatr. Clin. North Am. **22**:767, 1975.

Kirsner, J. B.: The challenges of ulcerative colitis, Postgrad. Med. **71**:109, 1971.

Klish, W. J., and Montandon, C. M.: Nutrition and upper gastro-intestinal disorders. In Halpern, S. L., editor: Quick reference to clinical nutrition, Philadelphia, 1979, J. B. Lippincott Co.

Larsen, D. M., Masters, S. S., and Spiro, H. M.: Medical and surgical therapy in diverticular disease, a comparative study, Gastroenterology **71**:734, 1976.

Levitt, M. D., Lasser, R. B., Schwartz, J. S., et al.: Studies of a flatulent patient, N. Engl. J. Med. **295**:260, July 29, 1976.

Mendeloff, A. I.: Dietary fiber, Nutr. Rev. **33**:321, 1975.

Mike, E. M.: Practical management of patients with the celiac syndrome, Am. J. Clin. Nutr. **35**:1184, 1959.

Newcomer, A. D.: Disaccharidase deficiencies, Mayo Clin. Proc. **48**:648, 1973.

Odell, A. C.: Ulcer dietotherapy: past and present, J. Am. Diet. Assoc. **58**:447, 1971.

Painter, N. S., Almeida, A. Z., and Colebourne, K. W.: Unprocessed bran in treatment of diverticular disease of the colon, Br. Med. J. **2**:137, 1972.

Plumley, P., and Francis, B.: Dietary management of diverticular disease, J. Am. Diet. Assoc. **63**:527, 1973.

Review: The lactose tolerance test and milk consumption, Nutr. Rev. **34**:302, 1976.

Rosensweig, N. S.: Diet and intestinal enzyme adaptation: implications for gastrointestinal disorders, Am. J. Clin. Nutr. **28**:648, 1975.

Schiff, L.: The Meulengracht diet in the treatment of bleeding peptic ulcer, J. Am. Diet. Assoc. **18**:298, 1942.

Sleisenger, M. H., and Fordtran, J. S., editors: Gastrointestinal disease: pathophysiology, diagnosis, management, ed. 2, Philadelphia, 1978, W. B. Saunders Co.

Soltoft, J., Kraz, B., Gudmand-Hoger, E., et al.: A double-blind trial of the effect of wheat bran on symptoms of irritable bowel syndrome, Lancet **1:**270, 1976.

Sturdevant, R. A., et al.: Antacid and placebo produced similar pain relief in duodenal ulcer patients, Gastroenterology **72:**1, 1977.

Taylor, K. B.: Gastroenterology. In Schneider, H. A., Anderson, C. E., and Coursin, D. B., editors: Nutritional support of medical practice, New York, 1977, Harper & Row, Publishers.

Thompson, W. G.: Constipation and catharsis, Can. Med. Assoc. J. **114:**927, 1976.

Trowell, H.: Definition of dietary fiber and hypotheses that it is a protective factor in certain diseases, Am. J. Clin. Nutr. **29:**417, 1976.

Wald, A. Back, C., and Bayless, T. M.: Effect of caffeine on the human small intestine, Gastroenterology **71:** 738, 1976.

Young, E. A., Heuler, N., Russell, P., and Weser, E.: Comparative nutritional analysis of chemically defined diets, Gastroenterology **69:**1338, 1975.

27 Diseases of the liver and gallbladder

METABOLIC FUNCTIONS OF THE LIVER

The liver is a highly active, vital metabolic organ. Through its vast network of biochemical reactions it controls a major portion of the body's internal environment, and its functions are intimately related to those of other organ systems. Therefore when the liver is diseased and its usual cellular activities do not proceed normally, repercussions of this diminished capacity are reflected in numerous metabolic difficulties and clinical manifestations.

Essentially the functions of the liver may be divided into three groups: (1) metabolic functions relating to the majority of the metabolic systems of the entire body, (2) secretory function of producing bile for the gastrointestinal tract, and (3) vascular functions for storing and filtering blood. The first two of these functional categories are of concern here. They bear a direct relationship to the nutritional therapy required by a patient with liver disease.

Therefore a careful review and clear understanding of the normal metabolic functions of the liver are essential first steps in establishing valid rationale for nutrient modifications in liver disease. These metabolic functions have been discussed at length in previous portions of this text. To guide a review, the outline here is given as a summary of the normal metabolic functions of the liver:

1. Carbohydrate metabolism (Chapter 2)
   a. Formation and storage of glycogen— glycogenesis
   b. Conversion of galactose and fructose to glucose
   c. Conversion of amino acid residues to glucose—gluconeogenesis
   d. Formation of many important chemical compounds from carbohydrate intermediates
2. Fat metabolism (Chapter 3)
   a. Fat conversion to transport form—formation of lipoproteins
   b. Oxidation of fatty acids to acetoacetic acid, hence to acetyl CoA (active acetate), and into the Krebs' cycle to yield energy
   c. Formation of cholesterol and phospholipids
   d. Formation of bile salts
   e. Conversion of carbohydrate and protein intermediates to fat—lipogenesis
3. Protein metabolism (Chapter 4)
   a. Deamination of amino acids
   b. Provision of lipotropic factor for fat conversion to lipoproteins
   c. Formation of plasma proteins
   d. Urea formation for removal of ammonia from body fluids
   e. Many amino acid interconversions; transamination, amination; synthesis of nonessential amino acids, purines, pyrimidines, creatine phosphate, and so on
4. Other related functions
   a. Vitamin storage—A, D, B_{12} and other B-complex vitamins, K

b. Blood coagulation factors—forms prothrombin in presence of vitamin K; also forms other blood factors such as fibrinogen, accelerator globulin, factor VII
d. Storage of iron as ferritin
e. Conjugation and excretion of steroid hormones
f. Detoxification of certain drugs—morphine, barbiturates

DISEASES OF THE LIVER
Hepatitis

Several types of hepatitis exist, mainly epidemic or infectious hepatitis (IH) and homologous serum or serum hepatitis (SH). However, the resulting clinical syndrome is much the same, and the two diseases may be considered essentially identical in terms of medical management.

Etiology. The exact organism responsible for hepatitis is not clearly defined. It is probably one of a group of related viruses. In infectious hepatitis the viral agent is transmitted by the oral-fecal route, a common one in many epidemic diseases. Thus the usual entry is through contaminated food or water. In serum hepatitis the organism is usually transmitted in infected blood (transfusions) or by contaminated instruments[1] (syringes, needles).

Clinical manifestations. The viral agents of hepatitis produce diffuse injury to liver cells, especially the parenchymal cells. In milder cases the tissue injury is largely reversible, but with increasing severity more extensive necrosis occurs. Massive necrosis in some cases leads to liver failure and death. Thus varying clinical manifestations appear depending on the degree of liver injury. *Jaundice,* the most obvious manifestation, serves as a rough index of the severity of the disease. However, jaundice is frequently not seen; 80% of the infected individuals in an outbreak of hepatitis may be nonicteric and thus go undiagnosed and untreated.[2]

After an incubation period of two to six weeks in infectious hepatitis and 10 to 17 weeks in serum hepatitis, manifestations develop. These include general malaise, lassitude, anorexia, diarrhea, headache, fever, enlarged and tender liver, and enlarged spleen. When jaundice develops, it usually follows a preicteric period of five to ten days, deepens for one to two weeks, then levels off and decreases. At this crisis point, sufficient recovery of injured cells has taken place to begin the convalescent period. Convalescence varies from three weeks to three months and is a significant period. Optimum care is essential to avoid relapse.

Treatment. The importance of *bed rest* in the treatment of acute hepatitis has been clearly demonstrated by observations during World War II among groups of infected soldiers.[3] Physical exercise increased both severity and duration of the disease.

A daily intake of 3,000 to 3,500 ml *fluid* guards against dehydration and gives a general sense of well-being and improved appetite.

Optimum nutrition provides the foundation for recovery of the injured liver cells and overall return of strength. It is the major therapy. The principles of diet therapy relate to the liver's function in the metabolism of each nutrient.

Principles of diet therapy

HIGH PROTEIN. Protein is essential for liver cell regeneration. It also provides lipotropic agents such as methionine and choline (p. 120) for the conversion of fats to lipoproteins and removal from the liver, thus preventing fatty infiltration. The diet should supply from 75 to 100 g of protein daily.

HIGH CARBOHYDRATE. Sufficient available glucose must be provided to restore protective glycogen reserves and meet the energy demands of the disease process. Also an adequate amount of glucose ensures the use of protein for vital tissue regeneration, the so-called protein-sparing action of carbohydrate. The diet

High-protein, moderate-fat, high-carbohydrate daily diet

1 L (1 qt) milk
1 to 2 eggs
224 g (8 oz) lean meat, fish, poultry
4 servings vegetables:
   2 servings potato or substitute
   1 serving green leavy or yellow vegetable
   1 to 2 servings of other vegetables, including 1 raw
3 to 4 servings fruit (include juices often)
   1 to 2 citrus fruits (or other good source of ascorbic acid)
   2 servings other fruit
6 to 8 servings bread and cereal (whole grain or enriched)
   1 serving cereal
   5 to 6 slices bread, crackers
2 to 4 tbsp butter or fortified margarine
Additional jam, jelly, honey, and other carbohydrate foods as patient desired and is able to eat them.
Sweetened fruit juices increase both carbohydrate and fluid.

Table 27-1. High-protein, high-calorie formula for milkshakes

Ingredients	Amount	Approximate food value	
Milk	1 cup	Protein	40 g
Eggs	2	Fat	30 g
Skim milk powder	6 to 8 tbsp	Carbohydrate	70 g
or Casec	2 tbsp	Calories	710
Sugar	2 tbsp		
Ice cream	2.5 cm (1 in) slice or 1 scoop		
Cocoa or other flavoring	2 tbsp		
Vanilla	Few drops, as desired		

should supply from 300 to 400 g of carbohydrate daily.

MODERATE FAT. An adequate amount of fat in the diet makes the food more palatable, and hence the anorexic patient will be more encouraged to eat. Former regimens limited the fat on the basis of preventing fat accumulation in the diseased liver. However, values of bet-

ter overall nutrition from improved food intake outweigh these concerns, and a moderate amount of easily utilizable fat (whole milk, cream, butter, margarine, vegetable oil, cooking fats) is beneficial. The diet should incorporate from 100 to 150 g of such fat daily.

HIGH CALORIE. From 2,500 to 3,000 calories are needed daily to furnish energy demands of the tissue regeneration process, to compensate for losses due to fever and general debilitation, and to renew strength and recuperative powers.

MEALS AND FEEDINGS. The problem of supplying a diet adequate to meet the increased nutritive demands to a patient whose illness makes food almost repellent to him is a delicate one calling for creativeness and supportive encouragement. The food may need to be in liquid form at first, using concentrated formulas such as the one in Table 27-1 for frequent feedings. As the patient can better tolerate solid food, every effort should be made to prepare and serve appetizing and attractive food. Nutritional therapy is the key to recovery. Therefore a major responsibility is the devising of ways to encourage an optimum food intake approximating the amount given on p. 595. The nurse and the dietitian will work closely together to achieve this goal.

Cirrhosis

Liver disease may advance to the chronic state of cirrhosis. The French physician Läennec first named the disease, from the Greek word *kirrhos,* meaning "orange," because the cirrhotic liver was a firm, fibrous mass with orange-colored nodules projecting from its surface. The nutritional or alcoholic form of cirrhosis bears his name, Läennec's cirrhosis.

Etiology. Some forms of cirrhosis result from biliary obstruction or liver necrosis from undetermined causes (idiopathic postnecrotic cirrhosis), or in some cases from previous viral hepatitis. The most common problem, however, is fatty cirrhosis associated with malnutrition. The associated malnutrition may develop from other causes but is usually the result of a long history of alcoholism. The fatty liver and early cirrhosis may appear within five years from the onset of the alcoholism, but more often 10 to 15 years is required. Increasingly poor food intake as the excessive drinking continues leads to multiple nutritional deficiencies.

However, alcoholism can cause cirrhosis and death not only because it promotes malnutrition but also because alcohol and its products disturb liver metabolism and hence damage liver cells directly.[4] Damage to the liver cells occurs as fatty infiltration causes cellular destruction and fibrotic tissue changes.

Clinical manifestations. Early signs include gastrointestinal disturbances such as nausea, vomiting, anorexia, distention, and epigastric pain. In time, jaundice may appear, with increasing weakness, edema, ascites, gastrointestinal bleeding tendencies, and iron-deficiency or hemorrhagic anemia. A macrocytic anemia from folic acid deficiency is also frequently observed.[5]

The protein deficiency produces multiple problems: (1) Low plasma protein levels lead to failure of the capillary fluid shift mechanism (p. 181), and the decreased colloidal osmotic pressure causes *ascites* to develop. (2) Lipotropic agents are not supplied to effect fat conversion to lipoproteins, and damaging fat accumulates in the liver tissue. (3) Blood clotting mechanisms are impaired, since factors such as prothrombin and fibrinogen are not adequately produced. (4) General tissue catabolism and negative nitrogen balance continue the overall degenerative process.

As the disease progresses, fibrous scar tissue increasingly impairs blood circulation through the liver, and portal hypertension develops. Contributing further to the problem is *ascites,* localization of edema fluid within the peritoneal cavity. The impaired portal circulation with increasing venous pressure may lead to *esophageal varices,* with danger of rupture and fatal massive hemorrhage.

Treatment. Treatment is difficult when alcoholism is the underlying problem. Each patient requires individual supportive care and approach (p. 498). Usually therapy is aimed at correction of fluid and electrolyte problems and at providing nutritional support to encourage hepatic repair as much as possible.

Principles of diet therapy

PROTEIN ACCORDING TO TOLERANCE. In the absence of impending hepatic coma the daily protein intake should be 80 to 100 g to correct the severe undernutrition, regenerate functional liver tissue, and replenish plasma proteins. However, if signs of hepatic coma appear, the protein is adjusted to individual tolerance.

LOW SODIUM. Sodium is usually restricted to 500 to 1,000 mg daily to reduce the fluid retention. Outlines of these low-sodium diet plans are given in Chapter 28, p. 618.

TEXTURE. If esophageal varices develop, it may be necessary to give soft foods that are smooth in texture to prevent the danger of rupture.

OPTIMUM GENERAL NUTRITION. The remaining overall diet principles outlined for hepatitis are continued for cirrhosis for the same reasons. Calories, carbohydrates, and vitamins are supplied according to individual need and deficiency. Moderate fat is used. Alcohol is strictly forbidden.

Hepatic coma

Etiology. As cirrhotic changes continue in the liver, and portal blood circulation diminishes, collateral circulation develops, bypassing the liver. The normal liver, by means of its urea cycle, is by far the most important organ in the body for the removal of ammonia from the blood, converting it to urea for excretion. In the diseased liver these normal reactions cannot take place. Ammonia-laden blood approaches the liver, cannot follow the usual portal pathways, and is detoured through the collateral circulation. It reenters the systemic blood flow still carrying its ammonia load and produces ammonia intoxication.

Ammonia is formed predominantly in the gastrointestinal tract as the result of enzymatic action on dietary protein. Gastrointestinal bleeding adds still another source, and intestinal bacteria produce more ammonia.

Thus three variables combine to produce hepatic coma: (1) hepatic functioning of the urea cycle, (2) extent of collateral circulation, and (3) the amount of nitrogenous material in the intestine from dietary protein, blood, and ammonia produced by bacteria.

Clinical manifestations. Typical response of the patient involves disorders of consciousness and alterations in motor function. There is apathy, mild confusion, inappropriate behavior, and drowsiness, progressing to coma. Facial expressions are described as an absent stare. The speech may be slurred and monotonous. A typical motor-system change is the coarse, flapping tremor (*asterixis*) observed in the outstretched hands. The breath may have a fecal odor (*fetor hepaticus*).

Treatment. The fundamental principle of therapy is the removal of the sources of excess ammonia. A Sengstaken-Blakemore tube may be used to depress varices and stop bleeding. Antibiotics such as neomycin as well as purgation by enema and a suitable laxative may be administered to reduce ammonia-producing bacteria. Diet adjustments will focus on reduced intake of protein and control of fluid and electrolytes.

Principles of diet therapy

LOW PROTEIN. Protein intake is reduced as individually necessary to restrict the exogenous source of nitrogen in amino acids. The amount of restriction will vary with the circumstances. The unconscious patient will receive no protein, but the usual amounts given range from 15 to 50 g depending on whether symptoms are severe or mild. A simple method for controlling the protein intake is given on p. 599. A base meal pattern containing approximately 15 g of protein is used, adding small items of protein foods according to the level of total protein desired.

CALORIES AND VITAMINS. The amounts of calories and vitamins are ordered according to need. About 1,500 to 2,000 calories are sufficient to prevent tissue catabolism (a source of more amino acids and available nitrogen). Carbohydrates and fats sufficient for energy needs are essential. Vitamin K is usually given parenterally, along with other vitamins that may be deficient.

FLUID INTAKE. Fluid is carefully controlled in relation to output.

DISEASES OF THE GALLBLADDER
Functions of the gallbladder

Bile produced by the hepatic cells is concentrated and stored in the gallbladder. Liver bile consists largely of bile salts, with additional amounts of bilirubin (a major end product of hemoglobin decomposition), cholesterol, fatty acids, and the usual plasma electrolytes (Na^+, K^+, Ca^{++}, Cl^-, HCO_3^-). When bile is concentrated in the gallbladder, water and most of the electrolytes are reabsorbed by the gallbladder mucosa, leaving the remaining ingredients, especially the bile salts, in a highly concentrated form in the gallbladder bile. The liver secretes about 600 to 800 ml of bile daily, which the gallbladder normally concentrates five- to ten-fold. Thus this constant concentrating power enables the gallbladder to accommodate the daily bile in its small 40 to 70 ml capacity. Through the cholecystokinin mechanism (p. 213) the presence of fat in the duodenum stimulates contraction of the gallbladder and the consequent release of bile into the common duct and then into the small intestine.

Cholecystitis and cholelithiasis

Cholecystitis is an inflammation of the gallbladder, usually resulting from a low-grade chronic infection. The infectious process produces changes in the gallbladder mucosa, which affect its absorptive powers. Normally the cholesterol in bile, which is insoluble in water, is kept in solution by the hydrotropic action of the other bile ingredients, especially the bile acids. However, when mucosal changes occur in cholecystitis, the absorptive powers of the gallbladder may be altered, affecting the solubility ratios of the bile ingredients. Excess water may

be absorbed, or excess bile acids may be absorbed.

Under these abnormal absorptive conditions cholesterol may precipitate, causing gallstones (almost pure cholesterol) to form, a condition called *cholelithiasis*. Also a high dietary fat intake over a long period of time predisposes to gallstone formation because of the constant stimulus to produce more cholesterol as a necessary bile ingredient to metabolize the fat.

Clinical manifestations. When inflammation, stones, or both are present in the gallbladder, contraction from the cholecystokinin mechanism causes pain. Sometimes the pain is severe. There is fullness and distention after eating, and difficulty particularly with fatty foods.

Treatment. Surgical removal of the gallbladder is usually indicated. However, the surgeon may wish to postpone surgery until the inflammation has subsided. If the patient is obese, as many persons with gallbladder disease are, some weight loss before surgery is advisable. Thus the supportive therapy is largely dietary.

Principles of diet therapy

FAT. Because fat is the principal cause of contraction of the diseased organ and the consequent pain, it should be greatly reduced. Calories should come principally from carbohydrate foods, especially during acute phases. The day's diet should be limited in fat to 20 to 30 g. Later the patient may tolerate 50 to 60 g, so that the diet may be made more palatable. A diet plan for a low-fat regimen is given on p. 600.

CALORIES. If weight loss is indicated, the calories will be reduced according to need. Principles of weight reduction regimens are given in Chapter 24. Usually such a low-calorie reduction diet will have a low-fat ratio and meet the needs of the patient with gallbladder disease for fat restriction.

CHOLESTEROL AND "GAS FORMERS." Two additional modifications usually found on traditional low-fat diets for gallbladder disease concern restriction of foods containing cholesterol and foods labeled "gas-formers." Neither modification has valid rationale; the body synthesizes daily several times more cholesterol than is present in an average diet. Thus restriction of exogenous cholesterol in food has no appreciable effect in reducing gallstone formation. Total dietary fat reduction is more to the point.

Blanket restriction on so-called gas-formers seems unwarranted also. Food tolerances are highly individual (p. 575). A survey of hospitalized patients failed to show any differences in food tolerances attributable to the presence of gastrointestinal disorders. Patients with gallbladder disease had no more incidence of specific food intolerances than patients without gastrointestinal disease.[6]

Low-protein diets—15 g, 30 g, 40 g, and 50 g protein

General description
1. The following diets are used when dietary protein is to be restricted.
2. The patterns limit foods containing a large percentage of protein, such as milk, eggs, cheese, meat, fish, fowl, and legumes.
3. Avoid meat extractives, soups, broth, bouillon, gravies, and gelatin desserts.

Basic meal patterns (contains approximately 15 g of protein)

Breakfast	Lunch	Dinner
½ cup fruit or fruit juice	1 small potato	1 small potato
½ cup cereal	½ cup vegetable	½ cup vegetable
1 slice toast	salad (vegetable or fruit)	salad (vegetable or fruit)
butter	1 slice bread	1 slice bread
jelly	butter	butter
sugar	1 serving fruit	1 serving fruit
2 tbsp cream	sugar	sugar
coffee	coffee or tea	coffee or tea

For 30 g protein
Add: 1 cup milk
28 g (1 oz) meat, 1 egg,
or equivalent

For 40 g protein
Add: 1 cup milk
70 g (2½ oz) meat or 1 egg and
42 g (1½ oz) meat

For 50 g protein
Add: 1 cup milk
112 g (4 oz) meat or 2 eggs and
56 g (2 oz) meat

Examples of meat portions

28 g (1 oz) meat = 1 thin slice roast—4 × 5 cm
(1½ × 2 in)
1 rounded tbsp cottage
cheese
1 slice American cheese

70 g (2½ oz) meat = Ground beef patty (5 from
448 g [1 lb])
1 slice roast

112 g (4 oz) meat = 2 lamb chops
1 average steak

Low-fat and fat-free diets

LOW-FAT DIET
General description
1. This diet contains foods that are low in fat.
2. Foods are prepared without the addition of fat.
3. Fatty meats, gravies, oils, cream, lard, and desserts containing eggs, butter, cream, nuts, and avocados are avoided.
4. Foods should be used in amounts specified and only as tolerated.
5. The sample pattern contains approximately 85 g protein, 50 g fat, 220 g carbohydrate, and 1,670 calories.

	Allowed	Not allowed
Beverages	Skim milk, coffee, tea, carbonated beverages, fruit juices	Whole milk, cream, evaporated and condensed milk
Bread and cereals	All kinds	Rich rolls or breads, waffles, pancakes
Desserts	Jell-O, sherbet, water ices, fruit whips made without cream, angel food cake, rice and tapioca puddings made with skim milk	Pastries, pies, rich cakes, and cookies, ice cream
Fruits	All fruits, as tolerated	Avocado
Eggs	3 allowed per week, cooked any way except fried	Fried eggs
Fats	3 tsp butter or margarine daily	Salad and cooking oils, mayonnaise
Meats	Lean meat such as beef, veal, lamb, liver, lean fish and fowl, baked, broiled, or roasted without added fat	Fried meats, bacon, ham, pork, goose, duck, fatty fish, fish canned in oil, cold cuts
Cheese	Dry or fat-free cottage cheese	All other cheese
Potato or substitute	Potatoes, rice, macaroni, noodles, spaghetti, all prepared without added fat	Fried potatoes, potato chips
Soups	Bouillon or broth, without fat; soups made with skimmed milk	Cream soups
Sweets	Jam, jelly, sugar, sugar candies without nuts or chocolate	Chocolate, nuts, peanut butter
Vegetables	All kinds as tolerated	The following should be omitted if they cause distress: broccoli, cauliflower, corn, cucumber, green pepper, radishes, turnips, onions, dried peas, and beans
Miscellaneous	Salt in moderation	Pepper, spices; highly spiced food, olives, pickles, cream sauces, gravies

Low-fat and fat-free diets—cont'd

Suggested menu pattern

Breakfast	Lunch and dinner
fruit	meat, broiled or baked
cereal	potato
toast, jelly	vegetable
1 tsp butter or margarine	salad with fat-free dressing
egg 3 times per week	bread, jelly
skim milk, 1 cup	1 tsp butter or margarine
coffee, sugar	fruit or dessert, as allowed
	skim milk, 1 cup
	coffee, sugar

FAT-FREE DIET
General description

The following additional restrictions are made to the low-fat diet to make it relatively fat free:
1. Meat, eggs, and butter or margarine are omitted.
2. A substitute for meat at the noon and evening meal is 84 g (3 oz) of fat-free cottage cheese.

CASE STUDY 20
The patient with infectious hepatitis

Jane Harris and Tom Blake, both aged 24, were excited as they made plans for their coming wedding. Jane worked in the community hospital as a staff clinical dietitian. She had met Tom at the hospital when he was working with the administrator in planning some new equipment for the renovations in the east wing. Tom and his brother owned and operated a hospital supply business. Jane and Tom had always wanted to make a trip to Mexico, but neither had gone before. They decided that this was the time to go. So they made reservations and plans for a trip to Mexico City, visiting a number of smaller towns along the way.

After the wedding they took a flight to Mexico City and engaged local transportation there to visit the adjoining areas. It was a glorious two weeks for them both. They enjoyed many new experiences, especially the Mexican food.

About three weeks after they had returned from their trip and were settled in their new apartment, Tom began to feel ill. He had little energy, no appetite, and complained of severe headaches. Nothing he ate seemed to agree with him. He felt nauseated and began to have diarrhea. When he developed a fever, Jane became alarmed, especially when she noticed that he was beginning to show evidence of jaundice. She called his physician, who admitted him to the hospital for tests and treatment.

Continued.

CASE STUDY 20

The patient with infectious hepatitis—cont'd

At the hospital the doctor ordered several liver function tests—serum bilirubin, BSP, hippuric acid, galactose tolerance, serum albumin, prothrombin time and response to vitamin K, cephalin-cholesterol flocculation, thymol turbidity, cholesterol-cholesterol ester ratio, LDH, transaminase (SGPT and SGOT). These tests indicated impaired function. The examinations also indicated an enlarged, tender liver and an enlarged spleen. Tom had infectious hepatitis, the doctor told them. When they told the doctor about their trip to Mexico and described some of the places they had been, she said it seemed fairly certain that the point of infectious contact had been there with some source of contaminated food or water.

In his initial days in the hospital, Tom felt pretty miserable. The doctor had ordered a diet high in proteins, carbohydrates, calories, and vitamins and moderately low in fats. But it was difficult for Tom to eat. He had no appetite, and food seemed to nauseate him even more. However, Jane came frequently to his room to help care for him and encouraged his intake of fluids and tolerated foods as much as possible. She explained to him something about the liver and its functions in handling nutrients and why it was so necessary therefore for him to get in as much needed nutrition as possible. At first he was only able to tolerate food in liquid form, so Jane helped to prepare for him concentrated beverages containing as much nourishment as possible. Gradually, as he began to improve somewhat, she added more food including some of the things he particularly liked. His appetite slowly improved, and he was able to eat a great deal more. Jane continued to help support his efforts to get well.

Finally the doctor told Tom he was able to go home but that he would have to rest there for some time before returning to his work. During the weeks that followed, Jane made every effort to see that Tom followed the diet that the doctor had discussed with him. It was difficult at times for her to keep him at home resting as he should, because he was anxious to get back to his business. However, he understood the importance of care during this convalescent period and cooperated with the plan of care that the doctor had discussed with Jane.

Questions to guide your inquiry

1. What significant metabolic functions of the liver relate to its handling of carbohydrates?
2. What are the functions of the liver in fat metabolism?
3. What are the functions of the liver in protein metabolism?
4. What other nutrient-related functions of the liver are there?
5. What is the relationship of these normal liver functions to effects or symptoms in infectious hepatitis?
6. What is infectious hepatitis? What are its symptoms?
7. Identify each of the liver function tests the doctor used to diagnose Tom's illness, giving the physiologic basis for each test, normal range, and significance in hepatitis.
8. What problems can you identify in Tom's nutritional care? What is the basis for them?
9. What solutions can you propose for meeting these problem?
10. What were the principles of diet therapy ordered for Tom when he was in the hospital?
11. Give the scientific basis for each of these dietary principles in the light of normal liver function in handling nutrients.
12. Why does nutritional therapy in liver disease such as hepatitis present such a challenge in care?
13. Outline the plan of action you would follow in caring for Tom. Give your reason for each of your actions.
14. Outline a day's food intake for Tom when he was in the hospital. Calculate the amount of calories and protein to ensure that he was getting an optimum intake.
15. What vitamins and minerals are significant aspects of nutritional therapy in hepatitis such as Tom's? Why?

CASE STUDY 21
The patient with cirrhosis

Manuel Martinez, aged 40, had been admitted to the hospital several times in the past few years with liver disease. His doctor had discussed with him the potential seriousness of his beginning cirrhosis, especially in relation to his long-standing drinking problem. But things seemed to get worse instead of better in the months that followed. Finally Maria had taken the children and left him. Their divorce was final. Now he lived alone in a dingy little upstairs flat. His meals were haphazard, if he ate at all. He hated to come home to the empty rooms, so after work on the swing shift at the plant he would drink with some of the other men to forget it all. Somehow he would manage to get himself together by the time he had to go to work the next afternoon.

But this time he did not get back to work. After the latest drinking bout over the weekend the pain had grown worse and the nausea and vomiting almost unbearable. He had managed to call a friend, who brought him to the hospital. Here the doctor found him jaundiced, weak, and his abdomen distended with fluid. He was anemic and generally malnourished and having gastrointestinal bleeding.

After initial correction of fluid and electrolyte problems the clinical nutritionist outlined a diet designed to provide optimum nutrition, especially one high in proteins, vitamins, minerals, and carbohydrates. Already much tissue damage had occurred from fatty infiltration. The liver function tests—serum bilirubin, SGOT, total serum proteins, serum thymol turbidity, cephalin flocculation, and BSP—were all abnormal.

Miss Rowan, the clinical nutritionist, knew that he would need rigorous nutritional support. When he began to respond and could take some oral feedings, she talked with him about his needs and explored different foods he would like, so that the necessary nourishment could be obtained. He told her what he really wanted was some of his Mexican food as soon as he could have it.

As the days passed, Manuel tried to eat because he knew it would help him to get well, but his strength did not return as rapidly as it had at other times. He still felt ill, and his condition remained poor.

The following week Manuel seemed more disoriented than usual. He was continually drowsy, and his speech was slurred. One day when the nurse spoke to him he failed to answer, only staring at her absently, so she called the doctor immediately. By evening he was semicomatose and bleeding internally from esophageal varices.

The doctor ordered a Sengstaken-Blakemore tube to control the bleeding, antibiotics, and vitamin therapy—K, B complex, and C. In consultation with the clinical nutritionist, he changed Manuel's diet to 20 g protein, 2,000 calories, 500 mg sodium, soft. His fluid intake was restricted to 800 ml.

Gradually Manuel began to improve. The bleeding stopped, and he became less confused. However, as the days went by, he failed to gain weight, and his intestinal problems increased. He still seemed to be jaundiced, and a fatty diarrhea—steatorrhea—persisted. He could not seem to tolerate his food, even though he tried to eat. The clinical nutritionist began to use MCT in his diet. When Manuel could not eat solid food, the nutritionist prepared for him a liquid formula made from Portagen or from a water dilution of Sustagen with added MCT. Miss Rowan also noted that Dr. Carter had ordered a triolein I^{131} test for the following day. In her plans for his care she would need to explain the test to Manuel and help him understand its purpose. Dr. Carter also requested a surgical consultation about possible treatment with a portacaval shunt.

Questions to guide your inquiry

1. What is cirrhosis?
2. What are the causes of cirrhosis? What was the apparent cause in Manuel's case?
3. Why did Manuel's alcoholism and subsequent malnutrition cause a fatty liver and eventually cirrhosis?
4. What problems from failures in normal liver metabolism does a protein deficiency cause?

Continued.

CASE STUDY 21
The patient with cirrhosis—cont'd

5. What were the metabolic reasons for each of the symptoms Manuel presented?
6. When Manuel first entered the hospital, what fluid and electrolyte problems did the doctor face that resulted from Manuel's prolonged vomiting and extreme malnutrition? Trace the chain of events that produced these fluid and electrolyte problems. (Compare the problems of edema, p. 196, and ketosis, p. 558.)
7. What form of initial feedings would Manuel probably need when he could take food orally?
8. After Manuel could eat solid food, what diet did the clinical nutritionist plan? Give the rationale for each dietary factor.
9. What particular problems did Miss Rowan face in planning for Manuel's nutritional care?
10. What solutions can you propose for meeting his problems? Give your reasons for each solution proposed.
11. When Manuel became disoriented, what was the cause?
12. What were all the possible sources of nitrogenous material in the blood?
13. What is a Sengstaken-Blakemore tube? What is its purpose?
14. Why were antibiotics ordered for Manuel? Why did he need vitamin therapy, especially vitamin K, vitamin B complex (particularly thiamin), and vitamin C?
15. Account for the changes made at this point in Manuel's diet. Give the rationale for each of the diet modifications.
16. What is steatorrhea? Why was this a complication in Manuel's case?
17. What is MCT? Portagen? Sustagen? Why were these substances used as therapy for Manuel at this time?
18. What is a triolein I 131 test? Why did Dr. Carter order this for Manuel at this time?
19. What is a portacaval shunt? Why might this surgical procedure be considered for Manuel?
20. What should Miss Rowan include in her plan of care for Manuel in view of his continued needs? Why would nutritional therapy have priority?
21. How could she involve other members of the health team in planning for his care?

REFERENCES
Specific

1. Capps, R. B., Sborov, V. M., and Scheiffley, C. H.: A syringe transmitted epidemic of infectious hepatitis, J.A.M.A. **136:**819, 1948.
2. Capps, R. B.: Acute hepatitis, Mod. Treatm. **1:**393, 1964.
3. Barker, M. H., Capps, R. B., and Allen, F. W.: Acute infectious hepatitis in the Mediterranean theater, J.A.M.A. **128:**997, 1945.
4. Lieber, C. S.: The metabolism of alcohol, Sci. Am. **234:**25, March, 1976.
5. Herbert, V., Zalusky, R., and Davidson, C. S.: Correlation of folate deficiency with alcoholism and associated macrocytosis anemia and liver disease, Ann. Intern. Med. **58:**977, 1963.
6. Koch, J. F., and Donaldson, R. M.: A survey of food intolerances of hospitalized patients, New Engl. J. Med. **271:**657, 1964.

General

Baraona, E., Leo, M. A., Borowsky, S. A., et al.: Alcoholic hepatomegaly: accumulation of protein in the liver, Science **190:**794, 1975.
Davidson, C. S.: Dietary treatment of hepatic disease, J. Am. Diet. Assoc. **68:**517, May, 1976.
Davidson, C. S.: Nutrition in diseases of the gastrointestinal tract: D. Diseases of the liver. In Goodhart, R. S., and Shils, M. E., editors: Modern nutrition in health and disease, Philadelphia, 1980, Lea & Febiger.

Dhar, P., Zamchech, N., and Broitman, S. A.: Nutrition in diseases of the GI tract: C. Nutrition in diseases of the pancreas. In Goodhart, R. S., and Shils, M. E., editors: Modern nutrition in health and disease, ed. 6, Philadelphia, 1980, Lea & Febiger.

Fischer, J. E., Rosen, H. M., Ebeid, O. M., et al.: The effect of normalization of plasma amino acids on hepatic encepholopathy in man, Surgery **80:**77, 1976.

Halstead, C. H.: Nutritional implications of alcohol. In Hegsted, D. M., editor: Nutrition reviews' present knowledge in nutrition, ed. 5, New York, 1976, The Nutrition Foundation, Inc.

Harper, H. A.: Protein intake in liver disease, J. Am. Diet. Assoc. **38:**350, April, 1961.

Iber, F. L.: In alcoholism the liver sets the pace, Nutr. Today **6**(1):2, 1971.

Isselbacher, K. J.: Metabolic and hepatic effects of alcohol, N. Engl. J. Med. **296:**612, 1977.

Krugman, S.: Etiology of viral hepatitis, Hosp. Pract. **70:** 45, 1970.

Leevy, C. M., Thompson, A., and Baker, H.: Vitamins and liver injury, Am. J. Clin. Nutr. **23:**493, 1970.

Lieber, C. S., editor: Metabolic aspects of alcoholism, Lancaster, England, 1977, MTP Press Ltd.

Quinlan, D. P., and Leevy, C. M.: Nutrition and liver disease. In Halpern, S. L., editor: Quick reference to clinical nutrition, Philadelphia, 1979, J. B. Lippincott Co.

Rudman, D., Smith, R. B., Salam, A. A., et al.: Ammonia content of food, Am. J. Clin. Nutr. **26:**487, 1973.

Symposium on nutrition and liver injury, Parts I and II, Am. J. Clin. Nutr. **23:**445; 579, 1970.

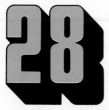

Cardiovascular diseases

Cardiovascular disease is a health problem of major proportion. Its incidence in the United States continues to increase, causing more deaths than all other diseases together and accounting for cardiac symptoms in about 75% of all adult patients under care in general hospitals. The pattern is the same in other developed countries. It is a problem of wide scope in all of Western society.

Although much has been learned by tremendous research efforts in many areas of the world, the precise etiology of cardiovascular disease is still obscure. Multiple factors have emerged as contributory such as hypercholesterolemia, obesity, hypertension, lack of exercise, cigarette smoking, and stress. These risk factors are grouped in Table 28-1 according to control approach. The National Heart and Lung Institute has recently conducted a six-year study, the Multiple-Risk Factor Intervention Trial (MRFIT), in some 20 clinical centers in the United States to determine the relation of some of these risk factors to heart disease.[1] Some prior studies[2-6] have suggested additional links with two other factors—heavy coffee drinking and insufficient sleep—although the association is unclear. Mayer[4] suggests the commonly observed relationship of heavy coffee use to heavy cigarette smoking and insufficient sleep to sedentary late night television habits.

Three of the established contributory factors have definite dietary relationships. Studies have linked hypercholesterolemia—or more generally, hyperlipidemia—to high-fat intake with a large percentage of it being animal (saturated) fat,[7] as well as to lack of exercise. The incidence of hypertension is related to high salt use with food. Obesity is the result of calorie intake, especially in carbohydrate foods, in excess of energy expenditure needs and lack of exercise. Therefore current diet therapy for patients with heart disease centers on modification of these three factors—fat, sodium, and calories.

The metabolism of these nutrients is associated with problems in atherosclerosis, congestive heart failure, hypertensive cardiovascular disease, and acute myocardial infarction.

THE PROBLEM OF ATHEROSCLEROSIS

Atherosclerosis, a basic pathologic process in coronary heart disease, remains an enigma in modern medicine. Fatty degeneration and thickening occur in arterial walls with plaque formations, narrowing of the vessel lumen, development of blood clots, and eventual occlusion of the involved artery. This tissue area serviced by the involved artery is deprived of its vital oxygen and nutrient supply (ischemia), and the cells die. The localized area of dying or dead tissue is called an *infarct*. When the artery is one supplying the cardiac muscle (myocardium), the result is an acute myocardial infarction.

Etiology—relation to general lipid metabolism

A search for the cause of atherosclerosis, the underlying disease process, has focused attention on *lipid metabolism* for two reasons: (1) the artery deposits and plaque formations are largely cholesterol and other fatty materials and (2) an elevated blood cholesterol level (hypercholesterolemia) and elevation of other serum lipids (hyperlipidemia, hypertriglyceridemia) are usually present. A number of large-scale studies have demonstrated a definite association between types of dietary fat and effect on elevated blood lipid levels. Dietary substitution of foods high in polyunsaturated fatty acids for foods high in saturated fatty acids produced a lowering of blood cholesterol. However, what the significance of lowered cholesterol levels is in terms of the disease process is unknown. If the serum cholesterol value returns to normal, is further atherosclerosis prevented? Is the disease process reversed?[8] These are the important questions to which full answers have not been found. But the mass of clinical and experimental data does suggest some disorder related to lipid metabolism.

Hyperlipoproteinemia

Increased concentrations of certain lipoproteins in the plasma have been associated in a number of studies with an increased risk of atherosclerotic heart and peripheral vascular disease.[9-12] Lipoproteins are the major vehicular forms of lipids in the blood. An increase in one or more of these plasma lipoproteins creates the condition called *hyperlipoproteinemia*. A more general term referring to elevation of one or more of the broad plasma lipid classes is *hyperlipidemia*.

The lipoproteins in the blood are produced in two places: (1) in the intestinal wall after initial ingestion, digestion, and absorption of exogenous fat in a meal and (2) in the liver from endogenous fat sources. The intestinal wall lipoproteins formed from exogenous fat sources are called *chylomicrons* (see p. 608). They have the highest lipid content of all the lipoproteins, containing mostly triglycerides with a small amount of protein as a carrier substance; hence they have the lowest density. The other major lipoproteins produced in the liver transport fat to the tissues for use in energy production and for interchange with other metabolites. These five basic types of lipoproteins may be grouped or classified according to their fat content and hence their density, those with the highest fat content having the lowest density. The five groups of lipoproteins, in order of lipid content, are the following:

1. *Chylomicrons*—highest lipid content,

Table 28-1. Multiple risk factors in cardiovascular disease

Personal characteristics (no control)	Learned behaviors (intervention-change)	Background conditions (screen-treat)
Sex	Stress-coping	Hypertension
Age	Smoking cigarettes	Diabetes mellitus
Family history	Sedentary life	Hyperlipidemia (especially hypercholesterolemia)
	Obesity	
	Food habits:	
	Excess fat	
	Excess sugar	
	Excess salt	

lowest density. Composed mostly of exogenous triglycerides (TG) with small amount of carrier protein, accumulating in portal blood following a meal and efficiently cleared from the blood by the specific enzyme, lipoprotein lipase.

2. *Prebeta lipoproteins*—very low-density lipoproteins (VLDL), still carrying large lipid content but including about 10% to 15% cholesterol, formed in the liver from endogenous fat sources.

3. *Broad-beta lipoproteins*—intermediate density lipoproteins (IDL), continuing the delivery of endogenous triglycerides (TG) to cells and carrying about 30% cholesterol.

4. *Beta lipoproteins*—low-density lipoproteins (LDL), carrying in addition to other lipids about two thirds or more of the total plasma cholesterol, formed in the liver from endogenous fat sources.

5. *Alpha lipoproteins*—high-density lipoproteins (HDL), carrying less total lipid and more protein carrier, also formed in the liver from endogenous fat sources. Since HDL carries cholesterol from the tissues to the liver for catabolism and excretion, higher serum levels are considered protective against cardiovascular disease. The "normal" (statistical) range for HDL-cholesterol is 30 to 80 mg/dl. Thus a value below 30 mg/dl implies significant risk, and a value of 75 or above contributes definite protection and decreased risk.

In brief the six types of lipid disorders and their respective lipid elevation and incidence are

Type I: Chylomicrons elevated, rare
Type IIa: LDL elevated, common
Type IIb: LDL and VLDL elevated, common
Type III: IDL elevated, uncommon
Type IV: VLDL elevated, common
Type V: VLDL and chylomicrons elevated, uncommon

A more detailed summary of the characteristics of these lipoproteins is given in Table 28-2. Note the comparative functions of LDL and HDL given in the table. Thus, since LDL carries cholesterol to the peripheral cells, it contributes the "cholesterol of concern" in type II lipid disorders and is a more valid measure of risk status than is the total cholesterol value. The LDL value may be calculated by the following formula:

LDL = Total cholesterol − (20% TG + HDL)

The causes of hyperlipoproteinemia are varied. Sometimes it is secondary to other diseases, for example, obstructive liver disease or pancreatitis, and hence treatment is directed toward the causative disorder. In other cases it may be primary without such obvious cause. In these instances it may be related to a disorder of lipid metabolism, to an abnormal diet or an abnormal response to a normal diet, or to some other more obscure cause. It is sometimes genetic in origin.

Types of abnormal blood lipid patterns. On the basis of the qualitative lipoprotein pattern on paper electrophoresis (a process by which the various blood lipid fractions are separated and identified; the respective colloidal particles suspended in the fluid medium migrate according to their density under the influence of an electric field and appear as resulting bands on special paper) and other clinical and laboratory data, six types of lipid disorders have been described. [10-15]

TYPE I. There is a marked increase in chylomicrons with normal or decreased beta and prebeta lipoproteins. This is a rare genetic type usually found in children, caused by a deficiency or absence of the specific enzyme *lipoprotein lipase,* which clears chylomicrons with their load of dietary triglycerides from the blood following intestinal absorption. [16] Therapy is aimed at keeping the diet low enough in fat to make the patient asymptomatic and free of recurrent bouts of pain. The fat is maintained at about 25 to 35 g a day, an ex-

Table 28-2. Characteristics of the classes of lipoproteins

	Chylo-microns	Very low density (VLDL)	Intermediate density (IDL)	Low density (LDL)	High density (HDL)
Composition					
Triglycerides (TG)	80%-95%; diet, exogenous	60%-80%; endogenous	40%; endogenous	10%-13%; endogenous	5%-10%; endogenous
Cholesterol	2%-7%	10%-15%	30%	45%-50%	20%
Phospholipid	3%-6%	15%-20%	20%	15%-22%	25%-30%
Protein	1%-2%	5%-10%	10%	20%-25%	45%-50%
Function	Transport dietary TG to plasma and tissues, cells	Transport endogenous TG to cells	Continue transport of endogenous TG to cells	Transport cholesterol to peripheral cells	Transport free cholesterol from membranes to liver for catabolism
Place of synthesis	Intestinal wall	Liver	Liver	Liver	Liver
Size, density					
Description	Largest, lightest	Next largest, lightest	Intermediate size, lighter	Smaller, heavier	Smallest, most dense, heaviest
Density	0.095	0.095-1.006	1.00-1.03	1.019-1.063	1.063-1.210
Size in nanometers (nm)	75-100	30-80	25-40	10-20	7.5-10
Electrophoretic equivalent	Origin (non-migrating)	Prebeta	Broad beta	Beta	Alpha

tremely low level, and the P/S (polyunsaturated fat/saturated fat) ratio is unimportant. There is no cholesterol restriction. Carbohydrate is increased, since it must serve as the major contributor of calories. Medium-chain triglycerides (MCT) in a commercially prepared oil form[17] may be used as a dietary supplement. This form of fat is absorbed directly into the portal vein and transported directly to the liver, without requiring chylomicron formation for transport.

TYPE IIa. There is an increase in serum beta lipoproteins. The prebeta form may be moderately increased or normal. The cholesterol is elevated—300 to 600 mg/dl—and the triglycerides may be moderately elevated or normal. This type is common and occurs at all ages. A familial form may occur in early life before age 1, and clinical symptoms are evident in young adult subjects. Treatment involves lowering the intake of cholesterol to less than 300 mg per day and decreasing the intake of saturated fats while increasing the intake of polyunsaturated fats. The familial type IIa is usually not as responsive to diet therapy as is the nonfamilial.

TYPE IIb. Type IIb is a common pattern with elevated beta lipoprotein, cholesterol, and triglycerides. The diet therapy for type IIb initially involves weight reduction to ideal body weight and control of both cholesterol and triglycerides. Then the maintenance diet is designed to reduce the cholesterol and elevate the unsaturated fatty acid content. Thus it is a diet balanced in fat and carbohydrates, about 40% of the calories coming from each.

TYPE III. Although displaying a similar lipid pattern to that of type IIb, type III is relatively

Table 28-3. Types of lipid disorders*

Type	Diet	Lipid pattern	Clinical signs	Genetic defect
I Rare Early childhood Familial	Low fat, 25-35 g; high carbohy- drate; MCT	Increased chylomicrons	Abdominal pain Lipemia, retinalis, xanthoma Hepatospleno- megaly	Deficient enzyme: lipoprotein lipase
IIa Common All ages Genetic autosomal dominant	Low cholesterol Low saturated fat High unsaturated fat	Increased beta LP (50% cholesterol), LDL Increased cholesterol	Xanthoma (tendon) Corneal arcus Vascular disease Accelerated atherosclerosis	Defective plasma clearing on catabolism of LDL
IIb and III III relatively uncommon Adult When genetic, recessive, sporadic	Weight reduction Low cholesterol High unsaturated fat	Increased inter- mediate broad beta LP (IDL) Increased triglycerides Increased cholesterol	Xanthoma (palmar) Vascular disease	Unclear
IV Most common Adult Familial	Weight reduction Low carbohydrate, no alcohol Low cholesterol High unsaturated fat	Increased prebeta LP, VLDL Increased triglycerides Sometimes carbohydrate induced	Usually no overt symptoms Abnormal glucose tolerance High uric acid Stress, obesity Accelerated atherosclerosis	Abnormal glucose tolerance Lipogenesis
V Uncommon Early adult Sporadic familial	Weight reduction Low fat and carbohydrate High protein	Increased chylomicrons Increased triglycerides Increased cholesterol	Abdominal pain Pancreatitis Hepatospleno- megaly	Unclear

*Data from Frederickson, D. S., Levy, R. I., and Lees, R. S.: Fat transport in lipoproteins—an integrated approach to mechanisms and disorders, N. Engl. J. Med. **276:**34, 1967; and Frederickson, D. S., et al.: Dietary management of hyperlipoproteinemia, DHEW Pub. No. (NIH) 76-110, Washington, D.C., 1975, Superintendent of Documents.

uncommon and is characterized by the elevation in the plasma of broad beta lipoprotein and by the presence of unique clinical xanthomas. There is also an increase in plasma cholesterol and triglycerides, with some elevation in the prebeta lipoprotein fraction. A characteristic diagnostic finding consists of orange-yellow streakings in the palmar creases of the hands (palmar xanthosis). Also in type III, male patients have an increased incidence of coronary and peripheral vascular disease, often before the age of 35, and female patients tend to develop these same manifestations 10 to 15 years later. This type is usually familial and apparently is transmitted as a recessive trait. The diet therapy is the same as that for type IIb.

TYPE IV. Type IV is a very common lipoprotein pattern, most frequently seen after the second decade of life and often associated with diabetes and glucose intolerance. It probably represents a form of premature atherosclerosis. The plasma triglycerides are elevated, sometimes to extremely high levels. The cholesterol may be normal, but increases usually in relation to the triglyceride level. About 50% of the patients with type IV patterns have abnormal glucose tolerance tests and may have hyperuricemia as well. This pattern may be familial also. It is usually compounded by obesity. Diet therapy is primarily aimed at weight reduction. With such a reduction to ideal weight the patient usually has lower triglyceride concentrations. Sometimes weight loss even returns the triglycerides to normal; therefore maintaining ideal body weight is an essential part of treatment. After weight reduction the maintenance diet is low in carbohydrate and cholesterol and high in unsaturated fatty acids. Alcohol intake is usually restricted, along with carbohydrate, since these materials tend to increase endogenous triglyceride concentrations.[18]

TYPE V. This pattern is often seen secondary to acute metabolic disorders such as diabetic acidosis, pancreatitis, alcoholism, and nephrosis. There is an elevation in the chylomicron fraction and in the prebeta fraction of lipoproteins. Usually the triglycerides and cholesterol are elevated. Patients with familial type V may have symptoms after age 20 and may have all the features of type I, that is, enlarged spleen, bouts of abdominal pain, and sometimes pancreatitis. They have varying degrees of intolerance to both dietary and endogenous fat. The diet concentrates on restricting calories and reducing weight to an ideal level. Sometimes weight reduction alone will return the plasma lipids to normal levels. After weight reduction the diet essentially involves a low-carbohydrate and low-fat intake. The protein content of the diet is usually high to supply energy and tissue needs, since both carbohydrate and fat must be restricted.

These lipid disorders and their treatment are summarized in Table 28-3.

Chapter 3 on fat metabolism should be reviewed carefully. The concepts of fatty acid saturation and unsaturation, essential fatty acid, and related fat substances such as cholesterol and lipoproteins should be clearly understood in theory and in terms of foods. Patients will need brief, concise explanations of their diet and its rationale, relating it to family food patterns and support.[19,20] Misunderstandings gained from lay articles or public advertising of food products may need to be corrected and clarified. The food fat spectrum, Fig. 3-2, will be a useful tool in teaching.

General principles of diet therapy— fat-controlled diets

Amount of fat. About half the calories of the average American's diet is contributed by fat. It is suggested that this be moderated to about 35% or lower if weight reduction is needed.

Kind of fat. About two thirds of the total fat in the American diet is of animal origin and therefore is mainly saturated fat. The remaining one third comes from vegetable sources

Table 28-4. Fat-controlled diets on three calorie levels

Diet plans	Total calories from fat	Total day's exchanges		
		1,200 calories P/S ratio 1.1:1	1,800 calories P/S ratio 1.3:1	2,400 calories P/S ratio 1.5:1
I. Modified fatty acid content	40%			
Milk		2	2	2
Vegetables A		As desired	As desired	As desired
Vegetables B		1	1	1
Fruits		3	5	5
Bread and cereals		4	6	8
Meat, fish, poultry		5	6	7
Eggs (if desired, as part of the meat exchange)		4 per week	4 per week	4 per week
Fat		5	9	15
Special margarine		1		3
Sugar, sweets		—	9	12
II. Moderate fat reduction	25%			
Milk		2	2	2
Vegetables A		As desired	As desired	As desired
Vegetables B		1	1	1
Fruits		6	8	10
Bread and cereals		3	5	6
Meat, fish, poultry		6	7	9
Eggs (if desired, as part of the meat exchange)		4 per week	4 per week	4 per week
Fat		3	6	8
Sugar, sweets		—	8	22
III. Severe fat reduction	10%			
Milk		2	2	2
Vegetables A		As desired	As desired	As desired
Vegetables B		1	1	1
Fruits		5	8	9
Bread and cereals		4	7	7
Meat, fish, poultry		6	7	9
Eggs (if desired, as part of the meat exchange)		4 per week	4 per week	4 per week
Fat		—	—	—
Sugar, sweets		8	15	36

*Adapted from The regulartion of dietary fat, Food and Nutrition Council, American Medical Association, J.A.M.A. **181:**411, 1962.

Food exchange lists for fat controlled diets*

List 1—Milk exchanges

Nonfat fried milk	¼ cup
Skim milk	1 cup
Buttermilk (made from skim milk)	1 cup

List 2—Vegetable exchanges

Vegetable A As desired

Asparagus	Okra	Escarole
Beans, string, young	Pepper	Eggplant
Broccoli	Radishes	Sauerkraut
Brussels sprouts	Cauliflower	Squash, summer
Cabbage	Celery	Tomatoes
Lettuce	Chicory	Watercress
Mushrooms	Cucumber	Greens (beet greens, chard, collard)

Vegetable B ½ cup per serving

Beets	Peas, green	Squash, winter
Carrots	Pumpkin	Turnip
Onions	Rutabaga	

List 3—Fruit exchanges

Apple (5 cm [2 in] diameter)	1	Grapes	12
Applesauce	½ cup	Honeydew melon (17.5 cm [7 in] diameter)	⅛
Apricots		Mango	½ small
Fresh	2 medium	Orange	1 small
Dried	4 halves	Orange juice	½ cup
Banana	½ small	Papaya	⅓ medium
Blackberries	1 cup	Peach	1 medium
Blueberries	⅔ cup	Pear	1 small
Cantaloupe (15 cm [6 in] diameter)	¼	Pineapple	½ cup
Cherries	10 large	Pineapple juice	⅓ cup
Dates	2	Plums	2 medium
Figs		Prunes, dried	2 medium
Fresh	2 large	Raisins	2 tbsp
Dried	2	Raspberries	1 cup
Grape juice	½ cup	Strawberries	1 cup
Grapefruit	½ small	Tangerine	1 large
Grapefruit juice	½ cup	Watermelon	1 cup

*Adapted from The regulation of dietary fat, Food and Nutrition Council, American Medical Association, J.A.M.A. **181**(5):411, 1962.

Continued.

Food exchange lists for fat controlled diets—cont'd

List 4—Bread exchanges

Bread	1 slice
*Biscuit, muffin, roll (5 cm [2 in] diameter)	1
*Cornbread (4 cm-[1½ in] cube)	1
Cereal, cooked	⅓ cup
Dry, flaked, or puffed	¾ cup
Rice, grits, cooked	½ cup
Spaghetti, noodles, cooked	½ cup
Macaroni, cooked	½ cup
Crackers, graham	2
Saltines	5
Soda	3
Beans, peas, dried, cooked	½ cup
Corn, sweet	⅓ cup
Corn on the cob, medium ear	½
Potatoes, white (5 cm diameter)	1
Potatoes, sweet	½ cup
Parsnips	⅔ cup

List 5—Meat, fish, and poultry exchanges†

(Select meat from this group for 3 meals a week)	
Beef, eye of round, top and bottom round, lean, ground round, lean rump, tenderloin	28 g (1 oz)
Lamb, leg only	28 g
Pork, lean loin	28 g
Ham, lean and well trimmed	28 g
(Make selections from this group for 11 meals a week)	
Chicken, no skin	28 g
Turkey, no skin	28 g
Veal	28 g
Fish	28 g
Shellfish	28 g
Meat substitute, cottage cheese, preferably uncreamed	¼ cup

List 6—Eggs

Four eggs per week allowed (as part of meat exchanges) in each diet plan at discretion of physician

*Made with corn or cottonseed oil. Diets planned according to American Diabetes Association exchange system.
†Meat exchanges were calculated as containing 3 g fat instead of ADA value of 5 g.

Food exchange lists for fat controlled diets—cont'd

List 7—Fat exchanges

50% polyunsaturated

Corn oil	1 tsp
Cottonseed oil	1 tsp
Safflower oil	1 tsp
Mayonnaise made with corn or cottonseed oil	1 tsp
French dressing made with corn or cottonseed oil	2 tsp

30% to 40% polyunsatured

Special margarines	1 tsp
Special shortenings	1 tsp

List 8—Sugar exchanges*

White, brown, or maple sugar	1 tsp
Corn syrup, honey, molasses	1 tsp
Candy (no chocolate)	
Gum drops	
Hard type	
Mints, cream	
Marshmallow, plain	
Jelly, jams, all varieties	
Sherbet	
Carbonated beverages	

*30 ml (1 oz) alcohol = 1 sugar exchange and may be substituted at discretion of physician.

and is mainly unsaturated fat. The fat-controlled diet reduces the animal fat and uses instead more plant fat, bringing the ratio of polyunsaturated fat calories to about half of the total fat calories.

American medical association fat-controlled diets. The Council on Foods and Nutrition of the American Medical Association has outlined a series of three fat-controlled diets, each one on three calorie levels with the ratio of polyunsaturated fatty acids to saturated fatty acids ranging from 1:1 to 1.5:1.[21] These diets may serve as guides for physicians who wish to use them with indicated patients:

1. Modified fatty acid content—40% of total calories
2. Moderate fat reduction—25% of total calories
3. Severe fat reduction—10% of total calories

The basic food exchange groups of the American Diabetes Association exchange system of dietary control (p. 546) are modified for fat content, and an additional list of sugar exchanges is outlined. These groups provide a basis for food choices on each of the three calorie levels—1,200 calories for weight reduction, 1,800 calories for reduction or maintenance, and 2,400 calories for maintenance. The day's food plan for each diet is given in Table 28-4. The modified food exchange groups are listed in the box on p. 613. A simplified fat-

Controlled fat diet—high polyunsaturated fatty acids diet

	Foods allowed	Foods not allowed
Soup	Bouillon cubes, vegetable soup, and broths from which fat has been removed. Cream soups made with nonfat milk	Meat soups, commercial cream soups, and cream soups made with whole milk or cream
Meat, fish, poultry	One or two servings daily (not to exceed a total of 112 g [4 oz]) lean muscle meat, broiled or roasted; beef, veal, lamb, pork, chicken, turkey, lean ham, organ meats (all visible fat should be trimmed from meat); all fish and shellfish	Bacon, pork sausage, luncheon meat, dried meat, and all fatty cuts of meat; weiners, fish roe, duck, goose, skin of poultry, and TV dinners
Milk and milk products	At least 2 cups nonfat milk or nonfat buttermilk daily; nonfat cottage cheese, Sap Sago cheese	Whole milk and cream; all cheeses (except nonfat cottage cheese), ice cream, imitation ice cream (except that containing safflower oil), ice milk, sour cream, commercial yogurt
Eggs	Egg whites only	Egg yolks
Vegetables	All raw or cooked as tolerated (leafy green and yellow vegetables are good sources of vitamin A)	No restrictions
Fruits	All raw, cooked, dried, frozen, or canned; use citrus or tomato daily; fruit juices	Avocado and olives
Salads	Any fruit, vegetable, or gelatin salad	
Cereals	All cooked and dry cereals; serve with nonfat milk or fruit; macaroni, noodles, spaghetti, and rice	
Bread	Whole wheat, rye, enriched white, French bread, English muffins, graham crackers, saltine crackers	Commercial pancakes, waffles, coffee cakes, muffins, doughnuts, and all other quick breads made with whole milk and fat; biscuit mixes and other commercial mixes, cheese crackers, pretzels
Desserts	Fruits; tapioca, cornstarch, rice, junket puddings all made with nonfat milk and without egg yolks; fruit whips made with egg whites, gelatin desserts, angel food cake, sherbet, water ices, and special imitation ice cream containing vegetable safflower oil; cake and cookies made with nonfat milk, oil, and egg white; fruit pie (pastry made with oil)	Omit desserts and candies made with whole milk, cream, egg yolk, chocolate, cocoa butter, coconut, hydrogenated shortenings, butter, and other animal fats

---

Controlled fat diet—high polyunsaturated fatty acids diet—cont'd

	Foods allowed	Foods not allowed
Concentrated fats	Corn oil, soybean oil, cottonseed oil, sesame oil, safflower oil, sunflower oil, walnuts and other nuts except cashew and those commercially fried or roasted	Butter, chocolate; coconut oil, hydrogenated fats and shortenings, cashew nuts; mineral oil, olive oil, margarine, except as specified; commercial salad dressings, except as listed; hydrogenated peanut butter; gravy, except as specified
	Margarine made from above oils, such as Award, Mazola, Emdee, Fleishmann's, and Kraft Corn Oil	
	Commercial French and Italian salad dressing if not made with olive oil	
	Gravy made from bouillon cubes or fat-free meat stock thickened with flour and added oil if desired	
	Freshly ground or old-fashioned peanut butter	
Sweets	Jelly, jam, honey, hard candy, and sugar	
Beverages	Tea, coffee, or coffee substitutes; tomato juice, fruit juice, cocoa prepared with non-fat milk	Beverages containing chocolate, ice cream, ice milk, eggs, whole milk or cream

If the diet is also to be high in unsaturated fat, it should include liberal amounts of
1. Oils allowed that can be incorporated in salad dressings or added to soups, to nonfat milk, to cereal, to vegetables
2. Walnuts, almonds, Brazil nuts, filberts, pecans
3. Extra margarine in or on foods

---

controlled diet list for general use without specific calorie modification is given on p. 616.

EDEMA CONTROL IN CONGESTIVE HEART FAILURE

In congestive heart failure the weakened myocardium is unable to maintain an adequate cardiac output to sustain a normal blood circulation. The resulting fluid imbalances cause edema to develop (p. 182), bringing problems in breathing and placing added stress on the laboring heart.

Etiology—relation to sodium and water metabolism

Imbalance in capillary fluid shift mechanism. As the heart fails to pump out the returning blood fast enough, the venous return is retarded and a disproportionate amount of blood accumulates in the vascular system concerned with the right side of the heart. The venous pressure rises, overcoming the balance of filtration pressures necessary to maintain the normal capillary fluid shift mechanism. (See Fig. 9-5 for a diagram of this mechanism.) Fluid that normally would flow between the interstitial spaces and the blood vessels is held in the tissue spaces rather than being returned to circulation.

Hormonal mechanisms. The *renin-angiotensin-aldosterone mechanism* (Fig. 9-8) compounds the edema problem. As the heart fails to propel the blood circulation forward, the deficient cardiac output effectively reduces the renal blood flow. The decreased renal blood pressure triggers the renin-angiotensin system[22] and the release of renin, an enzyme from the renal cortex that combines in the blood with its substrate, angiotensinogen, to produce angiotensin I and II. Angiotensin II acts as a stimulant to the adrenal gland. It causes the adrenals to produce aldosterone, the hormone that in turn effects a reabsorption of sodium in an ion exchange with potassium in the distal tubules of the nephrons, and water absorption follows. Ordinarily this is a life-saving mechanism to protect the body's water supply. In congestive heart failure, however, it only adds to the edema problem.

The ADH mechanism (Fig. 9-9) adds to the edema also. The cardiac stress and the reduced renal flow cause the release of *vasopressin,* the antidiuretic hormone, from the pituitary gland. This hormone stimulates still more water reabsorption in the distal tubules of the nephrons.

Increased cellular free potassium. As the reduced blood circulation depresses cellular metabolism, protein catabolism releases protein-bound potassium in the cell, increasing intracellular osmotic pressure from free potassium. Sodium ions in the surrounding extracellular fluid increase to prevent hypotonic dehydration (p. 181). The increased extracellular sodium in time adds to more water retention.

The metabolism of sodium, potassium, and water in Chapter 9 should be reviewed. These mechanisms are discussed there in greater detail with diagrams and will help clarify the abnormal shifts and balances involved in cardiac edema that produce a serious dislocation in the body water compartments.

Principles of diet therapy—sodium-restricted diets

Because of the role of sodium in water balance the diet used to treat cardiac edema restricts the sodium intake. Four levels of dietary sodium restriction have been outlined by the American Heart Association and are in common use throughout the United States. They may best be understood in reference to the usual range of dietary sodium and the common food items each level of restriction would affect.

Sodium in general diet. The taste for salt is an acquired one. Some persons salt food heavily and habituate their taste to high salt levels. Others acquire lighter tastes and use smaller amounts. Common daily adult intakes of sodium range widely from about 3 or 4 g with lighter tastes to as high as 10 to 12 g with heavy use.

Sodium-restricted diets. The main source of dietary sodium is in sodium chloride, common table salt. Many other lesser-used sodium compounds (baking powder, baking soda) contribute small amounts. Otherwise the remaining dietary source is sodium occurring in foods as a natural mineral. The four levels of sodium-restricted diets delete in turn an increasing number of food items or ways of food preparation.

MILD SODIUM RESTRICTION (2 TO 3 g SODIUM). Salt may be used *lightly* in cooking, but no *added* salt is allowed. Obviously, salty foods (salt used as a preservative or flavoring agent) are deleted such as pickles, olives, bacon, ham, and potato chips. A list for mild sodium restriction is shown (p. 619).

MODERATE SODIUM RESTRICTION (1,000 mg). There may be no salt in cooking, no added salt, and no salty foods. Beginning with this level, some control of natural sodium foods is evident. Higher sodium vegetables are limited in use, salt-free canned vegetables are substituted for regular canned ones, salt-free baked products are used, and meat and milk are used in moderate portions. The moderate sodium restriction list is shown on p. 620.

STRICT SODIUM RESTRICTION (500 mg). In addition to the deletions thus far, meat, milk, and eggs are allowed only in smaller portions. Milk is limited to 2 cups total in any form, meat to 140 to 168 g (5 to 6 oz) total, and no more than one egg. Higher sodium vegetables are

---

Restrictions for a mild low-sodium diet (2 to 3 g sodium)

Do not use

1. Salt at the table (use salt lightly in cooking)
2. Salt-preserved foods such as salted or smoked meat (bacon and bacon fat, bologna, dried or chipped beef, corned beef, frankfurters, ham, kosher meats, luncheon meats, salt pork, sausage, smoked tongue); salted or smoked fish (anchovies, caviar, salted and dried cod, herring, sardines; sauerkraut, olives)
3. Highly salted foods such as crackers, pretzels, potato chips, corn chips, salted nuts, salted popcorn
4. Spices and condiments such as bouillon cubes,* catsup,* chili sauce,* celery salt, garlic sauce, onion salt, monosodium glutamate, meat sauces, meat tenderizers,* pickles, prepared mustard, relishes, Worcestershire sauce, soy sauce
5. Cheese,* peanut butter*

*Dietetic low-sodium kind may be used.

---

deleted. A list of restrictions for a strict low-sodium diet is shown on p. 621.

SEVERE SODIUM RESTRICTION (250 mg). No regular milk may be used; low-sodium milk is substituted. Meat is limited to 56 to 112 g (2 to 4 oz) total, and eggs to about three a week. It becomes more important, therefore, to devise ways of incorporating adequate low-sodium milk to ensure adequate protein intake. The liquid beverage forms (whole and skim), available from processing plants in most larger urban centers, are acceptable if well chilled and served immediately upon thawing. Because these fresh milk products deteriorate rapidly after the sodium is removed, the milk is usually frozen and delivered to consumers in this form. If it is thawed just before using and consumed immediately while still icy, it is very palatable.

The lists of foods that should not be used for each sodium-restricted diet level have proved to be useful tools in patient education identifying key foods affected in maintaining a particular sodium intake. The lists also are helpful for general comparison of the diets when changes are made from one level to another.

HYPERTENSIVE CARDIOVASCULAR DISEASE

Hypertension alone is not a disease. It is a symptom complex that may be present in a number of disorders. It is a common clinical problem in cardiovascular disease. Little is known of its etiology. However, Dahl's[23,24] earlier studies linking hypertension to a sensitivity to high salt use have been reinforced by continued investigation related to renin-angiotensin sensitivity[25] in a variety of conditions.

Other early investigators have observed clinical improvement of hypertensive patients through use of a low-sodium dietary regimen. In 1944 Kempner[26] proposed a strict rice-fruit diet and administered it to his patients with beneficial effects to the hypertension. However, it was in reality a barren semistarvation regimen without realistic application in common use. Other clinicians[27] used a more liberal diet than Kempner's, but still the diet was a severe one, limiting sodium to 200 mg daily.

With the advent of effective antihypertensive drugs such as diuretics and others in the past two decades, severe diets are no longer necessary. However, the effectiveness of these

---

Restrictions for a moderate low-sodium diet (1,000 mg sodium)

Do not use
1. Salt in cooking or at the table
2. Salt-preserved foods such as salted or smoked meat (bacon and bacon fat, bologna, dried or chipped beef, brains, corned beef, frankfurters, ham, kosher meats, luncheon meats, salt pork, sausage, smoked tongue, kidneys); salted or smoked fish (anchovies, caviar, salted and dried cod, herring, sardines, frozen fish fillets, canned salmon,* tuna*); sauerkraut, olives
3. Highly salted foods such as crackers, pretzels, potato chips, corn chips, salted nuts, salted popcorn
4. Spices and condiments such as bouillon cubes,* catsup,* chili sauce,* celery salt, garlic salt, onion salt, monosodium glutamate, meat sauces, meat tenderizers,* pickles, prepared mustard, relishes, Worcestershire sauce, soy sauce
5. Cheese,* peanut butter*
6. Buttermilk (unsalted buttermilk may be used) instead of skim milk
7. Canned vegetables* or canned vegetable juices*
8. Frozen peas, frozen limas, frozen mixed vegetables, or any frozen vegetables to which salt has been added
9. More than one serving of any of these vegetables in one day—artichokes, beet greens, beets, carrots, celery, dandelion greens, kale, mustard greens, spinach, swiss chard, turnips (white)
10. Regular bread, rolls,* crackers*
11. Dry cereals,* except puffed rice, puffed wheat, and shredded wheat
12. Quick cooking Cream of Wheat
13. Shellfish—clams, crab, lobster, shrimp (oysters may be used)
14. Salted butter, salted margarine, commercial French dressings,* mayonnaise,* or other salad dressings*
15. Regular baking powder,* baking soda or anything containing them; self-rising flour
16. Prepared mixes—pudding,* gelatin,* cake, biscuit
17. Commercial candies

*Dietetic low-sodium kinds may be used.

---

drugs is enhanced and the hypertensive condition improved by moderate restriction of sodium from 500 to 1,000 mg, depending on individual need and response.[28] The 500 mg and 1,000 mg sodium diets given on pp. 622-624 may be used.

ACUTE CARDIOVASCULAR DISEASE

In the acute phase of cardiovascular disease, myocardial infarction, or congestive failure, additional dietary modifications are usually indicated. The basic therapeutic objective is cardiac rest. Hence all care is given to assure this requirement for restoring the damaged heart to adequate functioning. The diet will be modified, therefore, in energy value and texture.

Calories. A brief period of undernutrition during the first few days after the attack is advisable. The metabolic demands for digestion, absorption, and utilization of food require a generous cardiac output. Small intakes of food decrease the level of metabolic activity to one the weakened heart can accommodate. In 1866 a Russian physician recognized this principle and, during this acute period, fed his patients only four glasses of milk a day. Even today such a regimen is ordered by his name—the

Restrictions for a strict low-sodium diet (500 mg sodium)

Do not use

1. Salt in cooking or at the table
2. Salt-preserved foods such as salted or smoked meat—bacon and bacon fat, bologna, dried or chipped beef, brains, corned beef, frankfurters, ham, kosher meats, luncheon meats, salt pork, sausage, smoked tongue, kidneys; salted or smoked fish—anchovies, caviar, salted and dried cod, herring, sardines, frozen fish fillets, canned salmon,* tuna*; sauerkraut; olives
3. Highly salted foods such as crackers, pretzels, potato chips, corn chips, salted nuts, salted popcorn
4. Spices and condiments such as bouillon cubes,* catsup,* chili sauce,* celery salt, garlic salt, onion salt, monosodium glutamate (M.S.G., Accent, etc.), meat sauces, meat tenderizers,* pickles, prepared mustard, relishes, Worcestershire sauce, soy sauce
5. Cheese,* peanut butter*
6. Buttermilk (unsalted buttermilk may be used) instead of skim milk
7. More than 2 cups skim milk a day, including that used on cereal
8. Any commercial foods made of milk (ice cream, ice milk, milk shakes)
9. Canned vegetables* or canned vegetable juices*
10. Frozen peas, frozen limas, frozen mixed vegetables, or any frozen vegetables to which salt has been added
11. These vegetables—artichokes, beet greens, beets, carrots, celery, dandelion greens, kale, mustard greens, spinach, Swiss chard, turnips (white)
12. Regular bread,* rolls,* crackers*
13. Dry cereals,* except puffed rice, puffed wheat, and shredded wheat
14. Quick cooking cream of wheat
15. Shell fish—clams, crab, lobster, shrimp (oysters may be used)
16. Salted butter, salted margarine, commercial French dressings,* mayonnaise,* or other salad dressings*
17. Regular baking powder,* baking soda, or anything containing them; self-rising flour
18. Prepared mixes—pudding,* gelatin, cake, biscuit
19. Commercial candies

*Dietetic low-sodium kinds may be used.

Karell diet; or some physicians may simply request milk only for the first day or so and then progress to more food as the patient improves. During the recovery stages the calories may be limited to 800 to 1,200 to continue cardiac rest from metabolic loads. If the patient is obese, as is frequent, this caloric level may be continued for a longer period to effect desired weight loss.

Texture. Early feedings will be soft in nature or easily digested to avoid effort in eating. Smaller meals served more frequently may give needed nutrition without undue strain or pressure.

PATIENT EDUCATION

Since cardiovascular disease assumes more or less a chronic nature, an important responsibility of the health team is education of the patient and his family concerning continuing needs for health care.[19,20] Such teaching should not wait for discharge instructions but should begin early in convalescence, give the patient a clear knowledge of positive needs, and focus

Low-sodium diet (500 mg sodium)

General description
1. All foods are to be prepared and served without the addition of salt, baking powder, or baking soda.
2. Take only those foods that are tolerated and in the amounts specified.
3. Read all food labels for the *addition of salt or sodium in any form.*
4. Avoid medications and laxatives unless approved by your doctor.
5. The suggested menu pattern for 500 mg sodium contains approximately 275 g carbohydrate, 85 g protein, 130 g fat, and 2,300 calories. All menu patterns meet the recommended allowances of vitamins and minerals.

	Daily allowance	Foods to avoid
Milk	Limit to 2 cups milk daily—frozen, powdered, or canned or as 1 cup evaporated milk, used as beverage or in cooking; 2 tbsp cream (1 oz, or 30 ml)	Malted milk, sour cream, buttermilk, condensed milk, milk shakes, chocolate milk, fruit flavored beverage powders, whipped toppings
Eggs	One daily	
Meat, poultry,	Cooked daily, 168 g (6 oz); fresh beef, lamb, liver, pork, veal, rabbit, chicken, duck, goose, quail, turkey, cod, halibut, filet sole, tuna, salmon, or meats canned without salt; frozen meat containing no salt or sodium (beef or calf liver allowed not more than once in two weeks)	All meat, poultry, fish not listed; avoid meat, fish, or poultry that is smoked, cured, canned, frozen, containing salt or sodium, pickled, salted, or dried (bacon, ham, luncheon meats, sausages, salt pork, canned salmon and tuna, sardines), calms, crabs, lobsters, oysters (eastern), scallops, shrimp, anchovies, salted dried cod, frozen fish fillets, commercial meat pies, TV dinners
Cheese	Special dietetic low-sodium cheese may be used as a meat substitute as part of the daily allowance	Any other
Fruits	Three servings daily including one citrus fruit—½ cup per serving, fresh, canned, or frozen	Dried figs, raisins containing sodium sulfite
Vegetables	Four servings daily (fresh, frozen, or dietetic canned vegetables only)—½ cup per serving; asparagus, green beans, wax beans, lima beans, navy beans, broccoli, cauliflower, corn, cucumber, endive, egg plant, lentils, onions, parsnips, peppers, radishes, rutabagas, cabbage, brussels sprouts, lettuce, mushrooms, okra, soybeans, squash, tomatoes, unsalted tomato juice, turnip greens	Canned vegetables or juices containing salt (V-8 juice), sauerkraut, white turnip, beets, celery, carrot, artichoke; greens—beets, spinach, chard, dandelions, kalo, mustard greens; frozen peas, frozen lima beans, frozen mixed vegetables

Low-sodium diet (500 mg sodium)—cont'd

	Daily allowance—cont'd	Foods to avoid—cont'd
Potato or substitute	Two servings daily of potato, rice, macaroni, spaghetti, noodles, fresh sweet potatoes	Potato chips, corn chips
Cereals	One serving daily shredded wheat, puffed rice, puffed wheat, or cooked cereals that contain no added salt or sodium as regular Cream of Wheat, cornmeal, Maltomeal, rice, Wheatena, Pettijohns, Ralston, oatmeal	Quick-cooking Cream of Wheat and all other ready-to-eat cereals not listed; self-rising flour
Bread	Low-sodium bread or unsalted matzoth; low-sodium crackers	Potato chips, salted crackers, salted popcorn, pretzels, regular bread, rolls, biscuits, or muffins; waffles, commercial mixes
Fats	Sweet butter, lard, salad oils, shortening, low-sodium salad dressing as desired; unsalted margarine (check label and brand)	Salted nuts, salted butter, bacon fat, margarine, salted peanut butter, gravies, and commercial salad dressings
Soup	Homemade soup made with allowed meat, vegetables, and milk	Broth, bouillon, consommé, and canned soups
Sweets	Jelly, jam, sugar, honey, gumdrops, marshmallows as desired; small amounts of brown sugar	Any commercial jam and jelly containing a sodium preservative, molasses, candy, candy bars
Desserts	Fruit, gelatin dessert made with plain gelatin and fruit juice, fruit pie made without salt; rice, tapioca, or cornstarch pudding made with low-sodium milk or fruit and fruit juices; desserts made with sodium-free baking powder	All others, ice cream, sherbet, desserts made with regular baking powder, baking soda, rennet tablets, pudding mixes; commercial gelatin desserts, pudding and cake mixes
Beverages	Tea, coffee, postum, Sanka, cocoa (except Dutch process) made with low-sodium milk allowance, fruit juices	Instant cocoa mix, prepared beverage mixes
Condiments	Alspice, bay leaves, caraway seeds, cinnamon, curry powder, garlic, mace, marjoram, mustard powder, nutmeg, paprika, parsley, pimiento, rosemary, sage, sesame seeds, thyme, tumeric, ginger, pepper, vinegar; extracts of almond, lemon, vanilla, peppermint, walnut, maple	Celery salt, garlic salt, catsup, prepared mustard, salt, meat sauces, meat tenderizers, monosodium glutamate, soy sauce, pickles, relishes, olives, prepared horseradish, Worcestershire sauce, chili sauce, seasoning salts
Miscellaneous		Baking powder, baking soda, chewing tobacco

Continued.

Low-sodium diet (500 mg sodium)—cont'd

500 mg–sodium diet suggested menu pattern

Breakfast	Lunch	Dinner
1 fruit	84 g (3 oz) unsalted meat	84 g (3 oz) unsalted meat
1 egg	unsalted potato	unsalted potato
low-sodium cereal	low-sodium vegetable	low-sodium vegetable
1 low-sodium bread	low-sodium vegetable salad	low-sodium salad
1 unsalted butter	1 low-sodium bread	1 low-sodium bread
jelly	1 unsalted butter	1 unsalted butter
½ cup milk	jelly	jelly
coffee (1 oz, or 30 ml)	1 fruit	1 cup milk
2 tbsp cream (1 oz, or	½ cup milk	coffee
30 ml)	coffee	fruit

Modifications for a 250 mg sodium diet

The 250 mg sodium diet is essentially the same as the 500 mg sodium diet except
1. Use low-sodium milk (2 or more glasses) instead of regular milk
2. Use only 140 g (5 oz) of meat instead of 168 g (6 oz)
3. Omit the cream

Modifications for a 1,000 mg sodium diet

One of the three following modifications may be used to raise the sodium content in the 500 mg sodium diet to 1,000 mg.

Modification I
1. Two slices regular bread are allowed daily
2. Regular butter, 2 tsp only (above this amount, unsalted butter must be used)
3. One serving (½ cup) is allowed daily of spinach, celery, carrots, beets, artichoke, or white turnip

Modification II (high protein)
1. Meat, 28 g (10 oz) are allowed instead of 168 g (6 oz)
2. One serving of prepared or milk dessert, such as ice cream, custard, gelatin, or 1 cup milk
3. Two eggs instead of one
4. One serving of spinach, celery, carrots, beets, or artichoke is allowed

Modification III
1. Three slices regular bread may be used in place of the low-sodium bread (above this amount, unsalted bread must be used)

Low-sodium food exchange groups

Group A vegetables

Raw, cooked, or canned without salt or fat; may be eaten as desired; one serving contains little or no calories and 9 mg sodium

Foods permitted		Foods to avoid
Asparagus	Lettuce	Canned vegetables (unless canned without
Beans, green	Mushrooms	salt)
Broccoli	Okra	
Brussels sprouts	Parsley	The following vegetables are high in natural
Cauliflower	Peppers	salt and must be omitted from the diet:
Celery*	Radishes	Beet greens
Cabbage, fresh	Squash, summer	Chard
Chicory	Spinach*	Swiss kale
Cucumbers	Tomatoes	Sauerkraut
Eggplant	Salt-free tomato juice	
Endive	Watercress	
Escarole		

Group B vegetables

Only ½ cup of one of the following vegetables may be used per day; contains approximately 9 mg sodium per serving; 7 g carbohydrate, 2 g protein, and 35 calories

Foods permitted		Foods to avoid
Artichokes	Peas	White turnips
Beets*	Pumpkin	Frozen peas
Carrots*	Rutabagas	
Onions	Winter squash	

Fruits

Fresh, dried, cooked, or canned without added sugar; this list shows the amount of fruit to use for one serving; contains 2 mg sodium; one serving contains 10 g carbohydrate and 40 calories

Foods permitted		Foods to avoid
Apple	1 small	Canned tomato juice or vegetable juices
Applesauce	½ cup	Fruit or fruit products that contain sodium
Apricots, fresh	2 medium	benzoate, maraschino cherries; dried fruit
Apricots, dried	4 halves	sometimes has sodium sulfate added, these
Banana	½ small	should be avoided, read label (use only
Blackberries	1 cup	sundried fruits)
Raspberries	1 cup	
Blueberries	⅔ cup	
Strawberries	1 cup	
Cantaloupe	¼ medium	
Cherries	10 large	

*Vegetables allowed once a day if sodium allowance is 1,000 mg.

Low-sodium food exchange groups—cont'd

Fruits—cont'd

Foods permitted—cont'd		Foods to avoid—cont'd
Dates	2	
Figs, fresh	2 large	
Grapefruit juice	½ cup	
Grapes	12	
Grape juice	¼ cup	
Honeydew melon	⅛ medium	
Orange	1 small	
Orange juice	½ cup	
Peach	1 medium	
Pear	1 small	
Pineapple	½ cup	
Pineapple juice	⅓ cup	
Plums	2 medium	
Prunes, dried	2 medium	
Tangerine	1 large	
Watermelon	1 cup	

Bread

One serving contains 15 g carbohydrate, 2 g protein, 70 calories, 5 mg sodium (substitute the following for one slice salt-free bread)

Foods permitted		Foods to avoid
Salt-free Passover matzoth	½	Regular bread and rolls
Salt-free melba toast	3	Biscuits and popovers
Low-sodium toast (Nabisco)	2	Salted or soda crackers
Cooked cereals (without salt)	½ cup	Pastries and cakes
		Prepared muffins, waffles, cakes
Pearl barley, rice, noodles	½ cup	Self-rising flour
Macaroni, spaghetti	½ cup	Cornmeal
Lima beans, fresh	½ cup	Quick-cooking (5 minute) hot cereals
Navy beans, dried	½ cup	Dry cereals except those listed
Soybeans, cowpeas	½ cup	Pretzels, potato chips
Potato (white)	1 small	Salted popcorn
Potato (sweet)	¼ cup	Frozen lima beans
Parsnips	⅔ cup	
Corn (fresh, frozen, or canned unsalted, or 1 small ear)	⅔ cup	
Puffed wheat, puffed rice	¾ cup	
Shredded wheat	1 biscuit	
Popcorn, unsalted	1 cup	

Meat

Twenty-eight grams (1 oz) contains 7 g protein, 5 g fat, 25 mg sodium, 75 calories; substitute the following for 28 g salt-free meat (baked, broiled, stewed, or pan broiled):

Low-sodium food exchange groups—cont'd

Foods permitted		Foods to avoid
Fresh or frozen beef, lamb, liver, pork, rabbit, veal, or tongue	28 g	All smoked, processed or canned meats, fish, or fowl, such as anchovies, caviar, herring, salted dry cod, bacon, oysters
Fresh fish (except shellfish)	28 g	Cold cuts
Fresh or frozen chicken, duck, turkey, quail	28 g	Corned beef or chipped beef
		Frankfurters or sausages
Canned salt-free tuna or salmon	¼ cup	Brain, kidney
		Ham, smoked tongue, sausage
Salt-free peanut butter	1 tbsp	All cheese except salt-free cheese
Salt-free American cheese	28 g	Frozen fish fillets, clams, crab, lobster, shrimp, sardines, oysters, kosher meats
Salt-free cottage cheese (dry curd)	¼ cup	Peanut butter, except salt-free
Eggs	1 per day	

Fats

One serving contains 5 g fat, little or no sodium, and 45 calories; substitute the following for 1 tsp salt-free butter:

Foods permitted		Foods to avoid
Butter, salt-free	1 tsp	Salted butter, oleomargarine
Cream, light (sweet or sour)	2 tbsp	Commercial mayonnaise or French dressing
Cream, heavy	1 tbsp	Bacon fat and salty meat drippings and olives
Avocado	⅛	Salted nuts
French dressing, salt-free	1 tbsp	Salt pork
Mayonnaise, salt-free	1 tsp	
Oil or cooking fat	1 tsp	
Nuts, unsalted	6 small	

Seasonings

Foods permitted		Foods to avoid
Allspice	Paprika	Rennet tablets
Baking yeast	Parsley	Salt in any form
Caraway	Pepper, black	Baking soda and baking powder
Cinnamon	Pepper, red	Prepared mustard, ketchup, meat sauces, chili sauce, horseradish
Curry powder	Pepper, white	
Garlic	Peppermint extract	Bouillon or canned soups
Ginger	Sage	Olives and pickles and relishes
Herbs	Saccharine	Celery salt, celery seed, onion salt, garlic salt
Horseradish (fresh grated)	Thyme	
Lemon juice or extract	Turmeric	Accent, Zest, Tok
Mace	Vanilla extract	Salted meat tenderizers
Mustard, dry	Vinegar	Prepared horseradish
Nutmeg	Walnut extract	Worchestershire sauce
		Meat extracts
		Meat sauces

on positive behavior changes.[29] Such an approach will provide resources for sound and vigorous self-care within the limits of individual capacity and help avoid the negative apprehension of a cardiac cripple.

Many excellent resources for patient education are provided by the American Heart Association through their national and regional offices. Practical discussions need to center on food buying and preparation to make the diets palatable and acceptable to the patients. Many helpful suggestions are included in the American Heart Association booklets and in the listed cookbooks. A survey of local markets will give guidance concerning commercial products and label reading.

Modified low-sodium food exchange groups are listed on p. 625. These may be used to guide patients on calorie controlled low-sodium diets. The 800- to 1,500-calorie diet plans are on p. 538 and can be used to make food choices from these low-sodium food groups.

In the final analysis the wisest approach to the control of cardiovascular disease is that of prevention and positive health promotion and maintenance. Real prevention of cardiovascular problems begins in childhood with the building of sound health habits, food behaviors in relation to fat, sugar, and salt,[30,31] and an active life of physical activity.

CASE STUDY 22

The patient with a myocardial infarction

Walter Thomas, aged 47, was a successful corporation lawyer. He had been driving himself for some time to meet the increasing responsibilities and demands of his position with a large steel company. At his last physical checkup, which the company provided for all its executives, the doctor had cautioned him to slow his pace or his health would soon suffer. Already Walter was having some mild hypertension, the doctor reminded him. His blood cholesterol was elevated, and he was overweight.

"You don't get any consistent moderate physical exercise in your sedentary work situation," the doctor concluded. "If you could plan to include some simple exercise, like walking, for example, get your weight down, and learn to relax, you'd be a lot better off. When was the last time you had a real vacation anyway?"

Walter had thought about the doctor's words this past week since his physical examination. Now, driving home on the crowded freeway in the midst of the commuter crush, he realized that he was under increased pressure and that he was even chain smoking now. He crushed his cigarette in the ashtray with a vigorous push. He began to wonder about the purpose of it all. He thought of his wife, Martha, and their expensive home that she maintained with such great pride. He thought of their three children, two in college and one in graduate school, and the increasing problems he seemed to have communicating with them. He felt a tightness in his chest and a vague apprehension. He was glad when he finally made it to his own driveway. Martha had dinner ready when he came into the house, but he told her he didn't feel like eating anything and instead would lie down for a while.

The pain persisted in his chest, however, even as he rested, and it became increasingly severe. He broke out in a cold sweat and felt nauseated. When Martha came in to check on him a little later she found him in the bathroom vomiting and in evident distress. Despite his protest that it must be just some indigestion, she was alarmed at his pale appearance and called his physician. When she described Walter's symptoms, Dr. Owens said he would send an ambulance to bring Walter to the hospital without delay.

At the hospital Dr. Owens and the emergency room staff gave Walter immediate care to relieve his pain, aid his breathing, prevent shock, and give him complete rest. A number of laboratory tests were ordered, including SGOT, LDH, prothrombin time, lipid panel plus HDL-cholesterol, sedimentation rate, Lee-White coagulation time, FBS, BUN, and CBC. An EKG was also ordered. Walter was moved to the coronary care unit, where his condition could be closely monitored. The test results showed elevated SGOT, LDH, total cholesterol, triglycerides, glucose, prothrombin time, and white blood cell count, low HDL value, and increased sedimentation rate. The EKG revealed an infarction of the posterior wall of the myocardium.

In conference with Dr. Owens the clinical nutritionist outlined and directed Walter's nutritional therapy. At first he had only a liquid diet. After the first few days Walter's condition was beginning to stabilize, and his diet was increased to an 800-calorie soft diet, low saturated fat. By the end of the first week Walter's diet was further increased to 1,200 calories, full diet, low saturated fat. This time, however, the nutritionist specified that the calories from fat be only 25% of the total calories with a P/S ratio of 1.1 to 1. Walter's nurse, Miss Newman, noted these changes in his diet and discussed them with Dr. Owens and the nutritionist.

Walter gradually improved over the next few weeks and was finally able to go home in about a month. Dr. Owens discussed with him the need for care at home during a period of convalescence. He explained that Walter had an underlying lipid disorder—Type IIb hyperlipoproteinemia—and was to continue his weight loss with a modified fat and carbohydrate diet under the direction of the clinical nutritionist. The doctor told him he and the nutritionist would continue his follow-up care in the clinic later.

Continued.

CASE STUDY 22
The patient with a myocardial infarction—cont'd

Questions to guide your inquiry

1. What factors can you identify in Walter's background and personal and medical history that place him in a "high-risk category" for coronary disease?
2. Why would the doctor recommend moderate, consistent physical exercise to Walter?
3. Account for the initial symptoms of Walter's illness. What happens in a myocardial infarction?
4. Identify the laboratory tests Dr. Owens ordered. Relate these tests to cell metabolism. Why would they be elevated in Walter's case?
5. Why would Walter receive only a liquid diet at first?
6. What are the reasons for each of the modifications in Walter's first diet of solid food?
7. What occurs in the underlying disease process, atherosclerosis?
8. What relation does fat metabolism have to the disease?
9. What is the concept of saturation as applied to the structure of fats?
10. What food fats are saturated fats? Which are unsaturated? What does the term "polyunsaturated" mean?
11. When Walter's diet was changed, what was meant by "P/S ratio 1.1 to 1"?
12. Outline a day's menu for Walter on his increased diet of 1,200 calories as specified by the clinical nutritionist.
13. What problems can you identify that Walter may have with his hospital diet? Why?
14. What solutions can you propose? Why?
15. If you were Walter's nutritionist, what plan of action would you outline to meet his nutritional needs?
16. How would you involve other health team members in your plan of care?
17. How would you involve Walter's wife, Martha, in your plan of care?
18. What is a lipoprotein? What are the five classes of lipoproteins and their respective functions?
19. Interpret Walter's lipid panel results: total cholesterol 350, triglycerides 250, HDL-cholesterol 30. Calculate his LDL-cholesterol value and indicate its significance.
20. Compare the six types of lipid disorders. Describe the characteristics of Walter's type—Type IIb—and the diet therapy indicated.
21. What needs might Walter have when he goes home? What plan would you make for helping Walter prepare to go home?
22. Name some community resources you might use in helping Walter understand his illness and its care.
23. Describe some teaching materials, methods, and approaches you would plan to use with Walter and his wife.
24. What follow-up plans for care after discharge from the hospital can you suggest for Walter?

CASE STUDY 23
The patient with hypertensive cardiovascular disease

Sam Harris, aged 57, was a large black man—183 cm (6 ft, 1 in) tall, weighing 157 kg (348 lb). For a number of years he had worked as an aircraft mechanic at the Naval Air Station. Recently, however, because of his health problems, he had been worried about the security of his job. There had been a change of supervisors, and Mr. Harris was having some difficulty communicating his needs to the new foreman. He knew with his lack of education—he had had to stop school years ago after the seventh grade to help support his family—that changing jobs, finding a new one at his age, would be difficult if not impossible. He made a fairly adequate salary now, but it was becoming increasingly difficult to make ends meet.

For some 10 years Mr. Harris had had a history of hypertension, but with little consistent follow-through of medical care. Lately, however, as a result of his increasing concern about his health, he had begun to keep his regular monthly appointments in the hypertension clinic at the medical center with a greater degree of consistency. He did have some group insurance through his union that partly covered the cost of his care and medications.

Mr. Harris's most recent chest X-ray revealed an enlarged heart and left ventricular hypertrophy. His six-lead EKG was borderline. His FBS test was 158, placing him in a prediabetic category. Blood pressure readings at various clinic visits over the past year remained elevated: 202/130, 160/108, 182/110, 210/110, 158/100. His family history revealed that his mother had suffered from hypertension. His physician at the clinic had ordered for him Apresoline (hydralazine hydrochloride) and reserpine. He said that he tried to remember to take his medication faithfully, but his wife on one visit had indicated his inconsistency in this also.

Mr. Harris was being followed in the interim by the nurse practitioner in the hypertension clinic, Miss Martin, and the nutritionist at the health center, Mrs. Wright. The necessity of weight loss and for cutting down on his high salt intake had been impressed on him.

Changing food habits was difficult, however, for Mr. Harris. He was a big-hearted man. His wife's sister and mother had had various personal problems, and he had opened his home to them. Now, in addition to his two children, a boy 15 and a girl 10, and his wife, his family numbered six. And there always seemed to be extra friends or relatives around, especially at meal times, so food was important in his home. Also, there was little exercise on his job, and his leisure habits were sedentary.

Mr. Harris indicated to the nutritionist that he ate a large quantity of food containing much fat and salt. He was straightforward about his habits. He said that he usually skipped breakfast, had a doughnut and coffee at midmorning, and then ate soup and a sandwich that he purchased at a counter nearby for lunch. At home in the evening the family had a large dinner—fried foods, gravies, corn bread, and vegetables cooked in salt pork. There were usually baked goods such as pies and cakes always on hand.

At the clinic health team conference, Dr. Grant discussed Mr. Harris's case with the other staff members. Again he reviewed with them the seriousness of Mr. Harris's situation and repeated the need for vigorous therapy and support.

"We're sitting on a case here that may well blow at any minute," he concluded, "and we have reason to be concerned."

Continued.

CASE STUDY 23
The patient with hypertensive cardiovascular disease—cont'd

Questions to guide your inquiry

1. What is the nature of hypertensive cardiovascular disease? How is it usually treated?
2. Identify the problems involved in Mr. Harris's health care. What are the reasons for them?
3. What solutions would you propose? Why?
4. What goals would you establish in relation to these problems?
5. What are Mr. Harris's nutritional needs?
6. What diet—calories and sodium levels—do you think would be appropriate for the nutritionist to use in helping Mrs. Harris plan his meals? Why?
7. Outline a diet pattern to guide meal planning on the diet you have given in the previous question.
8. Plan a day's food for Mr. Harris following the prescribed diet pattern.
9. What personal factors would the nutritionist have to consider in planning Mr. Harris's diet? Why?
10. Why is it so important that Mr. Harris change his food habits? How would you go about helping him do so?
11. What resources, approaches, teaching materials, and methods can you suggest to help in your teaching plan for Mr. and Mrs. Harris?

REFERENCES
Specific

1. Multiple Risk Factor Intervention Trial, Nutr. Today **9**(3):28, 1974.
2. Bellet, S., et al.: Comparative human study; coffee linked to free fatty acid increase, J.A.M.A. **197**:37, 1966.
3. Jankelson, O. M., Beaser, S. B., Howard, F. M., et al.: Effect of coffee on glucose tolerance and circulating insulin in men with maturity-onset diabetes, Lancet **1**:527, 1967.
4. Mayer, L.: Obesity and cardiovascular disease, J. Am. Diet. Assoc. **52**:13, 1968.
5. Boston Collaborative Drug Surveillance Program: Coffee drinking and acute myocardial infarction, Lancet **2**:1278, 1973.
6. Klatsky, A. L., Friedman, G. D., and Siegelaub, A. B.: Coffee drinking prior to acute myocardial infarction: results from the Kaiser-Permanente epidemiologic study of myocardial infarction, J.A.M.A. **226**:540, 1973.
7. Anderson, J. T., Grande, F., and Keys, A.: Independence of the effects of cholesterol and degree of saturation of the fat in the diet on serum cholesterol in man, Am. J. Clin. Nutr. **29**:1184, 1976.
8. Gatto, A. M.: Is atherosclerosis reversible? J. Am. Diet. Assoc. **74**:551, May, 1979.
9. Kannel, W. B.: The disease of living, Nutr. Today **6**(3):2, 1971.

10. Kannel, W. B., Dawber, T. R., and Friedman, G. D.: Risk factors in coronary heart disease: the Framingham study, Ann. Intern. Med. **61**:888, 1964.
11. Fredrickson, D. S., Levy, R. I., and Lees, R. S.: Fat transport in lipoproteins—an integrated approach to mechanisms and disorders. N. Engl. J. Med. **276**:34, 1967.
12. Strisower, E. G., Adamson, G., and Strisower, B.: Treatment of hyperlipidemias, Am. J. Med. **45**:488, 1968.
13. Kannel, W. B., Castelli, W. P., Gordon, T., and McNamara, P. M.: Serum cholesterol, lipoproteins, and the risk of coronary heart disease, the Framingham study, Ann. Intern. Med. **74**:1, 1971.
14. Lees, R. S., and Wilson, D. E.: The treatment of hyperlipidemia, N. Engl. J. Med. **284**:186, 1971.
15. Ernst, N., and Levy, R. I.: Diet, hyperlipidemia, and atherosclerosis. In Goodhart, R. S., and Shils, M. E., editors: Modern nutrition in health and disease, Philadelphia, 1980, Lea & Febiger, p. 1058.
16. Ireton, C. L., Davidson, A. G., Applegarth, D. A., et al.: Case report: diagnosis and management of type I hyperlipoproteinemia, J. Am. Diet. Assoc. **66**:42, 1975.
17. Harkins, R. W., and Sarett, H. P.: Medium chain triglycerides, J.A.M.A. **203**(4):110, 1968.
18. Smith, L. K., Luepker, R. V., Rothchild, S. S., et al.: Management of type IV hyperlipoproteinemia, Ann. Intern. Med. **84**:22, 1976.

19. Buller, A. C.: Improving dietary education for patients with hyperlipidemia, J. Am. Diet. Assoc. **72**:277, March, 1978.

20. Witschi, J. C., Singer, M., Wu-Lee, M., and Starl, F. J.: Family cooperation and effectiveness in a cholesterol-lowering diet, J. Am. Diet. Assoc. **72**:384, April, 1978.

21. American Medical Association Council on Foods and Nutrition: The regulation of dietary fat, J.A.M.A. **181**:411, 1962.

22. Peart, S. W.: Renin-angiotensin system, N. Engl. J. Med. **292**:302, 1975.

23. Dahl, L. K.: Role of dietary sodium in essential hypertension, J. Am. Diet. Assoc. **34**:585, 1958.

24. Dahl, L. K.: Salt and hypertension, Am. J. Clin. Nutr. **25**:231, 1972.

25. Gant, N. F., Daley, G. L., Chand, S., et al.: A study of angiotensin II pressor response throughout primigravid pregnancy, J. Clin. Invest. **52**:2682, 1973.

26. Kempner, W.: Rice diet in the treatment of hypertension and vascular disease, N. C. Med. J. **5**:125, 1944.

27. Grollman, A., et al.: Sodium restriction in the diet for hypertension, J.A.M.A. **129**:533, 1945.

28. Dustan, H. R.: Diuretic and diet treatment of hypertension, Arch. Intern. Med. **133**:1007, 1974.

29. Pomerleau, O., Bass, F., and Crown, V.: Role of behavior modification in preventive medicine, N. Engl. J. Med. **292**:1277, 1975.

30. Mitchell, S. C.: Prevention of atherosclerosis at the pediatric level, Am. J. Cardiol. **31**:539, 1973.

31. American Academy of Pediatrics, Committee on Nutrition: Salt intake and eating patterns of infants and children in relation to blood pressure, Pediatrics **53**:115, 1974.

General

American Heart Association, Committee on Nutrition: Diet and coronary heart disease, New York, 1973.

American Medical Association, Council on Foods and Nutrition: Diet and the possible prevention of coronary atheroma, J.A.M.A. **194**:1149, 1965.

Baker, B. M., Frantz, I. D., Jr., Keys, A., et al.: The national diet-heart study. An initial report, J.A.M.A. **185**:105, 1963.

Bills, C. E., McDonald, F. G., Niedermeier, W., and Schwartz, M. C.: Sodium and potassium in foods and water, J. Am. Diet. Assoc. **25**:304, 1949.

Bine, R., Jr.: Cardiology. In Schneider, H. A., Anderson, C. E., and Coursin, D. B., editors: Nutritional support of medical practice, New York, 1977, Harper & Row, Publishers.

Bortz, W. M.: The pathogenesis of hypercholesterolemia, Ann. Intern. Med. **80**:738, 1974.

Braunwald, E., editor: The myocardium: failure and infarction, New York, 1974, H P Publishing Co.

Brown, H. B.: Food patterns that lower blood lipids in man, J. Am. Diet. Assoc. **58**:303, 1971.

Brown, H. B.: What a dietitian should know about hyperlipidemia, J. Am. Diet. Assoc. **63**:169, Aug., 1973.

Connor, W. E.: Dietary sterols: their relationship to atherosclerosis, J. Am. Diet. Assoc. **52**:202, 1968.

Cooper, T., and Mitchell, S. C.: Research in cardiovascular disease, J. Am. Diet. Assoc. **58**(5):401, 1971.

Ernst, N., and Levy, R. I.: Diet, hyperlipidemia, and atherosclerosis. In Goodhart, R. S., and Shils, M. E., editors: Modern nutrition in health and disease, Philadelphia, 1980, Lea & Febiger.

Freis, E. D.: Salt, volume, and the prevention of hypertension, Circulation **53**:589, 1976.

Fulton, L., and Davis, C.: Baked products for the fat-controlled, low-cholesterol diet, J. Am. Diet. Assoc. **73**:261, Sept., 1978.

Gotto, A. M., and Scott, L.: Dietary aspects of hyperlipidemia, J. Am. Diet. Assoc. **62**:617, 1973.

Hashim, S. A.: Medium-chain triglycerides—clinical and metabolic aspects, J. Am. Diet. Assoc. **51**:221, 1967.

Hill, P., and Wynder, E. I.: Dietary regulation of serum lipids in healthy, young adults, J. Am. Diet. Assoc. **68**:25, Jan., 1976.

Hodges, R. E., and Krehl, W. A.: The role of carbohydrates in lipid metabolism, Am. J. Clin. Nutr. **17**:334, 1965.

Holinger, B. W., Steinberg, R., and Gordon, R.: Analyzed sodium values in foods ready to serve, J. Am. Diet. Assoc. **48**:501, June, 1966.

Hurst, J. W., Logue, R. B., Schlant, R. C., and Wenger, N. K., editors: The heart, arteries, and veins, ed. 3, New York, 1974, McGraw-Hill Book Co.

Kannel, W. B., and Gordon, T., editors: The Framingham study: diet and regulation of serum cholesterol, Section 24, U.S. Dept. of HEW, 1970, Public Health Service.

Kark, R. M., and Oyama, J. H.: Nutrition, hypertension, and kidney diseases. In Goodhart, R. S., and Shils, M. E., editors: Modern nutrition in health and disease, Philadelphia, 1980, Lea & Febiger.

Klevay, L. M.: Coronary heart disease: the zinc/copper hypothesis, Am. J. Clin. Nutr. **28**:764, 1975.

Kuo, P. T.: Prevention and treatment of hyperlipidemia. In Halpern, S. L., editor: Quick reference to clinical nutrition, Philadelphia, 1979, J. B. Lippincott Co.

Kuo, P. T.: Hyperlipidemia and coronary artery disease, Med. Clin. North Am. **53**:351, 1974.

LaCroix, W. A., et al.: Cholesterol, fat, and protein in dairy products, J. Am. Diet. Assoc. **62**:275, March, 1973.

Lees, R. S., and Wilson, D. E.: The treatment of hyperlipoproteinemia, N. Engl. J. Med. **284**:186, 1971.

Levy, R. I., Bounell, M., and Ernst, N. D.: Dietary management of hyperlipoproteinemia, J. Am. Diet. Assoc. **58**(5):406, 1971.

Levy, R. I., and Fredrickson, D. S.: The current status of hypolipidemic drugs, Postgrad. Med. **70:**130, 1970.

Levy, R. I., Fredrickson, D. S., et al.: Dietary and drug treatment of primary hyperlipoproteinemia, Ann. Intern. Med. **77:**267, 1972.

Macdonald, I.: Ingested glucose and fructose in serum lipids in healthy men and after myocardial infarction, Am. J. Clin. Nutr. **21**(12):1366, 1968.

Mazlen, R. G.: Nutrition and cardiovascular disease. In Halpern, S. L., editor: Quick reference to clinical nutrition, Philadelphia, 1979, J. B. Lippincott Co.

Miljanich, P., and Ostwald, R.: Fatty acids in newer brands of margarine, J. Am. Diet. Assoc. **56**(1):29, 1970.

Moltulsky, A.: The genetic hyperlipidemias, N. Engl. J. Med. **294:**823, 1976.

Mueller, J. F.: A dietary approach to coronary artery disease, J. Am. Diet. Assoc. **62:**613, 1973.

Ostwald, R.: Fatty acids in eleven brands of margarine, J. Am. Diet. Assoc. **39:**313, 1961.

Page, I. H., et al.: The national diet-heart study final report, American Heart Association Monograph No. 18, New York, 1968, The American Heart Association.

Perry, M. H.: Minerals in cardiovascular disease, J. Am. Diet. Assoc. **62:**631, 1973.

Peterkin, B. B., Shore, C. J., and Kerr, R. L.: Some diets that meet the dietary goals for the United States, J. Am. Diet. Assoc. **74:**423, April, 1979.

Peterson, C. R.: Dietary counseling for patients admitted for coronary artery bypass surgery, J. Am. Diet. Assoc. **68:**158, Feb., 1976.

Ponsati, L. P., et al.: Comprehensive evaluation of fatty acids in foods, J. Am. Diet. Assoc. I. Dairy products **66:**482, 1975;·II. Beef products **67:**35, 1975; III. Eggs and egg products **67:**111, 1975; IV. Nuts, peanuts, and soups **67:**351, 1975; V. Unhydrogenated fats and oils **68:**224, 1976; VI. Cereal products **68:**335, 1976; VII. Pork products **69:**44, 1976; VIII. Finfish **69:**243, 1976; IX. Fowl **69:**517, 1976; X. Lamb and veal **70:**53, 1977; XI. Leguminous seeds **71:**412, 1977.

Raymond, T. L., et al.: The interaction of dietary fibers and cholesterol upon the plasma lipids and lipoproteins, sterol balance, and bowel function in human subjects, J. Clin. Invest. **60:**1429, 1977.

Schizas, A. A., Cremen, J. A., Larson, E., et al.: Medium-chain triglycerides—use in food preparation, J. Am. Diet. Assoc. **51:**228, Sept., 1967.

Scott, L. W., Foreyt, J. P., Young, J., et al.: Are low-cholesterol diets expensive? J. Am. Diet. Assoc. **74:** 558, May, 1979.

Seelig, M. S., and Heggrveit, H. A.: Magnesium interrelationships in ischemic heart disease: a review, Am. J. Clin. Nutr. **27:**59, 1974.

Standal, B. R., Bassett, D. R., Policar, P. B., et al.: Fatty acids, cholesterol, and proximate analyses of some ready-to-eat foods, J. Am. Diet. Assoc. **56:**392, May, 1970.

Trulson, M. F., et al.: Comparison of siblings in Boston and Ireland, J. Am. Diet. Assoc. **45:**225, 1964.

U.S. Senate, Select Committee on Nutrition and Human Needs: Dietary goals for the United States, Washington, D.C., 1977, U.S. Government Printing Office.

Vickrey, A. T. E.: The role of the dietitian in a screening/monitoring program for hypertension, J. Am. Diet. Assoc. **75:**45, July, 1979.

Whyte, H. M., and Havenstein, N.: A perspective view of dieting to lower the blood cholesterol, Am. J. Clin. Nutr. **29:**784, July, 1976.

Yudkin, J., and Morland, J.: Sugar intake and myocardial infarction, Am. J. Clin. Nutr. **20:**503, 1967.

Zilversmit, D. B.: Cholesterol index of foods, J. Am. Diet. Assoc. **74:**562, May, 1979.

PATIENT EDUCATION ASSESSMENT AND MATERIALS

American Heart Association: Heart book: a guide to prevention and treatment of cardiovascular diseases, New York, 1980, E. P. Dutton & Co., Inc.

American Heart Association: Cookbook, ed. 2, New York, 1976, David McKay Co., Inc.

American Heart Association: Fat, calorie, and sodium controlled diet booklets, 44 E. 23rd St., New York, N.Y., 10010, or local office.

Connor, W. E., et al.: The alternative diet book, Iowa City, 1976, University of Iowa Press.

Haferkorn, V.: Assessing individual learning needs as a basis for patient teaching, Nurs. Clin. North Am. **6**(1): 199, 1971.

Jones, J.: Diet for a happy heart, San Francisco, 1976, 101 Productions, Inc.

Keys, A., and Keys, M.: Eat well and stay well, Garden City, New York, 1963, Doubleday & Co., Inc.

National Institutes of Health, National Heart and Lung Institute: The dietary management of hyperlipoproteinemia, Bethesda, Md., rev. 1974.

Payne, A. S., and Callahan, D.: The low-sodium, fat-controlled cookbook, Boston, 1965, Little, Brown and Co.

Public Health Service: The food you eat and heart disease, Pub. 537, U.S. Dept. Health, Education, and Welfare, 1963, U.S. Government Printing Office.

Pye, O. F., Brooks, C. G., and Winston, M. M.: Developing a program of learning on the fat-controlled diet, J. Am. Diet. Assoc. **57**(5):428, 1970.

Stead, E. S., and Warren, G. K.: Low-fat cookery, New York, 1959, McGraw-Hill Book Co., Inc.

Waldo, M.: Cooking for your heart and health, New York, 1961, G. P. Putnam's Sons.

29 Renal disease

PHYSIOLOGY OF THE KIDNEY

Knowledge of the normal functions of the kidney forms an essential background for relating therapy in renal disorders to the organ's impaired functioning in disease. In Chapter 9 these functions are discussed in detail in relation to fluid and electrolyte balance. This basic section should be reviewed, and the diagram of the nephron in Fig. 9-6 should be carefully studied.

Basic renal functions

The nephron is an exquisite example of a highly complex, minute tissue unit, adapted in fine structural detail to its vital function—maintaining an internal fluid environment compatible with life. Through the successive sections of some 1 million nephrons in each kidney, important body fluid flows. The nephrons *filter* from the entering blood most of its constituents except red cells and protein, *reabsorb* needed substances as the filtrate continues along the winding tubules, *secrete* additional ions to maintain acid-base balance, and finally *excrete* unneeded materials in a concentrated urine.

Several nephron structures perform unique homeostatic and metabolic tasks.

Glomerulus. At the head of the nephron an entering arteriole breaks up into a group of collateral capillaries that rejoin to form the efferent or leaving arteriole. The tuft of collateral capillaries is held closely applied in a cupped membrane. This capsule is named for the young English physician Sir William Bowman, who in 1843 first clearly established the basis of plasma filtration and consequent urine secretion upon this intimate relationship of blood-filled glomeruli and enveloping membrane. The filtrate formed here is cell free and virtually protein free. Otherwise it carries the same constituents as does the entering blood.

Tubules. Continuous with the base of Bowman's capsule, the nephron's tubule winds in a series of convolutions toward its terminal in the kidney pelvis. Specific reabsorption functions are performed by the sections of the tubule.

PROXIMAL TUBULE. In the first section major nutrient reabsorption occurs. Essentially 100% of the glucose and amino acids, 80% to 85% of the water, sodium, potassium, chloride, and most other substances are absorbed. Only 15% to 29% of the filtrate remains to enter the loop of Henle.

LOOP OF HENLE. Midway, the tubule narrows, and its thin loop dips into the central renal medulla. Through a balanced system of water and sodium exchange in the limbs of the loop (the counter-current system, p. 186), important interstitial fluid densities are created in the medulla to concentrate the urine by osmotic pressure as it later passes through the environment in the collecting tubule.

DISTAL TUBULE. The later portion of the tubule functions primarily in acid-base balance through secretion of ionized hydrogen and in conservation of sodium through the influence of aldosterone.

COLLECTING TUBULE. In the final section of the tubule, water is absorbed under the influence of vasopressin (ADH) and the osmotic pressure of the surrounding interstitial fluid. The resulting volume of urine, now concentrated and excreted, is only 0.5% to 1.0% of the original filtered water.

• • •

Inflammatory and degenerative diseases of the kidney diffusely involve entire nephrons or nephron segments. In such conditions the normal functions of the nephron are disrupted, and nutritional disturbances in the metabolism of protein, electrolytes, and water follow. Several of these diseases are discussed here as representative of the correlation of diet therapy to impaired renal function and resulting clinical symptoms. These include acute glomerulonephritis, the nephrotic syndrome, acute renal failure, and chronic uremia.

ACUTE GLOMERULONEPHRITIS
Etiology

Usually some antecedent streptococcal infection is related to the onset of glomerulonephritis. It has a more or less sudden onset, and after a brief course, in the majority of cases (especially those among children) recovery is complete. In others the disease may progress or become latent only to develop later into chronic glomerulonephritis. There is some dispute as to whether acute and chronic glomerulonephritis are one continuous disease. The inflammatory process involves primarily the glomeruli; as a result of loss of glomerular function, degeneration of the conjoined tubules follows.

Clinical symptoms

Classic symptoms include hematuria, proteinuria, and varying degrees of edema, hyper-

tension, and renal insufficiency. There may be oliguria or anuria (acute renal failure) and chronic renal failure.

Diet therapy

Protein. Much controversy exists concerning the use of a low-protein diet. Studies seem to indicate, however, that no advantage is found in restricting protein.[1] In short-term acute cases in children, pediatricians in general favor overall optimum nutrition with adequate protein, unless oliguria or anuria develop. This complication usually lasts no more than two or three days and is managed by conservative treatment.

Sodium. Salt also is usually not restricted unless complications of edema, hypertension, or oliguria become dangers. In such cases a 500 to 1,000 mg sodium diet may be used (p. 622). In most patients, especially in children with acute poststreptococcal glomerulonephritis, diet modifications are not crucial. Treatment centers on bed rest and drugs.

Water. Intake should be adjusted to output, as a rule, including losses in vomiting or diarrhea. During periods of oliguria the intake of water may be 500 to 700 ml a day.

NEPHROTIC SYNDROME
Etiology

The nephrotic syndrome may result from many causes. Kark et al.[2,3] identify some of these causes as infective (syphilis, malaria, bacterial endocarditis), allergic (bee sting, serum sickness), mechanical (renal vein thrombosis, congestive heart failure), generalized disease processes (amyloidosis, systemic lupus erythematosus, diabetic glomerulosclerosis, arteriolar nephrosclerosis), and intrinsic renal disease (membranous or proliferative glomerulonephritis, tubular degeneration—lipoid nephrosis). However, in a number of cases no underlying cause is recognized. Whether the nephrotic syndrome represents a stage of chronic glomerulonephritis is unclear. Some patients do show progressive renal failure as in chronic glomerulonephritis. Others, however, respond to treatment with complete recoveries.

Formerly it was believed that the disease process in nephrosis affected primarily the tubular epithelium. Now it is recognized that the primary degenerative defect is in the capillary basement membrane of the glomerulus, which permits the escape of large amounts of protein into the filtrate. The tubular changes are probably secondary to the high protein concentration in the filtrate, with some protein uptake from the tubule lumen.

Clinical symptoms

The primary symptom in the nephrotic syndrome is massive albuminuria. Other findings include additional protein losses in the urine, including globulins, and specialized binding proteins for thyroid and iron, which sometimes produce signs of hypothyroidism and anemia. Blood levels of plasma proteins drop, and serum cholesterol levels rise.

As serum protein losses continue, tissue proteins are broken down, and general malnutrition ensues. There are fatty tissue changes in the liver, sodium retention, and edema. Severe ascites and pedal edema mask gross tissue wasting.

Diet therapy

Treatment is directed toward control of the major symptoms—edema and malnutrition—from the massive protein losses.

Protein. Replacement of the prolonged nitrogen deficit is a fundamental and immediate need. The plasma albumin level may have been reduced to 20% or less of its normal value. This is a major factor in the development of nephrotic ascites and edema. Daily protein allowances of 100 to 150 g or more will be needed.

Calories. To ensure protein use for tissue synthesis, sufficient calories must always be given. High-calorie intakes daily of 50 to 60 calories per kilogram body weight are essential. Every effort must be made to ensure that the patient consumes the diet. Since appetite is usually poor, much encouragement and support are needed. The food must be appetizing and in a form most easily tolerated.

Sodium. To combat the massive edema, sodium levels in the diet must be sufficiently low. Usually the 500 mg sodium diet (p. 622) is satisfactory to help initiate diuresis.

The dietary management is similar to that given for hepatitis (p. 594) with added need for sodium restriction. The use of low-sodium milk is indicated to help maintain the desired high-protein intake and yet restrict sodium to the more severe levels.

CHRONIC RENAL FAILURE— UREMIA
Etiology

Progressive degenerative changes in renal tissue bring marked depression of all renal functions. Few functioning nephrons remain, and these gradually deteriorate. Uremia is the term given the symptom complex of advanced renal insufficiency. Although the name derives from the common finding of elevated blood urea levels, the symptoms result not so much from urea concentrations as from disturbances in acid-base balance and in fluid and electrolyte metabolism and from accumulation of other obscure toxic substances not clearly identified.

Clinical symptoms

Individual patients vary in degree of symptoms and must be managed according to laboratory test indications of renal function. Usually there is anemia, lassitude, weakness, loss of weight, and hypertension. Sometimes aching and pain in bones and joints are present Later signs in progressive illness include skin, oral, and gastrointestinal bleeding from increased capillary fragility, muscular twitching, uremic convulsions, pericarditis, Cheyne-Stokes respiration (an irregular, cyclic type of breathing), ulceration of the mouth, and fetid breath. Resistance to infection is low.

Treatment

The variables of treatment center primarily on protein, sodium, potassium, and water. Levels of each nutrient will need to be individually adjusted according to progression of the illness, type of treatment being used, and the patient's response to treatment. In general, however, overall treatment has several basic objectives:

1. To reduce and minimize protein catabolism
2. To avoid dehydration or overhydration
3. To carefully correct acidosis
4. To correct electrolyte depletions and avoid excesses
5. To control fluid and electrolyte losses from vomiting and diarrhea
6. To maintain nutrition and weight
7. To maintain appetite and morale
8. To control complications such as hypertension, bone pain, and central nervous system abnormalities

Diet therapy

In many of these general therapy objectives, nutritional care plays a large role. Principles of therapeutic nutrition involve variable nutrient adjustments according to individual need.

Protein. The knotty problem is to provide sufficient protein to prevent tissue protein catabolism, yet avoid an excess that would elevate urea levels. A number of years ago Borst,[4] an English physician, proposed a nonprotein, nonpotassium regimen composed of butter, sugar, and cornstarch served as soup, pudding, or butterballs. However, the diet is drastic and intolerable and is rarely administered except in extreme cases (see p. 639).

With advances in the use of hemodialysis, some kidney treatment centers have outlined a more liberal but moderate protein intake for their patients undergoing intermittent dialysis for chronic uremia. Jordan et al.[5] recommend a carefully controlled 70 to 75 g protein diet. Bakke et al.[6] report the use of a 40 to 60 g pro-

tein diet at the Seattle Artificial Kidney Center. Mitchell and Smith[7] describe a protein intake adjusted according to weight: 0.2 to 0.5 g/kg body weight. Merrill[8] advises a diet of 35 to 50 g protein, chiefly of animal origin, for the average patient with advanced renal failure. Most renal treatment centers continue to follow similar diet therapy[9] and have developed innovative methods of teaching dialysis patients.[10]

Thus according to individual need and response to treatment, protein in any event will be closely controlled and will range in quantity from 30 to 70 g and have a high biologic value to supply essential amino acids.

Sodium. The recommendations for sodium intake vary also. Both severe restriction and excess are to be avoided. Since sodium is the chief determinant of extracellular fluid osmolarity, the dietary need is closely related to the patient's handling of water. Some patients may tolerate little sodium, whereas others waste salt excessively in their urine and require a high salt intake of 4 or 5 g daily to achieve balance. Usually, however, the sodium intake is controlled between 400 and 2,000 mg.

Potassium. In renal failure the patient's potassium levels may be depressed or elevated. Guided by blood potassium determinations, the potassium intake is adjusted to maintain normal levels. The damaged kidney cannot clear potassium adequately, so the daily dietary intake is kept at about 1,500 mg.

Water. Much care must be exercised to avoid water intoxication from overloading, or dehydration from too little water. The capacity of the damaged kidney to handle water is limited, and in many cases solids can be excreted better with a controlled amount of water. As little as 600 ml daily may be indicated for some patients to prevent dilution of sodium ions and further fall in the filtration rate. The usual recommendation is from 800 to 1,000 ml daily. Careful records of total fluid intake and output are necessary.

Carbohydrate and fat. The diet must sup-

Borst nonprotein, nonpotassium diet for renal shutdown (uremia)

I. Borst butter soup
150 g sugar
150 g salt-free butter
 20 gm flour
300 g water
Coffee extract, vanilla or lemon flavoring
Serve hot
Divide into 6 feedings

II. Borst pudding or soup
720 ml cold water
 85 g salt-free butter
 18 g cornstarch
 60 g sugar
  2 drops vanilla
May be served hot as a soup or cold as a pudding
Add peppermint extract when served as a pudding

III. Butterballs
168 g salt-free butter—1,250 calories
100 g powdered sugar—400 calories
Makes 60 butterballs

---

ply sufficient nonprotein calories to ensure protein use for tissue protein synthesis and to supply energy. Carbohydrate should always be given with protein food to increase utilization of the amino acids. About 300 to 400 g of carbohydrate is the average daily need. Sufficient fat is added (75 to 90 g) to give the patient 2,000 to 2,500 total calories daily.

**Summary of average dietary needs
in chronic renal failure**

Protein	30 to 50 g
Carbohydrate	300 to 400 g
Fat	70 to 90 g
Calories	2,000 to 2,500
Sodium	400 to 2,000 mg (4 g salt)
Potassium	1,300 to 1,900 mg

Dietary management

General protein and electrolyte control. New treatments, such as hemodialysis, have prolonged life in patients with chronic renal disease. Such treatment has also made necessary a more rigidly controlled diet to prevent serum electrolytes and the products of protein catabolism from reaching fatal heights during the intervals between treatments.[11] Therefore to achieve a twofold objective—rigid control and patient acceptance—diets for uremia patient are being organized on the exchange system of control. A basic daily food pattern is outlined, and food exchange groups are listed from which to make equivalent food choices. An example of such a plan is given in Table 29-1. Individual patient adjustments may be made from such a plan. For example, salt may be added if increased sodium chloride is needed; protein food allowances may be decreased and low-protein bread[12,13] used if less protein is desired; and carbohydrate foods may be increased if added calories and protein-sparing effect are required. Basic food exchange lists for use with this diet plan are given in Table 29-2.

The low protein–essential amino acid diet (modified Giordano-Giovannetti regimen). The separate work of two Italian physicians, Carmelo Giordano[14] at the University of Naples and Sergio Giovanetti[15] at the University of Pisa, has given an encouraging dietary base to sustain patients with uremia and alleviate many of their difficult symptoms. In 1963 Giordano

Table 29-1. Basic pattern for a controlled protein, sodium, and potassium diet*

Food	Protein g	Sodium mg	Potassium mg	Calories	Water ml
Breakfast					
Scrambled egg (1 med.)	6.0	61.0	64.5	80	36.9
Puffed wheat (28 g [1 oz] or substitute from cereal list)	4.0	1.1	95.2	102	1.0
Whole milk (⅓ cup)	3.0	40.5	117.1	53	71.1
Unsalted bread (1 slice)	2.0	5.2	7.2	60	8.2
Unsalted butter (2 tsp)	—	7.6	3.2	70	2.2
Jam or preserves (1 tbsp or substitute from sweets list)	—	2.4	17.6	54	5.8
Noon meal					
Roast beef (84 g [3 oz] or substitute from meat list)	22.0	51.0	314.5	245	46.5
Green beans, low sodium, canned (½ cup or substitute from vegetable list)	1.5	2.0	95.0	25	58.3
Rice, cooked (½ cup or substitute from rice list)	1.7	0.5	23.5	92	60.9
Unsalted bread (1 slice)	2.0	5.2	7.2	60	8.2
Unsalted butter (2 tsp)	—	7.6	3.2	70	2.2
Jelly (1 tbsp or substitute from sweets list)	—	3.4	15.0	55	5.8
Apricots, canned (4 halves or substitute from fruit list)	0.4	0.6	142.7	52	46.9
Evening meal					
Broiled chicken (84 g or substitute from meat list)	20.0	56.0	233.0	185	60.4
Mixed vegetables, frozen (½ cup or substitute from vegetable list)	2.4	40.5	146.0	48	63.2
Unsalted bread (1 slice)	2.0	5.2	7.2	60	8.2
Unsalted butter (2 tsp)	—	7.6	3.2	70	2.2
Apple, fresh (one 5 cm [2 in] diameter or substitute from fruit list)	0.2	1.0	110.0	70	126.6
Sugar (6 tsp)	—	0.2	0.4	92	Trace
Fat, cooking (4 tbsp)	—	—	—	442	—
TOTAL	67.2	298.6	1,405.7	1,985	614.6

*Jordan, W. L., Cimino, J. E., Grist, A. C., McMahon, G. E., and Doyle, M. M.: Basic pattern for a controlled protein sodium and potassium diet, J. Am. Diet. Assoc. **50**:138, Feb., 1967.

Table 29-2. Food exchange lists for use with controlled protein, sodium, and potassium diet*

Food	Protein g	Sodium mg	Potassium mg	Water ml
Meat list—select two items daily				
Beef				
Ground, commercial (56 g [2 oz])	14.0	26.7	255.1	30.4
Loin roast (84 g [3 oz])	20.0	51.0	314.5	37.3
Pot roast (84 g)	22.0	51.0	314.5	46.5
Rib roast (84 g)	17.0	51.0	314.5	34.0
Cheese, low sodium dietetic (56 g)	17.0	7.0	17.5	22.5
Chicken				
†Broiled (84 g)	20.0	56.0	233.0	60.4
Dark meat, boned, no skin (70 g [2½ oz])	22.0	62.3	233.8	45.1
White meat, no skin (56 g)	18.1	38.4	244.9	38.2
Lamb				
Leg, roast (84 g)	20.0	59.5	246.5	42.8
Loin chops, without bone (84 g)	16.5	58.5	243.6	35.0
Shoulder, roast (84 g)	18.0	59.5	246.5	39.3
†Perch, breaded (84 g)	17.0	57.8	195.5	50.0
Pork				
Chops, without bone (70 g)	16.0	45.5	272.9	29.4
Roast (56 g)	13.0	36.6	221.3	25.3
Turkey, roast (56 g)	17.4	42.0	147.0	31.0
Veal roast or cutlet (56 g)	15.0	45.3	283.3	32.9
Vegetable list—select two items daily				
Asparagus				
Canned, low sodium (42 g [1½ oz])	1.3	1.5	79.5	39.3
Fresh (42 g)	0.9	0.4	80.0	39.3
Frozen (42 g)	1.4	0.4	96.3	38.9
Beans				
Green, canned, low sodium (½ cup)	1.5	2.0	95.0	58.3
Lima, canned, low sodium (¼ cup)	2.3	1.6	88.8	30.2
Beets				
Canned, low sodium (½ cup)	0.7	37.9	138.0	74.1
Fresh, cooked (¼ cup)	0.5	17.8	85.8	37.5
Broccoli, fresh, cooked (¼ cup)	1.2	3.8	100.0	34.2
Brussels sprouts				
Fresh, cooked (¼ cup)	1.4	3.3	88.5	28.7
Frozen (¼ cup)	1.1	4.5	96.5	29.0
Cabbage				
†Cooked (½ cup)	0.9	11.0	128.0	80.2
Raw (½ cup)	0.7	10.0	117.0	46.0

*Jordan, W. L., Cimino, J. E., Grist, A. C., McMahon, G. E., and Doyle, M. M.: Basic pattern for a controlled protein, sodium and potassium diet, J. Am. Diet. Assoc. **50:**138, Feb., 1967.
†If these items (highest in fluid in each list) are selected, fluid intake for the day would be approximately 1,000 ml.

Continued.

Table 29-2. Food exchange lists for use with controlled protein, sodium, and potassium diet—cont'd

Food	Protein g	Sodium mg	Potassium mg	Water ml
Vegetable list—select two items daily—cont'd				
Carrots				
Canned, low sodium (½ cup)	0.6	28.3	87.0	67.4
Fresh, cooked (¼ cup)	0.4	11.9	81.0	33.1
Raw, (half, 28 g [1 oz])	0.3	11.7	85.5	24.7
Cauliflower				
Fresh, cooked (½ cup)	1.4	5.4	124.0	55.7
Frozen (½ cup)	1.1	6.0	124.0	56.4
Celery (1 stalk, 20 × 4 cm [8 × 1½ in])	0.4	50.4	136.0	37.6
Corn, fresh, cooked (¼ cup)	2.1	Trace	105.5	48.9
Cucumber, raw (42 g [1½ oz])	0.3	3.1	82.4	40.9
Endive or escarole (28 g [1 oz])	0.5	3.9	83.7	26.5
Kale, fresh, cooked (½ cup)	2.5	23.6	121.5	50.1
Lettuce (⅛ head, 28 g)	0.2	2.5	48.1	26.3
Mixed vegetables, frozen (½ cup)	2.4	40.5	146.0	63.2
Okra				
Fresh (8 pods, 84 g [3 oz])	1.7	1.7	147.9	77.4
Frozen (8 pods, 84 g)	1.9	1.7	139.4	75.1
*Onions, mature, cooked (½ cup)	1.3	7.4	115.5	96.4
Peas				
Early June, canned, low sodium (¼ cup)	3.0	1.9	60.0	50.1
Fresh (¼ cup)	2.2	0.4	78.4	32.6
Frozen (¼ cup)	2.0	46.0	54.0	32.8
Spinach, fresh, cooked (¼ cup)	1.3	22.5	146.0	41.4
Squash				
Summer, fresh, cooked (¼ cup)	0.5	0.5	74.0	50.1
Winter, fresh, cooked (¼ cup)	0.6	0.5	132.3	46.2
Tomatoes				
Canned, low sodium (¼ cup)	0.6	1.8	131.5	56.9
Raw (¼ of 5 × 6 cm [2 × 2½ in])	0.4	1.2	91.5	35.1
Turnips, fresh, cooked (½ cup)	0.6	26.0	145.7	73.0
Fruit list—select two items daily				
Apple				
Juice, canned (⅓ cup)	0.1	0.7	77.1	73.0
*Raw (1 small, 5 cm (2 in) diameter)	0.2	1.0	110.0	126.6
Apricots, canned, heavy syrup (4 halves)	0.4	0.6	142.7	46.9
Blackberries				
Canned, heavy syrup (½ cup)	1.0	1.3	136.0	92.6
Raw (½ cup)	0.9	0.7	122.4	60.8
Blueberries				
Canned, heavy syrup (½ cup)	0.5	1.3	68.8	72.3
Raw (½ cup)	0.5	0.7	56.7	58.2
Cherries				
Raw, sweet or sour (½ cup)	0.7	1.1	108.8	45.8
Royal Ann, canned, heavy syrup (¼ cup)	0.6	0.6	78.1	48.4

*If these items (highest in fluid in each list) are selected, fluid intake for the day would be approximately 1,000 ml.

Table 29-2. Food exchange lists for use with controlled protein, sodium, and potassium diet—cont'd

Food	Protein g	Sodium mg	Potassium mg	Water ml
Fruit list—select two items daily—cont'd				
Grapes				
Juice, canned (⅓ cup)	0.4	0.8	134.5	70.5
Raw (½ cup)	1.0	2.3	120.9	62.4
Grapefruit sections, syrup pack (¼ cup)	0.4	0.6	84.0	50.5
Peach, raw (1 small, 5 cm (2 in) diameter)	0.3	0.6	115.0	101.6
Pears				
Canned (2 halves)	0.2	1.2	98.3	93.4
*Raw (1 small 8 × 6 cm [3 × 2½ in])	0.6	1.8	118.0	151.4
Pineapple				
Canned, heavy syrup (2 slices)	0.4	1.2	117.0	97.5
Juice, canned (⅓ cup)	0.3	0.7	110.8	71.4
Raw (½ cup)	0.3	0.7	102.0	59.7
Plums				
Greengage, raw (½ cup)	0.5	1.3	105.0	99.1
Not Damson (1 raw, 5 cm (2 in) diameter)	0.3	0.6	102.0	51.9
Raisins, dried, seedless (2 tbsp)	0.4	4.0	144.0	1.8
Raspberries				
Black, raw (½ cup)	0.9	0.6	123.0	50.1
Red, raw (½ cup)	0.7	0.6	104.0	50.1
Strawberries				
Frozen (70 g [2½ oz])	0.3	0.7	74.0	49.9
Raw (½ cup)	0.5	0.7	122.2	66.9
Tangerine (1 small, 6 cm (2½ in) diameter, 140 g [5 oz])				
Cereal list—select one item daily				
Cornflakes (14 g [½ oz])	1.0	140.5	16.8	0.5
*Corn grits, cooked (1 cup)	3.0	—	26.6	210.8
Farina, enriched, uncooked, unsalted (28 g [1 oz])	3.4	0.6	24.9	23.4
Oatmeal, cooked, unsalted (¾ cup)	3.4	0.5	84.5	152.2
Puffed wheat, low sodium (28 g)	4.0	1.1	95.2	0.9
Shredded wheat, low sodium (28 g)	3.0	0.8	97.4	1.8
Rice list—select one item daily				
Macaroni, cooked, unsalted (½ cup)	2.5	0.7	42.7	50.4
Noodles, cooked, unsalted (½ cup)	3.5	1.6	35.2	56.3
Rice, cooked, unsalted (½ cup)	1.7	0.5	23.5	60.9
*Spaghetti, cooked, unsalted (½ cup)	2.5	0.7	42.7	82.8
Sweets list—select two items daily				
Cookie, plain assorted (one)	1.0	91.0	16.8	1.6
*Jams or preserves (1 tbsp)	Trace	2.4	17.6	5.8
*Jelly (1 tbsp)	0	3.4	15.0	5.8
*Honey (1 tbsp)	Trace	1.0	10.7	3.6
Sugar, powdered (¼ cup)	0	0.3	0.9	Trace

*If these items (highest in fluid in each list) are selected, fluid intake for the day would be approximately 1,000 ml.

reported an experiment with eight uremia patients using a synthetic diet of carbohydrate (starch and sugar) and fat (margarine or vegetable oil) made into a flavored pudding, served with an additional vegetable and fruit, and supplemented with a formula of essential amino acids. All the patients improved clinically, azotemia was lowered, and positive nitrogen balance was achieved. He formulated his approach on the principle of feeding only essential amino acids, which caused the body to use its own excess urea nitrogen to synthesize the nonessential amino acids needed for tissue protein production.

Using a similar principle, Giovannetti treated chronic uremia patients, some of whom were on dialysis, with a low-protein basal diet composed of bread and Italian pastes made with a special low-protein wheat starch, fats and sugars, selected low-protein vegetables, and fruit, supplemented with essential amino acids and small amounts of egg protein (selected because it has the highest biologic value of the protein foods, p. 67). His report in 1964 indicated the same positive effects. Blood urea concentrations decreased, nitrogen balance became positive and reached equilibrium, and clinical symptoms such as anorexia, vomiting, fatigue, and twitching disappeared or improved. The diet effectively reduced the production of protein catabolites and prevented wastage of body protein.

In 1965 confirmation of these original results of Giordano and Giovannetti was reported in England by Berlyne's group at the Manchester Royal Infirmary.[16-18] Adapting the Giovannetti diet to British tastes (milk for tea; a low-protein bread product and wafers instead of Italian pastes), they observed the same clinical improvement in chronic uremia patients treated with the modified diet of 18 to 20 g protein. The protein was of animal source—195 ml (6½ oz) of milk and one egg—and vegetable protein and included minimum requirements of all the essential amino acids except methionine. This one essential amino acid was added as a dietary supplement. In 1966 Schloerb[19] also reported confirmation of these results in studies at the University of Kansas with uremic patients using the low-protein (20 g), high-calorie (2,000) diet with amino acid supplementation.

A number of U.S. clinics have since used the modified Giovannetti diet for uremic patients and observed similar relief of clinical symptoms. Practical diet plans and food exchange lists, recipes and food preparation suggestions have helped to make the diet useful in the home situation. Careful instruction is given the patient and his family, with much follow-up help and support to carry out the plan. The basic diet pattern is given on pp. 645-646 and food lists on pp. 647-649.

RENAL CALCULI
Etiology

Although the basic cause of renal calculi is unknown, many factors contribute directly or indirectly to their formation. These factors relate to the nature of the urine itself or to the conditions of urinary tract environment.

Concentration of urinary constituents

Calcium. By far the majority of renal stones —about 96%—are composed of calcium compounds. The normal excretion of calcium on a relatively moderate calcium diet of about 400 mg daily is 100 to 175 mg each 24 hours. On an average adult intake of 800 mg or more of calcium, homeostatic mechanisms regulate the amount of calcium excretion. In some persons, however, hyperexcretion of calcium may occur, which produces supersaturation of the urine with crystalloid elements. Apparently in persons who form stones there is a greater precipitating tendency caused by the lack of substances in normal urine that prevent agglomeration of these crystals. Excessive urinary calcium may result from the following:

1. *Excess calcium intake*. Prolonged use of large amounts of milk and alkali therapy for peptic ulcer or of a hard water supply contribute to excess calcium loads.

Basic food plan for modified Giovannetti diet (20 g protein, 1,500 mg potassium)

Daily food plan

One egg

180 ml (6 oz) milk or one additional egg*

Low-protein bread: one loaf (225 g [½ lb]; approximately 650 calories and 1.5 g protein)

Fruit: 2 to 4 servings from fruit list

Vegetables: 2 to 4 servings from vegetable list (fruit and vegetable choices to total 3 to 12 g protein and 1,300 to 1,900 mg potassium)

Free food list: Use as desired for extra calories

Nutrient supplements as prescribed

*Amino acid supplement: Formula of minimum adult requirements of essential amino acids, or only methionine 0.5 g if additional food source given in milk or eggs

Multivitamin supplement

Iron supplement

Sample meal plan

Breakfast

Fruit or juice

One egg

Two slices low-protein bread,† butter, jelly

Amino acid supplement

Lunch

Vegetable

Rice (or substitute starch)

Pudding,* (wheat starch, fruit)

Two slices low-protein bread,† butter, jelly

Dinner

Clear broth (rice or pastes, if desired)

Vegetable salad

Cooked vegetable

Two slices low-protein bread,† butter, jelly

Fruit

Snacks

Tea with milk

Low-protein bread,† butter, jelly, fruit

Basic pudding and bread recipes for use with modified Giovannetti diet

Low-protein pudding* (makes six servings)

Ingredients	*Amount*
Butter or margarine	140 g (5 oz)
Sugar	¾ cup
Cornstarch (or tapioca)	2 tbsp
Water	1¼ cups
Lemon extract (see other variations of flavors below)	⅛ tsp

Method

Combine sugar and cornstarch.

Melt butter or margarine and add above mixture.

Stir well.

Add hot water, blend.

Cook until mixture is thick and clear.

Remove from heat and add flavoring.

Pour into individual cups and chill.

Variations

Instead of lemon extract use lemon juice, peppermint extract, rum extract, orange peel, vanilla extract, or a combination of two or three extracts.

*Paygel, P. General Mills, Inc., or Cellu.

†Steele, B. F., Hjortland, M. C., and Block, W. D.: A yeast-leavened, low-protein bread for research diets, J. Am. Diet. Assoc. **47:**405, Nov., 1965.

Continued.

Variations—cont'd

Instead of water, or instead of part of the water, substitute part of the fruit juice allowance for the day (examples: pineapple juice, drained fruit cocktail juice, apricot juice). Red, sour, pitted cherries are good with tapioca pudding.

Add to the pudding crushed peppermint stick candy, crushed pineapple, sliced peaches, fruit cocktail.

Garnish with gumdrops, 1 tbsp whipped cream (0.3 g protein), maraschino cherry, fruit cocktail. Serve in half a pear. Serve with a slice of candied ginger on top.

Low-protein bread*

Ingredients	Amount (g)	Ingredients	Amount (g)
Granulated sugar	12	Hydrogenated vegetable fat‡	5
Salt	3	Glyceryl monostearate	0.5
Water (38° C [100° F])	105	Glycerol, pure	2 drops
Yeast compressed†	9	Wheat starch§	150
Butter	5		

Method

The amount of each ingredient needed for one batch of rolls or one loaf of bread is given in above list. Procedures are as follows:

1. Place sucrose and sodium chloride in mixing bowl, add water.
2. Dissolve yeast in above solution.
3. Melt butter and vegetable fat together, add glyceryl monostearate to hot fat mixture and stir until dissolved. Add glycerol.
4. Add mixture (3) to (2).
5. Add wheat starch to (4), one half at a time, stirring gently at low speed with an automatic mixer until starch is well moistened.
6. Mix for five to seven minutes (use either a rotary beater or paddle) with automatic mixer. Scrape sides and bottom of bowl with spatula once during mixing. Do not scrape any material adhering to beaters into batter at end of mixing period.
7. Scrape mixture adhering to side of bowl into the mass of material at bottom of bowl. Cover bowl with a damp cloth, and allow mixture to ferment for 30 minutes at 28° C (82° F).
8. At end of 30-minute period stir mixture thoroughly by hand until batter returns to the fluid but plastic state it had before fermentation.
9. If making rolls, divide mixture equally between six heavy aluminum muffin cups (7.5 cm diameter × 4 cm deep [3 in × 1½ in]) greased with vegetable fat. Brush top of each roll with melted butter. If making a loaf, pour mixture into a heavy aluminum pan (19 × 9 × 6 cm [7½ × 3½ × 2½ in]) greased with vegetable fat. Brush top with melted butter.
10. Cover with a damp cloth and let rise for 45 minutes at 28° C (82° F).
11. Bake rolls at 204° C (400° F) for 20 minutes; place under broiler for two minutes to brown tops of rolls. Bake loaf at 287° C (550° F) for five minutes, then at 204° C for 30 to 35 minutes; place under broiler for two minutes to brown top of loaf.
12. Remove rolls or loaf from oven; remove from pan and cool on a wire rack.

*Steele, B. F., Hjortland, M. C., and Block, W. D.: A yeast-leavened, low-protein bread for research diets, J. Am. Diet. Assoc. **47**:405, Nov., 1965.
†Fleischmann's cake yeast.
‡Crisco.
§Paygel, P. General Mills, Inc., or Cellu.

Food exchange lists* for use with modified Giovannetti diet (1 g protein)

List 1—fruits and fruit juices

Food	Description	Amount containing 1 g protein	Potassium mg
Applesauce	Canned or fresh	1⅔ cups	325
Apricots	Fresh, medium	2-3	281
	Canned in heavy syrup, medium halves	5	390
Banana	Small, 15 cm (6 in)	1	370
Blackberries	Fresh	½ cup	136
	Canned	½ cup	215
	Frozen	½ cup	115
Blueberries	Fresh, canned, frozen	1 cup	128
Cantaloupe	Fresh, diced	⅔ cup	401
Sweet cherries	Fresh, large	13	165
	Fresh, small	21	161
	Canned in heavy syrup	½ cup	124
Maraschino cherries	Large	60	
Figs, fresh	Large	2	194
	Small	3	194
Fruit cocktail	Canned	1¼ cups	363
Grapefruit	White or pink, medium, 10 cm (4 in) diameter	1	270
Grapes	American type	½ cup	158
	Thompson seedless, canned or fresh	1 cup	220
Orange	Small	1	200
	Segments	½ cup	194
Papaya	Fresh	½ cup	290
Peaches	Fresh, sliced	1 cup	340
	Canned, heavy syrup, medium halves	5	325
Pears	Small halves	10	420
Pineapple	Fresh, diced	2 cups	390
	Canned, in heavy syrup, large slices	3	300
Strawberries	Fresh, stems removed, or sliced and frozen	1 cup	246-286
	Whole, frozen, sugar added, 300 ml (10 oz) carton	1	295
Tangerine	Large	1	126
	Small	2	126
Tomato	Small	1	244
Watermelon	Balls or cubes	1 cup	200
Fruit juice or nectar			
Apple juice		1 cup	250
Apricot juice		1 cup	
Apricot nectar		1¼ cups	469
Cranberry juice		5 cups	125
Grapefruit juice	Canned	1 cup	360
	Fresh	1 cup	405

*Figures from Bowes, A. D., and Church, C. F.: Food values of portions commonly used, ed. 11. Revised by Church, C. F., and Church, H. N., Philadelphia, 1975, J. B. Lippincott Co.

Continued.

Food exchange lists for use with modified Giovannetti diet (1 g protein)—cont'd

List 1—fruits and fruit juices—cont'd

Food	Description	Amount containing 1 g protein	Potassium mg
Grapefruit-orange juice		¾ cup	345
Grape juice		2 cups	580
Orange juice		¾ cup	375
Peach nectar		2 cups	390
Pear nectar		1¼ cups	125
Pineapple juice		1 cup	375
Prune juice		1 cup	600
Tangerine juice		1 cup	450
Tomato juice		½ cup	273

List 2—vegetables

Food	Description	Amount containing 1 g protein	Potassium mg
Beans	Green snap or yellow wax, cooked and drained	½ cup	114
Beets	Red, diced, canned, drained	½ cup	138
Cabbage	Head green, cooked	⅗ cup	163
Chinese cabbage	Raw, shredded	2¼ cups	253
	Cooked	½ cup	253
Carrots	Cooked, drained	⅔ cup	222
	Fresh, one large, two small		341
Celery	Diced	1 cup	341
Cucumber	Fresh, pared, medium	1½	240
Pickles	Dill or sweet, large	1½	300
Eggplant	Cooked, drained	½ cup	150
Lettuce	Large, outer leaves	2	264
	Coarsely broken	1¼ cups	264
	Finely cut	½ cup	264
Mushrooms	Canned and drained	⅓ cup	164
Pepper	Green: fresh or cooked, large, empty shell	1	213
Onion	Fresh, 4 cm (1½ in) diameter	1	104
	Cooked	½ cup	110
	Scallions 12.5 cm (5 in) long, 1 cm (½ in) diameter	5	231
Potatoes	Crisp chips, 5 cm (2 in) diameter	10	226
Rutabagas	Cooked cubes	½ cup	167
Sauerkraut	Drained	⅔ cup	140
Summer squash	Fresh, cooked	½ cup	202
Sweet potato	Canned, syrup pack	1 small with syrup	120
Tomato	Ripe, fresh, small	1	244
Turnip	Cooked, diced	⅔ cup	188

Food exchange lists for use with modified Giovannetti diet (1 g protein)—cont'd

List 3—vegetables and other foods containing 2 g protein in amounts listed

Food	Description	Amount containing 2 g protein	Potassium mg
Vegetables			
Asparagus	Cooked, cut pieces	½ cup	140
	Canned, medium spears	5	160
Beans	Green snap or yellow wax, fresh, canned, frozen, cooked and drained	1 cup	243
Red cabbage	Raw, shredded	1 cup	268
Corn	Canned, drained	½ cup (scant)	81
Okra	Cooked pods	8-9	174
Potato	Boiled or baked, 6 cm (2¼ in) diameter	1	285
	French fries: pieces 1 × 1 × 5 cm (½ × ½ × 2 in)	10	427
Other foods			
Bacon	Slice (28 g [1 oz] before cooking)	1	16
Bread	Average slice	1	20-30
Danish	Small sweet roll	1	39
Zweiback	Piece	2	
Melba toast	Slice	2	
Raspberries	Frozen, sugar added, 300 ml (10 oz) carton	1	284
Rice	Cooked, white or brown	⅔ cup	105
Spaghetti	Cooked, tender (not firm)	½ cup (scant)	50
Macaroni	Cooked, tender	⅓ cup	45
Noodles	Cooked	⅓ cup	25
Myost	Cheese product	28 g	—

List 4—free list (foods containing little or no protein)

Foods	Exceptions
Butter	
Oil	
Vinegar	
Jelly	No jams
Honey	
Alcoholic beverages	No beer or ale
Soy sauce	
Tea, coffee, Sanka, carbonated beverages	
Herbs and spices (pepper, oregano, cinnamon, etc.)	
Candy: hard candy, sour balls, butterscotch, cream mints (no chocolate coating), lollipops, jelly beans	No chocolate candy
Sugar: white, powdered, brown, sugar syrup, corn syrup	
Limeade	
Cornstarch	
Tapioca	

Food sources of oxalates

Fruits	Vegetables	Nuts	Beverages
Currants	Beans, green and wax	Almonds	Chocolate
Concord grapes	Beets	Cashew nuts	Cocoa
Figs	Beet greens		Tea
Gooseberries	Chard		
Plums	Endive		
Raspberries	Okra		
Rhubarb	Spinach		
	Sweet potato		
	Tomato		

2. *Hypervitaminosis D.* Excess Vitamin D may cause increased calcium absorption from the intestine as well as increased calcium withdrawal from bone.

3. *Prolonged immobilization.* Body casting or immobilization in illness or disability may lead to withdrawal of bone calcium and increased urine concentration (p. 489).

4. *Hyperparathyroidism.* Primary hyperparathyroidism causes excess calcium excretion (p. 138). About two thirds of the persons with this endocrine disorder have renal stones, but this disorder accounts for only a small number (about 5%) of the total calcium stones.

5. *Renal tubular acidosis.* Excess excretion of calcium is caused by defective ammonia formation.

6. *Idiopathic hypercalciuria.* Some persons even on a low-calcium diet and for unknown reasons may excrete as much as 500 mg of calcium daily.

7. *Oxalate.* Because of some error in handling oxalates, about half the calcium stones are compounds with these materials. For example, hyperoxaluria with stone formation has been observed in some patients following ileal resection or bypass surgery for morbid obesity.[20,21] Oxalates occur naturally in only a few food sources, such as rhubarb, spinach, tomatoes, and others. These foods are listed above.

8. *Uric acid.* Excess uric acid excretion may be caused by a derangement in the intermediary metabolism of purines, as in gout. It may also result from rapid tissue breakdown as in wasting diseases.

Cystine. A hereditary metabolic defect in renal tubular reabsorption of the amino acid cystine causes it to accumulate in the urine (cystinuria).

Urinary tract conditions

Physical changes in the urine. Physical changes in the urine may predispose susceptible persons to stone formation.

Concentration of urine may result from a lower water intake or from excess water loss, as in prolonged sweating, fever, vomiting, or diarrhea.

Changes in urinary pH from its mean of 5.85 to 6.00 may be influenced by diet or altered by the ingestion of acid or alkaline medications.

Organic stone matrix. Formation of an organic stone matrix provides the core or nucleus (nidus), which acts as a seed crystal for precipitation. This organic matrix is a mucoprotein-carbohydrate complex in which galactose and hexosamine are the principal carbohydrates. The source of these organic materials is obscure. Some possible factors include (1) bacteria masses from recurrent urinary tract infections, (2) renal epithelial tissue of urinary tract that has sloughed off, possibly because of vitamin A deficiency, and (3) calcified plaques (Randall's plaques) formed beneath the renal epithelium in hypercalcinuria. Irritation and ulceration of overlying tissue causes the plaques to slough off into the collecting tubules.

Clinical symptoms

Severe pain and numerous urinary symptoms may result. There is general weakness and sometimes fever. Laboratory examination of urine and chemical analysis of any stone that is passed help to determine treatment.

Treatment

Fluid intake. A large fluid intake produces a more dilute urine and helps to prevent concentration of stone constituents.

Urinary pH. An attempt to control the solubility factor is made by changing the urinary pH to an increased acidity or alkalinity, depending on the chemical composition of the stones formed.

Stone composition. Dietary constituents of the stone are controlled to reduce the amount of the substance available for precipitation.

Binding agents. Materials that bind the stone elements and prevent their absorption in the intestine cause fecal excretion. For example, sodium phytate is used to bind calcium, and aluminum gels are used to bind phosphate. Glycine and calcium may have a similar effect on oxalates.

Diet therapy

Diet therapy is directly related to the stone chemistry.

Calcium stones. A low-calcium diet of about 400 mg daily is usually given. This amount is about half that of an average adult intake of 800 mg. The lower level is achieved mainly by removal of milk and dairy products. Other calcium food sources affected are leafy vegetables and whole grains. An outline for a low-calcium diet is given on p. 652. If the stone is calcium phosphate, phosphorus foods will be low (p. 653). Diets with other calcium levels may occasionally be used. Shorr[22] has recommended a moderately lowered calcium and phosphorus intake (700 mg calcium and 1,200 mg phosphorus) to be used with aluminum hydroxide gels in the management of calcium-phosphate stones. A test diet of 200 mg calcium may be used also to rule out hyperparathyroidism as an etiologic factor. Such a test diet is given on p. 654.

Since calcium stones have an alkaline chemistry, an acid ash diet may also be used to create a urinary enviornment less conducive to precipitation of the basic stone elements. On p. 655 the classification of food groups is given according to pH of the metabolic ash produced. An acid ash diet would increase the amounts of meat, grains, eggs, and cheese used and limit the amounts of vegetables, milk, and fruits. An alkaline ash diet would outline the opposite use of these foods. An acid ash diet pattern applying these classifications is shown on p. 655. Cranberry juice seems to have a strong urinary acidifying effect on bacteriostatic value and is frequently used as a dietary adjunct.

Uric acid stones. About 4% of the total incidence of renal calculi are uric acid stones. Since uric acid is a metabolic product of purines, dietary control of this precursor is indicated. Purines are nucleoproteins (p. 52) found in active tissue such as glandular meat, other lean meat, meat extractives, and in lesser amounts in plant sources such as whole grains and legumes. A low-purine diet is outlined on p. 656. An effort to produce an alkaline ash would be made.

Cystine stones. About 1% of the total stones produced are cystine. Its occurrence is relatively rare. Cystine is a nonessential amino acid produced from the essential amino acid methionine. A diet low in methionine has been suc-

cessfully used by Smith, Kolb, and Harper[23] at the University of California Medical Center in San Francisco as part of their program for managing cystinuria and cystine-stone disease. The low-methionine diet is outlined on pp. 658-659. It is used extensively with high-fluid and alkali therapy.

A summary of the diet theory principles in renal stone disease is outlined on p. 659.

Low-calcium diet (approximately 400 mg calcium)

	Foods allowed	Foods not allowed
Beverage*	Carbonated beverage, coffee, tea	Chocolate flavored drinks, milk, milk drinks
Bread	White and light rye bread or crackers	
Cereals	Refined cereals	Oatmeal, whole grain cereals
Desserts	Cake, cookies, gelatin desserts, pastries, pudding, sherbets, all made without chocolate, milk or nuts. If egg yolk is used, it must be from one egg allowance.	
Fat	Butter, cream, 2 tbsp daily; French dressing, margarine, salad oil, shortening	Cream (except in amount allowed), mayonnaise
Fruits	Canned, cooked or fresh fruits or juice except rhubarb	Dried fruit, rhubarb
Meat, eggs	224 g (8 oz) daily of any meat, fowl or fish except clams, oysters, or shrimp; not more than one egg daily including those used in cooking	Clams, oysters, shrimp, cheese
Potato or substitute	Potato, hominy, macaroni, noodes, refined rice, spaghetti	Whole grain rice
Soup	Broth, vegetable soup made from vegetables allowed	Bean or pea soup, cream or milk soup
Sweets	Honey, jam, jelly, sugar	
Vegetables	Any canned, cooked, or fresh vegetables or juice except those listed	Dried beans, broccoli, green cabbage, celery, chard, collards, endive, greens, lettuce, lentils, okra, parsley, parsnips, dried peas, rutabagas
Miscellaneous	Herbs, pickles, popcorn, relishes, salt, spices, vinegar	Chocolate, cocoa, milk gravy, nuts, olives, white sauce

*Depending on calcium content of local water supply. In instances of high calcium content, distilled water may be indicated.

Low-phosphorus diet (approximately 1 g phosphorus and 40 g protein)

	Foods allowed	Foods not allowed
Milk	Not more than 1 cup daily; whole, skim, or buttermilk or 3 tbsp powdered including the amount used in cooking	
Beverages	Fruit juices, tea, coffee, carbonated drinks, Postum	Milk and milk drinks except as allowed
Bread	White only. Enriched commercial, French, hard rolls, soda crackers, rush	Rye and whole grain breads, cornbread, biscuits, muffins, waffles
Cereals	Refined cereals, such as Cream of Wheat, Cream of Rice, rice, cornmeal, dry cereals, cornflakes, spaghetti and noodles	All whole grain cereals
Desserts	Berry or fruit pies, cookies, cakes in average amounts; Jell-O, gelatin, angel food cake, sherbet, meringues made with egg whites; puddings if made with one egg or milk allowance	Desserts with milk and eggs, unless made with the daily allowance
Eggs	Not more than one egg daily including those used in cooking; extra egg whites may be used	
Fats	Butter, margarine, oils, shortening	
Fruits	Fresh, frozen, canned, as desired	Dried fruits such as raisins, prunes, dates, figs, apricots
Meat	One large serving or two small servings daily of beef, lamb, veal, pork, rabbit, chicken, or turkey	Fish, shellfish (crab, oyster, shrimp, lobster, etc.), dried and cured meats (bacon, ham, chipped beef, etc.), liver, kidney, sweetbreads, brains
Cheese	None	Avoid all cheese and cheese spreads
Vegetables	Potatoes as desired; at least 2 servings per day of any of the following: asparagus, carrots, beets, green beans, squash, lettuce, rutabagas, tomatoes, celery, peas, onions, cucumber, corn. No more than 1 serving daily of either cabbage, spinach, broccoli, cauliflower, brussels sprouts, or artichokes	Dried vegetables such as peas, mushrooms, lima beans
Miscellaneous	Sugar, jams, jellies, syrups, salt, spices, seasonings, condiments in moderation	Chocolate, nuts, and nut products such as peanut butter; cream sauces

Continued.

Low-phosphorus diet (approximately 1 g phosphorus and 40 g protein)—cont'd

Sample menu pattern

Breakfast	*Lunch*	*Dinner*
Fruit juice	Meat 56 g (2 oz)	Meat 56 g
Refined cereal	Potato	Potato
Egg	Vegetable	Vegetable
White toast	Salad	Salad
Butter	Bread, white	Bread, white
½ cup milk	Butter	Butter
Coffee or tea	½ cup milk	Dessert
	Dessert	Coffee or tea
	Coffee or tea	

Low-calcium test diet (200 mg calcium)

	g		mg calcium
Breakfast			81.22
Orange juice, fresh	100	19.00	
Bread (toast), white	25	19.57	
Butter	15	3.00	
Rice Krispies	15	3.70	
Cream, 20% butterfat	35	33.95	
Sugar	7	0.00	
Jam	20	2.00	
Distilled water, coffee, or tea*		0.00	
Lunch			56.57
Beef steak, cooked	100	10.00	
Potato	100	11.00	
Tomatoes	100	11.00	
Bread	25	19.57	
Butter	15	3.00	
Honey	20	1.00	
Applesauce	20	1.00	
Distilled water, coffee, or tea		0.00	
Dinner			60.89
Lamb chop, cooked	90	10.00	
Potato	100	11.00	
Frozen green peas	80	10.32	
Bread	25	19.57	
Butter	15	3.00	
Jam	20	2.00	
Peach sauce	100	5.00	
Distilled water, coffee, or tea		0.00	
TOTAL MG CALCIUM			198.68

*Use distilled water only for cooking and for beverages.

Acid and alkaline ash food groups

Acid ash	Alkaline ash	Neutral
Meat	Milk	Sugars
Whole grains	Vegetables	Fats
Eggs	Fruits (except cranberries, prunes,	Beverages (coffee and tea)
Cheese	and plums)	
Cranberries		
Prunes		
Plums		

Acid ash diet

The purpose of this diet is to furnish a well-balanced diet in which the total acid ash is greater than the total alkaline ash each day. It lists

   I. Unrestricted foods
  II. Restricted foods
 III. Foods not allowed
 IV. Sample of a day's diet

I. Unrestricted foods: Eat as much as desired of the following foods.
1. Bread: any, preferably whole grain; crackers, rolls
2. Cereals: any, preferably whole grain
3. Desserts: angel food or sunshine cake; cookies made without baking powder or soda; cornstarch pudding, cranberry desserts, custards, gelatin desserts, ice cream, sherbet, plum or prune desserts; rice or tapioca pudding
4. Fats: any, as butter, margarine, salad dressings, Crisco, Spry, lard, salad oils, olive oil, etc.
5. Fruits: cranberries, plums, prunes
6. Meat, eggs, cheese; any meat, fish or fowl, 2 servings daily; at least one egg daily
7. Potato substitutes: corn, hominy, lentils, macaroni, noodles, rice, spaghetti, vermicelli
8. Soup: broth as desired; other soups from foods allowed
9. Sweets: cranberry or plum jelly; sugar, plain sugar candy
10. Miscellaneous: cream sauce, gravy, peanut butter, peanuts, popcorn, salt, spices, vinegar, walnuts

II. Restricted foods: Do not eat any more than the amount allowed each day.
1. Milk: 2 cups daily (may be used in other ways than as beverage)
2. Cream: ⅓ cup or less daily
3. Fruits: 1 serving of fruit daily (in addition to the prunes, plums, and cranberries); certain fruits listed below in group IV are not allowed at any time
4. Vegetables including potato: 2 servings daily; certain vegetables listed below in group III are not allowed at any time

III. Foods not allowed:
1. Carbonated beverages, such as ginger ale, cola, root beer
2. Cakes or cookies made with baking powder or soda
3. Fruits: dried apricots, bananas, dates, figs, raisins, rhubarb
4. Vegetables: dried beans, beet greens, dandelion greens, carrots, chard, lima beans
5. Sweets; chocolate or other candies than those in group I; syrups
6. Miscellaneous: other nuts, olives, pickles

Continued.

Acid ash diet—cont'd

IV. Sample menu:

Breakfast	*Lunch*	*Dinner*
Grapefruit	Creamed chicken	Broth
Wheatena	Steamed rice	Roast beef, gravy
Scrambled eggs	Green beans	Buttered noodles
Toast, butter, plum jam	Stewed prunes	Sliced tomato
Coffee, cream, sugar	Bread, butter	Mayonnaise
	Milk	Vanilla ice cream
		Bread, butter

Low-purine diet (approximately 125 mg purine)

General directions
1. During acute stages use only list 1.
2. After acute stage subsides and for chronic conditions, use the following schedule:
   a. Two days a week, not consecutive, use list 1 entirely
   b. The remaining days add foods from list 2 and 3 as indicated
   c. Avoid list 4 entirely
3. Keep diet moderately low in fat.

Typical meal pattern

Breakfast	**Lunch**	**Dinner**
Fruit	Egg or cheese dish	Egg or cheese dish
Refined cereal and/or egg	Vegetables, as allowed	Cream of vegetable soup, if
White toast	(cooked or salad)	desired
Butter, 1 tsp	Potato or substitute	Starch (potato or substitute)
Sugar	White bread	Colored vegetable, as allowed
Coffee	Butter 1 tsp	White bread, butter, 1 tsp (if
Milk, if desired	Fruit or simple dessert	desired)
	Milk	Salad, as allowed
		Fruit or simple dessert
		Milk

Food list 1—may be used as desired; foods that contain an insignificant amount of purine bodies

Beverages	Eggs	Celery
Carbonated	Fats of all kinds*	Corn
Chocolate	(moderation)	Cucumber
Cocoa	Fruits of all kinds	Eggplant

*High in fat.

Low-purine diet (approximately 125 mg purine)—cont'd

Coffee
Fruit juices
Postum
Tea
Butter*
Bread: white and crackers,
  cornbread
Cereals and cereal products
  Corn
  Rice
  Tapioca
  Refined wheat
  Macaroni
  Noodles
Cheese of all kinds*

Gelatin, Jell-O
Milk: buttermilk,
  evaporated, malted, sweet
Nuts of all kinds*
  Peanut butter*
Pies* (except mincemeat)
Sugar and sweets
Vegetables
  Artichokes
  Beets
  Beet greens
  Broccoli
  Brussels sprouts
  Cabbage
  Carrots

Endive
Kohlrabi
Lettuce
Okra
Parsnips
Potato—white and sweet
Pumpkin
Rutabagas
Sauerkraut
String beans
Summer squash
Swiss chard
Tomato
Turnips

Food list 2—one item four times a week; foods that contain a moderate amount (up to 75 mg) of purine bodies in 100 g serving

Asparagus
Bluefish
Bouillon
Cauliflower
Chicken
Crab
Finnan haddie
Ham

Herring
Kidney beans
Lima beans
Lobster
Mushrooms
Mutton
Navy beans
Oatmeal

Oysters
Peas
Salmon
Shad
Spinach
Tripe
Tuna fish
Whitefish

Food list 3—one item once a week; foods that contain a large amount (75-150 mg) of purine bodies in 100 g serving

Bacon
Beef
Calf tongue
Carp
Chicken soup
Codfish
Duck
Goose
Halibut

Lentils
Liver sausage
Meat soups
Partridge
Perch
Pheasant
Pigeon
Pike
Pork

Quail
Rabbit
Sheep
Shellfish
Squab
Trout
Turkey
Veal
Venison

Food list 4—avoid entirely; foods that contain very large amounts (150 to 1,000 mg) of purine bodies in 100 g serving

Sweetbreads	825 mg	Kidneys (beef)	200
Anchovies	363 mg	Brains	195 mg
Sardines (in oil)	295 mg	Meat extracts	160-400 mg
Liver (calf, beef)	233 mg	Gravies	Variable

*High in fat

Low-methionine diet*

	Foods allowed	Foods not allowed
Soup	Any soup made without meat stock or addition of milk	Rich meat soups, broths, canned soups made with meat broth
Meat or meat substitute	Peanut butter sandwich, spaghetti or macaroni dish made without addition of meat, cheese or milk; 1 serving per day: chicken, lamb, veal, beef, pork, crab, or bacon (3)	Fish and those not listed above
Beverages	Soy milk, tea, coffee	Milk in any form
Vegetables	Asparagus, artichoke, beans, beets, carrots, chicory, cucumber, eggplant, escarole, lettuce, onions, parsnips, potatoes, pumpkin, rhubarb, tomatoes, turnips	Those not listed as allowed
Fruits	Apples, apricots, bananas, berries, cherries, fruit cocktail, grapefruit, grapes, lemon juice, nectarines, oranges, peaches, pears, pineapple, plums, tangerines, watermelon, cantaloupe	Those not listed as allowed
Salads	Raw or cooked vegetable or fruit salad	
Cereals	Macaroni, spaghetti, noodles	
Bread	Whole wheat, rye, white	
Nuts	Peanuts	
Desserts	Fresh or cooked fruit, ices, fruit pies	
Eggs		In any form
Cheese		All varieties
Concentrated sweets	Sugar, jams, jellies, syrup, honey, hard candy	
Concentrated fats	Butter, margarine, cream	
Miscellaneous	Pepper, mustard, vinegar, garlic, oil, herbs, spices	

Meal pattern

Breakfast	Lunch	Dinner
1 cup fruit juice	1 serving soup	56 g (2 oz) meat
½ cup fruit	1 serving sandwich	1 med starch
1 slice toast	1 cup fruit	½ cup vegetable
1½ pats butter	240 ml (8 oz) soy milk†	1 serving salad
2 tsp jelly	3 tsp sugar	1 tbsp dressing
1 tbsp sugar	1 tbsp cream	1 slice bread
Beverage	Beverage	1 serving dessert
1 tbsp cream		1 tbsp sugar
		1 tbsp cream
		1½ pats butter
		Beverage

*Smith, D. R., Kolb, F. O., and Harper, H. A.: The management of cystinuria and cystine-stone disease, J. Urol. **81**:61, 1959.

†Optional; use in children to include protein intake. Omit if urine calcium is elevated in adults.

Low-methionine diet—cont'd

Sample menu

Breakfast	Lunch	Dinner
Orange juice	Vegetable soup, vegetarian	Chicken, roast
Applesauce	Peanut butter sandwich	Baked potato
Whole wheat toast	Canned peaches	Artichoke
Butter	Soy milk*	Sliced tomatoes
Jelly	Sugar	French dressing
Sugar	Cream	Whole wheat bread
Coffee	Coffee or tea	Fruit ice
Cream		Sugar
		Cream
		Butter
		Coffee or tea

*Optional; use in children to include protein intake. Omit if urine calcium is elevated in adults.

Summary of diet therapy principles in renal stone disease

Stone chemistry	Nutrient modification	Diet ash (urinary pH)
Calcium	Low calcium (400 mg)	Acid ash
Phosphate	Low phosphorus (1,000 to 1,200 mg)	
Oxalate	Low oxalate	
Uric acid	Low purine	Alkaline ash
Cystine	Low methionine	Alkaline ash

CASE STUDY 24

The patient with chronic renal failure and uremia

Norman Taylor, aged 47, was an active man, employed by a large municipal government as city planner. He was creative and energetic. His wife, Mary, worked as an administrative secretary for a business executive. She was capable and skilled. They had three healthy, vigorous children, a boy 18 and two girls 16 and 14. They were a close, busy family, enjoying many activities such as summer camping together.

Over a period of time Norman began to tire more easily. He had no appetite and felt nauseated and ill a great part of the time. He began to notice some ankle swelling and hematuria. Finally, at Mary's insistence, he decided to see his physician.

Dr. Roberts gave Norman a thorough examination and workup. He learned that Norman had suffered a severe case of influenza, accompanied by throat infection, during an epidemic within his company when he was overseas in the army. Other than that there had been no major illnesses, and he had been well until these symptoms started. Dr. Roberts had a number of laboratory tests done, and he asked Norman to return to follow-up in two weeks or sooner if his symptoms changed. When the laboratory tests returned, the doctor noted that they showed albumin, casts, red and white cells in the urine, and an elevated BUN. A PSP test had indicated a reduced filtration rate. The urine showed a high specific gravity. There were hypertension, edema, and other symptoms such as headache, occasional blurred vision, and a low-grade fever.

On Norman's return visit, Dr. Roberts discussed with him the findings. They indicated chronic renal failure, probably the result of the previous infectious illness he had had some years before. The physician indicated the serious prognosis of the disease process, and he explored with Norman the alternatives of medical management with dialysis when needed and of kidney transplant surgery. He began Norman's medications to control the hypertension and to ease his growing discomforts and symptoms.

Norman's symptoms increased as time went by. He lost more weight, was anemic, and was having increased aching in his bones and joints. He had numerous public meetings to conduct in which he made speeches, and he had reached the point where he could not stand at these conferences but would sit as often as he could. There was also increased gastrointestinal bleeding and nausea, with occasional muscular twitching or spasms. Numerous small mouth ulcers made eating a painful effort. He and Mary discussed candidly the prospects before him. They decided they would prefer to have the kidney transplant surgery that Dr. Roberts had suggested as a possible therapy.

Dr. Roberts consulted with the clinical nutritionist about Norman's needs. Mary had told the doctor that she wanted to take a leave of absence from her job and to keep Norman at home if at all possible. Since they decided to have the surgery, she wanted to help build Norman up as much as possible to withstand the surgery and make it a success. Also, she told Dr. Roberts that the family simply wanted Norman at home so that they could be together for as long a time as they might have.

Dr. Roberts and the health team discussed Norman's needs. The decision was made to use a modified Giordano-Giovannetti diet to help improve Norman's nutritional state and control his debilitating symptoms. The nutritionist arranged several clinic appointments for Mary so that she could learn how to care for Norman at home. Mary was eager to learn all she could. The principles of diet and their relation to the disease process were carefully reviewed. The nutritionist outlined a definite meal pattern and food selection lists providing precise control of protein, sodium, and potassium. She gave Mary many practical suggestions for obtaining and preparing foods that Norman needed.

Mary planned Norman's diet carefully and followed through with excellent control. Norman too cooperated fully and ate only what Mary planned. In a short while Dr. Roberts found that Norman's

CASE STUDY 24
The patient with chronic renal failure and uremia—cont'd

condition improved. There was a dramatic cessation of his major symptoms. For example, his blood pressure even came down within normal limits so that Dr. Roberts discontinued his hypertension medication. Norman began to gain weight, and his nutritional status improved markedly.

Finally a donor was located, and the kidney transplant was performed. Norman withstood the surgery well. It was a success. After Norman returned home from the hospital and was convalescing, Mary wrote a note of appreciation to the nutritionist and, in turn, to the other members of the health team. In it she expressed her appreciation for the dietary control, guidance, and support that had enabled them to cope with Norman's illness.

Questions to guide your inquiry

1. What metabolic imbalances in chronic renal failure account for the characteristic symptoms Norman displayed?
2. What are the objectives of treatment in chronic renal failure?
3. Why is there a problem in controlling dietary protein? What levels of protein have been advocated? What is the general principle of protein control?
4. What is the problem with sodium control? What amounts are usually used?
5. Why is potassium control vital? What amount is usually used in the diet?
6. What problem exists with water balance? Why are careful intake and output records necessary? What is the usual amount of water limitation?
7. Why are sufficient amounts of carbohydrates and fat necessary in the diet? What amount is usually used?
8. What is the basic principle of the modified Giordano-Giovannetti dietary regimen? Describe this type of diet.
9. How is the diet managed on the modified Giordano-Giovannetti regimen?
10. What practical problems would the nutritionist face in teaching Norman's dietary program to his wife Mary? Outline a teaching plan that you would use for them.

CASE STUDY 25

The patient with renal calculi

Bill Harris, aged 25, lived in a small walk-up studio apartment in Manhattan, where he taught school with a group of other young teachers in a hard-core urban ghetto school. He had sought this teaching position after his return from the Peace Corps because he was concerned about the problems in the inner-city ghetto and felt that reaching children at the elementary school level was an important and significant work. He had been in the city for two years working with this group of teachers. He was a warm, outgoing young man, single, and with many friends. For the past year he had been regularly dating one of his fellow teachers in the same school, a girl from the Midwest, Ruth Kramer, who had also been with the Peace Corps. Bill's family lived on the West Coast, and he had no relatives nearby.

Bill had group medical coverage through his employment in the city school system. He had been well during the past year, save for several bouts with a recurrent urinary tract infection. On one occasion, he had suffered some renal colic and passed several small stones. At that time the physician had given Bill a specific low-calcium screening diet to follow for a few days and then had Bill return for some laboratory tests.

Bill ate sporadically, getting very little for breakfast before he left the apartment, eating a sandwich for lunch at school, and eating irregularly in the evening at dinner time. Sometimes he would get involved in some reading or study and skip dinner altogether, getting snacks through the evening, drinking several glasses of milk. Occasionally he would have dinner at a small neighborhood restaurant near his apartment. He drank a great deal of milk, a carry-over habit from his childhood. His mother had always told him it was a "perfect food" and, besides, it was easy to keep on hand and was filling. Most days he would drink about 2L (2 qt) at least. He was also fond of ice cream and could eat as much as a liter (quart) at a time.

During the past month or so, Bill had been feeling an increasing pain through his right flank and back. He had mentioned this to Ruth, who had encouraged him to see a physician. However, as the pain passed he would put off checking into it. One day, however, the pain became so severe that he could not go to school. He telephoned the principal to report his illness. He began to have chills, and when he took his temperature his fever was 38° C (100° F).

When Ruth came by Bill's apartment after school to see how he was, she found him nauseous and vomiting and in severe pain. She called his physician and drove him immediately to the hospital as Dr. Rowan requested. After his hospital examination, Dr. Rowan decided to keep Bill in the hospital for several days for studies to determine what treatment would be needed. He ordered tests, including KUB, IVP, PSP, Sulkowitch test, serum creatinine, BUN, serum calcium, phosphorus, and uric acid. He also asked the nurse to be sure that all urine passed was strained in order to retrieve any possible stone fragments for chemical analysis.

The results of the studies indicated normal kidney function and normal uric acid levels. The previous low-calcium test diet had already helped to rule out parathyroidism as a factor. However, there was some elevation of urinary calcium and serum calcium and phosphorus. The X-ray studies indicated the presence of a large stone in the kidney pelvis on the left side. Dr. Rowan discussed with the clinical dietitian a diet of 400 mg calcium and 1,000 mg phosphorus, acid ash. He also asked the nurse to force fluids.

As Bill's pain diminished and he was feeling better, Dr. Rowan had him ambulate as much as possible. He discussed his findings and the possible need for surgery with Bill. After a few more days of observation, the decision was made to remove the kidney stone surgically. Bill was prepared for surgery, and a pyelolithotomy was performed. Bill tolerated the surgery well, and his recovery was rapid. After a week the physician indicated he could go home. The dietitian discussed with Bill his continuing needs following the diet initiated in the hospital.

CASE STUDY 25
The patient with renal calculi—cont'd

Questions to guide your inquiry

1. What conditions predispose to the formation of renal calculi? Which of these factors may have been operative in Bill's case?
2. What is a low-calcium test diet? Why is it used? Outline such a diet, indicating how Bill might manage such a test diet over a five-day period in his school job situation.
3. What was the purpose of each of the tests the doctor ordered to diagnose Bill's difficulty?
4. What do the results of these tests indicate that the probable chemistry of Bill's renal calculi was? What kind of stone do the tests results rule out?
5. Give the rationale for the diet ordered for Bill. Indicate the reasons for each factor.
6. Outline a day's menu on this special diet. Calculate the amount of protein, calories, calcium, and phosphorus to ensure proper amounts of each factor.
7. Identify Bill's nutritional needs—his personal needs and those incurred by his illness.
8. What solutions can you propose to meet Bill's needs? Why? What factors would you need to consider in planning his diet?
9. When Bill was ready to go home, what suggestions would you have given him to plan his diet at home? What problems would he face in carrying it out? What solutions would you propose?
10. Suppose the hospital nurse had retrieved at the hospital several small, smooth, *yellow* stones from Bill's urine. Identify the probable stone chemistry and its cause. Indicate in such a case the diet that would be used for treatment. Why? Outline a day's diet pattern for such a dietary need.
11. If the uric acid levels had been elevated in Bill's case and if his renal calculi had been of uric acid composition, what diet would have been indicated for his treatment? Why? Outline a day's diet for such a pattern.
12. What does the term "urinary ash" mean? What foods produce an alkaline ash? What foods produce an acid ash? What is the value of such dietary considerations in cases of renal calculi or urinary tract infections?

REFERENCES
Specific

1. Illingworth, R. S., Philpott, M. G., and Rendle-Short, J.: Controlled investigation of effect of diet on acute nephritis, Arch. Dis. Child. **29:**551, Dec., 1954.
2. Kark, R. M., et al.: The nephrotic syndrome in adults: a common disorder with many causes, Ann. Intern. Med. **49:**751, 1958.
3. Kark, R. M., and Oyama, J. H.: Nutrition, hypertension, and kidney disease. In Goodhart, R. S., and Shils, M. E., editors: Modern nutrition in health and disease, ed. 6, Philadelphia, 1980, Lea & Febiger.
4. Borst, J. C. G.: Protein katabolism in uraemia, effects of protein-free diets, infections, and blood transfusions, Lancet **1:**824, 1948.
5. Jordan, W. L., Cimino, J. E., Grist, A. C., et al.: Basic pattern for a controlled protein, sodium, and potassium diet, J. Am. Diet. Assoc. **50:**137, Feb., 1967.
6. Bakke, J., Goodwin, L., and Okiyama, T.: Sodium-restricted diets for dialysis patients, Hospitals **40:**76, 1966.
7. Mitchell, M. C., and Smith, E. J.: Dietary care of the patient with chronic oliguria, Am. J. Clin. Nutr. **19:**163, 1966.
8. Merrill, A. J.: Nutrition in chronic renal failure, J.A.M.A. **173:**905, 1960.
9. Burton, B. T.: Current concepts of nutrition and diet in diseases of the kidney, J. Am. Diet. Assoc. **65:**623, 1974.
10. Lawson, V. K., Traylor, M. N., and Gram, M. R.: An audio-tutorial aid for dietary instruction in renal dialysis, J. Am. Diet. Assoc. **69:**390, Oct., 1976.
11. Spinozzi, N. S.: Teaching nutritional management to children on chronic hemodialysis, J. Am. Diet. Assoc. **75:**157, Aug., 1979.
12. Steele, B. F., Hiortland, M. C., and Block, W. D.: A

yeast-leavened, low-protein bread for research diets, J. Am. Diet. Assoc. **47:**405, Nov., 1965.

13. Nishita, K. D.: A yeast-leavened, rice-flour bread, J. Am. Diet. Assoc. **70:**397, April, 1977.

14. Giordano, C.: Use of exogenous and endogenous urea for protein synthesis in normal and uremic subjects, J. Lab. Clin. Med. **62:**231, Aug., 1963.

15. Giovannetti, S., and Maggior, Q.: A low-nitrogen diet with proteins of high biological value for severe chronic uraemia, Lancet **1:**1000, 1964.

16. Berlyne, G. M., and Shaw, A. B.: Giordano-Giovannetti diet in terminal renal failure, Lancet **2:**7, 1965.

17. Berlyne, G. M., Shaw, A. B., and Nilwarangkur, S.: Dietary treatment of chronic renal failure: experiences with a modified Giovanetti diet, Nephron **2:**129, 1965.

18. Shaw, A. B., Bazzard, F. J., Booth, E. M., et al.: The treatment of chronic renal failure by a modified Giovannetti diet, Quart. J. Med. **34:**237, April, 1965.

19. Schloerb, P. R.: Essential L-amino acid administration in uremia, Am. J. Med. Sci., **252:**650, Dec., 1966.

20. Stauffer, J. Q., Humphreys, M. H., and Weir, G. J.: Acquired hyperozaluria with regional enteritis after ileal resection, Ann. Intern. Med. **79:**383, 1973.

21. Chadwick, V. S., Modha, K., and Dowling, R. H.: Mechanism for hyperozaluria in patients with ileal dysfunction, N. Engl. J. Med. **289:**172, 1973.

22. Shorr, E.: Aluminum hydroxide gels in the management of renal stone, J. Urol. **53:**507, 1945.

23. Smith, D. R., Kolb, F. O., and Harper, H. A.: The management of cystinuria and cystine-stone disease, J. Urol. **81:**61, 1959.

General

Anderson, C. F., et al.: Nutritional therapy for adults with renal disease. In Nutrition reviews' present knowledge in nutrition, ed. 4, New York, 1976, The Nutrition Foundation, Inc.

Anderson, C. F., Nelson, R. A., Morgie, J. D., et al.: Nutritional therapy for adults with renal disease, J.A.M.A. **223:**68, 1973.

Aronson, A. S., Fürst, P., Kuylenstierna, B., et al.: Essential amino acids in the treatment of advanced uremia: twenty-two months' experience in a 5-year-old girl, Pediatrics **56:**538, Oct., 1975.

Ashburn, B. H.: Acceptance of recipes adopted for patients with renal disease, J. Am. Diet. Assoc. **64:**287, March, 1974.

Atkin-Thor, E., Goddard, B. W., O'Nion, J., Stephen, R. L., and Kolff, W. J.: Hypogeusia and zinc depletion in chronic dialysis patients, Am. J. Clin. Nutr. **31:**1948, Oct., 1978.

Berger, M.: Dietary management of children with uremia, J. Am. Diet. Assoc. **70:**498, May, 1977.

Berlyne, G. M., editor: Nutrition in renal disease, Baltimore, 1968, The Williams & Wilkins Co.

Brenner, B. M., and Rector, F. S., Jr., editors: The kidney, Philadelphia, 1976, W. B. Saunders Co.

Burton, B. T.: Current concepts of nutrition and diet in diseases of the kidney, J. Am. Diet. Assoc. **65:**623, 1974.

Burton, B. T.: Nutritional implications of renal disease. I. Current overview and general principles, J. Am. Diet. Assoc. **70:**479, May, 1977.

Close, J. H.: The use of amino acid precursors in nitrogen accumulation diseases, N. Engl. J. Med. **290:**663, 1974.

Cost, J. S.: Diet in chronic renal disease: a focus on calories, J. Am. Diet. Assoc. **64:**186, Feb., 1974.

Cost, J. S.: Dietary management of renal disease, Thorofare, N. J., 1975, Charles B. Slack, Inc.

Davis, M., Comty, C., and Shapiro, F.: Dietary management of patients with diabetes treated by hemodialysis, J. Am. Diet. Assoc. **75:**265, Sept., 1979.

Gokal, R., Mann, J. I., Oliver, D. O., and Ledingham, J. G.: Dietary treatment of hyperlipidemia in chronic hemodialysis patients, Am. J. Clin. Nutr. **31:**1915, Oct., 1978.

Hansen, G. L., editor: Caring for patients with chronic renal disease, Philadelphia, 1972, J. B. Lippincott Co.

Hughes, J., Coppridge, W. M., Roberts, L. C., and Mann, V. I.: Oxalate urinary tract stones, J.A.M.A. **172:**774, 1960.

Ing, T. S., and Kark, R. M.: Renal disease. In Schneider, H. A., Anderson, C. E., and Coursin, D. B., editors: Nutritional support of medical practice, New York, 1977, Harper & Row, Publishers.

Kark, R. M., and Oyama, J. H.: Nutrition, hypertension, and kidney diseases. In Goodhart, R. A., and Shils, M. E., editors: Modern nutrition in health and disease, ed. 6, Philadelphia, 1980, Lea & Febiger.

Karp, N. R. S.: Electrodialyzed whey-based foods for use in chronic uremia, J. Am. Diet. Assoc. **59**(6):568, 1971.

Kopple, J. E.: Dietary requirements. In Massry, S. G., and Sellars, A. L., editors: Clinical aspects of uremia and dialysis, Springfield, Ill., 1976, Charles C. Thomas, Publisher.

Kopple, J. D., et al.: Controlled comparison of 20-g. and 40-g. protein diets in the treatment of chronic uremia, Am. J. Clin. Nutr. **21:**553, 1978.

Massry, S. G., and Kopple, J. D.: Diet therapy of renal failure. In Halpern, S. L., editor: Quick reference in clinical nutrition, Philadelphia, 1979, J. B. Lippincott Co.

Nishita, K. D.: A yeast-leavened, rice-flour bread, J. Am. Diet. Assoc. **70:**397, April, 1977.

Overly, V. A., and Greenwood, M. L.: Developing wafers and biscuits of varying protein content, J. Am. Diet. Assoc. **45:**342, 1964.

Pitts, R. F.: Physiology of the kidney and body fluid: an

introductory test, ed. 4, Chicago, 1974, Year Book Medical Publishers, Inc.

Reichman, S., and Guttmann, N.: Providing a "brown bag" lunch for ambulatory hemodialysis patients, J. Am. Diet. Assoc. **70:**394, April, 1977.

Robinson, L. G., and Paulbitski, A. H.: Diet therapy and educational program for patients with chronic renal failure, J. Am. Diet. Assoc. **61:**531, Nov., 1972.

Sargent, J. A., and Gotch, F. A.: Mass balance: a quantitative guide to clinical nutritional therapy. I. The predialysis patient with renal disease, J. Am. Diet. Assoc. **75:**547, Nov., 1979.

Sargent, J. A., Gotch, F. A., Henry, R. R., and Bennett, N.: Mass balance: a quantitative guide to clinical nutritional therapy. II. The dialyzed patient, J. Am. Diet. Assoc. **75:**551, Nov., 1979.

Sargent, J., Gotch, F., Borah, M., et al.: Urea kinetics: a guide to nutritional management of renal failure, Am. J. Clin. Nutr. **31:**1696, Sept., 1978.

Schoolwerth, A. C., and Engle, J. E.: Calcium and phosphorus in diet therapy of uremia, J. Am. Diet. Assoc. **66:**460, 1975.

Smith, E. B.: Gluten-free breads for patients with uremia, J. Am. Diet. Assoc. **59**(6):572, 1971.

Smith, E. B.: Development of recipes for low protein gluten-free bread, J. Am. Diet. Assoc. **65:**50, July, 1974.

Smith, E. B., and Hill, P. A.: Protein in diets of dialyzed and non-dialyzed uremic patients, J. Am. Diet. Assoc. **60**(5):389, 1972.

Smith, H. W.: Kidney, structure and function in health and disease, New York, 1951, Oxford University Press, Inc.

Spinozzi, N. S., and Grupe, W. E.: Nutritional implications of renal disease. IV. Nutritional aspects of chronic renal insufficiency in childhood, J. Am. Diet. Assoc. **70:**493, May, 1977.

Stein, P. G., and Winn, N. J.: Diet controlled in sodium, potassium, protein, and fluid: use of points for dietary calculation, J. Am. Diet. Assoc. **61:**538, Nov., 1972.

Swendseid, M. E.: Nutritional implications of renal disease. III. Nutritional needs of patients with renal disease, J. Am. Diet. Assoc. **70:**488, May, 1977.

Vander, A. J.: Renal physiology, New York, 1975, McGraw-Hill Book Co.

Williams, H. E.: Nephrolithiasis, N. Engl. J. Med. **290:**33, 1974.

Wineman, R. J., Sargent, J. A., and Piercy, L.: Nutritional implications of renal disease. II. The dietitian's key role in studies of dialysis therapy, J. Am. Diet. Assoc. **70:**483, May, 1977.

PATIENT EDUCATION

de St. Jeor, S. T., et al.: Low protein diets for the treatment of chronic renal failure, Salt Lake City, 1970, University of Utah Press.

Jones, O.: Diet guide for patients on chronic dialysis, DHEW Pub. No. (NIH) 76-685, Bethesda, Md., 1976, National Institutes of Health.

Kidney Foundation of Illinois: Fun with food for dialysis patients, 1977, Illinois Council on Renal Nutrition, 127 N. Dearborn, Chicago, Ill. 60602.

Margie, J. D., et al.: The Mayo Clinic renal diet cookbook, Racine, Wis., 1974, Golden Press/Western Publishing Co., Inc.

Spinozzi, N. S.: Teaching nutritional management to children on chronic hemodialysis, J. Am. Diet. Assoc. **75:**157, Aug., 1979.

Spitzer, M. E., et al.: A renal failure diet manual utilizing the food exchange system, Springfield, Ill., 1976, Charles C Thomas, Publisher.

U.S. Public Health Service: Living with end-stage renal failure: a book for patients, Washington, D.C., 1976, U.S. Government Printing Office.

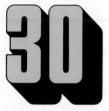

Care of the surgery patient

The physiologic stress of surgery places added nutritional demands on the patient. Deficiencies can accrue easily and sooner or later may lead to serious clinical manifestations. Careful attention to preoperative preparation of the patient and to postoperative therapeutic needs reduces complications and provides resources for better wound healing and a more rapid recovery period.

PREOPERATIVE NUTRITION

Nutrient stores. When time permits, nutritional preparation of the patient for surgery should correct any nutrient deficiencies and provide optimum reserves for the period of surgery itself and the time following until oral feedings can be resumed.

PROTEIN. The most common nutritional deficiency related to surgery is that of protein. Tissue and plasma reserves are imperative to fortify the patient for blood losses during surgery and tissue catabolism in the immediate postoperative period.

CALORIES. Sufficient calories should be provided to build up any weight deficit. Carbohydrate is needed for glycogen stores and to spare protein for tissue synthesis. If the patient is overweight, some weight reduction is indicated to reduce surgical risks.

VITAMINS AND MINERALS. Tissue stores of vitamins are needed for metabolism of carbohydrate and protein. Any deficiency state, such as anemia, should be corrected. Electrolytes and

fluid should be in balance, with any dehydration, acidosis, or alkalosis corrected.

Immediate preoperative period. Nothing is given by mouth for at least eight hours prior to surgery, so that the stomach will have no retained food at the time of the operation. Food in the stomach may be vomited and aspirated during anesthesia or recovery from anesthesia. Also, any food present may increase the possibility of postoperative gastric retention and gastric dilatation or may interfere with the surgical procedure itself.

MINIMUM RESIDUE. Prior to gastrointestinal surgery a low-residue (p. 583) or residue-free diet (p. 668) may be followed for two to three days to clear the operative site of any fecal residue.

POSTOPERATIVE NUTRITION
Therapeutic nutritional needs

In health the body tissues undergo continuous turnover, with small physiologic losses being constantly replenished with nutrients in food eaten. In disease, however, especially surgical disease, losses are greatly increased while at the same time replacement from food is diminished or even absent for a period of time. Therapeutic nutrition becomes all the more significant as a means of aiding recovery.

Protein. Adequate protein intake in the postoperative recovery period is of primary therapeutic concern to replace losses and supply increased needs.

Progressively increasing protein deficiency is common in surgical patients. Negative nitrogen balances of as much as 20 g per day may occur. This amount of nitrogen loss represents an actual loss of tissue protein of over a pound a day. In addition to protein losses from tissue catabolism, there is loss of plasma proteins through hemorrhage, wound bleeding, and exudates. Increased metabolic losses result also from extensive tissue inflammation or from infection and trauma. If any degree of prior malnutrition or chronic infection existed, the patient's protein deficit may become severe and cause serious complications to develop. The following are the body's protein needs:

1. *Tissue synthesis in wound healing.* Tissue proteins can be synthesized only by amino acids brought to the tissue by the circulating blood (p. 60). These necessary amino acids must come either from ingested protein or by intravenous injection. Tissue protein deficiencies are best met by oral feedings. When appetite is poor, often palatable concentrated liquid drinks are useful. Examples of oral nutrient feedings and high-protein beverages are given in Table 27-1 (p. 593). During early feeding periods, or with the extremely malnourished patient, a daily intake of 50 to 75 g of protein may be all that can be tolerated. However, this amount should be increased as early as possible to achieve the 100 to 200 g daily that is needed to restore lost protein tissues and synthesize new tissue at the wound site. Although tissue protein is broken down more rapidly during stress, it is also built up more rapidly—provided sufficient amino acids are present to supply the demand.

2. *Avoidance of shock.* A reduction in blood volume, a loss of plasma proteins, and a decrease in circulating red blood cell volume contribute to the potential danger of shock. Where protein deficiencies exist, this danger is enhanced.

3. *Control of edema.* When the serum protein level is low, edema develops due to loss of colloidal osmotic pressure to maintain the normal shift of fluid between capillaries and surrounding interstitial tissues (p. 182). Considerable excess fluid may collect in the interstitial spaces before clinical edema is evident and may affect heart and lung action. Local edema at the surgical site also delays closure of the wound and hinders the normal healing process.

4. *Bone healing.* In orthopedic surgery, where extensive bone healing is involved, protein is also essential for proper callus formation and calcification. A sound protein matrix must be present for the anchoring of mineral matter in the bone.

5. *Resistance to infection.* Amino acids are necessary constituents of the proteins involved in body defense mechanisms—antigens, antibodies, blood cells, hormones, enzymes. Tissue integrity itself is a bulwark against infection.

6. *Lipid transport.* Proteins are necessary for the transportation of lipids in the body and therefore for the protection of the liver, a main site of fat metabolism, from damage by fatty infiltration. Protein provides essential lipotropic agents to form lipoproteins, the transport form of fat in the body (p. 45).

Effect of inadequate protein. It is evident therefore that multiple clinical problems may easily develop where protein deficiencies exist. There may be poor wound healing and dehiscence, delayed healing of fractures, anemia, failure of gastrointestinal stomas to function, depressed pulmonary and cardiac function, reduced resistance to infection, extensive weight loss, liver damage, and increased mortality risks.

Calories. *Carbohydrate* must be supplied in adequate quantities to ensure the use of protein for necessary tissue protein synthesis and to supply the energy required for increased metabolic demands. As protein is increased, the total calories must be increased also. The studies of Calloway and Spector[1] have indi-

Nonresidue diet

General description

1. This diet includes only those foods free from fiber, seeds, and skins, and with the minimum amount of residue.
2. Fruits and vegetables are omitted except for strained fruit juices.
3. Milk is omitted.
4. The diet is adequate in protein and calories, containing approximately 75 g protein, 110 g fat, 250 g carbohydrate, and 2,260 calories. It is likely to be inadequate in vitamin A, calcium, riboflavin.
5. If patients are to remain for a long length of time on this diet, supplementary vitamins and minerals should be given.

	Allowed	Not allowed
Beverages	Carbonated beverages, coffee, tea	Milk and milk drinks
Bread	Crackers, melba or rusks	Whole grain bread
Cereals	Refined as Cream of Wheat, Farina, fine corn-meal, Malt-o-Meal, pablum, rice, strained oatmeal, corn flakes, puffed rice, Rice Krispies	Whole grain and other cereals
Cheese		None allowed
Desserts	Plain cakes and cookies, gelatin desserts, water ices, angel food cake, arrowroot cookies, tapioca puddings made with fruit juice only	Pastries and all others
Eggs	As desired, preferably hard cooked	Fried eggs
Fats	Butter or substitute, small amount cream	None
Fruits	Strained fruit juices	All others
Meat, fish, poultry	Tender beef, chicken, fish, lamb, liver, veal, and crisp bacon	Fried or tough meat, pork
Potatoes or substitute	Only macaroni, noodles, spaghetti, refined rice	Potatoes, corn, hominy, unrefined rice
Soup	Bouillon and broth only	All others
Sweets	Hard candy, fondant, gumdrops, jelly, marsh-mallows, sugar, syrup, and honey	Other candy, jam, marmalade
Vegetables	Tomato juice	All others
Miscellaneous	Salt	Pepper

NOTE: *Fruit juices and hard candies may be taken between meals to increase caloric intake.*

POSTSURGICAL NONRESIDUE DIET
General description

1. This diet is slightly higher in residue but has greater variety, including potatoes, white bread products, processed cheese, sauces, and desserts made with milk, and cream for coffee and cereal.
2. The average daily menu will contain 85 g protein, 2,300 calories, and is slightly higher in vitamins and minerals.

Nonresidue diet—cont'd

Selection of foods
To the above add
Cheese: Processed cheese, mild cream cheeses
Potatoes: Prepared any way, no skin
Bread: Any kind without bran, white bread, rolls, pancakes, waffles
Fats: Two ounces of cream or half and half per meal, cream sauce, cream gravy
Desserts: All desserts except those containing fruit and nuts
Condiments: As desired

Table 30-1. Daily water requirements of the surgical patient

Type of case and fluid needs	Average fluid required (ml)
Uncomplicated cases	
For vaporizations	1,000-1,500
For urine	1,000-1,500
	2,000-3,000 TOTAL
Complicated cases (sepsis, elevation of temperature, humid weather, renal damage)	
For vaporization	2,000-2,500
For urine	1,000-1,500
	3,000-4,000 TOTAL
Seriously ill patients with drainage	
For vaporization	2,000
For urine	1,000
For replacement of body fluid losses	
1,000 ml bile drainage	1,000
3,000 ml Wangensteen drainage	3,000
	7,000 TOTAL

Adapted from Zintel, H. A.: Nutrition in the care of the surgical patient. In Wohl, M., and Goodhart, R., editors: Modern nutrition in health and disease, ed. 3, Philadelphia, 1964, Lea & Febiger, p. 1055.

cated that a minimum of 2,800 calories per day must be provided before protein can be used for tissue repair and not be converted in part to provide energy. In acute stress, as in extensive radical surgery or burns, where protein needs are as high as 250 g daily, 4,000 to 6,000 calories are required. In addition to its protein-sparing action, carbohydrate also helps to avoid liver damage from depletion of glycogen reserves.

Fat calories must be adequate but not excessive. Excessive body fat is to be avoided since fatty tissue heals poorly and is more susceptible to infections, hematomas, and serum collections.

Fluid. Adequate fluid therapy is of paramount importance to ensure the patient against dehydration. During the postoperative period there may be large fluid losses from vomiting, hemorrhage, exudates, diuresis, or fever. Where drainage is involved, more fluid loss is incurred. Table 30-1 indicates the magnitude of water requirements for surgical patients. Intravenous therapy will supply initial needs, but oral intake should begin as soon as possible and be maintained in sufficient quantity.

Minerals. Replacement of mineral deficiencies and insurance of continued adequacy is essential. In tissue catabolism, potassium and phosphorus are lost. Electrolyte imbalances in sodium and chloride result from fluid losses. Iron-deficiency anemia may develop from blood loss or from faulty iron absorption.

Vitamins. Vitamin C is imperative for wound healing. Its presence is necessary for formation of cementing material in the ground substance of connective tissue, in capillary walls, and in the building up of new tissue (p. 124). Extensive tissue regeneration as in burns or mastectomy may require as much as 1 g daily, about 15 to 20 times the normal requirement. As calories and protein are increased, the B vitamins—thiamin, riboflavin, and niacin—must also be increased to provide essential coenzyme factors to metabolize car-

bohydrate and protein. Other B-complex vitamins—folic acid, B_{12}, pyridoxine, pantothenic acid—also have important metabolic roles in stress situations. Vitamin K is essential to the blood-clotting mechanism (p. 97).

The occasions for therapeutic increases in vitamin intake have been well-defined by the National Research Council in the pamphlet *Therapeutic Nutrition:*

1. A healthy person having minor surgery or an illness expected to last less than ten days and who is ambulatory and eating well and has no history of previous malnutrition has no need for special consideration as to vitamin therapy.

2. If the qualifications above are not met, the patient needs one to two times the normal daily requirement of vitamins.

3. If the patient is being fed entirely by the intravenous route, he should receive one to two times the minimum requirement for parenteral injection together with additional amounts of vitamin C.

4. If serious illness or severe trauma or burn is present, the vitamin requirement for the first few days is five to ten times the usual daily requirement. Thereafter the patient will require two to three times the basic need until recovery is complete.

Dietary management

Oral vs. parenteral feeding. In a number of patients the gastrointestinal tract cannot be used, and parenteral feeding is the only way to sustain the patient. In such cases solutions of hydrolyzed proteins (amino acids and polypeptides) and dextrose are used. A basic fat emulsion is also available for intravenous therapy.[2,3]

However, the majority of patients can and should progress to oral feeding as soon as possible to provide adequate nutrition. In generally used postoperative intravenous solutions 1 L of a 5% dextrose solution contains 50 g of sugar with an energy value of 200 calories. Therefore 3 L a day at best can supply only 600 calories, and the *basal* energy requirement is about 700 calories, to say nothing of the increased metabolic demands of the stress of surgical illness. Ordinary postsurgical intravenous therapy therefore cannot supply nutrient needs or compete with oral feedings; *it can only compete with starvation!* Therefore a rapid return to regular eating should be encouraged and maintained.

Hyperalimentation. In cases of major tissue trauma or damage or when a patient is unable to obtain sufficient nutrients orally, hyperalimentation is used as a feeding process. It provides parenteral nutritional support with solutions containing high-percentage glucose (20% to 50%), hydrolysates of amino acids, electrolytes, minerals, and vitamins. Intravenous hyperalimentation is usually done in the inferior or superior vena cava because there is danger of thrombosis if the concentrated nutrient solution is injected into peripheral veins.[4] A number of products are available for use in hyperalimentation programs, and the team approach to patient care ensures optimal nutritional and personal support.[5-7]

With the rapidly expanding development of parenteral and enteral feeding techniques and materials for specific clinical nutrition needs, malnutrition in surgical patients need not occur. In Chapter 31 these nutritional care procedures are discussed in greater detail.

Postoperative diets

Clear liquids. As soon as intestinal peristalsis returns, water and clear liquids—tea, coffee, broth, juice—may be given to help supply important fluids and some sodium and chloride. These liquids also help stimulate normal gastrointestinal function and early return to a full diet.

Full liquids. Since clear liquids have little other nutrient value, progression to full liquids should soon follow. Milk and milk products—puddings, cream soups, high protein beverages,

ice cream—supply much vital protein and carbohydrate.

Soft to regular diet. Each patient will progress to solid foods according to his individual tolerance, but encouragement and help should be supplied to enable oral intake of solid foods as soon as possible. The usual diet pattern of postoperative feeding is outlined in Table 23-1.

NUTRITIONAL CARE OF PATIENT WITH GASTROINTESTINAL SURGERY
Mouth, throat, or neck surgery

Surgery involving the mouth, throat, or neck will require modification in manner of feeding, since the patient usually cannot chew or swallow in the normal way.

Oral liquid feedings. Concentrated feedings in liquid form will need to be planned, using protein hydrolysates and added carbohydrate. Milk-based beverages, soups, fruit juices with lactose or other sugar, and eggnogs can supply frequent reinforced nourishment. A milk-shake formula, for example, supplemented with skim milk powder or a protein concentrate such as Casec, can supply 20 g of protein and 400 calories (p. 593).

Tube feedings. If a patient is comatose, severely debilitated, or has undergone radical neck or facial surgery, he may require tube feeding. Usually a nasogastric tube is used. However, in cases of esophagus obstruction the tube is inserted into an opening made in the abdominal wall—a gastrostomy. The formula will be prescribed according to the need and tolerance of the individual patient. Small amounts are used at first and gradually increased. Usually 2 L of formula are sufficient for a 24-hour period, and the feeding should not exceed 240 to 360 ml (8 to 12 oz) in each three- to four-hour interval. Two general types of formula may be used:

1. Nutrient preparations in powdered or liquid form, such as Sustagen, a protein hydrolysate, or Lonolac, a low-sodium product,

Table 30-2. Sample tube feeding formula (2,500 ml, 3,000 calories)

Ingredients	Amount	Protein	Fat	Carbohydrate
Homogenized milk	1 L	32	40	48
Eggs	3	21	16	
Apple juice	400 ml			55
Vegetable oil	30 ml		30	
Strained baby food (112 g [4 oz] jars)				
Beef liver	4 jars	56	12	14
Beets	2 jars	3		20
Peaches	2 jars	1	1	59
Sustagen	1½ cups (225 g)	52	7	150
(Water as needed to total 2,500 ml)				
TOTALS		165	106	346
TOTAL CALORIES			2,998	

or any one of a number of commercial products can be used according to need. These preparations, mixed with water as needed in the desired proportions, are simple to prepare. However, in the higher calorie formula requirements the amount of the nutrient material needed to fill the calorie requirement sometimes renders too concentrated an amount of carbohydrate, and diarrhea results. In such cases a planned formula of balanced ingredients would achieve a more desirable ratio of nutrients. For example, a 3,000-calorie formula using Sustagen alone would require about 5 cups to 2,500 ml of water and would render a nutrient ratio of 180 g protein, 500 g carbohydrate, and 30 g fat. A planned food formula used instead, such as the example given in Table 30-2, would give a more balanced ratio and probably be better tolerated. This formula may be compared with other sample mixtures given in Table 30-3.

2. Blenderized food mixtures are preferred by many patients because they feel they are getting regular food. Any foods that will liquefy in a high-speed blender can be used, or strained baby food may be used to simplify the mixing. Usual ingredients include a milk base, with ad-

ditions of egg, strained meat, vegetable, fruit, fruit juices, nonfat dry milk, cream, brewer's yeast, and ascorbic acid.

A broad range of oral and tube feedings designed to achieve a high nutrient density for patients at nutritional risk is discussed in detail in the following chapter.

Gastric resection

A number of nutritional problems may develop following gastric surgery, depending on the type of surgical procedure and the patient's individual response. A partial gastrectomy may create little postoperative difficulty. However, a total gastrectomy, in which there is complete excision of the stomach and establishment of an anastomosis between the jejunum and the remaining portion of the esophagus, may, without care in planning the diet, produce serious nutritional deficits. When a vagotomy is performed, there may be increased gastric fullness and distention. The stomach becomes atonic and empties poorly, so that food fermentation follows, producing flatus and diarrhea. After gastric surgery about 50% of the patients fail to regain weight to optimum levels.

Table 30-3. Types of tube feedings

Ingredients	Calories	Protein (g)	Fat (g)	Carbohydrate (g)
Regular tube feeding				
6 eggs	452	36.6	33.0	—
1 L homogenized milk	666	34.2	38.1	47.8
1 cup nonfat milk solids	434	42.7	1.2	121.3
½ cup Karo syrup	469			62.4
1 tablet brewer's yeast				
75 mg ascorbic acid				
¼ tsp salt				
1,500 ml				
TOTAL	2,021	113.5	72.3	231.5
Sustagen				
3 cups Sustagen	1,755	105.0	15.0	300.0
4 cups water				
1,200 ml				
600 g Sustagen (4 cups)	2,300	140.0	20.0	400.0
1,200 ml water				
1,400 ml				
Add for banana Sustagen:				
2 tsp banana flakes	88	1.2	—	23.0
or				
1 mashed banana				
Low-calcium tube feeding				
6 cans strained meat	540	80.4	25.2	0
1 L fruit juice	432	0	2.0	108.0
Karo syrup, ¼ cup	234			61.0
ascorbic acid				
brewer's yeast				
1,800 ml				
TOTAL	1,206	80.4	27.2	169.0
Low-sodium tube feeding				
1 L low-sodium milk	666	34.2	38.1	47.8
Casec 90 g—3 oz, 18 tbsp	306	75.0		
Karo syrup ¼ cup	234			61.0
1,000 ml				
TOTAL	1,206	109.2	38.1	108.8

By and large the nutritional care of patients who have had gastric surgery falls into the following two areas.

The immediate postoperative period. Following surgery there is a very gradual resumption of oral feedings, according to the individual patient's tolerance. A typical pattern of dietary progression will cover about a two-week period:

First 24 to 48 hours — Nothing by mouth; intravenous therapy

Days 2 to 4 — Ice chips, sips of water (temperature adjusted to patient response; some tolerate warm water better)

Gastrectomy diets

No. 1	No. 2	No. 3	No. 4
Breakfast	*Breakfast*	*Breakfast*	*Breakfast*
Soft cooked egg	Soft cooked egg or	Same as No. 2	Egg, not fried
Salt	poached egg		Cereal
Sugar	Butter		Toast
	White toast		Butter
	Strained cereal		Canned fruit
	Cream		Cream
10:00 a.m.	*10:00 a.m.*	*10:00 a.m.*	*10:00 a.m.*
Jell-O with cream	Same as No. 1	Same as No. 1	Same as No. 1
Luncheon	*Luncheon*	*Luncheon*	*Luncheon*
Mashed potato	Sliced turkey or	Roast beef	Tender meat
with butter	plain tender meat	Mashed potatoes	Potato or substitute
Salt	Baked potato with	Pureed vegetable	Whole vegetables
Sugar	butter	White bread	Bread, butter
	Salt, sugar	Butter	Dessert (no fresh fruit)
		Plain pudding	
2:00 p.m.	*2:00 p.m.*	*2:00 p.m.*	*2:00 p.m.*
Baked custard	Same as No. 1	Same as No. 1	Same as No. 1
Dinner	*Dinner*	*Dinner*	*Dinner*
Baked potato	Small tender steak	Small tender steak	Tender meat
	Baked potato with	Baked potato	Potato or substitute
	butter	Pureed vegetable	Whole vegetables
	White toast	White bread	Bread, butter
	Butter	Butter	Dessert (no fresh fruit)
		Vanilla ice cream	
8:00 p.m.	*8:00 p.m.*	*8:00 p.m.*	*8:00 p.m.*
Plain pudding	Same as No. 1	Plain pudding with cookie	Same as No. 3

NOTE: *All meals are small in portions. Fluids, such as soup, milk, fruit juices, and other beverages, should be taken in moderation.*

Diet for postoperative gastric dumping syndrome

General description
1. Five or six small meals daily.
2. Relatively high fat content to retard passage of food and help maintain weight.
3. High protein content (meat, egg, cheese) to rebuild tissue and maintain weight.
4. Relatively low carbohydrate content to prevent rapid passage of quickly utilized foods.
5. No milk; no sugar, sweets, or desserts; no alcohol or sweet carbonated beverages.
6. Liquids between meals only; avoid fluids for at least one hour before and after meals.
7. Relatively low roughage foods. Raw foods as tolerated.

Meal pattern

Breakfast	2 scrambled eggs with 1 or 2 tbsp butter or margarine
	½ to 1 slice bread or small serving cereal with butter or margarine
	2 crisp bacon
	1 serving solid fruit*
Midmorning	
sandwich of:	1 slice bread
	butter or margarine
	56 g (2 oz) lean meat
Lunch	112 g (4 oz) lean meat with 1 or 2 tbsp butter or margarine
	green or colored vegetable* with butter or margarine
	½ to 1 slice bread with butter or margarine
	½ banana or other solid fruit*
Midafternoon	Same snack as midmorning
Dinner	112 g lean meat with 1 or 2 tbsp butter or margarine
	green or colored vegetable† with butter or margarine
	½ to 1 slice bread with butter or margarine (or small serving starchy vegetable substitute)
	1 serving solid fruit*
Bedtime	56 g meat or 2 eggs or 56 g cheese or cottage cheese
	1 slice bread or 5 crackers
	butter or margarine

*Fruit choice: applesauce, baked apple, canned fruit (drained), banana, orange or grapefruit sections.
†Vegetable choice: asparagus, spinach, green beans, squash, beets, carrots, green peas.

Day 5	30 to 60 ml (1 to 2 oz) of water every even hour, and 30 to 60 ml milk each odd hour between
Day 6	Same feedings—increase to 90 ml (3 oz) each
Day 7	Same feedings—increase to 120 ml (4 oz) each
Day 8	Same feedings—add a soft egg at 8 AM and 6 PM feedings
Days 9 to 16	Water as desired; progress to a six-feeding ulcer-type diet
Day 16	Full bland diet; small meals with interval snacks

PRINCIPLES OF DIET THERAPY. The basic principles of diet therapy for the postgastrectomy period are (1) size of meals, small, frequent, and (2) type of food, simple, easily digested, mild, and low in bulk. A progressive gastrectomy diet in four stages is outlined on p. 674.

The later "dumping syndrome." After the patient has recovered from the surgery and begins to eat food in greater volume and variety, he may begin to experience increasing discomfort following meals. About 10 to 15 minutes after he has eaten, he has a cramping, full feeling. His pulse is rapid, and he feels a wave of weakness, cold sweating, and dizziness. Frequently he becomes nauseated and vomits. Such distressing reactions to food intake increase his anxiety, and he eats less and less. He continues to lose weight and becomes increasingly malnourished.

This postgastrectomy complex of symptoms is commonly called the "dumping syndrome," although the more precise term used by Lieber[8] is the *jejunal hyperosmolic syndrome*. This difficulty is more likely to occur in patients who have had total gastrectomy. The symptoms of shock result when a meal containing a high proportion of readily hydrolyzed carbohydrate rapidly enters the jejunum. This entering food mass is a concentrated hyperosmolar solution in relation to the surrounding extracellular fluid. To achieve an osmotic balance, water is drawn from the blood into the intestine, causing a rapid decrease in the vascular fluid compartment. The blood pressure drops, and signs of cardiac insufficiency appear—rapid pulse, sweating, weakness, and tremors.

A second sequence of events may follow about two hours later. The concentrated solution of carbohydrate is rapidly digested and absorbed, causing a postprandial rise in the blood glucose. The glucose load stimulates an overproduction of insulin, which in turn leads to an eventual drop in the blood sugar below normal fasting levels. Symptoms of mild hypoglycemia result.

PRINCIPLES OF DIET THERAPY. Careful control of the diet often brings dramatic relief of the distressing symptoms and leads to a gradual regaining of lost weight. Carbohydrate intake, especially simple sugars, is kept to a minimum to prevent rapid passage of food and formation of a concentrated, hyperosmolar solution. Protein and fat are increased to provide tissue building material and retard emptying of the food mass into the intestine. Meals are small, frequent, and dry, with fluid only between meals. There is less bulk to stimulate motility and less water to form rapid nutrient solutions. A summary of the dietary regimen is given on p. 675. Several follow-up studies of postgastrectomy patients on this regimen have indicated a good recovery of lost weight and correction of nutritional deficiencies.[9,10]

Cholecystectomy

For patients suffering from acute cholecystitis and cholelithiasis the treatment is usually surgical removal of the gallbladder. The discussion of gallbladder disease in Chapter 27, p. 598, should be reviewed.

Following surgery, control of fat in the diet remains essential to wound healing and comfort. The presence of fat in the duodenum continues to stimulate the cholecystokinin mechanism, which causes contraction and pain in the surgical area. There is also a period of adjustment to the more aqueous supply of liver bile for the preparation of fats for digestion. Depending on individual toleration and response, a relatively low-fat diet may need to be followed for as long as a month with moderate habits of fat use thereafter. The low-fat regimen outlined on p. 600 for gallbladder disease may serve as a guide.

Ileostomy and colostomy

In cases of intestinal lesion or obstruction or when chronic ulcerative colitis involves the entire colon, the treatment of choice is usually resection of the intestine and establishment of a permanent *ileostomy,* with removal of the diseased colon. The end of the remaining small intestine, the ileum, is attached to an opening in the abdominal wall, and a stoma is formed to provide for discharge of intestinal contents. In a *colostomy* the left side of the colon is resected, and a stoma is made with the proximal sigmoid or descending colon.

Therefore an ileostomy and a colostomy produce different problems in management. The intestinal contents at the point of the ileus are unformed, irritating, even erosive to the skin. The ileostomy drains freely, almost continuously, and should never be irrigated. Thus establishment of controlled functioning is difficult, although many patients do develop a reasonable degree of regularity in relation to meals. Some sort of appliance is necessary to hold the discharge.

A colostomy is more manageable. The normal contents of the intestine at this point in the colon are solid, or semisolid, because of absorption of water and electrolytes by the proximal colon. The consistency of the discharge and its less irritating nature create fewer control problems. Often the sigmoid colostomy can be adequately controlled by simple dietary measures and periodic irrigation, so that in many cases no protective appliance is required.

A low-residue diet (p. 583) is usually used in the immediate postoperative period. However, as soon as possible the diet should be advanced to a regular pattern of food to (1) provide optimum nutrition and physical rehabilitation and (2) provide an additional means of psychologic support. Diet counseling with the patient and his family will help to establish the most successful pattern of meals for him and avoid those foods that may cause individual discomfort.

Rectal surgery

For a brief period following rectal surgery (hemorrhoidectomy) a clear fluid or nonresidue diet may be indicated to delay initial bowel movement until healing has begun. The basic foods used are almost completely digested and absorbed in the small intestine, leaving minimal residue for elimination by the colon. An outline of foods allowed is given on p. 668.

NUTRITIONAL CARE OF PATIENT WITH BURNS

A major aspect of therapy for the patient with extensive burns is rigorous nutritional care. Tremendous loss of tissue results from the burn itself, and in the catabolic period following, additional tissue destruction and nitrogen loss continue. To ensure adequate nutritional therapy for patients with major burns a formula for calculating dietary requirements has been developed.[11] Artz has described studies in eight burned patients in whom the average daily protein loss for a catabolic period of one month was 166 g and has provided a useful guide to assessment and management of burns.[12,13] Fluid and electrolyte imbalances create management problems. Feeding the burned child presents special problems and is a constant challenge.[14]

The nutritional care of the burned patient is adjusted to the individual patient's needs and responses over three distinct periods following the injury.

Immediate shock period—days 1 to 3 (4 or 5)

Initial fluid and electrolyte problems (days 1 to 2). A massive flooding edema occurs at the burn site during the first hours to about the second day. Loss of enveloping skin surface and exposure of extracellular fluids leads to immediate loss of interstitial water and electrolytes, mainly sodium, and large protein depletion. In an effort to balance the loss, water shifts from extracellular spaces in other parts of the body, only to add to the continuous loss at the burn site.

As a result of the initial shifts and losses, vascular fluid is decreased in volume and pressure, and there is hemoconcentration and diminished urine output. Cellular (hypertonic) dehydration (p. 181) follows as intracellular water is drawn out to balance extracellular fluid losses. Cell potassium is also withdrawn, and circulating serum potassium levels rise.

Fluid therapy. Immediate intravenous fluid therapy seeks to replace the following:

1. Colloid (protein) through blood or plasma transfusion or by use of plasma expanders —Dextran
2. Electrolytes sodium and chlorine by use of a saline solution—lactated Ringer's solution
3. Water (dextrose solution) to cover additional insensible losses

The amount of fluid given is calculated by the "rule of nines" and the Brooke formula[15] or by a formula such as that of Evans[16] (1 ml colloid plus 1 ml electrolyte solution for each 1% of surface burned and each kilogram of body weight). The rate of flow should be carefully controlled. Half the calculated fluid and electrolyte needs should be given during the first eight hours, one quarter during the second eight hours, and one quarter during the third eight hours. During the second 24-hour period the patient will require about half the amount of fluid given the first 24 hours. Throughout there must be constant individual checks and adjustments.

Recovery period—days 3 to 5

As the fluid and electrolytes are gradually reabsorbed into the general circulation, balance is reestablished, and the pattern of massive tissue loss is reversed. At this point there is a sudden diuresis. Intravenous therapy may be discontinued and oral solutions such as Holdrane's used:

Holdrane's solution (oral fluid and electrolyte replacement)
3 to 4 g (½ tsp) salt
1.5 to 2 g (1½ tsp) sodium bicarbonate (baking soda)
1,000 ml (1 qt) water
Flavor with lemon juice and chill

A careful check of fluid intake and output is essential, with constant checks for signs of dehydration or overhydration.

Secondary feeding period—days 6 to 15

Factors demanding optimum nutritional therapy. Despite the patient's depression and anorexia his life may well depend on rigorous nutritional therapy during the secondary feeding period. Several factors necessitate this increased intake.

1. Tissue destruction by the burn with large losses of protein and electrolytes
2. Tissue catabolism following with continuing nitrogen losses
3. Increased metabolic demands of *infection* or *fever* make extra calories necessary; for energy, extra carbohydrate and B vitamins are needed; tremendously increased basal needs as body resources are mobilized; *tissue regeneration* requires extra protein and vitamin C
4. Optimum tissue health necessary for subsequent grafting to be successful

Principles of diet therapy

High protein. Individual needs will vary from 150 g to as high as 400 g. Concentrated protein foods must be planned with follow-through support to see that they are consumed.

High calories. From 3,500 to 5,000 calories with a high percentage of carbohydrate is necessary to spare protein essential for tissue regeneration and to supply the greatly increased metabolic demands for energy.

High vitamins. From 1 to 2 g of vitamin C are needed for tissue regeneration. Increased thiamin, riboflavin, and niacin are necessary to supply oxidative enzyme systems to metabolize extra carbohydrate and protein.

Intake record. Since the nutritional needs are so vital, a careful record of protein and calorie value in the amount of food consumed is a necessary tool for planning care.

Dietary management

1. Initial tube feeding may be required to ensure adequate intake. Formulas such as those in Tables 30-2 and 30-3 may be used.

2. Concentrated oral liquids must be given using protein hydrolysates to ensure adequate intake. Milk shakes such as those on p. 595 supply large amounts of nourishment.

3. Soft to regular diet will probably be taken by the second week or so.

4. Continuous individual support and encouragement are necessary to help the patient to eat the food he requires. Every effort should be made to make the foods as attractive and appetizing as possible, supplying items particularly liked and respecting disliked foods.

Follow-up reconstruction period—weeks 2 to 5 and following

Grafting and plastic surgery. Continued optimum nutrition is essential to maintain tissue integrity for successful skin grafting or plastic reconstructive surgery.

Rehabilitation. The principles of rehabilitation nursing discussed in Chapter 21 apply here. The patient will need not only physical rebuilding of his body's resources but also much emotional and social support to rebuild his spirit and his will. There may be disfigurement and disability. Health team members can do much to help instill the courage and confidence the patient must have to face the future again. Whatever his future demands, however, optimum physical stamina gained through persistent, supportive care—medical, nutritional, and nursing—will give him the personal resources to cope.

CASE STUDY 26
Ralph Gregory has a gastrectomy (continued from Case 14, p. 587)

After Ralph Gregory's initial episode of gastric bleeding and subsequent hospitalization, he returned home full of good intentions, at the insistence of his wife, to take things a little easier. But as time passed and he returned to his work, the old pressures and his responses to them resumed. Over the months that followed there were repeated episodes of the pain and several other hospitalizations for bleeding. The physician discussed surgery with Ralph and called in a surgeon for consultation. The decision was made to perform a total gastrectomy, and Ralph entered the hospital for this procedure.

The following day the surgeon performed a total gastrectomy and established an anastomosis between the jejunum and the remaining portion of the esophagus. Ralph withstood the surgery well. Gradually, over the next two-week period immediately following surgery, a refeeding program was initiated. In the first 24 to 48 hours immediately after the surgery Ralph received nothing by mouth but was fed by intravenous therapy, with close attention given to maintaining fluid and electrolyte balances. When he received his initial bit of water in the form of ice chips or sips of water adjusted in temperature for the best tolerance, the nurse observed carefully to see what Ralph's responses were.

Since Ralph tolerated the initial water by mouth very well, the next few days he received 30 to 60 ml (1 to 2 oz) of milk between the small amounts of water. Gradually the amount of milk was increased a bit, and a single soft food item added at one or two of the feedings during the day. Soft foods such as eggs, soft-cooked cereal, baked custard, baked potatoes, or plain puddings were used. By the end of the second week Ralph was tolerating a full soft diet in small feedings about six times during the day. The clinical dietitian cautioned him to use his fluids, such as milk, soup, fruit juice, and other beverages, in moderation.

After Ralph recovered from the surgery and was improved enough to go home, he gradually felt his strength returning. The dietitian had emphasized that he should observe his tolerances, eat smaller amounts at a time, and emphasize the use of protein foods. When Ralph had recovered from the surgery itself and began to resume more and more of his usual activities, his food intake increased. He began to eat a greater volume of food and in greater variety. Friends invited the Gregory family out for meals, and they began to do more entertaining themselves, because Mrs. Gregory felt it would be good for Ralph to get out more. Also, as he began to become involved in more of his old business activities, he was engaged in business luncheon conferences with more food and alcohol included.

As time went by, Ralph began to experience increasing discomfort following his meals. About 10 or 15 minutes after he had eaten he would have a cramping full feeling. He felt his heart begin to beat more rapidly, and a wave of weakness would suddenly come over him. He would break out in a cold sweat and feel extremely dizzy. Often he would become nauseated and vomit. As these episodes increased, his anxiety concerning himself increased accordingly. As a result he began to eat less and less. His weight began to drop. He was already fairly thin, and this increased weight loss only made him look more emaciated and debilitated. Soon he was in a general state of malnutrition.

Ralph went to his physician when these symptoms did not subside. Dr. Black referred him to the clinical nutrition specialist, Mrs. Rowan, who initiated a change in his eating habits. She explained the diet in detail to Mr. and Mrs. Gregory and worked out a new food plan that would be acceptable in his situation. The diet seemed to be a strange one to Ralph, but he began to follow it carefully because he felt so ill that he was glad to make any change that would be helpful. He found to his pleased surprise that the symptoms he had experienced before almost completely disappeared. Because he felt so much better on the new diet plan, he formed his new eating habits around it. His wife commented that she had never seen him watch what he ate so closely.

CASE STUDY 26
Ralph Gregory has a gastrectomy (continued from Case 14, p. 587)—cont'd

As Ralph began to improve and concentrated on the increase of protein and calories in his new diet plan, his weight gradually increased and his general state of nutrition improved markedly. The nutritionist followed his progress closely and indicated to him that he would always fare better if his permanent habits became those of a "nibbler" rather than ever consuming a large heavy meal at one time. Ralph began to take food from home to the office to eat during the day, and he kept snack foods in his desk drawer so that he could eat frequently during the day and never a great deal at any one time. He avoided sweets, but this was no special problem because he had never been very fond of them, and he used liquid foods only between the feedings of dry food. On the whole, with his new habits well learned by now, along with an adjustment in his business and home life for the better, Ralph made a good recovery and maintained a far better state of general nutrition and health.

Questions to guide your inquiry

1. Why do you think the physician decided to intervene with surgical therapy in Ralph's case?
2. Identify Ralph's nutritional needs immediately following surgery and in the next two weeks. Why was it necessary for his feedings to be resumed cautiously?
3. What observations would be important during this period?
4. Why would there be an emphasis on protein intake following Ralph's surgery as he began to tolerate food? Why is a negative nitrogen balance a usual follow-up to surgical procedures?
5. Why does the body need protein following surgery? What are its functions during this period?
6. Why should sufficient calories be consumed as soon as tolerated?
7. Why is fluid therapy of paramount importance following surgery?
8. What minerals and vitamins should be increased following surgery?
9. When Ralph began to feel better and resumed heavier eating habits, why did he experience the symptoms he did after consuming a meal? What is this response called? Why?
10. Account for the symptoms that followed eating, according to the physiologic changes that had been produced by the surgery and the fluid and electrolyte imbalances incurred.
11. Why would a still later symptom in the sequence of symptoms be a hypoglycemic reaction from a lowered blood sugar level?
12. What principles of diet therapy would be followed in the corrective diet suggestions given to Ralph by the nutritionist? Give the rationale for each of these principles.
13. Outline a day's meal pattern for Ralph on his newly adjusted diet pattern.
14. What practical problems might Ralph encounter on his new diet plan? What solutions can you propose to help meet these problems?

CASE STUDY 27

Margaret has surgery—an ileostomy (continued from Case 19, p. 588)

For a while after Margaret went home from the hospital following her latest siege with her ulcerative colitis, she seemed to improve. But some weeks later her condition worsened. The diarrhea increased, as well as the symptoms that had bothered her before. Dr. Towers admitted her to the hospital again. He talked a long time with Margaret and Ray, after her latest X-rays, and called in a surgeon for consultation. It seemed that by now the chronic ulcerative colitis had involved the entire colon, and the treatment that seemed indicated at this point was surgery. Finally the decision was made to resect the intestine and remove the involved colon. An ileostomy was to be done.

The next few days Dr. Towers tried to prepare Margaret for surgery as much as possible. When she went to surgery the surgeon removed the involved intestine and attached the end of the remaining small intestine, the ileum, to an opening in the abdominal wall on the right, forming a stoma to provide for discharge of the intestinal contents.

In the days following the surgery Margaret responded gradually. She found great difficulty in accepting the results of the surgery and was depressed. The nurses on the surgery ward were kind and understanding, however, and gave her a great deal of support in helping her to learn about her surgery and how to take care of herself. At first Margaret did not want to participate in changing the appliance used over her stoma, but gradually she realized that this was something she would be living with and that she would, in the long run, be feeling a great deal better as a result of the surgery.

One day shortly before Margaret was to be discharged, her nurse came into the room accompanied by a young woman about Margaret's age. She was an attractive person with a bright smile. The nurse explained that this was a friend of hers who had had the same surgery as Margaret and who would be glad to help her after she got home and to introduce her to the local chapter of the United Ostomy Association.

After Margaret was able to go home she recovered slowly from the surgery. She had been underweight and generally malnourished for so long that it took some time for her to rebuild herself. As her physical strength returned, however, her spirits brightened also. She called the nurse's friend and invited her to visit. They talked a long while about their common experiences, and in the months that followed, Margaret became an active member of the Ostomy Association. She learned a great deal through this active group of people with whom she shared a significant life experience.

Margaret was also following many of the diet suggestions that the dietitian had discussed with her. Her appetite was greatly improved, and she was finding that with care she could eat many of the things that she had enjoyed before. She had learned how to handle her ileostomy with skill.

Perhaps the thing that helped Margaret most, however, was the opportunity she received through the Ostomy Association to be of help, in turn, to another young woman who had also undergone the same surgery. Somehow, it gave her a good feeling to think that she was being asked to help another human being. It had seemed so long since she had felt of use to anyone.

Questions to guide your inquiry

1. Describe the surgical procedure in an ileostomy.
2. What problems of care does an ileostomy present to the body's handling of food and residue material? Why?
3. Identify Margaret's postoperative nutritional needs. What is the basis for each?
4. What plan of action would you use in meeting these needs? Why?
5. What dietary management would be indicated? Why?
6. How would you help Margaret plan for follow-up care?
7. What is the United Ostomy Association? Obtain information about a possible local chapter in your own community. Investigate its activities.
8. What factors do you think contributed to Margaret's improvement and changed attitude and outlook?

CASE STUDY 28
Care of the burned patient

Ann Rodriquez, aged 18, was excited about taking the first big step toward her goal. She had decided that she wanted to be a nurse, and although she did not know how she would manage it, she was determined. Now she was enrolled in the state university to begin her study on an academic scholarship.

As she began her first basic course in the physical and behavioral sciences, her interest grew. Her awareness of some of the tremendous human problems facing society had grown in the past few years, and she felt a serious challenge to help find answers and to be a part of the solutions.

Ann's family lived some distance from her school. She had a large family, and although there was little material resource, there was much love, mutual understanding, and support. Ann was the first child to go to college, to bring in new ideas and new hope for the future. When she had graduated from high school as the top student in her class, not only Ann's family but also her whole Mexican community was very proud of her. All of them were following Ann's plans with great interest.

At the university Ann became part of a group of students interested in campus and community problems. One evening when she was returning with another student in the group, John Reed, following a meeting at a nearby community center, an oncoming car went out of control. It crossed over the freeway's center divider strip and crashed into John's car. The gasoline tank exploded, and Ann was caught in the fire. John managed to free himself and pull Ann to the edge of the road, rolling her over and over on the grass to put out the flames on her clothing. An ambulance was summoned and brought Ann and John to the nearest emergency hospital.

At the hospital the emergency team found that somehow John had escaped serious injury. But Ann was seriously burned. The nurse and resident cut away Ann's clothing and called in medical specialists, who instituted immediate care. Ann was still responsive and able to give her age, height, and weight— 162.5 cm, 54 kg (5 ft, 5 in, 120 lb). Morphine was given and stat orders for blood tests, including BUN, hematocrit, CO_2-combining power, serum sodium, potassium and chlorides, and a urinalysis. Type and cross-match for blood was also ordered, as well as careful measures and control of intake and output of fluid. The examination by the team of physicians revealed extensive burns over 60% of Ann's body. She was moved to the hospital's burn unit.

Careful calculation of fluid and electrolyte needs in the first critical 48-hour period was made. Initial intravenous therapy included whole blood, Ringer's lactate solution, albumin, dextran, and 5% dextrose in water. Later Berocca-C was added to the intravenous infusion.

By the third day after the accident, Ann's urine output improved. The burn team was relieved to observe a sudden diuresis. At this point they decided to begin 60 to 120 ml (2 to 4 oz) feedings of Holdrane's solution in dilute orange juice every hour Ann was awake. Careful checks of fluid intake and urinary output were continued.

Since Ann tolerated the initial oral liquids well, the burn team decided to begin a careful feeding program and consulted with the clinical nutrition specialist. Together they planned a high-protein, high-calorie, high-vitamin diet, working with Ann to provide foods she desired and in the form she could best tolerate. The nurse and dietitian kept a close record of her food intake and the nutrients involved, especially protein, calories, and key vitamins and minerals. By the third week Ann's nutritional status had greatly improved. The physicians began a projected program of skin grafting and eventual plastic surgery.

Many problems faced Ann, her family, and the health team during the months that followed. Long patient work with rehabilitation therapy was needed, during which the team worked closely together. These were truly testing times for Ann, and although there were periods of depression, her courage and determination prevailed. She was a strong young woman with physical and personal resources.

Finally, the following year, she was able to reenter school and continue her education. Now she possessed even more insight into human need as the result of her own personal experiences.

Continued.

CASE STUDY 28
Care of the burned patient—cont'd

Questions to guide your inquiry

1. What immediate fluid and electrolyte problems faced the burn team when Ann was brought in to the hospital? Why?
2. What purpose did the physician have in ordering each of the initial blood and urine tests? What results of these tests would you expect to find? Why?
3. On what basis would the burn team calculate Ann's initial fluid and electrolyte therapy?
4. Using the Evans formula (p. 678, check primary reference given) calculate the approximate amount of colloid and electrolyte solution Ann would require.
5. Indicate the rate of flow at which these intravenous fluids would be given during the first 24 hours. Why?
6. In comparison, about how much intravenous fluid would Ann require during the second 24-hour period?
7. Why is a careful measure of fluid intake and output, as well as a constant check on serum electrolyte levels, essential during these early periods?
8. Why did Ann experience a sudden diuresis on the third day? What did this indicate? Why was the burn team relieved?
9. What is Holdrane's solution? How would this help Ann at this point?
10. What were Ann's nutritional problems at the end of the second week, when she could begin to eat? What nutritional therapy was essential? Why was this rigorous nutritional care needed at this stage?
11. What increases in specific nutrients would be necessary? Give your reasons for increasing each one.
12. What personal factors do you think would be important for the dietitian to consider in planning Ann's diet? How would you involve Ann and her family in your planning?
13. Outline a day's food plan for Ann to meet her needs.
14. What were Ann's needs during her rehabilitation period? During grafting and plastic surgery?
15. What factors do you think contributed to Ann's recovery?
16. How do you think Ann's experience would influence her own future practice as a professional nurse?
17. Ann was deeply concerned with community problems. With what community problems do you think health care is bound up? What solutions and alternatives can you propose to meet these problems? On what basis? How do you see persons on the health team helping in these new solutions?

REFERENCES
Specific

1. Calloway, D., and Spector, H.: Nitrogen balance as related to caloric and protein intake in active young men, Am. J. Clin. Nutr. **2:**405, 1954.
2. Zohrab, W. J., McHattie, J. D., and Jeejeebhoy, K. N.: Total parenteral alimentation with lipid, Gastroenterology **64:**583, 1973.
3. Deitel, M., and Kaminsky, V.: Total nutrition by peripheral vein—the lipid system, Can. Med. Assoc. J. **111:**152, July 20, 1974.
4. Dudrick, S. J., Wilmore, D. W., and Vors, H. M.: Long term total parenteral nutrition with growth, development, and positive nitrogen balance, Surgery **64:**134, July, 1968.
5. Dudrick, S. J., and Rhoads, J. E.: Total intravenous feeding, Sci. Am. **226:**73, May, 1972.
6. Shils, M. E.: Guidelines for total parenteral nutrition, J.A.M.A. **220**(3):14, 1972.
7. Johnson, E. Q.: The therapeutic dietitian's role in the alimentation group, J. Am. Diet. Assoc. **62:**648, June, 1973.
8. Lieber, H.: The jejunal hyperosmolic syndrome (dumping) and its prophylaxis, J.A.M.A. **176:**208, 1961.

9. Pittman, A. C., and Robinson, F. W.: Dumping syndrome—control by diet, J. Am. Diet. Assoc. **34:**596, 1958.

10. Pittman, A. C., and Robinson, F. W.: Dietary management of the "dumping" syndrome, J. Am. Diet. Assoc. **40:**108, Feb., 1962.

11. Curreri, P. W., Richmond, D., Marvin, J., et al.: Dietary requirements of patients with major burns, J. Am. Diet. Assoc. **65:**415, Oct., 1974.

12. Artz, C. P., et al.: Some recent developments in oral feedings for optimal nutrition in burns, Am. J. Clin. Nutr. **4:**642, 1956.

13. Artz, C. P.: Guide to assessment and management of burns, Hosp. Med. **13:**105, 1977.

14. Holli, B. B., and Oakes, J. B.: Feeding the burned child, J. Am. Diet. Assoc. **67:**240, Sept., 1975.

15. Callentine, G. E., Jr.: How to calculate fluids for burned patients, Am. J. Nurs. **62:**77, 1962.

16. Evans, I. E.: The early management of the severely burned patient, Surg. Gynecol. Obstet. **94:**273, 1952.

General

Alexander, H. C.: A protein dietary supplement for the severe dumping syndrome, Surg. Gynecol. Obstet. **141:**863, 1975.

Ames, F. C., et al.: Fatty metamorphosis of the liver complicating small bowel bypass for obesity. Nonoperative treatment with parenteral hyperalimentation, J.A.M.A. **235:**1249, 1976.

Ballinger, W. F., editor: Manual of surgical nutrition, Philadelphia, 1975, W. B. Saunders Co.

Barron, J., and Fallis, L. S.: Tube feeding with natural foods in elderly patients, J. Am. Geriat. Soc. **4:**400, 1956.

Barron, J., Prendergast, J. J., and Jocz, M. W.: Food pump: new approach to tube feeding, J.A.M.A. **161:**621, 1956.

Blackburn, G. L., and Bistrian, B. R.: Nutritional care of the injured and/or septic patient, Surg. Clin. North Am. **56:**1195, 1976.

Blackburn, G. L., et al.: Surgical nutrition. In Halpern, S. L., editor: Quick reference to clinical nutrition, Philadelphia, 1979, J. B. Lippincott Co.

Bury, K.: Carbohydrate digestion and absorption after massive resection of the small intestine, Surgery **135:**177, 1972.

Carter, L. H., and Goldsmith, G. A.: The ordeal of Donald Boone, Nutr. Today **5**(3):2, 1970.

Dietschy, J. M., and Sanford, J. P., editors: Disorders of the gastrointestinal tract, disorders of the liver, nutritional disorders, New York, 1976, Grune & Stratton, Inc.

Dudrick, S. J., and Duke, J. H., Jr.: Nutritional complications in the surgical patient. In Artz, C. P., and Hardy, J. D., editors: Complications in surgery and their management, ed. 3, Philadelphia, 1974, W. B. Saunders Co.

Freeman, J. B., Stegnick, L. D., Meyer, P. D., et al.: Metabolic effects of amino acids vs. dextrose infusion in surgical patients, Arch. Surg. **110:**916, 1975.

Ghadimi, H., editor: Total parenteral nutrition: premises and promises, New York, 1975, John Wiley & Sons, Inc.

Glotzer, D. J., Boyle, P. L., and Silen, W.: Preoperative preparation of the colon with an elemental diet, Surgery **74:**703, 1973.

Gordon, P. H.: The chemically defined diet and anorectal procedures, Can. J. Surg. **19:**511, 1976.

Gormican, A., Liddy, E., and Thrush, L. B., Jr.: Nutritional status of patients after extended tube feeding, J. Am. Diet. Assoc. **63:**247, Sept., 1973.

Greenberg, G. R., Morliss, E. B., Anderson, G. H., et al.: Protein-sparing therapy in post operative patients: effect of added hypocaloric glucose or lipid, N. Engl. J. Med. **294:**1411, 1976.

Hill, E. L.: Ileostomy: surgery, physiology, and management, New York, 1976, Grune & Stratton, Inc.

Kaminsky, V.: Enteral hyperalimentation, Surg. Gynecol. Obstet. **143:**12, 1976.

Kark, R. M.: Liquid formula and chemically defined diets, J. Am. Diet. Assoc. **64:**476, May, 1974.

Law, D. K., Dudrick, S. J., and Abdou, N. I.: Effects of protein-calorie malnutrition on immune competence of the surgical patient, Surg. Gynecol. Obstet. **139:**257, 1974.

Lee, P. W. R., Green, M. A., Long, W. B., III, et al.: Zinc and wound healing, Surg. Gynecol. Obstet. **143:**549, 1976.

MacFadyen, B. V., Jr., Copeland, E. M., III, and Dudrick, S. J.: Surgery. In Schneider, H. A., Anderson, C. E., and Coursin, D. B., editors: Nutritional support of medical practice, New York, 1977, Harper & Row, Publishers.

Mason, E. E.: Fluid, electrolyte and nutrient therapy in surgery, Philadelphia, 1974, Lea & Febiger.

Review: Stimulus for hyperplasia of the small bowel, Nutr. Rev. **34:**345, 1976.

Rhodes, M. J., Gruendemann, B. J., and Ballinger, W. F.: Alexander's care of the patient in surgery, ed. 6, St. Louis, 1978, The C. V. Mosby Co.

Scheflan, M., Galli, S. J., Perrotto, J., et al.: Intestinal adaptation after extensive resection of the small intestine and prolonged administration of parenteral nutrition, Surg. Gynecol. Obstet. **143:**757, 1976.

Schwartz, P. L.: Ascorbic acid in wound healing—a review, J. Am. Diet. Assoc. **56:**497, June, 1970.

Shils, M. E., and Randall, H. T.: Diet and nutrition in the care of the surgical patient. In Goodhart, R. S., and Shils, M. E., editors: Modern nutrition in health and disease, ed. 6, Philadelphia, 1980, Lea & Febiger.

Stahl, W.: Supportive care of the surgical patient, New York, 1972, Grune & Stratton, Inc.

Vanamee, P.: Parenteral nutrition. In Hegsted, D. M.,

editor: Nutrition reviews' present knowledge in nutrition, ed. 4, New York, 1976, The Nutrition Foundation, Inc.

Webster, M. W., and Corey, L. C.: Fistulae of the intestinal tract, Curr. Probl. Surg. **13**(6):1976.

White, P. L., and Nagy, M. E., editors: Total parenteral nutrition, Acton, Mass., 1974, Publishing Science Group.

Wright, H. K., and Tilson, M. S.: Postoperative disorders of the gastrointestinal tract, New York, 1973, Grune & Stratton, Inc.

BURNS

Artz, C. P.: Guide to assessment and management of burns, Hosp. Med. **13**:105, 1977.

Curreri, P. W., Richmond, D., Marvin, J., et al.: Dietary requirements of patients with major burns, J. Am. Diet. Assoc. **65**:415, Oct., 1974.

Feller, I., Jones, C. A., Koepke, G., et al.: The team approach to total rehabilitation of the severely burned patient, Heart Lung **2**:701, 1973.

Holli, B. B., and Oakes, J. B.: Feeding the burned child, J. Am. Diet. Assoc. **67**:240, Sept., 1975.

Larkin, J. M., and Moylon, J. A.: Complete enteral support of thermally injured patients, Am. J. Surg. **131**:722, 1976.

McAlhany, J. C., Czja, A. J., and Pruitt, B. A.: Antacid control of complications from acute gastroduodenal disease after burns, J. Trauma **16**:645, 1976.

Moncrief, J. A.: Burns, N. Engl. J. Med. **288**:444, 1973.

Newsome, T. W., Mason, A. D., Jr., and Pruitt, B. A., Jr.: Weight loss following thermal injury, Ann. Surg. **178**:215, 1973.

Wilmore, D. W., Long, J. M., Mason, A. D., Jr., et al.: Catecholamines: mediator of the hypermetabolic response to thermal injury, Ann Surg. **180**:653, 1974.

Zitzka, C.: Nutritional support of hospitalized burn patients, J. Am. Diet. Assoc. **75**:458, Oct., 1979.

31 Nutrition and cancer— care of the hypermetabolic or malnourished patient

The role of nutritional factors in the pathogenesis and treatment of cancer and the care of hypermetabolic or malnourished patients are drawing increased attention and concern among nutrition practitioners and researchers. It is clear from current studies and practice that important nutritional relationships exist in two fundamental areas: (1) *prevention* in relation to the environment and to the body's defense system and (2) *therapy* in relation to nutritional support for medical treatment and rehabilitation. To understand these relationships it is necessary to clarify them in terms of the general nature of cancer as a growth process, its physiologic basis in the structure and function of cells, and the body's defense systems, both in immunity and in the healing process.

The *increasing incidence of cancer* has thrust it into the role of a major health problem in the United States, giving impetus to the study of its nature, etiology, and treatment. Its incidence has nearly tripled since 1900 and has continued to increase approximately 1% each year since 1933.[1] This increasing rate of occurrence is no doubt due in part to our increased life expectancy, since cancer is generally associated with the aging process, as well as to better diagnostic techniques and screening programs. However, it is also apparently related in large measure to the rapid changes in our environment in conjunction with our rapidly expanding industrial technology without equally developed environmental safeguards. Cancer has become the second cause of death in the United States, claiming about 20% of the total, close on the heels of the number one killer, heart disease, with about 50% of the total. Each year there are about 665,000 new cancer patients, more than 1 million under treatment, and some 365,000 deaths. It has indeed become a major public health problem in the United States.

At the outset, in attempting to understand the nature of cancer, we are confronted with the related problems of definition and study. There are multiple forms of cancer varying worldwide and changing with population migrations, multiple etiologies, and conflicting research results. We find immediately that we are not dealing with a single entity. We are dealing rather with a wide range of malignant tumors or neoplasms (''new growths'') collectively known as cancer. More correctly, therefore, we should use the plural term ''cancers.''

CANCER PATHOGENESIS AND NUTRITION

Since the term ''cancer'' refers to the process of forming inappropriate malignant neoplasms or ''new growths'' in various body tissue sites, for a beginning understanding of the relation of nutritional factors we need to recall briefly the basic physiologic nature of cells and their normal growth pattern. Then we can compare the growth of the ''misguided cell'' in cancer to that of the normal cell in health.

687

The normal cell

The basic biologic unit of life is the cell. Recognition of this basis of life was established and accepted only in the early part of the nineteenth century when two German physiologists, Theodor Schwann and Matthias Schleiden, described the cell theory in 1839. Later, in 1853, Rudolf Virchow developed the theory further by demonstrating that cells arise from preexisting cells by division. Studies of the cell contents led to clarification of its colloidal nature, a protein network existing in interchanging fluid-gel states within a cell wall boundary held by interweaving internal structural scaffolding. The name "protoplasm" was given to this gel-like substance in 1839 by a Prague physiologist, Johannes Purkinje, from "protoplastus," a liturgical term of the day with reference to Adam. Subsequent studies have led to identification of the characteristic properties of protoplasm: irritability, motility, metabolism, growth, and reproduction. Continuing scientific work in molecular biology has further developed knowledge of cell organization at the molecular level and the formation and function of differentiated tissue.

Cell structure

Two main parts make up the cell structure. These are the central nucleus and the surrounding cytoplasm.

Cell nucleus. The nucleus, the central body of the cell, serves as the cell's master control site. It contains the specific genetic material that regulates synthesis of cell parts and substances as well as transmission of individual inherited traits. The components of this nuclear material, chromosomes and genes, hold the controlling agent, deoxyribonucleic acid (DNA).

CHROMOSOMES AND GENES. The genetic control material inside the nucleus, DNA, is packaged and protected in a substance called chromatin, a large mass of molecules made up of about two-thirds protein and one-third DNA. When cells prepare to divide, the chromatin arranges itself into discrete groupings of 23 pairs forming chromosomes ("stained bodies"). Specific sections or points along the chromosome threads are called genes. Each gene site carries specific unique genetic information, controlling the synthesis of the specific protein for which it is coded or transmitting specific hereditary traits. A single chromosome thread is made up of hundreds of genes end to end, and each gene of DNA is made up of some 600 to several thousand small molecular subunits of the DNA structure called nucleotides.

DEOXYRIBONUCLEIC ACID (DNA). Nucleic acids were so named because they were originally isolated from cell nuclei. It was assumed for many years that they were not found elsewhere, a view that was not seriously challenged until 1940 when new techniques for studying the structural elements of cells were devised. The two types of nucleic acids, deoxyribonucleic acid (DNA) and ribonucleic acid (RNA), differ in that DNA has one less oxygen molecule (carbon atom number 2) in its component sugar ribose, as the name implies, and is a double strand.

Based on the work of M. H. F. Wilkins with X-ray crystallography, reported in 1950, and the working model developed by J. D. Watson and F. H. C. Crick in 1953, the structure of DNA has been identified. These three scientists shared the Nobel Prize for physiology and medicine in 1962 for their work, which has been confirmed and extended by subsequent studies and has provided a pivotal development in molecular biology, giving a basis for understanding how this complex molecule carries genetic specifications and instructs the cell to produce more DNA, RNA, and protein.[2]

These discoveries of the structure of DNA have shown it to be a large polynucleotide with constituent mononucleotides composed of three parts: a sugar (deoxyribose), phosphate, and a specific nitrogenous base—adenine, cytosine, guanine, or thymine (Fig. 31-1). Its molecular weight may be as high as 2 billion, made up of

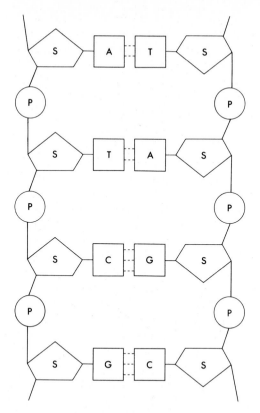

Fig. 31-1. Diagram of a portion of DNA structure. Note the components. The sugar deoxyribose and phosphate form the parallel bars of the ladderlike structure (a double helix); the connecting nitrogenous bases (the pyrimidines thymine and cytosine and the purines adenine and guanine) form the rungs (*A*, adenine; *T*, thymine; *C*, cytosine; *G*, guanine; *S*, sugar—deoxyribose; *P*, phosphate). The dotted lines represent the hydrogen bonding between the nitrogenous bases.

as many as 1 billion or more of the nitrogenous bases arranged in a continuous line. Its structure is that of a double strand helix (''spiral''), appearing as a twisted ladder or spiral staircase, with the sugar-phosphate chain providing the parallel side bars and the nitrogenous bases providing the rungs or steps. The spiral makes one complete turn for every 10 nucleotides, or steps. Two of these connecting nitrogenous bases, adenine and guanine, are purines; the

two others, cytosine and thymine, are pyrimidines (Fig. 31-1). According to the ''pairing rule,'' with the parallel side bars of the chain running in opposite directions, the bases in each chain are so arranged that an adenine of one chain is always opposite a thymine of the other chain and vice versa, and a guanine in one chain is always opposite a cytosine of the other chain and vice versa. The two parallel chains are held together by hydrogen bonding between these base pairs (Fig. 31-2). This specific pairing of the nitrogenous bases, A—T, C—G, provides the essential foundation of the Watson-Crick working model of DNA and explains how it can transmit ''messages'' to guide specific protein synthesis through a triplet code written in multiple combinations of these four letters—A, T, C, G—and how genes can thus replicate their precise structures when their copies are synthesized. Moreover, it also explains how mutational changes in the genes are produced.

RIBONUCLEIC ACID (RNA). The DNA companion nucleic acid, ribonucleic acid (RNA), provides the transmission link for carrying the genetic code message of the master pattern in the DNA. RNA occurs in the cell in three types: messenger RNA, ribosomal RNA, and transfer RNA.

1. *Messenger RNA* (mRNA) is a single strand molecule with a molecular weight of about 1 million. It is made in the cell nucleus as a copy of one strand of the DNA, except that the pyrimidine base uracil substitutes in RNA for the thymine base in DNA. Thus mRNA transcribes the coded information stored in the DNA to determine the exact amino acid sequence for synthesis of a specific protein in the cell. This sequence of amino acids for a specific protein is guided by the triplet code combinations of the four nitrogenous bases: adenine (A), uracil (U) translated from the thymine (T) of the DNA, cytosine (C), and guanine (G). For example, the triplet code for the amino acid leucine is CUA, and for the amino acid valine, GUU.

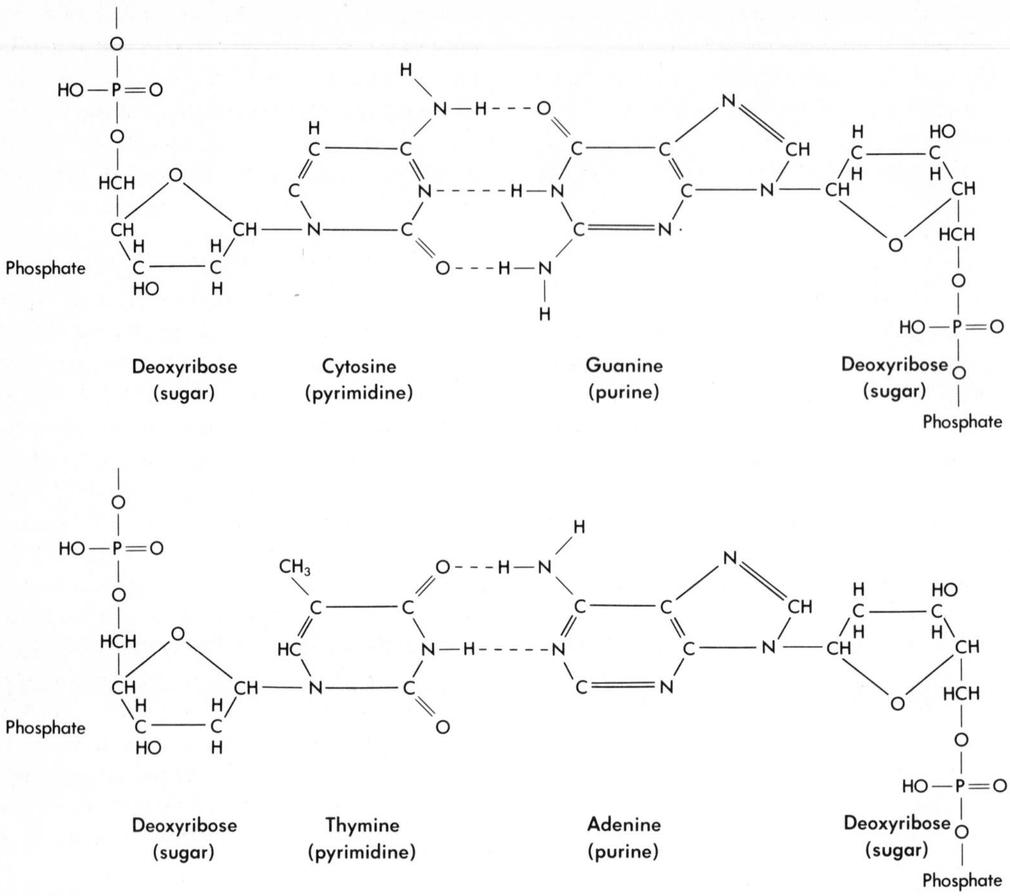

Fig. 31-2. Pairing of the nitrogenous bases in forming the specific DNA structure. Note the double and triple hydrogen bonding connecting the specific pairs of bases: adenine with thymine and guanine with cytosine.

2. *Ribosomal RNA* (rRNA) is constituent material associated with the ribosomes of the endoplasmic reticulum in the cell cytoplasm. The ribosomes are the sites for protein synthesis in the cell.

3. *Transfer RNA* (tRNA) is formed of triplet code sections of RNA matching the primary mRNA template from the original DNA pattern. These coded sections of RNA serve to transport the respective amino acids that make up a specific protein into the necessary sequence of amino acids to form the polypeptide linkage of that particular protein. A detailed description of this process of protein synthesis

is given in Chapter 4 and can be reviewed there. *Specificity* therefore is the critical hallmark of protein synthesis, guided by the master pattern code of DNA as transmitted by RNA, and provides the base for the central dogma sine qua non of modern molecular biology: DNA—RNA—AA—protein.

Cell cytoplasm. The cell cytoplasm surrounds the nucleus and fills the remainder of the cell. It is a gelatinous fluid, a protoplasmic ground substance containing nutrient material and numerous ultrastructures or organelles. These organelles include the following:

Ribosomes: sites of protein synthesis located

on the threadlike *endoplasmic reticulum* clustered around the nucleus.

Golgi apparatus: named for the Italian histologist Camillo Golgi, structures that receive the packaged proteins and other materials from the endoplasmic reticulum and prepare them for distribution.

Lysosomes: so-called suicide bags of the cell containing small packets of powerful enzymes for hydrolysis of proteins into their constituent parts that can then be used by the cell to help maintain a state of dynamic equilibrium, particularly in the face of environmental stress such as temperature, chemical imbalance, or varying digestive states.

Mitochondria: elliptical bodies containing the series of enzymes comprising the Krebs cycle for energy metabolism and formation of the high-energy compound ATP (see p. 27).

Cell function

Two fundamental physiologic tasks of the body are essential to life: tissue building and rebuilding, and energy "production." Many types of specialized cells carry on particular functions to contribute to the whole of life. Thus two major cell characteristics make this infinite variety of life functions possible: variation and differentiation. The human body is made up of a wide range of cell sizes and types to meet specialized needs. These cells differentiate early in embryonic life and become modified in structure and function according to the division of labor necessary to sustain life.

The various cell structures and functions operate in health in an orderly manner under gene control, directing the cell's specific processes of protein synthesis. Gene action can be switched on and off, depending on the position of a cell in the body, the stage of body development, and the external environment. Specific regulator genes control function by producing a repressor substance as needed to regulate operator genes and structural genes. This order-

ly regulation of induction and repression of cell activity can be lost with mutation of the regulatory genes. The human body is a highly complex system composed of many types of cells and tissues, each of which interacts with the others and with the environment in a precise manner.

Cell growth and reproduction

The growth and reproductive process in the cell is important to an understanding of the relationships between nutrition and cancer. Details of the cell cycle were described by two British scientists, Alma Howard and Stephen Pele, based on their work at Hammersmith Hospital in London and built on the contributions of numerous other investigators.[3] Four distinct stages have been identified in the cell life cycle. Although different cells have various life cycle time periods, the four stages can be related in time on the clock face of 12 hours (Fig. 31-3).

1. *Growth period (G_1):* the longest period in the cycle, formerly thought to be a resting stage but now known to be a period of intense growth in cell size primarily by synthesis of proteins. This initial growth period would take up the first six hours on the clock face.

2. *Synthesis period (S):* the stage of chromosome reproduction through DNA duplication in preparation for cell division. This second period, setting up the four-letter DNA triplet code, would take up the next three and one-half hours on the clock face.

3. *Growth period (G_2):* the second growth period covers the time required for the cell to arrange itself for splitting into two daughter cells. This final period of preparation for cell division would take up the next two hours on the clock face.

4. *Division period (D):* the final brief period of cell division by mitosis (Gr. *mitos*, "thread"). This final period of mitosis would take up the remaining half hour on the clock face. This final rapid period of

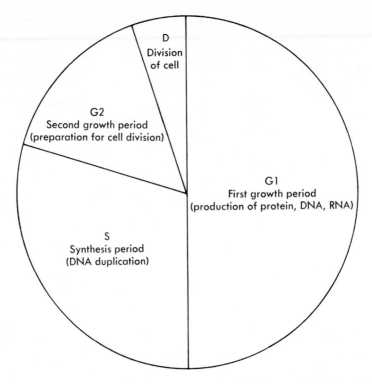

Fig. 31-3. Cell life cycle illustrating the four stages and relative time periods. The final brief cell division stage (*D*, mitosis) is made up of the four rapid phases: prophase, metaphase, anaphase, and telophase. The remaining periods *(G1, S, G2)* make up the interphase.

cell division is accomplished through four distinct phases:

a. *Prophase:* each of the cell's 46 chromosomes coil as springs into tight packages. Thus shortened and thickened they are now visible by microscope.

b. *Metaphase:* the packaged chromosomes, doubled as the result of DNA duplication during the prior synthesis (S) period, arrange for separation. The cell nucleus membrane disappears, and the attached threads of chromosomes form a central line across the cell with attachment points at the equator.

c. *Anaphase:* the chromosome attachment points break, forming two independent identical daughter chromosomes. These copies move to opposite sides, and a cleavage in the central cell area divides it into two parts, forming two daughter cells. Special spindle fibers act like muscles to pull the nucleus in half.

d. *Telophase:* the packaged chromosomes uncoil and disperse to form daughter cell nuclei. Each daughter cell now forms its own intact new cell in all its parts, ready to repeat the same life cycle again.

The first three periods of the cell cycle—the first growth period (G_1), the synthesis period (S), and the second growth period (G_2)—are collectively called the *interphase* between each rapid cell division period.

The cancer cell

In adult humans some 3 to 4 million cells complete the normal life-sustaining process of cell division every second, largely without mistake, guided by the genetic code. The central question in cell biology has been, How is the process and rate of cell reproduction maintained so precisely in normal cells? The question in cancer research, based on the increased knowledge of normal cell physiology, follows: How and why is this normal precise regulation of cell reproduction and function lost in cancer cells, and why do cancer cells then remain mutant and malformed, functionally immature and imperfect, incapable of normal cell life?

Principles of cancer pathogenesis

As indicated before, in 1853 the German physiologist and physician Virchow was the first scientist to realize and demonstrate that cells arise only from preexisting cells by division and to apply this knowledge to disease. Since then, continuing application of the cell theory to problems in pathology has followed. From such studies in relation to cancer pathogenesis, key summary principles have emerged:

1. The cancer cell is a derivative of a normal cell that has lost control over cell reproduction and is thereby transformed from a normal cell to a cancer cell.
2. Based on cell nature and differentiation, it is possible to classify cancer tumor types according to (a) originating tissue, for example, those arising from connective tissue are called *sarcomas* (Gk. *sarkoma*, "fleshy growth"), those arising from epithelial tissue are called *carcinomas* (Gk. *karkinos*, "crab") and (b) extent or degree of cell tissue change and differentiation as to rate of growth, degree of autonomy, and invasiveness.
3. Since the incidence of cancer increases with age, a relationship exists between cancer genesis and the aging process in cells, tissues, and organ systems.

Causes of cancer cell development

It seems evident, therefore, that the basic underlying cause of cancers is a fundamental loss of control over normal cell reproduction. Several contributory causes of this loss of cell control have been brought forward by research and are interrelated.

Mutations. Mutations are due to loss of one or more regulatory genes of the cell nucleus. Such a mutant gene may come by inheritance, a factor in some cancers but not in all. However, even where it is a factor, inheritance alone may not be enough to cause disease; there must also be exposure to some environmental agent to bring it out. For example, skin cancer may be related to inherited skin color and thickness, not only to exposure rate to sunlight.

Chemical carcinogens. Chemical carcinogens (hydrocarbons) interfere with the structure or function of regulatory genes. Exposure to such agents may be by individual choice as in cigarette smoking or by general environmental exposure. Some of these environmental factors are related to industrial development and its effect on general environmental changes in water, air, and food supplies. Others are related more specifically to an individual's work setting in key occupations such as those surrounding asbestos, oils, tars, petroleum products, plastics, and dyestuffs. Still others are related to food such as pesticides, additives, and natural agents such as cycasin in cycad nuts. Possible causative actions of such substances may be mutation, effect on regulation of gene function, or activation of a dormant virus.

Radiation. Radiation that is sufficient to damage DNA causes chromosome breakage and incorrect rejoining. These radiations may be ionizing such as from X-ray, radioactive materials, or atomic exhausts and wastes or nonionizing as from sunlight.

Oncogenic viruses. Oncogenic viruses, which interfere with the function of regulatory genes, have been identified in animals but not clearly in humans. A virus is a mass of small chromosomes (DNA or RNA) with a relatively small number of genes, six or less, and a coat of protein or conjugated protein. Generally when they produce disease, they act as parasites, taking over the cell machinery to replicate themselves.

Epidemiologic factors

Answers to the enigma of cancer have also been sought in epidemiologic studies of distribution and occurrence in relation to such factors as race, diet, region, sex, age, heredity, and occupation, with variable and conflicting results.[4] For example, until the 1950s a racial genetic transmission was assumed in several cancers, but in two instances epidemiologic surveys have revealed extrinsic correlations instead: (1) frequent stomach cancer in Icelanders was found to be related to the hydrocarbons in the smoke they use to cure fish and meat and (2) frequent liver cancer among Bantu tribesmen in Africa seems more related to severe malnutrition, since the incidence was found to drop sharply when they started eating nutritionally adequate diets. Also, observations have been made that racial incidence of some cancers fades when migration occurs, and the group takes on the cancer characteristics of the new population.[5] For example, several studies have shown significant changes in the incidence of colon cancer among population groups migrating from rural areas where their diet was largely of primary foods with high-fiber content to more urban areas where their diet changed to one largely made up of low-fiber refined foods, indicating a significant relationship between colon cancer and a low-fiber diet.[6-8]

Stress factors

The idea that emotions may play a part in malignancy is not new. Galen, a second century Greek physician, wrote of such relationships, as have many different kinds of "healers" since that time. With our great technologic and scientific advance, however, the paradigm of Western medicine is held fast to the scientific method and its basic tenet that a thing must be measurable under controlled conditions to be said to exist. However, increasing observations are being made of relationships of cancer and less measurable stress factors. Clinicians and researchers such as Selye,[9] Simonton and Simonton,[10] LeShan,[11] and Thomas and Greenstreet[12] have reported that psychic trauma, especially the loss of a central relationship, does seem to bear a strong cancer correlation. The answer to such a possible relationship to cancer may lie in two physiologic areas: (1) damage to the thymus and the immune system and (2) hormonal effect mediated through the hypothalamus, pituitary, and adrenal cortex. Such effects may provide the neurologic currency that converts anxiety to malignancy. Such a state may also make a person more vulnerable to other factors present, influencing the integrity of the immune system, food behaviors, and the nutritional status.

The body's defense system

The human body maintains a remarkably efficient and profoundly complex defense system. This normal immune response has long been thought of as concerned only with providing protection against organisms such as bacteria and viruses that invade the body from without. However, more recent evidence indicates that this is too narrow a view. The same system comes into play to protect against "alien" malignant cells from tumors that develop within the body as well. It has been shown, for example, that children born congenitally lacking part of the immune surveillance mechanism, especially the thymus-dependent T cell or cellular immunity, develop cancer some 10,000 times more frequently than normal children.[13]

Components of the immune system

The immune system consists of primary surveillance or "police" mechanisms to detect and destroy malignant cells arising in our bodies daily. Two major populations of lymphoid cells are involved, which in turn mediate specific *cellular* and *humoral* immunity as well as supportive backup biologic systems. These two populations of lymphoid cells, or lymphocytes, a type of white blood cell, arise early in life from a common stem cell in fetal liver and bone marrow, differentiating and populating the peripheral lymphoid organs during the later stages of gestation. They are called T cells (from thymal lymphoid tissue) and B cells (from bursal lymphoid gut tissue).

T cells. The T cell population of lymphoid cells is differentiated in the thymus gland, which lies posterior to the sternum and anterior to the great vessels partly covering the trachea. The thymus is a small organ, weighing about 14 g (½ oz) at birth, reaching its largest size of 37 g (1⅓ oz) at puberty, and reducing in older age to a weight of 7 g (¼ oz). The T cells represent the majority of the circulating pool of small lymphocytes, a form of white cells, in blood and lymph and in certain areas of the lymph nodes and spleen. When these T cells contact an antigen (foreign intruder, "nonself," or alien substance such as abnormal cancer cells), they proliferate and initiate specific cellular immune responses: (1) they activate the phagocytes, special cells of the reticuloendothelial system that have intracellular killing and degrading mechanisms for destroying invaders, and (2) they initiate the inflammatory response through chemical mediators released by the antigen-stimulated T cells.

B cells. The B cell population is differentiated in the bursal lymphoid tissue of the gut. They are responsible for synthesis and secretion of antibodies. When the B cells contact an antigen, they proliferate, differentiate, and initiate specific humoral immune responses: (1) they start production of specific antibodies or immunoglobulins of the five major molecular classes (IgG, IgA, IgM, IgD, IgE) in blood and (2) they produce a specific form of IgA in secretions of the bowel and upper respiratory mucosa. A subsequent combination of antigen and antibody activates the complement system, which attracts phagocytes and initiates inflammation.

Integrity of the body's immune system requires nutritional support. Observations of severely malnourished populations have shown changes in the structure and function of the immune system with atrophy of liver, bowel wall, bone marrow, spleen, and lymphoid tissue. This condition has been called "nutritional thymectomy" by health workers in these depressed areas.[13] Thus the role of nutrition in maintaining normal immunity and in combating sustained attacks in malignancy is evident.

Tissue integrity through protein synthesis. An added component of the body's overall defense system is the integrity of body tissue and its capacity to maintain the healing process. These functions of tissue protein synthesis require optimum nutritional intake to support cell function and structure involving DNA, RNA, amino acids, and proteins. Tissue protein synthesis maintains the structure and function of all components of the immune system as well as the healing process and require nutritional support. Specific nutrients must be supplied—protein and key vitamins and minerals—as well as sufficient energy from nonprotein calorie sources.

CANCER THERAPY AND NUTRITION
Methods of cancer therapy

Current cancer therapy takes three major forms: surgery, radiation, and chemotherapy. A fourth form, immunotherapy, is under study. Nutritional support for any form of cancer therapy enhances its potential success.

Surgery

Early diagnosis of operable tumors has led to successful surgical treatment of a large number of cancer patients. As with any surgery, and especially with cancer patients, optimum nutritional status preoperatively and maximum nutritional support postoperatively are fundamental to the healing process. Nutrition has both general and specific relationships: (1) support of the general healing process and overall body metabolism and (2) specific modification of nutrient factors, texture, or feeding modality according to the surgical site and organ function involved. A detailed discussion of the relation of nutrition and surgery is presented in Chapter 30 and may be reviewed there.

Prevention of problems through early detection and surgical treatment has increased cure rates significantly. Surgical treatment may also be used with other forms of therapy, for removal of single metastases or for prevention and alleviation of symptoms.

Radiation

Following the discovery of radiation in the nineteenth century, scientists soon found that it could damage body tissue. However, continued study of its use and control revealed that normal tissue could largely withstand an amount of radiation that would damage or destroy cancer tissue. The subsequent role of radiation in cancer treatment has developed around controlled use with two types of tumors: (1) tumors that are responsive within a dose level tolerable to health of normal tissue and (2) tumors that can be targeted without damage to overlying vital organ tissue.

Forms of radiation therapy. Radiation used in cancer therapy is produced from three main sources: X-ray, gamma rays emitted by radioactive isotopes, and atomic particles derived from radioactive materials.

X-RAY. The oldest form of cancer treatment is X-ray. These are electromagnetic waves similar to heat and light rays. Their penetration varies with the speed at which the electrons strike the target.

RADIOACTIVE ISOTOPES. A number of elements, some occurring in nature as radioactive materials such as radium and uranium and others made radioactive by bombardment with

high-velocity atomic particles, have been used for radiation therapy. Radioactive isotopes of these materials produce gamma rays as the unstable elements are broken down. One of the most common radioisotopes in use at present is cobalt 60.

ATOMIC PARTICLES. Other high-speed atomic particles such as neutrons, protons, and electrons produced by accelerators are being used to treat some cancers resistant to conventional types of radiation. These more recent developments of physics have enabled physicians to treat a larger number of cancer patients more effectively.

Effects of radiotherapy in cancer management. Radiotherapy has become increasingly important in cancer management in the past few years. At present it is used either alone or in conjunction with other therapies, both for curative and for palliative care, for some 50% of all cancer patients at some time during the course of their disease. Depending on site and intensity of treatment, radiation effects will influence nutritional status and therapy a great deal. Radiation to the head, neck, or esophagus will affect the oral mucosa and the salivary secretions. It will also influence taste sensations and sensitivity to food temperature and texture. Abdominal radiation may produce denuded bowel mucosa, loss of villi and absorbing surface area, vascular changes from intimal thickening, thrombosis, ulcer formation, or inflammation. Obstruction, fistula formation, or strictures may further contribute to general malabsorption compounded by curtailment of food due to anorexia and nausea.

Chemotherapy

Of the three major forms of cancer therapy, chemotherapy is a relatively recent practice and has developed into a specialty area in medicine for the oncologist. Although it has been recognized as a valid therapy over the past 20 to 30 years, the most effective agents currently in use have been developed only within the past five years or so. However, the attempt to treat tumors by caustic agents is an ancient practice, going back to early Egyptian civilization; later in 400 BC the Greek physician Hippocrates was treating tumors with such materials. Over the centuries numbers of agents were tried, but no effective ones were found until more modern times.

During World War I and later during and after World War II two basic observations gave rise to the development of modern chemical compounds, natural and synthetic, which have provided an array of highly effective agents for cancer chemotherapy.

1. During World War I soldiers exposed to the poisonous mustard gas used in chemical warfare, before it was later outlawed for such purposes, were observed to suffer severe damage to bone marrow and lymphoid tissue with resulting deterioration of white blood cells. Subsequent animal studies with the nitrogen mustards led to development of these agents in controlled use to treat such lymphoid cancers as lymphomas and Hodgkin's disease, which cause an overproduction of certain white blood cells.

2. After World War II leukemic children were observed to worsen after folic acid was added to their diets. Based on the reasoning that a reduced amount of folic acid would diminish the disease, a strenuous effort was made to develop an agent that would inhibit folic acid synthesis or activation. The result in 1948 was the first breakthrough in the development of effective chemotherapeutic agents for cancer when methotrexate, a folic acid antagonist, was created for the treatment of leukemia.

Principles of action. Intensive research in the years since 1948 have resulted in the development of a bewildering array of some 80 effective antineoplastic drugs. Their therapeutic use is based on two general principles in relation to rate and mode of action.

1. *Rate of action.* The so-called cell or log (logarithm) kill hypothesis[14] of the action of chemotherapeutic agents on tumors indicates that a single dose can only be as much as 99.9% effective in killing the tumor cells. Thus if as large a tumor as is compatible with life consisting of about 10^{12} cancer cells (1 trillion) and weighing about 1 kg (2.2 lbs) can be treated with a drug tolerable at a toxicity level that is 99.9% effective, the tumor is reduced to a size of 10^9 cells (1 billion), a 1 cm tumor. Through successive doses causing this rate of "fractional killing" the tumor is reduced to less than 10^5 cells and brought within the capability of the body's own immune system to take over and make the final kill and cure. The smaller the tumor, either by early detection or by initial treatment by surgery or radiation, the greater the possible effectiveness of the chemotherapeutic agents. Also, two other principles of dosage rate for greater effectiveness are (a) aggressive use of maximum tolerable doses in repeated series and (b) use of several drugs together for synergistic effect.

2. *Mode of action.* The cell cycle relation to mode of action of the various chemotherapy agents accounts for their combined effectiveness in controlling tumor growth as well as for their side effects. According to the "central dogma" of cell biology (p. 690), nucleic acids provide the material essential for life of the cell: DNA produces RNA, which in turn guides amino acids into specific protein synthesis. Through the exquisitely interbalanced and regulated stages of the cell growth and reproduction cycle through cell division these materials carry out their orderly processes (p. 691). The cancer chemotherapeutic agents achieve their goal of arresting the tumors by disrupting these cell processes. Some agents interfere with the production of the necessary nitrogenous bases of nucleic acids for normal DNA synthesis. Others disrupt the normal DNA structure and RNA replication. Still others prevent normal mitosis or cell division, or cause hormonal imbalances, or make specific amino acids necessary for protein synthesis unavailable. These modes of

action help to provide a basis for grouping agents into classes as indicated below. Those cells that reproduce most rapidly, such as cancer cells, are most responsive to these agents.

Toxic effects of chemotherapy. Chemotherapeutic agents have the same effects on rapidly reproducing normal cells as they do on rapidly reproducing cancer cells. These normal cells where interference with normal function is most apparent include those of the bone marrow, the gastrointestinal tract, and the hair follicles, accounting for a number of the toxic side effects and problems in nutritional management:

Bone marrow effects: interference with production of red cells (anemia), white cells (infections), platelets (bleeding).

Gastrointestinal effects: nausea and vomiting, stomatitis, anorexia, ulcers, diarrhea.

Hair follicle effects: alopecia (baldness), general hair loss.

Classes of chemotherapy agents. According to their chemical nature or mode of action, the most commonly used cancer chemotherapy agents may be divided into six main classes.[15]

1. *Alkaloids (plant)* interfere with cell division, mitosis, by disorganizing the chromosome spindles. Examples: the *Vinca* alkaloids vincristine and vinblastine, derived from the periwinkle plant *(Vinca rosea).*

2. *Alkylating agents* interefere with cell division by binding to DNA, RNA, and certain cell enzymes, preventing their normal actions in control of cell reproduction. Examples: nitrogen mustard, cyclophosphamide.

3. *Antibiotics* interfere with DNA structure or function, disrupting cell organization and actions. Examples: doxorubicin (Adriamycin), bleomycin, mithramycin.

4. *Antimetabolites* interfere with DNA synthesis by blocking reactions that provide necessary precursors. Examples: methotrexate (limits the availability of folic

acid), 6-mercaptopurine, 5-fluorouracil, cytosine arabinoside.

5. *Enzymes* interfere with reactions that make necessary amino acids available for protein synthesis. Example: L-asparaginase.

6. *Hormones* interfere with cell metabolism by altering the hormonal balance of the body with probable effects on the cell membrane. Examples: prednisone, estrogens, androgens, progestins.

The cancer chemotherapy agents are usually used in one of two ways:

1. *Combined therapy:* employing combinations of drugs in a coordinated and sequential manner allowing time between series for normal tissue recovery. Example: the so-called ''MOPP'' therapy (combination of mechlorethamine [mustard], Oncovin [vincristine], procarbazine, and prednisone) used for Hodgkin's disease.

2. *Adjuvant therapy:* employing chemotherapy in conjunction with other treatment such as surgery or radiation to increase the cure rate.

Immunotherapy

A fourth form of cancer treatment, immunotherapy, holds promise of adding another mode of attack. Its therapeutic base is the specificity of the body's natural immune response system and the hope that this approach can target cancer cells and spare normal ones. Host resistance to cancer cells does play an important role in the incidence and clinical course of cancer. Thus this area of research to find control agents is a natural outgrowth of this relationship, and the effort to find a relevant vaccine for cancers has followed. Although a polyvalent vaccine may be impossible, given the multiple forms of cancers, at least there is a research effort to use immunotherapy to strengthen the body's own preexisting natural immune system, in conjunction with other treatment modalities.

An example of such an immunotherapeutic agent being used in clinical trials presently is bacillus Calmette-Guerin (BCG).[16] Researchers using the technique in controlled studies with a group of lung cancer patients report results showing a statistically significant decrease in rates of recurrence and increase in survival. These results and those of other studies seem to indicate that immunotherapy holds some promise of keeping the large bulk of the neoplastic cell population under control, especially when used in conjunction with other forms of treatment—surgery, radiation, chemotherapy. Another avenue of research has centered on the possible benefits of a form of passive immunotherapy achieved through a sort of "transplantation" of immunologically active extract, a process in which a "transfer factor" of lymphocyte extract could be given from a donor to a cancer patient. However, this approach does not seem too feasible, and interest in it has waned. Given the complexities of the immune system, work in this direction has as yet been inconclusive.

Nutritional therapy

Numerous problems present needs for nutritional therapy in the care of patients with cancer. Important contributions are beginning to accrue from research and clinical experience of nutritionists working on oncology teams or from practitioners working with nutritional support teams using alternative feeding modalities such as total parenteral nutrition (TPN).[17] It is clear at this point from many studies that optimum nutritional support bears a direct positive relationship to the outcome of the medical treatment for cancer.[18]

In general, nutritional therapy deals with two types of problems: (1) those related to the disease process itself and (2) those related to treatment of the disease process. The basic objectives, therefore, of nutritional therapy in cancer are (1) to meet the increased metabolic demands of the disease and prevent catabolism as much as possible and (2) to alleviate symptoms resulting from the disease and its treatment through adaptations of food and the feeding process.

Problems related to the disease process

Problems forming the basic challenge to nutritional therapy are caused by general systemic effects of the neoplastic disease process and by specific responses related to the type of cancer.

General systemic reactions to neoplastic disease. Nutritional therapy in cancer is not so much concerned with specific nutrient etiologies and subsequent manipulations of these factors as it is with the body's overall systemic reactions to the neoplastic disease process. Neoplastic disease is commonly associated with three basic systemic effects: anorexia, a hypermetabolic state, and a negative nitrogen balance, often accompanied by increasing weight loss. These effects may vary widely with individual patients according to the type and stage of the disease, from mild, scarcely discernible responses to the extreme forms of debilitating cachexia seen in advanced disease. The anorexia is frequently accompanied by depression or discomfort from normal eating, which contributes to a limited nutrient intake at the very time the disease process causes an increased basal metabolic rate and nutrient demand. Often this imbalance of decreased intake and increased demand creates a negative nitrogen balance, an indication of body tissue wasting. Sometimes a true tissue loss of protein is masked by outward nitrogen equilibrium as the growing tumor retains nitrogen at the expense of the host, further compounding the problem (see p. 59).

Specific responses related to type of cancer. Interrelated functional and metabolic problems arise from specific types of cancer and their effects on the body, further contributing to nutritional depletion. In addition to the primary nutritional deficiencies induced by the disease process, these secondary specific difficulties in ingestion and utilization of nutrients relate to specific tumors that cause obstructions or lesions in the gastrointestinal tract or adjacent tissue, curtailing the intake of adequate amounts of nutrients. These nutritional problems may stem from such conditions as malabsorption, intestinal bypass, fluid-electrolyte imbalances, hormonal imbalances, and anemia.

MALABSORPTION. If the malignancy involves the pancreas, the pancreatic duct, or the common bile duct, there may be subsequent curtailment of normal function and secretion of digestive enzymes and related materials such as bile salts. Biliary obstruction can also produce a deficiency of prothrombin, leading to blood clotting problems, and a deficiency of bile flow, leading to interference with normal digestion and absorption of fats and fat-soluble vitamins. A resulting vitamin D deficiency, for example, can lead to further decreased calcium absorption and metabolism with subsequent osteomalacia. Protein and electrolyte absorption, as well as that of other nutrients, may also be diminished by solid tumor infiltration of the small intestine or by dissemination to lymph nodes.

BYPASS PROBLEMS. Abdominal tumors may also cause either gastrocolic or jejunocolic fistulas. This results in a bypass of the small intestine and contributes to the subsequent malabsorption. Diarrhea and steatorrhea as well as protein loss follow. Extensive protein may also be lost in exudates associated with various gastrointestinal enteropathies.

FLUID-ELECTROLYTE IMBALANCES. Gastrointestinal lesions leading to general malabsorption can also contribute to fluid and electrolyte losses. Ensuing vomiting and diarrhea not only bring loss of water but also cause loss of water-soluble vitamins. Tumors of the liver or metastasis involving heart muscle may bring liver or cardiac failure and consequent ascites and cardiac edema. Any urinary tract obstruction or renal involvement brings additional water im-

balance. Any general obstruction of venous circulation or of the lymphatic drainage brings further edema. Villous adenoma and adenocarcinoma of the colon can contribute to severe electrolyte imbalance.

HORMONAL IMBALANCES. Medullary carcinoma of the thyroid with associated excess secretion of calcitonin and increased urinary sodium and phosphorus contributes to the problem of hyponatremia. Intestinal malignancy and hyperadrenocorticism contribute to the problem of hypokalemia. Osseous cancer and breast cancer with bone metastases contribute to hypercalcemia.

ANEMIA. The underlying problem of anemia may be compounded by a number of factors. These include anorexia with curtailment of dietary nutrients necessary for hemoglobin synthesis—iron, protein, folic acid, vitamin B_{12}, vitamin C— as well as malabsorption of these materials. Additional contributory factors may be increased hemolysis, bleeding of ulcerated lesions, or presence of gastrointestinal fistulas.

Problems related to the cancer treatment

Each of the treatments for cancer entails physiologic stress or toxic tissue effects or change in normal body function. Thus the benefit achieved is not without attendant problems caused by the surgery, the radiation, or the chemotherapy, which nutritional therapy seeks to alleviate.

Problems related to surgical treatment. Beyond the regular nutritional needs surrounding any surgical procedure and its healing process, gastrointestinal surgery poses special problems for normal ingestion, digestion, and absorption of food nutrients. Head and neck surgery, or resections in the oropharyngeal area, are frequently necessitated by cancer. Food intake is greatly affected in such cases, and a variety of food forms and textures as well as modes of feeding must be devised.[19] Often the mechanical problems of food ingestion make long-term tube feeding necessary.

Vagotomy contributes to gastric stasis, and gastrectomy causes numerous postgastrectomy "dumping" and "jejunal hyperosmolic" problems requiring frequent, small, low-carbohydrate feedings (p. 676). There may also be steatorrhea due to bacterial overgrowth in the afferent intestinal loop (blind loop syndrome), general malabsorption, fistulas, or stenosis from various intestinal resections for tumor excisions. Pancreatectomy contributes to loss of digestive enzymes, induced diabetes mellitus, and general weight loss. The preceding chapter on surgery (Chapter 30) provides numerous dietary guides for reference and may be reviewed for additional background.

Problems related to radiotherapy. Radiation to the oropharyngeal area often produces a loss of taste sensation with increasing anorexia, nausea, and consequent decreased incentive to eat. Other means of tempting appetite through food appearance and aroma must be developed. Abdominal radiation may cause intestinal damage with tissue edema and congestion, decreased peristalsis, or endarteritis in small blood vessels. In the intestinal wall there may be fibrosis, stenosis, necrosis, or ulceration. If this condition continues over time, it may lead to hemorrhage, obstruction, fistulas, diarrhea, or malabsorption, all contributing to nutritional problems. The liver is somewhat more resistant to damage from radiation in adults, but children are more vulnerable.

Problems related to chemotherapy. The major problem areas of nutritional support during chemotherapy relate to the gastrointestinal symptoms caused by the effect of the chemotherapeutic agents on the rapidly developing mucosal cells, the anemia associated with bone marrow effects, and the general systemic toxicity. The stomatitis, nausea, diarrhea, and malabsorption contribute to many food intolerances, although this response is not true in all cases. Frequently before the chemotherapy is started for each series of treatments an antiemetic drug such as prochlorperazine (Compazine) is used. This drug acts on the chemoreceptor trigger zone (CTZ) in the ventral surface of the fourth ventricle to inhibit stimulus of the "vomiting center" located in the lateral reticular formation of the brain. Prolonged vomiting seriously affects fluid and electrolyte balance, especially in the elderly, and needs to be controlled. Certain chemotherapeutic drugs also have special individual effects. For example, monoamine oxidase (MAO) inhibitors, such as tranylcypromine (Parnate) and phenelzine (Nardil), may be used for pretreatment relief of mental or emotional depression or for palliative therapy. These antidepressant drugs cause well-known pressor effects when used with tyramine-rich foods (p. 702); thus these foods should be avoided with these drugs.

Principles of nutritional therapy

Two important principles of nutritional therapy, vital in any sound nutrition practice but especially essential in care of patients with cancer, provide the basis for planning nutritional care of each individual patient: (1) personal nutrition assessment and (2) optimum nutritional therapy to maintain good nutritional status and thus support medical treatment.

Nutritional assessment. The primary goal in nutritional care for cancer patients is to maintain a high level of body nutrition and prevent states of malnutrition. Since it is more difficult to replenish a malnourished patient, initial assessment is imperative to determine individual status with vigorous follow-up care to maintain good nutrition. Therefore both initial assessment for baseline data and regular monitoring thereafter for close surveillance of progress are necessary. Assessment procedures should include all four areas of data: (1) anthropometric measures, (2) biochemical data, (3) clinical observations, and (4) dietary evaluations. An outline and description of all these procedures is given in Chapter 23 and can be reviewed there. By and large these basic assessment procedures being followed currently in

Tyramine-restricted diet*

General directions

1. Designed for patients on monoamine oxidase (MOA) inhibitors, drugs that have been reported to cause hypertensive crises when used with tyramine-rich foods. These include foods in which aging, protein breakdown, and putrefaction are used to increase flavor. Studies indicate that as little as 5 to 6 mg tyramine can produce a response, and 25 mg is a danger dose.
2. Food sources of other pressor amines such as histamine, dihydroxyphenylalanine, and hydroxytyramine are also avoided.
3. Avoid all foods listed. Limited amounts of foods with a lower tyramine amount such as yeast bread may be included in a specific diet.
4. Avoid over-the-counter drugs such as decongestants, cold remedies, and antihistamines.

Foods to avoid (Representative tyramine values in μg/g or ml)

Cheeses	
N.Y. state cheddar	1416
Gruyère	516
Stilton	466
Emmentaler	225
Brie	180
Camembert	86
Processed American	50
Wines	
Chianti	25.4
Sherry	3.6
Riesling	0.6
Sauterne	0.4
Beer, ale	
Varies with brand	
Highest	4.4
Average	2.3
Least	1.8

Additional foods to avoid

Other aged cheeses
  Blue
  Boursault
  Brick
  Cheddars (other)
  Gouda
  Mozzarella
  Parmesan
  Provolone
  Romano
  Roquefort
Yeast and products made with yeast
  Homemade bread
  Yeast extracts such as soup cubes, canned meats, and marmite
Italian broad beans with pod (fava beans)
Meat
  Aged game
  Liver
  Canned meats with yeast extracts
Fish (salted dried)
  Herring, cod, capelin
  Pickled herring
Other
  Cream, especially sour
  Yogurt
  Soy sauce, vanilla, chocolate
  Salad dressings

*See references for a tyramine-restricted diet.

many medical care centers have been developed in the main by Blackburn and co-workers,[20] based on the World Health Organization protocols adapted to hospital settings, protocols established through the early significant work of Jelliffe in international nutrition.[21]

Nutritional therapy and plan of care. Based on careful individual nutritional assessment, a plan for optimum nutritional therapy can be developed for each patient according to identified needs. Since *early* vigorous attention to maintaining an optimum state of nutrition has proved to be essential to rates of success with medical treatment, primary care by the clinical nutritionist on a regular basis is a necessary part of the oncology team practice. Thus this clinical nutrition specialist can assess needs, determine nutritional requirements, plan and manage nutritional care, monitor progress and responses to therapy, and make adjustments in care according to status and tolerances.

Nutritional needs

Each of the nutrient factors related to tissue protein synthesis and energy metabolism requires careful attention. The increased needs for energy, protein, vitamins and minerals, and fluid are based on demands made by the disease and its treatment. Individual needs vary, but guidelines include the following.

Energy. To prevent excessive weight loss and meet increased metabolic demands the total caloric value of the diet must be increased. Caloric density sufficient to counter catabolic or hypermetabolic states and support necessary anabolism is necessary. Of this total caloric value of the diet there must be sufficient carbohydrate and fat to spare protein for vital tissue synthesis. For an adult patient in good nutritional status, about 2,000 calories will provide for maintenance needs. A more malnourished patient will require 3,000 to 4,000 calories or more, depending on the degree of malnutrition and body trauma.

Protein. Additional protein is required to provide essential amino acids and nitrogen necessary for tissue regeneration, healing, and rehabilitation. A protein-calorie ratio sufficient to allow efficient utilization of protein and to prevent body protein wastage is important. An adult patient in good nutritional status will need about 80 to 100 g to meet maintenance needs and to ensure anabolism. A malnourished patient will need 100 to 200 g to replenish tissues and to ensure positive nitrogen balance.

Vitamins and minerals. The need for key vitamins and minerals controlling efficient protein and amino acid metabolism and energy metabolism is basic. For example, the B-complex vitamins in general serve as necessary coenzyme agents in energy and protein metabolism. Vitamins A and C are important tissue-structuring materials. Vitamin D exerts hormonelike activity to ensure proper calcium and phosphorus metabolism in bone and in blood serum. Vitamin E protects the integrity of cell wall materials and hence tissue integrity. Many minerals function in structural or enzyme roles in vital metabolic and tissue-building processes. Thus an optimum intake of vitamins and minerals, at least at recommended dietary allowances (RDA) levels and frequently augmented with supplements according to nutritional status, is indicated.

Fluid. Fluids are increased to counteract losses from gastrointestinal problems as well as any additional loss due to infections and fever. Also, sufficient fluid intake is necessary to help the kidneys rid the body of the breakdown products from destroyed cancer cells as well as from the drugs themselves. Increased fluid also helps to protect the urinary tract from irritation and inflammation. For example, the use of some chemotherapeutic agents, such as cyclophosphamide (Cytoxan), requires 2 to 3 L of forced fluids daily to prevent hemorrhagic cystitis.

Nutritional management

The classic dictum of nutritional management is fundamental here: *"If the gut works, use it!''* Oral and enteral feeding modalities pose fewer problems than do alternative means, by and large. However, faced with the need for increased nutrition in cancer therapy and attendant problems in food tolerances, the nutritionist does have a wide spectrum of feeding methods and materials from which to select the most appropriate nutritional therapy for each patient, always basing clinical judgments on individual needs and circumstances. This spectrum of feeding modalities includes an oral diet amplified with nutrient supplements for increased protein, calories, vitamins, and minerals; enteral tube feeding with several routes of entry; and parenteral nutrition through central and peripheral veins.

Oral diet and nutrient supplementation

If at all possible, of course, use of the normal ingestion of food with nutrient supplements as needed is most desirable. This should be a high-protein and high-calorie diet with optimum total nutrition as outlined above. Based on individual nutrition assessment, a personal food plan should be developed with the patient, incorporating desired food forms and family food patterns. Often the diet of the hospitalized patient can be supplemented with foods from home as the clinical nutritionist plans with the family. Food tolerances will vary with individual patients according to current treatment and nature of disease. A number of adjustments in food texture, temperature, amount, timing, taste, appearance, and form can be made to help alleviate symptoms stemming from common problems in successive parts of the gastrointestinal tract.

Food ingestion problems. Difficulties in eating may be due to loss of appetite, problems in the mouth, or swallowing problems.

1. *Loss of appetite* is frequently a major problem and curtails food intake when it is needed most. It is a common side effect of the cancer disease process and its treatment, progressively enhanced by the consequent anxiety, depression, and stress of the illness. Such a vicious cycle, if not countered by much effort, can lead to more malnutrition with ever increasing anorexia. A program of eating, not dependent on appetite for stimulus, must be planned with the patient and family. It is helpful sometimes to develop protein and calorie goals with discussions of the role of nutrients and key foods in combating the disease and providing support for therapy, thus building a mental attitude toward the diet as an integral part of the treatment and a means of accepting self-responsibility for this aspect of therapy as much as possible. Often this positive attitude and view of the vital role patients can play in their own treatment is a means of gaining some sense of control of their own lives, a sense frequently lost in the bewildering world of cancer and its therapy. Many of the food suggestions provided for a variety of specific symptoms can help to improve appetite. The overall goal is to provide food with as much nutrient density as possible so that "every bite will count," with varied texture as tolerated, and with appeal to sensory perceptions of color, aroma, and taste to enhance desire to eat and to provide food in many minimeals by use of a wide variety of items. Some exercise before meals and surroundings that reduce stress may also help.

2. *Mouth problems* may include sore mouth, stomatitis, taste blindness, or dental problems. Sore mouth often results from chemotherapy or from radiation treatments to the head and neck area and would be increased from any state of malnutrition or from infections such as candidiasis ("thrush") with numerous ulcerations of the oral and throat mucosa. Frequent small meals and snacks, soft in texture, bland in nature, and cool to cold in temperature are often better tolerated. Medications such as anesthetic liquids (lidocaine) used as sprays or mouth gels or washes help to relieve pain so that the patient may eat. Other simple water solutions with baking soda or salt help to control irritation. Chemotherapy or head and neck radiation may

also cause alterations in the tongue's taste buds, causing taste distortion and inability to distinguish the basic tastes of salt, sweet, sour, or bitter and consequent food aversions. Since the aversion is often toward basic protein foods, a high-protein liquid supplement may be needed. Preparation of foods appealing in odor and appearance and in small amounts should be continued. Since zinc deficiency is related to diminished taste, sometimes a zinc supplement may be indicated. Dental problems may also contribute to mouth difficulties. If brushing the teeth is painful, they may be cleaned with cotton swabs dipped in a 3% hydrogen peroxide solution diluted with warm water. Glycerin flavored with a few drops of lemon juice may be helpful as a mouth freshener, and sponge-tipped sticks impregnated with dentifrice are available. Attention to any dental work needed and avoidance of concentrated sweets will help to prevent tooth decay. Salivary secretions are also affected by cancer therapy, so foods with a high liquid content should be used, and solid foods may be swallowed more easily with use of sauces, gravies, broths, yogurt, or salad dressings. The food processor or blender can render foods to semisolid or liquid forms easier to swallow. If the swallowing problem is especially severe because of tumor growth or therapy, a special swallowing training program including progressive food textures, exercises, and positions, such as that outlined by Rosenbaum's team, is very useful. A number of excellent suggestions and resources are given in their guide, *Nutrition for the Cancer Patient*.[22]

3. *Upper gastrointestinal problems* include nausea and vomiting, general indigestion, bloating, or specific surgery responses such as the postgastrectomy dumping syndrome (see p. 676). Nausea is often enhanced by foods that are hot, sweet, fatty, or spicy, so these can be avoided according to individual toleration. Frequent small feeding of cold foods may be more appealing, soft to liquid in texture, eaten slowly with rest between. Dry foods such as crackers

and dry toast upon arising may be helpful. The physician may prescribe an antinausea drug such as Compazine to help with food toleration. Also, practitioners are frequently asked questions about the use of marijuana to reduce nausea as it has been found by many persons to be effective. It is imperative, however, because of the legal implications, to secure sound background information before discussing it. Reliable information and recipes for its use are available.[23]

4. *Lower gastrointestinal problems* include general diarrhea, constipation, flatulence, and specific lactose intolerance or surgery responses such as with intestinal resections and various ostomies. A helpful resource book for patients with colostomies, ileostomies, and urostomies has been provided by Mullen.[24] Lactose intolerance due to deficiency of the enzyme lactase (see p. 450) may necessitate avoidance of milk and milk products. The effect of chemotherapy or radiation treatment on the mucosal cells secreting lactose may also cause the condition. In such cases a nutrient supplement with a nonmilk protein base may be used. To control diarrhea a diet of liquid and low-residue food with low-residue nutrient supplements is useful. As the condition improves, foods with more bulk may gradually be added in small frequent meals. Constipation is helped by high-fiber foods, increased fluids, and naturally laxative foods such as prunes or prune juice.

Nutrient supplements. A number of commercial nutrient supplement products are available and should be studied carefully as to nutrient ratios to make wise selections among them according to specific need. They come in a variety of forms and flavors and may be used in different ways. They may be high-protein supplements used as snacks between meals of regular food to add extra protein and calories. They may be high-calorie supplements added to foods prepared. They may be so-called elemental diets, nutritionally complete, for use when only clear liquids can be used. A comparative review of these products has been provided by Shils, Bloch, and Chernoff and will be a helpful resource for the practitioner.[25] A food processor or blender can produce creative solid and liquid food combinations from regular foods for interval liquid nutrient supplementation.

Enteral tube feeding

When a patient is unable to eat but the gastrointestinal tract can be used, tube feedings may provide the needed nutritional support. The route of entry may vary from the traditional nasogastric method to alternate surgical placements of esophagostomy, gastrostomy, or jejunostomy tubes. In practical usage many patients have negative attitudes toward nasogastric tubes. However, there is better acceptance with the newer small-caliber feeding tubes, and some highly motivated patients will even learn to pass the tube themselves. Patients can be fed in some instances by slow drip, pump monitored, during the night and freed from the tube during the day.

Osmolality is an important consideration in selecting a tube feeding formula, as well as its specific composition of nutrients. The osmolality of blood is about 300 mosmol/kg solvent (water), and an ideal tube feeding formula should have a similar osmolality so as not to draw an undue amount of fluid into the intestine by osmotic pressure created. However, most commercial products are hyperosmolar having an osmolality greater than that of blood serum. These products can range from about 500 mosmol/kg water to over 1,000 mosmol/kg water in some elemental formulas. Careful attention, therefore, must be given to formula selection (that it meet the specifically defined nutritional problem), to proper dilution, and to rate of administration. Delivery systems that ensure a controlled, slow drip are helpful. Jejunostomy feedings given by gavage must be administered very slowly to prevent dumping symptoms.

Types of formulas. Formulas may be of two basic types: (1) formulas prepared from food and nutrient items and calculated according to individual need and mixed in a blender or food processor and (2) commercial formulas with "fixed" composition, ready to use liquids or powders for mixing with water or milk.

1. *Home or hospital prepared formula.* These formulas have the advantage of being less costly and more flexible in nutritional composition according to individual patient therapeutic needs and tolerances. They are made up of food items such as cooked meat, vegetables, starch, a fat source such as vegetable oil, additional carbohydrate such as syrup, fruit juice, additional protein such as nonfat milk powder and egg (cooked), water or vegetable juice for dilution, salt as needed, and added liquid vitamins and minerals. Such formulas have the added advantage for patients when used over long periods of time, not only of cost control but also of emotional support from knowledge that they are receiving regular food. An example of such a blended food formula is given on p. 672. Of course careful attention must be given to sanitary mixing procedures, refrigeration, and disposal of left over formula.

2. *Commercial formula products.* In recent years the market has been filled with a complex array of commercial formula products that require careful study if wise use of them is to be made. They are "fixed" formulas at present, leaving the user no control over formulation. If manufacturers prepared these formulas in modules or parts, enabling the consumer to add or delete certain critical items such as fat or type of carbohydrate or sodium-potassium salts, this disadvantage would be overcome. Also, they are more costly items, a large consideration in long-term use. However, they do have the advantages of convenience, being ready to use, and of providing specific nutrient modifications for a variety of therapeutic requirements, with standardization of ingredients and composition. They are simple to order, store,

and administer to patients. However, if they are to be used with patients having metabolic problems making them incapable of tolerating specific nutrients in the formulation, especially in the amounts frequently included to achieve increased nutrient intakes, the clinical nutritionist must modify the formula by adding desired ingredients while diluting to lower others or calculate an entirely different formula from specific nutrients. Individual formula ingredients are available and can be combined according to indicated individual prescription by trained clinical nutritionists.

The booklet by Shils, Bloch, and Chernoff[25] presents a comprehensive, up-to-date comparative listing of commercial formula products available according to the following categories:

1. Complete defined-formula diet preparations with intact protein containing milk (lactose), some with moderate residue and others with low residue.
2. Complete diet formulas of intact protein, protein isolates, low lactose, and low residue.
3. Complete diet formulas of hydrolyzed protein, amino acids, low lactose, and low residue.
4. Defined formula diets for special metabolic needs, such as in renal disease, hepatic disease, and aminoaciduria in children.
5. Supplementary feedings for special nutritional needs such as protein, calories, specific carbohydrates and fats, and electrolytes.

To clarify differences in these products and to use them more wisely, such a guide as this can be used for study. A wide variety can be obtained for testing, by taste if for oral use, and for comparison by nutritional objective and cost. Then a relatively short list of the types of major selections can be drawn up to meet specific requirements and used with a variety of patients, and careful observation of reactions can be made. Protocols based on these selected formula products can be established to meet specific patient situations and nutritional needs to simplify and coordinate patient management.

Parenteral feeding

The term "parenteral" comes from two Greek roots, the prefix *para* meaning "beside" and *enteron* meaning "intestine." Applied to nutritional therapy, it is used to mean any feeding method other than by the intestine. In current usage it refers to the feeding modality using central and peripheral veins to achieve necessary nutritional support when the gastrointestinal tract cannot be used. Since development of the basic surgical technique involved over the past decade, it has provided a major advance in the care of critical patients and will be discussed in the following section.

TOTAL PARENTERAL NUTRITION— CARE OF THE MALNOURISHED AND HYPERMETABOLIC PATIENT

When illness from cancer or other trauma creates malnutrition (present or potential) and hypermetabolic nutritional demands and the patient cannot eat or be fed by tube, nutritional status can be improved and maintained over extended periods of time solely through intravenous means of feeding. Hypertonic solutions of essential nutrients can be fed into large central veins, avoiding vascular inflammation and thrombosis and delivering large amounts of life-sustaining nourishment that would otherwise not be available. This complete sustaining of increased nutritional requirements through intravenous feeding has been termed *total parenteral nutrition* (TPN), or *intravenous hyperalimentation* (IVH), by its developers.

The idea of feeding by vein is not new. Intravenous glucose in isotonic 5% solutions, although not sustaining overall nutritional needs but supplying fluid and electrolyte sources, has been used since the late 1890s. Later in 1935 an attempt was made to obtain needed calories by the intravenous feeding of fat emulsions. Again the effort was made with the use of protein hydrolysates in 1939, but results with the products available at that time were unsatisfactory. Another effort was made with fat emulsions in the 1950s and early 1960s using a 15% cottonseed oil emulsion (Lipomul), but adverse effects were encountered with long-term use.

The current era of parenteral nutrition found its direction in the late 1960s, largely through the work of Dudrick and others who in 1968 were able to develop and demonstrate a technique for introducing highly concentrated nutrient solutions into larger blood vessels capable of handling its osmotic density by rapidly diluting it into central circulation.[26,26a] This new surgical technique involved the feeding of a solution of protein hydrolysate and concentrated glucose with added vitamins and minerals through an indwelling catheter into the superior vena cava by way of a large central vein, usually the subclavian vein. In the following decade development of the technique and of nutrient solutions to meet the increased nutritional requirements of catabolic illness has led to widespread use of the procedure. It has helped to prevent complications of malnutrition, sepsis, and general tissue breakdown in patients denied the normal use of gastrointestinal feeding pathways by critical illness or injury or requiring excess calories and protein because of hypermetabolic conditions. Many studies in the past few years have substantiated the effectiveness of carefully administered total parenteral nutrition to selected patients and of supplementary parenteral nutrition (SPN) used to support other feeding means such as oral intake or tube feeding.[27] The clinical nutritionist and the physician now have available to them a wide spectrum of feeding modalities from which to plan individual nutritional therapy according to the clinical problem presented by each patient situation.

General principles of nutritional therapy with TPN include the following:

1. *Indications for use:* general rules governing consideration of TPN and patient candidates.
2. *Nutrition assessment:* initial assessment to identify and select patients for its use and to serve as a basis for calculation of the formula to meet nutritional requirements.
3. *Formula solution preparation:* products and materials available to form solutions and method of mixing.
4. *Route of feeding:* general technique, central vs. peripheral vein, and rigid protocols to avoid complications.
5. *Duration of use:* nutritional support during hospital medical care, longer term use with home TPN, concept of the "artificial gut."

Indications for use of TPN

Intravenous hyperalimentation, or TPN, provides a highly effective alternative means of sustaining necessary nutritional support for severely debilitated or injured patients for whom the normal oral means of eating is limited or impossible.

General considerations

Three basic considerations govern decisions concerning the use of TPN. Since there are risks involved in this feeding procedure, assessment of each of these factors is imperative.

Availability of gastrointestinal tract. If the gut has been rendered totally unavailable for use by major abdominal injury, an alternative means of sustaining nutrition is an obvious emergent necessity. In other cases the gut may be unavailable because of obstruction, fistulas, or malignant disease. In still other cases the patient may be unable to eat because of coma, severe anorexia, or mental disturbance.

Degree of malnutrition. If a patient is in a state of malnutrition, any medical treatment attempted will have less chance of success. Studies in the past few years have indicated that there is far more general malnutrition among hospitalized patients than was assumed before. In addition, it is now clear that disease states impose an even greater threat to positive nutritional status. Thus the assessment of nutritional status becomes an important part of overall care, especially for hospitalized patients. For the more severely malnourished patient, more serious consideration of TPN is indicated.

Degree of hypermetabolism or catabolism. If a patient is suffering from major trauma or severe sepsis or from malignant disease, the rate of catabolism may take a devastating toll on the body resources. This toll may be measured by nitrogen balance studies, with a loss ranging up to 15 g of nitrogen over a 24-hour period. Catabolic periods seem inevitable following surgery, the more extensive surgery bringing the greatest losses of body resources, and malignant disease or critical illness places additional demands on the body's metabolic functions. The extent of these increased demands can be seen in the increased nutritional requirements, especially in energy demand, listed below.

Basic rules for use of TPN

Using the three basic considerations above, most clinicians have formed general rules to guide the choice of TPN as the preferred means of therapy. Combinations of these factors indicating need for TPN are given in Table 31-1. In essence, two basic rules for use of TPN may be stated as follows.

The "rule of 5." If a patient has had no food for five days and is likely not to be able to eat for at least another week, TPN must be considered *then* rather than waiting until malnutrition has ensued. It is an easier task to maintain positive nutrition than to replenish body stores from malnutrition losses. Starvation effects on the body are well documented, even during relatively brief periods.[28] The 50 to 75 g of glucose stored in the liver as hepatic glycogen is a small but crucial energy source able to maintain the body's normal blood sugar levels for only a few hours. Further, the 200 g of glucose stored as muscle glycogen could satisfy basal calorie demands for only about 12 hours. During the early days of starvation, amino acids of the body's tissue proteins are deaminated to provide blood glucose (gluconeogenesis) and substrate for needed metabolic functions, with a urinary nitrogen loss of 10 to 15 g daily. As starvation is prolonged, fatty acids are mobilized from the body's adipose tissues to provide keto acids as the principal fuel for heart, brain, and other vital organ function.

Weight loss rule. Any patient who has lost 7% of his usual body weight over two months or who is deprived of oral nutrition for 5 to 7 days or longer is a candidate for TPN.

Table 31-1. Patient situations imposing need for TPN

Patient with limited or impossible use of gut	Metabolic rate, degree of catabolism (nitrogen loss per 24 hr)	Degree of malnutrition*
Situation 1	Normal (0-8 g)	Severe
Situation 2	Moderate (8-15 g)	Moderate
Situation 3	Severe (15 g)	Normal

*In terms of percent of normal standards by nutritional assessment.

Patient candidates for TPN

Based on the three general considerations discussed, a number of types of patient situations present needs for vigorous nutritional therapy through TPN.

1. Preoperative preparation of severely malnourished patients
   a. Congenital anomalies creating gastrointestinal disorders
   b. Stricture or cancer of esophagus, swallowing difficulties
   c. Cancer of the stomach
   d. Severe peptic ulcer disease, gastric obstruction
2. Postoperative surgical complications
   a. Prolonged ileus, obstruction
   b. Stomal dysfunction
   c. Short bowel syndrome
   d. Fistulas—enterocutaneous, biliary, pancreatic
   e. Peritoneal sepsis
3. Inflammatory bowel disease
   a. Intractable gastroenteritis
   b. Regional enteritis
   c. Acute Crohn's disease
   d. Ulcerative colitis
   e. Extensive diverticulitis
   f. Radiation enteritis
4. Inadequate oral intake or malabsorption
   a. Malignant neoplasms, chemotherapy, or radiation
   b. Acute and chronic relapsing pancreatitis
   c. Hypermetabolic states, major trauma, burns
   d. Coma, hepatic insufficiency and encephalopathy
   e. Chronic malnutrition, anorexia nervosa

Nutrition assessment

Initial individual nutrition assessment is necessary to identify those patients requiring special nutritional therapy and their type and degree of malnutrition. It is also needed to provide the basis for calculating nutritional requirements and selecting the specific nutrient formula to meet these requirements. Once therapy is begun, continued careful monitoring of nutritional and metabolic parameters is essential to maintaining optimum therapy and avoiding metabolic complications.

In addition to clinical judgment concerning the medical problem, a key to selection of appropriate patients for TPN is the careful diagnosis of varying degrees of protein-calorie malnutrition.

Guidelines for nutrition assessment

Necessary nutrition assessment data for selection of patients for TPN according to their degree of protein-calorie malnutrition are collected by standard assessment methods: anthropometric measures, biochemical laboratory data, clinical observations, and dietary evaluations. These methods are described in detail in Chapter 23 (see p. 511) and can be reviewed there for specific procedural instructions. According to individual patient needs and clinical situations, guidelines for TPN nutritional assessment include the following procedures.

1. *Classify degree of weight loss.* Using measures of current body weight and height, interpret current weight in terms of ideal body weight for height, usual body weight, and amount of recent weight change:

$$\text{Percent ideal body weight} = \frac{\text{Actual weight}}{\text{Ideal weight}} \times 100$$

$$\text{Percent usual body weight} = \frac{\text{Actual weight}}{\text{Usual weight}} \times 100$$

$$\text{Percent weight change} =$$
$$\frac{\text{Usual weight} - \text{actual weight}}{\text{Usual weight}} \times 100$$

Compare patient's amount of recent weight change with the values indicating malnutrition given in Table 31-2.

2. *Estimate body fat stores and skeletal muscle mass.* Using caliper measures of triceps skinfold (TSF) and standard reference tables for TSF data, estimate the patient's body fat stores.

Using the midarm circumference measure (MAC), calculate the midarm muscle circumference (MAMC) and compare with the standard reference tables for MAMC data. This gives an estimate of the patient's muscle mass, interpreted as percentage of standard:

$$\text{MAMC (cm)} = \text{MAC (cm)} - (0.314 \times \text{TSF [mm]})$$

3. *Estimate lean body mass.* Use the creatinine-height index (CHI) as an estimate of overall lean body mass. Compute the patient's CHI by using the patient's daily urinary creatinine excretion value, determined by laboratory analysis of a 24-hour urine collection, and comparison of this value with the ideal creatinine excretion value for the patient's height (cm) from standard tables (see p. 515). This gives an effective index of the patient's overall muscle mass and total lean body mass.

4. *Calculate degree of catabolism.* A measure of degree of catabolism may be obtained by calculation of the daily nitrogen balance. Using an accurate record of the patient's protein intake for the day (food or formula) and the laboratory analysis of the urinary urea nitrogen in a careful 24-hour collection of urinary output, calculate the nitrogen balance for that day:

$$\text{N balance} = \text{N intake} \left(\frac{\text{Protein intake}}{6.25} \right) - \\ \text{N loss (urinary urea N} + 4)$$

5. *Estimate immune function.* Use total lymphocyte count or percentage of lymphocytes in total white blood cell count to determine general function of the patient's immune system. Compare with values in Table 31-3.

$$\text{Total lymphocyte count} = \frac{\% \text{ lymphocytes} \times \text{WBC}}{100}$$

Skin testing for sensitivity to common recall antigens (PPD, streptokinase (SK)/streptodornase (SD), etc.) can provide additional immune function data.

6. *Measure plasma protein compartment.* Using laboratory analysis of total iron-binding capacity (TIBC), calculate the value for transferrin, the body's iron transport protein compound:

$$\text{Transferrin (mg/dl)} = (\text{TIBC } [\mu\text{g/dl}] \times 0.8) - 43$$

Table 31-2. Indications of severe protein-calorie malnutrition according to percentage of recent weight loss

% body weight loss	Time period
2%	1 week
5%	1 month
7.5%	3 months
10%	6 months

Table 31-3. Determination of protein-calorie malnutrition by plasma values

Laboratory data	Normal values	Degree of malnutrition	
		Moderate	Severe
Serum albumin (g/dl)	3.5	2.1-3.0	<2.1
Serum transferrin (mg/dl)	180-260	100-150	<100
Total lymphocyte count			
Per mm³	1,500-4,000	800-1,200	<800
% WBC	20%-53%		

The serum albumin will provide additional data concerning the body's visceral protein mass. However, a decreased transferrin value is a more sensitive manifestation of recent malnutrition than serum albumin because transferrin has a shorter half-life and is depleted faster. Compare these serum protein values obtained for the patient with the values in Table 31-3.

Baseline and monitoring assessment for TPN

At the initiation of TPN it is important to gather a broad assessment of nutritional and metabolic data as a baseline by which to measure progress. Then at designated time periods during therapy, repetition of certain tests is imperative to monitor the patient's course and to avoid metabolic complications. Specific protocols vary in different medical centers. However, a general guide for such monitoring data is summarized in the boxed material on p. 713.

Careful charting of all the initial baseline nutrition assessment data should be entered in the patient's record when instituting TPN. Then throughout therapy all monitoring data should be recorded along with TPN solution orders.

Nutrition requirements: TPN prescription

Calculation of basic nutritional requirements plus additional needs due to patient's degree of catabolism and malnutrition and any activity form the basis of the individual patient's TPN prescription and plan of care. This is the same principle of all nutritional therapy in any modality. Fundamental nutritional needs center on requirements for energy, protein, electrolytes, vitamins, and minerals.

Energy requirements. The calorie needs of the critically ill patient are great, even as high as 5,000 to 6,000 calories per day in the case of major trauma and sepsis, as in burns. These calorie requirements are necessary to meet basal energy expenditures (BEE) plus additional needs to cover the energy cost of catabolism, fever, malnutrition, and any physical activity.

1. *Basal energy expenditure (BEE).* The adult patient's energy needs for basal tissue metabolism may be calculated by the following formulas:

Men: $BEE = 66 + (13.7 \times \text{Weight in kg}) + (5 \times \text{Height in cm}) - (6.8 \times \text{Age})$

Women: $BEE = 655 + (9.6 \times \text{Weight in kg}) + (1.7 \times \text{Height in cm}) - (4.7 \times \text{Age})$

2. *Added energy requirements.* In addition to basal energy needs, the patient's total caloric requirements will reflect the large energy drain of the illness. This physiologic stress of the illness will demand calories to combat the hypermetabolism and its resulting catabolic state and weight loss. If any large degree of malnutrition exists, even more calorie input is necessary. Also, there will be a need to cover any muscular or physical activity, which will vary considerably depending on the patient's condition, respiratory status, presence of delirium tremens, and extent of mobility. The presence of fever will call for still more calories.

Adequate energy input is essential to meet all these requirements if the patient's treatment is to be supported. About 1,700 to 1,800 calories per day on the average are required to support basal tissue metabolism needs for biochemical functions. If the calorie intake is less than 1,000, gradual starvation and general malnutrition will ensue. If the patient is febrile, an additional 950 to 1,000 calories are required for every degree Celsius of fever (500 to 600 calories for every degree Fahrenheit of fever). In general, about 3,000 calories are required daily for most of the patients on TPN. In the catabolic stress of severe trauma the need may well rise to 5,000 to 7,000 calories. The great difference is seen in comparing health and illness needs. In health about 35 calories per kilogram are required for maintenance, whereas in catabolic illness it is 50 to 60 calories per kilogram.

Protein requirements. Several factors are

Monitoring protocol for TPN

Baseline tests

CBC: Hgb		Nitrogen balance	SGOT	
	Hct	Fe and TIBC	Alkaline phosphatase	
	RBC indexes	FBS	Serum osmolality	
	WBC differential count	BUN	Cholesterol	
	Platelets	Creatinine	Triglycerides	
Na^+	Ca^{++}	Uric acid	Urinalysis	
K^+	PO_4	PT	Chest X-ray	
Cl^-	Mg^{++}	PTT	ECG	
Co_2		Albumin	Body weight (kg)	
Skin tests (PPD, mumps, cocci)		Total protein	Height (cm)	
		Bilirubin		

Stabilization tests (daily first 5-7 days)

Fractional urines (sugar and acetone) every six hours; simultaneous blood sugars first and second days
Body weight
Intake and output record
Nitrogen balance
Serum electrolytes
Blood glucose

Follow-up routine

Daily	Fractional urines (sugar and acetone)
	Body weight
	Intake and output
Three times a week	Electrolytes (Na^+, K^+, Cl^-, CO_2)
Once a week	CBC: platelets PT Mg^{++}
	RBC indexes Ca^{++}
	Creatinine PO_4
	BUN
Once a month	Repeat baseline tests
	Add serum B_{12}, folate, Zn^{++}

involved in determinations of protein requirements to meet the stress of catabolic illness.

1. *Nitrogen balance*. The function of protein in health is to sustain tissue growth and maintenance. In adults this ideal state in normal persons is reflected in nitrogen equilibrium. In illness, however, catabolism is reflected by a state of negative nitrogen balance—more nitrogen loss than intake—indicating wasting of tissue protein. The goal of nutritional therapy in illness, therefore, is to maintain a state of positive nitrogen balance to counter the catabolic deterioration.

2. *Essential amino acids*. The quality of the protein intake in terms of equivalent essential amino acids is fundamental to tissue synthesis. Not only must all the essential amino acids be present, but they must also be present in the opti-

mum ratio for best utilization of individual amino acids. One amino acid, methionine, can even be toxic in large amounts.

3. *Ratio of nitrogen to nonprotein calories.* To protect the nitrogen sources, amino acids, and make them available for tissue synthesis, sufficient nonprotein energy sources must be present to meet the large calorie demand. Carbohydrate is necessary to promote incorporation of plasma amino acids in muscle tissue protein. For optimum utilization the normal adult diet sustains a ratio of 150 nonprotein calories per 1 g nitrogen. To meet the metabolic stress of critical illness with minimum activity this ratio should be 150 to 200 calories per 1 g nitrogen.

In terms of protein, the requirements in illness reflect these increased needs:

Health: Weight (kg) $\times$ 0.8-1.0 g protein
Catabolic states: Weight (kg) $\times$ 1.2-1.5$^+$ g protein

Electrolyte requirements. Specific electrolyte profiles are required in intracellular and extracellular fluid for all tissues (see Chapter 9). In illness these balances must be maintained in the face of metabolic imbalances. For example, active tissue synthesis requires phosphate and potassium and is also influenced by available sodium and chloride ions. Monitoring of individual electrolyte status will supply the data needed to determine daily electrolyte requirements. In general, the basic electrolyte needs for a 3,000 calorie intake (3 L solution) would be approximately the following meq: 120 to 150 Na, 120 K, 150 Cl, 24 to 36 Mg, 6 to 15 Ca, 60 to 75 HPO_4. This will vary according to metabolic needs of the individual patient.

Vitamin and mineral requirements. Needs for vitamins and minerals are based on normal requirements (see Chapters 6 to 8 and current RDAs in Appendix M) with added needs to cover increased metabolism and depletion states according to individual patient condition. Attention to necessary trace minerals is especially important. The TPN solutions will reflect these additions.

Preparation of TPN solutions

With the development of the TPN technique, products for use in the TPN nutrient solutions have also been developing. A number are now available for use by the TPN team in formulating nutritional needs for each patient, based on the nutritional requirements listed above for protein, calories, electrolytes, vitamins, and minerals.

Protein-nitrogen source. (6.25 g protein, amino acids, = 1 g N). Originally protein hydrolysates were used in TPN solutions as the source of nitrogen for tissue synthesis. These products included casein derivatives such as those found in the commercial formulas Amigen, CPH, Hyprotigen, or the fibrin products such as Aminosol. However, in clinical use over time these hydrolysate products have proved to have problems and are not now recommended or available and are being withdrawn from production. Currently the nitrogen source of choice is crystalline amino acids, essential and nonessential. A number of commercial products are available in a variety of compositions and dilutions, for example, Travasol, Freamine, Aminosyn, and Nephramine. It is an important task of the pharmacist on the TPN team to know the composition of these solutions to formulate accurate solutions for each patient according to individual need. A usual amino acid need is supplied by a 4.25% dilution, achieved by use of 1 L of a standard 8.5% amino acid solution mixed with 1L of dextrose solution.

Nonprotein energy source—calories. Nonprotein calories to protect protein for tissue synthesis demands are supplied by glucose and fat solutions.

GLUCOSE (DEXTROSE). Dextrose solutions range from the 5% solution used traditionally in peripheral intravenous support of fluid and electrolytes postsurgically to the hypertonic 70% solutions available for TPN formulations. When 1 L of dextrose is mixed with 1 L of amino acid solution for TPN use, the dextrose concentration is halved per liter of formula resulting. For example, the usual solution used for TPN is 50% dextrose, which when mixed with amino acid solution renders a 25% dextrose solution in the formula. Dextrose solutions given by IV route do not deliver the classic 4 calories per gram; they are 91% calorigenic, providing 3.75 calories per gram. Thus a final solution of 25% dextrose would provide 850 calories. A liter of 25% glucose per 2.75% amino acid (Travasol) would provide 4.63 g nitrogen and a calorie per nitrogen ratio of 183:1. This ratio will vary with different solutions.

FAT. Fat emulsions provide a concentrated source of nonprotein calories as well as ensure a necessary supply of essential fatty acid (linoleic, see p. 37). The current commercial product available in the United States is Intralipid. This is a 10% fat emulsion derived from soybean oil, containing neutral triglycerides of predominantly unsaturated fatty acids and supplying the necessary essential fatty acids. It is supplied in 500 ml bottles that provide 550 calories (1.1 calories per milliliter). It is usually used as a supplement to the main TPN solution, provided separately in the amount of one to two bottles a week for adults.

Table 31-4. Example of basic TPN formula components

Components	Amounts
Basic solution	
Crystalline amino acids	2.75%
Dextrose	25%
Additives	
Electrolytes	
Na	50 meq/L
Cl	50 meq/L
K	40 meq/L
HPO_4	25 meq/L
Ca	5 meq/L
Mg	8 meq/L
Vitamins	
Multiple (MVI)	1.7 ml conc./L
Vitamin C (day)	500 mg
Trace elements solution (day)	
Zn	3 mg
Cu	1.6 mg
Cr	2 μg
Se	120 μg
Mn	2 mg
I	120 μg
Fe	1.5 mg
Other additives (as needed)	
Regular insulin	0-25 units per liter
Heparin	1,000 units per liter

ELECTROLYTES. The formulation of electrolytes is based on the usual requirements for normal electrolyte balance with adjustments according to individual patient monitoring. Some electrolytes are present in amino acid solutions and must be taken into account when calculating additions for a specific patient requirement. A general ratio of electrolytes is shown in Table 31-4.

VITAMINS. Multiple vitamin formulas are available for use in TPN solutions as well as individual vitamins for formulation of solution as needed. Multiple formulas such as MVI (multiple vitamin injection) supply water-soluble B-complex vitamins and vitamin C as well as water-soluble forms of vitamins A, D, and E. Since vitamins B_{12}, folate, and K may alter their form when added to the rest of the vitamin formula, they are added separately, not on a daily basis, as indicated in Table 31-4.

MINERALS. Caution is exercised in adding minerals to the TPN solution because incompatibilities of certain electrolytes and other components may result in the formation of an insoluble precipitate, depending on factors such as ion concentration and solution pH. For example, phosphate equilibrium is pH dependent; thus mixing of large amounts of calcium ions with phosphate or sulfate ions may produce such a precipitate. Attention must be given to phosphate addition if a patient is receiving a phosphate-free solution, as hypophosphatemia may develop in seven to ten days. This is due to the decreased levels of 2,3-DPG (diphosphoglycerate), a product of glycolysis in erythrocytes associated with the oxygen-carrying capacity of these red blood cells. More attention has been given recently to the need for added trace minerals such as zinc, copper, iron, chromium, and manganese, but such use is still investigational at this time, and caution should be exercised. A helpful guideline for trace mineral use in TPN formulas has been provided by the *Journal of the American Medical Association*.[29]

The various components of the specific TPN solution for an individual patient's needs are mixed according to rigid protocol by the pharmacist on the TPN team. A laminar flow hood provides an aseptic environment in which the solutions, open medication vials, and other materials can be handled safely. To ensure stability, the individual solution formulas are ordered and mixed on a daily basis.

Administration of TPN

The surgical procedure for insertion of the central vein TPN line and its careful maintenance by rigid protocol to avoid infection has been well developed, and in the hands of a well-trained TPN team its risks have been minimized. Complications in the three categories of insertion, sepsis, and metabolism can be controlled by such team effort. This has been clearly shown in control studies, such as that by Nehme.[30]

Home TPN for long-term use

Experience with home use of other long-term medical care equipment such as that for renal dialysis has led to the concept of self-infusion of parenteral nutrients at home. Self-infusion at home can greatly reduce the cost of such treatment, and in the hands of selected, well-trained patients and their families it can allow mobility and travel. This has led to the term "artificial gut" for such long-term parenteral nutrition procedures.[31] Indeed it has offered special promise in long-term management of such conditions as severe abdominal injury or chronic severe Crohn's disease.[32] Special equipment and solutions have been developed and successfully used in a number of cases.[33]

CASE STUDY 30

The patient requiring tube feeding

Mr. and Mrs. Wilson, both aged 70, lived on their small farm in a rural area of the county. They had no family, as their two sons had been killed in World War II. Mr. Wilson had tended his small farm as long as he was able to do so, but now he was unable to work. They had gradually sold off parcels of their land until they had only the farmhouse and a small plot of land remaining. Their income was small, and they could scarcely meet the taxes for the land. They were both in poor health and worried about their future care. Their closest relationship was with the small church in the community where they had been members most of their lives, but they now were unable to attend. The present pastor of the church was a young man with several small children whose wife was a dietitian. The pastor's family had a warm affection for Mr. and Mrs. Wilson and visited frequently in their small home.

Mrs. Wilson began to have some symptoms of difficulty in swallowing and pain in the area of her throat and neck. It developed, eventually, that it was cancer. Finally radical neck surgery became necessary. After the surgery she was unable to take food in the normal manner and had to be fed through a tube.

The first formula used was a water dilution of a commercial-defined formula product to provide 2,000 calories a day. Mrs. Wilson tolerated this feeding fairly well and gradually improved. As her need for protein and calories was increased, the formula diet was increased to 3,000 calories. At first this increase in calories was also attained by use of the commercial formula, but Mrs. Wilson began to have gastrointestinal difficulties and diarrhea. To counteract this problem, the formula was changed to a calculated food mixture yielding a better balance of nutrients at the same calorie level. She needed to have 2,500 to 3,000 ml of the formula each day.

In the days that followed, Mrs. Wilson continued to improve and regain her strength. Her pastor and his wife visited frequently and brought Mr. Wilson with them. Soon the day came when the doctor indicated that Mrs. Wilson would be able to go home. He discussed her needs for home care with the pastor's wife who was a clinical nutrition specialist and could assume responsibility for her continued nutritional therapy. They both felt reasonably sure that after a period of continued use of the tube feeding, Mrs. Wilson would be able to gradually resume small liquid to soft textured oral feedings. Her need for optimum nutrition was evident.

The day Mrs. Wilson was to go home the pastor and his wife and Mr. Wilson came to get her. The doctor discussed her overall needs with all of them, and the pastor and his wife assured him they would do what was necessary to see that she had the care she needed.

Questions to guide your inquiry (Refer also to Chapter 23.)

1. What nutritional needs did Mrs. Wilson have in preparing her for surgery? What solutions to these needs can you propose? How would you involve the physician, the clinic nurse, and the pastor and his wife in your solutions?
2. What are some of the indications for tube feeding?
3. What are the implications of such a method of feeding for Mrs. Wilson? What are her needs? Her husband's needs?
4. Make a list of some of the commercial-defined formulas and elemental diets available on the market. Compare their nutrient composition and characteristics, as well as costs. Indicate situations in which they would be used.
5. Why do gastrointestinal difficulties sometimes result when tube feeding using a commercial product alone is increased to 3,000 calories?
6. What solution was found for meeting this problem? Why was the calculated mixed tube feeding better tolerated? Outline such a tube feeding: 3,000 calories, 165 g protein, and not more than 350 g carbohydrate.
7. In planning for Mrs. Wilson's home care, what problems do you see? What solutions can you propose? What persons would you involve?

CASE STUDY 31

The patient with enterocutaneous fistula requiring TPN

Grace Silver lay back on the pillow of her hospital bed, weak and spent, as new tears gathered and spilled over her cheeks. "And I'm only 35 years old!" she thought as her mind went back over the rapid events of the past few months. She remembered so sharply the day her physician had told her about the cancer and the need for surgery. First there had been the radiation treatment and chemotherapy with the periods of nausea and lack of appetite. Then with the recurrence of the invasive carcinoma of the cervix the first surgery had followed—a hysterectomy—and she had felt as if she were only half a woman.

Now she was back in the hospital again for more pelvic surgery and had developed multiple enterocutaneous fistulas. Her physician had explained all the problems to her and to her husband, Bill, and this had helped some to enable her to cope. For about two weeks now she had been unable to eat solid food, taking only some clear liquids. The fistulas continued to drain, so today the physician had given her some intravenous feeding in her arm of a solution of 10% glucose per 0.45 normal saline to try to supplement her fluid and calorie needs. This was now her third week since surgery, and more complications had developed. She had peritonitis, a fever of 39° C (102° F), and the fistulas were not healing. She now weighed only 41 kg (90 lb). The drainage from the fistulas was odorous, and she was in isolation.

Grace thought about her family and wondered how they were holding up in the face of all this. She had been divorced a few years ago and had lived with her three children since, that is, until she had married again just before this illness began. She had always been proud of her trim figure, even after the children had come, but now she felt thin, bony, and ugly, afraid to face her husband and worried about her sexual functioning. And why was that nurse testing her urine sample for sugar? . . . oh, no, not diabetes, too! Grace pressed her hand to her face to try to hold back the tears as the jumbled thoughts kept coming . . . not like that neighbor, only 27, who was already blind from diabetes she had developed as a teenager . . .

Grace's thoughts were interrupted by the arrival of her physician. He explained to her that the nutritional support team had decided to start her on more complete feeding through a larger vein up around her neck. He had called it TPN, total parenteral nutrition, and said it would help to build up her weight and nutritional state. They would be doing some more tests to see what her progress was. After he left, Grace felt her anxiety about the new procedure rising, but hopeful also that it would help her to get well.

Questions to guide your inquiry (Refer also to Chapter 15.)

1. Using a nutritional assessment data summary sheet for a patient on TPN, list all the available data for Mrs. Silver. What additional data are needed, to which the physician referred? Anthropometric? Biochemical laboratory tests? Clinical observations? Other?
2. Explain each of these tests and its significance in relation to Mrs. Silver's condition.
3. Calculate her energy and protein requirements and account for the increased needs.
4. Why was the decision made to start Mrs. Silver on TPN therapy?
5. Why did Mrs. Silver find difficulties with eating during her prior radiation and chemotherapy treatments? What nutrition counseling would you as her nutritionist have provided for her? What nutrition supplements would you have used? Why?
6. If during her prior outpatient care Mrs. Silver had asked about her cancer, what cancer is, and what radiation and chemotherapy do for it, how would you have answered her? Outline your response. What resources would you have used in your overall plan of nutritional care?
7. Why was Mrs. Silver concerned about the urine sugar tests and diabetes? Why were the tests being done?
8. What personal needs can you identify from her social history? What solutions or emotional support would you propose? What staff persons or family or working colleagues (she had worked for some years as a highly skilled legal administrative assistant in a large law firm in the city) would you involve in your plan of care?

REFERENCES
Specific

1. Department of Health, Education, and Welfare: Cancer questions, No. (NIH) 77-1040, Washington, D.C., 1975.
2. Watson, J. D.: Molecular biology of the gene, ed. 3, New York, 1976, W. A. Benjamin, Inc.
3. Richards, V.: Cancer: the wayward cell, its origins, nature, and treatment, ed. 2, Berkeley, Calif., 1978, University of California Press.
4. Wynder, E. L., editor: Symposium: nutrition in the causation of cancer, Cancer Res. vol. 35, pt. 2, Nov., 1975.
5. Wynder, E. L.: The dietary environment and cancer, J. Am. Diet. Assoc. **71:**385, Oct., 1977.
6. Burkitt, D. P.: Epidemiology of cancer of the colon and rectum, Cancer **28:**3, 1971.
7. Hill, M. J., Crowther, J. S., Draser, B. S., et al.: Bacteria and aetiology of cancer of the large bowel, Lancet **1:**95, 1971.
8. Dales, L. G., Friedman, G. D., Ury, H. K., Grossman, S., and Williams, S. R.: A case-control study of relationships of diet and other traits to colorectal cancer in American blacks, Am. J. Epidemiol. **109**(2): 132, 1978.
9. Selye, H.: The stress of life, New York, 1978, McGraw-Hill Book Co.
10. Simonton, C., and Simonton, S.: Getting well again, Los Angeles, 1978, J. P. Tarcher, Inc.
11. LeShan, L.: You can fight for your life: emotional factors in the causation of cancer, New York, 1978, Harcourt Brace Jovanovich, Inc.
12. Thomas, C. B., and Greenstreet, R. I.: Psychological characteristics in youth as predictors of five disease states: suicide, mental illness, hypertension, coronary heart disease, and tumor, Johns Hopkins Med. J. **132:**16, 1973.
13. Jose, D. G.: The cancer connection with immunity and nutrition, Nutr. Today **8:**4, March-April, 1973.
14. Rubin, P., editor: Clinical oncology for medical students and physicians, ed. 5, New York, 1978, American Cancer Society, p. 43.
15. Carter, S. K., Bakowski, M. T., and Hellmann, K.: Chemotherapy of cancer, New York, 1977, John Wiley & Sons, Inc.
16. Pilch, Y.: Research in cancer immunotherapy. In Renneker, M., and Leib, S., editors: Understanding cancer, Palo Alto, Calif., 1979, Bull Publishing Co., p. 210.
17. Copeland, E. M., III, MasFadyen, B. V., Jr., Lanzotti, V. J., and Dudrick, S. J.: Intravenous hyperalimentation as an adjunct to cancer chemotherapy, Am. J. Surg. **129:**167, 1975.
18. Munro, H. N.: Tumor-host competition for nutrients in the cancer patient, J. Am. Diet. Assoc. **71:**380, Oct., 1977.
19. Fleming, S. M., Weaver, A. W., and Brown, J. M.: The patient with cancer affecting the head and neck: problems in nutrition, J. Am. Diet. Assoc. **70:**391, April, 1977.
20. Blackburn, G. L., Bistrian, B. R., Maini, B. S., Schlamm, H. T., and Smith, M. F.: Nutritional and metabolic assessment of the hospitalized patient, J.P.E.N. **1**(1):11, 1977.
21. Jelliffe, D. B.: The assessment of the nutritional status of the community, World Health Organization Monograph Service No. 53, 1966.
22. Rosenbaum, E. H., Stitt, C. N., Drasin, H., and Rosenbaum, I. R.: Nutrition for the cancer patient, Palo Alto, Calif., 1980, Bull Publishing Co.
23. Raffman, R.: Using marijuana in the reduction of nausea associated with chemotherapy, Seattle, 1979, Murray Publishing Co.
24. Mullen, B. D.: The ostomy book: living comfortably with colostomies, ileostomies, and urostomies, Palo Alto, Calif., 1980, Bull Publishing Co.
25. Shills, M. E., Bloch, A. S., and Chernoff, R.: Liquid formulas for oral and tube feeding, New York, 1979, Memorial Sloan-Kettering Cancer Center.
26. Dudrick, S. J., Wilmore, D. W., Vars, H. M., and Rhoads, J. E.: Long-term parenteral nutrition with growth, development, and positive nitrogen balance, Surgery **64:**134, 1968.
26a. Dudrick, S. J., and Rhoads, J. E.: New horizons for intravenous feeding, J.A.M.A. **215:**939, 1971.
27. Shils, M. E.: Parenteral nutrition. In Goodhart, R. S., and Shils, M. E., editors: Modern nutrition in health and disease, ed. 6, Philadelphia, 1980, Lea & Febiger, p. 1125.
28. Cahill, G. F., Jr.: Starvation in man, N. Engl. J. Med. **282:**668, 1970.
29. Review: Guidelines for essential trace element preparations for parenteral use, J.A.M.A. **241:**2051, 1979.
30. Nehme, A. E.: Nutritional support of the hospitalized patient: the team concept, J.A.M.A. **243:**1906, 1980.
31. Scribner, B. H., Cole, J. J., Christopher, T. G., et al.: Long term total parenteral nutrition: the concept of an artificial gut, J.A.M.A. **212:**457, 1970.
32. Rault, R. M. J., and Scribner, B. H.: Treatment of Crohn's disease with home parenteral nutrition, Gastroenterology **72:**1249, 1977.
33. Scribner, B. H., and Cole, J. J.: Evolution of the technique of home parenteral nutrition, J.P.E.N. **3**(2): 58, March-April, 1979.

General

Ballinger, W. F., et al., editors: Manual of surgical nutrition, Philadelphia, 1975, W. B. Saunders Co.
Bistrian, B. R.: Nutritional assessment and therapy of

protein-calorie malnutrition in the hospital, J. Am. Diet. Assoc. **71:**393, Oct., 1977.

Bistrian, B. R., Blackburn, G. L., Vitale, J., et al.: Prevalence of malnutrition in general medical patients, J.A.M.A. **235:**1567, 1976.

Blackburn, G. L., and Bistrian, B. R.: Nutritional support resources in hospital practice. In Schneider, H. A., Anderson, C. E., and Coursin, D. B., editors: Nutritional support of medical practice, New York, 1977, Harper & Row, Publishers, p. 139.

Blackburn, G. L., Flatt, J. P., Clawes, G. H. A., and O'Donnell, T. E.: Peripheral intravenous feeding with isotonic amino acid solutions, Am. J. Surg. **125:**447, April, 1973.

Chernoff, R., and Bloch, A. S.: Liquid feedings: considerations and alternatives, J. Am. Diet. Assoc. **70:**389, 1977.

Cline, M. J., and Haskell, C. M.: Cancer chemotherapy, Philadelphia, 1975, W. B. Saunders Co.

Cooper, W. C., Good, R. A., and Mariani, T.: Effect of protein insufficiency on immune responsiveness, Am. J. Clin. Nutr. **27:**647, 1974.

Costa, G., and Donaldson, S. S.: Current concepts in cancer: effects of cancer and cancer treatment on the nutrition of the host, N. Engl. J. Med. **300:**1471, June 28, 1979.

Cairns, J.: The cancer problem, Sci. Am. **233:**64, Nov., 1975.

Cairns, J.: Mutation, selection and cancer, Nature **255:** 197, 1975.

Carson, J. A. S.: Nutrition in a team approach to rehabilitation of the patient with cancer, J. Am. Diet. Assoc. **72:**407, April, 1978.

Carson, J. A. S., and Gormican, A.: Taste acuity and food attitudes of selected patients with cancer, J. Am. Diet. Assoc. **70:**361, April, 1977.

Carter, S. K., Bakowski, M. T., and Hellmann, K.: Chemotherapy of cancer, New York, 1977, John Wiley & Sons, Inc.

Deitel, M., and Kaminsky, V.: Total nutrition by peripheral vein—the lipid system, Can. Med. Assoc. J. **111:**152, July 20, 1974.

DeWys, W. D., and Walters, K.: Abnormalities of taste sensation in cancer patients, Cancer **36:**1888, 1975.

Faulk, W. P., and Vitale, J. J.: Immunology. In Schneider, H. A., Anderson, C. E., and Coursin, D. B., editors: Nutritional support of medical practice, New York, 1977, Harper & Row, Publishers, p. 341.

Fiore, N.: Fighting cancer—one patient's perspective, N. Engl. J. Med. **300:**284, Feb. 8, 1979.

Fischer, J. E., editor: Total parenteral nutrition, Boston, 1976, Little, Brown and Co.

Fleming, C. R., Hodges, R. E., and Hurley, L. S.: A prospective study of serum copper and zinc levels in patients receiving total parenteral nutrition, Am. J. Clin. Nutr. **29:**70, 1976.

Food and Nutrition Board, National Research Council: Recommended dietary allowances, ed. 9, Washington, D.C., 1980, National Academy of Sciences.

Goodhart, R. S., and Shils, M. E., editors: Modern nutrition in health and disease, ed. 6, New York, 1980, Lea & Febiger.

Gori, G. B.: Diet and cancer, J. Am. Diet. Assoc. **71:** 375, Oct., 1977.

Grant, A.: Nutritional assessment guidelines, Seattle, 1979, NP.

Heird, W. C., and Winters, R. W.: Parenteral nutrition. In Schneider, H. A., Anderson, C. E., and Coursin, D. B., editors: Nutritional support of medical practice, New York, 1977, Harper & Row, Publishers, p. 184.

Herlihy, P., Stanaszek, W. F., and Covington, T. R.: Total parenteral nutrition, J. Am. Diet. Assoc. **70:**279, March, 1977.

Heymsfield, S. B., Bethel, R. A., Ansley, J. D., et al.: Enteral hyperalimentation: an alternative to central venous hyperalimentation, Ann. Intern. Med. **90:**63, Jan., 1979.

Johnson, E. Q.: The therapeutic dietitian's role in the alimentation group, J. Am. Diet. Assoc. **62:**648, June, 1973.

Krakoff, I. H.: Cancer chemotherapeutic agents, New York, 1977, American Cancer Society.

Krakoff, I. H.: Principles of cancer chemotherapy, Drug Ther. **10:**40, 1980.

Law, D. K., Dudrick, S. J., and Abdou, N. I.: Immunocompetence of patients with protein-calorie malnutrition: the effects of nutritional repletion, Ann. Intern. Med. **79:**545, 1973.

Lee, H. A., editor: Parenteral nutrition in acute metabolic illness, New York, 1974, Academic Press, Inc.

Mazia, D.: The cell cycle, Sci. Am. **230:**54, Jan., 1974.

Meng, H. C.: Parenteral nutrition: principles, nutrient requirements, techniques, and clinical applications. In Schneider, H. A., Anderson, C. E., and Coursin, D. B., editors: Nutritional support of medical practice, New York, Harper & Row, Publishers, p. 152.

Mitchison, J. M.: The biology of the cell cycle, Cambridge, England, 1971, Cambridge University Press.

Munro, H. N.: Tumor-host competition for nutrients in the cancer patient, J. Am. Diet. Assoc. **71:**380, Oct., 1977.

Ochsner, A.: Cancer of the lung, J. Am. Diet. Assoc. **62:** 249, March, 1973.

Review: Vitamin A, tumor initiation and tumor promotion, Nutr. Rev. **37:**153, May, 1979.

Richards, V.: Cancer: the wayward cell, ed. 2, Berkeley, Calif., 1978, University of California Press.

Roitt, I. M.: Essential immunology, London, 1977, Blackwell Scientific Publications Ltd.

Rubin, P., editor: Clinical oncology for medical students and physicians, ed. 5, New York, 1978, American Cancer Society.

Russell, R. I.: Progress report: elemental diets, Gut **16:**68, 1975.

Schneider, P. D., and Buchwald, H.: Total parenteral nutrition and elemental diets. In Halpern, S. L., editor: Quick reference to clinical nutrition, Philadelphia, 1979, J. B. Lippincott Co., p. 295.

Shils, M. E.: Guidelines for total parenteral nutrition, J.A.M.A. **220:**1721, 1972.

Shils, M. E.: A program for total parenteral nutrition at home, Am. J. Clin. Nutr. **28:**1429, 1975.

Shils, M. E., editor: Defined formula diets for medical purposes, Chicago, 1977, American Medical Association.

Silver, R. T., Lauper, R. D., and Jarowsi, C. I.: A synopsis of cancer chemotherapy, New York, 1977, Dun-Donnely Pub. Corp.

Theologides, A.: Nutrition in cancer. In Halpern, S. L., editor: Quick reference to clinical nutrition, Philadelphia, 1979, J. B. Lippincott Co., p. 258.

Thorn, G. W., editor: Harrison's principles of internal medicine, ed. 8, New York, 1977, McGraw-Hill Book Co.

Wang, R. I. H.: Practical drug therapy, Philadelphia, 1979, J. B. Lippincott Co.

White, P. L., and Nagy, M. E., editors: Total parenteral nutrition, Acton, Mass., 1974, Publishing Sciences Group Inc.

Wilmore, D. W.: The metabolic management of the critically ill, New York, 1977, Plenum Medical Book Co.

Wynder, E. L.: The dietary environment and cancer, J. Am. Diet. Assoc. **71:**385, Oct., 1977.

CANCER: PATIENT EDUCATION MATERIALS

Achterberg, J., Simonton, C., and Simonton, S., editors: Stress, psychological factors, and cancer, Fort Worth, Tex., 1976, New Medicine Press.

Aker, S., and Lenssen, P.: A guide to good nutrition during and after chemotherapy and radiation, ed. 2, Seattle, 1979, Fred Hutchinson Cancer Research Center.

American Cancer Society: Unproven methods of cancer management, New York, 1971.

American Cancer Society: Nutrition for persons receiving chemotherapy and radiation treatment, New York, 1974.

Benson, H.: The relaxation response, New York, 1975, William Morrow and Co.

Biofeedback and self-control, an Aldine annual on the regulation of bodily processes and consciousness, Chicago, Aldine Publishing Co. Published annually: annual highlights of scientific research in the field of self-regulation.

Cannon, W. B.: The wisdom of the body, New York, 1963, W. W. Norton & Co., Inc.

Epstein, S. S.: The politics of cancer, San Francisco, 1978, Sierra Club Books.

Fink, D. H.: Release from nervous tension, New York, 1962, Simon & Schuster, Inc. (relaxation exercises).

Fiore, N.: Fighting cancer—one patient's perspective, N. Engl. J. Med. **300:**284, Feb. 8, 1979.

Fiore, N.: Fighting cancer, Sci. Dig. **85:**62, June, 1979.

Helsel, J. E.: Food for those who hesitate . . . tips that they might tolerate, Durham, N.C., 1976, Duke University Comprehensive Cancer Center.

Hofer, J.: Total massage, New York, 1976, Grosset & Dunlap, Inc.

Israel, L.: Conquering cancer, New York, 1978, Random House, Inc.

Keith, R. L., Shore, H. C., Coates, H. L. C., and Devine, K. D.: Looking forward: a guidebook for the laryngectomee, Rochester, Minn., 1977, Mayo Foundation.

Klinger, J. L., editor: Mealtime manual for people with disabilities and the aging, Ronks, Pa., Mealtime Manual, ND.

Kubler-Ross, E.: Death: the final stage of growth, Englewood Cliffs, N.J., 1975, Prentice-Hall, Inc.

LeShan, L.: You can fight for your life, New York, 1978, Harcourt Brace Jovanovich, Inc.

Levin, A.: Talk back to your doctor, New York, 1975, Doubleday & Co., Inc.

Levitt, P. M., Guralnick, E. S., Kagan, A. R., and Gilbert, H.: The cancer reference book, New York, 1979, Paddington Press Ltd.

Mullen, B. D.: The ostomy book: living comfortably with colostomies, ileostomies, and urostomies, Palo Alto, Calif., 1980, Bull Publishing Co.

National Cancer Institute: Nutrition for the cancer patient: selected annotations of educational materials, Bethesda, Md., 1977.

National Cancer Institute: Cancer questions and answers about risks, rates, Bethesda, Md., 1978.

Pelletier, K.: Mind as healer, mind as slayer, New York, 1977, Delacorte Press.

Prescott, D. M.: Cancer: the misguided cell, Indianapolis, 1973, The Bobbs-Merrill Co., Inc.

Raffman, R.: Using marijuana in the reduction of nausea associated with chemotherapy, Seattle, 1979, Murray Publishing Co. (recipes).

Renneker, M., and Leib, S.: Understanding cancer, Palo Alto, Calif., 1979, Bull Publishing Co.

Rosenbaum, E. H., and Rosenbaum, I. R.: A comprehensive guide for cancer patients and their families, Palo Alto, Calif., 1980, Bull Publishing Co.

Rosenbaum, E. H., Stitt, C. N., Drasin, H., and Rosenbaum, I. R.: Nutrition for the cancer patient, Palo Alto, Calif., 1980, Bull Publishing Co.

Samuels, M., and Samuels, N.: Seeing with the mind's eye,

Berkeley, Calif., 1975, Bookworks (Random House, Inc.).

Sherman, M.: Feeding the sick child, Bethesda, Md., 1976, National Cancer Institute.

Simonton, C.: Relaxation and mental imagery as it applies to cancer therapy (audio tape recordings), Saratoga, Calif., 1974, Cognetics.

Simonton, C., and Simonton, S.: Getting well again, Los Angeles, 1978, J. P. Tarcher, Inc.

TYRAMINE-RESTRICTED DIET

Blackwell, B., Mabbitt, L. A., and Marley, E.: Histamine and tyramine content of yeast products, J. Food Sci. **34:**47, Jan., 1969.

Horowitz, D., et al.: Monoamine oxidase inhibitors, tyramine, and cheese, J.A.M.A. **188:**1108, 1964.

Price, K., and Smith, S. E.: Cheese reaction and tyramine, Lancet **1:**130, Jan. 16, 1971.

Review: Headache, tyramine, serotonin and migraine, Nutr. Rev. **26:**40, Feb., 1968.

Sen, N. P.: Analysis and significance of tyramine in food, J. Food Sci. **34:**22, Jan., 1969.

Wurtman, R. J.: Catecholamines, Boston, 1966, Little, Brown and Co.

APPENDIXES

Nutritive values of the edible part of foods[1]

Food, approximate measure, and weight (in grams)			Food energy (calo-ries)	Pro-tein (g)	Fat (total lipid) (g)	Fatty acids			Carbo-hydrate (g)	Cal-cium (mg)	Iron (mg)	Vita-min A value (IU)	Thia-min (mg)	Ribo-flavin (mg)	Niacin (mg)	Ascor-bic acid (mg)
						Satu-rated (total) (g)	Unsaturated									
							Oleic (g)	Linoleic (g)								
Milk, cream, cheese (related products)																
Milk, cow's																
Fluid, whole (3.5% fat)	1 cup	244	160	9	9	5	3	Trace	12	288	0.1	350	0.08	0.42	0.1	2
Fluid, nonfat (skim)	1 cup	246	90	9	Trace	—	—	—	13	298	.1	10	.10	.44	.2	2
Buttermilk, cultured, from skim milk	1 cup	246	90	9	Trace	—	—	—	13	298	.1	10	.09	.44	.2	2
Evaporated, unsweet-ened, undiluted	1 cup	252	345	18	20	11	7	1	24	635	.3	820	.10	.84	.5	3
Condensed, sweetened, undiluted	1 cup	306	980	25	27	15	9	1	166	802	.3	1,090	.23	1.17	.5	3
Dry, whole	1 cup	103	515	27	28	16	9	1	39	936	.5	1,160	.30	1.50	.7	6
Dry, nonfat, instant	1 cup	70	250	25	Trace	—	—	—	36	905	.4	20	.24	1.25	.6	5
Milk, goat's																
Fluid, whole	1 cup	244	165	8	10	6	2	Trace	11	315	.2	390	.10	.27	.7	2
Cream																
Half-and-half (cream and milk)	1 cup	242	325	8	28	16	9	1	11	261	.1	1,160	.08	.38	.1	2
	1 tbsp.	15	20	Trace	2	1	1	Trace	1	16	Trace	70	Trace	.02	Trace	Trace
Light, coffee or table	1 cup	240	505	7	49	27	16	1	10	245	.1	2,030	.07	.36	.1	2
	1 tbsp.	15	30	Trace	3	2	1	Trace	1	15	Trace	130	Trace	.02	Trace	Trace
Whipping, unwhipped (volume about double when whipped)																
Light	1 cup	239	715	6	75	41	25	2	9	203	.1	3,070	.06	.30	.1	2
	1 tbsp.	15	45	Trace	5	3	2	Trace	1	13	Trace	190	Trace	.02	Trace	Trace
Heavy	1 cup	238	840	5	89	49	29	3	7	178	.1	3,670	.05	.26	.1	2
	1 tbsp.	15	55	Trace	6	3	2	Trace	Trace	11	Trace	230	Trace	.02	Trace	Trace

Cheese															
Blue or Roquefort type	1 oz.	28	105	6	9	5	3	Trace	1	89	.1	350	.01	.17	.1	0
Cheddar or American																
Ungrated	1 inch cube	17	70	4	5	3	2	Trace	Trace	128	.2	220	Trace	.08	Trace	0
Grated	1 cup	112	445	28	36	20	12	1	2	840	1.1	1,470	.03	.51	.1	0
	1 tbsp.	7	30	2	2	1	1	Trace	Trace	52	.1	90	Trace	.03	Trace	0
Cheddar, process	1 oz.	28	105	7	9	5	3	Trace	1	219	.3	350	Trace	.12	Trace	0
Cheese foods, Cheddar	1 oz.	28	90	6	7	4	2	Trace	2	162	.2	280	.01	.16	Trace	0
Cottage cheese, from skim milk																
Creamed	1 cup	225	240	31	9	5	3	Trace	7	212	0.7	380	0.07	0.56	0.2	0
	1 oz.	28	30	4	1	1	Trace	Trace	1	27	.1	50	.01	.07	Trace	0
Uncreamed	1 cup	225	195	38	1	Trace	Trace	—	6	202	.9	20	.07	.63	.2	0
	1 oz.	28	25	5	Trace	Trace	Trace	—	1	26	.1	Trace	.01	.08	Trace	0
Cream cheese	1 oz.	28	105	2	11	6	4	Trace	1	18	.1	440	Trace	.07	Trace	0
	1 tbsp.	15	55	1	6	3	2	Trace	Trace	9	Trace	230	Trace	.04	Trace	0
Swiss (domestic)	1 oz.	28	105	8	8	4	3	Trace	1	262	.3	320	Trace	.11	Trace	0
Milk beverages																
Cocoa	1 cup	242	235	8	11	6	4	Trace	26	286	.9	390	.09	.45	.4	2
Chocolate-flavored milk drink (made with skim milk)	1 cup	250	190	8	6	3	2	Trace	27	270	.4	210	.09	.41	.2	2
Malted milk	1 cup	270	280	13	12	—	—	—	32	364	.8	670	.17	.56	.2	2
Milk desserts																
Cornstarch pudding, plain (blanc mange)	1 cup	248	275	9	10	5	3	Trace	39	290	.1	390	.07	.40	.1	2
Custard, baked	1 cup	248	285	13	14	6	5	1	28	278	1.0	870	.10	.47	.1	1
Ice cream, plain, factory packed																
Slice or cut brick, ⅛ of quart brick	1 slice or cut brick	71	145	3	9	5	3	Trace	15	87	.1	370	.03	.13	.1	1
Container	3½ fld. oz.	62	130	2	8	4	3	Trace	13	76	.1	320	.03	.12	.1	1
Container	8 fld. ozs.	142	295	6	18	10	6	1	29	175	.1	740	.06	.27	.1	1
Ice milk	1 cup	187	285	9	10	6	3	Trace	42	292	.2	390	.09	.41	.2	2
Yogurt, from partially skimmed milk	1 cup	246	120	8	4	2	1	Trace	13	295	.1	170	.09	.43	.2	2

Continued.

[1]Reprinted from Nutritive value of foods, U.S. Department of Agriculture, Home and Garden Bulletin No. 72.

Dashes show that no basis could be found for imputing a value although there was some reason to believe that a measurable amount of the constituent might be present.

Food, approximate measure, and weight (in grams)		Food energy (calories)	Protein (g)	Fat (total lipid) (g)	Fatty acids			Carbohydrate (g)	Calcium (mg)	Iron (mg)	Vitamin A value (IU)	Thiamin (mg)	Riboflavin (mg)	Niacin (mg)	Ascorbic acid (mg)
					Saturated (total) (g)	Unsaturated Oleic (g)	Linoleic (g)								
Eggs															
Eggs, large, 24 ounces per dozen															
Raw															
Whole, without shell	1 egg	50	80	6	6	2	3	Trace	Trace	27	1.1	590	.05	.15	Trace	0
White of egg	1 white	33	15	4	Trace	—	—	—	Trace	3	Trace	0	Trace	.09	Trace	0
Yolk of egg	1 yolk	17	60	3	5	2	2	Trace	Trace	24	.9	580	.04	.07	Trace	0
Cooked															
Boiled, shell removed	2 eggs	100	160	13	12	4	5	1	1	54	2.3	1,180	.09	.28	.1	0
Scrambled, with milk and fat	1 egg	64	110	7	8	3	3	Trace	1	51	1.1	690	.05	.18	Trace	0
Meat, poultry, fish, shellfish (related products)															
Bacon, broiled or fried, crisp	2 slices	16	100	5	8	3	4	1	1	2	.5	0	.08	.05	.8	—
Beef, trimmed to retail basis[2], cooked															
Cuts braised, simmered, or pot-roasted															
Lean and fat	3 oz.	85	245	23	16	8	7	Trace	0	10	2.9	30	.04	.18	3.5	—
Lean only	2.5 oz.	72	140	22	5	2	2	Trace	0	10	2.7	10	.04	.16	3.3	—
Hamburger (ground beef), broiled															
Lean	3 oz.	85	185	23	10	5	4	Trace	0	10	3.0	20	.08	.20	5.1	—
Regular	3 oz.	85	245	21	17	8	8	Trace	0	9	2.7	30	.07	.18	4.6	—
Roast, oven-cooked, no liquid added															
Relatively fat, such as rib															
Lean and fat	3 oz.	85	375	17	34	16	15	1	0	8	2.2	70	.05	.13	3.1	—
Lean only	1.8 oz.	51	125	14	7	3	3	Trace	0	6	1.8	10	.04	.11	2.6	—
Relatively lean, such as heel of round															
Lean and fat	3 oz.	85	165	25	7	3	3	Trace	0	11	3.2	10	.06	.19	4.5	—
Lean only	2.7 oz.	78	125	24	3	1	1	Trace	0	10	3.0	Trace	.06	.18	4.3	—
Steak, broiled															
Relatively fat, such as sirloin															
Lean and fat	3 oz.	85	330	20	27	13	12	1	0	9	2.5	50	.05	.16	4.0	—
Lean only	2.0 oz.	56	115	18	4	2	2	Trace	0	7	2.2	10	.05	.14	3.6	—
Relatively lean, such as round															
Lean and fat	3 oz.	85	220	24	13	6	6	Trace	0	10	3.0	20	.07	.19	4.8	—
Lean only	2.4 oz.	68	130	21	4	2	2	Trace	0	9	2.5	10	.06	.16	4.1	—

Food	Measure	Grams													
Beef, canned															
Corned beef	3 oz.	85	185	22	10	5	4	Trace	0	17	3.7	20	.01	.20	2.9	—
Corned beef hash	3 oz.	85	155	7	10	5	4	Trace	9	11	1.7	—	.01	.08	1.8	—
Beef, dried or chipped	2 oz.	57	115	19	4	2	2	Trace	0	11	2.9	—	.04	.18	2.2	—
Beef and vegetable stew	1 cup	235	210	15	10	5	4	Trace	15	28	2.8	2,310	.13	.17	4.4	15
Beef potpie, baked: individual pie, 4¼-inch diameter, weight before baking about 8 oz.	1 pie	227	560	23	33	9	20	2	43	32	4.1	1,860	.25	.27	4.5	7
Chicken, cooked															
Flesh only, broiled	3 oz.	85	115	20	3	1	1	1	0	8	1.4	80	0.05	0.16	7.4	—
Breast, fried, ½ breast															
With bone	3.3 oz.	94	155	25	5	1	2	1	1	9	1.3	70	.04	.17	11.2	—
Flesh and skin only	2.7 oz.	76	155	25	5	1	2	1	1	9	1.3	70	.04	.17	11.2	—
Drumstick, fried															
With bone	2.1 oz.	59	90	12	4	1	2	1	Trace	6	.9	50	.03	.15	2.7	—
Flesh and skin only	1.3 oz.	38	90	12	4	1	2	1	Trace	6	.9	50	.03	.15	2.7	—
Chicken, canned, boneless	3 oz.	85	170	18	10	3	4	2	0	18	1.3	200	.03	.11	3.7	3
Chicken potpie—See Poultry potpie															
Chile con carne, canned															
With beans	1 cup	250	335	19	15	7	7	Trace	30	80	4.2	150	.08	.18	3.2	—
Without beans	1 cup	255	510	26	38	18	17	1	15	97	3.6	380	.05	.31	5.6	—
Heart, beef, lean, braised	3 oz.	85	160	27	5	—	—	—	1	5	5.0	20	.21	1.04	6.5	1
Lamb, trimmed to retail basis,[2] cooked															
Chop, thick, with bone, broiled	1 chop, 4.8 oz.	137	400	25	33	18	12	1	0	10	1.5	—	.14	.25	5.6	—
Lean and fat	4.0 oz.	112	400	25	33	18	12	1	0	10	1.5	—	.14	.25	5.6	—
Lean only	2.6 oz.	74	140	21	6	3	2	Trace	0	9	1.5	—	.11	.20	4.5	—
Leg, roasted															
Lean and fat	3 oz.	85	235	22	16	9	6	Trace	0	9	1.4	—	.13	.23	4.7	—
Lean only	2.5 oz.	71	130	20	5	3	2	Trace	0	9	1.4	—	.12	.21	4.4	—
Shoulder, roasted															
Lean and fat	3 oz.	85	285	18	23	13	8	1	0	9	1.0	—	.11	.20	4.0	—
Lean only	2.3 oz.	64	130	17	6	3	2	Trace	0	8	1.0	—	.10	.18	3.7	—
Liver, beef, fried	2 oz.	57	130	15	6	—	—	—	3	6	5.0	30,280	.15	2.37	9.4	15

Continued.

[2]Outer layer of fat on the cut was removed to within approximately ½ inch of the lean. Deposits of fat within the cut were not removed.

Food, approximate measure, and weight (in grams)		Food energy (calories)	Protein (g)	Fat (total lipid) (g)	Fatty acids Saturated (total) (g)	Unsaturated Oleic (g)	Linoleic (g)	Carbohydrate (g)	Calcium (mg)	Iron (mg)	Vitamin A value (IU)	Thiamin (mg)	Riboflavin (mg)	Niacin (mg)	Ascorbic acid (mg)
Pork, cured, cooked															
Ham, light cure, lean and fat, roasted	3 oz. 85	245	18	19	7	8	2	0	8	2.2	0	.40	.16	3.1	—
Luncheon meat															
Boiled ham, sliced	2 oz. 57	135	11	10	4	4	1	0	6	1.6	0	.25	.09	1.5	—
Canned, spiced or unspiced	2 oz. 57	165	8	14	5	6	1	1	5	1.2	0	.18	.12	1.6	—
Pork, fresh, trimmed to retail basis,[2] cooked															
Chop, thick, with bone	1 chop, 3.5 oz. 98	260	16	21	8	9	2	0	8	2.2	0	.63	.18	3.8	—
Lean and fat	2.3 oz. 66	260	16	21	8	9	2	0	8	2.2	0	.63	.18	3.8	—
Lean only	1.7 oz. 48	130	15	7	2	3	1	0	7	1.9	0	.54	.16	3.3	—
Roast, oven-cooked, no liquid added															
Lean and fat	3 oz. 85	310	21	24	9	10	2	0	9	2.7	0	.78	.22	4.7	—
Lean only	2.4 oz. 68	175	20	10	3	4	1	0	9	2.6	0	.73	.21	4.4	—
Cuts, simmered															
Lean and fat	3 oz. 85	320	20	26	9	11	2	0	8	2.5	0	.46	.21	4.1	—
Lean only	2.2 oz. 63	135	18	6	2	3	1	0	8	2.3	0	.42	.19	3.7	—
Poultry potpie (based on chicken potpie). Individual pie, 4¼-inch diameter, weigh before baking	1 pie 227	535	23	31	10	15	3	42	68	3.0	3,020	.25	.26	4.1	5
Sausage															
Bologna, slice, 4.1 by 0.1 inch	8 slices 227	690	27	62	—	—	—	2	16	4.1	—	.36	.49	6.0	—
Frankfurter, cooked	1 51	155	6	14	—	—	—	1	3	.8	—	.08	.10	1.3	—
Pork, links or patty, Cooked	4 oz. 113	540	21	50	18	21	5	Trace	8	2.7	0	.89	.39	4.2	—
Tongue, beef, braised	3 oz. 85	210	18	14	—	—	—	Trace	6	1.9	—	.04	.25	3.0	—
Turkey potpie. See Poultry potpie															
Veal, cooked															
Cutlet, without bone, broiled	3 oz. 85	185	23	9	5	4	Trace	—	9	2.7	—	.06	.21	4.6	—
Roast, medium fat, medium done; lean and fat	3 oz. 85	230	23	14	7	6	Trace	0	10	2.9	—	.11	.26	6.6	—

Food	Measure	Weight (g)	Food energy (cal)	Protein (g)	Fat (g)	Fatty acids — Saturated (total) (g)	Fatty acids — Unsaturated Oleic (g)	Fatty acids — Unsaturated Linoleic (g)	Carbohydrate (g)	Calcium (mg)	Iron (mg)	Vitamin A (IU)	Thiamin (mg)	Riboflavin (mg)	Niacin (mg)	Ascorbic acid (mg)
Fish and shellfish																
Bluefish, baked or broiled	3 oz.	85	135	22	4	—	—	—	0	25	.6	40	.09	.08	1.6	—
Clams																
Raw, meat only	3 oz.	85	65	11	1	—	—	—	2	59	5.2	90	.08	.15	1.1	8
Canned, solids and liquid	3 oz.	85	45	7	1	—	—	—	2	47	3.5	—	.01	.09	.9	—
Crabmeat, canned	3 oz.	85	85	15	2	—	—	—	1	38	.7	—	.07	.07	1.6	—
Fish sticks, breaded, cooked, frozen; stick 3.8 by 1.0 by 0.5 inch	10 sticks or 8 oz. package	227	400	38	20	5	4	10	15	25	.9	—	.09	.16	3.6	—
Haddock, fried	3 oz.	85	140	17	5	1	3	—	5	34	1.0	—	0.03	0.06	2.7	2
Mackerel																
Broiled, Atlantic	3 oz.	85	200	19	13	—	—	—	0	5	1.0	450	.13	.23	6.5	—
Canned, Pacific, solids and liquid[3]	3 oz.	85	155	18	9	—	—	—	0	221	1.9	20	.02	.28	7.4	—
Ocean perch, breaded (egg and bread-crumbs), fried	3 oz.	85	195	16	11	—	—	—	6	28	1.1	—	.08	.09	1.5	—
Oysters, meat only. Raw, 13-19 medium selects	1 cup	240	160	20	4	—	—	—	8	226	13.2	740	.33	.43	6.0	—
Oyster stew, 1 part oysters to 3 parts milk by volume, 3-4 oysters	1 cup	230	200	11	12	—	—	—	11	269	3.3	640	.13	.41	1.6	—
Salmon, pink, canned	3 oz.	85	120	17	5	1	1	Trace	0	[4]167	.7	60	.03	.16	6.8	—
Sardines, Atlantic, canned in oil, drained solids	3 oz.	85	175	20	9	—	—	—	0	372	2.5	190	.02	.17	4.6	—
Shad, baked	3 oz.	85	170	20	10	—	—	—	0	20	.5	20	.11	.22	7.3	—
Shrimp, canned, meat only	3 oz.	85	100	21	1	—	—	—	1	98	2.6	50	.01	.03	1.5	—
Swordfish, broiled with butter or margarine	3 oz.	85	150	24	5	—	—	—	0	23	1.1	1,780	.03	.04	9.3	—
Tuna, canned in oil, drained solids	3 oz.	85	170	24	7	—	—	—	0	7	1.6	70	.04	.10	10.1	—
Mature dry beans and peas, nuts, peanuts (related products)																
Almonds, shelled	1 cup	142	850	26	77	6	52	15	28	332	6.7	0	.34	1.31	5.0	Trace

[2]Outer layer of fat on the cut was removed to within approximately 1/2 inch of the lean. Deposits of fat within the cut were not removed.

[3]Vitamin values based on drained solids.

[4]Based on total contents of can. If bones are discarded, value will be greatly reduced.

Continued.

Food, approximate measure, and weight (in grams)		Food energy (calories)	Protein (g)	Fat (total lipid) (g)	Fatty acids			Carbohydrate (g)	Calcium (mg)	Iron (mg)	Vitamin A value (IU)	Thiamin (mg)	Riboflavin (mg)	Niacin (mg)	Ascorbic acid (mg)
					Saturated (total) (g)	Unsaturated									
						Oleic (g)	Linoleic (g)								
Beans, dry															
Common varieties, such as Great Northern, navy, and others, canned:															
Red	1 cup	256	230	15	1	—	—	—	42	74	4.6	Trace	.13	.10	1.5	—
White, with tomato sauce																
With pork	1 cup	261	320	16	7	3	3	1	50	141	4.7	340	.20	.08	1.5	5
Without pork	1 cup	261	310	16	1	—	—	—	60	177	5.2	160	.18	.09	1.5	5
Lima, cooked	1 cup	192	260	16	1	—	—	—	48	56	5.6	Trace	.26	.12	1.3	Trace
Brazil nuts	1 cup	140	915	20	94	19	45	24	15	260	4.8	Trace	1.34	.17	2.2	—
Cashew nuts, roasted	1 cup	135	760	23	62	10	43	4	40	51	5.1	140	.58	.33	2.4	—
Coconut																
Fresh, shredded	1 cup	97	335	3	34	29	2	Trace	9	13	1.6	0	.05	.02	.5	3
Dried, shredded, sweetened	1 cup	62	340	2	24	21	2	Trace	33	10	1.2	0	.02	.02	.2	0
Cowpeas or blackeye peas, dry, cooked	1 cup	248	190	13	1	—	—	—	34	42	3.2	20	.41	.11	1.1	Trace
Peanuts, roasted, salted																
Halves	1 cup	144	840	37	72	16	31	21	27	107	3.0	—	.46	.19	24.7	0
Chopped	1 tbsp.	9	55	2	4	1	2	1	2	7	.2	—	.03	.01	1.5	0
Peanut butter	1 tbsp.	16	95	4	8	2	4	2	3	9	.3	—	.02	.02	2.4	0
Peas, split, dry, cooked	1 cup	250	290	20	1	—	—	—	52	28	4.2	100	.37	.22	2.2	—
Pecans																
Halves	1 cup	108	740	10	77	5	48	15	16	79	2.6	140	.93	.14	1.0	2
Chopped	1 tbsp.	7.5	50	1	5	Trace	3	1	1	5	.2	10	.06	.01	.1	Trace
Walnuts, shelled																
Black or native, chopped	1 cup	126	790	26	75	4	26	36	19	Trace	7.6	380	.28	.14	.9	—
English or Persian																
Halves	1 cup	100	650	15	64	4	10	40	16	99	3.1	30	.33	.13	.9	3
Chopped	1 tbsp.	8	50	1	5	Trace	1	3	1	8	.2	Trace	.03	.01	.1	Trace
Vegetables and vegetable products																
Asparagus																
Cooked, cut spears	1 cup	175	35	4	Trace	—	—	—	6	37	1.0	1,580	.27	.32	2.4	46
Canned spears, medium																
Green	6 spears	96	20	2	Trace	—	—	—	3	18	1.8	770	.06	.10	.8	14
Bleached	6 spears	96	20	2	Trace	—	—	—	4	15	1.0	80	.05	.06	.7	14

Food	Measure															
Beans																
Lima, immature, cooked	1 cup	160	180	12	1	—	—	—	32	75	4.0	450	.29	.16	2.0	28
Snap, green																
Cooked																
In small amount of water, short time	1 cup	125	30	2	Trace	—	—	—	7	62	.8	680	.08	.11	.6	16
In large amount of water, long time	1 cup	125	30	2	Trace	—	—	—	7	62	0.8	680	0.07	0.10	0.4	13
Canned																
Solids and liquid	1 cup	239	45	2	Trace	—	—	—	10	81	2.9	690	.08	.10	.7	9
Strained or chopped (baby food)	1 oz.	28	5	Trace	Trace	—	—	—	1	9	.3	110	.01	.02	.1	Trace
Bean sprouts. See Sprouts																
Beets, cooked, diced	1 cup	165	50	2	Trace	—	—	—	12	23	.8	40	.04	.07	.5	11
Broccoli spears, cooked	1 cup	150	40	5	Trace	—	—	—	7	132	1.2	3,750	.14	.29	1.2	135
Brussels sprouts, cooked	1 cup	130	45	5	1	—	—	—	8	42	1.4	680	.10	.18	1.1	113
Cabbage																
Raw																
Finely shredded	1 cup	100	25	1	Trace	—	—	—	5	49	.4	130	.05	.05	.3	47
Coleslaw	1 cup	120	120	1	9	2	2	5	9	52	.5	180	.06	.06	.3	35
Cooked																
In small amount of water, short time	1 cup	170	35	2	Trace	—	—	—	7	75	.5	220	.07	.07	.5	56
In large amount of water, long time	1 cup	170	30	2	Trace	—	—	—	7	71	.5	200	.04	.04	.2	40
Cabbage, celery or Chinese																
Raw, leaves and stalk, 1-inch pieces	1 cup	100	15	1	Trace	—	—	—	3	43	.6	150	.05	.04	.6	25
Cabbage, spoon (or pakchoy), cooked	1 cup	150	20	2	Trace	—	—	—	4	222	.9	4,650	.07	.12	1.1	23
Carrots																
Raw																
Whole, 5½ by 1 inch, (25 thin strips)	1	50	20	1	Trace	—	—	—	5	18	.4	5,500	.03	.03	.3	4
Grated	1 cup	110	45	1	Trace	—	—	—	11	41	.8	12,100	.06	.06	.7	9
Cooked, diced	1 cup	145	45	1	Trace	—	—	—	10	48	.9	15,220	.08	.07	.7	9
Canned, strained or chopped (baby food)	1 oz.	28	10	Trace	Trace	—	—	—	2	7	.1	3,690	.01	.01	.1	1
Cauliflower, cooked, flowerbuds	1 cup	120	25	3	Trace	—	—	—	5	25	.8	70	.11	.10	.7	66

Continued.

Food, approximate measure, and weight (in grams)		Food energy (calories)	Protein (g)	Fat (total lipid) (g)	Fatty acids			Carbo-hydrate (g)	Cal-cium (mg)	Iron (mg)	Vita-min A value (IU)	Thia-min (mg)	Ribo-flavin (mg)	Niacin (mg)	Ascor-bic acid (mg)
					Satu-rated (total) (g)	Unsaturated									
						Oleic (g)	Linoleic (g)								
Celery, raw															
Stalk, large outer, 8 by about 1½ inches, at root end	1 stalk	40	5	Trace	Trace	—	—	—	2	16	.1	100	.01	.01	.1	4
Pieces, diced	1 cup	100	15	1	Trace	—	—	—	4	39	.3	240	.03	.03	.3	9
Collards, cooked	1 cup	190	55	5	1	—	—	—	9	289	1.1	10,260	.27	.37	2.4	87
Corn, sweet																
Cooked, ear 5 by 1¾ inches[5]	1 ear	140	70	3	1	—	—	—	16	2	.5	[6]310	.09	.08	1.0	7
Canned, solids and liquid	1 cup	256	170	5	2	—	—	—	40	10	1.0	[6]690	.07	.12	2.3	13
Cowpeas, cooked, imma-mature seeds	1 cup	160	175	13	1	—	—	—	29	38	3.4	560	.49	.18	2.3	28
Cucumbers, 10 oz., 7½ by about 2 inches																
Raw, pared	1	207	30	1	Trace	—	—	—	7	35	.6	Trace	.07	.09	.4	23
Raw, pared, center slice ⅛-inch thick	6 slices	50	5	Trace	Trace	—	—	—	2	8	.2	Trace	.02	.02	.1	6
Dandelion greens, cooked	1 cup	180	60	4	1	—	—	—	12	252	3.2	21,060	.24	.29	—	32
Endive, curly (including escarole)	2 oz.	57	10	1	Trace	—	—	—	2	46	1.0	1,870	.04	.08	.3	6
Kale, leaves including stems, cooked	1 cup	110	30	4	1	—	—	—	4	147	1.3	8,140	—	—	—	68
Lettuce, raw																
Butterhead, as Boston types; head, 4-inch diameter	1 head	220	30	3	Trace	—	—	—	6	77	4.4	2,130	.14	.13	.6	18
Crisphead, as Iceberg; head, 4¾-inch diameter	1 head	454	60	4	Trace	—	—	—	13	91	2.3	1,500	.29	.27	1.3	29
Looseleaf, or bunching varieties, leaves	2 large	50	10	1	Trace	—	—	—	2	34	.7	950	.03	.04	.2	9
Mushrooms, canned, solids and liquid	1 cup	244	40	5	Trace	—	—	—	6	15	1.2	Trace	.04	.60	4.8	4
Mustard greens, cooked	1 cup	140	35	3	1	—	—	—	6	193	2.5	8,120	.11	.19	.9	68
Okra, cooked, pod 3 by ⅝ inch	8 pods	85	25	3	Trace	—	—	—	5	78	.4	420	.11	.15	.8	17

Onions															
Mature															
Raw, onion 2½-inch diameter	1	110	40	2	Trace	—	—	10	30	0.6	40	0.04	0.04	0.2	11
Cooked	1 cup	210	60	3	Trace	—	—	14	50	.8	80	.06	.06	.4	14
Young green, small, without tops	6	50	20	1	Trace	—	—	5	20	.3	Trace	.02	.02	.2	12
Parsley, raw, chopped	1 tbsp.	3.5	1	Trace	Trace	—	—	Trace	7	.2	300	Trace	.01	Trace	6
Parsnips, cooked	1 cup	155	100	2	1	—	—	23	70	.9	50	.11	.13	.2	16
Peas, green															
Cooked	1 cup	160	115	9	1	—	—	19	37	2.9	860	.44	.17	3.7	33
Canned, solids and liquid	1 cup	249	165	9	1	—	—	31	50	4.2	1,120	.23	.13	2.2	22
Canned, strained (baby food)	1 oz.	28	15	1	Trace	—	—	3	3	.4	140	.02	.02	.4	3
Peppers, hot, red, without seeds, dried (ground chili powder, added seasonings)	1 tbsp.	15	50	2	2	—	—	8	40	2.3	9,750	.03	.17	1.3	2
Peppers, sweet															
Raw, medium, about 6 per pound															
Green pod without stem and seeds	1 pod	62	15	1	Trace	—	—	3	6	.4	260	.05	.05	.3	79
Red pod without stem and seeds	1 pod	60	20	1	Trace	—	—	4	8	.4	2,670	.05	.05	.3	122
Canned, pimentos, medium	1 pod	38	10	Trace	Trace	—	—	2	3	.6	870	.01	.02	.1	36
Potatoes, medium (about 3 per pound raw)															
Baked, peeled after baking	1	99	90	3	Trace	—	—	21	9	.7	Trace	.10	.04	1.7	20
Boiled															
Peeled after boiling	1	136	105	3	Trace	—	—	23	10	.8	Trace	.13	.05	2.0	22
Peeled before boiling	1	122	80	2	Trace	—	—	18	7	.6	Trace	.11	.04	1.4	20
French-fried, piece 2 by ½ by ½ inch															
Cooked in deep fat	10 pieces	57	155	2	7	2	2	4	20	9	.7	Trace	.07	.04	1.8	12
Frozen, heated	10 pieces	57	125	2	5	1	1	2	19	5	1.0	Trace	.08	.01	1.5	12
Mashed															
Milk added	1 cup	195	125	4	1	—	—	25	47	.8	50	.16	.10	2.0	19
Milk and butter added	1 cup	195	185	4	8	4	3	Trace	24	47	.8	330	.16	.10	1.9	18

Continued.

[5]Measure and weight apply to entire vegetable or fruit including parts not usually eaten.

[6]Based on yellow varieties; white varieties contain only a trace of cryptoxanthin and carotenes, the pigments in corn that have biological activity.

Food, approximate measure, and weight (in grams)		(grams)	Food energy (calories)	Protein (g)	Fat (total lipid) (g)	Fatty acids			Carbohydrate (g)	Calcium (mg)	Iron (mg)	Vitamin A value (IU)	Thiamin (mg)	Riboflavin (mg)	Niacin (mg)	Ascorbic acid (mg)
						Saturated (total) (g)	Unsaturated Oleic (g)	Linoleic (g)								
Potato chips, medium, 2-inch diameter	10 chips	20	115	1	8	3	2	4	10	8	.4	Trace	.04	.01	1.0	3
Pumpkin, canned	1 cup	228	75	2	1	—	—	—	18	57	.9	14,590	.07	.12	1.3	12
Radishes, raw, small, without tops	4	40	5	Trace	Trace	—	—	—	1	12	.4	Trace	.01	.01	.1	10
Sauerkraut, canned, solids and liquid	1 cup	235	45	2	Trace	—	—	—	9	85	1.2	120	.07	.09	.4	33
Spinach																
Cooked	1 cup	180	40	5	1	—	—	—	6	167	4.0	14,580	.13	.25	1.0	50
Canned, drained solids	1 cup	180	45	5	1	—	—	—	6	212	4.7	14,400	.03	.21	.6	24
Canned, strained or chopped (baby food)	1 oz.	28	10	1	Trace	—	—	—	2	18	.2	1,420	.01	.04	.1	2
Sprouts, raw																
Mung bean	1 cup	90	30	3	Trace	—	—	—	6	17	1.2	20	.12	.12	.7	17
Soybean	1 cup	107	40	6	2	—	—	—	4	46	.7	90	.17	.16	.8	4
Squash																
Cooked																
Summer, diced	1 cup	210	30	2	Trace	—	—	—	7	52	.8	820	.10	.16	1.6	21
Winter, baked, mashed	1 cup	205	130	4	1	—	—	—	32	57	1.6	8,610	.10	.27	1.4	27
Canned, winter, strained and chopped (baby food)	1 oz.	28	10	Trace	Trace	—	—	—	2	7	.1	510	.01	.01	.1	1
Sweetpotatoes																
Cooked, medium, 5 by 2 inches, weight raw about 6 oz.																
Baked, peeled after baking	1	110	155	2	1	—	—	—	36	44	1.0	8,910	.10	.07	.7	24
Boiled, peeled after boiling	1	147	170	2	1	—	—	—	39	47	1.0	11,610	.13	.09	.9	25
Candied, 3½ by 2¼ inches	1	175	295	2	6	2	3	1	60	65	1.6	11,030	.10	.08	.8	17
Canned, vacuum or solid pack	1 cup	218	235	4	Trace	—	—	—	54	54	1.7	17,000	.10	.10	1.4	30

Food	Measure	Weight (g)	Food energy (cal)	Protein (g)	Fat (g)	Saturated (g)	Oleic (g)	Linoleic (g)	Carbohydrate (g)	Calcium (mg)	Iron (mg)	Vitamin A (IU)	Thiamine (mg)	Riboflavin (mg)	Niacin (mg)	Ascorbic acid (mg)
Tomatoes																
Raw, medium, 2 by 2½ inches, about 3 per pound	1	150	35	2	Trace	—	—	—	7	20	.8	1,350	.10	.06	1.0	[7]34
Canned	1 cup	242	50	2	Trace	—	—	—	10	15	1.2	2,180	.13	.07	1.7	40
Tomato juice, canned	1 cup	242	45	2	Trace	—	—	—	10	17	2.2	1,940	.13	.07	1.8	39
Tomato catsup	1 tbsp.	17	15	Trace	Trace	—	—	—	4	4	.1	240	.02	.01	.3	3
Turnips, cooked, diced	1 cup	155	35	1	Trace	—	—	—	8	54	.6	Trace	.06	.08	.5	33
Turnip greens, Cooked																
In small amount of water, short time	1 cup	145	30	3	Trace	—	—	—	5	267	1.6	9,140	.21	.36	.8	100
In large amount of water, long time	1 cup	145	25	3	Trace	—	—	—	5	252	1.4	8,260	.14	.33	.8	68
Canned, solids and liquid	1 cup	232	40	3	1	—	—	—	7	232	3.7	10,900	.04	.21	1.4	44
Fruits and fruit products																
Apples, raw, medium, 2½-inch diameter, about 3 per pound[5]	1	150	70	Trace	Trace	—	—	—	18	8	.4	50	.04	.02	.1	3
Apple brown betty	1 cup	230	345	4	8	4	3	Trace	68	41	1.4	230	.13	.10	.9	3
Apple juice, bottled or canned	1 cup	249	120	Trace	Trace	—	—	—	30	15	1.5	—	.01	.04	.2	2
Applesauce, canned																
Sweetened	1 cup	254	230	1	Trace	—	—	—	60	10	1.3	100	.05	.03	.1	3
Unsweetened or artificially sweetened	1 cup	239	100	Trace	Trace	—	—	—	26	10	1.2	100	.04	.02	.1	2
Applesauce and apricots, canned, strained or junior (baby food)	1 oz.	28	25	Trace	Trace	—	—	—	6	1	.1	170	Trace	Trace	Trace	1
Apricots																
Raw, about 12 per pound[5]	3 apricots	114	55	1	Trace	—	—	—	14	18	.5	2,890	.03	.04	.7	10
Canned in heavy syrup																
Halves and syrup	1 cup	259	220	2	Trace	—	—	—	57	28	.8	4,510	.05	.06	.9	10
Halves (medium) and syrup	4 halves; 2 tbsp. syrup	122	105	1	Trace	—	—	—	27	13	.4	2,120	.02	.03	.4	5

Continued.

[5]Measure and weight apply to entire vegetable or fruit including parts not usually eaten.

[7]Year-round average. Samples marketed from November through May average around 15 milligrams per 150-gram tomato; from June through October, around 39 milligrams.

Food, approximate measure, and weight (in grams)			Food energy (calories)	Protein (g)	Fat (total lipid) (g)	Fatty acids			Carbohydrate (g)	Calcium (mg)	Iron (mg)	Vitamin A value (IU)	Thiamin (mg)	Riboflavin (mg)	Niacin (mg)	Ascorbic acid (mg)
						Saturated (total) (g)	Unsaturated Oleic (g)	Linoleic (g)								
Apricots—cont'd																
Dried																
Uncooked, 40 halves, small	1 cup	150	390	8	1	—	—	—	100	100	8.2	16,350	.02	.23	4.9	19
Cooked, unsweetened, fruit and liquid	1 cup	285	240	5	1	—	—	—	62	63	5.1	8,550	.01	.13	2.8	8
Apricot nectar, canned	1 cup	250	140	1	Trace	—	—	—	36	22	.5	2,380	.02	.02	.5	7
Avocados, raw																
California varieties, mainly Fuerte																
10-ounce avocado, about 3½ by 4¼ inches, peeled, pitted	½	108	185	2	18	4	8	2	6	11	.6	310	.12	.21	1.7	15
½-inch cubes	1 cup	152	260	3	26	5	12	3	9	15	.9	440	.16	.30	2.4	21
Florida varieties																
13 oz. avocado, about 4 by 3 inches, peeled, pitted	½	123	160	2	14	3	6	2	11	12	.7	360	.13	.24	2.0	17
½-inch cubes	1 cup	152	195	2	17	3	8	2	13	15	.9	440	.16	.30	2.4	21
Bananas, raw, 6 by 1½ inches, about 3 per pound[5]	1	150	85	1	Trace	—	—	—	23	8	.7	190	.05	.06	.7	10
Blackberries, raw	1 cup	144	85	2	1	—	—	—	19	46	1.3	290	.05	.06	.5	30
Blueberries, raw	1 cup	140	85	1	1	—	—	—	21	21	1.4	140	.04	.08	.6	20
Cantaloups, raw; medium, 5-inch diameter, about 1⅔ pounds[5]	½	385	60	1	Trace	—	—	—	14	27	.8	[8] 6,540	.08	.06	1.2	63
Cherries																
Raw, sweet, with stems[5]	1 cup	130	80	2	Trace	—	—	—	20	26	.5	130	.06	.07	.5	12
Canned, red, sour, pitted, heavy syrup	1 cup	260	230	2	1	—	—	—	59	36	.8	1,680	.07	.06	.4	13
Cranberry juice cocktail, canned	1 cup	250	160	Trace	Trace	—	—	—	41	12	.8	Trace	.02	.02	.1	(⁹)

Food	Measure															
Cranberry sauce, sweetened, canned, strained	1 cup	277	405	Trace	1	—	—	—	104	17	.6	40	.03	0.3	.1	5
Dates, domestic, natural and dry, pitted, cut	1 cup	178	490	4	1	—	—	—	130	105	5.3	90	.16	.17	3.9	0
Figs																
Raw, small, 1½-inch diameter, about 12 per pound	3 figs	114	90	1	Trace	—	—	—	23	40	.7	90	.07	.06	.5	2
Dried, large, 2 by 1 inch	1 fig	21	60	1	Trace	—	—	—	15	26	.6	20	.02	.02	.1	0
Fruit cocktail, canned in heavy syrup, solids and liquid	1 cup	256	195	1	1	—	—	—	50	23	1.0	360	.04	.03	1.1	5
Grapefruit																
Raw, medium, 4¼-inch diameter, size 64																
White[5]	½	285	55	1	Trace	—	—	—	14	22	.6	10	.05	.02	.2	52
Pink or red[5]	½	285	60	1	Trace	—	—	—	15	23	.6	640	.05	.02	.3	52
Raw sections, white	1 cup	194	75	1	Trace	—	—	—	20	31	.8	20	.07	.03	.3	72
Canned, white																
Syrup pack, solids and liquid	1 cup	249	175	1	Trace	—	—	—	44	32	.7	20	.07	.04	.5	75
Water pack, solids and liquid	1 cup	240	70	1	Trace	—	—	—	18	31	.7	20	.07	.04	.5	72
Grapefruit juice																
Fresh	1 cup	246	95	1	Trace	—	—	—	23	22	.5	([10])	.09	.04	.4	92
Canned, white																
Unsweetened	1 cup	247	100	1	Trace	—	—	—	24	20	1.0	20	.07	.04	.4	84
Sweetened	1 cup	250	130	1	Trace	—	—	—	32	20	1.0	20	.07	.04	.4	78
Frozen, concentrate, unsweetened																
Undiluted, can, 6 fluid oz.	1 can	207	300	4	1	—	—	—	72	70	.8	60	.29	.12	1.4	286
Diluted with 3 parts water, by volume	1 cup	247	100	1	Trace	—	—	—	24	25	.2	20	.10	.04	.5	96
Frozen, concentrate, sweetened																
Undiluted, can, 6 fluid oz.	1 can	211	350	3	1	—	—	—	85	59	.6	50	.24	.11	1.2	245
Diluted with 3 parts water, by volume	1 cup	249	115	1	Trace	—	—	—	28	20	.2	20	.08	.03	.4	82

Continued.

[5]Measure and weight apply to entire vegetable or fruit including parts not usually eaten.

[8]Value based on varieties with orange-colored flesh; for green-fleshed varieties value is about 540 I.U. per ½ melon.

[9]About 5 milligrams per 8 fluid ounces is from cranberries. Ascorbic acid is usually added to approximately 100 milligrams per 8 fluid ounces.

[10]For white-fleshed varieties value is about 20 I.U. per cup; for red-fleshed varieties, 1,080 I.U. per cup.

Food, approximate measure, and weight (in grams)		Food energy (calories)	Protein (g)	Fat (total lipid) (g)	Fatty acids Saturated (total) (g)	Fatty acids Unsaturated Oleic (g)	Fatty acids Unsaturated Linoleic (g)	Carbohydrate (g)	Calcium (mg)	Iron (mg)	Vitamin A value (IU)	Thiamin (mg)	Riboflavin (mg)	Niacin (mg)	Ascorbic acid (mg)
Grapefruit juice—cont'd															
Dehydrated															
Crystals, can, net weight 4 oz.	1 can	114	430	5	1	—	—	—	103	99	1.1	90	.41	.18	2.0	399
Prepared with water (1 pound yields about 1 gal.)	1 cup	247	100	1	Trace	—	—	—	24	22	.2	20	.10	.05	.5	92
Grapes, raw															
American type (slip skin), such as Concord, Delaware, Niagara, Catawba, and Scuppernong[5]	1 cup	153	65	1	1	—	—	—	15	15	.4	100	.05	.03	.2	3
European type (adherent skin), such as Malaga, Muscat, Thompson Seedless, Emperor, and Flame Tokay[5]	1 cup	160	95	1	Trace	—	—	—	25	17	.6	140	.07	.04	.4	6
Grape juice, bottled or canned	1 cup	254	165	1	Trace	—	—	—	42	28	.8	—	.10	.05	.6	Trace
Lemons, raw, medium, 2½-inch diameter, size 150[5]	1 lemon	106	20	1	Trace	—	—	—	6	18	.4	10	.03	.01	.1	38
Lemon juice															
Fresh	1 cup	246	60	1	Trace	—	—	—	20	17	.5	40	.08	.03	.2	113
	1 tbsp.	15	5	Trace	Trace	—	—	—	1	1	Trace	Trace	Trace	Trace	Trace	7
Canned, unsweetened	1 cup	245	55	1	Trace	—	—	—	19	17	.5	40	.07	.03	.2	102
Lemonade concentrate, frozen, sweetened															
Undiluted, can, 6 fluid oz.	1 can	220	430	Trace	Trace	—	—	—	112	9	.4	40	.05	.06	.7	66
Diluted with 4⅓ parts water, by volume	1 cup	248	110	Trace	Trace	—	—	—	28	2	.1	10	.01	.01	.2	17
Lime juice															
Fresh	1 cup	246	65	1	Trace	—	—	—	22	22	.5	30	.05	.03	.03	80
Canned	1 cup	246	65	1	Trace	—	—	—	22	22	.5	30	.05	.03	.3	52

Food	Measure															
Limeade concentrate, frozen, sweetened																
Undiluted, can, 6 fluid oz.	1 can	218	410	Trace	Trace	—	—	—	108	11	.2	Trace	Trace	Trace	.3	26
Diluted with 4⅓ parts water, by volume	1 cup	248	105	Trace	Trace	—	—	—	27	2	Trace	Trace	Trace	Trace	Trace	6
Oranges, raw																
California, Navel (winter), 2⁴/₅-inch diameter, size 88[5]	1 orange	180	60	2	Trace	—	—	—	16	49	.5	240	.12	.05	.5	75
Florida, all varieties, 3-inch diameter[5]	1	210	75	1	Trace	—	—	—	19	67	.3	310	.16	.06	.6	70
Orange juice																
Fresh																
California, Valencia (summer)	1 cup	249	115	2	1	—	—	—	26	27	.7	500	.22	.06	.9	122
Florida varieties																
Early and mid-season	1 cup	247	100	1	Trace	—	—	—	23	25	.5	490	.22	.06	.9	127
Late season, Valencia	1 cup	248	110	1	Trace	—	—	—	26	25	.5	500	.22	.06	.9	92
Canned, unsweetened	1 cup	249	120	2	Trace	—	—	—	28	25	1.0	500	.17	.05	.6	100
Frozen concentrate																
Undiluted, can, 6 fluid oz.	1 can	210	330	5	Trace	—	—	—	80	69	.8	1,490	.63	.10	2.4	332
Diluted with 3 parts water, by volume	1 cup	248	110	2	Trace	—	—	—	27	22	.2	500	.21	.03	.8	112
Dehydrated																
Crystals, can, net weight 4 oz.	1 can	113	430	6	2	—	—	—	100	95	1.9	1,900	.76	.24	3.3	406
Prepared with water, 1 lb. yields about 1 gal.	1 cup	248	115	1	Trace	—	—	—	27	25	.5	500	.20	.06	.9	108
Orange and grapefruit juice																
Frozen concentrate																
Undiluted, can, 6 fluid oz.	1 can	209	325	4	1	—	—	—	78	61	.8	790	.47	.06	2.3	301
Diluted with 3 parts water, by volume	1 cup	248	110	1	Trace	—	—	—	26	20	.3	270	.16	.02	.8	102
Papayas, raw, ½-inch cubes	1 cup	182	70	1	Trace	—	—	—	18	36	.5	3,190	.07	.08	.5	102

Continued.

[5]Measure and weight apply to entire vegetable or fruit including parts not usually eaten.

Food, approximate measure, and weight (in grams)		(grams)	Food energy (calories)	Protein (g)	Fat (total lipid) (g)	Fatty acids			Carbohydrate (g)	Calcium (mg)	Iron (mg)	Vitamin A value (IU)	Thiamin (mg)	Riboflavin (mg)	Niacin (mg)	Ascorbic acid (mg)
						Saturated (total) (g)	Unsaturated Oleic (g)	Linoleic (g)								
Peaches																
Raw																
Whole, medium, 2-inch diameter, about 4 per pound[5]	1	114	35	1	Trace	—	—	—	10	9	.5	[11]1,320	.02	.05	1.0	7
Sliced	1 cup	168	65	1	Trace	—	—	—	16	15	.8	[11]2,230	.03	.08	1.6	12
Canned, yellow-fleshed, solids and liquid																
Syrup pack, heavy																
Halves or slices	1 cup	257	200	1	Trace	—	—	—	52	10	.8	1,100	.02	.06	1.4	7
Halves (medium) and syrup	2 halves and 2 tbsp. syrup	117	90	Trace	Trace	—	—	—	24	5	.4	500	.01	.03	.7	3
Water pack	1 cup	245	75	1	Trace	—	—	—	20	10	.7	1,100	.02	.06	1.4	7
Strained or chopped (baby food)	1 oz.	28	25	Trace	Trace	—	—	—	6	2	.1	140	Trace	.01	.2	1
Dried																
Uncooked	1 cup	160	420	5	1	—	—	—	109	77	9.6	6,240	.02	.31	8.5	28
Cooked, unsweetened, 10-12 halves and 6 tbsp. liquid	1 cup	270	220	3	1	—	—	—	58	41	5.1	3,290	.01	.15	4.2	6
Frozen																
Carton, 12 oz., not thawed	1 carton	340	300	1	Trace	—	—	—	77	14	1.7	2,210	.03	.14	2.4	[12]135
Can, 16 oz., not thawed	1 can	454	400	2	Trace	—	—	—	103	18	2.3	2,950	.05	.18	3.2	[12]181
Peach nectar, canned	1 cup	250	120	Trace	Trace	—	—	—	31	10	.5	1,080	.02	.05	1.0	1
Pears																
Raw, 3 by 2½-inch diameter[5]	1	182	100	1	1	—	—	—	25	13	.5	30	.04	.07	.2	7
Canned, solids and liquid																
Syrup pack, heavy																
Halves or slices	1 cup	255	195	1	1	—	—	—	50	13	.5	Trace	.03	.05	.3	4
Halves (medium) and syrup	2 halves and 2 tbsp. syrup	117	90	Trace	Trace	—	—	—	23	6	.2	Trace	.01	.02	.2	2

Water pack	1 cup	243	80	Trace	Trace	—	—	—	20	12	.5	Trace	.02	.05	.3	4
Strained or chopped (baby food)	1 oz.	28	20	Trace	Trace	—	—	—	5	2	.1	10	Trace	.01	.1	1
Pear nectar, canned	1 cup	250	130	1	1	—	—	—	33	8	.2	Trace	.01	.05	Trace	1
Persimmons, Japanese or kaki, raw, seedless, 2½-inch diameter[5]	1	125	75	1	1	—	—	—	20	6	.4	2,740	.01	.02	.1	11
Pineapple																
Raw, diced	1 cup	140	75	1	Trace	—	—	—	19	24	.7	100	.12	.04	.3	24
Canned, heavy syrup pack, solids and liquid																
Crushed	1 cup	260	195	1	1	—	—	—	50	29	.8	120	.20	.06	.5	17
Sliced, slices and juice	2 small or 1 large and 2 tbsp. juice	122	90	Trace	Trace	—	—	—	24	13	.4	50	.09	.03	.2	8
Pineapple juice, canned	1 cup	249	135	1	1	—	—	—	34	37	.7	120	.12	.04	.5	22
Plums, all except prunes																
Raw, 2-inch diameter, about 2 ounces[5]	1	60	25	Trace	Trace	—	—	—	7	7	.3	140	.02	.02	.3	3
Canned, syrup pack (Italian prunes)																
Plums (with pits) and juice[5]	1 cup	256	205	1	1	—	—	—	53	22	2.2	2,970	.05	.05	.9	4
Plums (without pits) and juice	3 plums and 2 tbsp. juice	122	100	Trace	Trace	—	—	—	26	11	1.1	1,470	.03	.02	.5	2
Prunes, dried, "softenized," medium																
Uncooked[5]	4	32	70	1	Trace	—	—	—	18	14	1.1	440	.02	.04	.4	1
Cooked, unsweetened, 17-18 prunes and ⅓ cup liquid[5]	1 cup	270	295	2	1	—	—	—	78	60	4.5	1,860	.08	.18	1.7	2
Prunes with tapioca, canned, strained or junior (baby food)	1 oz.	28	25	Trace	Trace	—	—	—	6	2	.3	110	.01	.02	.1	1
Prune juice, canned	1 cup	256	200	1	Trace	—	—	—	49	36	10.5	—	.02	.03	1.1	4
Raisin, dried	1 cup	160	460	4	Trace	—	—	—	124	99	5.6	30	.18	.13	.9	2

Continued.

[5] Measure and weight apply to entire vegetable or fruit including parts not usually eaten.

[11] Based on yellow-fleshed varieties; for white-fleshed varieties value is about 50 I.U. per 114-gram peach and 80 I.U. per cup of sliced peaches.

[12] Average weighted in accordance with commercial freezing practices. For products without added ascorbic acid, value is about 37 milligrams per 12-ounce carton and 50 milligrams per 16-ounce can; for those with added ascorbic acid, 139 milligrams per 12 ounces and 186 milligrams per 16 ounces.

Food, approximate measure, and weight (in grams)		Food energy (calories)	Protein (g)	Fat (total lipid) (g)	Fatty acids			Carbohydrate (g)	Calcium (mg)	Iron (mg)	Vitamin A value (IU)	Thiamin (mg)	Riboflavin (mg)	Niacin (mg)	Ascorbic acid (mg)
					Saturated (total) (g)	Unsaturated Oleic (g)	Unsaturated Linoleic (g)								
Raspberries, red															
Raw	1 cup	123	70	1	1	—	—	—	17	27	1.1	160	.04	.11	1.1	31
Frozen, 10 oz. carton, not thawed	1 carton	284	275	2	1	—	—	—	70	37	1.7	200	.06	.17	1.7	59
Rhubarb, cooked, sugar added	1 cup	272	385	1	Trace	—	—	—	98	212	1.6	220	.06	.15	.7	17
Strawberries															
Raw, capped	1 cup	149	55	1	1	—	—	—	13	31	1.5	90	.04	.10	1.0	88
Frozen, 10-oz. carton, not thawed	1 carton	284	310	1	1	—	—	—	79	40	2.0	90	.06	.17	1.5	150
Frozen, 16-ounce can, not thawed	1 can	454	495	2	1	—	—	—	126	64	3.2	150	.09	.27	2.4	240
Tangerines, raw, medium, 2½-inch diameter, about 4 per pound[5]	1	114	40	1	Trace	—	—	—	10	34	.3	350	.05	.02	.1	26
Tangerine juice															
Tangerine juice															
Canned, unsweetened	1 cup	248	105	1	Trace	—	—	—	25	45	.5	1,040	.14	.04	.3	56
Frozen concentrate															
Undiluted, can, 6 fluid oz.	1 can	210	340	4	1	—	—	—	80	130	1.5	3,070	.43	.12	.9	202
Diluted with 3 parts water, by volume	1 cup	248	115	1	Trace	—	—	—	27	45	.5	1,020	.14	.04	.3	67
Watermelon, raw, wedge, 4 by 8 inches (1/16 of 10 by 16-inch melon, about 2 pounds with rind)[5]	1 wedge	925	115	2	1	—	—	—	27	30	2.1	2,510	.13	.13	.7	30
Barley, pearled, light, uncooked	1 cup	203	710	17	2	Trace	1	1	160	32	4.1	0	.25	.17	6.3	0
Biscuits, baking powder with enriched flour, 2½-inch diameter	1	38	140	3	6	2	3	1	17	46	.6	Trace	.08	.08	.7	Trace
Bran flakes (40 percent bran) added thiamine	1 oz.	28	85	3	1	—	—	—	23	20	1.2	0	.11	.05	1.7	0

Food	Measure															
Bread																
Boston brown bread, slice, 3 by ¾ inch	1 slice	48	100	3	1	—	—	—	22	43	.9	0	.05	.03	.6	0
Cracked-wheat bread																
Loaf, 1-pound, 20 slices	1 loaf	454	1,190	39	10	2	5	2	236	399	5.0	Trace	.53	.42	5.8	Trace
Slice	1	23	60	2	1	—	—	—	12	20	.3	Trace	.03	.02	.3	Trace
French or Vienna bread																
Enriched, 1-pound loaf	1 loaf	454	1,315	41	14	2	8	3	251	195	10.0	Trace	1.26	.98	11.3	Trace
Unenriched, 1-pound loaf	1 loaf	454	1,315	41	14	2	8	3	251	195	3.2	Trace	.39	.39	3.6	Trace
Italian bread																
Enriched, 1-pound loaf	1 loaf	454	1,250	41	4	2	1	Trace	256	77	10.0	0	1.31	.93	11.7	0
Unenriched, 1-pound loaf	1 loaf	454	1,250	41	4	2	1	Trace	256	77	3.2	0	.39	.27	3.6	0
Raisin bread																
Loaf, 1-pound, 20 slices	1 loaf	454	1,190	30	13	2	8	3	243	322	5.9	Trace	.24	.42	3.0	Trace
Slice	1	23	60	2	1	—	—	—	12	16	.3	Trace	.01	.02	.2	Trace
Rye bread																
American, light (⅓ rye, ⅔ wheat)																
Loaf, 1-pound, 20 slices	1 loaf	454	1,100	41	5	—	—	—	236	340	7.3	0	.81	.33	6.4	0
Slice	1	23	55	2	Trace	—	—	—	12	17	.4	0	.04	.02	.3	0
Pumpernickel, loaf, 1 pound	1 loaf	454	1,115	41	5	—	—	—	241	381	10.9	0	1.05	.63	5.4	0
White bread, enriched																
1 to 2 percent nonfat dry milk																
Loaf, 1-pound, 20 slices	1 loaf	454	1,225	39	15	2	8	3	229	318	10.9	Trace	1.13	.77	10.4	Trace
Slice	1	23	60	2	1	Trace	Trace	Trace	12	16	.6	Trace	.06	.04	.5	Trace
3 to 4 percent nonfat dry milk[13]																
Loaf, 1-pound	1	454	1,225	39	15	2	8	3	229	381	11.3	Trace	1.13	.95	10.8	Trace
Slice, 20 per loaf	1	23	60	2	1	Trace	Trace	Trace	12	19	.6	Trace	.06	.05	.6	Trace
Slice, toasted	1	20	60	2	1	Trace	Trace	Trace	12	19	.6	Trace	.05	.05	.6	Trace
Slice, 26 per loaf	1	17	45	1	1	Trace	Trace	Trace	9	14	.4	Trace	.04	.04	.4	Trace

Continued.

[5]Measure and weight apply to entire vegetable or fruit including parts not usually eaten.

[13]When the amount of nonfat dry milk in commercial white bread is unknown, values for bread with 3 to 4% nonfat dry milk are suggested.

Food, approximate measure, and weight (in grams)		Food energy (calories)	Protein (g)	Fat (total lipid) (g)	Fatty acids			Carbohydrate (g)	Calcium (mg)	Iron (mg)	Vitamin A value (IU)	Thiamin (mg)	Riboflavin (mg)	Niacin (mg)	Ascorbic acid (mg)
					Saturated (total) (g)	Unsaturated Oleic (g)	Unsaturated Linoleic (g)								
Bread—cont'd															
White bread, enriched—cont'd															
5 to 6 percent nonfat dry milk															
Loaf, 1-pound, 20 slices	1 loaf	454	1,245	41	17	4	10	2	228	435	11.3	Trace	1.22	.91	11.0	Trace
Slice	1	23	65	2	1	Trace	Trace	Trace	12	22	.6	Trace	.06	.05	.6	Trace
White bread, unenriched															
1 to 2 percent nonfat dry milk															
Loaf, 1-pound, 20 slices	1 loaf	454	1,225	39	15	3	8	2	229	318	3.2	Trace	.40	.36	5.6	Trace
Slice	1	23	60	2	1	Trace	Trace	Trace	12	16	.2	Trace	.02	.02	.3	Trace
3 to 4 percent nonfat dry milk[13]															
Loaf, 1-pound	1 loaf	454	1,225	39	15	3	8	—	229	381	3.2	Trace	.31	.39	5.0	Trace
Slice, 20 per loaf	1 slice	23	60	2	1	Trace	Trace	Trace	12	19	.2	Trace	.02	.02	.3	Trace
Slice, toasted	1 slice	20	60	2	1	Trace	Trace	Trace	12	19	.2	Trace	.01	.02	.3	Trace
Slice, 26 per loaf	1 slice	17	45	1	1	Trace	Trace	Trace	9	14	.1	Trace	.01	.01	.2	Trace
5 to 6 percent nonfat dry milk															
Loaf, 1-pound, 20 slices	1 loaf	454	1,245	41	17	4	10	2	228	435	3.2	Trace	.32	.39	4.1	Trace
Slice	1	23	65	2	1	Trace	Trace	Trace	12	22	.2	Trace	.02	.03	.2	Trace
Whole-wheat bread, made with 2 percent nonfat dry milk															
Loaf, 1-pound, 20 slices	1 loaf	454	1,105	48	14	3	6	3	216	449	10.4	Trace	1.17	.56	12.9	Trace
Slice	1	23	55	2	1	Trace	Trace	Trace	11	23	.5	Trace	.06	.03	.7	Trace
Slice, toasted	1	19	55	2	1	Trace	Trace	Trace	11	22	.5	Trace	.05	.03	.6	Trace
Breadcrumbs, dry, grated	1 cup	88	345	11	4	1	2	1	65	107	3.2	Trace	.19	.26	3.1	Trace
Cakes[14]															
Angelfood cake; sector, 2-inch (1/12 of 8-inch-diameter cake)	1 sector	40	110	3	Trace	—	—	—	24	4	.1	0	Trace	.06	.1	0
Chocolate cake, chocolate icing; sector, 2-inch (1/16 of 10-inch-diameter layer cake)	1 sector	120	445	5	20	8	10	1	67	84	1.2	[15]190	.03	.12	.3	Trace

Food	Measure	Weight	Food energy	Protein	Fat	Saturated	Oleic	Linoleic	Carbohydrate	Calcium	Iron	Vitamin A	Thiamine	Riboflavin	Niacin	Ascorbic acid
Fruitcake, dark (made with enriched flour); piece, 2 by 2 by ½ inch	1 piece	30	115	1	5	1	3	1	18	22	.8	[15]40	.04	.04	.2	Trace
Gingerbread (made with enriched flour); piece, 2 by 2 by 2 inches	1 piece	55	175	2	6	1	4	Trace	29	37	1.3	50	.06	.06	.5	0
Plain cake and cupcakes, without icing																
Piece, 3 by 2 by 1½ inches	1	55	200	2	8	2	5	1	31	35	.2	[15]590	.01	.05	.1	Trace
Cupcake, 2¾-inch diameter	1	40	145	2	6	1	3	Trace	22	26	.2	[15]570	.01	.03	.1	Trace
Plain cake and cupcakes, with chocolate icing																
Sector, 2-inch (1/16 of 10-inch-layer cake)	1	100	370	4	14	5	7	1	59	63	.6	[15]180	.02	.09	.2	Trace
Cupcake, 2¾-inch diameter	1	50	185	2	7	2	4	Trace	30	32	.3	[15]590	.01	.04	.1	Trace
Poundcake, old-fashioned (equal weights flour, sugar, fat, eggs); slice, 2¾ by 3 by ⅝ inch	1 slice	30	140	2	9	2	5	1	14	6	.2	[15]580	.01	.03	.1	0
Sponge cake; sector, 2-inch (1/12 of 8-inch-diameter cake)	1	40	120	3	2	1	1	Trace	22	12	.5	180	.02	.06	.1	Trace
Cookies																
Plain and assorted, 3-inch diameter	1 cooky	25	120	1	5	—	—	—	18	9	.2	20	.01	.01	.1	Trace
Fig bars, small	1	16	55	1	1	—	—	—	12	12	.2	20	.01	.01	.1	Trace
Corn, rice and wheat flakes, mixed, added nutrients	1 oz.	28	110	2	Trace	—	—	—	24	11	.5	0	.11	—	.9	0
Corn flakes, added nutrients																
Plain	1 oz.	28	110	2	Trace	—	—	—	24	5	.4	0	.12	.02	.6	0
Sugar-covered	1 oz.	28	110	1	Trace	—	—	—	26	3	.3	0	.12	.01	.5	0

Continued.

[13]When the amount of nonfat dry milk in commercial white bread is unknown, values for bread with 3 to 4% nonfat dry milk are suggested.

[14]Unenriched cake flour and vegetable cooking fat used unless otherwise specified.

[15]If the fat used in the recipe is butter or fortified margarine, the vitamin A value for chocolate cake with chocolate icing will be 490 I.U. per 2-inch sector; 100 I.U. for fruitcake; for plain cake without icing, 300 I.U. per piece; 220 I.U. per cupcake; for plain cake with icing, 440 I.U. per 2-inch sector; 220 I.U. per cupcake; and 300 I.U. for poundcake.

Food, approximate measure, and weight (in grams)		Food energy (calories)	Protein (g)	Fat (total lipid) (g)	Fatty acids			Carbohydrate (g)	Calcium (mg)	Iron (mg)	Vitamin A value (IU)	Thiamin (mg)	Riboflavin (mg)	Niacin (mg)	Ascorbic acid (mg)
					Saturated (total) (g)	Unsaturated Oleic (g)	Linoleic (g)								
Corn grits, degermed, cooked															
Enriched	1 cup	242	120	3	Trace	—	—	—	27	2	[16].7	[17]150	[16].10	[16].07	[16]1.0	0
Unenriched	1 cup	242	120	3	Trace	—	—	—	27	2	.2	[17]150	.05	.02	.5	0
Cornmeal, white or yellow, dry															
Whole ground, unbolted	1 cup	118	420	11	5	1	2	2	87	24	2.8	[17]600	.45	.13	2.4	0
Degermed, enriched	1 cup	145	525	11	2	Trace	1	1	114	9	[16]4.2	[17]640	[16].64	[16].38	[16]5.1	0
Corn muffins, made with enriched degermed cornmeal and enriched flour; muffin, 2¾-inch diameter	1 muffin	48	150	3	5	2	2	Trace	23	50	.8	[18]80	.09	.11	.8	Trace
Corn, puffed, pre-sweetened, added nutrients	1 oz.	28	110	1	Trace	—	—	—	26	3	.5	0	.12	.05	.6	0
Corn, shredded, added nutrients	1 oz.	28	110	2	Trace	—	—	—	25	1	.7	0	.12	.05	.6	0
Crackers															
Graham, plain	4 small or 2 medium	14	55	1	1	—	—	—	10	6	.2	0	.01	.03	.2	0
Saltines, 2 inches squares	2 crackers	8	35	1	1	—	—	—	6	2	.1	0	Trace	Trace	.1	0
Soda Cracker, 2½ inches square	2 crackers	11	50	1	1	Trace	1	Trace	8	2	.2	0	Trace	Trace	.1	0
Oyster crackers	10 crackers	10	45	1	1	Trace	1	Trace	7	2	.2	0	Trace	Trace	.1	0
Cracker meal	1 tbsp.	10	45	1	1	Trace	1	Trace	7	2	.1	0	Trace	Trace	.1	0
Doughnuts, cake type	1 doughnut	32	125	1	6	1	4	Trace	16	13	[19].4	30	[19].05	[19].05	[19].4	0
Farina, regular, enriched, cooked	1 cup	238	100	3	Trace	—	—	—	21	10	[16].7	0	[16].11	[16].07	[16]1.0	0
Macaroni, cooked Enriched															
Cooked, firm stage (8 to 10 minutes; undergoes additional cooking in a food mixture)	1 cup	130	190	6	1	—	—	—	39	14	[16]1.4	0	[16].23	[16].14	[16]1.9	0

	Measure															
Cooked until tender Unenriched	1 cup	140	155	5	1	—	—	—	32	11	1.3[16]	0	.19[16]	.11[16]	1.5[16]	0
Cooked, firm stage (8 to 10 minutes; undergoes additional cooking in a food mixture)	1 cup	130	190	6	1	—	—	—	39	14	.6	0	.02	.02	.5	0
Cooked until tender	1 cup	140	155	5	1	—	—	—	32	11	.6	0	.02	.02	.4	0
Macaroni (enriched) and cheese, baked	1 cup	220	470	18	24	11	10	1	44	398	2.0	950	.22	.44	2.0	Trace
Muffins, with enriched white flour; muffin, 2¾-inch diameter	1	48	140	4	5	1	3	Trace	20	50	.8	50	.08	.11	.7	Trace
Noodles (egg noodles), cooked																
Enriched	1 cup	160	200	7	2	1	1	Trace	37	16	1.4[16]	110	.23[16]	.14[16]	1.8[16]	0
Unenriched	1 cup	160	200	7	2	1	1	Trace	37	16	1.0	110	.04	.03	.7	0
Oats (with or without corn) puffed, added nutrients	1 oz.	28	115	3	2	Trace	1	1	21	50	1.3	0	.28	.05	.5	0
Oatmeal or rolled oats, regular or quick-cooking, cooked	1 cup	236	130	5	2	Trace	1	1	23	21	1.4	0	.19	.05	.3	0
Pancakes (griddlecakes), 4-inch diameter																
Wheat, enriched flour (home recipe)	1 cake	27	60	2	2	Trace	1	Trace	9	27	.4	30	.05	.06	.3	Trace
Buckwheat (buckwheat pancake mix, made with egg and milk)	1 cake	27	55	2	2	1	1	Trace	6	59	.4	60	.03	.04	.2	Trace
Piecrust, plain, baked Enriched flour																
Lower crust, 9-inch shell	1	135	675	8	45	10	29	3	59	19	2.3	0	.27	.19	2.4	0
Double crust, 9-inch pie	1	270	1,350	16	90	21	58	7	118	38	4.6	0	.55	.39	4.9	0

Continued.

[16] Iron, thiamine, riboflavin, and niacin are based on the minimum levels of enrichment specified in standards of identity promulgated under the Federal Food, Drug, and Cosmetic Act.

[17] Vitamin A value based on yellow product. White product contains only a trace.

[18] Based on recipe using white cornmeal; if yellow cornmeal is used, the vitamin A value is 140 I.U. per muffin.

[19] Based on product made with enriched flour. With unenriched flour, approximate values per doughnut are: Iron, 0.2 milligram; thiamine, 0.01 milligram; riboflavin, 0.03 milligram; niacin, 0.2 milligram.

Food, approximate measure, and weight (in grams)		weight (in grams)	Food energy (calories)	Protein (g)	Fat (total lipid) (g)	Fatty acids Saturated (total) (g)	Unsaturated Oleic (g)	Unsaturated Linoleic (g)	Carbohydrate (g)	Calcium (mg)	Iron (mg)	Vitamin A value (IU)	Thiamin (mg)	Riboflavin (mg)	Niacin (mg)	Ascorbic acid (mg)
Piecrust, plain, baked—cont'd																
Unenriched flour																
Lower crust, 9-inch shell	1	135	675	8	45	10	29	3	59	19	.7	0	.04	.04	.6	0
Double crust, 9-inch pie	1	270	1,350	16	90	21	58	7	118	38	1.4	0	.08	.07	1.3	0
Pies (piecrust made with unenriched flour); sector, 4-inch, 1/7 of 9-inch-diameter pie																
Apple	1 sector	135	345	3	15	4	9	1	51	11	.4	40	.03	.02	.5	1
Cherry	1 sector	135	355	4	15	4	10	1	52	19	.4	590	.03	.03	.6	1
Custard	1 sector	130	280	8	14	5	8	1	30	125	.8	300	.07	.21	.4	0
Lemon meringue	1 sector	120	305	4	12	4	7	1	45	17	.6	200	.04	.10	.2	4
Mince	1 sector	135	365	3	16	4	10	1	56	38	1.4	Trace	.09	.05	.5	1
Pumpkin	1 sector	130	275	5	15	5	7	1	32	66	.6	3,210	.04	.13	.6	Trace
Pizza (cheese); 5½-inch sector; 1/8 of 14-inch-diameter pie	1 sector	75	185	7	6	2	3	Trace	27	107	.7	290	.04	.12	.7	4
Popcorn, popped, with added oil and salt	1 cup	14	65	1	3	2	Trace	Trace	8	1	.3	—	—	.01	.2	0
Pretzels, small stick	5 sticks	5	20	Trace	Trace	—	—	—	4	1	0	0	Trace	Trace	Trace	0
Rice, white (fully milled or polished), enriched, cooked																
Common commercial varieties, all types	1 cup	168	185	3	Trace	—	—	—	41	17	[20] 1.5	0	[20] .19	[20] .01	[20] 1.6	0
Long grain, parboiled	1 cup	176	185	4	Trace	—	—	—	41	33	[20] 1.4	0	[20] .19	[20] .02	[20] 2.0	0
Rice, puffed, added nutrients (without salt)	1 cup	14	55	1	Trace	—	—	—	13	3	.3	0	.06	.01	.6	0
Rice flakes, added nutrients	1 cup	30	115	2	Trace	—	—	—	26	9	.5	0	.10	.02	1.6	0
Rolls																
Plain, pan; 12 per 16 ounces																
Enriched	1 roll	38	115	3	2	Trace	1	Trace	20	28	.7	Trace	.11	.07	.8	Trace
Unenriched	1 roll	38	115	3	2	Trace	1	Trace	20	28	.3	Trace	.02	.03	.3	Trace
Hard, round; 12 per 22 oz.	1 roll	52	160	5	2	Trace	1	Trace	31	24	.4	Trace	.03	.05	.4	Trace
Sweet, pan; 12 per 18 oz.	1 roll	43	135	4	4	1	2	Trace	21	37	.3	30	.03	.06	.4	Trace

Food	Measure	Grams													
Rye wafers, whole-grain, 1⅞ by 3½ inches	2 wafers	13	45	2	Trace	—	—	—	10	7	.5	0	.04	.03	.2	0
Spaghetti																
Cooked, tender stage (14 to 20 minutes)																
Enriched	1 cup	140	155	5	1	—	—	—	32	11	[16] 1.3	0	[16] .19	[16] .11	[16] 1.5	0
Unenriched	1 cup	140	155	5	1	—	—	—	32	11	.6	0	.02	.02	.4	0
Spaghetti with meat balls in tomato sauce (home recipe)	1 cup	250	335	19	12	4	6	1	39	125	3.8	1,600	.26	.30	4.0	22
Spaghetti in tomato sauce with cheese (home recipe)	1 cup	250	260	9	9	2	5	1	37	80	2.2	1,080	.24	.18	2.4	14
Waffles, with enriched flour, ½ by 4½ by 5½ inches	1	75	210	7	7	2	4	1	28	85	1.3	250	.13	.19	1.0	Trace
Wheat, puffed																
With added nutrients (without salt)	1 oz.	28	105	4	Trace	—	—	—	22	8	1.2	0	.15	.07	2.2	0
With added nutrients, with sugar and honey	1 oz.	28	105	2	1	—	—	—	25	7	.9	0	.14	.05	1.8	0
Wheat, rolled; cooked	1 cup	236	175	5	1	—	—	—	40	19	1.7	0	.17	.06	2.1	0
Wheat, shredded, plain (long, round, or bite-size)	1 oz.	28	100	3	1	—	—	—	23	12	1.0	0	.06	.03	1.2	0
Wheat and malted barley flakes, with added nutrients	1 oz.	28	110	2	Trace	—	—	—	24	14	.7	0	.13	.03	1.1	0
Wheat flakes, with added nutrients	1 oz.	28	100	3	Trace	—	—	—	23	12	1.2	0	.18	.04	1.4	0
Wheat flours																
Whole-wheat, from hard wheats, stirred	1 cup	120	400	16	2	Trace	1	1	85	49	4.0	0	.66	.14	5.2	0
All-purpose or family flour																
Enriched, sifted	1 cup	110	400	12	1	Trace	Trace	Trace	84	18	[16] 3.2	0	[16] .48	[16] .29	[16] 3.8	0
Unenriched, sifted	1 cup	110	400	12	1	Trace	Trace	Trace	84	18	.9	0	.07	.05	1.0	0
Self-rising, enriched	1 cup	110	385	10	1	Trace	Trace	Trace	82	292	[16] 3.2	0	[16] .49	[16] .29	[16] 3.9	0
Cake or pastry flour, sifted	1 cup	100	365	8	1	Trace	Trace	Trace	79	17	.5	0	.03	.03	.7	0
Wheat germ, crude, commercially milled	1 cup	68	245	18	7	1	2	4	32	49	6.4	0	1.36	.46	2.9	0

Continued.

[16] Iron, thiamine, riboflavin, and niacin are based on the minimum levels of enrichment specified in standards of identity promulgated under the Federal Food, Drug, and Cosmetic Act.

[20] Iron, thiamine, and niacin are based on the minimum levels of enrichment specified in standards of identity promulgated under the Federal Food, Drug, and Cosmetic Act. Riboflavin is based on unenriched rice. When the minimum level of enrichment for riboflavin specified in the standards of identity becomes effective the value will be 0.12 milligram per cup of parboiled rice and of white rice.

Food, approximate measure, and weight (in grams)		Food energy (calories)	Protein (g)	Fat (total lipid) (g)	Fatty acids			Carbohydrate (g)	Calcium (mg)	Iron (mg)	Vitamin A value (IU)	Thiamin (mg)	Riboflavin (mg)	Niacin (mg)	Ascorbic acid (mg)
					Saturated (total) (g)	Unsaturated Oleic (g)	Unsaturated Linoleic (g)								
Fats, oils															
Butter, 4 sticks per pound															
Sticks, 2	1 cup	1,625	1	184	101	61	6	1	45	0	[21]7,500	—	—	—	0
Stick, 1/8	1 tbsp.	100	Trace	11	6	4	Trace	Trace	3	0	[21]460	—	—	—	0
Pat or square (64 per pound)	1	50	Trace	6	3	2	Trace	Trace	1	0	[21]230	—	—	—	0
Fats, cooking															
Lard	1 cup	1,985	0	220	84	101	22	0	0	0	0	0	0	0	0
Lard	1 tbsp.	125	0	14	5	6	1	0	0	0	0	0	0	0	0
Vegetable fats	1 cup	1,770	0	200	46	130	14	0	0	0	—	0	0	0	0
Vegetable fats	1 tbsp.	110	0	12	3	8	1	0	0	0	—	0	0	0	0
Margarine, 4 sticks per pound															
Sticks, 2	1 cup	1,635	1	184	37	105	33	1	45	0	[22]7,500	—	—	—	0
Stick, 1/8	1 tbsp.	100	Trace	11	2	6	2	Trace	3	0	[22]460	—	—	—	0
Pat or square (64 per pound)	1 pat	50	Trace	6	1	3	1	Trace	1	0	[22]230	—	—	—	0
Oils, salad or cooking															
Corn	1 tbsp.	125	0	14	1	4	7	0	0	0	—	0	0	0	0
Cottonseed	1 tbsp.	125	0	14	4	3	7	0	0	0	—	0	0	0	0
Olive	1 tbsp.	125	0	14	2	11	1	0	0	0	—	0	0	0	0
Soybean	1 tbsp.	125	0	14	2	3	7	0	0	0	—	0	0	0	0
Salad dressings															
Blue cheese	1 tbsp.	80	1	8	2	2	4	1	13	Trace	30	Trace	.02	Trace	Trace
Commercial, mayonnaise type	1 tbsp.	65	Trace	6	1	1	3	2	2	Trace	30	Trace	Trace	Trace	—
French	1 tbsp.	60	Trace	6	1	1	3	3	2	.1	—	—	—	—	—
Home cooked, boiled	1 tbsp.	30	1	2	1	1	Trace	3	15	.1	80	.01	.03	Trace	Trace
Mayonnaise	1 tbsp.	110	Trace	12	2	3	6	Trace	3	.1	40	Trace	.01	Trace	Trace
Thousand island	1 tbsp.	75	Trace	8	1	2	4	2	2	.1	50	Trace	Trace	Trace	Trace
Sugars, sweets															
Candy															
Caramels	1 oz.	115	1	3	2	1	Trace	22	42	.4	Trace	.01	.05	Trace	Trace
Chocolate, milk, plain	1 oz.	150	2	9	5	3	Trace	16	65	.3	80	.02	.09	.1	Trace
Fudge, plain	1 oz.	115	1	3	2	1	Trace	21	22	.3	Trace	.01	.03	.1	Trace

Note: The "weight (in grams)" values for each row: Sticks, 2 = 227; Stick, 1/8 = 14; Pat = 7; Lard (cup) = 220; Lard (tbsp.) = 14; Vegetable fats (cup) = 200; Vegetable fats (tbsp.) = 12.5; Margarine Sticks, 2 = 227; Margarine Stick, 1/8 = 14; Margarine pat = 7; Corn/Cottonseed/Olive/Soybean = 14 each; Blue cheese = 16; Commercial = 15; French = 15; Home cooked, boiled = 17; Mayonnaise = 15; Thousand island = 15; Caramels = 28; Chocolate, milk, plain = 28; Fudge, plain = 28.

Food	Measure	Grams	Food energy (calories)	Protein (g)	Fat (g)	Saturated fatty acids (g)	Oleic (g)	Linoleic (g)	Carbohydrate (g)	Calcium (mg)	Iron (mg)	Vitamin A (I.U.)	Thiamine (mg)	Riboflavin (mg)	Niacin (mg)	Ascorbic acid (mg)
Hard candy	1 oz.	28	110	0	Trace	—	—	—	28	6	.5	0	0	0	0	0
Marshmallows	1 oz.	28	90	1	Trace	—	—	—	23	5	.5	0	0	Trace	Trace	0
Chocolate sirup, thin type	1 tbsp.	20	50	Trace	Trace	—	—	—	13	3	.3	—	Trace	.01	.1	0
Honey, strained or extracted	1 tbsp.	21	65	Trace	0	—	—	—	17	1	.1	0	Trace	.01	.1	Trace
Jams and preserves	1 tbsp.	20	55	Trace	Trace	—	—	—	14	4	.2	Trace	Trace	.01	Trace	Trace
Jellies	1 tbsp.	20	55	Trace	Trace	—	—	—	14	4	.3	Trace	Trace	.01	Trace	1
Molasses, cane																
Light (first extraction)	1 tbsp.	20	50	—	—	—	—	—	13	33	.9	—	.01	.01	Trace	—
Blackstrap (third extraction)	1 tbsp.	20	45	—	—	—	—	—	11	137	3.2	—	.02	.04	.4	—
Sirup, table blends (chiefly corn, light and dark)	1 tbsp.	20	60	0	0	—	—	—	15	9	.8	0	0	0	0	0
Sugars (cane or beet)																
Granulated	1 cup	200	770	0	0	—	—	—	199	0	.2	0	0	0	0	0
	1 tbsp.	12	45	0	0	—	—	—	12	0	Trace	0	0	0	0	0
Lump, 1⅛ by ¾ by ⅜	1 lump	6	25	0	0	—	—	—	6	0	Trace	0	0	0	0	0
Powdered, stirred before measuring	1 cup	128	495	0	0	—	—	—	127	0	.1	0	0	0	0	0
	1 tbsp.	8	30	0	0	—	—	—	8	0	Trace	0	0	0	0	0
Brown, firm-packed	1 cup	220	820	0	0	—	—	—	212	187	7.5	0	.02	.07	.4	0
	1 tbsp.	14	50	0	0	—	—	—	13	12	.5	0	Trace	Trace	Trace	0
Miscellaneous items																
Beer (average 3.6 percent alcohol by weight)	1 cup	240	100	1	0	—	—	—	9	12	Trace	—	.01	.07	1.6	—
Beverages, carbonated																
Cola type	1 cup	240	95	0	0	—	—	—	24	—	—	0	0	0	0	0
Ginger ale	1 cup	230	70	0	0	—	—	—	18	—	—	0	0	0	0	0
Bouillon cube, ⅝ inch	1 cube	4	5	1	Trace	—	—	—	Trace	—	—	—	—	—	—	—
Chili powder. See Vegetables, peppers																
Chili sauce (mainly tomatoes)	1 tbsp.	17	20	Trace	Trace	—	—	—	4	3	.1	240	.02	.01	.3	3
Chocolate																
Bitter or baking	1 oz.	28	145	3	15	8	6	Trace	8	22	1.9	20	.01	.07	.4	0
Sweet	1 oz.	28	150	1	10	6	4	Trace	16	27	.4	Trace	.01	.04	.1	Trace
Cider. See Fruits, apple juice																

Continued.

[21] Year-round average.
[22] Based on the average vitamin A content of fortified margarine. Federal specifications for fortified margarine require a minimum of 15,000 I.U. of vitamin A per pound.

Food, approximate measure, and weight (in grams)			Food energy (calories)	Protein (g)	Fat (total lipid) (g)	Fatty acids			Carbohydrate (g)	Calcium (mg)	Iron (mg)	Vitamin A value (IU)	Thiamin (mg)	Riboflavin (mg)	Niacin (mg)	Ascorbic acid (mg)
						Saturated (total) (g)	Unsaturated Oleic (g)	Linoleic (g)								
Gelatin, dry																
Plain	1 tbsp.	10	35	9	Trace	—	—	—	—	—	—	—	—	—	—	—
Dessert powder, 3-oz. package	½ cup	85	315	8	0	—	—	—	75	—	—	—	—	—	—	—
Gelatin dessert, ready-to-eat																
Plain	1 cup	239	140	4	0	—	—	—	34	—	—	—	—	—	—	—
With fruit	1 cup	241	160	3	Trace	—	—	—	40	—	—	—	—	—	—	—
Olives, pickled																
Green	4 medium or 3 extra large or 2 giant	16	15	Trace	2	Trace	2	Trace	Trace	8	.2	40	—	—	—	—
Ripe: Mission	3 small or 2 large	10	15	Trace	2	Trace	2	Trace	Trace	9	.1	10	Trace	Trace	—	—
Pickles, cucumber																
Dill, large, 4 by 1¾ inches	1	135	15	1	Trace	—	—	—	3	35	1.4	140	Trace	.03	Trace	8
Sweet, 2¾ by ¾ inches	1	20	30	Trace	Trace	—	—	—	7	2	.2	20	Trace	Trace	Trace	1
Popcorn. See Grain products																
Sherbet, orange	1 cup	193	260	2	2	—	—	—	59	31	Trace	110	.02	.06	Trace	4
Soups, canned; ready-to-serve (prepared with equal volume of water)																
Bean with pork	1 cup	250	170	8	6	1	2	2	22	62	2.2	650	.14	.07	1.0	2
Beef noodle	1 cup	250	70	4	3	1	1	1	7	8	1.0	50	.05	.06	1.1	Trace

Food	Measure	Grams	Food energy	Protein	Fat	Saturated	Oleic	Linoleic	Carbohydrate	Calcium	Iron	Vitamin A	Thiamine	Riboflavin	Niacin	Ascorbic acid
Beef bouillon, broth, consomme	1 cup	240	30	5	0	0	0	0	3	Trace	.5	Trace	Trace	.02	1.2	—
Chicken noodle	1 cup	250	65	4	2	Trace	1	1	8	10	.5	50	.02	.02	.8	Trace
Clam chowder	1 cup	255	85	2	3	—	—	—	13	36	1.0	920	.03	.03	1.0	—
Cream soup (mushroom)	1 cup	240	135	2	10	1	3	5	10	41	.5	70	.02	.12	.7	Trace
Minestrone	1 cup	245	105	5	3	—	—	—	14	37	1.0	2,350	.07	.05	1.0	—
Pea, green	1 cup	245	130	6	2	Trace	1	Trace	23	44	1.0	340	.05	.05	1.0	7
Tomato	1 cup	245	90	2	2	Trace	1	1	16	15	.7	1,000	.06	.05	1.1	12
Vegetable with beef broth	1 cup	250	80	3	2	—	—	—	14	20	.8	3,250	.05	.02	1.2	—
Starch (cornstarch)	1 cup	128	465	Trace	Trace	—	—	—	112	0	0	0	0	0	0	0
	1 tbsp.	8	30	Trace	Trace	—	—	—	7	0	0	0	0	0	0	0
Tapioca, quick-cooking granulated, dry, stirred before measuring	1 cup	152	535	1	Trace	—	—	—	131	15	.6	0	0	0	0	0
	1 tbsp.	10	35	Trace	Trace	—	—	—	9	1	Trace	0	0	0	0	0
Vinegar	1 tbsp.	15	2	0	0	—	—	—	1	1	.1	—	—	—	—	—
White sauce, medium	1 cup	265	430	10	33	18	11	1	23	305	.5	1,220	.12	.44	.6	Trace
Yeast																
Baker's																
Compressed	1 oz.	28	25	3	Trace	—	—	—	3	4	1.4	Trace	.20	.47	3.2	Trace
Dry active	1 oz.	28	80	10	Trace	—	—	—	11	12	4.6	Trace	.66	1.53	10.4	Trace
Brewer's, dry, debittered	1 tbsp.	8	25	3	Trace	—	—	—	3	17	1.4	Trace	1.25	.34	3.0	Trace
Yogurt. See Milk, cream, cheese; related products																

B Amino acid content of foods, 100 g, edible portion[1]

Protein content and nitrogen conversion factor	Trypto-phan (g)	Threo-nine (g)	Iso-leucine (g)	Leucine (g)	Lysine (g)	Methi-onine (g)	Cystine (g)	Phenyl-alanine (g)	Tyro-sine (g)	Valine (g)	Argi-nine (g)	Histi-dine (g)
Milk; milk products												
Milk (Protein, N × 6.38)												
Cow												
fluid, whole and non-fat (3.5% protein)	0.049	0.161	0.223	0.344	0.272	0.086	0.031	0.170	0.178	0.240	0.128	0.092
canned												
evaporated, unsweetened (7.0% protein)	0.099	0.323	0.447	0.688	0.545	0.171	0.063	0.340	0.357	0.481	0.256	0.185
condensed, sweetened (8.1% protein)	0.114	0.374	0.518	0.796	0.631	0.198	0.072	0.393	0.413	0.557	0.296	0.214
dried												
whole (25.8% protein)	0.364	1.191	1.648	2.535	2.009	0.632	0.231	1.251	1.316	1.774	0.944	0.680
nonfat (35.6% protein)	0.502	1.641	2.271	3.493	2.768	0.870	0.318	1.724	1.814	2.444	1.300	0.937
Goat (3.3% protein)	0.039	0.217	0.087	0.278	0.312	0.065	—	0.121	—	0.139	0.174	0.068
Human (1.4% protein)	0.023	0.062	0.075	0.124	0.090	0.028	0.027	0.060	0.071	0.086	0.055	0.030
Indian buffalo (4.2% protein)	0.059	0.212	0.204	0.420	0.331	0.112	0.058	0.177	—	0.255	0.136	0.086
Milk products												
Buttermilk (3.5% protein, N × 6.38)	0.038	0.165	0.219	0.348	0.291	0.082	0.032	0.186	0.137	0.262	0.168	0.099
Casein (100% protein, N × 6.29)	1.335	4.277	6.550	10.048	8.013	3.084	0.382	5.389	5.819	7.393	4.070	3.021
Cheese (protein, N × 6.38)												
blue mold (21.5% protein)	0.293	0.799	1.449	2.096	1.577	0.559	0.121	1.153	1.028	1.543	0.785	0.701
Camembert (17.5% protein)	0.239	0.650	1.179	1.706	1.284	0.455	0.099	0.938	0.837	1.256	0.639	0.571
Cheddar (25.0% protein)	0.341	0.929	1.685	2.437	1.834	0.650	0.141	1.340	1.195	1.794	0.913	0.815
Cheddar processed (23.2% protein)	0.316	0.862	1.563	2.262	1.702	0.604	0.131	1.244	1.109	1.665	0.847	0.756
cheese foods, Cheddar (20.5% protein)	0.280	0.761	1.382	1.998	1.504	0.533	0.116	1.099	0.980	1.472	0.749	0.668
cottage (17.0% protein)	0.179	0.794	0.989	1.826	1.428	0.469	0.147	0.917	0.917	0.978	0.802	0.549
cream cheese (9.0% protein)	0.080	0.408	0.519	0.923	0.721	0.229	0.085	0.547	0.408	0.538	0.313	0.278
Limburger (21.2% protein)	0.289	0.788	1.429	2.067	1.555	0.552	0.120	1.136	1.014	1.522	0.774	0.691
Parmesan (36.0% protein)	0.491	1.337	2.426	3.510	2.641	0.937	0.203	1.930	1.721	2.584	1.315	1.174

Food												
Swiss (27.5% protein)	0.375	1.021	1.853	2.681	2.017	0.715	0.155	1.474	1.315	1.974	1.004	0.896
Swiss processed (26.4% protein)	0.360	0.981	1.779	2.574	1.937	0.687	0.149	1.415	1.262	1.895	0.964	0.861
Lactalbumin (100% protein, N × 6.49)	2.203	5.239	6.209	12.342	9.060	2.250	3.405	4.360	3.806	5.686	3.498	1.911
Whey (protein, N × 6.49)												
fluid (0.9% protein)	0.010	0.048	0.052	0.074	0.055	0.013	0.018	0.023	0.009	0.045	0.017	0.011
dried (12.7% protein)	0.147	0.677	0.734	1.043	0.769	0.188	0.250	0.323	0.131	0.640	0.235	0.159

Eggs, chicken (protein, N × 6.25)

Food												
Fresh or stored												
whole (12.8% protein)	0.211	0.637	0.850	1.126	0.819	0.401	0.299	0.739	0.551	0.950	0.840	0.307
whites (10.8% protein)	0.164	0.477	0.698	0.950	0.648	0.420	0.263	0.689	0.449	0.842	0.634	0.233
yolks (16.3% protein)	0.235	0.827	0.996	1.372	1.074	0.417	0.274	0.717	0.756	1.121	1.132	0.368
Dried												
whole (46.8% protein)	0.771	2.329	3.108	4.118	2.995	1.468	1.093	2.703	2.014	3.474	3.070	1.123
whites (85.9% protein)	1.306	3.793	5.553	7.559	5.154	3.340	3.089	5.484	3.573	6.693	5.044	1.855
yolks (31.2% protein)	0.449	1.582	1.907	2.626	2.057	0.799	0.524	1.373	1.448	2.147	2.167	0.704

Meat; poultry; fish and shellfish (their products)

Meat (protein, N × 6.25)

Food												
Beef carcass or side												
thin (18.8% protein)	0.220	0.830	0.984	1.540	1.642	0.466	0.238	0.773	0.638	1.044	1.212	0.653
medium fat (17.5% protein)	0.204	0.773	0.916	1.434	1.529	0.434	0.221	0.720	0.594	0.972	1.128	0.608
fat (16.3% protein)	0.190	0.720	0.853	1.335	1.424	0.404	0.206	0.670	0.553	0.905	1.051	0.566
very fat (13.7% protein)	0.160	0.605	0.717	1.122	1.197	0.340	0.173	0.563	0.465	0.761	0.883	0.476
medium fat, trimmed to retail basis (18.2% protein)	0.213	0.804	0.952	1.491	1.590	0.451	0.230	0.748	0.617	1.010	1.174	0.632
Beef cuts, medium fat												
chuck (18.6% protein)	0.217	0.821	0.973	1.524	1.625	0.461	0.235	0.765	0.631	1.033	1.199	0.646
flank (19.9% protein)	0.232	0.879	1.041	1.630	1.738	0.494	0.252	0.818	0.675	1.105	1.283	0.691
hamburger (16.0% protein)	0.187	0.707	0.837	1.311	1.398	0.397	0.202	0.658	0.543	0.888	1.032	0.556
porterhouse (16.4% protein)	0.192	0.724	0.858	1.343	1.433	0.407	0.207	0.674	0.556	0.911	1.057	0.569
rib roast (17.4% protein)	0.203	0.768	0.910	1.425	1.520	0.432	0.220	0.715	0.590	0.966	1.122	0.604
round (19.5% protein)	0.228	0.861	1.020	1.597	1.704	0.484	0.246	0.802	0.661	1.083	1.257	0.677
rump (16.2% protein)	0.189	0.715	0.848	1.327	1.415	0.402	0.205	0.666	0.550	0.899	1.045	0.562
sirloin (17.3% protein)	0.202	0.764	0.905	1.417	1.511	0.429	0.219	0.711	0.587	0.960	1.116	0.601
Beef, canned (25.0% protein)	0.292	1.104	1.308	2.048	2.184	0.620	0.316	1.028	0.848	1.388	1.612	0.868
Beef, dried or chipped (34.3% protein)	0.401	1.515	1.795	2.810	2.996	0.851	0.434	1.410	1.163	1.904	2.212	1.191

Continued.

Courtesy Orr, M. L., and Watt, B. K.: Amino acid content of foods. Home Economics Research Report No. 4, U.S. Department of Agriculture, 1966. This selected listing reprinted here is taken from the original report of the Agricultural Research Service which contains data on 18 amino acids in 202 food items.

Protein content and nitrogen conversion factor	Trypto-phan (g)	Threo-nine (g)	Iso-leucine (g)	Leucine (g)	Lysine (g)	Methi-onine (g)	Cystine (g)	Phenyl-alanine (g)	Tyro-sine (g)	Valine (g)	Argi-nine (g)	Histi-dine (g)
Lamb carcass or side												
thin (17.1% protein)	0.222	0.782	0.886	1.324	1.384	0.410	0.224	0.695	0.594	0.843	1.114	0.476
medium fat (15.7% protein)	0.203	0.718	0.814	1.216	1.271	0.377	0.206	0.638	0.545	0.774	1.022	0.437
fat (13.0% protein)	0.168	0.595	0.674	1.007	1.052	0.312	0.171	0.528	0.451	0.641	0.847	0.362
Lamb cuts, medium fat												
leg (18.0% protein)	0.233	0.824	0.933	1.394	1.457	0.432	0.236	0.732	0.625	0.887	1.172	0.501
rib (14.9% protein)	0.193	0.682	0.772	1.154	1.206	0.358	0.195	0.606	0.517	0.734	0.970	0.415
shoulder (15.6% protein)	0.202	0.714	0.809	1.208	1.263	0.374	0.205	0.634	0.542	0.769	1.016	0.434
Pork, packer's carcass or side												
thin (14.1% protein)	0.183	0.654	0.724	1.038	1.157	0.352	0.165	0.555	0.503	0.733	0.864	0.487
medium fat (11.9% protein)	0.154	0.552	0.611	0.876	0.977	0.297	0.139	0.468	0.425	0.619	0.729	0.411
Fat (9.8% protein)	0.127	0.455	0.503	0.721	0.804	0.245	0.114	0.386	0.350	0.510	0.601	0.339
Pork cuts, medium fat, fresh												
ham (15.2% protein)	0.197	0.705	0.781	1.119	1.248	0.379	0.178	0.598	0.542	0.790	0.931	0.525
loin (16.4% protein)	0.213	0.761	0.842	1.207	1.346	0.409	0.192	0.646	0.585	0.853	1.005	0.567
miscellaneous lean cuts (14.5% protein)	0.188	0.673	0.745	1.067	1.190	0.362	0.169	0.571	0.517	0.754	0.889	0.501
Pork, cured												
bacon, medium fat (9.1% protein)	0.095	0.306	0.399	0.728	0.587	0.141	0.106	0.434	0.234	0.434	0.622	0.246
fat back or salt pork (3.9% protein)	0.006	0.141	0.110	0.367	0.317	0.055	0.043	0.157	0.052	0.168	0.379	0.035
ham (16.9% protein)	0.162	0.692	0.841	1.306	1.420	0.411	0.273	0.646	0.652	0.879	1.068	0.544
luncheon meat												
boiled ham (22.8% protein)	0.219	0.934	1.135	1.762	1.915	0.554	0.368	0.872	0.879	1.186	1.441	0.733
canned, spiced (14.9% protein)	0.143	0.610	0.741	1.161	1.252	0.362	0.241	0.570	0.575	0.775	0.942	0.479
Rabbit, domesticated, flesh only (21.9% protein)	—	1.021	1.082	1.636	1.818	0.541	—	0.793	—	1.021	1.176	0.474
Veal, carcass or side												
thin (19.7% protein)	0.258	0.854	1.040	1.444	1.645	0.451	0.233	0.801	0.709	1.018	1.283	0.634
medium fat (19.1% protein)	0.251	0.828	1.008	1.400	1.595	0.437	0.226	0.776	0.688	0.987	1.244	0.614
Fat (18.5% protein)	0.243	0.802	0.977	1.356	1.545	0.423	0.219	0.752	0.666	0.956	1.205	0.595
Veal cuts, medium fat												
round (19.5% protein)	0.256	0.846	1.030	1.429	1.629	0.446	0.231	0.792	0.702	1.008	1.270	0.627
shoulder (19.4% protein)	0.255	0.841	1.024	1.422	1.620	0.444	0.230	0.788	0.698	1.003	1.263	0.624
stew meat (18.3% protein)	0.240	0.793	0.966	1.341	1.528	0.419	0.217	0.744	0.659	0.946	1.192	0.589
Poultry (protein, N × 6.25)												
Chicken, flesh only												
broilers or fryers (20.6% protein)	0.250	0.877	1.088	1.490	1.810	0.537	0.277	0.811	0.725	1.012	1.302	0.593
hens (21.3% protein)	0.259	0.907	1.125	1.540	1.871	0.556	0.286	0.838	0.750	1.046	1.346	0.613

	1	2	3	4	5	6	7	8	9	10	11	12
Ducks, domesticated, flesh only (21.4% protein)	—	0.935	1.109	1.657	1.842	0.531	—	0.842	—	1.027	1.301	0.486
Turkey, flesh only (24.0% protein)	—	1.014	1.260	1.836	2.173	0.664	0.330	0.960	—	1.187	1.513	0.649
Fish and shellfish (protein, N × 6.25)												
Bluefish (20.5% protein)	0.203	0.889	1.040	1.548	1.797	0.597	0.276	0.761	0.554	1.092	1.155	—
Cod												
fresh (16.5% protein)	0.164	0.715	0.837	1.246	1.447	0.480	0.222	0.612	0.446	0.879	0.929	—
dried (81.8% protein)	0.811	3.547	4.149	6.178	7.172	2.382	1.099	3.036	2.212	4.358	4.607	—
Croaker (17.8% protein)	0.177	0.772	0.903	1.344	1.561	0.518	0.239	0.661	0.481	0.948	1.002	—
Eel (18.6% protein)	0.185	0.806	0.943	1.405	1.631	0.542	0.250	0.690	0.503	0.991	1.048	—
Flounder (14.9% protein)	0.148	0.646	0.756	1.125	1.306	0.434	0.200	0.553	0.403	0.794	0.839	—
Haddock (18.2% protein)	0.181	0.789	0.923	1.374	1.596	0.530	0.245	0.676	0.492	0.970	1.025	—
Halibut (18.6% protein)	0.185	0.806	0.943	1.405	1.631	0.542	0.250	0.690	0.503	0.991	1.048	—
Herring												
Atlantic (18.3% protein)	0.182	0.793	0.928	1.382	1.605	0.533	0.246	0.679	0.495	0.975	1.031	—
lake (18.5% protein)	0.184	0.802	0.938	1.397	1.622	0.539	0.249	0.687	0.500	0.986	1.042	—
Pacific (16.6% protein)	0.165	0.720	0.842	1.254	1.455	0.483	0.223	0.616	0.449	0.884	0.935	—
Mackerels												
raw, common Atlantic (18.7% protein)	0.186	0.811	0.948	1.412	1.640	0.545	0.251	0.694	0.506	0.996	1.053	—
canned, solids and liquid Atlantic (19.3% protein)	0.191	0.837	0.979	1.458	1.692	0.562	0.259	0.716	0.522	1.028	1.087	—
Pacific (21.1% protein)	0.209	0.915	1.070	1.593	1.850	0.614	0.284	0.783	0.571	1.124	1.188	—
Salmon												
raw, Pacific (Chinook or King) (17.4% protein)	0.173	0.754	0.883	1.314	1.526	0.507	0.234	0.646	0.470	0.927	0.980	—
canned, solids and liquid (sockeye or red) (20.2% protein)	0.200	0.876	1.025	1.526	1.771	0.588	0.271	0.750	0.546	1.076	1.138	—
Sardines, canned, solids and liquid Atlantic type (21.1% protein)	0.209	0.915	1.070	1.593	1.850	0.614	0.284	0.783	0.571	1.124	1.188	—
Pacific type (17.7% protein)	0.176	0.767	0.898	1.337	1.552	0.515	0.238	0.657	0.479	0.943	0.997	—
Shrimp, canned, solids and liquid (18.7% protein)	0.186	0.811	0.948	1.412	1.640	0.545	0.251	0.694	0.506	0.996	1.053	—
Products from meat, poultry, and fish (protein, N × 6.25)												
Brains (10.4% protein)	0.138	0.494	0.504	0.845	0.760	0.220	0.145	0.506	0.433	0.536	0.614	0.278
Chitterlings (8.6% protein)	0.094	0.398	0.308	0.457	0.670	0.193	0.109	0.359	0.228	0.462	1.406	0.169
Fish flour (76.0% protein)	0.754	4.378	4.232	6.189	7.381	2.019	—	2.845	—	3.916	5.204	1.289
Gelatin (85.6% protein, N × 5.55)	0.006	1.912	1.357	2.930	4.226	0.787	0.077	2.036	0.401	2.421	7.866	0.771
Gizzard, chicken (23.1% protein)	0.207	1.072	1.094	1.689	1.567	0.554	0.218	0.968	0.680	1.116	1.741	0.480

Continued.

Protein content and nitrogen conversion factor	Tryptophan (g)	Threonine (g)	Isoleucine (g)	Leucine (g)	Lysine (g)	Methionine (g)	Cystine (g)	Phenylalanine (g)	Tyrosine (g)	Valine (g)	Arginine (g)	Histidine (g)
Products from meat, poultry and fish—cont'd												
Heart												
beef or pork (16.9% protein)	0.219	0.776	0.857	1.509	1.387	0.403	0.168	0.765	0.627	0.973	1.068	0.433
chicken (20.5% protein)	0.266	0.941	1.040	1.830	1.683	0.489	0.203	0.928	0.761	1.181	1.296	0.525
Kidney												
beef (15.0% protein)	0.221	0.665	0.730	1.301	1.087	0.307	0.182	0.706	0.557	0.876	0.934	0.377
pork (16.3% protein)	0.240	0.722	0.793	1.414	1.181	0.334	0.198	0.767	0.605	0.952	1.015	0.409
sheep (16.6% protein)	0.244	0.736	0.807	1.440	1.203	0.340	0.202	0.781	0.616	0.969	1.033	0.417
Liver												
beef or pork (19.7% protein)	0.296	0.936	1.031	1.819	1.475	0.463	0.243	0.993	0.738	1.239	1.201	0.523
calf (19.0% protein)	0.286	0.903	0.994	1.754	1.423	0.447	0.234	0.958	0.711	1.195	1.158	0.505
chicken (22.1% protein)	0.332	1.050	1.156	2.040	1.655	0.520	0.272	1.114	0.827	1.390	1.347	0.587
sheep or lamb (21.0% protein)	0.316	0.998	1.099	1.939	1.572	0.494	0.259	1.058	0.786	1.320	1.280	0.558
Pancreas												
beef (13.5% protein)	0.175	0.626	0.683	1.054	0.996	0.244	—	0.562	0.590	0.724	0.771	0.266
pork (14.5% protein)	0.188	0.673	0.733	1.132	1.070	0.262	—	0.603	0.633	0.777	0.828	0.285
Pork or beef, canned (14.3% protein)	0.151	0.618	0.730	1.190	1.345	0.327	0.261	0.579	0.570	0.810	1.050	0.460
Potted meat (16.1% protein)	0.149	0.662	0.641	1.203	1.061	0.361	—	0.641	—	0.943	1.002	0.322
Sausage												
Bologna (14.8% protein)	0.126	0.606	0.718	1.061	1.191	0.313	0.185	0.540	0.481	0.744	1.028	0.398
Braunschweiger (15.4% protein)	0.172	0.668	0.754	1.291	1.200	0.320	0.187	0.700	0.471	0.956	0.954	0.458
frankfurters (14.2% protein)	0.120	0.582	0.688	1.018	1.143	0.300	0.177	0.518	0.461	0.713	0.986	0.382
head cheese (15.0% protein)	0.079	0.418	0.509	0.946	0.907	0.250	0.209	0.569	0.569	0.617	1.075	0.278
liverwurst (16.7% protein)	0.187	0.724	0.818	1.400	1.301	0.347	0.203	0.759	0.510	1.037	1.034	0.497
pork, links or bulk, raw (10.8% protein)	0.092	0.442	0.524	0.774	0.869	0.228	0.135	0.394	0.351	0.543	0.750	0.290
pork, bulk, canned (15.4% protein)	0.131	0.631	0.747	1.104	1.239	0.325	0.192	0.562	0.500	0.774	1.069	0.414
salami (23.9% protein)	0.203	0.979	1.159	1.713	1.923	0.505	0.298	0.872	0.776	1.201	1.660	0.642
Vienna sausage, canned (15.8% protein)	0.134	0.647	0.766	1.133	1.272	0.334	0.197	0.576	0.513	0.794	1.097	0.425
Tongue												
beef (16.4% protein)	0.197	0.708	0.792	1.286	1.364	0.357	0.207	0.661	0.548	0.840	1.065	0.412
pork (16.8% protein)	0.202	0.726	0.812	1.317	1.398	0.366	0.212	0.677	0.562	0.860	1.091	0.422
Veal and pork loaf, canned (17.2% protein)	0.198	0.627	0.859	1.236	1.258	0.418	0.209	0.619	0.468	0.958	0.916	0.388

Legumes (dry seed), common nuts, other nuts and dry seeds (their products)

Legume seeds and their products

Beans (*Phaseolus vulgaris*) (N × 6.25)												
pinto and red Mexican (23.0% protein)	0.213	0.997	1.306	1.976	1.708	0.232	0.228	1.270	0.887	1.395	1.384	0.655
red kidney												
raw (23.1% protein)	0.214	1.002	1.312	1.985	1.715	0.233	0.229	1.275	0.891	1.401	1.390	0.658
canned, solids and liquid (5.7% protein)	0.053	0.247	0.324	0.490	0.423	0.057	0.057	0.315	0.220	0.346	0.343	0.162
other common beans including navy, pea-bean, white marrow												
raw (21.4% protein)	0.199	0.928	1.216	1.839	1.589	0.216	0.212	1.181	0.825	1.298	1.287	0.609
baked with pork, canned (5.8% protein)	0.057	0.274	0.291	0.486	0.354	0.059	0.018	0.333	0.165	0.312	0.251	0.186
Black gram, raw (23.6% protein, N × 6.25)	0.242	0.801	1.390	2.062	1.510	0.332	0.287	1.242	0.551	1.450	1.552	0.559
Broadbeans, raw (25.4% protein, N × 6.25)	0.236	0.829	1.593	2.211	1.426	0.106	0.179	1.057	0.687	1.276	1.780	0.748
Chickpeas (20.8% protein, N + 6.25)	0.170	0.739	1.195	1.538	1.434	0.276	0.296	1.012	0.692	1.025	1.551	0.559
Cowpeas (22.9% protein, N × 6.25	0.220	0.901	1.110	1.715	1.491	0.352	0.297	1.198	0.678	1.293	1.473	0.692
Dolichos, twinflower (21.6% protein, N × 6.25)	0.221	0.836	1.448	1.707	1.700	0.294	0.480	1.486	0.560	1.286	1.230	0.650
Lentils, whole (25.0% protein, N × 6.25)	0.216	0.896	1.316	1.760	1.528	0.180	0.294	1.104	0.664	1.360	1.908	0.548
Lima beans (20.7% protein, N × 6.25)	0.195	0.980	1.199	1.722	1.378	0.331	0.311	1.222	0.543	1.298	1.315	0.669
Lupine (32.3% protein, N × 6.25)	—	1.101	1.618	1.964	1.447	0.114	—	1.271	—	1.328	2.718	0.811
Moth beans (24.4% protein, N × 6.25)	0.164	—	1.093	1.484	1.202	0.191	0.109	1.003	1.245	0.695	—	0.722
Mung beans (24.4% protein, 6.25)	0.180	0.765	1.351	2.202	1.667	0.265	0.152	1.167	0.390	1.444	1.370	0.543
Peanuts (26.9% protein, N × 5.46)	0.340	0.828	1.266	1.872	1.099	0.271	0.463	1.557	1.104	1.532	3.296	0.749
Peanut flour (51.2% protein, N × 5.46)	0.647	1.575	2.410	3.563	2.091	0.516	0.881	2.963	2.100	2.916	6.273	1.425
Peanut butter (26.1% protein, N × 5.46)	0.330	0.803	1.228	1.816	1.066	0.263	0.449	1.510	1.071	1.487	3.198	0.727
Peas (*Pisum sativum*) (N × 6.25)												
entire seeds (23.8% protein)	0.251	0.918	1.340	1.969	1.744	0.286	0.308	1.200	0.960	1.333	2.102	0.651
split (24.5% protein)	0.259	0.945	1.380	2.027	1.795	0.294	0.318	1.235	0.988	1.372	2.164	0.670
Pigeonpeas, without seed coat (21.9% protein, N × 6.25)	0.119	0.834	1.346	1.717	1.580	0.256	0.308	1.875	0.725	1.153	1.489	0.617
Soybeans, whole (34.9% protein, N × 5.71)	0.526	1.504	2.054	2.946	2.414	0.513	0.678	1.889	1.216	2.005	2.763	0.911
Soybean flour, flakes, and grits (protein, N × 5.71)												
low fat (44.7% protein)	0.673	1.926	2.630	3.773	3.092	0.658	0.869	2.419	1.558	2.568	3.538	1.166
medium fat (42.5% protein)	0.640	1.831	2.501	3.588	2.940	0.625	0.826	2.300	1.481	2.441	3.364	1.109
full fat (35.9% protein)	0.541	1.547	2.112	3.030	2.483	0.528	0.698	1.943	1.251	2.062	2.842	0.937
Soybean curd (7.0% protein, N × 5.71)	—	—	—	—	—	0.081	0.091	—	—	—	—	—
Soybean milk (3.4% protein, N × 5.71)	0.051	0.176	0.175	0.305	0.269	0.054	0.071	0.195	0.193	0.186	0.302	0.121
Vetch (28.8% protein, N × 6.25)	0.203	0.899	2.198	2.290	1.898	0.346	0.336	1.014	0.369	1.442	2.249	0.659

Continued.

Protein content and nitrogen conversion factor	Trypto-phan (g)	Threo-nine (g)	Iso-leucine (g)	Leucine (g)	Lysine (g)	Methi-onine (g)	Cystine (g)	Phenyl-alanine (g)	Tyro-sine (g)	Valine (g)	Argi-nine (g)	Histi-dine (g)
Common nuts and their products												
Almonds (18.6% protein, N × 5.18)	0.176	0.610	0.873	1.454	0.582	0.259	0.377	1.146	0.618	1.124	2.729	0.517
Brazil nuts (14.4% protein, N × 5.46)	0.187	0.422	0.593	1.129	0.443	0.941	0.504	0.617	0.483	0.823	2.247	0.367
Cashews (18.5% protein, N × 5.30)	0.471	0.737	1.222	1.522	0.792	0.353	0.527	0.946	0.712	1.592	2.098	0.415
Coconut (3.4% protein, N × 5.30)	0.033	0.129	0.180	0.269	0.152	0.071	0.062	0.174	0.101	0.212	0.486	0.069
Coconut meal (20.3% protein, N × 5.30)	0.199	0.770	1.076	1.605	0.908	0.421	0.372	1.038	0.605	1.268	2.899	0.414
Filberts (12.7% protein, N × 5.30)	0.211	0.415	0.853	0.939	0.417	0.139	0.165	0.537	0.434	0.934	2.171	0.288
Peanuts. See Legumes.												
Pecans (9.4% protein, N × 5.30)	0.138	0.389	0.553	0.773	0.435	0.153	0.216	0.564	0.316	0.525	1.185	0.273
Walnuts (English or Persian) (15.0% protein, N × 5.30)	0.175	0.589	0.767	1.228	0.441	0.306	0.320	0.767	0.583	0.974	2.287	0.405
Other nuts and seeds and their products (protein N × 5.30)												
Acorns (10.4% protein)	0.126	0.434	0.561	0.808	0.636	0.139	0.184	0.473	—	0.718	0.722	0.251
Amaranth (14.6% protein)	0.149	0.832	0.882	1.209	1.074	0.372	0.521	1.141	—	0.849	1.747	0.441
Balsam pear seed meal (41.9% protein)	—	—	—	—	1.265	—	—	2.609	0.617	—	5.914	0.917
Breadnut tree, Ramon (9.6% protein)	0.261	0.373	0.543	1.041	0.418	0.056	—	0.453	—	0.927	0.884	0.147
Chinese tallow tree-nut flour (57.6% protein)	0.837	2.174	3.510	4.347	1.587	0.924	0.696	2.847	2.011	4.510	10.031	1.587
Chocolate tree, Nicaragua (38.5% protein)	0.588	1.496	2.092	3.952	2.223	0.276	0.814	2.630	1.365	2.404	4.220	0.683
Cottonseed flour and meal (42.3% protein)	0.591	1.764	1.884	2.945	2.139	0.686		2.610		2.458	5.603	1.325
Earpod tree, Guanacaste (34.1% protein)	0.444	1.165	2.213	4.581	1.930	0.360	—	1.325	—	1.570	2.857	1.004
Lead tree (24.1% protein)	0.191	0.828	1.651	1.787	1.164	0.055	—	0.855	—	0.864	2.410	0.564
Pumpkin seed (30.9% protein)	0.560	0.933	1.737	2.437	1.411	0.577	—	1.749	—	1.679	4.810	0.711
Safflower seed meal (42.1% protein)	0.675	1.462	1.914	2.740	1.525	0.731	—	2.605	—	2.446	4.623	0.985
Sesame												
seed (19.3% protein)	0.331	0.707	0.951	1.679	0.583	0.637	0.495	1.457	0.951	0.885	1.992	0.441
meal (33.4% protein)	0.573	1.223	1.645	2.905	1.008	1.103	0.857	2.521	1.645	1.531	3.447	0.763
Sunflower												
kernel (23.0% protein)	0.343	0.911	1.276	1.736	0.868	0.443	0.464	1.220	0.647	1.354	2.370	0.586
meal (39.5% protein)	0.589	1.565	2.191	2.981	1.491	0.760	0.797	2.094	1.110	2.325	4.069	1.006
Grains and their products												
Barley (12.8% protein, N × 5.83)	0.160	0.433	0.545	0.889	0.433	0.184	0.257	0.661	0.466	0.643	0.659	0.239
Bread, white (4% non-fat dry milk, flour basis) (8.5% protein, N × 5.70)	0.091	0.282	0.429	0.668	0.225	0.142	0.200	0.465	0.243	0.435	0.340	0.192

Buckwheat flour												
dark (11.7% protein, N × 6.25)	0.165	0.461	0.440	0.683	0.687	0.206	0.228	0.442	0.240	0.607	0.930	0.256
light (6.4% protein, N × 6.25)	0.090	0.252	0.241	0.374	0.376	0.113	0.125	0.242	0.131	0.332	0.509	0.140
Canihua (14.7% protein, N × 6.25)	0.118	0.706	1.000	0.851	0.882	0.263	0.162	0.529	0.294	0.677	1.162	0.367
Cereal combinations												
corn and soy grits (18.0% protein, N × 6.25)	0.161	0.792	0.841	1.656	0.772	0.271	0.311	0.832	0.562	1.054	0.982	0.472
infant food, precooked, mixed cereals with non-fat dry milk and yeast (19.4% protein, N × 6.25)	0.118	—	—	—	0.273	0.310	0.137	0.543	0.447	—	0.447	0.233
oat-corn-rye mixture, puffed (14.5% protein, N × 5.83)	0.172	0.545	0.841	1.368	0.343	0.388	0.234	0.933	0.622	0.900	0.776	0.326
Corn, field (10.0% protein, N × 6.25)	0.061	0.398	0.462	1.296	0.288	0.186	0.130	0.454	0.611	0.510	0.352	0.206
Corn flour (7.8% protein, N × 6.25)	0.047	0.311	0.361	1.011	0.225	0.145	0.101	0.354	0.477	0.398	0.275	0.161
Corn grits (8.7% protein, N × 6.25)	0.053	0.347	0.402	1.128	0.251	0.161	0.113	0.395	0.532	0.444	0.306	0.180
Cornmeal												
whole ground (9.2% protein, N × 6.25)	0.056	0.367	0.425	1.192	0.265	0.171	0.119	0.418	0.562	0.470	0.324	0.190
de-germed (7.9% protein, N × 6.25)	0.048	0.315	0.365	1.024	0.228	0.147	0.102	0.359	0.483	0.403	0.278	0.163
Corn products												
flakes (8.1% protein, N × 6.25)	0.052	0.275	0.306	1.047	0.154	0.135	0.152	0.354	0.283	0.386	0.231	0.226
germ (14.5% protein, N × 6.25)	0.144	0.622	0.578	1.030	0.791	0.232	0.130	0.483	0.343	0.789	1.134	0.464
gluten (10.0% protein, N × 6.25)	0.059	0.344	0.443	1.563	0.179	0.282	0.141	0.558	0.582	0.512	0.322	0.200
hominy (8.7% protein, N × 6.25)	0.084	0.316	0.349	0.810	0.358	0.099	—	0.333	0.331	0.398	0.444	0.203
masa (2.8% protein, N × 6.25)	0.010	—	—	—	0.103	0.108	0.030	—	—	—	—	—
pozol (5.9% protein, N × 6.25)	0.042	0.336	0.304	0.591	0.234	0.087	—	0.254	—	0.267	0.197	0.122
tortilla (5.8% protein, N × 6.25)	0.031	0.235	0.345	0.939	0.145	0.111	—	0.252	—	0.304	0.223	0.128
zein (16.1% protein, N × 6.25)	0.010	0.495	0.822	3.184	—	0.281	0.162	1.664	0.981	0.654	0.286	0.216
Job's tears (13.8% protein, N × 5.83)	0.066	0.620	1.065	3.506	0.362	0.459	0.265	0.703	—	—	0.518	0.317
Millets												
foxtail millet (9.7% protein, N × 5.83)	0.103	0.323	0.790	1.737	0.218	0.291	—	0.697	—	0.717	0.374	0.218
little millet (7.2% protein, N × 5.83)	0.047	0.262	0.517	0.841	0.138	0.178	—	0.370	—	0.471	0.363	0.147
pearl millet (11.4% protein, N × 5.83)	0.248	0.456	0.635	1.746	0.383	0.270	0.152	0.506	—	0.682	0.524	0.240
ragimillet (6.2% protein, N × 5.83)	0.085	0.270	0.398	0.620	0.202	0.270	0.187	0.263	—	0.473	0.100	0.079
Oatmeal and rolled oats (14.2% protein, N × 5.83)	0.183	0.470	0.733	1.065	0.521	0.209	0.309	0.758	0.524	0.845	0.935	0.261
Quinoa (11.0% protein, N × 6.25)	0.120	0.523	0.722	0.781	0.729	0.278	0.107	0.394	0.253	0.447	0.820	0.297
Rice												
brown (7.5% protein, N × 5.95)	0.081	0.294	0.352	0.646	0.296	0.135	0.102	0.377	0.343	0.524	0.432	0.126
white and converted (7.6% protein, N × 5.95)	0.082	0.298	0.356	0.655	0.300	0.137	0.103	0.382	0.347	0.531	0.438	0.128

Continued.

Protein content and nitrogen conversion factor	Trypto-phan (g)	Threo-nine (g)	Iso-leucine (g)	Leucine (g)	Lysine (g)	Methi-onine (g)	Cystine (g)	Phenyl-alanine (g)	Tyro-sine (g)	Valine (g)	Argi-nine (g)	Histi-dine (g)
Rice products												
flakes or puffed (5.9% protein, N × 5.95)	0.046	—	—	—	0.056	—	0.044	0.286	0.124	—	0.137	0.137
germ (14.2% protein, N × 5.95)	0.270	2.177	0.630	0.838	1.707	0.420	0.169	0.750	0.929	0.938	1.559	0.430
Rye (12.1% protein, N × 5.83)	0.137	0.448	0.515	0.813	0.494	0.191	0.241	0.571	0.390	0.631	0.591	0.276
Rye flour												
light (9.4% protein, N × 5.83)	0.106	0.348	0.400	0.632	0.384	0.148	0.187	0.443	0.303	0.490	0.459	0.214
medium (11.4% protein, N × 5.83)	0.129	0.422	0.485	0.766	0.465	0.180	0.227	0.538	0.368	0.594	0.557	0.260
Sorghum (11.0% protein, N × 6.25)	0.123	0.394	0.598	1.767	0.299	0.190	0.183	0.547	0.303	0.628	0.417	0.211
Teosinte (22.0% protein, N × 6.25)	0.049	—	—	—	0.348	0.496	—	—	—	—	—	—
Wheat, whole grain												
hard red spring (14.0% protein, N × 5.83)	0.173	0.403	0.607	0.939	0.384	0.214	0.307	0.691	0.523	0.648	0.670	0.286
hard red winter (12.3% protein, N × 5.83)	0.152	0.354	0.534	0.825	0.338	0.188	0.270	0.608	0.460	0.570	0.589	0.251
soft red winter (10.2% protein, N × 5.83)	0.126	0.294	0.443	0.684	0.280	0.156	0.224	0.504	0.382	0.472	0.488	0.208
white (9.4% protein, N × 5.83)	0.116	0.271	0.408	0.630	0.258	0.143	0.206	0.464	0.351	0.435	0.450	0.192
durum (12.7% protein, N × 5.83)	0.157	0.366	0.551	0.852	0.348	0.194	0.279	0.627	0.475	0.588	0.608	0.259
Wheat flour												
whole grain (13.3% protein, N × 5.83)	0.164	0.383	0.577	0.892	0.365	0.203	0.292	0.657	0.497	0.616	0.636	0.271
intermediate extraction (12.0% protein, N × 5.70)	—	0.392	0.619	0.924	0.356	0.198	0.320	0.732	0.335	0.583	0.549	0.286
white (10.5% protein, N × 5.70)	0.129	0.302	0.483	0.809	0.239	0.138	0.210	0.577	0.539	0.453	0.466	0.210
Wheat products												
bran (12.0% protein, N × 6.31)	0.196	0.342	0.485	0.717	0.491	0.145	0.270	0.434	0.259	0.552	0.742	0.280
burghul (12.4% protein, N × 5.83)	0.070	—	—	—	0.430	0.300	0.319	—	—	—	—	—
farina (10.9% protein, N × 5.70)	0.124	—	—	—	0.199	0.143	0.184	0.579	0.447	—	0.424	0.268
flakes (10.8% protein, N × 5.70)	0.121	0.356	0.496	0.891	0.360	0.127	0.191	0.478	0.311	0.572	0.559	0.231
germ (25.2% protein, N × 5.80)	0.265	1.343	1.177	1.708	1.534	0.404	0.287	0.908	0.882	1.364	1.825	0.687
gluten, commercial (80.0% protein, N × 5.70)	0.856	2.119	3.677	5.993	1.530	1.389	1.726	4.351	2.596	3.789	3.481	1.825
gluten flour (41.4% protein, N × 5.70)	0.443	1.097	1.903	3.101	0.792	0.719	0.893	2.252	1.344	1.961	1.801	0.944
macaroni or spaghetti (12.8% protein, N × 5.70)	0.150	0.499	0.642	0.849	0.413	0.193	0.243	0.669	0.422	0.728	0.582	0.303
noodles, containing egg solids (12.6% protein, N × 5.70)	0.133	0.533	0.621	0.834	0.411	0.212	0.245	0.610	0.312	0.745	0.621	0.301
Shredded Wheat (10.1% protein, N × 5.83)	0.085	0.405	0.449	0.684	0.331	0.139	0.204	0.481	0.236	0.577	0.523	0.236
whole wheat with added germ (12.8% protein, N × 5.83)	0.136	—	—	—	0.466	—	0.246	0.755	0.481	—	0.742	0.371

Food												
Fruits (protein, N × 6.25)												
Abiu (1.7% protein)	0.028	—	—	—	0.085	0.013	—	—	—	—	—	—
Avocados (1.3% protein)	0.014	—	—	—	0.074	0.012	—	—	—	—	—	—
Bananas, ripe												
common (1.2% protein)	0.018	—	—	—	0.055	0.011	—	—	—	—	—	—
dwarf (1.2% protein)	0.012	—	—	—	0.049	0.004	—	—	—	—	—	—
Dates (2.2% protein)	0.061	0.074	0.077	—	0.065	0.027	—	0.063	0.031	0.094	0.094	0.049
Grapefruit (0.5% protein)	0.001	—	—	—	0.006	0.000	—	—	—	—	—	—
Guavas, common (1.0% protein)	0.010	—	—	—	0.030	0.010	—	—	—	—	—	—
Limes (0.8% protein)	0.003	—	—	—	0.015	0.002	—	—	—	—	—	—
Mamey (0.5% protein)	0.006	—	—	—	0.040	0.007	—	—	—	—	—	—
Mangos (0.7% protein)	0.014	—	—	—	0.093	0.008	—	—	—	—	—	—
Muskmelons (0.6% protein)	0.001	—	—	—	0.015	0.002	—	—	—	—	—	—
Oranges, sweet (0.9% protein)	0.003	—	—	—	0.024	0.003	—	—	—	—	—	—
Orange juice (0.8% protein)	0.003	—	—	—	0.021	0.002	—	—	—	—	—	—
Oranges, mandarin, including tangerines (0.8% protein)	0.005	—	—	—	0.028	0.004	—	—	—	—	—	—
Papayas (0.6% protein)	0.012	—	—	—	0.038	0.002	—	—	—	—	—	—
Pineapple (0.4% protein)	0.005	—	—	—	0.009	0.001	—	—	—	—	—	—
Plantain or baking banana (1.1% protein)	0.010	0.027	0.056	0.059	0.050	0.005	0.016	0.049	—	0.065	0.045	—
Soursop (1.0% protein)	0.011	—	—	—	0.060	0.007	—	—	—	—	—	—
Sugarapple (1.8% protein)	0.009	—	—	—	0.071	0.008	—	—	—	—	—	—
Vegetables												
Immature seeds (protein, N × 6.25)												
Corn, sweet, white or yellow												
raw (3.7% protein)	0.023	0.151	0.137	0.407	0.137	0.072	0.062	0.207	0.124	0.231	0.174	0.095
canned, solids and liquid (2.0% protein)	0.012	0.082	0.074	0.220	0.074	0.039	0.033	0.112	0.067	0.125	0.094	0.052
Cowpeas (9.4% protein)	0.099	0.353	0.465	0.653	0.617	0.131	—	0.523	—	0.513	0.615	0.310
Lima beans												
raw (7.5% protein)	0.097	0.338	0.460	0.605	0.474	0.080	0.083	0.389	0.259	0.485	0.454	0.247
canned, solids and liquid (3.8% protein)	0.049	0.171	0.233	0.306	0.240	0.041	0.042	0.197	0.131	0.246	0.230	0.125
Peas												
raw (6.7% protein)	0.056	0.245	0.308	0.418	0.316	0.054	0.073	0.257	0.163	0.274	0.595	0.109
canned solids and liquid (3.4% protein)	0.028	0.125	0.156	0.212	0.160	0.027	0.037	0.131	0.083	0.139	0.302	0.055
Leafy vegetables, raw (protein, N × 6.25)												
Amaranth (3.5% protein)	0.038	0.056	0.164	0.206	0.141	0.025	0.024	0.096	0.105	0.136	0.134	0.069
Beet greens (2.0% protein)	0.024	0.076	0.084	0.129	0.108	0.034	—	0.116	—	0.101	0.083	0.026
Brussels sprouts (4.4% protein)	0.044	0.153	0.186	0.194	0.197	0.046	—	0.148	—	0.193	0.279	0.106
Cabbage (1.4% protein)	0.011	0.039	0.040	0.057	0.066	0.013	0.028	0.030	0.030	0.043	0.105	0.025
Chard (1.4% protein)	0.014	0.058	0.060	0.076	0.055	0.004	—	0.046	—	0.055	0.035	0.018

Continued.

Protein content and nitrogen conversion factor	Trypto-phan (g)	Threo-nine (g)	Iso-leucine (g)	Leucine (g)	Lysine (g)	Methi-onine (g)	Cystine (g)	Phenyl-alanine (g)	Tyro-sine (g)	Valine (g)	Argi-nine (g)	Histi-dine (g)
Leafy vegetables, raw (protein, N × 6.25)—cont'd												
Chicory (1.6% protein)	0.024	—	—	—	0.052	0.016	0.006	—	0.040	—	—	0.024
Collards (3.9% protein)	0.055	0.114	0.121	0.218	0.202	0.046	0.059	0.124	0.151	0.195	0.258	0.087
Kale (3.9% protein)	0.042	0.139	0.133	0.252	0.121	0.035	0.036	0.158	—	0.184	0.202	0.062
Lettuce (1.2% protein)	0.012	—	—	—	0.070	0.004	—	—	—	—	—	—
Mustard greens (2.3% protein)	0.037	0.060	0.075	0.062	0.111	0.024	0.035	0.074	0.121	0.108	0.167	0.041
Parsley, curly garden (2.5% protein)	0.050	—	0.107	0.176	0.160	0.012	0.046	0.099	0.073	0.126	0.116	0.049
Spinach (2.3% protein)	0.037	0.102	0.107	0.207	0.142	0.039	0.045	0.146	0.105	0.149	0.167	0.051
Turnip greens (2.9% protein)	0.045	0.125	0.107	0.207	0.129	0.052	0.045	—	—	—	—	—
Watercress (1.7% protein)	0.028	0.084	0.076	0.131	0.091	0.010	—	0.062	0.036	0.084	0.053	0.034
Starchy roots and tubers (protein, N × 6.25)												
Apio arracacia (1.2% protein)	0.008	—	—	—	0.042	0.003	—	—	—	—	—	—
Cassava												
flour (1.6% protein)	0.021	0.044	0.045	0.066	0.066	0.010	0.018	0.045	0.030	0.049	0.159	0.025
root (1.1% protein)	0.014	0.030	0.031	0.045	0.045	0.007	0.012	0.031	0.021	0.033	0.110	0.017
Potatoes												
raw (2.0% protein)	0.021	0.079	0.088	0.100	0.107	0.025	0.019	0.088	0.036	0.107	0.099	0.029
canned, solids and liquid (1.7% protein)	0.018	0.067	0.075	0.085	0.091	0.021	0.016	0.075	0.030	0.091	0.084	0.024
flour (7.1% protein)	0.076	0.279	0.311	0.353	0.378	0.089	0.068	0.314	0.127	0.379	0.350	0.102
Sweet potatoes (Ipomaea batatas)												
raw (1.8% protein)	0.031	0.085	0.087	0.103	0.085	0.033	0.029	0.100	0.081	0.135	0.094	0.036
dehydrated (5.0% protein)	0.087	0.235	0.241	0.286	0.236	0.093	0.080	0.278	0.225	0.374	0.261	0.099
Taro (1.9% protein)	0.035	0.089	0.099	0.169	0.110	0.021	—	0.099	—	0.114	0.118	0.032
Yam (Dioscorea spp.) (2.1% protein)	0.035	—	—	—	0.110	0.034	—	—	—	—	—	—
Yautia malanga (1.7% protein)	0.023	—	—	—	0.067	0.016	—	—	—	—	—	—
Other vegetables (protein, N × 6.25)												
Asparagus												
raw (2.2% protein)	0.027	0.066	0.080	0.096	0.103	0.032	—	0.069	—	0.106	0.123	0.036
canned, solids and liquid (1.9% protein)	0.023	0.057	0.069	0.083	0.089	0.027	—	0.060	—	0.092	0.106	0.031
Beans, snap												
raw (2.4% protein)	0.033	0.091	0.109	0.139	0.126	0.035	0.024	0.057	0.050	0.115	0.101	0.045
canned, solids and liquid (1.0% protein)	0.014	0.038	0.045	0.058	0.052	0.014	0.010	0.024	0.021	0.048	0.042	0.019
Beets												
raw (1.6% protein)	0.014	0.034	0.051	0.055	0.086	0.006	—	0.027	—	0.049	0.028	0.022
canned, solids and liquid (0.9% protein)	0.008	0.019	0.029	0.031	0.048	0.003	—	0.015	—	0.028	0.016	0.012
Broccoli (3.3% protein)	0.037	0.122	0.126	0.163	0.147	0.050	—	0.119	—	0.170	0.192	0.063

Carrots												
raw (1.2% protein)	0.010	0.043	0.046	0.065	0.052	0.010	0.029	0.042	0.020	0.056	0.041	0.017
canned, solids and liquid (0.5% protein)	0.004	0.018	0.019	0.027	0.022	0.004	0.012	0.018	0.008	0.023	0.017	0.007
Cauliflower (2.4% protein)	0.033	0.102	0.104	0.162	0.134	0.047	—	0.075	0.034	0.144	0.110	0.048
Celery (1.3% protein)	0.012	—	—	—	0.021	0.015	0.006	—	0.016	—	—	—
Chayote (0.6% protein)	0.008	—	—	—	0.038	0.001	—	—	—	—	—	—
Cowpeas, yardlong, immature pod												
(3.4% protein)	0.034	—	—	—	0.203	0.021	—	—	—	—	—	—
Cucumbers (0.7% protein)	0.005	0.019	0.022	0.030	0.031	0.007	—	0.016	—	0.024	0.053	0.001
Cushaw (1.5% protein)	0.014	—	—	—	0.044	0.008	—	—	—	—	—	—
Eggplant (1.1% protein)	0.010	0.038	0.056	0.068	0.030	0.006	—	0.048	—	0.065	0.037	0.019
Mallow (3.7% protein)	0.144	0.155	—	0.259	0.155	0.030	—	0.166	—	0.181	0.189	0.063
Mushrooms												
(*Agaricus campestris*)[2]	0.006	—	0.532	0.281	—	0.167	—	—	—	0.378	0.235	—
(*Lactarius* spp.)[3]	0.006	0.156	0.201	0.139	0.088	0.021	—	0.018	—	0.116	0.021	00.27
Okra (1.8% protein)	0.018	0.066	0.069	0.101	0.076	0.022	0.017	0.065	0.079	0.091	0.093	0.030
Onions, mature (1.4% protein)	0.021	0.022	0.021	0.037	0.064	0.013	—	0.039	0.046	0.031	0.180	0.014
Peppers (1.2% protein)	0.009	0.050	0.046	0.046	0.051	0.016	—	0.055	—	0.033	0.024	0.014
Prickly pears (1.1% protein)	0.009	0.053	0.044	0.057	0.044	0.008	—	0.059	—	0.041	0.032	0.016
Pumpkin (1.2% protein)	0.016	0.028	0.044	0.063	0.058	0.011	—	0.032	0.016	0.045	0.043	0.019
Radishes (1.2% protein)	0.005	0.059	—	—	0.034	0.002	—	—	—	0.030	—	—
Seepweed (2.6% protein)	0.027	0.089	0.113	0.152	0.089	0.013	—	0.116	—	0.091	0.062	0.036
Soybean sprouts (6.2% protein)	—	0.159	0.225	0.265	0.211	0.045	—	0.186	—	0.225	0.225	0.133
Squash, summer (0.6% protein)	0.005	0.014	0.019	0.027	0.023	0.008	—	0.016	—	0.022	0.027	0.009
Tomatoes and cherry tomatoes (1.0%												
protein)	0.009	0.033	0.029	0.041	0.042	0.007	—	0.028	0.014	0.028	0.029	0.015
Turnips (1.1% protein)	—	—	0.020	—	0.057	0.012	—	0.020	0.029	—	—	—
Waxgourd, Chinese (0.4% protein)	0.002	—	—	—	0.009	0.003	—	—	—	—	—	—
Miscellaneous food items												
Vegetable patty or steak (principally wheat												
protein) (15% protein, N × 5.70)	0.142	0.411	0.884	1.079	0.321	0.253	—	0.811	—	0.705	0.597	0.321
Yeast												
baker's, compressed[4] (N × 6.25)	0.122	0.655	0.655	1.151	0.914	0.248	0.120	0.607	0.580	0.840	0.536	0.353
brewer's, dried[5] (N × 6.25)	0.710	2.353	2.398	3.226	3.300	0.836	0.548	1.902	1.902	2.723	2.250	1.251
primary, dried												
(*Saccharomyces cerevisiae*)[5] (N × 6.25)	0.636	2.353	2.708	3.300	3.337	0.851	0.444	1.813	2.472	2.553	1.931	1.103
(*Torulopsis utilis*)[5] (N × 6.25)	0.636	2.331	3.323	3.707	3.648	0.710	0.422	2.361	2.464	2.901	3.337	1.251

[2]Total nitrogen is 0.58%. This is equivalent to 2.4% protein on the basis that two-thirds of the nitrogen is protein nitrogen. If total nitrogen is used for the calculation, the protein content is 3.6%.
[3]Total nitrogen is 0.69%. This is equivalent to 2.9% protein on the basis that two-thirds of the nitrogen is protein nitrogen. If total nitrogen is used for the calculation, the protein content is 4.3%.
[4]Total nitrogen is 2.1%. This is equivalent to 10.6% protein on the basis that four-fifths of the nitrogen is protein nitrogen. If total nitrogen is used for the calculation, the protein content is 13.1%.
[5]Total nitrogen is 7.4%. This is equivalent to 36.9% protein on the basis that four-fifths of the nitrogen is protein nitrogen. If total nitrogen is used for the calculation, the protein content is 46.1%.

Sodium and potassium content of foods, 100 g, edible portion[1]

Food and description	Sodium (mg)	Potassium (mg)
Almonds		
dried	4	773
roasted and salted	198	773
Apples		
raw, pared	1	110
frozen, sliced, sweetened	14	68
Apple brown betty	153	100
Apple butter	2	252
Apple juice, canned or bottled	1	101
Applesauce, canned, sweetened	2	65
Apricots		
raw	1	281
canned, syrup pack, light	1	239
dried, sulfured, cooked, fruit, and liquid	8	318
Apricot nectar, canned (approx. 40% fruit)	Trace	151
Asparagus		
cooked spears, boiled, drained	1	183
canned spears, green		
regular pack, solids and liquid	236[2]	166
special dietary pack (low-sodium), solids and liquids	3	166
frozen		
cuts and tips, cooked, boiled, drained	1	220
spears, cooked, boiled, drained	1	238
Avocados, raw, all commercial varieties	4	604
Bacon, cured, cooked, broiled or fried, drained	1,021	236
Bacon, Canadian, cooked, broiled or fried, drained	2,555	432
Baking powders		
home use		
straight phosphate	8,220	170
special low-sodium preparations	6	10,948
Bananas, raw, common	1	370
Barbecue sauce	815	174
Bass, black sea, raw	68	256

[1] Numbers in parentheses denote values inputed—usually from another form of the food or from a similar food. Dashes denote lack of reliable data for a constituent believed to be present in measurable amount. Values are selected from Watt, B. K., and Merrill, A. L.: Composition of foods—raw, processed, prepared, U.S. Department of Agriculture, Agriculture Handbook No. 8, December, 1963.

[2] Estimated average based on addition of salt in the amount of 0.6% of the finished product.

Food and description	Sodium (mg)	Potassium (mg)
Beans, common, mature seeds, dry		
white		
cooked	7	416
canned, solids and liquid, with pork and tomato sauce	463	210
red, cooked	3	340
Beans, lima		
immature seeds		
cooked, boiled, drained	1	422
canned		
regular pack, solids and liquid	236[2]	222
special dietary pack (low-sodium), solids and liquid	4	222
frozen, thin-seeded types, commonly called baby limas, cooked,		
boiled, drained	129	394
mature seeds, dry, cooked	2	612
Beans, mung, sprouted seeds, cooked, boiled, drained	4	156
Beans, snap		
green		
cooked, boiled, drained	4	151
canned		
regular pack, solids and liquid	236[2]	95
special dietary pack (low sodium), solids and liquid	2	95
frozen, cut, cooked, boiled, drained	1	152
yellow or wax		
cooked, boiled, drained	3	151
canned		
regular pack, solids and liquid	236[2]	95
special dietary pack (low-sodium), solids and liquid	2	95
frozen, cut, cooked, boiled, drained	1	164
Beans and frankfurters, canned	539	262
Beef		
retail cuts, trimmed to retail level		
round	60	370
rump	60	370
hamburger, regular ground, cooked	47	450
Beef and vegetable stew, canned	411	174
Beef, corned, boneless		
cooked, medium-fat	1,740	150
canned corned-beef hash (with potato)	540	200
Beef, dried, cooked, creamed	716	153
Beef potpie, commercial, frozen, unheated	366	93
Beets, common, red		
canned		
regular pack, solids and liquid	236[2]	167
special dietary pack (low-sodium), solids and liquid	46	167
Beet greens, common, cooked, boiled, drained	76	332
Beverages, alcoholic		
beer, alcohol 4.5% by volume (3.6% by weight)	7	25
gin, rum, vodka, whisky		
80-proof (33.4% alcohol by weight)	1	2
86-proof (36.0% alcohol by weight)	1	2
90-proof (37.9% alcohol by weight)	1	2
94-proof (39.7% alcohol by weight)	1	2
100-proof (42.5% alcohol by weight)	1	2
wines		
dessert, alcohol 18.8% by volume (15.3% by weight)	4	75
table, alcohol 12.2% by volume (9.9% by weight)	5	92

[2]Estimated average based on addition of salt in the amount of 0.6% of the finished product.

Continued.

Food and description	Sodium (mg)	Potassium (mg)
Biscuits, baking powder, made with enriched flour	626	117
Biscuit dough, commercial, frozen	910	86
Biscuit mix, with enriched flour, and biscuits baked from mix		
mix, dry form	1,300	80
biscuits, made with milk	973	116
Blackberries, including dewberries, boysenberries, and young-		
berries, raw	1	170
Blackberries, canned, solids and liquid		
water pack, with or without artificial sweetener	1	115
syrup pack, heavy	1	109
Blueberries		
raw	1	81
frozen, not thawed, sweetened	1	66
Bluefish, cooked		
baked or broiled	104	—
fried	146	—
Boston brown bread	251	292
Bouillon cubes or powder	24,000	100
Boysenberries, frozen, not thawed, sweetened	1	105
Bran, added sugar and malt extract	1,060	1,070
Bran flakes (40% bran), added thiamine	925	—
Bran flakes with raisins, added thiamine	800	—
Brazil nuts	1	715
Breads		
cracked-wheat	529	134
French or vienna, enriched	580	90
Italian, enriched	585	74
raisin	365	233
rye, American (1/3 rye, 2/3 clear flour)	557	145
white, enriched, made with 3%-4% non-fat dry milk	507	105
whole-wheat, made with 2% non-fat dry milk	527	273
Bread crumbs, dry, grated	736	152
Bread stuffing mix and stuffings prepared from mix		
mix, dry form	1,331	172
Broccoli		
cooked spears, boiled, drained	10	267
frozen, spears, cooked, boiled, drained	12	220
Brussels sprouts, frozen, cooked, boiled, drained	14	295
Buffalo fish, raw	52	293
Bulgur (parboiled wheat)		
canned, made from hard red winter wheat		
unseasoned[3]	599	87
seasoned[4]	460	112
Butter[5]	987	23
Buttermilk, fluid, cultured (made from skim milk)	130	140
Cabbage		
common varieties (Danish, domestic, and pointed types)		
raw	20	233
cooked, boiled until tender, drained, shredded, cooked in small		
amount of water	14	163
red, raw	26	268

[3] Processed, partially debranned, whole-kernel wheat with salt added.

[4] Processed, partially debranned, whole-kernel wheat with chicken fat, chicken stock base, dehydrated onion flakes, salt, monosodium glutamate, and herbs.

[5] Values apply to salted butter. Unsalted butter contains less than 10 mg of either sodium or potassium per 100 grams. Value for vitamin A is the year-round average.

Food and description	Sodium (mg)	Potassium (mg)
Cabbage, Chinese (also called celery cabbage or petsai)	23	253
Cakes		
baked from home recipes		
angelfood	283	88
fruitcake, made with enriched flour, dark	158	496
gingerbread, made with enriched flour	237	454
plain cake or cupcake, without icing	300	79
pound, modified	178	78
frozen, commercial, devil's food, with chocolate icing	420	119
Candy		
caramels, plain or chocolate	226	192
chocolate, sweet	33	269
chocolate-coated, chocolate fudge	228	193
gum drops, starch jelly pieces	35	5
hard	32	4
marshmallows	39	6
peanut bars	10	448
Carp, raw	50	286
Carrots		
raw	47	341
canned		
regular pack, solids and liquid	236[2]	120
special dietary pack (low-sodium), solids and liquid	39	120
Cashew nuts	15[6]	464
Catfish, freshwater, raw	60	330
Cauliflower		
cooked, boiled, drained	9	206
frozen, cooked, boiled, drained	10	207
Caviar, sturgeon, granular	2,200	180
Celery, all, including green and yellow varieties		
raw	126	341
cooked, boiled, drained	88	239
Chard, Swiss, cooked, boiled, drained	86	321
Cheese straws	721	63
Cheeses		
natural cheeses		
cheddar (domestic type, commonly called American)	700	82
cottage (large or small curd)		
creamed	229	85
uncreamed	290	72
cream	250	74
parmesan	734	149
Swiss (domestic)	710	104
pasteurized process cheese, American	1,136[7]	80
pasteurized process cheese spread, American	1,625[7]	240

[2] Estimated average based on addition of salt in the amount of 0.6% of the finished product.

[6] Applies to unsalted nuts. For salted nuts, value is approximately 200 mg per 100 grams.

[7] Values for phosphorus and sodium are based on use of 1.5% anhydrous disodium phosphate as the emulsifying agent. If emulsifying agent does not contain either phosphorus or sodium, the content of these two nutrients in milligrams per 100 grams is as follows:

	P	Na
American process cheese	444	650
Swiss process cheese	540	681
American cheese food	427	—
American cheese spread	548	1,139

Continued.

Food and description	Sodium (mg)	Potassium (mg)
Cherries		
raw, sweet	2	191
canned		
sour, red, solids and liquid, water pack	2	130
sweet, solids and liquid, syrup pack, light	1	128
frozen, not thawed, sweetened	2	130
Chicken		
all classes		
light meat without skin, cooked, roasted	64	411
dark meat without skin, cooked, roasted	86	321
Chicken potpie, commercial, frozen, unheated	411	153
Chicory, Witloof (also called French or Belgian endive), bleached head (forced), raw	7	182
Chili con carne, canned, with beans	531	233
Chocolate, bitter or baking	4	830
Chocolate syrup, fudge type	89	284
Chop suey, with meat, canned	551	138
Chow mein, chicken (without noodles), canned	290	167
Citron, candied	290	120
Clams, raw		
soft, meat only	36	235
hard or round, meat only	205	311
Clams, canned, including hard, soft, razor, and unspecified solids and liquid	—	140
Cocoa and chocolate-flavored beverage powders		
cocoa powder with non-fat dry milk	525	800
mix for hot chocolate	382	605
Cocoa, dry powder		
high-fat or breakfast		
plain	6	1,522
processed with alkali	717	651
Coconut cream (liquid expressed from grated coconut meat)	4	324
Coconut meat, fresh	23	256
Cod		
cooked, broiled	110	407
dehydrated, lightly salted	8,100	160
Coffee, instant, water-soluble solids		
dry powder	72	3,256
beverage	1	36
Coleslaw, made with French dressing (commercial)	268	205
Collards, cooked, boiled, drained, leaves, including stems, cooked in small amount of water	25	234
Cookies		
assorted, packaged, commercial	365	67
butter, thin, rich	418	60
gingersnaps	571	462
molasses	386	138
oatmeal with raisins	162	370
sandwich type	483	38
vanilla wafer	252	72
Cookie dough, plain, chilled in roll, baked	548	48
Corn, sweet		
cooked, boiled, drained, white and yellow, kernels, cut off cob before cooking	Trace	165

Food and description	Sodium (mg)	Potassium (mg)
Corn, sweet—cont'd		
canned		
regular pack, cream style, white and yellow, solids and liquid	236[2]	(97)
special dietary pack (low-sodium), cream style, white and yellow, solids and liquid	2	(97)
frozen, kernels cut off cob, cooked, boiled, drained	1	184
Corn fritters	477	133
Corn grits, degermed, enriched, dry form	1	80
Corn products used mainly as ready-to-eat breakfast cereals		
corn flakes, added nutrients	1,005	120
corn, puffed, added nutrients	1,060	—
corn, rice, and wheat flakes, mixed, added nutrients	950	—
Cornbread, baked from home recipes, southern style, made with degermed cornmeal, enriched	591	157
Cornbread mix and cornbread baked from mix, cornbread, made with egg, milk	744	127
Cornmeal, white or yellow, degermed, enriched, dry form	1	120
Cornstarch	Trace	Trace
Cowpeas, including blackeye peas		
immature seeds, canned, solids and liquid	236[2]	352
young pods, with seeds, cooked, boiled, drained	3	196
Crab, canned	1,000	110
Crackers		
butter	1,092	113
graham, plain	670	384
saltines	(1,100)	(120)
sandwich type, peanut-cheese	992	226
soda	1,100	120
Cranberries, raw	2	82
Cranberry juice cocktail, bottled (approx. 33% cranberry juice)	1	10
Cranberry sauce, sweetened, canned, strained	1	30
Cream, fluid, light, coffee, or table, 20% fat	43	122
Cream substitutes, dried, containing		
cream, skim milk (calcium reduced), and lactose	575	—
Cream puffs with custard filling	83	121
Cress, garden, raw	14	606
Croaker, Atlantic, cooked, baked	120	323
Cucumbers, raw, pared	6	160
Custard, baked	79	146
Dates, domestic, natural and dry	1	648
Doughnuts, cake type	501	90
Duck, domesticated, raw, flesh only	74	285
Eggs, chicken		
raw		
whole, fresh and frozen	122	129
whites, fresh and frozen	146	139
yolks, fresh	52	98
Eggplant, cooked, boiled, drained	1	150
Endive (curly endive and escarole), raw	14	294
Farina		
enriched		
regular		
dry form	2	83
cooked	144	9
quick-cooking, cooked	165	10
instant-cooking, cooked	188	13
unenriched, regular, dry form	2	83

[2]Estimated average based on addition of salt in the amount of 0.6% of the finished product.

Continued.

Food and description	Sodium (mg)	Potassium (mg)
Figs, canned, solids and liquid, syrup pack, light	2	152
Flatfishes (flounders, soles, and sand dabs), raw	78	342
Fruit cocktail, canned, solids and liquid, water pack, with or without artificial sweetener	5	168
Garlic, cloves, raw	19	529
Ginger root, fresh	6	264
Gizzard, chicken, all classes, cooked, simmered	57	211
Goose, domesticated, flesh only, cooked, roasted	124	605
Gooseberries, canned, solids and liquid, syrup pack, heavy	1	98
Grapefruit		
raw, pulp, pink, red, white, all varieties	1	135
canned, juice, sweetened	1	162
Grapefruit juice and orange juice blended, canned, sweetened	1	184
Grapes, raw, American type (slip skin) such as Concord, Delaware, Niagara, Catawba, and Scuppernong	3	158
Grapejuice, canned or bottled	2	116
Guavas, whole, raw, common	4	289
Haddock, cooked, fried	177	348
Hake, including Pacific hake, squirrel hake, and silver hake or whiting; raw	74	363
Halibut, Atlantic and Pacific, cooked, broiled	134	525
Ham croquette	342	83
Heart, beef, lean, cooked, braised	104	232
Herring		
raw, Pacific	74	420
smoked, hard	6,231	157
Honey, strained or extracted	5	51
Horse-radish, prepared	96	290
Ice cream and frozen custard		
regular, approximately 10% fat	63[8]	181
Ice cream cones	232	244
Ice milk	68[8]	195
Jams and preserves	12	88
Kale, cooked, boiled, drained, leaves including stems	43	221
Kingfish; southern, gulf, and northern (whiting); raw	83	250
Lake herring (cisco), raw	47	319
Lamb, retail cuts	70	290
Lemon juice, canned or bottled, unsweetened	1	141
Lettuce, raw crisphead varieties such as Iceberg, New York, and Great Lakes strains	9	175
Lime juice, canned or bottled, unsweetened	1	104
Liver, beef, cooked, fried	184	380
Lobster, northern, canned or cooked	210	180
Loganberries, canned, solids and liquid, syrup pack, light	1	111
Macadamia nuts	—	164
Macaroni, unenriched, dry form	2	197
Macaroni and cheese, canned	304	58
Margarine[9]	987	23
Marmalade, citrus	14	33
Milk, cow		
fluid (pasteurized and raw)		
whole, 3.7% fat	50	144
skim	52	145
canned, evaporated (unsweetened)	118	303

[8] Value for product without added salt.

[9] Values apply to salted margarine. Unsalted margarine contains less than 10 mg. per 100 grams of either sodium or potassium. Vitamin A value based on the minimum required to meet federal specifications for margarine with vitamin A added, namely 15,000 I.U. of vitamin A per pound.

Food and description	Sodium (mg)	Potassium (mg)
Milk, cow—cont'd		
dry, skim (non-fat solids), regular	532	1,745
malted		
dry powder	440	720
beverage	91	200
chocolate drink, fluid, commercial		
made with skim milk	46	142
made with whole (3.5% fat) milk	47	146
Molasses, cane		
first extraction or light	15	917
third extraction or blackstrap	96	2,927
Muffin mixes, corn, and muffins baked from mixes		
muffins, made with egg, milk	479	110
muffins, made with egg, water	346	104
Mushrooms		
raw	15	414
canned, solids and liquid	400	197
Muskmelons, raw, cantaloupes, other netted varieties	12	251
Mussels, Atlantic and Pacific, raw, meat only	289	315
Mustard greens, cooked, boiled, drained	18	220
Mustard, prepared		
brown	1,307	130
yellow	1,252	130
Nectarines, raw	6	294
New Zealand spinach, cooked, boiled, drained	92	463
Noodles, egg noodles, enriched, cooked	2	44
Oat products used mainly as hot breakfast cereals		
oatmeal or rolled oats		
dry form	2	352
cooked	218	61
Oat products used mainly as ready-to-eat breakfast cereals		
oats (with or without corn), puffed, added nutrients	1,267	—
Ocean perch, Atlantic (redfish)		
raw	79	269
cooked, fried	153	284
Ocean perch, Pacific, raw	63	390
Oils, salad or cooking	0	0
Okra		
raw	3	249
cooked, boiled, drained	2	174
Olives, pickled; canned or bottled		
green	2,400	55
ripe, Ascolano (extra large, mammoth, giant jumbo)	813	34
ripe, salt-cured, oil-coated, Greek style	3,288	—
Onions, mature (dry), raw	10	157
Onions, young green (bunching varieties), raw		
bulb and entire top	5	231
Oranges, raw, peeled fruit, all commercial varieties	1	200
Orange juice		
raw, all commercial varieties	1	200
canned, unsweetened	1	199
frozen concentrate, unsweetened, diluted with 3 parts water, by volume	1	186
Oysters		
raw, meat only, Eastern	73	121
cooked, fried	206	203
frozen, solids and liquid	380	210

Continued.

Food and description	Sodium (mg)	Potassium (mg)
Oyster stew, commercial frozen, prepared with equal volume of milk	366	176
Pancake and waffle mixes and pancakes baked from mixes		
plain and buttermilk, made with egg, milk	564	154
Parsnips, cooked, boiled, drained	8	379
Peaches		
raw	1	202
canned, solids and liquid, water pack, with or without artificial		
sweetener	2	137
frozen, sliced, sweetened, not thawed	2	124
Peanuts		
roasted with skins	5	701
roasted and salted	418	674
Peanut butters made with small amounts of added fat, salt	607	670
Pears		
raw, including skin	2	130
canned, solids and liquid, syrup pack, light	1	85
Peas, green, immature		
cooked, boiled, drained	1	196
canned, Alaska (Early or June peas)		
regular pack, solids and liquid	236[2]	96
special dietary pack (low-sodium), solids and liquid	3	96
frozen, cooked, boiled, and drained	115	135
Peas, mature seeds, dry, whole, raw	35	1,005
Peas and carrots, frozen, cooked, boiled, drained	84	157
Pecans	Trace	603
Peppers, hot, chili, mature, red, raw, pods excluding seeds	25	564
Peppers, sweet, garden varieties, immature, green, raw	13	213
Perch, yellow, raw	68	230
Pickles, cucumber, dill	1,428	200
Pies		
baked, piecrust made with unenriched flour		
apple	301	80
cherry	304	105
mince	448	178
pumpkin	214	160
Piecrust or plain pastry, made with enriched flour, baked	611	50
Pike, walleye, raw	51	319
Pineapple		
raw	1	146
frozen chunks, sweetened, not thawed	2	100
Pizza, with cheese, from home recipe, baked		
with cheese topping	702	130
with sausage topping	729	168
Plate dinners, frozen, commercial, unheated		
beef pot roast, whole oven-browned potatoes, peas, and corn	259	244
chicken, fried; mashed potatoes; mixed vegetables (carrots, peas,		
corn, beans)	344	112
meat loaf with tomato sauce, mashed potatoes, and peas	393	115
turkey, sliced; mashed potatoes; peas	400	176
Plums		
raw, Damson	2	299
canned, solids and liquid, purple (Italian prunes), syrup pack,		
light	1	145
Popcorn, popped		
plain	(3)	—
oil and salt added	1,940	—

[2] Estimated average based on addition of salt in the amount of 0.6% of the finished product.

Food and description	Sodium (mg)	Potassium (mg)
Pork, fresh		
retail cuts, trimmed to retail level		
loin	65	390
Pork, cured, light-cure, commercial, ham, medium-fat class, separable		
lean, cooked, roasted	930	326
Pork, cured, canned		
ham, contents of can	(1,100)	(340)
Potatoes		
cooked, boiled in skin	3[10]	407
dehydrated mashed		
flakes without milk		
dry form	89	1,600
prepared, water, milk, table fat added	231	286
Pretzels	1,680[11]	130
Prunes		
dried, "softenized," cooked (fruit and liquid), with added sugar	3	262
Pudding mixes and puddings made from mixes		
with starch base		
pudding made with milk, cooked	129	136
pudding made with milk, without cooking	124	129
Pumpkin, canned	2	240
Radishes, raw, common	18	322
Raisins, natural (unbleached)		
cooked, fruit and liquid, added sugar	13	355
Raspberries		
canned, solids and liquid, water pack, with or without artificial		
sweetener, red	1	114
frozen, red, sweetened, not thawed	1	100
Rennin products		
tablet (salts, starch, rennin enzyme)	22,300	—
dessert mixes and desserts prepared from mixes		
chocolate, dessert made with milk	52	125
other flavors (vanilla, caramel, fruit flavorings)		
mix, dry form	6	—
dessert, made with milk	46	128
Rhubarb, cooked, added sugar	2	203
Rice		
brown		
raw	9	214
cooked	282	70
white (fully milled or polished)		
enriched		
common commercial varieties, all types		
raw	5	92
cooked	374	28
Rice products used mainly as ready-to-eat breakfast cereals		
rice flakes, added nutrients	987	180
rice, puffed; added nutrients, without salt	2	100
rice, puffed or open-popped, presweetened, honey and added		
nutrients	706	—
Rockfish, including black, canary, yellowtail, rasphead, and bocaccio,		
cooked, oven-steamed	68	446

[10] Applies to product without added salt. If salt is added, an estimated average value for sodium is 236 mg. per 100 grams.

[11] Sodium content is variable. For example, very thin pretzel sticks contain about twice the average amount listed.

Continued.

Food and description	Sodium (mg)	Potassium (mg)
Roe, cooked, baked or broiled, cod and shad[12]	73	132
Rolls and buns		
commercial		
ready-to-serve		
Danish pastry	366	112
hard rolls, enriched	625	97
plain (pan rolls), enriched	506	95
sweet rolls	389	124
Rusk	246	161
Rutabagas, cooked, boiled, drained	4	167
Rye, flour, medium	(1)	203
Rye wafers, whole-grain	882	600
Salad dressings, commercial[13]		
Blue and Roquefort cheese		
regular	1,094	37
special dietary (low-calorie)		
low-fat (approx. 5 cal. per tsp.)	1,108	34
French		
regular	1,370	79
special dietary (low-calorie)		
low-fat (approx. 5 cal. per tsp.)	787	79
mayonnaise	597	34
Thousand island		
regular	700	113
special dietary (low-calorie, approx. 10 cal. per tsp.)	700	113
Salmon		
Coho (silver)		
raw	48[15]	421
canned, solids and liquid	351[14]	339
Salt pork, raw	1,212	42
Salt sticks, regular type	1,674	92
Sandwich spread (with chopped pickle)		
regular	626	92
special dietary (low-calorie, approx. 5 cal. per tsp.)	626	92
Sardines, Atlantic, canned in oil, drained solids	823	590
Sardines, Pacific, in tomato sauce, solids and liquid	400	320
Sauerkraut, canned, solids and liquid	747[16]	140
Sausage, cold cuts, and luncheon meats		
bologna, all samples	1,300	230
frankfurters, raw, all samples	1,100	220
luncheon meat, pork, cured ham or shoulder, chopped, spiced or unspiced, canned	1,234	222
pork sausage, links or bulk, cooked	958	269
Scallops, bay and sea, cooked, steamed	265	476
Soups, commercial, canned		
beef broth, bouillon, and consomme, prepared with equal volume of water	326	54
chicken noodle, prepared with equal volume of water	408	23
tomato		
prepared with equal volume of water	396	94
prepared with equal volume of milk	422	167
vegetable beef, prepared with equal volume of water	427	66

[12] Prepared with butter or margarine, lemon juice or vinegar.

[13] Values apply to products containing salt. For those without salt, sodium content is low, ranging from less than 10 mg. to 50 mg. per 100 grams; the amount usually is indicated on the label.

[14] For product canned without added salt, value is approximately the same as for raw salmon.

[15] Sample dipped in brine contained 215 mg. sodium per 100 grams.

[16] Values for sauerkraut and sauerkraut juice are based on salt content of 1.9 and 2.0 per cent, respectively, in the finished products. The amounts in some samples may vary significantly from this estimate.

Food and description	Sodium (mg)	Potassium (mg)
Soy sauce	7,325	366
Spaghetti, enriched, cooked, tender stage	1	61
Spaghetti, in tomato sauce with cheese, canned	382	121
Spinach		
cooked, boiled, drained	50	324
canned		
regular pack, drained solids	236[2]	250
special dietary pack (low-sodium), solids and liquid	34	250
frozen, chopped, cooked, boiled, drained	52	333
Squash, summer, all varieties, cooked, boiled, drained	1	141
Squash, frozen		
summer, yellow crookneck, cooked, boiled, drained	3	167
winter, heated	1	207
Strawberries		
raw	1	164
frozen, sweetened, not thawed, sliced	1	112
Sturgeon, cooked, steamed	108	235
Succotash (corn and lima beans), frozen		
cooked, boiled, drained	38	246
Sugars, beet or cane, brown	30	344
Sweet potatoes		
cooked, all, baked in skin	12	300
canned, liquid pack, solids and liquid, regular pack in syrup	48	(120)
dehydrated flakes, prepared with water	45	140
Tangerines, raw (Dancy variety)	2	126
Tapioca, dry	3	18
Tapioca desserts, tapioca cream pudding	156	135
Tartar sauce, regular	707	78
Tea, instant (water-soluble solids), carbohydrate added		
dry powder	—	4,530
beverage	—	25
Tomatoes, ripe		
raw	3	244
canned, solids and liquid, regular pack	130	217
Tomato catsup, bottled	1,042[17]	363
Tomato juice		
canned or bottled		
regular pack	200	227
special dietary pack (low-sodium)	3	227
Tomtato juice cocktail, canned or bottled	200	221
Tomtato puree, canned		
regular pack	399	426
special dietary pack (low-sodium)	6	426
Tongue, beef, medium-fat, cooked, braised	61	164
Tuna, canned		
in oil, solids and liquid	800	301
in water, solids and liquid	41[18]	279[18]
Turkey, all classes		
light meat, cooked, roasted	82	411
dark meat, cooked, roasted	99	398
Turkey potpie, commercial, frozen, unheated	369	114
Turnips, cooked, boiled, drained	34	188

[2]Estimated average based on addition of salt in the amount of 0.6% of the finished product.   *Continued.*

[17]Applies to regular pack. For special dietary pack (low sodium), values range from 5 to 35 mg. per 100 grams.

[18]One sample with salt added contained 875 mg. of sodium per 100 grams and 275 mg. of potassium.

Food and description	Sodium (mg)	Potassium (mg)
Turnip greens, leaves, including stems		
canned, solids and liquid	236[2]	243
frozen, cooked, boiled, drained	17	149
Veal, retail cuts, untrimmed	80	500
Vinegar, cider	1	100
Waffles, frozen, made with enriched flour	644	158
Walnuts		
black	3	460
Persian or English	2	450
Watercress leaves including stems, raw	52	282
Watermelon, raw	1	100
Wheat flours		
whole (from hard wheats)	3	370
patent		
all-purpose or family flour, enriched	2	95
self-rising flour, enriched (anhydrous monocalcium phosphate used as a baking acid)[19]	1,079	— [20]
Wild rice, raw	7	220
Yeast		
baker's, compressed	16	610
brewer's, debittered	121	1,894
Yogurt, made from whole milk	47	132
Zweiback	250	150

[2] Estimated average based on addition of salt in the amount of 0.6% of the finished product.

[19] The acid ingredient most commonly used in self-rising flour. When sodium acid pyrophosphate in combination with either anhydrous monocalcium phosphate or calcium carbonate is used, the value for calcium is approximately 120 mg. per 100 grams; for phosphorus, 540 mg.; for sodium, 1,360 mg.

[20] 90 mg. of potassium per 100 grams contributed by flour. Small quantities of additional potassium may be provided by other ingredients.

D Cholesterol content of foods[1]

Item	Amount of cholesterol in		Refuse from item as purchased (%)
	100 g edible portion[2] (mg)	Edible portion of 450 g (1 lb) as purchased (mg)	
Beef, raw			
with bone[3]	70	270	15
without bone[3]	70	320	0
Brains, raw	> 2,000	> 9,000	0
Butter	250	1,135	0
Cavier or fish roe	> 300	> 1,300	0
Cheese			
cheddar	100	455	0
cottage, creamed	15	70	0
cream	120	545	0
other (25% to 30% fat)	85	385	0
Cheese spread	65	295	0
Chicken, flesh only, raw	60	—	0
Crab			
in shell[3]	125	270	52
meat only[3]	125	565	0
Egg, whole	550	2,200	12
Egg white	0	0	0
Egg yolk			
fresh	1,500	6,800	0
frozen	1,280	5,800	0
dried	2,950	13,380	0
Fish			
steak[3]	70	265	16
fillet[3]	70	320	0
Heart, raw	150	680	0
Ice cream	45	205	0
Kidney, raw	375	1,700	0
Lamb, raw			
with bone[3]	70	265	16
without bone[3]	70	320	0
lard and other animal fat	95	430	0

[1]From Watt, B. K., and Merrill, A. L.: Composition of foods—raw, processed, prepared, U.S. Department of Agriculture, Agriculture Handbook, No. 8, December, 1963.

[2]Data apply to 100 grams of edible portion of the item, although it may be purchased with the refuse indicated and described or implied in the first column.

[3]Designate items that have the same chemical composition for the edible portion but differ in the amount of refuse.

Continued.

Item	Amount of cholesterol in		Refuse from item as purchased (%)
	100 g edible portion[2] (mg)	Edible portion of 450 g (1 lb) as purchased (mg)	
Liver, raw	300	1,360	0
Lobster			
whole[3]	200	235	74
meat only[3]	200	900	0
Margarine			
all vegetable fat	0	0	0
two-thirds animal fat, one-third vegetable fat	65	295	0
Milk			
fluid, whole	11	50	0
dried, whole	85	385	0
fluid, skim	3	15	0
Mutton			
with bone[3]	65	250	16
without bone[3]	65	295	0
Oysters			
in shell[3]	> 200	> 90	90
meat only[3]	> 200	> 900	0
Pork			
with bone[3]	70	260	18
without bone[3]	70	320	0
Shrimp			
in shell[3]	125	390	31
flesh only[3]	125	565	0
Sweetbreads (thymus)	250	1,135	0
Veal			
with bone[3]	90	320	21
without bone[3]	90	410	0

[3]Designates items that have the same chemical composition for the edible portion but differ in the amount of refuse.

Calorie values of some common snack foods

Food	Weight (g)	Approximate measure	Calories
Beverages			
Carbonated, cola type	180	1 bottle, 6 ounces	70
Malted milk	405	1 regular (1½ cups)	420
Chocolate milk (made with skim milk)	250	1 cup	190
Cocoa	200	1 cup	235
Soda, vanilla ice cream	242	1 regular	260
Cake			
Angel food	40	2-inch sector	110
Cupcake, chocolate, iced	50	1 cake, 2¾ inches in diameter	185
Fruit cake	30	1 piece, 2 by 2 by ½ inch	115
Candy and popcorn			
Butterscotch	15	3 pieces	60
Candy bar, plain	57	1 bar	295
Caramels	30	3 medium	120
Chocolate coated creams	30	2 average	130
Fudge	28	1 piece	115
Peanut brittle	30	1 ounce	125
Popcorn with oil added	14	1 cup	65
Cheese			
Camembert	28	1 ounce	85
Cheddar	28	1 ounce	105
Cream	28	1 ounce	105
Swiss (domestic)	28	1 ounce	105
Cookies			
Brownies	30	1 piece, 2 by 2 by ¾ inch	140
Cookies, plain and assorted	25	1 cooky, 3 in. in diameter	120
Crackers			
Cheese	18	5 crackers	85
Graham	14	2 medium	55
Saltines	16	4 crackers	70
Rye	13	2 crackers	45
Dessert type cream puff and doughnuts			
Cream puff—custard filling	105	1 average	245
Doughnut, cake type, plain	32	1 average	125
Doughnut, jelly	65	1 average	225
Doughnut, raised	30	1 average	120

Continued.

Food	Weight (g)	Approximate measure	Calories
Miscellaneous			
Hamburger and bun	96	1 average	330
Ice cream, vanilla	62	3½ ounce container	130
Sherbet	96	½ cup	120
Jams, jellies, marmalades, preserves	20	1 tablespoon	55
Syrup, blended	80	¼ cup	240
Waffles	75	1 waffle, 4½ by 5½ by ½ inch	210
Nuts			
Mixed, shelled	15	8-12	95
Peanut butter	16	1 tablespoon	95
Peanuts, shelled, roasted	144	1 cup	840
Pie			
Apple	135	4-inch sector	345
Cherry	135	4-inch sector	355
Custard	130	4-inch sector	280
Lemon meringue	120	4-inch sector	305
Mince	135	4-inch sector	365
Pumpkin	130	4-inch sector	275
Potato chips			
Potato chips	20	10 chips, 2 inches in diameter	115
Sandwiches			
Bacon, lettuce, tomato	150	1 sandwich	280
Egg salad	140	1 sandwich	280
Ham	80	1 sandwich	280
Liverwurst	90	1 sandwich	250
Peanut butter	85	1 sandwich	330
Soups, commercial canned			
Bean with pork	250	1 cup	170
Beef noodle	250	1 cup	70
Chicken noodle	250	1 cup	65
Cream (mushroom)	240	1 cup	135
Tomato	245	1 cup	90
Vegetable with beef broth	250	1 cup	80

Composition of beverages—alcoholic and carbonated nonalcoholic per 100 g[1]

	Food energy	Protein	Carbo- hydrate	Calcium	Phos- phorus	Iron	Thiamin	Ribo- flavin	Niacin
Beverages, alcoholic and carbonated non-alcoholic									
Alcoholic									
Beer, alcohol 4.5% by volume (3.6% by weight)	42	.3	3.8	5	30	Trace	Trace	.03	.6
Gin, rum, vodka, whisky:									
80-proof (33.4% alcohol by weight)	231	—	Trace	—	—	—	—	—	—
86-proof (36.0% alcohol by weight)	249	—	Trace	—	—	—	—	—	—
90-proof (37.9% alcohol by weight)	263	—	Trace	—	—	—	—	—	—
94-proof (39.7% alcohol by weight)	275	—	Trace	—	—	—	—	—	—
100-proof (42.5% alcohol by weight)	295	—	Trace	—	—	—	—	—	—
Wines									
Dessert, alcohol 18.8% by volume (15.3% by weight)	137	.1	7.7	8	—	—	.01	.02	.2
Table, alcohol 12.2% by volume (9.9% by weight)	85	.1	4.2	9	10	4	Trace	.01	.1
Carbonated, non-alcoholic									
Carbonated waters:									
sweetened (quinine sodas)	31	—	8	—	—	—	—	—	—
unsweetened (club sodas)	—	—	—	—	—	—	—	—	—
Cola type	39	—	10	—	—	—	—	—	—
Cream sodas	43	—	11	—	—	—	—	—	—
Fruit-flavored sodas (citrus, cherry, grape, strawberry, Tom Collins mixer, other) (10%-13% sugar)	46	—	12	—	—	—	—	—	—
Ginger ale, pale dry and golden	31	—	8	—	—	—	—	—	—
Root beer	41	—	10.5	—	—	—	—	—	—
Special dietary drinks with artificial sweetener (less than 1 calorie per ounce)	—	—	—	—	—	—	—	—	—

[1]From Watt, B. K., and Merrill, A. L.: Composition of foods—raw, processed, prepared, U. S. Department of Agriculture, Agriculture Handbook, No. 8, December, 1963.

Suggested patterns of daily food intake to supply adequate nutrition in various groups[1]

	Age (yr)	Weight		Height		Basic foods in exchange list portions						
		kg	lb	cm	in	Milk	Veg. A	Veg. B	Fruit	Bread	Meat	Fat
Children	1-3	12	27	87	34	3	1	1	3	5	1	2
	4-6	18	40	109	43	3	1	1	3	6	2	2
	7-9	27	60	129	51	3	1	1	3	8	3	3
	10-12	36	79	144	57	3	1	1	4	10	4	4
Boys	13-15	49	108	163	64	3	1	1	4	12	5	5
	16-19	63	139	175	69	3	1	1	4	16	6	6
Girls	13-15	49	108	160	63	3	1	1	4	8	6	4
	16-19	54	120	162	64	3	1	1	4	8	5	3
Men	20-34	70	154	175	69	2	1	1	4	12	6	6
	35-54	70	154	175	69	2	1	1	4	10	5	5
	55-74	70	154	175	69	2	1	1	4	10	5	5
	75-	68	150	175	69	2	1	1	4	8	5	4
Women	20-34	58	128	163	64	2	1	1	4	6	5	4
	35-54	58	128	163	64	2	1	1	4	6	5	4
	55-74	58	128	163	64	2	1	1	4	5	5	3
	75-	56	123	163	64	2	1	1	4	4	4	3
Pregnant (second half)						3	1	1	5	6	6	4
Lactating						4	1	1	5	10	6	4

[1]Based on the Recommended Daily Allowances, National Research Council (1964 rev.), Family Food Plan at Moderate Cost, U.S. Department of Agriculture, 1964, and the Basic Food Exchange Groups. These patterns are adequate in protein, minerals and vitamins, but relatively low in carbohydrate, fat, and total calories. When more calories are needed, bread or fruit exchanges may be added. Many authorities recommend keeping the fat intake near the minimum. (Reprinted from Church, C. F., and Church, H. N.: Food values of portions commonly used, ed. 9, Philadelphia, 1963, J. B. Lippincott Co., p. 122.)

Height and weight tables for adults

DESIRABLE WEIGHTS FOR PERSONS AGE 25 and OVER[1] (weight in pounds according to frame [in indoor clothing])

Men					Women[2]			
Height (with shoes on) 1-inch heels		Small frame lb	Medium frame lb	Large frame lb	Height (with shoes on) 2-inch heels		Small frame lb	Medium frame lb	Large frame lb
ft	in				ft	in			
5	2	112-120	118-129	126-141	4	10	92- 98	96-107	104-119
5	3	115-123	121-133	129-144	4	11	94-101	98-110	106-122
5	4	118-126	124-136	132-148	5	0	96-104	101-113	109-125
5	5	121-129	127-139	135-152	5	1	99-107	104-116	112-128
5	6	124-133	130-143	138-156	5	2	102-110	107-119	115-131
5	7	128-137	134-147	142-161	5	3	105-113	110-122	118-134
5	8	132-141	138-152	147-166	5	4	108-116	113-126	121-138
5	9	136-145	142-156	151-170	5	5	111-119	116-130	125-142
5	10	140-150	146-160	155-174	5	6	114-123	120-135	129-146
5	11	144-154	150-165	159-179	5	7	118-127	124-139	133-150
6	0	148-158	154-170	164-184	5	8	122-131	128-143	137-154
6	1	152-162	158-175	168-189	5	9	126-135	132-147	141-158
6	2	156-167	162-180	173-194	5	10	130-140	136-151	145-163
6	3	160-171	167-185	178-199	5	11	134-144	140-155	149-168
6	4	164-175	172-190	182-204	6	0	138-148	144-159	153-173

[1]Metropolitan Life Insurance Company, New York.
[2]For girls between 18 and 25, subtract 1 pound for each year under 25.

Average height and weight tables for children

HEIGHT-WEIGHT TABLES FOR GIRLS (juvenile and adolescent ages)*

Height (in)	5 yr	6 yr	7 yr	8 yr	9 yr	10 yr	11 yr	12 yr	13 yr	14 yr	15 yr	16 yr	17 yr	18 yr
38	33	33												
39	34	34												
40	36	36	36											
41	37	37	37											
42	39	39	39											
43	41	41	41	41										
44	42	42	42	42										
45	45	45	45	45	45									
46	47	47	47	48	48									
47	49	50	50	50	50	50								
48		52	52	52	52	53	53							
49			54	55	55	56	56							
50			56	57	58	59	61	62						
51			59	60	61	61	63	65						
52			63	64	64	64	65	67						
53			66	67	67	68	68	69	71					
54				69	70	70	71	71	73					
55				72	74	74	74	75	77	78				
56					76	78	78	79	81	83				
57					80	82	82	82	84	88	92			
58						84	86	86	88	93	96	101		
59						87	90	90	92	96	100	103	104	
60						91	95	95	97	101	105	108	109	111
61							99	100	101	105	108	112	113	116
62							104	105	106	109	113	115	117	118
63								110	110	112	116	117	119	120
64								114	115	117	119	120	122	123
65								118	120	121	122	123	125	126
66									124	124	125	128	129	130
67									128	130	131	133	133	135
68									131	133	135	136	138	138
69										135	137	138	140	142
70										136	138	140	142	144
71										138	140	142	144	145

*Prepared by Bird T. Baldwin, Ph.D., and Thomas D. Wood, M.D. Published originally by American Child Health Association.

HEIGHT-WEIGHT TABLES FOR BOYS (juvenile and adolescent ages)*

Height (in)	5 yr	6 yr	7 yr	8 yr	9 yr	10 yr	11 yr	12 yr	13 yr	14 yr	15 yr	16 yr	17 yr	18 yr	19 yr
38	34	34													
39	35	35													
40	36	36													
41	38	38	38												
42	39	39	39	39											
43	41	41	41	41											
44	44	44	44	44											
45	46	46	46	46	46										
46	47	48	48	48	48										
47	49	50	50	50	50	50									
48		52	53	53	53	53									
49		55	55	55	55	55	55								
50		57	58	58	58	58	58	58							
51			61	61	61	61	61	61	61						
52			63	64	64	64	64	64	64						
53			66	67	67	67	67	68	68						
54				70	70	70	70	71	71	72					
55				72	72	73	73	74	74	74					
56				75	76	77	77	77	78	78	80				
57					79	80	81	81	82	83	83				
58					83	84	84	85	85	86	87				
59						87	88	89	89	90	90	90			
60						91	92	92	93	94	95	96			
61							95	96	97	99	100	103	106		
62							100	101	102	103	104	107	111	116	
63							105	106	107	108	110	113	118	123	127
64								109	111	113	115	117	121	126	130
65								114	117	118	120	122	127	131	134
66									119	122	125	128	132	136	139
67									124	128	130	134	136	139	142
68										134	134	137	141	143	147
69										137	139	143	146	149	152
70										143	144	145	148	151	155
71										148	150	151	152	154	159
72											153	155	156	158	163
73											157	160	162	164	167
74											160	164	168	170	171

*Prepared by Bird T. Baldwin, Ph.D., and Thomas D. Wood, M.D. Published originally by American Child Health Assocation.

Normal constituents of the blood in the adult

Physical measurements

Specific gravity		1.025-1.029
Viscosity (water as unity)		4.5
Bleeding time (capillary)	minutes	1-3
Prothrombin time (plasma) (Quick)	seconds	10-20
Sedimentation rate (Wintrobe method)		
Men	mm/hr	0-9
Women	mm/hr	0-20

Hematologic studies

Cell volume	%	39-50
Red blood cells	million per mm^3	4.25-5.25
White blood cells	per mm^3	5000-9000
Lymphocytes	%	25-30
Neutrophils	%	60-65
Monocytes	%	4-8
Eosinophils	%	0.5-4
Basophils	%	0-1.5
Platelets	per mm^3	125,000-300,000

Proteins

Total protein (serum)	g/dl	6.5-7.5
Albumin (serum)	g/dl	4.5-5.5
Globulin (serum)	g/dl	1.5-2.5
Albumin: globulin ratio		1.8-2.5
Fibrinogen (plasma)	g/dl	0.2-0.5
Hemoglobin		
Males	g/dl	14-17
Females	g/dl	13-16

Nitrogen constituents

Nonprotein N (serum)	mg/dl	20-36
(whole blood)	mg/dl	25-40
Urea (whole blood)	mg/dl	18-38
Urea N (whole blood)	mg/dl	8-18
Creatinine (whole blood)	mg/dl	1-2
Uric acid (whole blood)	mg/dl	2.5-5.0
Amino acid N (whole blood)	mg/dl	3-6

Carbohydrates and lipids

Glucose (whole blood)	mg/dl	70-90
Ketones—as acetone (whole blood)	mg/dl	1.5-2

Carbohydrates and lipids—cont'd

Fats (total lipids) (serum)	mg/dl	570-820
Cholesterol (serum)	mg/dl	100-230
Bilirubin (serum)	mg/dl	0.1-0.25
Icteric index (serum)	units	4-6

Blood gases

CO_2 content (serum)	vol %	55-75
	mmol/L	(24.5-33.5)
CO_2 content (whole blood)	vol %	40-60
	mmol/L	(18.0-27.0)
Oxygen capacity (whole blood)		
Males	vol %	18.7-22.7
Females	vol %	17.0-21.0
Oxygen saturation		
Arterial blood	%	94-96
Venous blood	%	60-85

Acid-base constituents

Base, total fixed (serum)	meq/L	142-150
Sodium (serum)	mg/dl	320-335
	meq/L	(139-146)
Potassium (serum)	mg/dl	16-22
	meq/L	(4.1-5.6)
Calcium (serum)	mg/dl	9.0-11.5
	meq/L	(4.5-5.8)
Magnesium (serum)	mg/dl	1.0-3.0
	meq/L	(1.0-2.5)
Phosphorus, inorganic (serum)	mg/dl	3.0-5.0
	meq/L	(1.0-1.6)
Chlorides, expressed as Cl (serum)	mg/dl	352-383
	meq/L	(99-108)
As NaCl (serum)	mg/dl	580-630
	meq/L	(99-108)
Sulfates, inorganic as SO_4 (serum)	mg/dl	2.5-5.0
	meq/L	(0.5-1.0)
Lactic acid (venous blood)	mg/dl	10-20
	meq/L	(1.1-2.2)
Serum protein base binding power	meq/L	(15.5-18.0)
Base bicarbonate HCO_3 (serum)	meq/L	(19-30)
pH (blood or plasma at 38° C)		7.3-7.45

Miscellaneous

Phosphatase (serum)	Bodansky units per deciliter	5
Iron (whole blood)	mg/dl	46-55
Ascorbic acid (whole blood)	mg/dl	0.75-1.50
Carotene (serum)	μg/dl	75-125

Abbreviations and conversion factors:

dl = deciliter

ml = milliliter

μg = microgram

$$meq/L = \frac{mg/L}{Equivalent\ weight}$$

$$Equivalent\ weight = \frac{Atomic\ weight}{Valence\ of\ element}$$

g = gram

mm^3 = cubic millimeter

meq = milliequivalent

$$mmol\ (millimole)/L = \frac{mg/L}{Molecular\ weight}$$

vol % (volumes percent) = mmol/L × 2.24

Normal constituents of the urine of the adult

Urine constituents	g/24 hr
Total solids	55-70
Nitrogenous constituents	
Total nitrogen	10-17
Ammonia	0.5-1.0
Amino acid N	0.4-1
Creatine	None
Creatinine	1-1.5
Protein	None
Purine bases	0.016-0.060
Urea	20-35
Uric acid	0.5-0.7
Acetone bodies	0.003-0.015
Bile	None
Calcium	0.2-0.4
Chloride (as NaCl)	10-15
Glucose	None
Indican	0-0.030
Iron	0.001-0.005
Magnesium (as MgO)	0.15-0.30
Phosphate, total (as phosphoric acid)	2.5-3.5
Potassium (as K_2O)	2.0-3.0
Sodium (as Na_2O)	4.0-5.0
Sulfates, total (as sulfuric acid)	1.5-3.0
Physical measurements	
Specific gravity	1.010-1.025
Reaction (pH)	5.5-8.0
Volume (ml/24 hr)	800-1600

Tools for use in calculating diets and planning meals for children with phenylketonuria

RECOMMENDED ALLOWANCES FOR PHENYLALANINE, PROTEIN, AND CALORIES FOR PKU CHILDREN OF VARIOUS AGES[1]

Age	Phenylalanine mg/0.5 kg (1 lb) body weight	Protein g	Calories per 0.5 kg body weight
Birth-3 mo	20-22	1¾-2 g/0.5 kg	60-65
4-12 mo	18-20	1½ g/0.5 kg	55-60
1-3 yr	16-18	40 g	50-55
4-7 yr	10-16	50 g	40-50

[1]A low-phenylalanine formula preparation (Lofenalac) is given to infants. Solid foods as permitted on the diet, chosen from the low-phenylalanine food lists, are introduced at the usual ages.

Lofenalac

Lofenalac (Mead Johnson and Company, Evansville, Indiana)—a balanced low-phenylalanine food—has the following composition:

		Powder	Normal dilution
Total nitrogen (equivalent to approximately 15% protein)		2.4%	0.36%
Fat		18.0	2.7
Carbohydrate		57.0	8.5
Minerals (ash)		5.0	0.75
including: Calcium	0.65%		0.1%
Phosphorus	0.50		0.07
Iron	0.01		0.0015
Sodium	0.4 (17.4 meq)		0.06
Potassium	1.0 (25.6 meq)		0.15
Chlorine	0.65		0.1
Moisture		2.0	86.0

Caloric distribution
15% of the calories of Lofenalac are derived from protein, 35% from fat, and 50% from carbohydrate.
Phenylalanine content
Lofenalac powder contains not more than 0.1% nor less than 0.06% phenylalanine (average, about 0.08%).

Vitamin content
A liter of Lofenalac in normal dilution (1 measure to 60 ml [2 oz] water) contains the following vitamins: Vitamin A, 1500 USP units; Vitamin D, 400 USP units; Vitamin E, 5 IU; ascorbic acid, 30 mg; thiamin hydrochloride, 0.46 mg; riboflavin, 1.8 mg, niacinamide, 4 mg; pyridoxine hydrochloride, 0.5 mg; calcium pantothenate, 3.2 mg; Vitamin B_{12}, 4.5 μg; folic acid, 0.5 mg; biotin, 0.03 mg; and choline chloride, 150 mg.

CALORIES, PROTEIN, AND PHENYLALANINE SUPPLIED BY TYPICAL QUANTITIES OF LOFENALAC

Lofenalac	Approx. calories	Approx. protein equiv. g	Average phenylalanine mg
100 g (⅔ cup)	450	15	80
1 packed level measure (9.5 g)	43	1.4	7.5
1 standard 8 oz measuring cup (150 g: 16 packed level measures)	680	22	120
30 ml (1 oz) of normal dilution	20	0.6	3.5
120 ml (4 oz) of normal dilution	80	2.4	14
240 ml (8 oz) of normal dilution	160	5	28
960 ml (32 oz) of normal dilution	640	19	110

Directions for mixing Lofenalac

Make a paste of the Lofenalac with a small amount of boiling water before adding the total water. Sprinkle the Lofenalac on top of the water and beat with an eggbeater or mix in a blender.

PHENYLALANINE, PROTEIN, AND CALORIE CONTENT OF SERVING LISTS OF FOODS USED ON RESTRICTED PHENYLALANINE DIETS[1]

Food	Measure	Phenylalanine mg	Protein g	Calories
Lofenalac	1 measure (1 tbsp)	7.5	1.5	43
Vegetables	1 serving	15	0.3	5
Fruit	1 serving	15	0.2	80
Bread, cereals	1 serving	30	0.5	20
Fats	1 serving	5	0.1	45
Desserts (special recipes)	1 serving	30	2.0	270
Free foods		0	0.0	Varies
Milk	30 ml (1 oz)	55	1.1	20

[1]Acosta, P. B.: Nutritional aspects of phenylketonuria. In The clinical team looks at phenylketonuria, rev., Children's Bureau, U.S. Department of Health, Education, and Welfare, 1964, p. 40. (See p. 440 of this text for listings of these food exchange groups for use with the low–phenylalanine diet.)

GUIDELINES FOR LOW-PHENYLALANINE DIETS FOR INFANTS AND CHILDREN[1]

Weight, kg	1 mo, 3.5 kg (8 lb)	8 mo, 8 kg (18 lb)	2 yr, 12 kg (26 lb)	4 yr, 16 kg (36 lb)
Diet prescription				
Phenylalanine, mg	160-176	324-360	416-468	360-576
Protein, g	14-16	27	32	40
Calories	440	810	1,300	1,700
Lofenalac, measures	10	18	19	23
Water to make, ml	720 (24 oz)	960 (32 oz)	720	720
Milk as necessary, ml	45 (1½ oz)	30 (1 oz)	—	—
Vegetables, servings	—	2	4	4
Fruit, servings	1	1	4	4
Bread, servings	—	3	5	4
Fats, servings	—	—	1	1
Desserts (special recipes)	—	—	—	1
Free foods	—	—	As desired	As desired
Nutritive values				
Phenylalanine, mg	172	325	417	447
Protein, g	16.8	30.4	33.1	40.6
Calories	540	944	1,302	1,724

[1]Acosta, P. B.: Nutritional aspects of phenylketonuria. In The clinical team looks at phenylketonuria, rev., Children's Bureau, U.S. Department of Health, Education, and Welfare, 1964, p. 52. (1 measure of Lofenalac equals 1 tbsp. Special recipes are required for the desserts. Excess amounts of the free foods should be avoided so the child will consume proper amounts of other foods.)

Food and Nutrition Board, National Academy of Sciences–National Research Council recommended daily dietary allowances, revised 1980

MEAN HEIGHTS AND WEIGHTS AND RECOMMENDED ENERGY INTAKE*

Category	Age (years)	Weight kg	Weight lb	Height cm	Height in	Energy needs (with range) kcal		Energy needs (with range) MJ
Infants	0.0-0.5	6	13	60	24	kg × 115	(95-145)	kg × .48
	0.5-1.0	9	20	71	28	kg × 105	(80-135)	kg × .44
Children	1-3	13	29	90	35	1300	(900-1800)	5.5
	4-6	20	44	112	44	1700	(1300-2300)	7.1
	7-10	28	62	132	52	2400	(1650-3300)	10.1
Males	11-14	45	99	157	62	2700	(2000-3700)	11.3
	15-18	66	145	176	69	2800	(2100-3900)	11.8
	19-22	70	154	177	70	2900	(2500-3300)	12.2
	23-50	70	154	178	70	2700	(2300-3100)	11.3
	51-75	70	154	178	70	2400	(2000-2800)	10.1
	76+	70	154	178	70	2050	(1650-2450)	8.6
Females	11-14	46	101	157	62	2200	(1500-3000)	9.2
	15-18	55	120	163	64	2100	(1200-3000)	8.8
	19-22	55	120	163	64	2100	(1700-2500)	8.8
	23-50	55	120	163	64	2000	(1600-2400)	8.4
	51-75	55	120	163	64	1800	(1400-2200)	7.6
	76+	55	120	163	64	1600	(1200-2000)	6.7
Pregnancy						+300		
Lactation						+500		

*From: Recommended Dietary Allowances, Revised 1979. Food and Nutrition Board National Academy of Sciences-National Research Council, Washington, D.C.

The data in this table has been assembled from the observed median heights and weights of children together with desirable weights for adults for the mean heights of men (70 in) and women (64 in) between the ages of 18 and 34 years as surveyed in the U.S. population (HEW/NCHS data).

The energy allowances for the young adults are for men and women doing light work. The allowances for the two older age groups represent mean energy needs over these age spans, allowing for a 2% decrease in basal (resting) metabolic rate per decade and a reduction in activity of 200 kcal per day for men and women between 51 and 75 years, 500 kcal for men over 75 years, and 400 kcal for women over 75. The customary range of daily energy output is shown for adults in parentheses and is based on a variation in energy needs of ±400 kcal at any one age, emphasizing the wide range of energy intakes appropriate for any group of people.

Energy allowances for children through age 18 are based on median energy intakes of children these ages followed in longitudinal growth studies. The values in parentheses are 10th and 90th percentiles of energy intake, to indicate the range of energy consumption among children of these ages.

ESTIMATED SAFE AND ADEQUATE DAILY DIETARY INTAKES OF ADDITIONAL SELECTED VITAMINS AND MINERALS*

	Age (years)	Vitamins			Trace elements†							Electrolytes		
		Vitamin K (μg)	Biotin (μg)	Panto-thenic acid (mg)	Copper (mg)	Man-ganese (mg)	Fluoride (mg)	Chromium (mg)	Selenium (mg)	Molyb-denum (mg)	Sodium (mg)	Potas-sium (mg)	Chloride (mg)
Infants	0-0.5	12	35	2	0.5-0.7	0.5-0.7	0.1-0.5	0.01-0.04	0.01-0.04	0.03-0.06	115-350	350-925	275-700
	0.5-1	10-20	50	3	0.7-1.0	0.7-1.0	0.2-1.0	0.02-0.06	0.02-0.06	0.04-0.08	250-750	425-1275	400-1200
Children and adolescents	1-3	15-30	65	3	1.0-1.5	1.0-1.5	0.5-1.5	0.02-0.08	0.02-0.08	0.05-0.1	325-975	550-1650	500-1500
	4-6	20-40	85	3-4	1.5-2.0	1.5-2.0	1.0-2.5	0.03-0.12	0.03-0.12	0.06-0.15	450-1350	775-2325	700-2100
	7-10	30-60	120	4-5	2.0-2.5	2.0-3.0	1.5-2.5	0.05-0.2	0.05-0.2	0.1 -0.3	600-1800	1000-3000	925-2775
	11+	50-100	100-200	4-7	2.0-3.0	2.5-5.0	1.5-2.5	0.05-0.2	0.05-0.2	0.15-0.5	900-2700	1525-4575	1400-4200
Adults		70-140	100-200	4-7	2.0-3.0	2.5-5.0	1.5-4.0	0.05-0.2	0.05-0.2	0.15-0.5	1100-3300	1875-5625	1700-5100

*Because there is less information on which to base allowances, these figures are not given in the main table of the RDA and are provided here in the form of ranges of recommended intakes.

†Since the toxic levels for many trace elements may be only several times usual intakes, the upper levels for the trace elements given in this table should not be habitually exceeded.

DESIGNED FOR THE MAINTENANCE OF GOOD NUTRITION OF PRACTICALLY ALL HEALTHY PEOPLE

	Age (years)	Weight		Height		Protein (g)	Minerals					
		kg	lb	cm	in		Calcium (mg)	Phos- phorus (mg)	Mag- nesium (mg)	Iron (mg)	Zinc (mg)	Iodine (μg)
Infants	0.0-0.5	6	13	60	24	kg × 2.2	360	240	50	10	3	40
	0.5-1.0	9	20	71	28	kg × 2.0	540	360	70	15	5	50
Children	1-3	13	29	90	35	23	800	800	150	15	10	70
	4-6	20	44	112	44	30	800	800	200	10	10	90
	7-10	28	62	132	52	34	800	800	250	10	10	120
Males	11-14	45	99	157	62	45	1200	1200	350	18	15	150
	15-18	66	145	176	69	56	1200	1200	400	18	15	150
	19-22	70	154	177	70	56	800	800	350	10	15	150
	23-50	70	154	178	70	56	800	800	350	10	15	150
	51+	70	154	178	70	56	800	800	350	10	15	150
Females	11-14	46	101	157	62	46	1200	1200	300	18	15	150
	15-18	55	120	163	64	46	1200	1200	300	18	15	150
	19-22	55	120	163	64	44	800	800	300	18	15	150
	23-50	55	120	163	64	44	800	800	300	18	15	150
	51+	55	120	163	64	44	800	800	300	10	15	150
Pregnant						+30	+400	+400	+150	†	+5	+25
Lactating						+20	+400	+400	+150	†	+10	+50

* The allowances are intended to provide for individual variations among most normal persons as they live in the United States under usual
have been less well defined. See table (preceding page) for weights and heights by individual year of age.
† The increased requirement during pregnancy cannot be met by the iron content of habitual American diets nor by the existing iron stores of many
those of nonpregnant women, but continued supplementation of the mother for 2-3 months after parturition is advisable in order to replenish
‡ Retinol equivalents. 1 Retinol equivalent = 1 μg retinol or 6 μg β carotene.
§ As cholecalciferol. 10 μg cholecalciferol = 400 IU vitamin D.
‖ α tocopherol equivalents. 1 mg d-α-tocopherol = 1 α TE.
¶ 1 NE (niacin equivalent) is equal to 1 mg of niacin or 60 mg of dietary tryptophan.
** The folacin allowances refer to dietary sources as determined by *Lactobacillus casei* assay after treatment with enzymes ("conjugases") to make
†† The RDA for vitamin B_{12} in infants is based on average concentration of the vitamin in human milk. The allowances after weaning are based on

IN THE U.S.A.*

Fat-soluble vitamins			Water-soluble vitamins						
Vitamin A (μg RE)‡	Vitamin D (μg)§	Vitamin E (mg α TE)‖	Vitamin C (mg)	Thiamin (mg)	Ribo-flavin (mg)	Niacin (mg NE)¶	Vitamin B_6 (mg)	Folacin** (μg)	Vitamin B_{12} (μg)
420	10	3	35	0.3	0.4	6	0.3	30	0.5††
400	10	4	35	0.5	0.6	8	0.6	45	1.5
400	10	5	45	0.7	0.8	9	0.9	100	2.0
500	10	6	45	0.9	1.0	11	1.3	200	2.5
700	10	7	45	1.2	1.4	16	1.6	300	3.0
1000	10	8	50	1.4	1.6	18	1.8	400	3.0
1000	10	10	60	1.4	1.7	18	2.0	400	3.0
1000	7.5	10	60	1.5	1.7	19	2.2	400	3.0
1000	5	10	60	1.4	1.6	18	2.2	400	3.0
1000	5	10	60	1.2	1.4	16	2.2	400	3.0
800	10	8	50	1.1	1.3	15	1.8	400	3.0
800	10	8	60	1.1	1.3	14	2.0	400	3.0
800	7.5	8	60	1.1	1.3	14	2.0	400	3.0
800	5	8	60	1.0	1.2	13	2.0	400	3.0
800	5	8	60	1.0	1.2	13	2.0	400	3.0
+200	+5	+2	+20	+0.4	+0.3	+2	+0.6	+400	+1.0
+400	+5	+3	+40	+0.5	+0.5	+5	+0.5	+100	+1.0

environmental stresses. Diets should be based on a variety of common foods in order to provide other nutrients for which human requirements

women; therefore the use of 30-60 mg of supplemental iron is recommended. Iron needs during lactation are not substantially different from stores depleted by pregnancy.

polyglutamyl forms of the vitamin available to the test organism.
energy intake (as recommended by the American Academy of Pediatrics) and consideration of other factors such as intestinal absorption.

Index

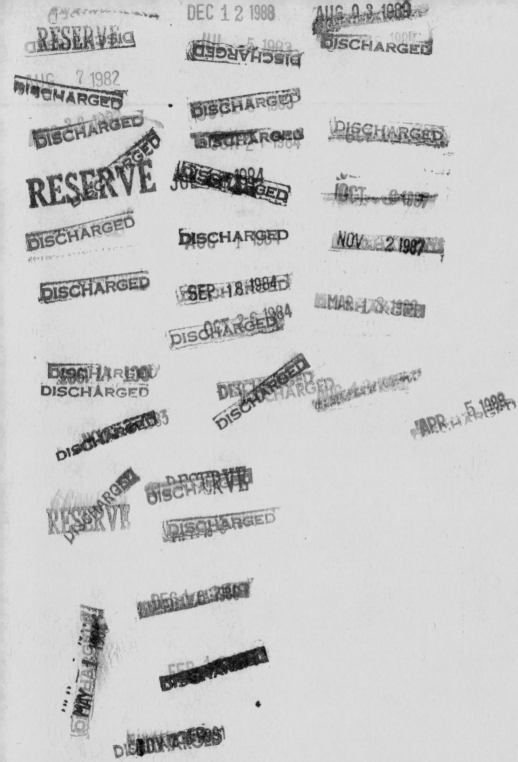